CT and MRI of Skull Base Lesions

Igor Pronin • Valery Kornienko

CT and MRI of Skull Base Lesions

A Diagnostic Guide

Springer

Igor Pronin
Department of Neuroradiology
Burdenko Neurosurgery Institute
Moscow, Russia

Valery Kornienko
Department of Neuroradiology
Burdenko Neurosurgery Institute
Moscow, Russia

ISBN 978-3-319-65956-5 ISBN 978-3-319-65957-2 (eBook)
https://doi.org/10.1007/978-3-319-65957-2

Library of Congress Control Number: 2017958789

Printed on acid-free paper

This Springer imprint is published by Springer Nature
The registered company is Springer International Publishing AG
The registered company address is: Gewerbestrasse 11, 6330 Cham, Switzerland

Preface

The skull base is a complex anatomical region that has a set of unique features, complex inner and outer surface and internal structure through which pass both the vascular and the nervous structures. All of this creates difficulties first in adequate visualization of pathological lesions located in this area and even more so in delineating them from the healthy anatomical tissue. Moreover, the skull base, being the most complicated part of modern neurosurgery, maxillofacial surgery, surgical otorhinolaryngology and ophthalmology, differs from other areas of the intracranial space with its histobiological variety of neoplasms, among which malignant forms are frequently encountered. Poor clinical symptoms and rapid aggressive growth of most tumours often lead to late diagnostics and unsatisfactory results of surgical or combined treatment.

Another feature of the skull base is that quite often there could be found structural changes that do not require any surgical treatment. The recognition and correct interpretation of those changes avoid misdiagnosis and unjustified surgical intervention or radiation therapy.

When examining the skull base, the presence of boundaries of tissues with different density, physical properties, chemical structure and magnetic characteristics leads to numerous artefacts on the diagnostic images. On CT, there are artefacts from the petrous bone (Hounsfield's artefact) which complicate the visualization of the posterior cranial fossa and artefacts from metal dental implants that sometimes make the examination completely noninformative. MRI is not devoid of artefacts either. The massive bone structure of the skull base does not fully use the unique capabilities of the modern MRI sequences such as diffusion-weighted imaging, MR spectroscopy, etc. Spatial distortion, caused by the proximity of the skull base bones, significantly reduces the quality of MR perfusion protocols based on intravenous administration of MR contrast medium. All of these factors reduce the diagnostic quality of the images of the skull base, making it difficult to identify tumours on an early stage.

It is important to emphasize that in the diagnosis of tumours in both the skull base and the brain, CT and MRI are used as complementary methods. That is the reason why we recommend a complex approach in the assessment of lesions of this region using the advantages of each method.

Modern neurosurgical approaches impose high requirements on neuroradiologist in the assessment of the location, extension and differential diagnosis of lesions in the region of the skull base. In order to plan surgical or radiation treatment, it has become essential to apply navigation technology with ultra-thin slices, which provides a high quality of 2D reformation and 3D reconstruction. Among the main issues concerning the diagnosis of skull base tumours, neuroradiologists pay special attention to the accurate topical diagnosis of lesions, their attitude towards meninges, the extension into bony and soft tissues, assessment of vessels and nerves of the skull base, the degree of tumour blood supply and, of course, the presumable pathological nature of tumours. The latter is particularly important, but as practice shows, it is the most difficult part in forming the final diagnosis. The solutions to all these difficulties could be found in a complex clinical-diagnostic approach in determining pathology, which may include direct angiography, CT, MRI, SPECT and PET.

New possibilities in the evaluation of vascular lesions of the skull base emerged with the introduction of dynamic CT angiography in the clinical setting. It is now possible to study tumour blood flow, without a highly invasive direct angiography. The combination of high spatial and time resolution, and various tools for the skull base bones' removal from the image, has led to a very good visualization of all blood flow stages in the tumour tissue.

CT perfusion plays a special role in the diagnosis of skull base tumours. The lack of spatial distortion (common in MR perfusion of this region), high spatial resolution, automatic removal of bone structures on perfusion maps and the ability to monitor dynamics of contrast agent bolus passage through different tissues and lesions – all of these ensured the leading position of the CT perfusion method among all other methods of perfusion in evaluation of haemodynamic characteristics of benign and malignant tumours of the skull base. Today, we consider CT perfusion to be the method of "non-invasive biopsy" of some vascular tumours of the petrous bone (e.g. paraganglioma) and craniofacial regions (e.g. juvenile angiofibroma of nasopharynx).

The algorithms of MR diagnosis of the skull base tumours are slightly different from those used in imaging of tumours of other regions of the brain. First of all, it should be noted that MRI can better evaluate and distinguish soft-tissue structures located under the skull base in comparison with CT scanning. The use of different pulse sequences and scan modes opens up new opportunities in the non-invasive diagnosis of lesions in this area. And despite the rather long total scanning time compared to CT, we consider MRI an integral part of the diagnostic protocol. In the evaluation of skull base tumours, MR technology to suppress MR signal from fat, so-called Fat-Sat modes, acts as the key element in the examination of this anatomical region. Here, we use suppression of the signal from fat on T2-weighted images, T2-FLAIR and, of course, on T1-weighted images (spin echo, SPGR, etc.).

We consider it is obligatory to use intravenous contrast enhancement for all MRI studies of skull base tumours. So the pulse sequences with T1-weighted images + Fat-Sat technology + contrast enhancement should present the final step in any MRI study of skull base lesions.

Another distinctive feature of MRI in comparison with CT scan is the ability of blood vessels imaging (arteries and veins) without contrast enhancement. Among the non-contrast angiographic MR techniques, 3D TOF technology is the best in the imaging of arteries. With the use of 3T MRI has significantly expanded its capacity in the assessment of microvascular pattern of the tumours' blood supply of the anterior, middle and posterior cranial fossae. Nowadays, we rarely use direct angiography in our clinical practice, replacing it with MR angiography with high spatial resolution on 3T MR scanners.

2D TOF angiography method in the skull base and upper cervical spine imaging is being gradually replaced by the new technology of imaging of mixed vascular picture (arteries and veins displaying on the same MR image) – a variation of phase contrast angiography – INHANCE (GE). The main advantages of the latter are a high spatial resolution and the possibility of manipulating the velocity encoding parameters (VENC) at rather short scanning time (about 5–6 min). This method is more sensitive in the diagnosis of complete or partial thrombosis of the skull base sinuses.

Enhanced techniques of MR angiography, bolus MRA and dynamic MRA (TRICKS, GE), have opened a new direction in the study of tumour blood supply, previously available only with direct angiography. Ultrashort scanning time (½–1 ½ min) allows visualizing the vascular architectonics of the skull base tumours with the arterial and venous components separately from each other.

Among the MR perfusion methods, the arterial spin labelling (ASL) technique should be emphasized as the most promising in the assessment of haemodynamics of intra- and extracranial lesions, including tumours in the skull base region. This method does not require intravenous contrast enhancement, can be easily repeated in the clinic and is especially applicable in paediatric practice. Unlike the widely used T2* MR perfusion, in ASL there are no artefacts from the skull base bones, and the blood flow parameters are characterized by absolute values.

Unfortunately, new pulse sequences based on magnetic susceptibility (SWI, SWAN, etc.) that in recent years are often applied in the diagnosis of various intracranial pathologies are still used to a limited extent in the assessment of skull base lesions. The main problem is the spatial distortion and artefacts caused by massive bone structures of the skull base. Furthermore, the bones themselves initially have low MR signal in these modes.

The unique diagnostic ability of modern 3.0 T MR scanners, specifically the combination of high resolution rates and signal-to-noise ratio that obtains ultra-thin slices (up to 0.6 mm) and 3D reconstructions, is reflected in the diagnosis of skull base pathology. With MRI, it has become possible to scan with isotropic voxel, which greatly reduced the total scanning time. It is sufficient to obtain images only in one plane, and the subsequent reformates are reconstructed separately without any loss of quality. In our everyday practice in the study of skull base anatomy, we prefer the following programmes: BRAVO (T1 MRI), CUBE (T2 MRI) and FIESTA (T2 MRI). A main and important feature of FIESTA (GE) sequence is the combination of the thin "hard" T2-weighted slices with "artefact suppression" technology from the pulsation of the cerebrospinal fluid. One of the important indications for the use of this programme was to study the location of cranial nerves in the skull base cisterns and their relationship with the surrounding vessels at suspicion of neurovascular conflict.

Due to the large amount of fat tissue not only in the extracranial space under the skull base but also in the bony structures, the majority of patients with lesions in this region require the use of different methods of MR signal suppression of fat tissue. In MRI, fat has a high MR signal in both most frequently used T1- and T2-weighted sequences, which creates difficulties in the pathology assessment. Today, there are several ways to suppress the signal from fat. The most commonly used method is a technology based on the effect of chemical shift. The saturation signal from the fat tissue (Fat-Sat method) with the use of special RF pulse is commonly applied. Another widely used sequence is an inversion-recovery sequence, in which the MR signal from fat can be selectively saturated (STIR method). T1 and T2 MRI technologies with suppresion of fat signal obtain a more accurate contrast enhancement in the anatomical areas surrounded by fat tissue or tissue with fat components and evaluate the changes in their signal characteristics. The suppression of MR signal from fat significantly distinguishes a subacute haemorrhage (with methaemoglobin) or cyst formations with high concentration of proteins from fat tissue. Fat-Sat mode is irreplaceable in the studies of the orbital and maxillofacial region. Diagnostic accuracy significantly increases with the combination of the Fat-Sat mode and intravenous contrast enhancement.

Recently, we have successfully tested a new method for MR signal suppression from fat based on the Dixon method. The new technology provides stronger suppression of high MR signal from fat tissue even in the presence of metal implants or metal fixation systems in the upper cervical spine after reconstructive surgery (IDEAL, GE). The second main task of the fat suppression technology is to improve the visualization of the lesions that accumulate contrast medium (tumours, lymph nodes, etc.).

The authors sincerely thank the staff of the ***Burdenko Neurosurgery Institute***, especially L. V. Shishkina, S. V. Tanyashin, A. B. Kadasheva and A. I. Belov, who helped in selecting material for this book.

Igor Pronin
Moscow, Russia Valery Kornienko

Contents

Part I

Orbital Disorders

1 Introduction to Orbital Disorders

The eye, oculus, consists of an eyeball, *bulbus oculi*, and surrounding accessory structures.

The eyeball is a spherical body located in the orbit. The eyeball has an anterior pole corresponding to the most prominent point of the cornea and a posterior pole located laterally to the exit of the optic nerve.

The oculomotor system consists of six striated muscles: superior, inferior, medial, and lateral muscles (TT. *recti superior, inferior, medialis et lateralis, respectively)* as well as superior and inferior oblique muscles (TT. *obliquus superior et inferior, respectively*). All these muscles, except for the inferior oblique muscle, originate deep in the orbit, in the vicinity of the optic canal and the adjacent part of the superior orbital fissure *(fissura orbitalis superior)* from the common tendinous ring *(anulus tendineus communis)* located here, which has a funnel shape and encloses the optic nerve and the ophthalmic artery (*a. ophthalmica*), as well as the oculomotor, nasociliary, and abducent nerves (*nn. oculomotorius, nasociliaris et abducens*, respectively). *The rectus muscles* attach with their anterior ends in front of the equator of the eyeball on the four sides of the latter, fusing with the sclera via tendons. *The superior oblique muscle* passes through the fibrocartilaginous ring (*trochlea*) attached to the trochlear fovea (*fovea trochlearis*) of the frontal bone, turns at an acute angle back and laterally and attaches to the eyeball on its superolateral side behind the equator. *The inferior oblique muscle* originates from the lateral circumference of the lacrimal fossa and goes under the eyeball laterally and posteriorly, below the anterior end of the inferior rectus muscle; its tendon is attached to the sclera on the side of the eyeball behind the equator.

Innervation of the extraocular muscles: the rectus muscles, except for the lateral rectus muscle, and the lower oblique muscle are innervated by the oculomotor nerve (*n. oculomotorius*); the superior oblique muscle is innervated by the trochlear nerve (*n. trochlearis*); and the lateral rectus muscle is innervated by the abducent nerve (*n. abducens*). The ophthalmic nerve (*n. ophthalmicus)* provides sensory innervation of the eye muscles.

Orbit is lined with a periosteum (*periorbita*), which merges with the dura mater at the optic canal (*canalis opticus*) and the superior orbital fissure.

Behind the eyeball lies the adipose tissue (orbital fat body, *corpus adiposum orbitae*), which occupies the entire space between the structures lying in the orbit. The adipose tissue, adhering to the eyeball, is separated from the latter by an adjacent connective tissue layer (Tenon's capsule, *vagina bulbi*) surrounding the eyeball. Tendons of the eyeball, running towards their attachment areas in the sclera, pass through the Tenon's capsule, which forms their sheaths becoming the fascia of individual muscles.

All orbital diseases and lesions are typically divided into five categories, depending on the localization in the orbital cavity in relation to the extraocular muscles that form a so-called muscle cone: outside the muscle cone—extraconal lesions (1); within the muscle cone—intraconal lesions with involvement of the optic nerve and its membranes (2) and without involvement of the optic nerve (3); lesions of the extraocular muscles themselves (conal) (4); eyeball diseases (5) (Fig. 1.1). Tumors that grow into the orbital cavity and may simultaneously involve several anatomical areas of the orbit are regarded as a separate category.

According to publications, more than 100 different types of diseases occur in the orbit (Rootman 1988; Baert and Sartor 2006; Muller-Forell 2006). The major role in the diagnosis of orbital diseases plays the analysis of medical history and clinical manifestations, with only a small percentage of cases requiring a neuroradiological examination to specify the diagnosis. An ophthalmic examination should precede the neuroradiological diagnosis and include an assessment of visual acuity, evaluation of mobility of the eyeballs, exophthalmometry, examination of pupillary function, eye lens transparency, eye fundus abnormalities, and visual field deficit (Ducrey and Spahn 2002). A patient age is also very important in prediction tumor etiology—in older adult patients malignant orbital tumors occur in 63% and benign in 27% (Demirci 2002). All this information has a significant

I. Pronin, V. Kornienko, *CT and MRI of Skull Base Lesions*, https://doi.org/10.1007/978-3-319-65957-2_1

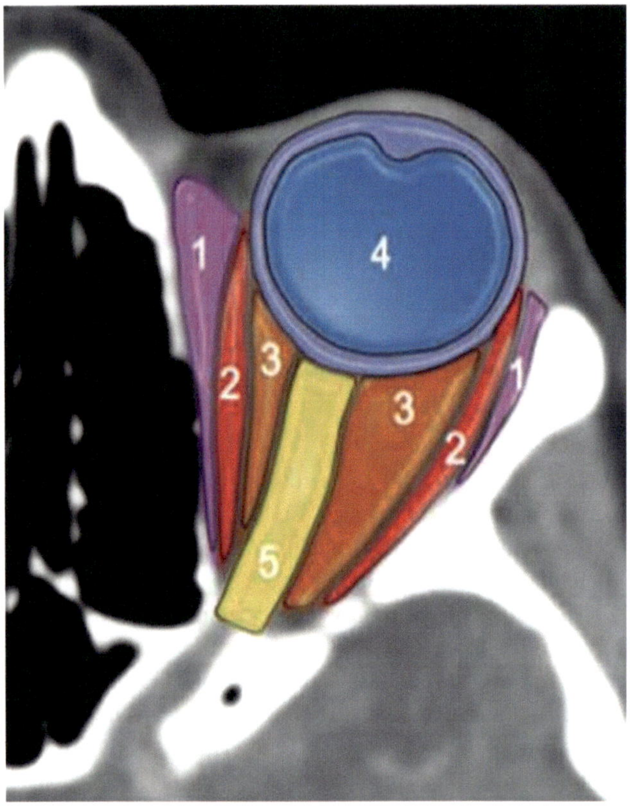

Fig. 1.1 Schematic divisions of the orbital cavity. Intraorbital spaces: 1—extraconal, 2—conal, 3—intraconal, without optic nerve, 4—eyeball, 5—optic nerve and membranes (intraconal)

impact on the choice of sequences and techniques for orbital imaging studies (MRI and/or CT).

CT and MRI are the most frequently used diagnostic methods for orbital diseases assessment. Orbital ultrasound is a more available, but less specific method, especially in evaluating the retro-orbital area. The use of SPECT and PET is limited due to their low spatial resolution in the imaging of the orbit components and their lower availability. Orbital MRI imaging is distinguished by the mandatory use of fat suppression techniques, both before and after intravenous contrast enhancement. Preference is given to T2- and T1-weighted sequences with 3 mm thin slices, directed along the course of the optic nerves in the axial, sagittal, and oblique sections. Coronal sections should be oriented perpendicular to the optic nerve. Orbital CT examinations use mainly thin-slice helical scanning with reformations in the plane of interest. The use of CT-perfusion imaging became a new approach in the diagnosis of orbital lesions, which opened a new era in the evaluation of hemodynamics of orbital tumors.

Intraconal Lesions Without Involvement of the Optic Nerve

2

Contents

2.1 Vascular Disorders

Vascular malformations of the orbit, involving the venous system, are rare diseases of the orbital area (Arat et al. 2004). Among these, the most important disorders are orbital venous varix and venous angiomas. These disorders are usually characterized by intermittent exophthalmos, often associated with active physical activities and movements followed by an increase in the venous pressure, such as cough or Valsalva maneuver. The absence of any valves in the internal jugular vein and orbital veins does not prevent free transmission of a pressure increase to the orbital venous system, which results in periodic exophthalmos in case of vascular venous malformations.

2.1.1 Orbital Venous Varix

Lloyd et al. (1971) distinguished two types of these lesions: primary and secondary. The classical definition of primary orbital venous varix is a venous malformation with uni- or bilateral dilatation of one or more orbital veins. Secondary (also known as acquired) venous varix often occurs as a result of an injury of the orbit or is associated with an invasion of the foreign body into the orbit. Secondary varix belongs to a group of extraorbital lesions such as carotid-cavernous fistula and cerebral AVM. Primary orbital varix is usually manifested in infants or in early childhood, but may also occur in the first or second decade of life. Infants or children may often have vascular stigmata on the face, forehead, eyelids, and buccal cavity. Later, venous changes may develop in the conjunctiva, the eyelid of the affected eye. In elderly, orbital varices can probably be secondary to or associated with some other orbital or extraorbital vascular disorders.

Intermittent proptosis is the main clinical symptom of orbital varices. Exophthalmos in children is easily induced by crying or straining, and, at the early stages, it may result from sudden movements or certain maneuvers that increase

I. Pronin, V. Kornienko, *CT and MRI of Skull Base Lesions*, https://doi.org/10.1007/978-3-319-65957-2_2

intraocular vascular pressure. In older children and adolescents, it may occur when pressing on the jugular vein or be caused by forced expiration with the pinched mouth and the nose, as well as by the Valsalva maneuver. Dilated venous channels in the orbit are characterized by a slow blood flow. Venous dilation is often manifested in active tests and actions related to an elevation in venous blood pressure in the orbit, this is why imaging techniques are often unable to detect lesions in the patient at rest. In such cases, in order to confirm the presumptive diagnosis, namely, venous varix, by clinical symptoms, it is recommended to conduct diagnostic tests at rest and during Valsalva maneuver or, as an alternative, with the patient lying face down, dropping his/her head to the chin in order to increase the orbital venous pressure. This is easily performed on CT scanners. Venous thrombosis or hemorrhage may lead to acute painful exophthalmos, sometimes with reduced mobility of the eyeball (De Potter et al. 1995).

2.1.1.1 Diagnosis

Craniography indirectly confirming congenital orbital varices (by the presence of phleboliths as an example) is mainly replaced by CT, MRI, and ultrasound imaging.

CT examination in most cases detects twisted and dilated venous channels located in the area of the superior ophthalmic vein, their walls being sometimes calcified. Orbital veins are easily dilated when the jugular vein is compressed or during the Valsalva maneuver (deep inspiration and holding the breath for 20–30 s). Varicose superior or inferior ophthalmic veins also respond in a similar way, but they are twisted or plexiform on the CT images. Dilated veins homogeneously accumulate contrast agents in the absence of a thrombus inside. In case of an expected thrombosis or a hemorrhage, MRI is preferred to CT. Osborn (2004a) demonstrated that the best way to visualize orbital varices on MRI is using T1-weighted sequences, showing a much lower MR signal intensity from varices than the surrounding orbital structures. Nevertheless, a high signal intensity of the orbital fat partially impairs the visualization of varicose veins, thus, we recommend the inclusion of a fat suppression sequence in the study protocol. In case of a rapid turbulent blood flow in dilated venous channels, a significant loss of MR signal (flow-void) can be observed. Conducting an MR angiography based on 2D time-of-flight or PC methods is acceptable for better visualization of the venous flow.

On T2-weighted images, the signal intensity may be heterogeneous due to the presence of a hemorrhage or thrombi (Fig. 2.1). Although direct contrast-enhanced venography of the orbit is superseded by non-invasive methods of CT and MRI, its use in rare cases may be justified. During venography, the filling of dilated venous structures occurs in the late venous phase and more precisely than in other diagnostic techniques the visible size and branched nature of varicose veins can be seen (Fig. 2.2). In all our cases with changing of patient position (face up and down) CT and MRI demonstrated the increase in volume of venous channels in dropping patient's head to the chin (Figs. 2.2 and 2.3). Recently, for detection of orbital varix time-resolved contrast-enhanced MR-angiography can be easily applied in clinical setting. This technology is very useful even in small orbital varices detection (Figs. 2.4 and 2.5) and helps to distinguish orbital varix from cavernous hemangiomas as a varix fills in completely by the venous phase, whereas cavernous hemangiomas show very little and patchy contrast enhancement during MR-angiography (Kahana et al. 2007).

2.1.1.2 Differential Diagnosis

Lymphangioma involving the venous blood flow, cavernous and capillary hemangioma, inflammation of the orbit. True venous varix has to be distinguished from orbital varices that arise secondary to AVM (Trombly et al. 2006) and cavernous sinus thrombosis (Fig. 2.6).

2.1.2 Carotid-cavernous fistula (CCF)

Carotid-cavernous fistula (CCF) usually has a traumatic origin and is formed between the cavernous part of internal carotid artery (rarely between branches of the external carotid artery) and the cavernous sinus. The carotid siphon passes through the cavernous sinus and a rupture of the wall at this site results in the formation of a fistula (Serbinenko 1974). A fistula is usually located in the middle or posterior portion of the cavernous sinus. In most cases, venous drainage runs anteriorly into the ophthalmic vein, increasing intraocular venous pressure, or there is combination drainage into the sphenoparietal sinus and other veins. In some cases, fistula may occur spontaneously or as a result of a ruptured arterial aneurysm of the cavernous segment of the internal carotid artery, or due to communicants between the dural branches of the external carotid artery and the cavernous sinus (dural arteriovenous malformation or indirect arteriovenous fistula). Serbinenko (1968) identified six types of CCF depending on a shunt and arterial blood supply of cerebral hemisphere: from full to partial shunting of the internal carotid artery blood flow into the cavernous sinus, taking into account the circle of Willis variants. The author also studied and described more than ten drainage pathways from the cavernous sinus. Djindjian et al. (1973) based the classification on the differences in the venous outflow from DAVF and identified three types of venous drainage. The classification based on whether the fistula is spontaneous or traumatic is also applicable, even if there are some overlapping symptoms. Spontaneous fistula occurs predominantly in women compared to men at a ratio of 4.5:1, these fistulae may occur in all age groups, but most of them are detected after the age of 50.

2.1.2.1 Clinical Manifestations

An elevation in the venous pressure in the orbit causes clinical symptoms, including exophthalmos (3 mm or more), pulsating noise over the orbit and temporal area, reduced mobility of the eyeball, swollen eyelids.

2.1.2.2 Diagnosis

Methods of ultrasound diagnostics detect an abnormally dilated superior ophthalmic vein and thickened extraocular muscles. Among them, the method of color flow mapping of the orbit can play an important role in the diagnosis of CCF.

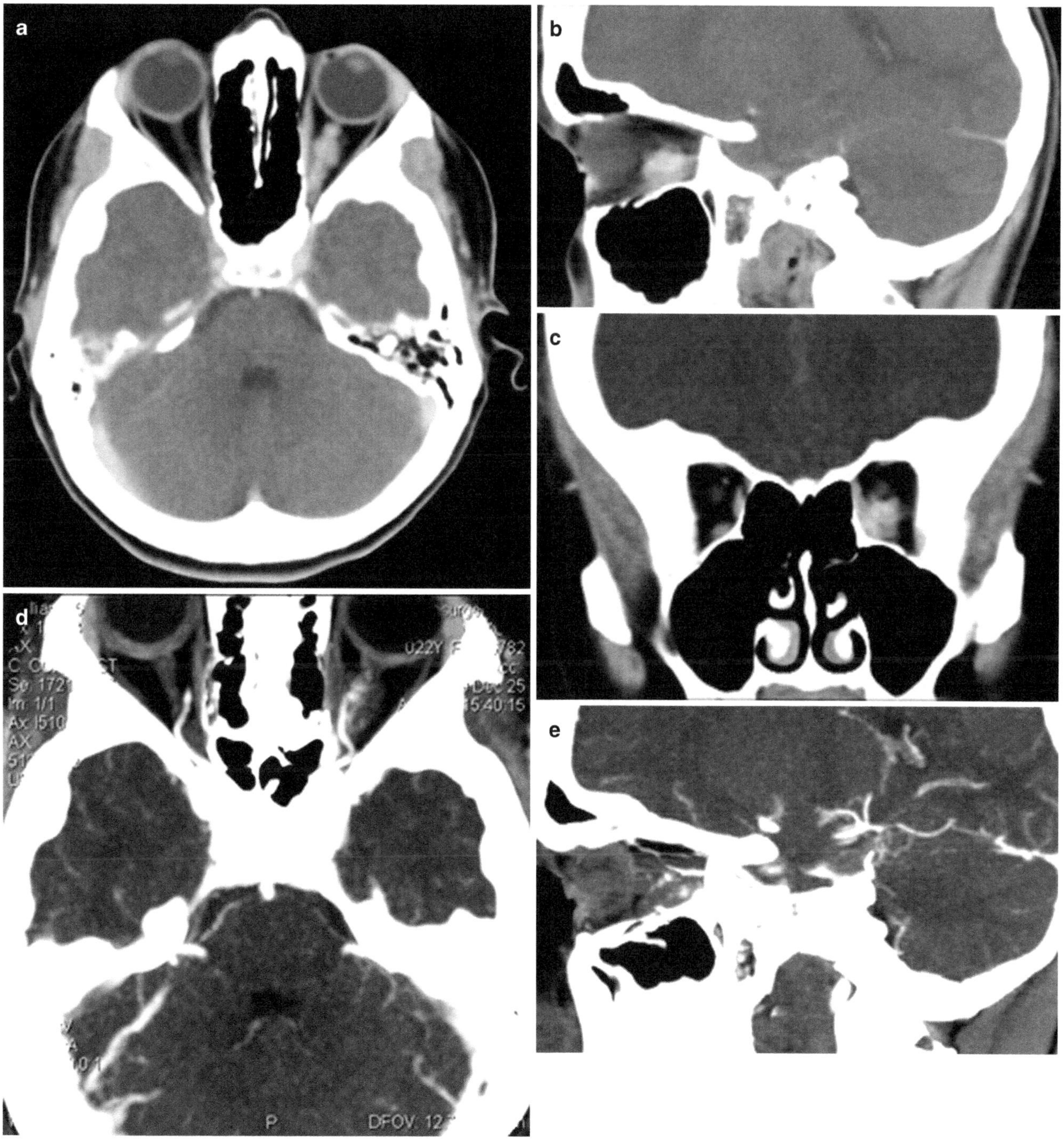

Fig. 2.1 Venous varix of the left orbit. CT scans before (**a**) and after contrast enhancement (**b**, **c**) in sagittal and coronal planes detect the lesion with homogeneous contrast enhancement involving the low medial orbital region. CT angiography (**d**–**f**) demonstrates the lesion with partial enhancement in projection of the inferior orbital vein. T1-weighted MRI before (**g**) and after contrast enhancement (**h** - fat saturation technique, **i** - without fat saturation technique) - there is the lesion with marked enhancement that can be better delineated with fat saturation

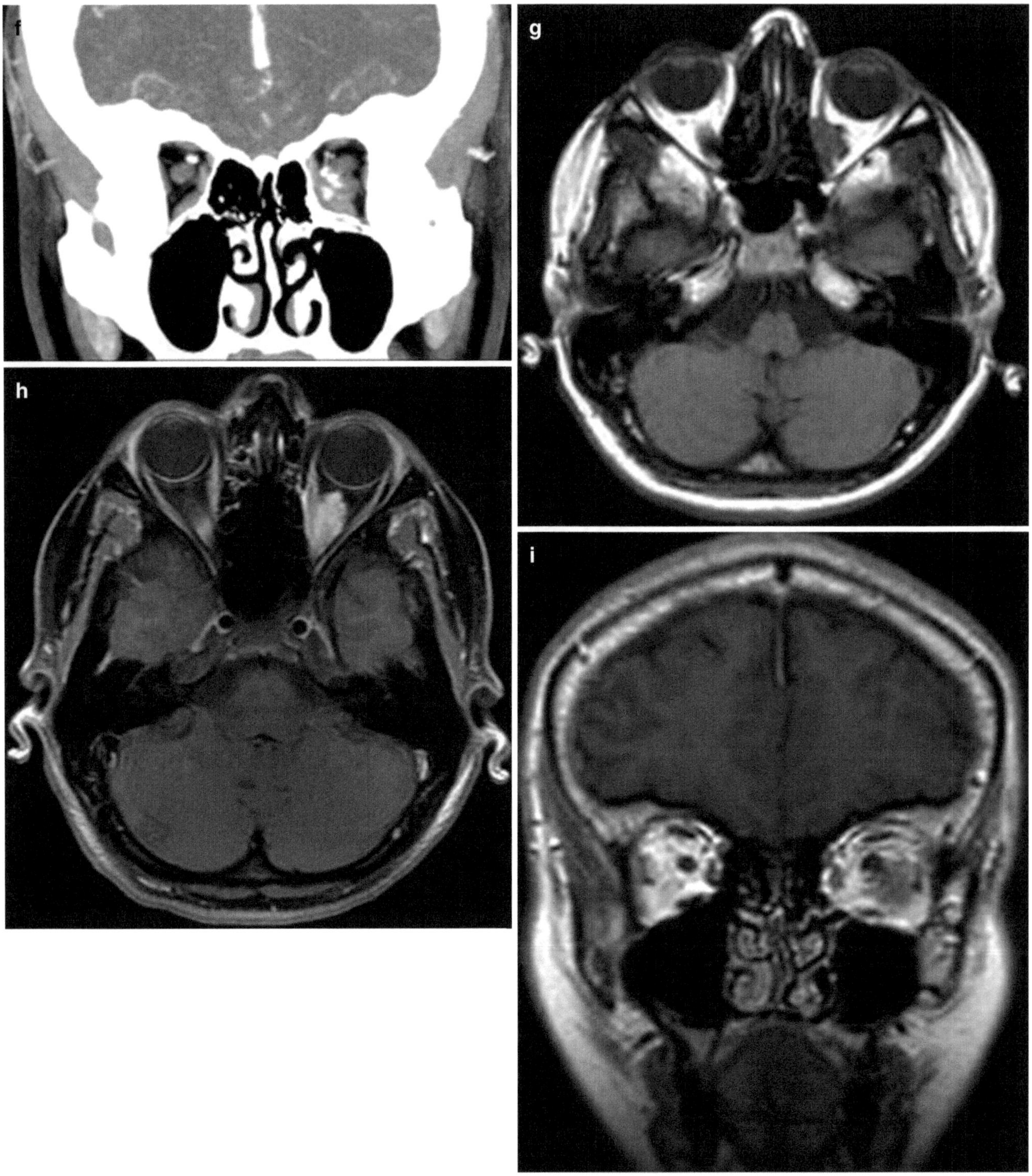

Fig. 2.1 (continued)

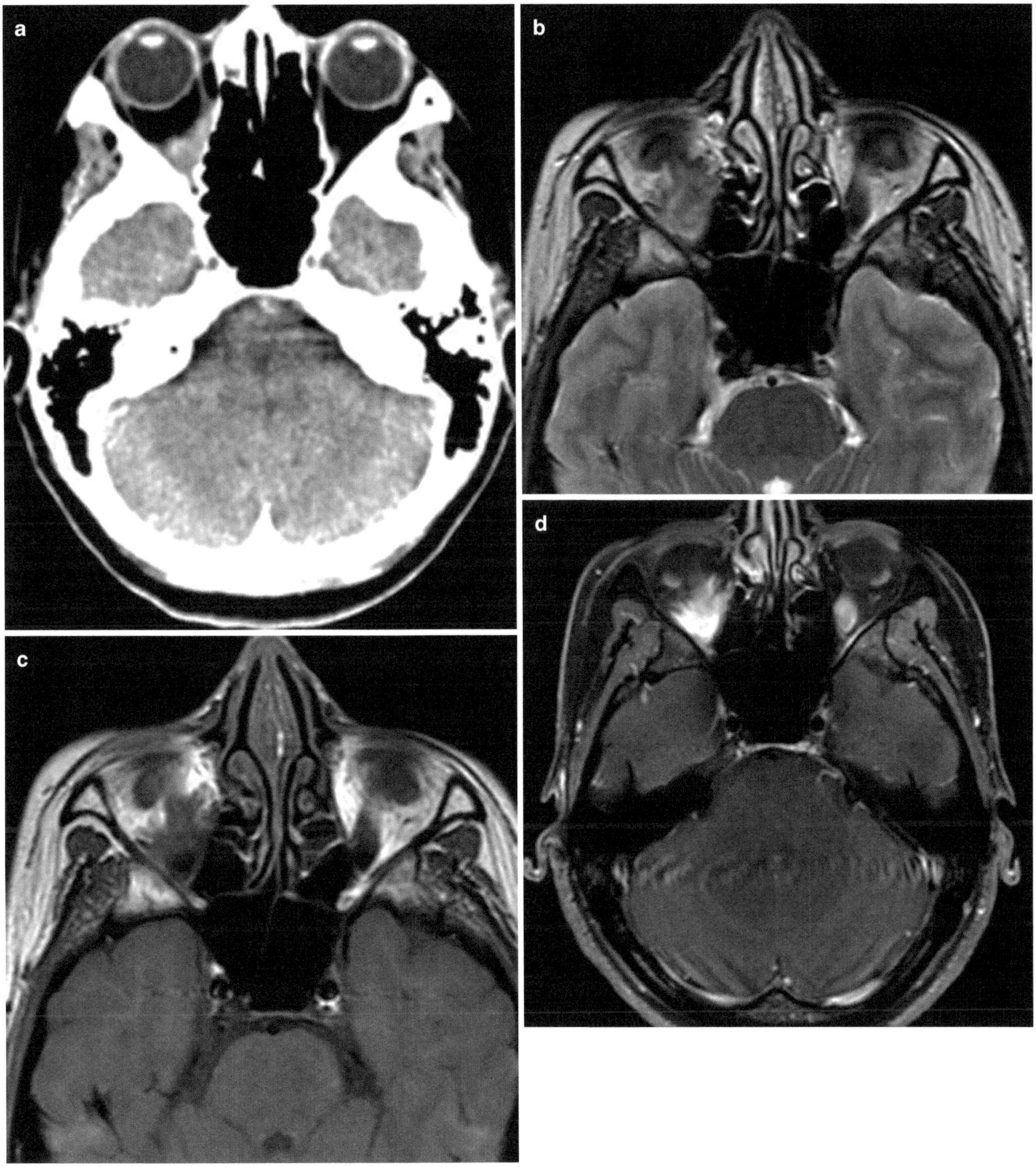

Fig. 2.2 Venous varix of the right orbit. CT scan (**a**), T2 (**b**), and T1 (**c**) MRI demonstrate the mass lesion in orbital apex. After i/v contrast medium injection with Fat-Sat technology venous varix shows marked enhancement (**d**). When a patient is in position «face down» (**e**, **f**) orbital varices increase in size. Enlarged pathologic venous vessels clearly visible on superselective digital subtraction angiography using intravenous approach (**g**–**i**)

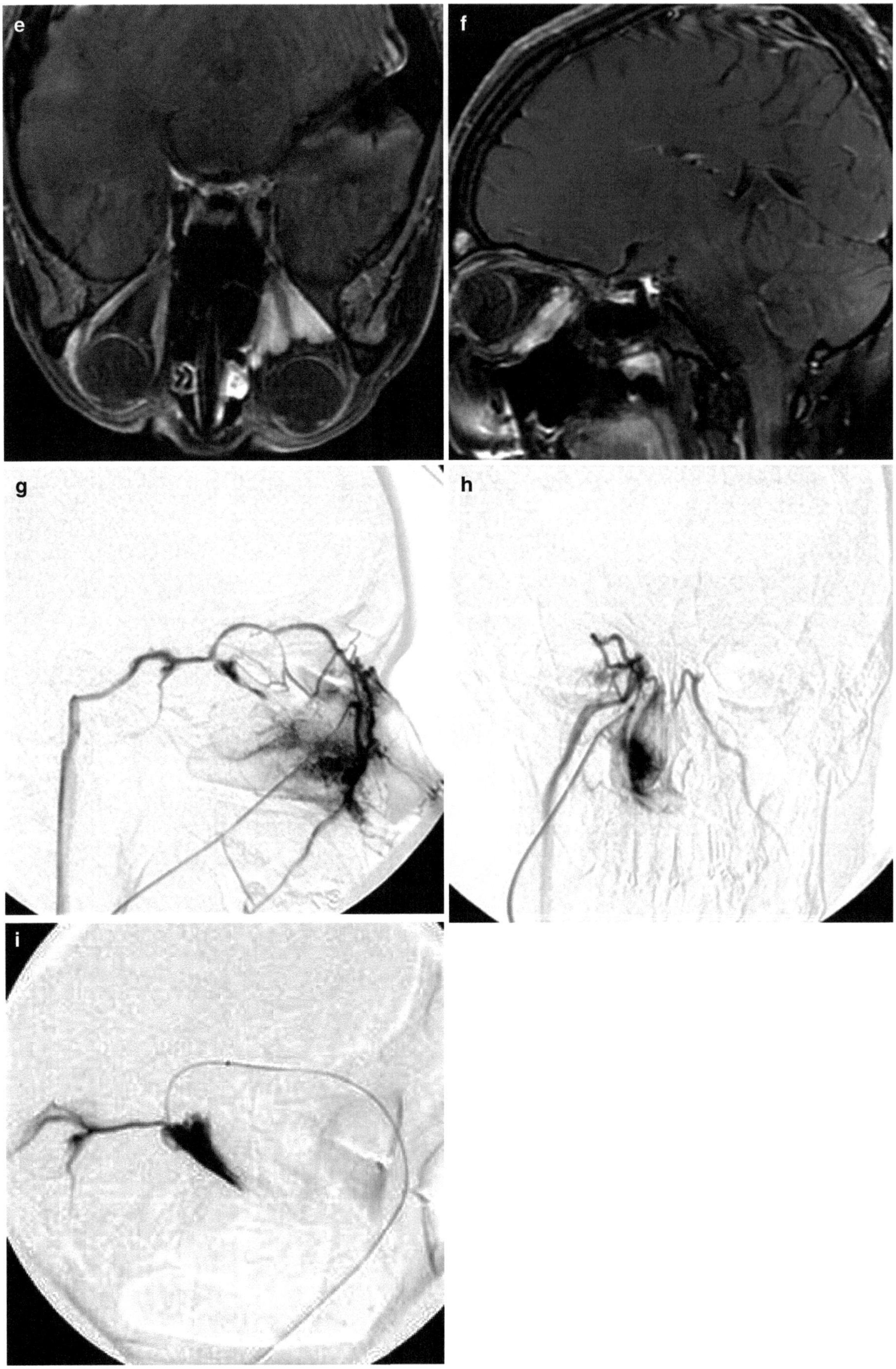

Fig. 2.2 (continued)

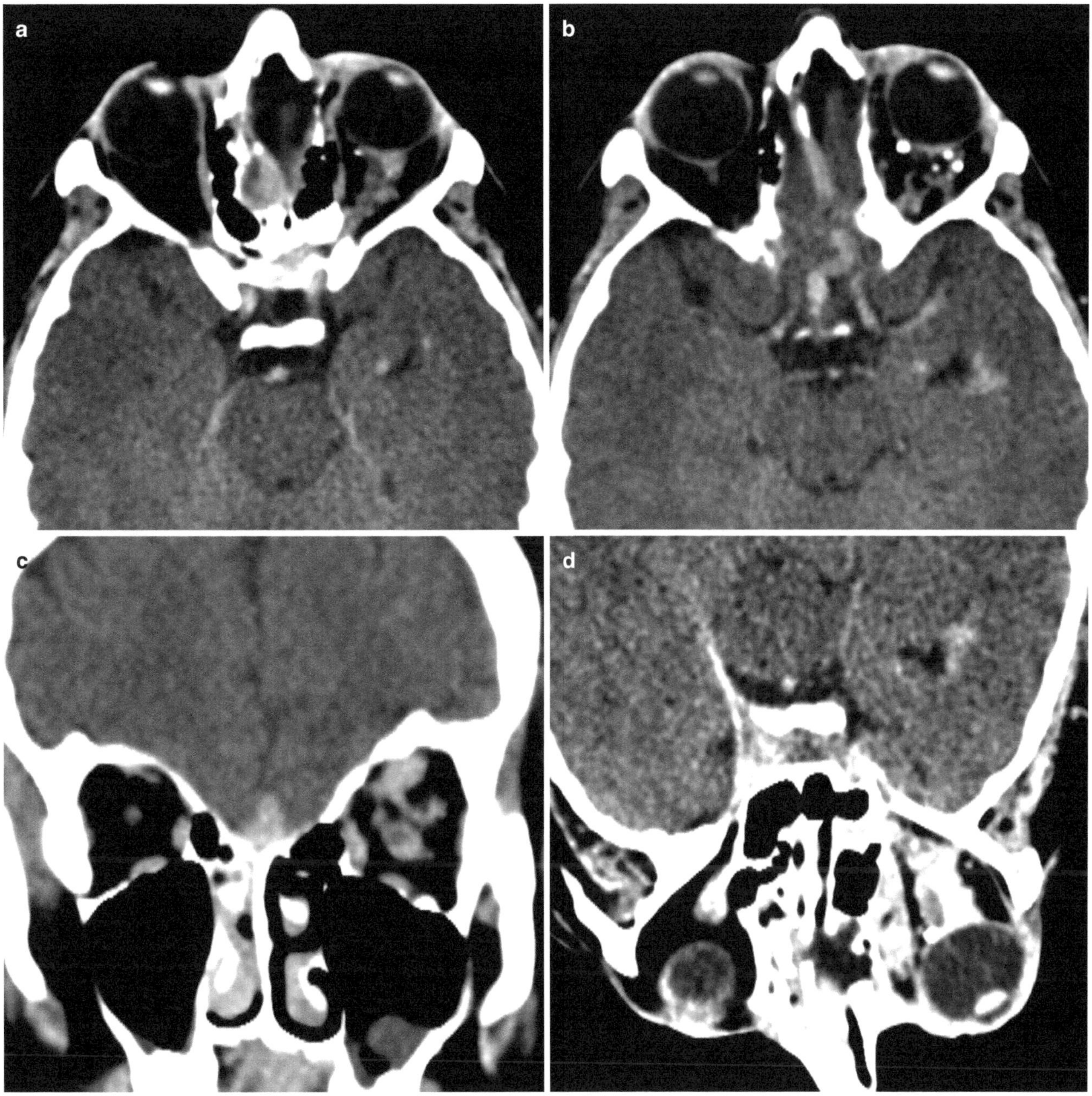

Fig. 2.3 Venous varix of the left orbit. CT scans in axial (**a**, **b**) plane and after coronal reformation (**c**) after i/v contrast enhancement show orbital varix with small around shape calcifications. When a patient is in position «face down» (**d**, **e**) the lesion demonstrates enlargement in size and occupies the whole orbital cavity with appearing of exophthalmos. T2-weighted MR images in axial (**f**, **g**) projection show heterogeneous pathologic structure involving the whole orbit and causing proptosis. There are a lot of small serpentine vessels with dark T2 MR-signal in retroorbital region. MR-angiography (3D TOF with CE) visualizes multiple giant venous angiomas in fronto-temporal areas of the left brain hemisphere additionally (**h**, **i**)

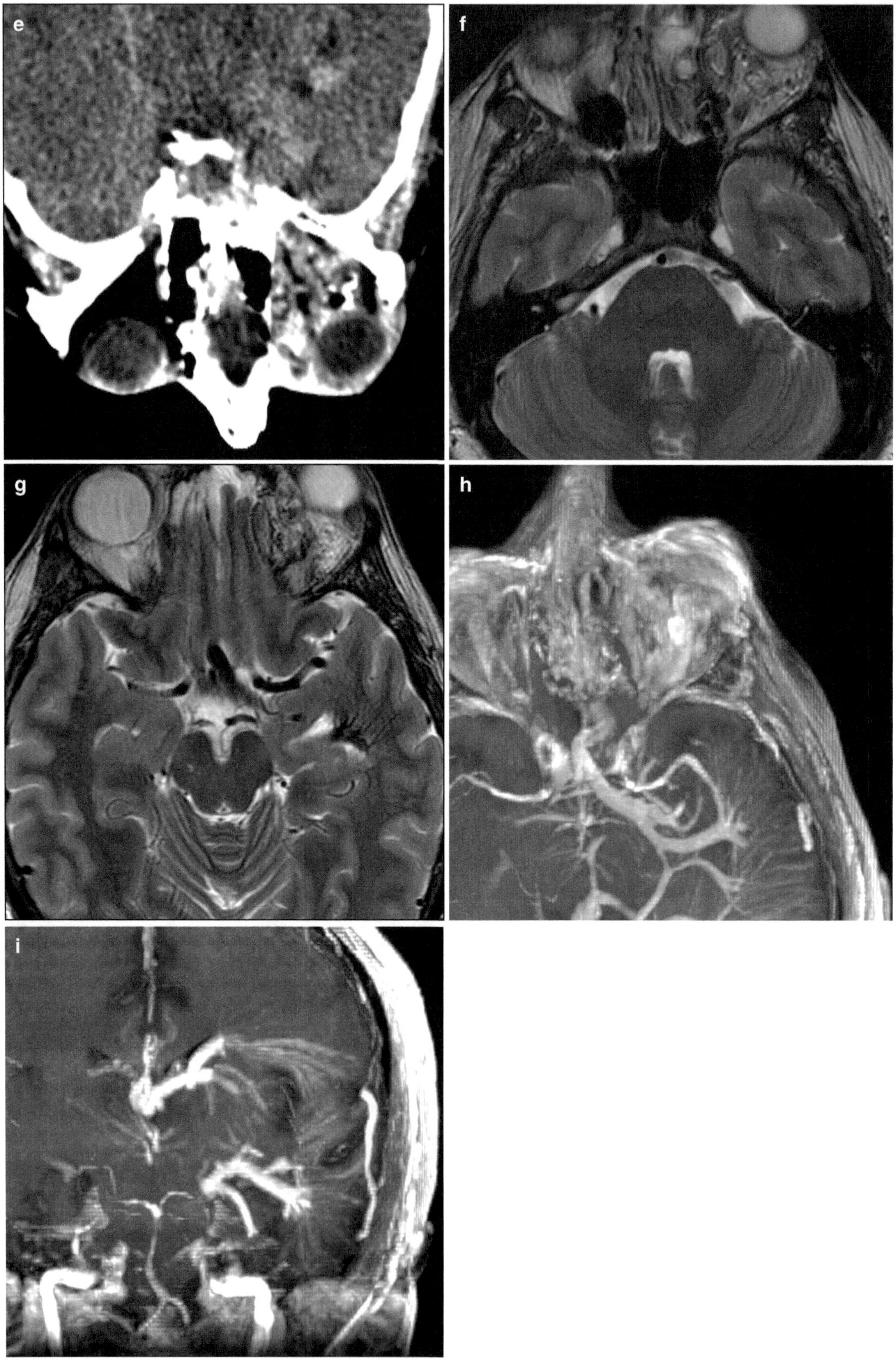

Fig. 2.3 (continued)

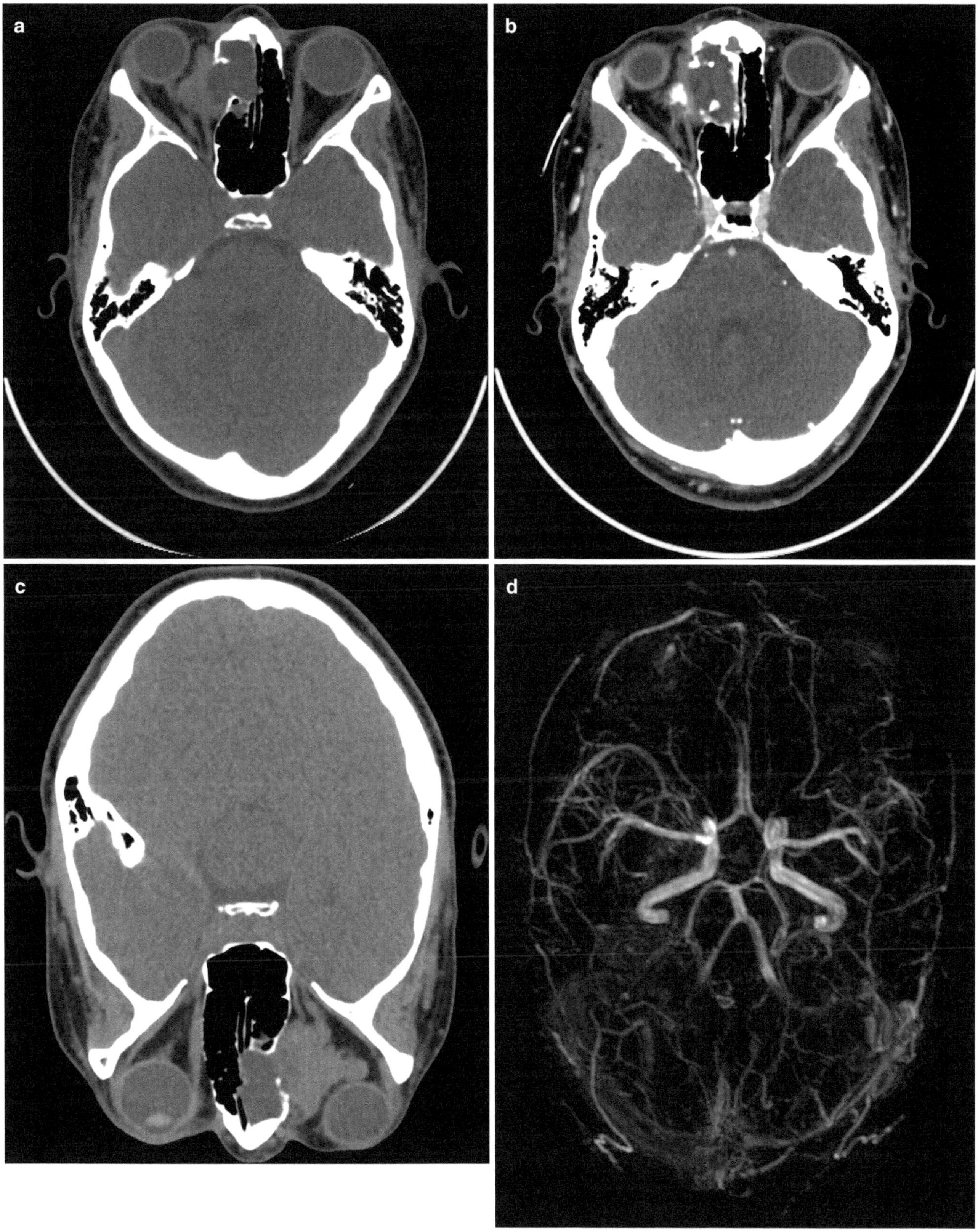

Fig. 2.4 Venous varix of the right orbit. CT scans before (**a**) and after (**b**) i/v contrast enhancement show orbital varix associated with fronto-nasal encephalocele due to bone destruction. In position "face-down" the size of the varix became large (**c**). Time-resolved contrast-enhanced MR-angiography presented in different time-points after contrast agent bolus injection (**d**–**f**) demonstrates the gradual contrast enhancement inside the dilated venous channels

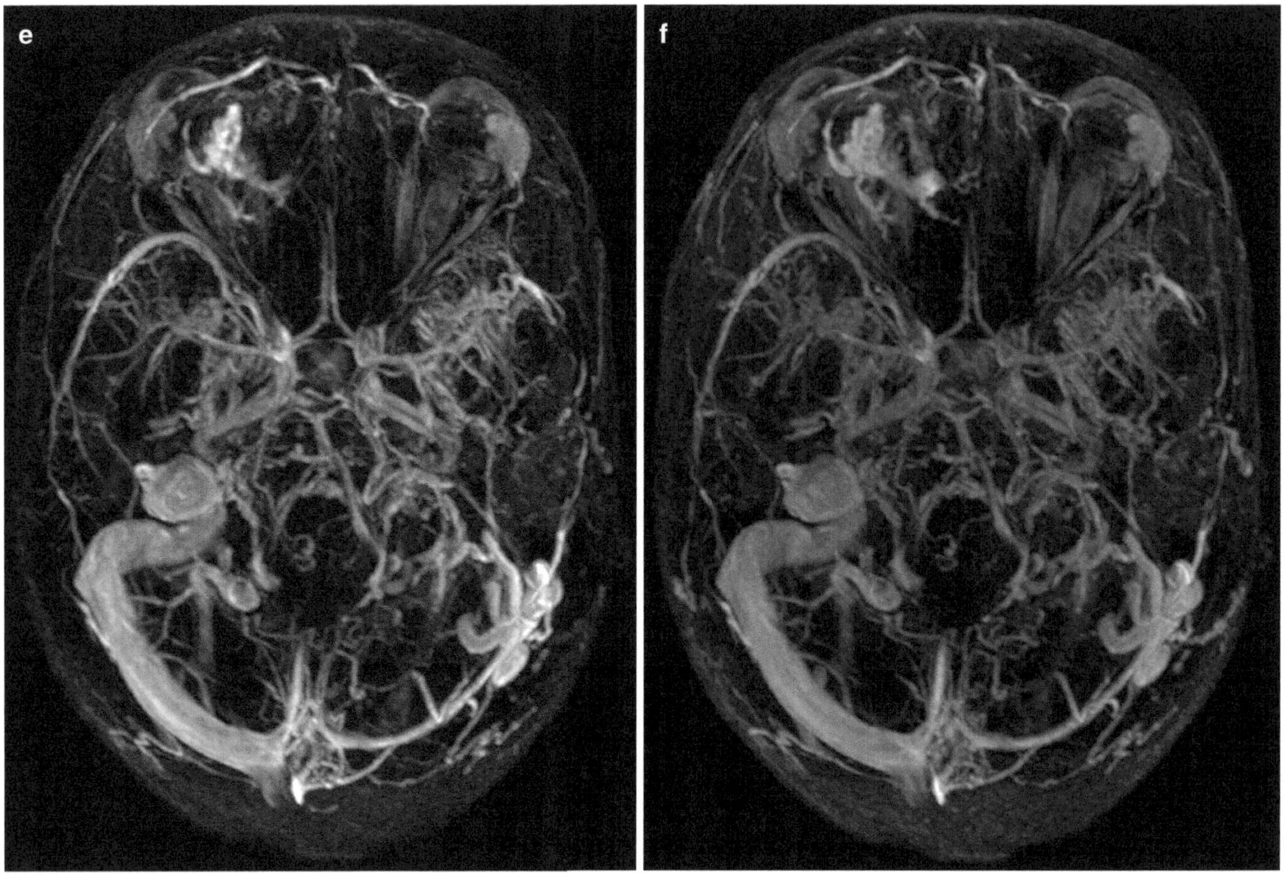

Fig. 2.4 (continued)

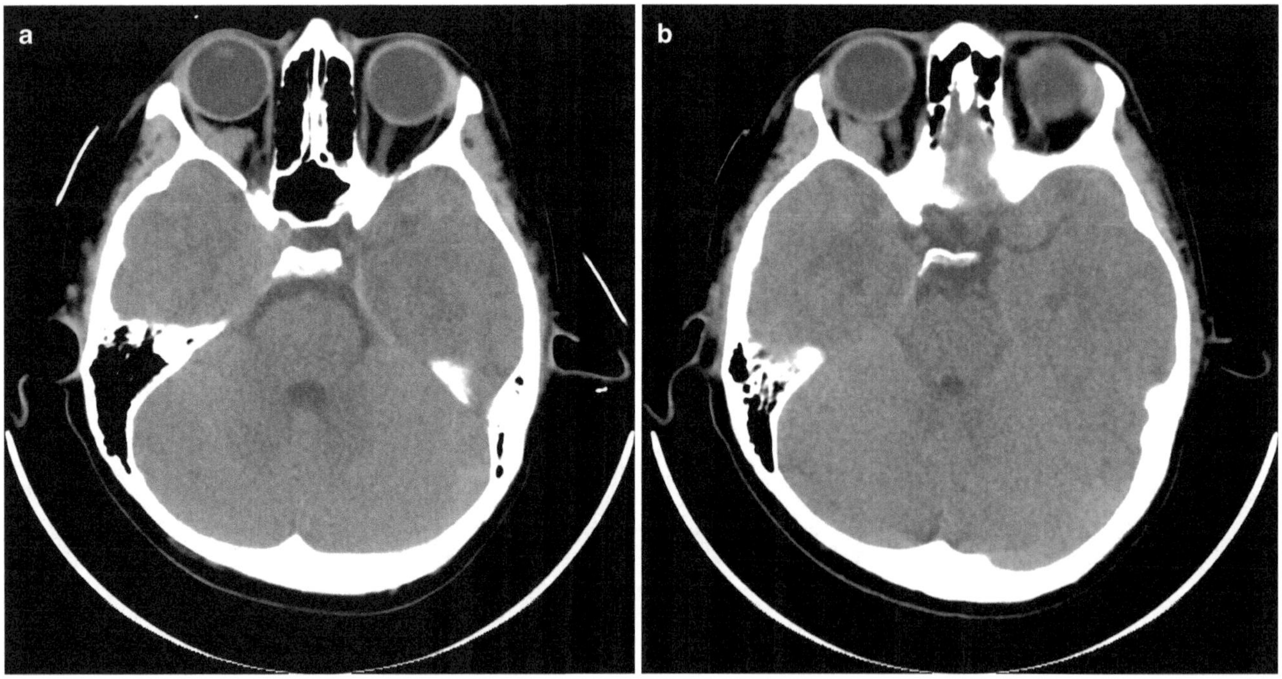

Fig. 2.5 Venous varix of the right orbit. CT scans before (**a**, **b**) and after (**c**, **d**) i/v injection of the contrast agent show orbital varix with partial enhancement in central part of the lesion. Time-resolved contrast-enhanced MR-angiography presented in different time-points after contrast agent bolus injection (**e**, **f**) demonstrates the irregular patchy contrast enhancement inside the dilated venous channels

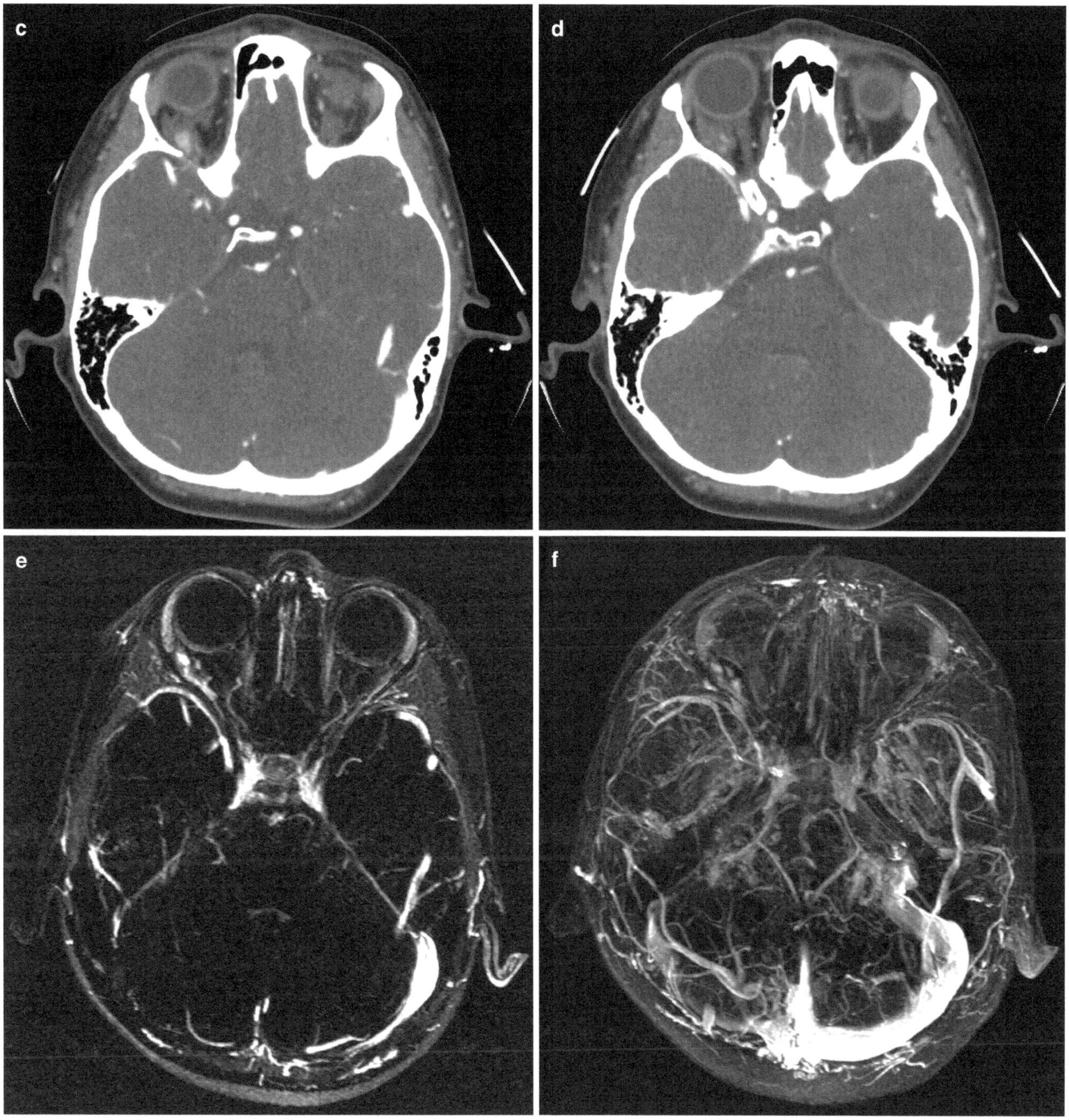

Fig. 2.5 (continued)

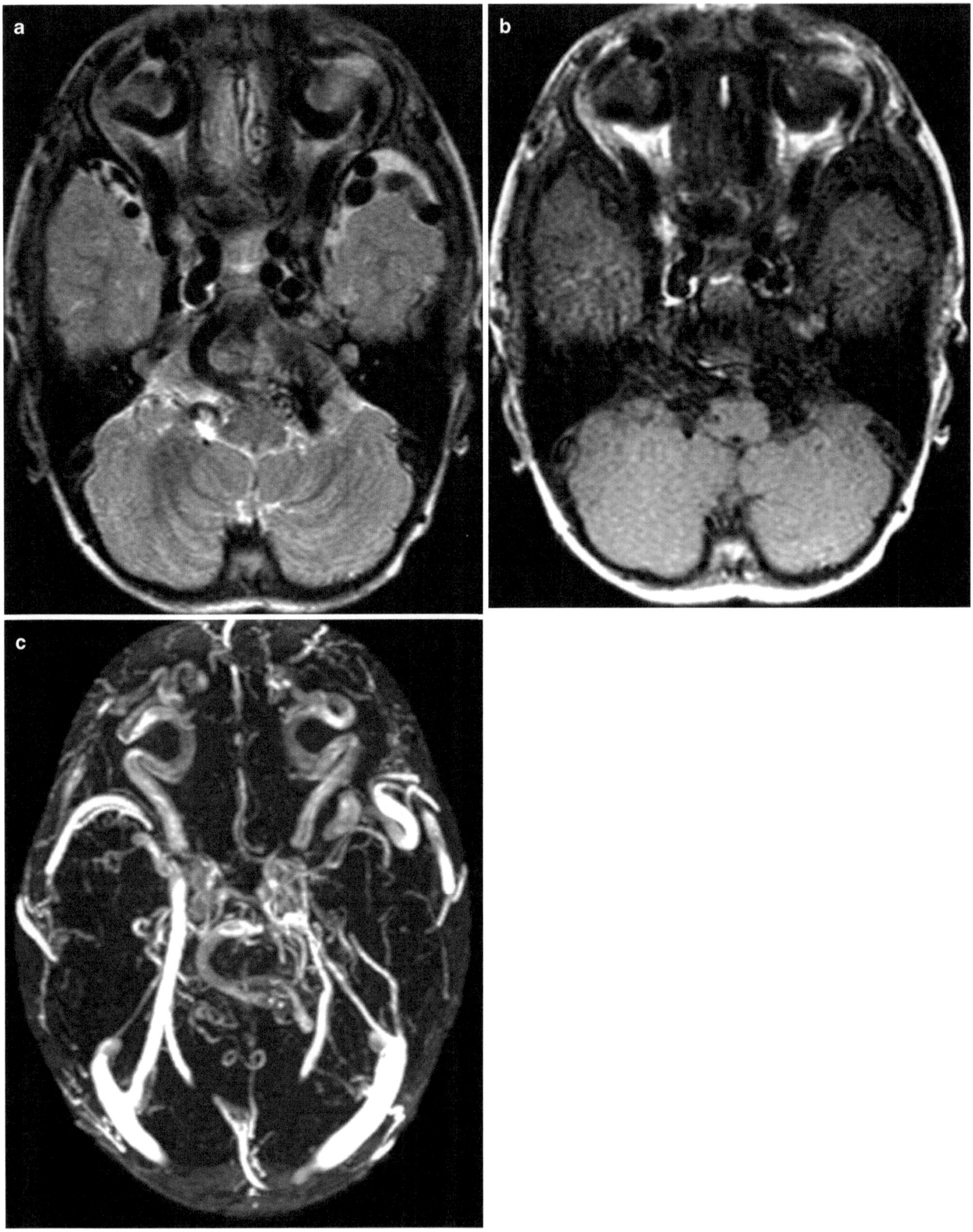

Fig. 2.6 Secondary venous varix of the orbits. A child with vein of Galen arteriovenous malformation. T2 (**a**), T1 (**b**) MRI and MR-angiography (**c**) demonstrate serpentine and enlarged intracranial and intraorbital veins with unusual shape

In case of carotid-cavernous fistula, the arterial blood flow dilates the sinus and produces the retrograde blood flow in the superior ophthalmic vein, dilating the latter. This is clearly visualized with Doppler ultrasound.

On MRI, rapidly flowing blood in the dilated ophthalmic vein and cavernous sinus causes a loss of signal on all standard sequences, allowing to clearly visualize the fistula and make an accurate diagnosis (Fig. 2.7).

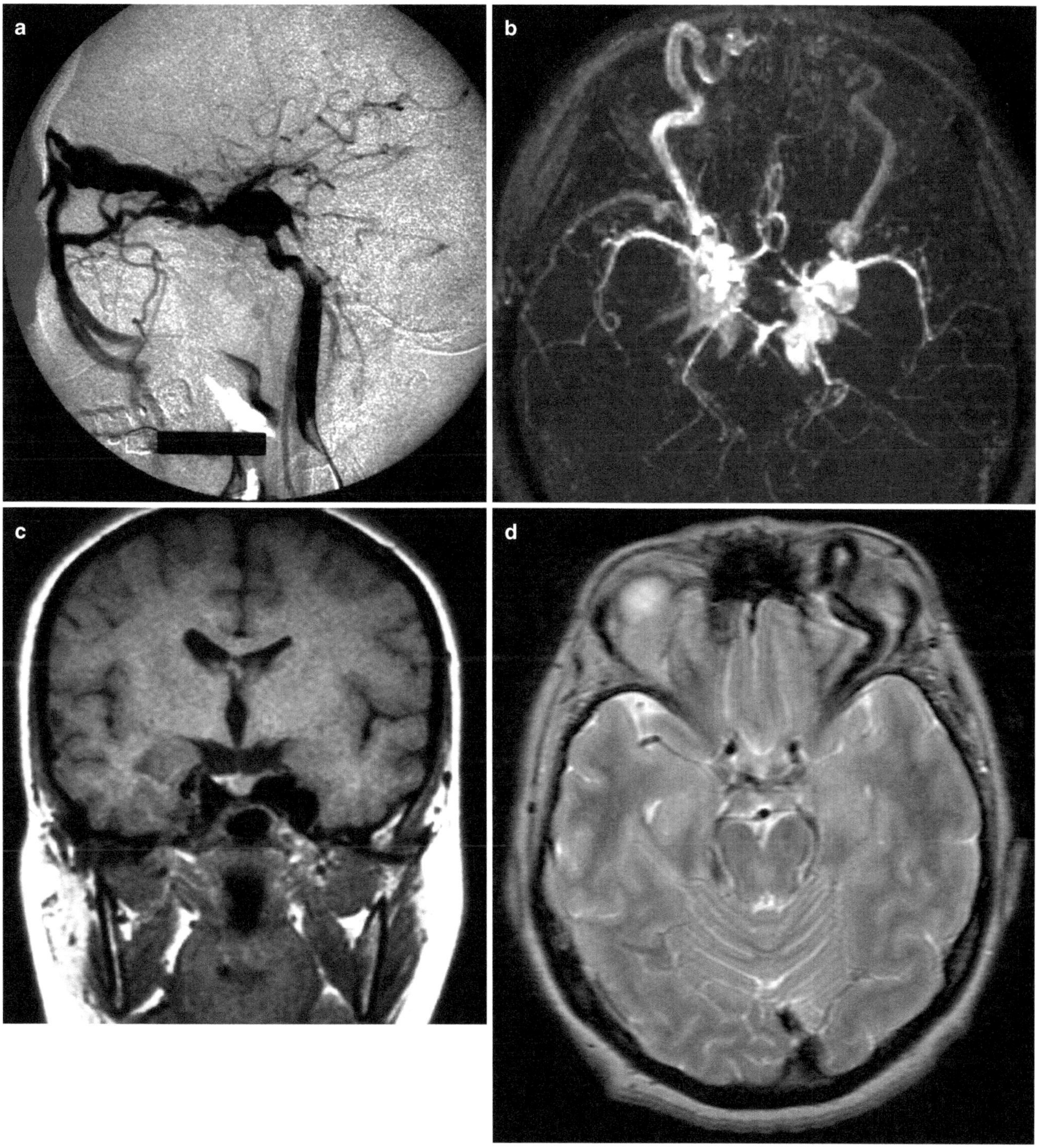

Fig. 2.7 Posttraumatic carotid–cavernous fistula (different cases). Case 1. DSA (**a**) depicts fistula in location of right cavernous sinus with retrograde flow into superior ophthalmic vein and facial veins. MR-angiography in 3DTOF (**b**) demonstrates bilateral carotid–cavernous fistula and dilatation orbital venous system including right spheno-parietal sinus. Both cavernous sinuses show flow-void phenomenon on MRI in T1 (**c**). Case 2. Left-side carotid–cavernous fistula can be clearly detected in the left orbit on T2 (**d**), T1 (**e**) and T1+ FatSat (**f**) MRI

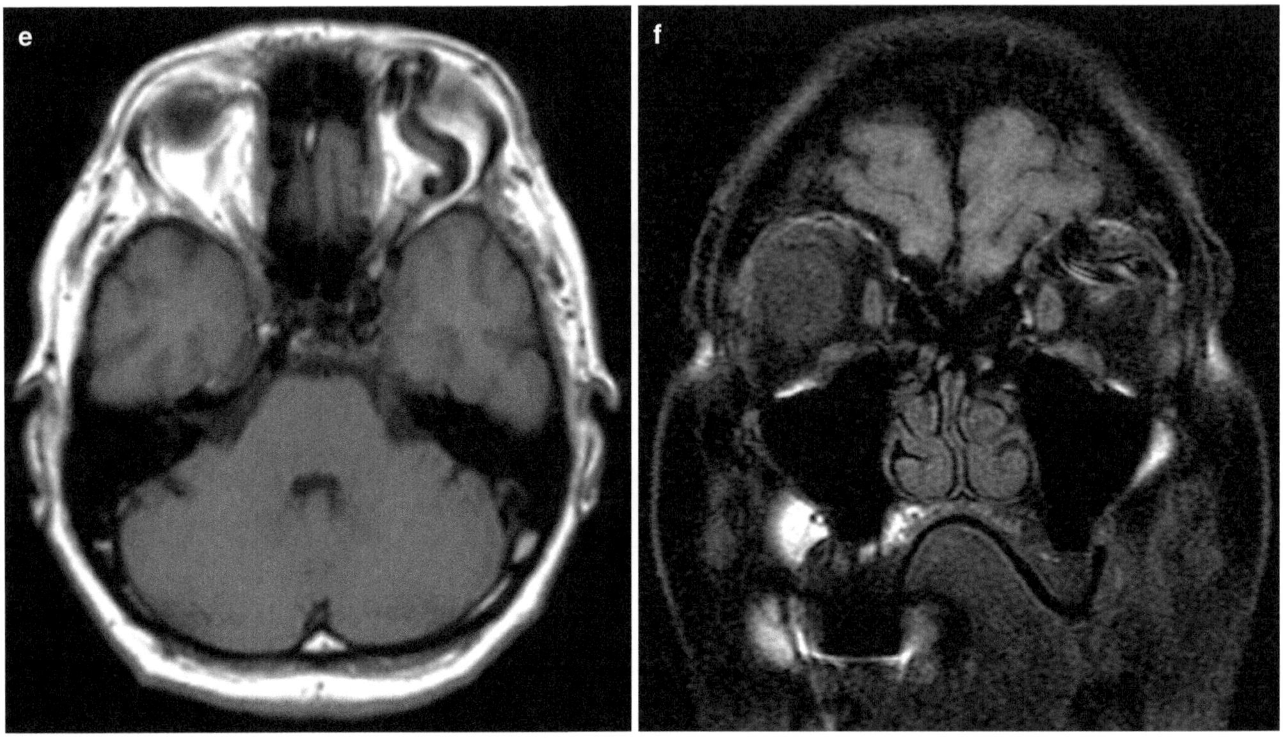

Fig. 2.7 (continued)

CT is useful in the imaging of dilated venous channels and enlarged veins in the orbit. CT angiography is the most informative method in the identification of all peculiarities of CCFs (Fig. 2.8). Coronal and sagittal CT reformations are especially useful for demonstrating the symmetric thickening of the extraocular muscles, in contrast to the asymmetric enlargement of these muscles in Grave's ophthalmopathy. However, the described changes can be visualized only with intravenous contrast enhancement. The use of MR angiography provides important additional information in the evaluation of vascular disorders in the cavernous sinus, especially those with slow blood flow. Relationship between fistula and cavernous sinus can be estimated based on MR angiography very precisely. For this purpose 2D–TOF or 3D–TOF techniques, or TRICKS can be applied. The latter method allowing to obtain high quality contrast-enhanced MR angiograms identical to direct angiography with estimation of contrast bolus movement in different phases can be used (Kornienko and Pronin 2009). Furthermore, the comprehensive analysis of MR images with standard sequences and MR angiograms allows evaluating the evolution of thrombosis in the venous drainage channels, which can occur either during treatment or after endovascular embolization. In case of venous thrombosis, a previously low MR signal from venous channels is replaced with an increased intensity signal proportional to the "age" of the thrombus. The MR signal reverses to hypointense at the stage of thrombus recanalization. In any case, MRI can replace direct monitoring angiography in assessing changes in the disease course.

Despite the use of non-invasive methods in the diagnosis of carotid-cavernous fistulae, direct angiography remains the gold standard in the primary diagnosis of this disease, verification of the affected side, topical localization of collateral circulation and its causes. Small fistulae are poorly detected with MRI and are revealed on DSA by a selective contrast agent injection into the external and internal carotid arteries. This allows visualizing the dilated venous channels that drain the fistula in details. Over the period of 1975–1999, more than 900 patients with direct CCF were examined at the N. N. Burdenko Institute of Neurosurgery, Moscow. They accounted for 21% of all patients with vascular neurosurgical pathology. Traumatic origin was responsible for development of majority of CCFs. Spontaneous CCFs were diagnosed only in 2.8%. In all cases, in order to confirm the diagnosis of CCF and affected sides, a direct selective angiography of all brain circulation regions should be performed on the side of the fistula, as well as on the contralateral side of the carotid and vertebral arteries with carotid artery cross-clamping on the fistula side in order to control the collateral circulation.

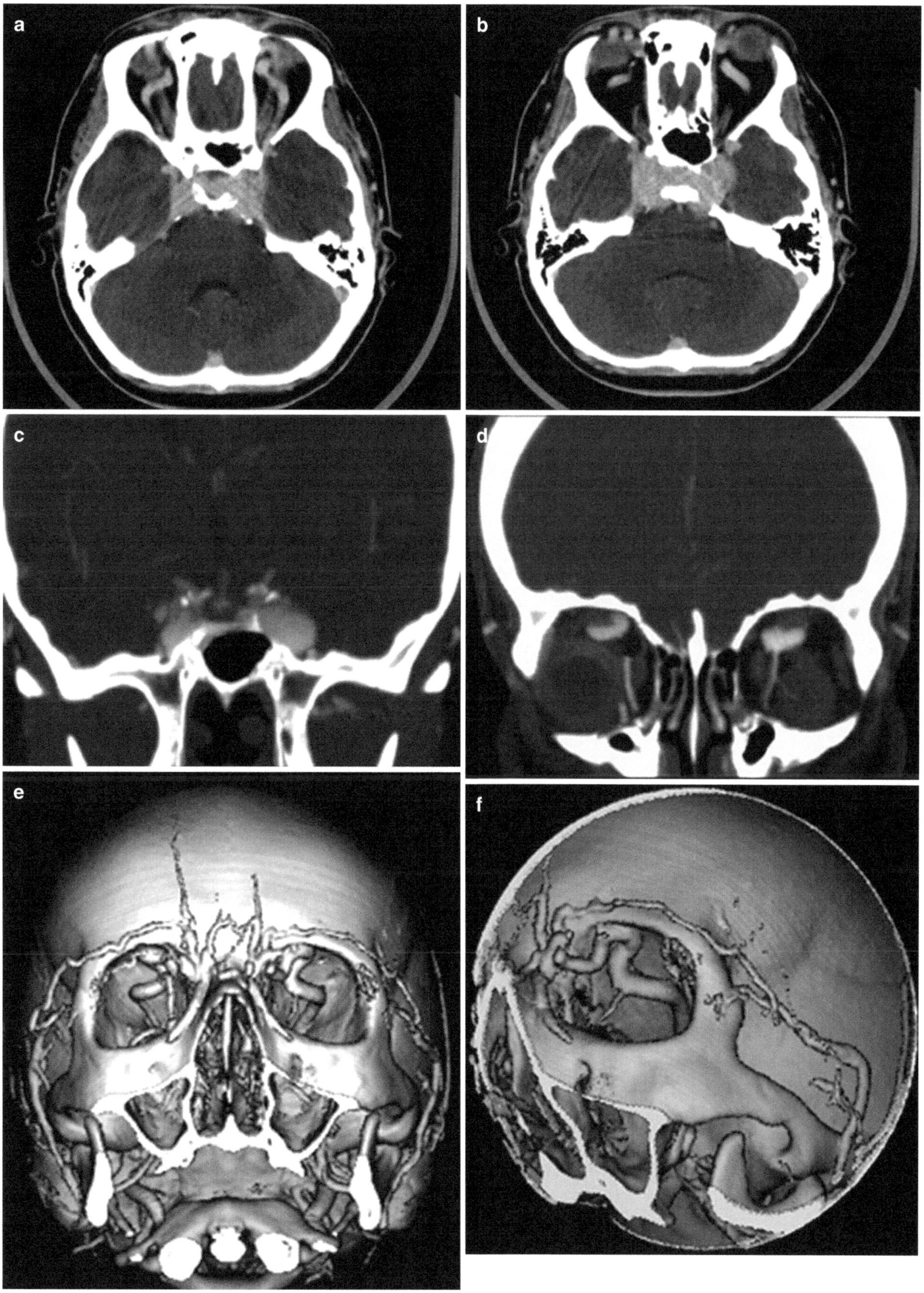

Fig. 2.8 Bilateral carotid–cavernous fistula. Raw data of CT angiography demonstrate that the cavernous sinuses and superior ophthalmic veins are abnormally increased (**a**, **b**). MIP reformats in the coronal plane define better the extension of venous structures of the skull base and orbits (**c**, **d**). Oblique views (**e**, **f**) of 3D processing of the data

2.1.2.3 Differential Diagnosis

Orbital tumor, lymphangioma, metastasis, sarcoidosis, venous malformation, venous thrombosis, cavernous sinus tumors, ICA aneurysm.

2.1.3 Ophthalmic Vein Thrombosis

The most common cause of unilateral ophthalmic vein thrombosis is an infection process (most often otogenic, odontogenic, or sinogenic) affecting the orbit. Despite the relative isolation of the orbit, it may be the area invaded by an infection process from the paranasal sinuses. The lack of valves and a large number of venous anastomoses is the main way of infection transmission to the orbit. The anastomosis connecting the venous plexus in the pterygopalatine fossa with the inferior ophthalmic vein can also serve as a port for infection (Tarasova and Drozdova 2005).

2.1.3.1 Clinical Manifestations

The disease is accompanied by exophthalmos, pain in the affected orbit, chemosis, symptoms of general intoxication.

2.1.3.2 Diagnosis

Orbital veins thrombosis is characterized by the presence of intravascular masses in the projection of the superior ophthalmic vein. Their characteristics differ depending on the imaging technique. On CT, before contrast agent administration, varicose superior ophthalmic veins are visualized as a hyperdense lesion with prolonged shape. MRI picture depends on the stage of thrombosis and paramagnetic properties of hemoglobin derivatives (Fig. 2.9). In case of deoxyhemoglobin

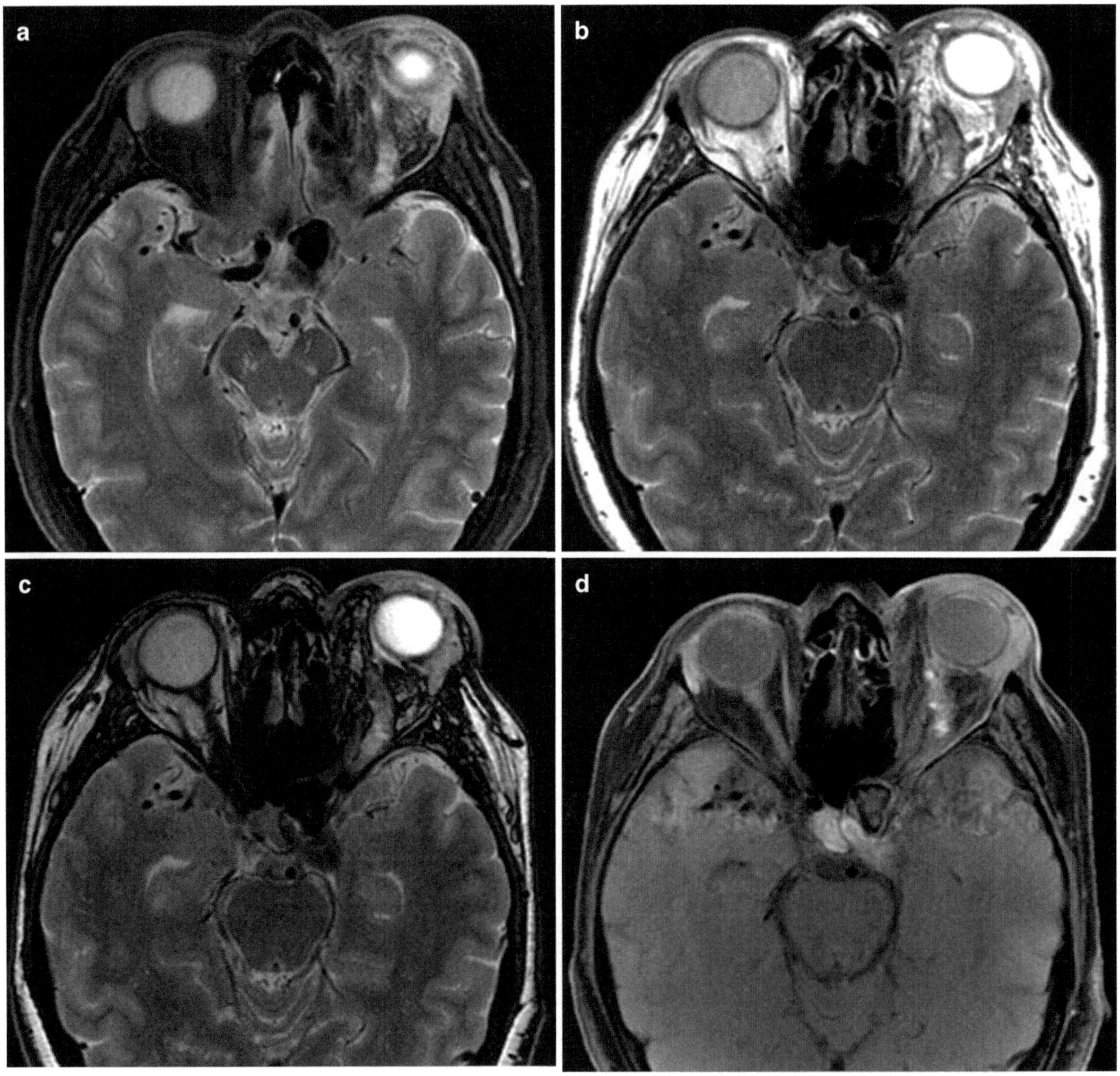

Fig. 2.9 Venous thrombosis of the left orbit. MRI in T2-WI (**a**–**c**) and T1-WI after intravenous contrast enhancement (**d**, **e**), with the technology Fat-Sat (**d**), demonstrate partially thrombosed the saccular aneurysm supraclinoid segment of ICA, complicated with thrombosis of the superior orbital vein of the left orbit. On MRI—3D PC angiography (**f**) clearly seen functioning part of left side ICA aneurysm and absent visualization of thrombosed vein

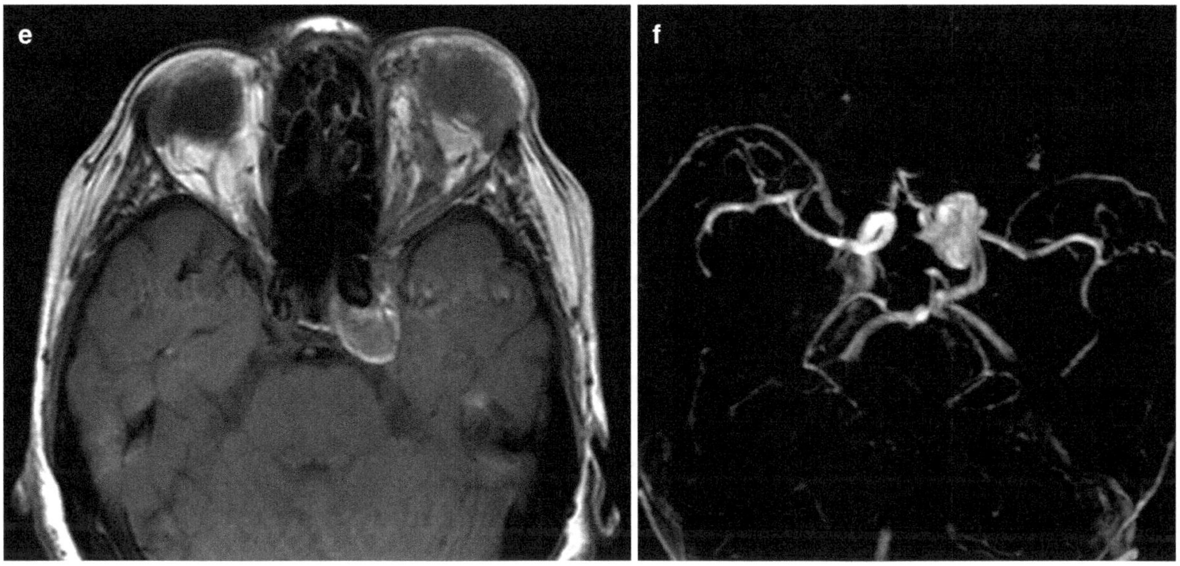

Fig. 2.9 (continued)

presence, the signal on T1- and T2-weighted images is hypointense, and becomes hyperintense when free methemoglobin appears (De Potter et al. 1995).

2.2 Tumors

2.2.1 Orbital Cavernous Hemangioma (OCH)

Orbital cavernous hemangioma (OCH) is a vascular space-occupying lesion that develops as a result of abnormal formation of the vascular system and is found in almost 70% of patients with vascular orbital lesions (Brovkina 2002). They account for 5–7% of all orbital tumors (Yan et al. 2004; Muller-Frell 2006). OCH is usually diagnosed at the age of 12–65 years old, mean age of 42 years old. Women suffer 2.5 folds more often than men. Cavernous hemangioma is usually localized within the inner surgical space (orbital space within the rectus muscles of the eye). Up to 80% of tumors are located intraconally. In most cases, OCH is a unilateral lesion with bilateral localization being rarely observed. Tumor sizes vary widely from a few millimeters to several centimeters, with a pronounced mass effect (Meyer and Hahn 2011).

2.2.1.1 Clinical Manifestations

Gradually increasing exophthalmos (axial in 60% of cases). The eye repositioning is difficult, early changes occur in the fundus. Tumor localization at the apex of the orbit is accompanied by pain in the orbit and headache.

2.2.1.2 Diagnosis

On CT, it is a round or oval, well-defined space-occupying lesion located mainly in the orbital apex. Large tumors may have a lobular structure and be surrounded by a pseudocapsule with compression of the surrounding tissues. In relation to CT density, it is a homogeneous, isodense, or hyperdense (with the presence of microcalcifications) lesion. Sometimes there is excavation of the orbit walls in case of a large tumor. A CT-perfusion study showed a low TBV, TBF values from the main part of the tumor with presence of small hyperperfusion spots within the lesion. All these structural and functional characteristics allow to differentiate capillary hemangioma from many other histological types of the orbital tumors, especially from orbital glioma or meningioma, with great accuracy (Figs. 2.10, 2.11, and 2.12).

Based on T1-weighted MR-images, it is homogeneous and isointense lesion with the pseudocapsule that is looking like a hypointense rim. On T2-weighted images, OCH usually has a hyperintense MR-signal, often internal septa are visible, mainly in large tumors. Contrast enhancement is heterogeneous in nature: when using a dynamic study (time-resolved CE MRA), at early stages, mainly the central part is enhanced, while the contrast agent is distributed to the peripheral regions at later stages (Tanaka et al. 2004; Kahana et al. 2007). A standard MR-study shows homogeneous moderate enhancement (Tanaka et al. 2004; Bertelmann et al. 2011). The most optimal study protocol for OCH visualization with MR imaging is the sequence with fat suppression and intravenous contrast enhancement (Figs. 2.13, 2.14, 2.15, and 2.16). Novel MR-technologies (T1-IDEAL, T2-IDEAL) can more clearly detect the pseudocapsule of the OCH as a hypointense rim (Fig. 2.17).

2.2.1.3 Differential Diagnosis

Meningioma of the optic nerve sheath, optic nerve glioma, hemangiopericytoma, schwannoma, lymphoma, metastasis.

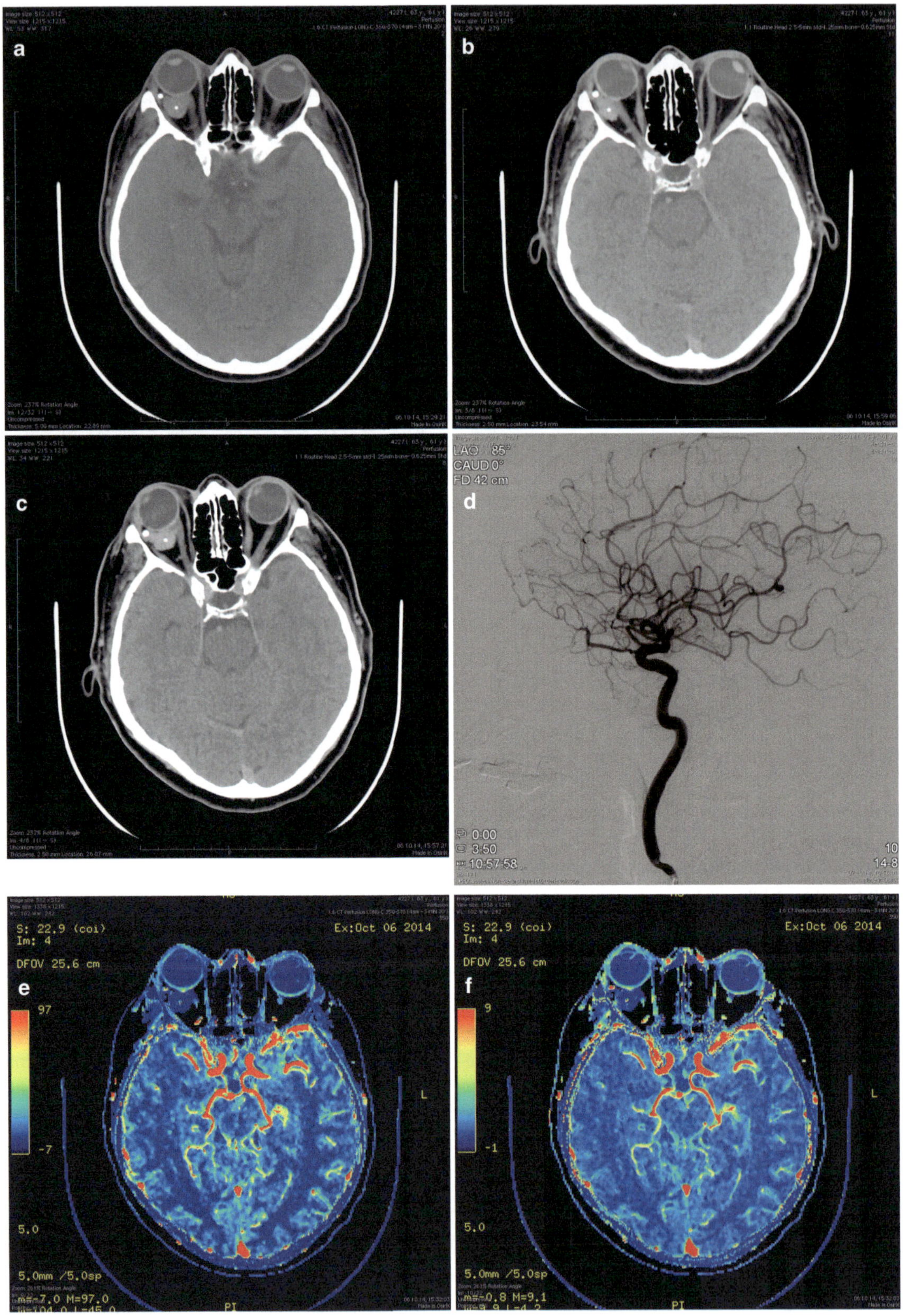

Fig. 2.10 Cavernous hemangioma of the right orbit. Axial CT scans (**a**) in standard eye position as well as with turn to *left* (**b**) and to *right* (**c**) sides show small retro eye ball lesion with calcifications (within and out) without involvement of rectus muscle of the orbit. DSA didn't find in this case feeding arteries (**d**). CT-perfusion CBF (**e**) and CBV (**f**) maps demonstrate intraorbital lesion with low perfusion from main part of the tumor, except small central hyperperfused spot

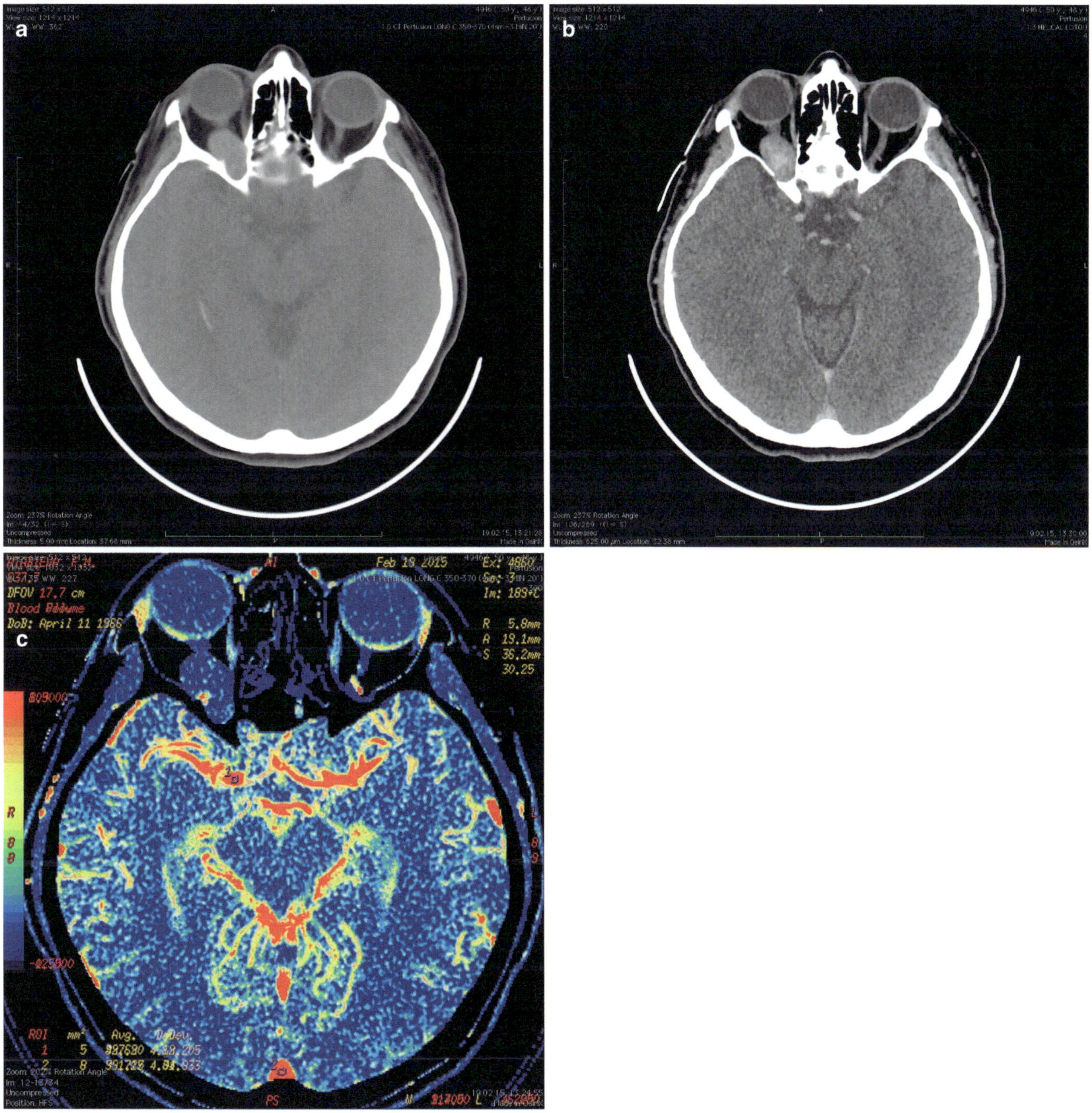

Fig. 2.11 Cavernous hemangioma of the right orbit. Axial CT scans before (**a**) and after (**b**) contrast enhancement demonstrate lesion in orbital apex with homogeneous enhancement and surrounding bone excavation. CT-perfusion CBV map (**c**) reveals lesion with low tumoral blood volume value from the most part of the hemangioma

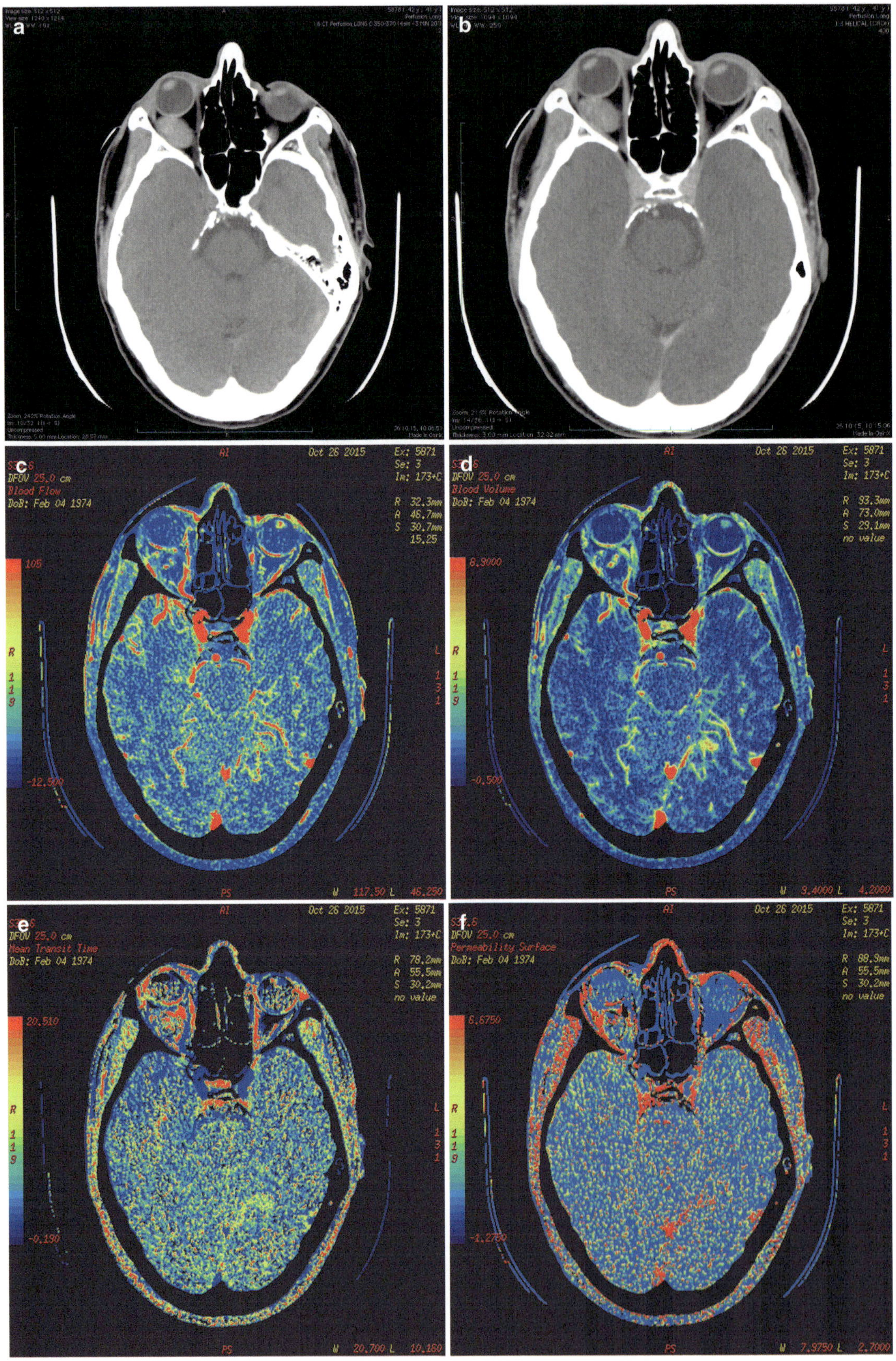

Fig. 2.12 Cavernous hemangioma of the right orbit. Axial CT scans before (**a**) and after (**b**) contrast enhancement demonstrate lesion in lateral part of the orbit with homogeneous enhancement. CT-perfusion (CBF (**c**), CBV (**d**), MTT (**e**) and PS (**f**) maps) reveals lesion with low tumoral blood flow and volume values from the most part of the hemangioma. The small central hyperperfused spots can be detected in this case. MTT parameter is typically prolonged. Permeability is characterized the low values within the lesion

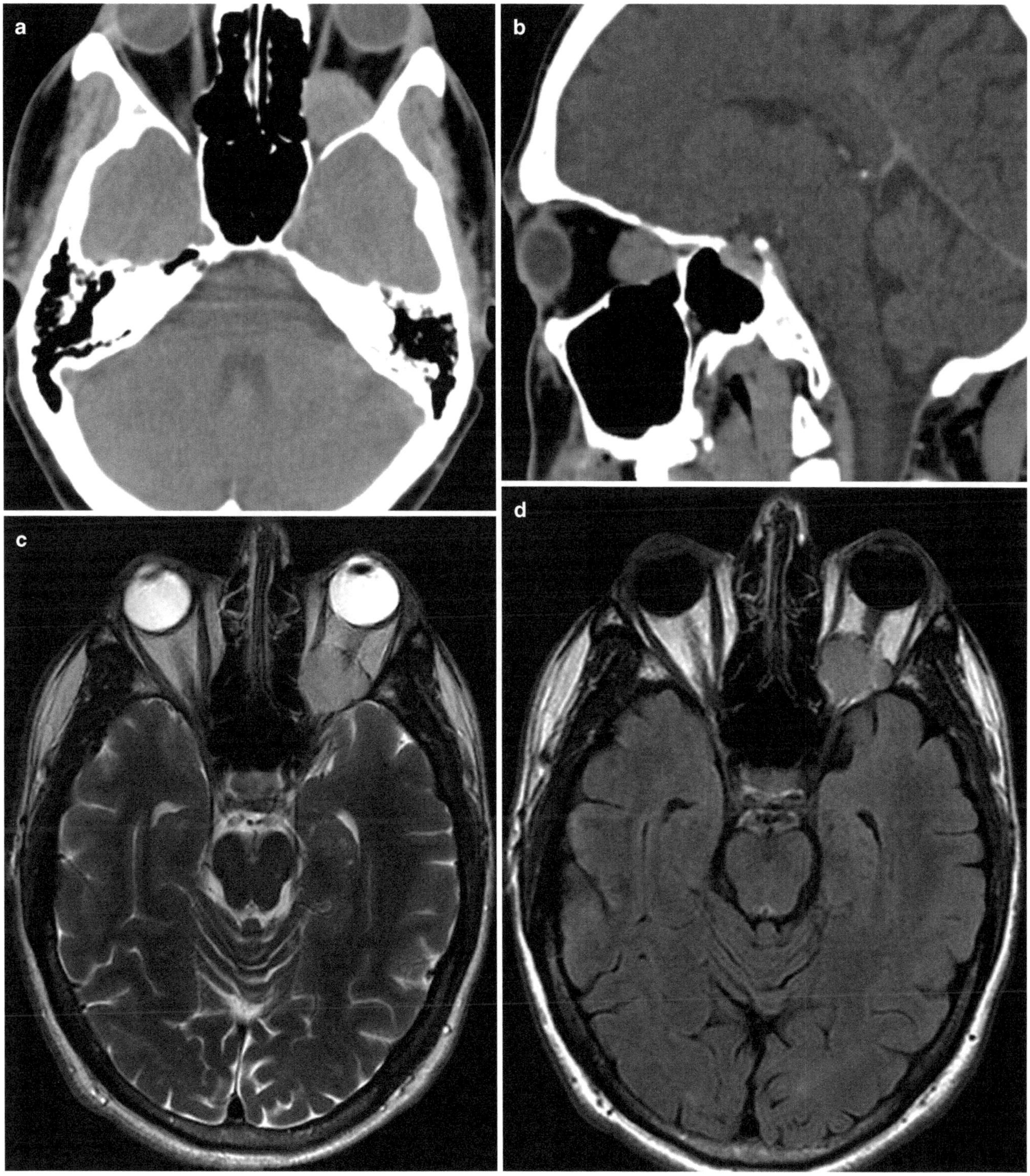

Fig. 2.13 Cavernous hemangioma of the left orbit. Axial CT scan (**a**) and sagittal reformat (**b**) show the homogeneously enhanced lesion located in orbital apex. There is no bone destruction on CT scans. Hemangioma has homogeneous hyperintense MR-signal on T2 (**c**), T2-FLAIR (**d**) and isointense MR-signal on T1 WI (**e**) images comparing to the rectus muscle of the orbit. MRI T2 weighted image in sagittal projection (**f**) reveals hemangioma with sharp edges in the top of the left orbit, which compresses the optic nerve

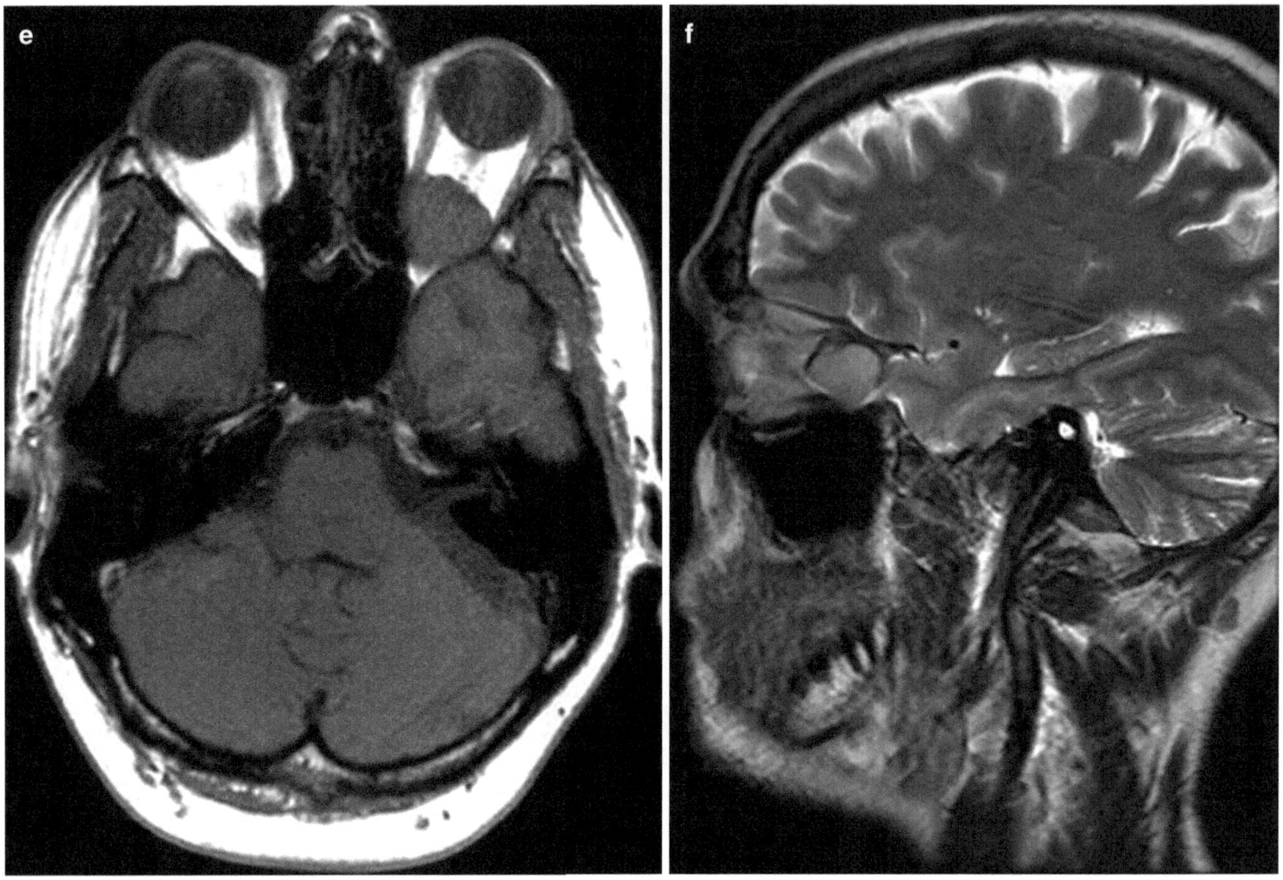

Fig. 2.13 (continued)

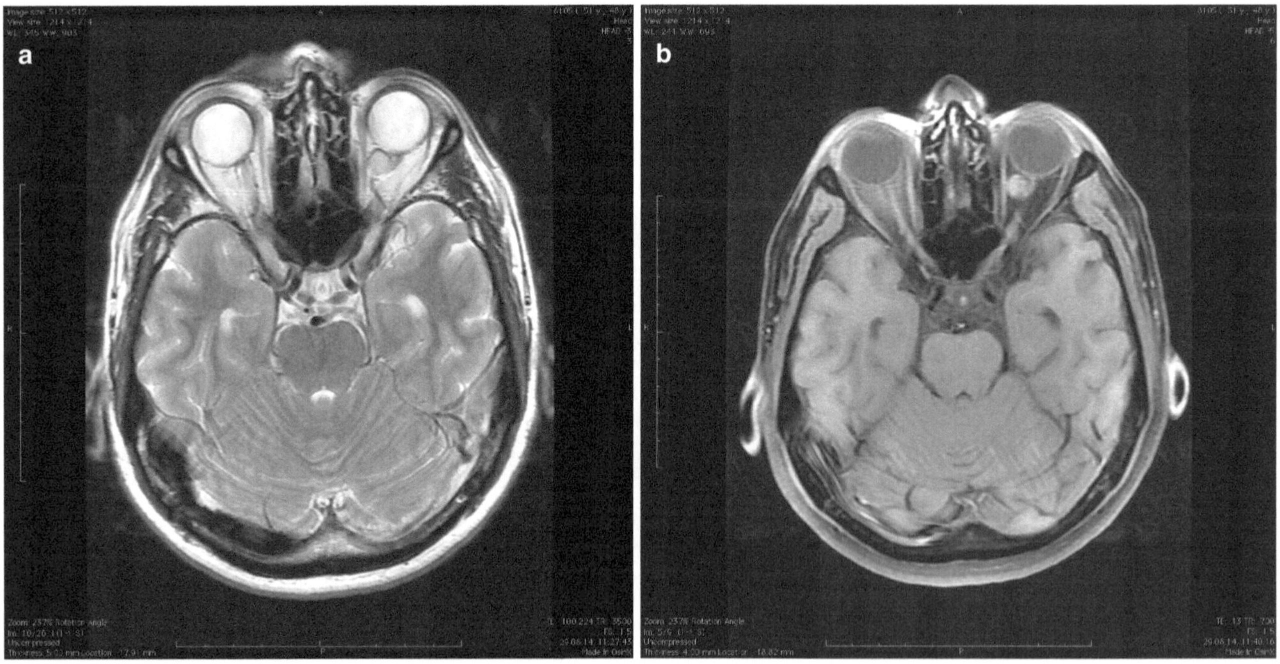

Fig. 2.14 Cavernous hemangioma of the left orbit. Axial MR scans in T2 (**a**) and T1 + FS (**b**) show the slightly hyperintense to the rectus muscle and homogeneous in structure retro globe small size lesion with hypointense ring (probably, due to chemical shift artifact). Lesion is characterized isointense compared to brain tissue MR-signal on DWI (**c**). Hemangioma shows lobular marked contrast enhancement on post-contrast T1 in axial (**d**), sagittal (**e**), and coronal (**f**) images

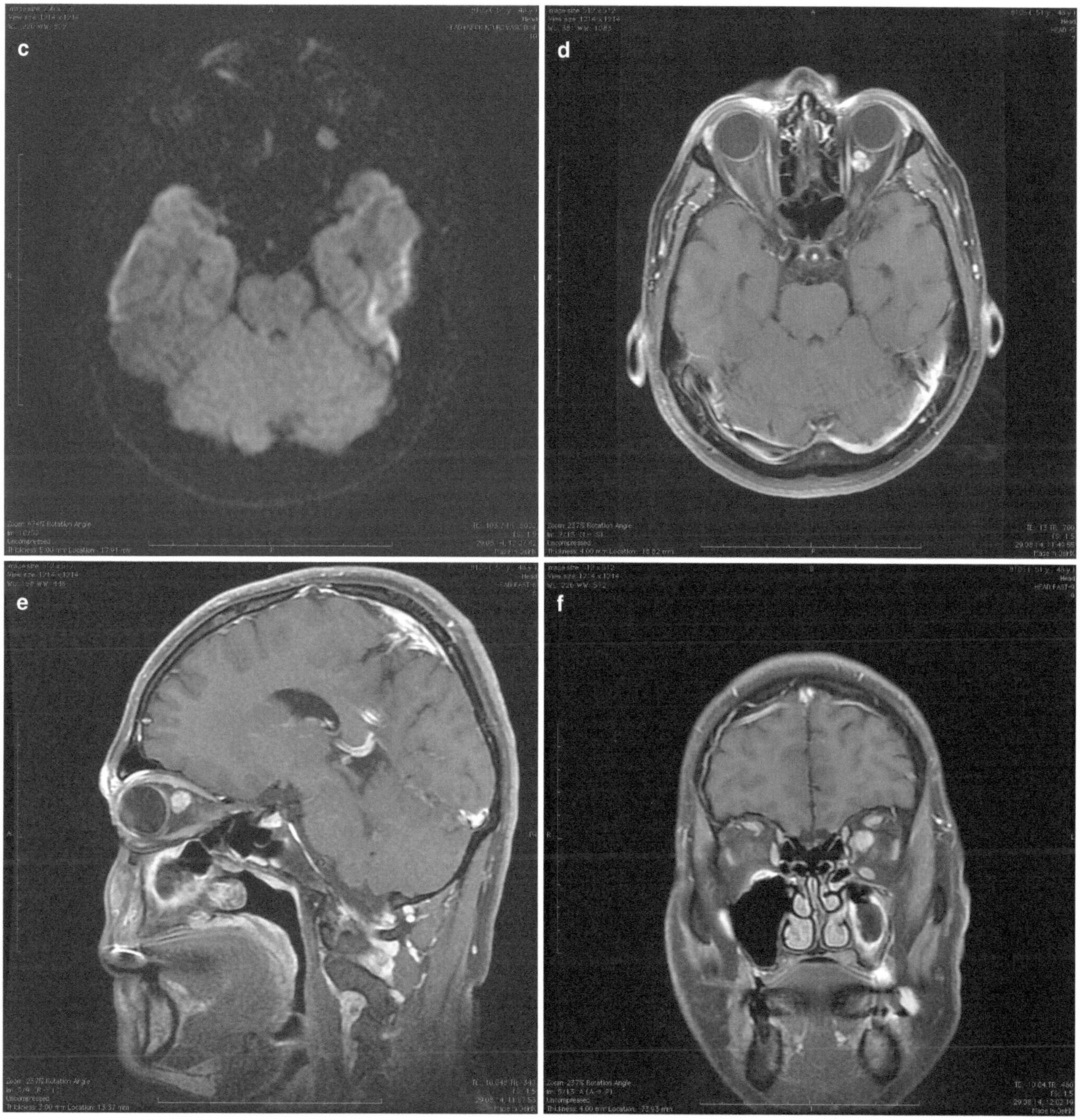

Fig. 2.14 (continued)

2.2.2 Lymphoma

Lymphoma is the most common malignant tumor of the orbit (10–15% of all orbital tumors (Valvassori et al. 1999; Coupland et al. 2002)) and up to 24% among older adult population (Demirci 2002), which belongs to hematopoietic tissue tumors of unknown pathogenesis; it ranks third among primary tumors of the orbit and is the most common multifocal lesion. Lymphoproliferative disorders, including lymphomas account for 8.1–10% of the total number of pediatric orbital tumors. In common, patients' age is 50–70 years, males being prevalent. The risk of primary lymphoma is increased in patients with HIV infection, drug-induced immunosuppression, systemic connective tissue diseases, chronic viral infections, in particular, association with Epstein-Barr virus is noted (Abramson et al. 2003; Jiltsova and Kaplina 2010). The majority of non-Hodgkin's lymphomas of the orbit are extranodular marginal-zone

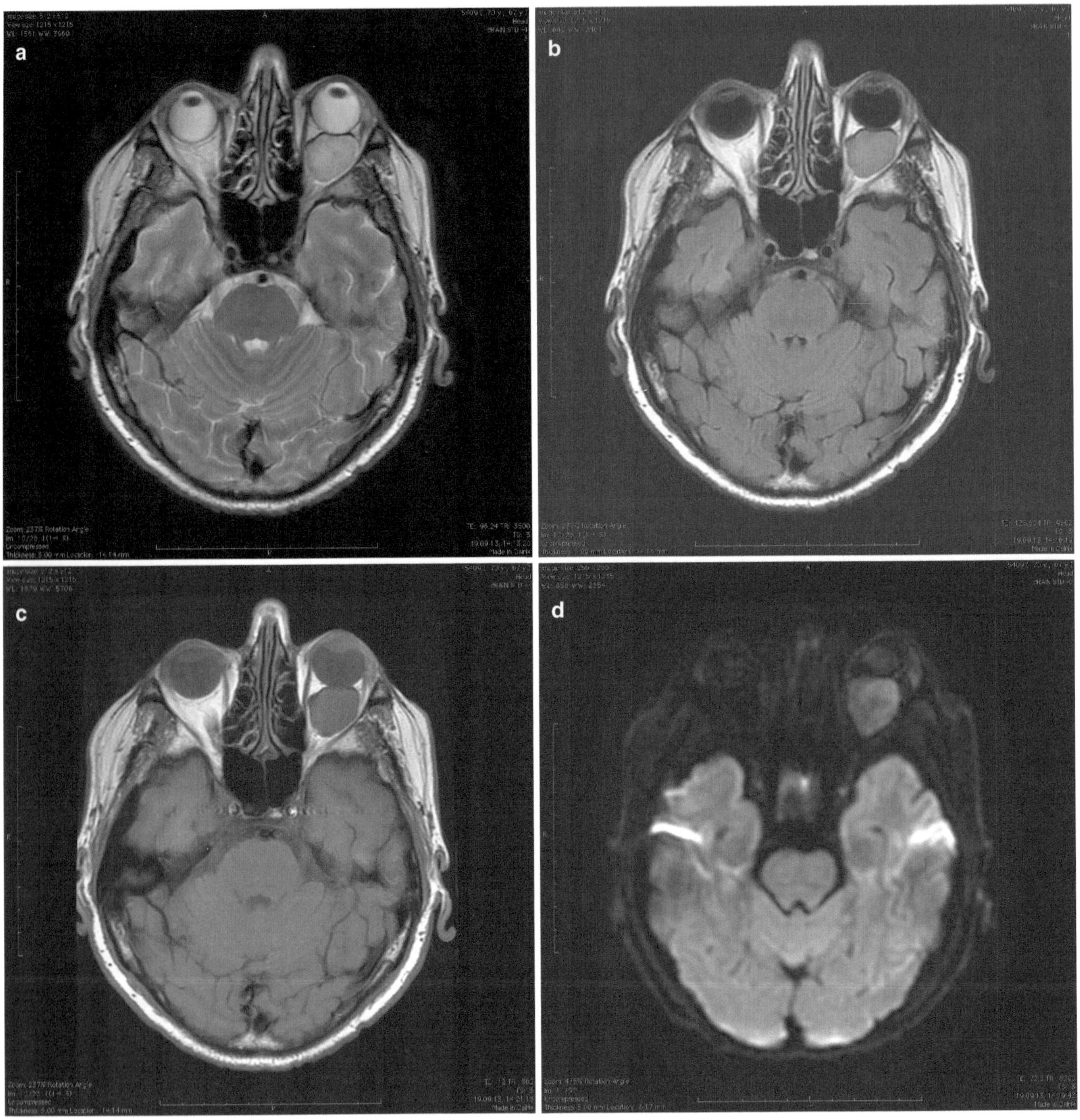

Fig. 2.15 Cavernous hemangioma of the left orbit. There is a large space occupied lesion retro eye ball location. Tumor has typical for hemangioma hyperintense MR-signal with hypointense ring on axial T2 (**a**) and T2-FLAIR (**b**) images. On T1 (**c**) and DWI (**d**) lesion shows isointense signal compared to brain tissue. After i/v contrast enhancement hemangioma demonstrates heterogeneous pattern of contrast enhancement with presence of small dark spots within the tumor structure ("pepper-salt" pattern) (**e**, **f**)

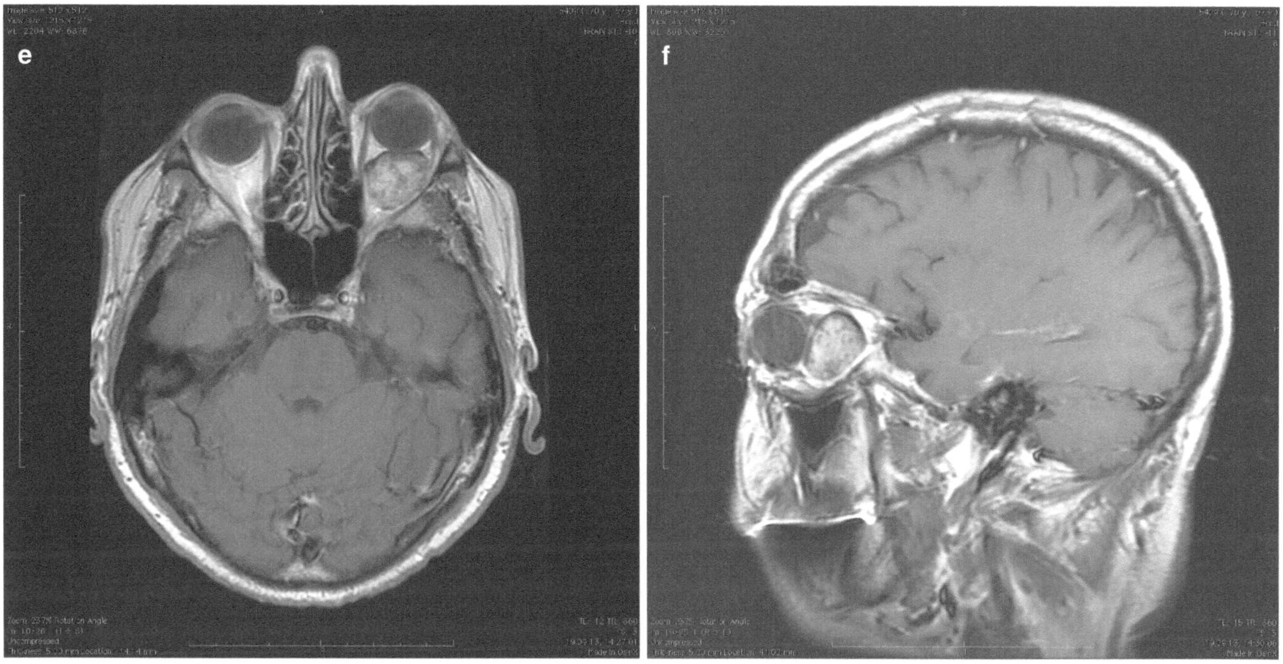

Fig. 2.15 (continued)

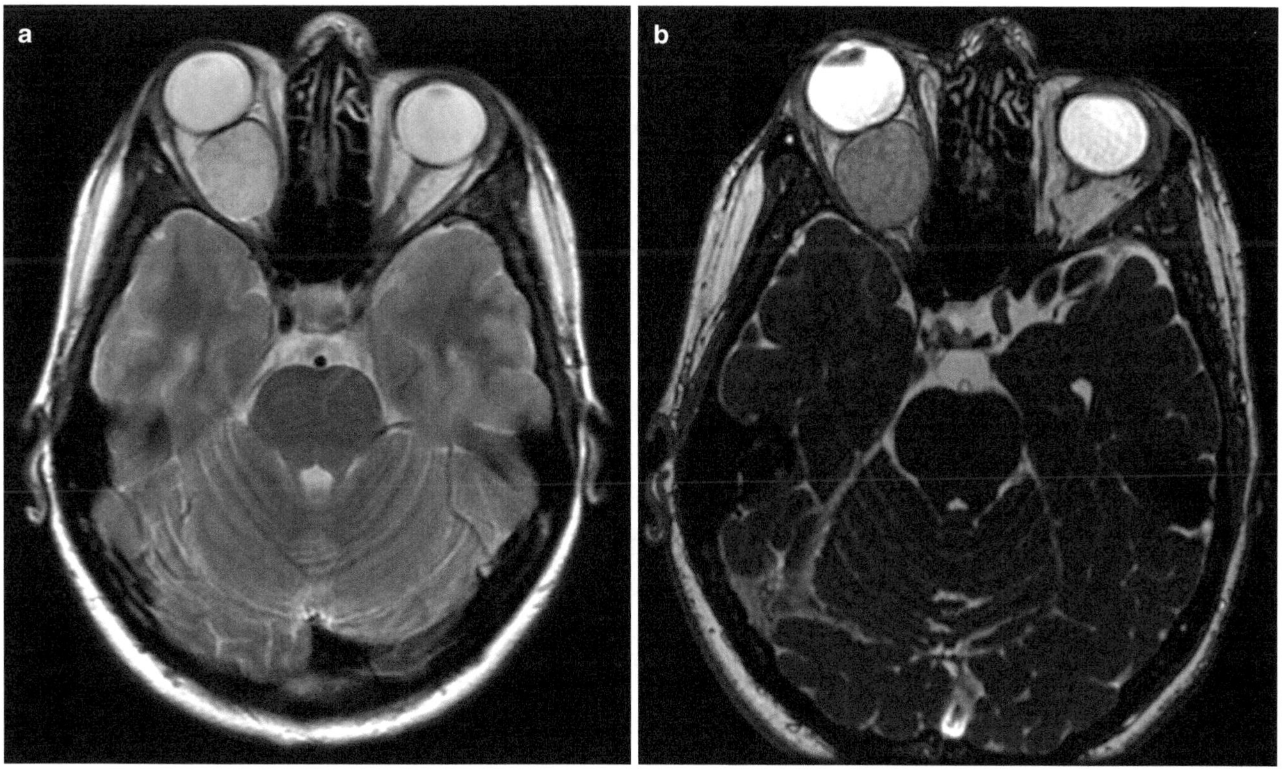

Fig. 2.16 Cavernous hemangioma of the right orbit. MR scans in T2 SE (**a**) and FIESTA (**b**) pulse sequences and in T2-FLAIR-WI (**c**) show the slightly hyperintense to the brain tissue and rather homogeneous in structure retro globe lesion with hypointense ring (due to chemical shift artifact). Lesion is characterized isointense signal compared to brain tissue on T1-WI (**d**). Hemangioma shows heterogeneous marked contrast enhancement on post-contrast T1-WI (**e**) and becomes more homogeneous on delayed post-contrast image (**f**)

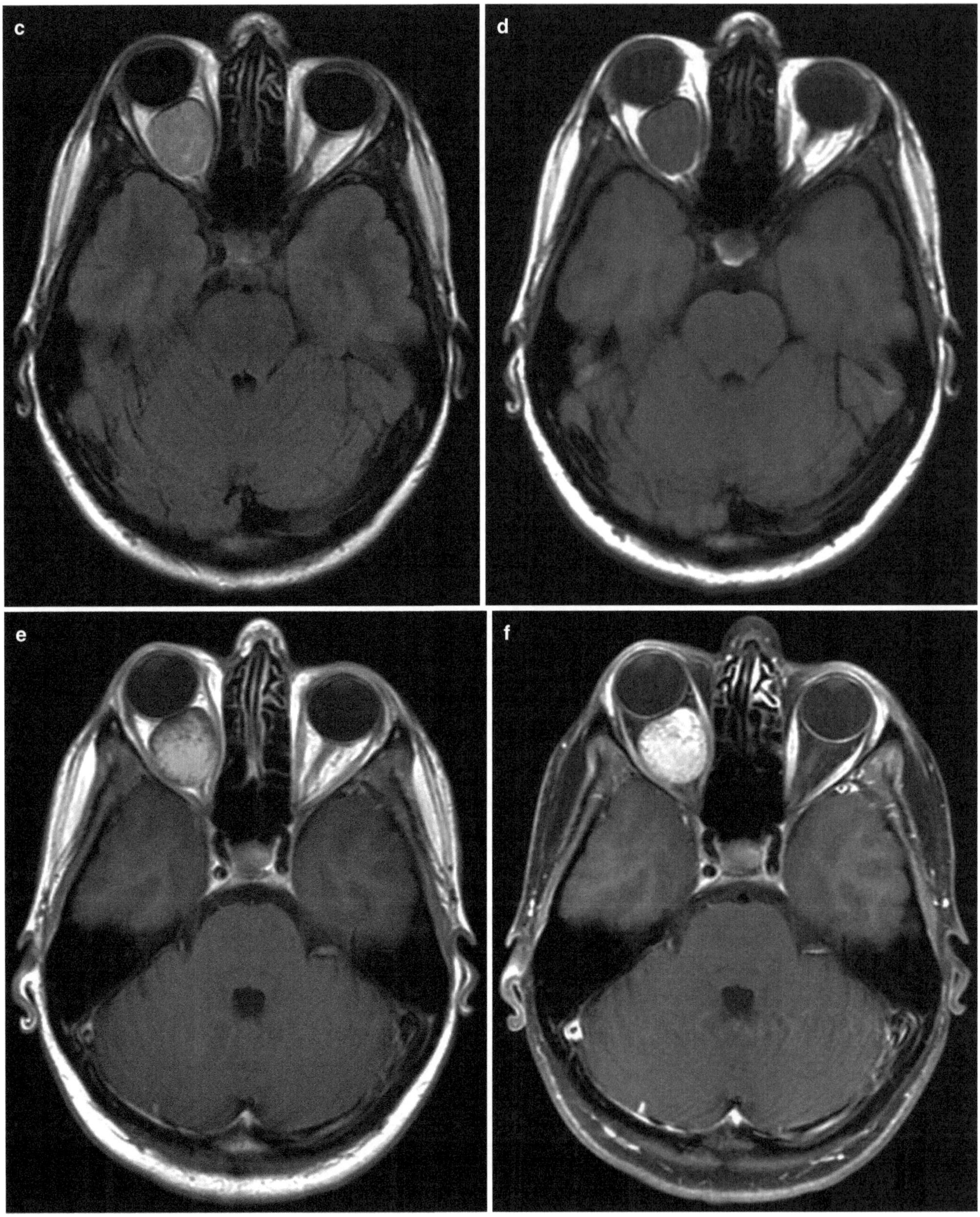

Fig. 2.16 (continued)

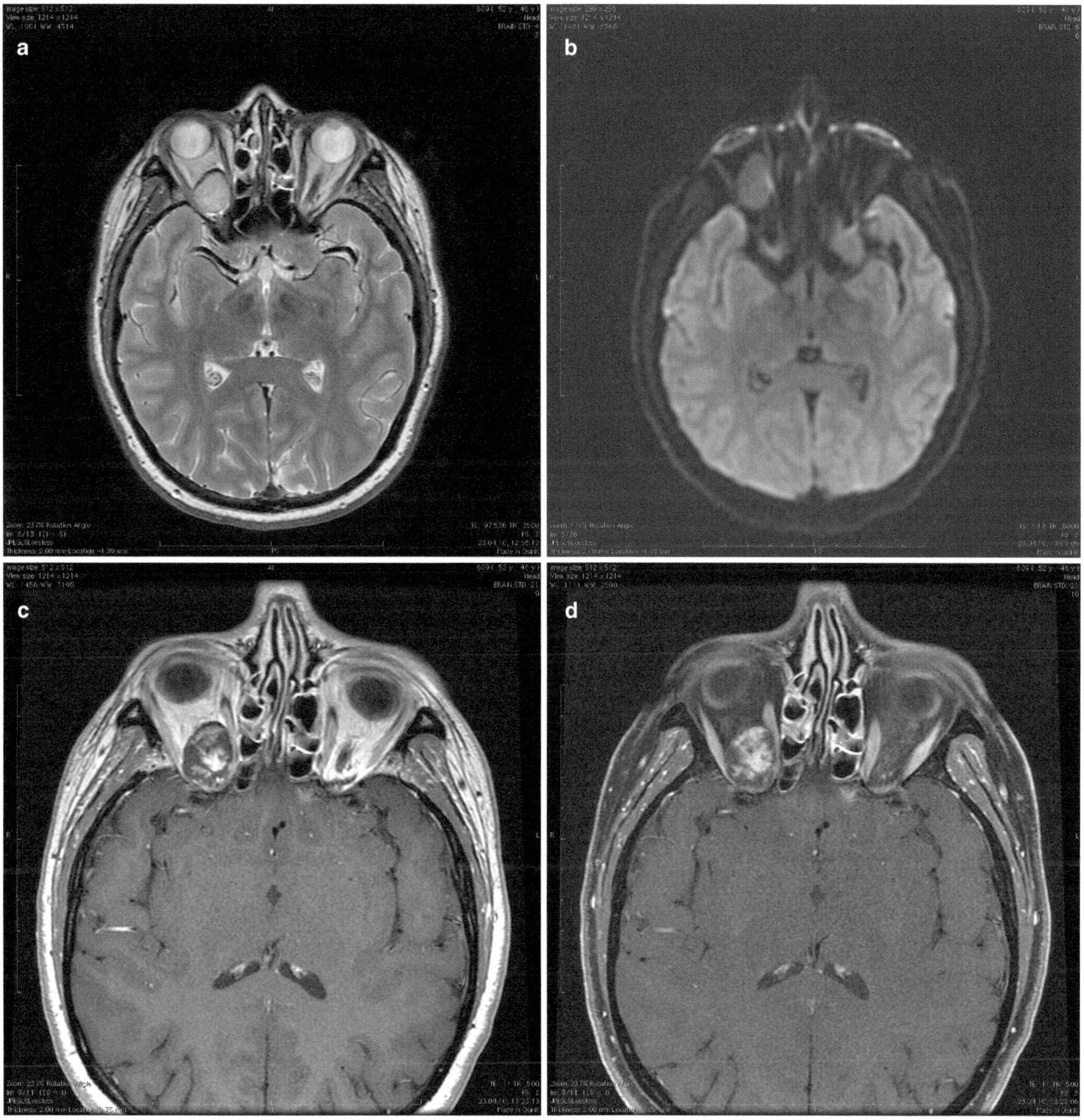

Fig. 2.17 Cavernous hemangioma of the right orbit. MR scan in T2 SE (**a**) shows the slightly hyperintense to the brain tissue and rather homogeneous in structure lesion located in orbital apex with hypointense ring (due to chemical shift artifact). Lesion is characterized isointense signal compared to brain tissue on DWI (**b**). Hemangioma shows heterogeneous partial lobular contrast enhancement on post-contrast T1-WI (**c**) with extantion this contrast enhancement within tumor structure with time on delayed post-contrast (10 min) image (**d**). Novel pulse sequences (T1(T2) IDEAL, GE) demonstrate advantages over the standard fat-sat technologies in assessment orbital region especially in cases with metal objects presence (T1 WI with FS (**e**) and T1 IDEAL / water (**f**) scans).

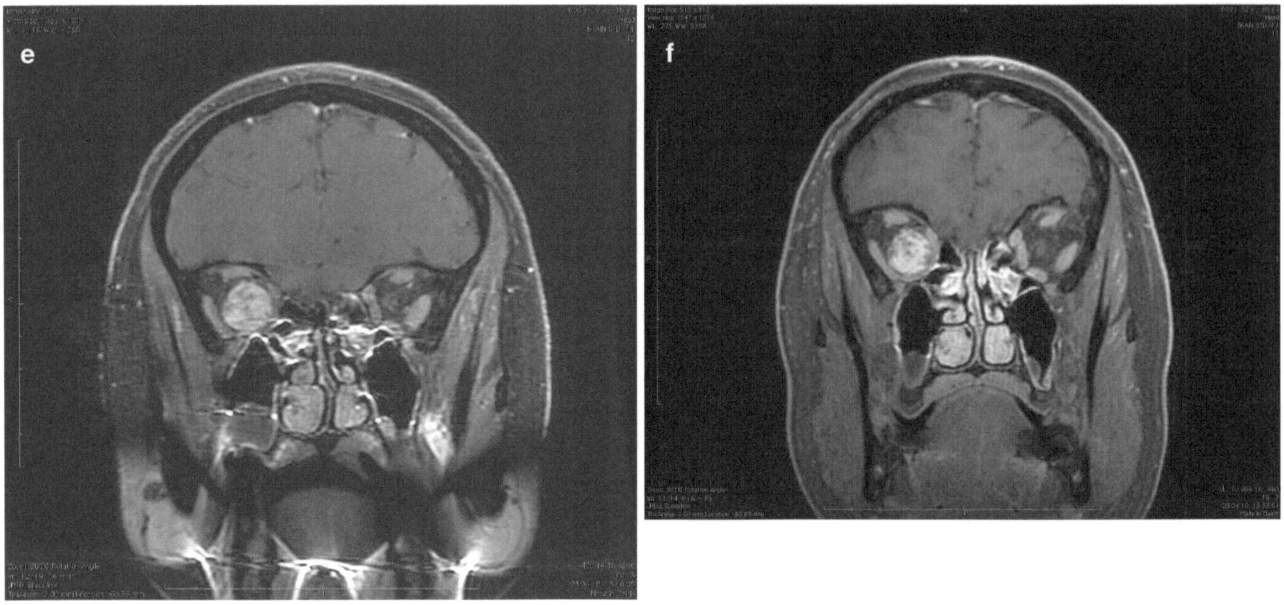

Fig. 2.17 (continued)

B-cell lymphomas of mucosa-associated lymphoid tissue type (Xu et al. 2010; Eckardt et al. 2013).

Lymphomas are referred to as orbital, if located only within the orbit, and extraorbital, the latter most often affect paranasal sinuses with involvement of the orbital cavity. The lesions that are disseminated at the time of diagnosis of orbital lymphoma are referred to as multifocal, which is 70% of patients with lymphomas (Harnsberger et al. 2004a).

2.2.2.1 Clinical Manifestations

Painless exophthalmos occurring without any prodromal syndrome, usually with a lateral displacement of the eye, non-inflammatory edema of the periorbital tissues. Early ptosis, diplopia are possible. The process is steadily progressing with development of chemosis and changes in the fundus with papilledema.

2.2.2.2 Diagnosis

On CT, tumors are visualized as homogeneous, initially hyperdense lesions, almost always intensely accumulating the contrast agent (Figs. 2.18 and 2.19). While being located in the peripheral orbital space or in the lacrimal gland area, lymphomas do not cause bone erosion. These lesions typically have a homogeneous structure, if there is a necrosis area in the center of the tumor, it has a relatively lower density as compared to the tumor stroma. Lymphomas tend to grow along orbital structures, outline solid structures such as the eyeball and the intraorbital portion of the optic nerve. In areas, where the lesion is adjacent to the soft tissue structures with increased density, the tumor margins become more distinguished. Perfusion parameters obtained in vast majority of intracranial lymphoma demonstrate a slight elevation in CBV, a moderate prolongation of MTT with a relatively low blood flow values and high level of permeability. In general, lymphomas are characterized by low levels of perfusion, and, thus, differ from malignant gliomas, metastases, and meningiomas. Data about intraorbital lymphomas according to their hemodynamic are unknown. In our case with intraorbital lymphoma we faced to lesion with atypical hyperperfusion, probably due to high malignancy status of this tumor (Fig. 2.20).

Lymphomas are visualized as isointense lesions comparing to the orbital muscles on T1-weighed images, and as hypointense or isointense lesions relative to the adipose tissue on T2-weighed images. If there is a cavity with necrosis, this area is characterized by a high signal on T2- and low signal on T1-weighted MR images. When using a contrast agent, intense homogeneous contrast enhancement is typically observed. On diffusion-weighted MRI images lymphomas are characterized by a high signal and the values of the apparent diffusion coefficient (ADC) close to those of the normal gray matter of the brain, or they have a slightly increased ADC (Henderson 1994; Yan et al. 2004; Kapur et al. 2009; Sepahdari et al. 2014).

Distinguishing atypical lymphoid infiltrates from malignant lymphoma in the orbit is very complicated task. Lymphoma is more common in the lacrimal gland area and often affects both orbits. Malignant lymphomas are characterized by more pronounced contrast enhancement and higher perfusion parameters than those for the extraorbital muscles. In case of atypical lymphoid infiltrates, pronounced heterogeneous contrast enhancement is observed (Xu et al. 2010).

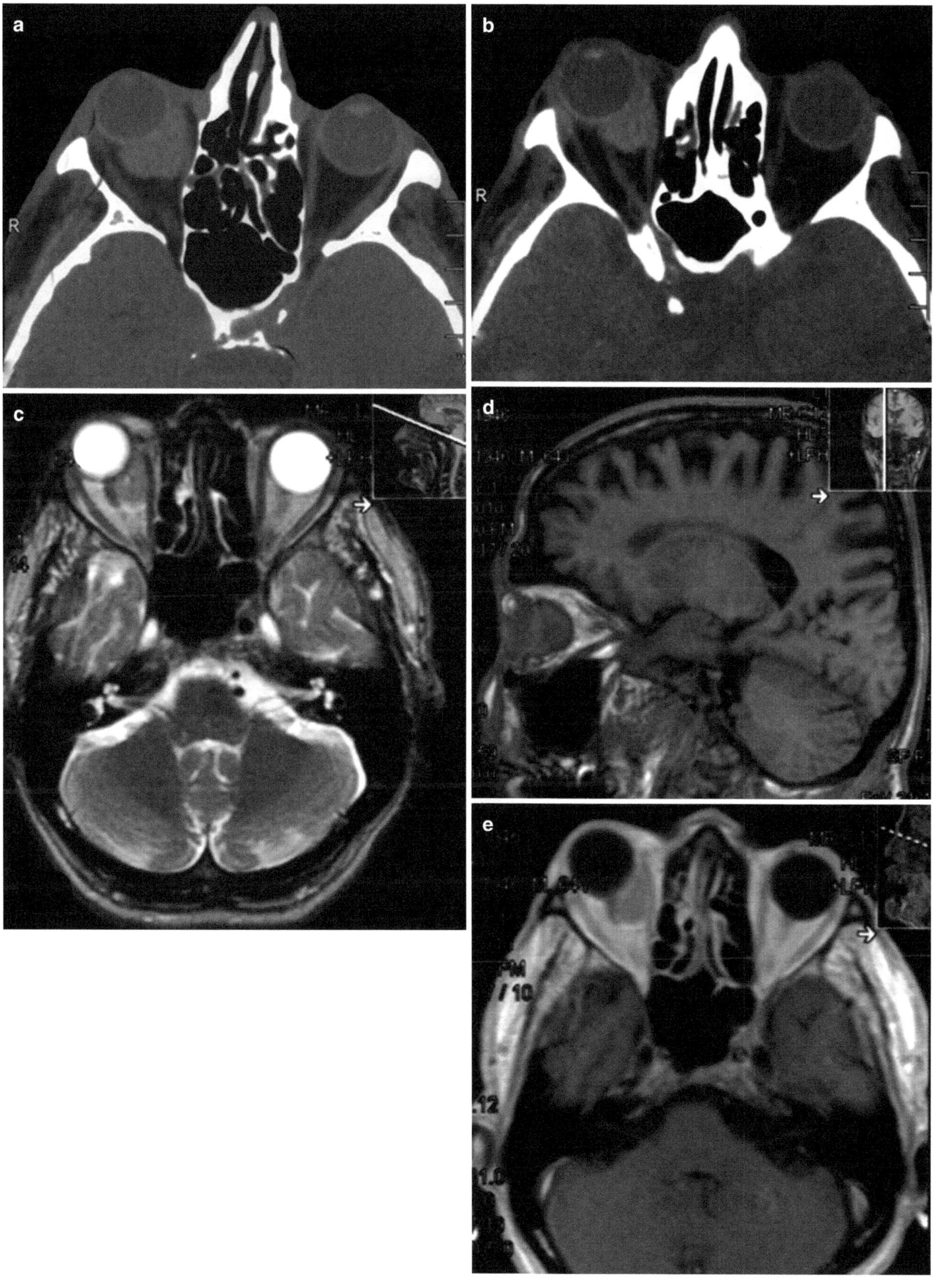

Fig. 2.18 Lymphoma. Axial CT scans (**a**, **b**) show hyperdense tumor in medial parts of the right orbit retroglobe location. There is wide scleral invasion and there is no bone destruction. The tumor is visible on axial T2-WI (**c**) and T1-WI (**d**) MR scans. The tumor locates between the optical nerve (laterally) and the medial rectus muscle (medially). Tumor is characterized marked and homogeneous contrast enhancement (**e**)

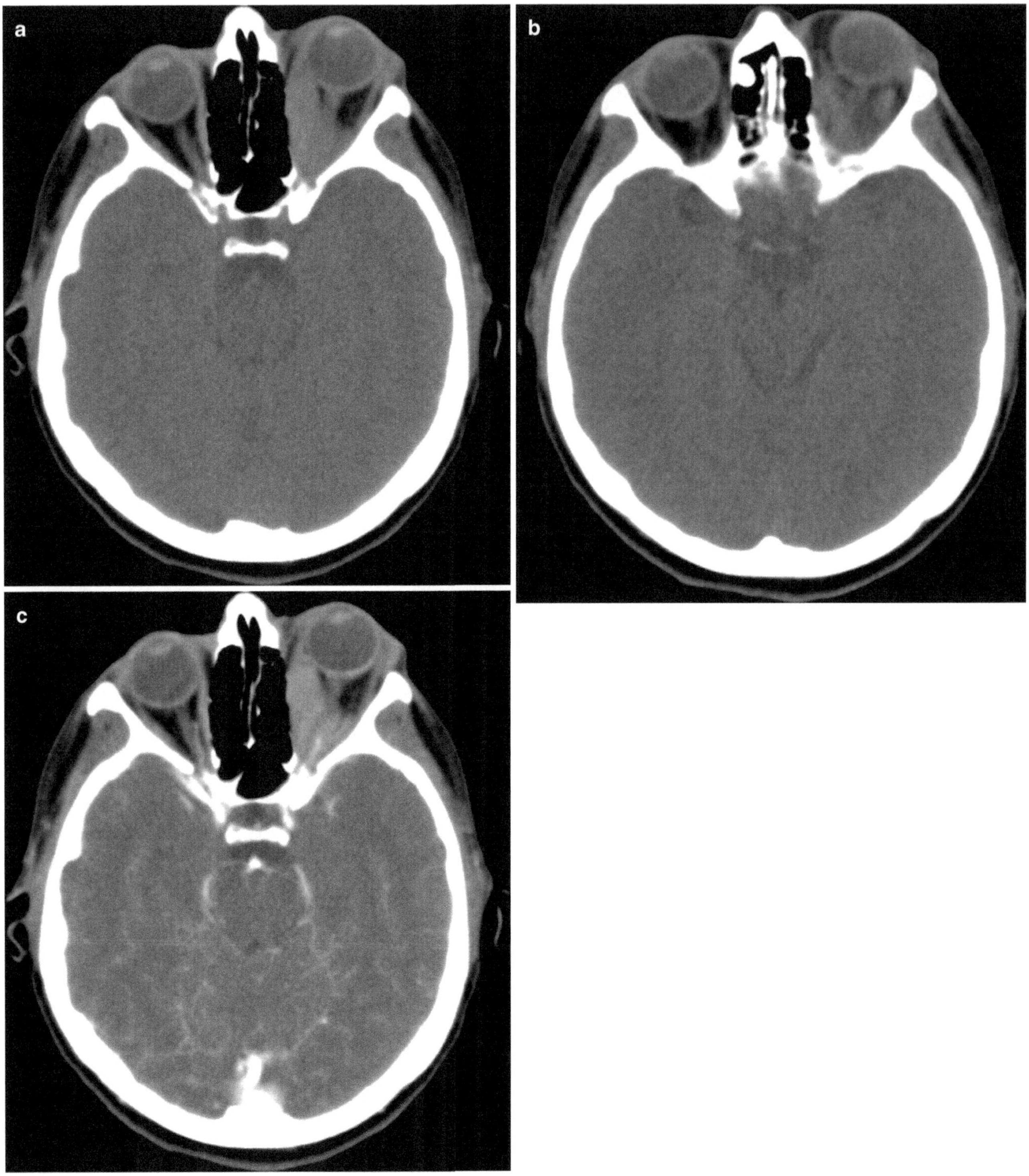

Fig. 2.19 Lymphoma of the left orbit. CT-scans before (**a**, **b**) and after (**c**) contrast agent i/v injection. The tumor involves the apex and lateral part of the orbit with infiltration of the medial rectus muscle. Tumor is characterized marked and homogeneous contrast enhancement (**c**)

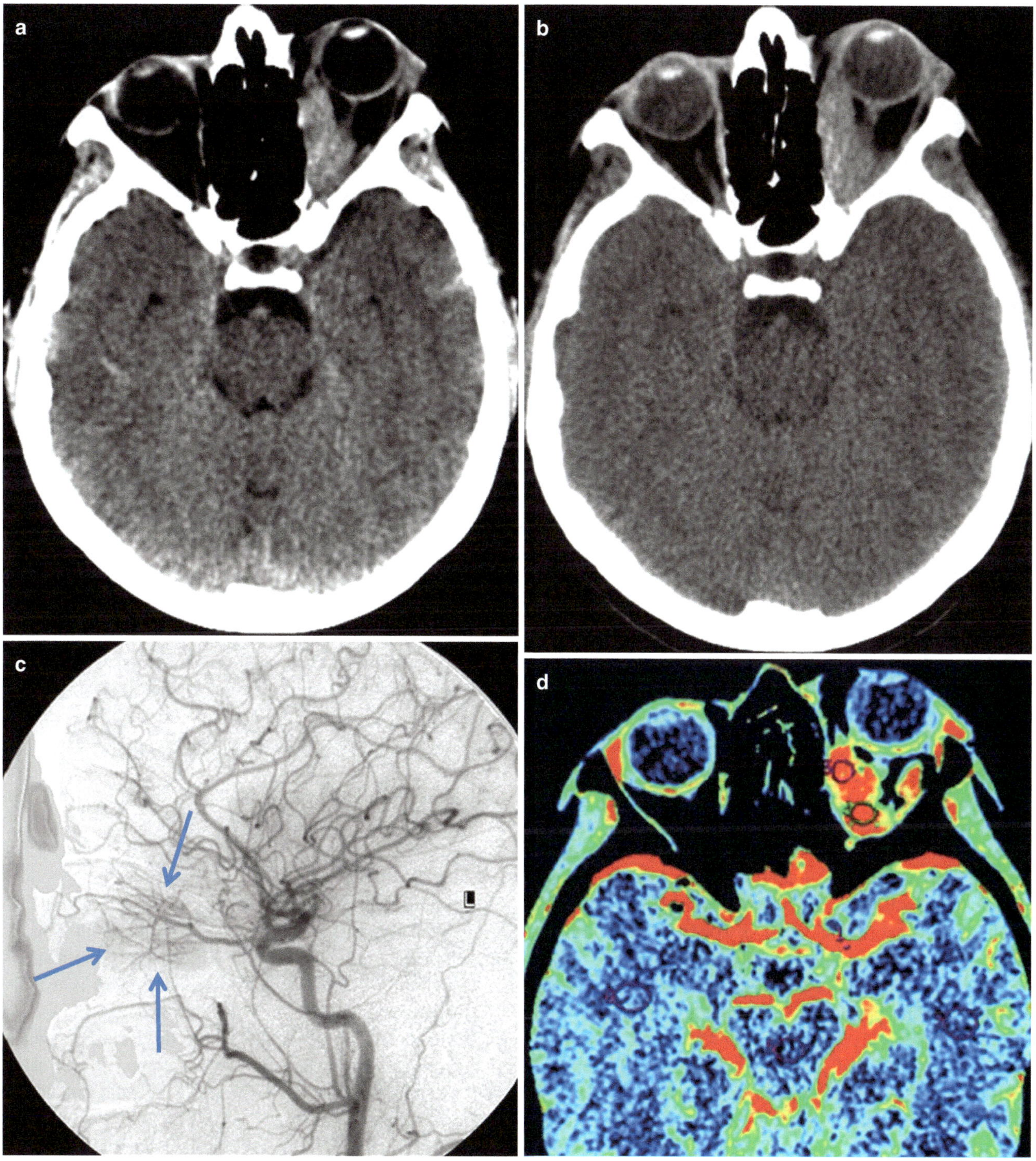

Fig. 2.20 Lymphoma of the left orbit. Axial CT scans with contrast enhancement (**a**, **b**) demonstrate tumor with irregular shape, which is located near the medial orbital wall and fills the apex of the orbit. Direct digital angiography of the common carotid artery reveals tiny tumoral vascular net with blood supply from the branches of the ophthalmic artery (**c**, *arrows*). Perfusion CT in this case in the contrary to intracranial lymphoma showed high values of CBF and CBV (**d**, **e**) in tumor tissue. There were similar to brain parameters of MTT (**f**)

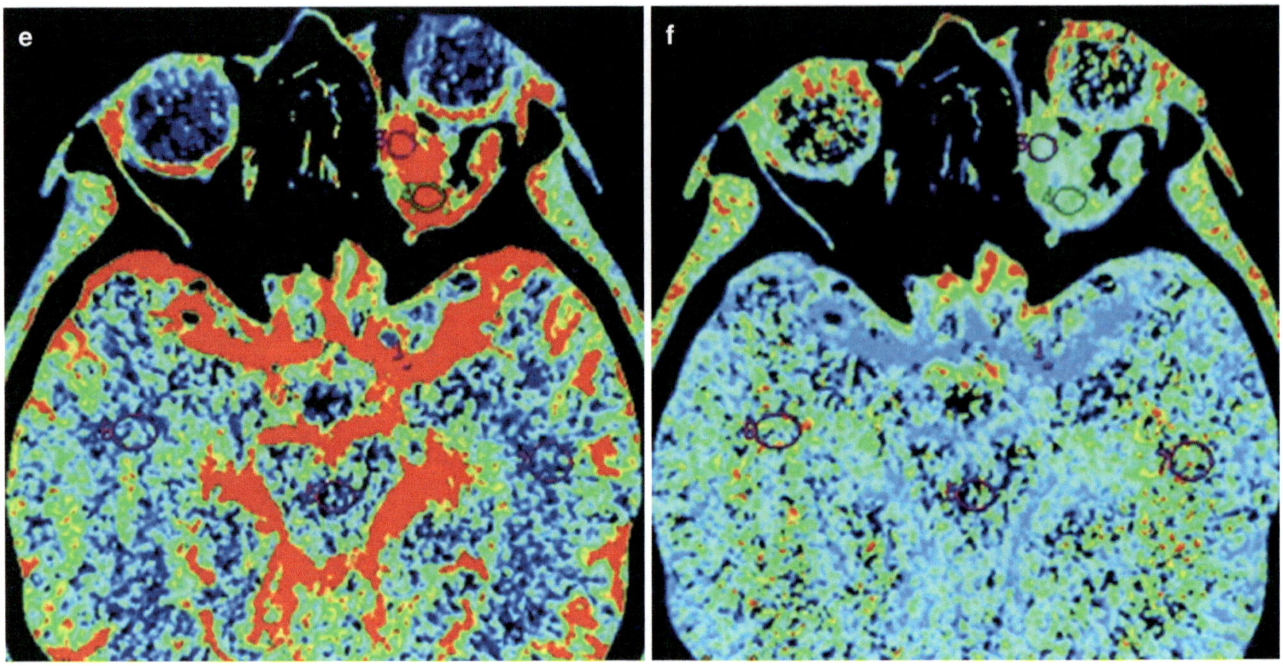

Fig. 2.20 (continued)

2.2.2.3 Differential Diagnosis

Glioma, metastasis, meningioma.

2.2.3 Lymphangioma

The lymphangioma term that was previously used has now been replaced by the term "lymphatic venous malformation" (LVM), as it more accurately describes the vascular anomaly (Harris 1999; Shields et al. 2004). Its prevalence is 0.3–4% of all orbital tumors (Shields et al. 2004). It mainly affects children, rarely young adults and slightly prevails in women. This malformation can be found in both the intraconal and extraconal orbit. It usually manifests within the first 10 years of life. LVM is represented by an encapsulated mass comprising mainly thin-walled bloodless vascular and lymphatic channels with smooth endothelium and multiple cystic inclusions of different sizes. There are two classifications in literature: the first one is based on the size of dysplastic channels, the second one is based on the localization of the lesion. According to the first classification, LVMs are divided into simple, cavernous, and cystic. By localization, they are divided into superficial (eyelid conjunctiva), deep-seated (retrobulbar orbital space), mixed (with superficial and deep-seated components), and complex (involving the orbit and a part of the face) (Baert and Sartor 2006).

2.2.3.1 Clinical manifestations

Clinical manifestations resemble those of capillary hemangioma with diffuse growth without regression. A spontaneous bleeding may trigger exophthalmos, decreased eye mobility, sometimes leading to compression of the optic nerve. The process begins in the mucosa of the eyelids and the eyes with possible development of lymphangiomatous nodes on the mucosa of the hard palate. The most frequent symptoms include increasing pain, exophthalmos, diplopia, restriction of the eyeball mobility, optic nerve compression.

2.2.3.2 Diagnosis

CT demonstrates a space-occupying polycystic hypodense lesion with hyperdense areas of hemorrhages. In case of large lesions, bone deformation is possible. Calcifications and phleboliths are rare. Contrast enhancement is usually inhomogeneous with presence of cystic structures and varying enhancement of the capsule, more diffuse enhancement of the venous component of lymphangioma. CT-perfusion study demonstrates the low CBV and CBF values in all five our clinical cases (Fig. 2.21).

The MRI signal from the lesion is isointense as compared to the brain on T1-weighted images and hyperintense on T2-weighted and proton-density-weighted images. MRI clearly visualizes multicystic structure of lymphangioma, showing lobular morphology with a weak defined capsule. Since thrombosis and hemorrhage are typical for this pathology, the MRI can demonstrate a heterogeneous area with hyperintense MR-signal. Following contrast enhancement, the contrast agent accumulation is usually inhomogeneous, more pronounced in the dilated venous channels (Figs.2.22 and 2.23). MR angiography does not usually visualize these lesions. It is characterized by slow long-term growth.

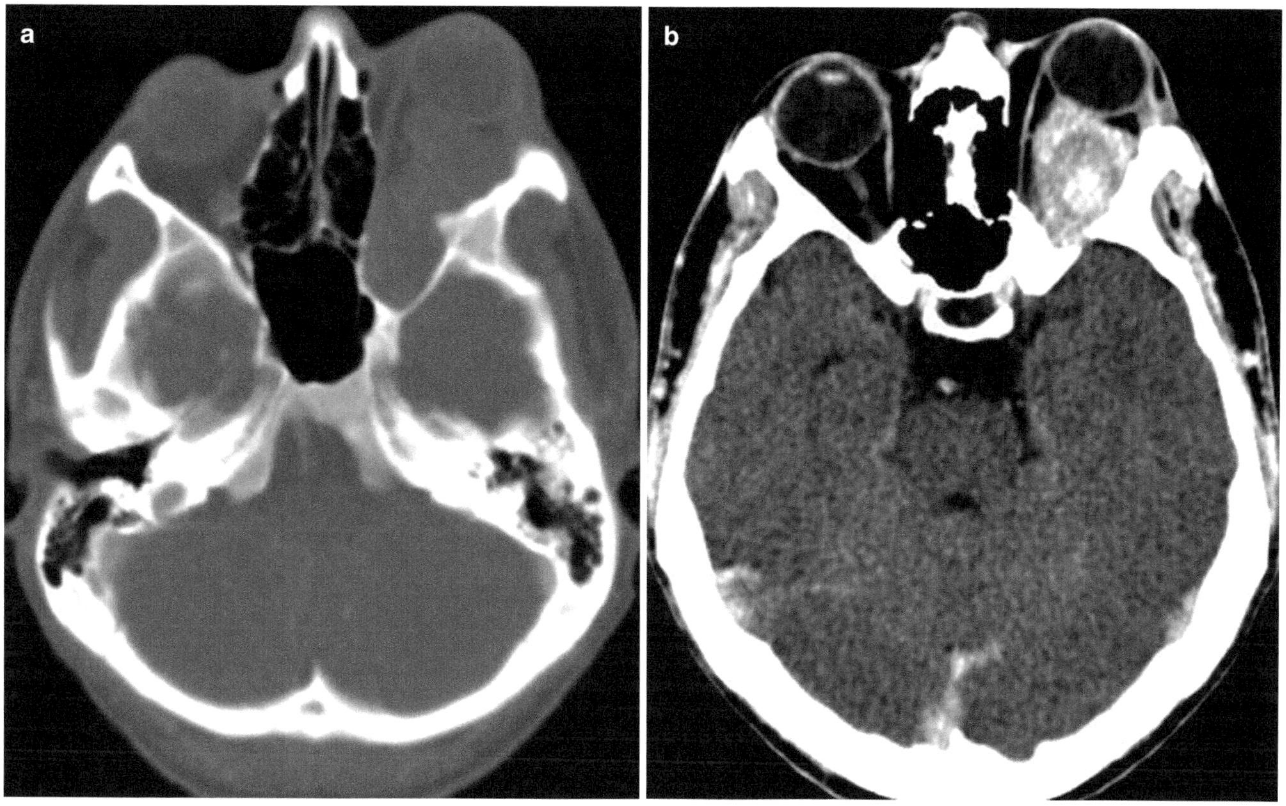

Fig. 2.21 Lymphangioma of the left orbit. Axial CT in "bone window" without contrast enhancement (**a**) and multiplanar CT scans with contrast enhancement (**b**–**d**) demonstrate tumor, which fills almost whole left orbit and heterogeneously accumulates contrast medium. There are expansive bone changes without signs of the destruction. Perfusion CT maps reveal low values of blood flow within the lesion (CBV—**e**, CBF–**f**)

2.2.3.3 Differential Diagnosis

Capillary hemangioma, plexiform neurofibroma, idiopathic orbital pseudotumor, rhabdomyosarcoma, lymphoma, Langerhans' cell histiocytosis.

2.2.4 Pseudotumor (Idiopathic Orbital Inflammation)

Idiopathic orbital inflammation is commonly considered as orbital pseudotumor (Jacobs and Galetta 2002; Yuen and Rubin 2003; Cunnane et al. 2011). But this terminology causes some confusion in description the diseases that are lead to appear these types of orbital pathology, so ophthalmologists prefer to use another designation of this disease and call it as idiopathic orbital inflammatory syndrome. According to the new classification approach, there are six distinct clinical forms of nonspecific inflammation: (1) anterior orbital inflammation, (2) diffuse orbital inflammation, (3) primary idiopathic myositis, (4) apical orbital inflammation, (5) dacryoadenitis, and (6) perineuritis (Yuen and Rubin 2003; Cunnane et al. 2011). Orbital fibrosis (or sclerosis) should be considered as the final stage of all three forms of the disease (Brovkina 2008).

The incidence of pseudotumor among orbital diseases, according to various estimates, ranges between 5 and 12%. The disease ranks third among orbital tumors. Pseudotumor develops in the 3rd–5th decade of life, but can also occur at an earlier age. Pediatric orbital pseudotumor represents from 6% up to 16% of orbital idiopathic inflammation. It mostly affects women. In ¼ cases it is a bilateral lesion of the orbits (Weber and Romo 1999; Gordon 2003).

2.2.4.1 Clinical Findings

Characterized by the rapid development of severe visual and oculomotor disorders, severe pain, exophthalmos; pain in the affected orbit, uveitis, in some cases retinal damage. Remission in the majority of the patients is induced by steroids.

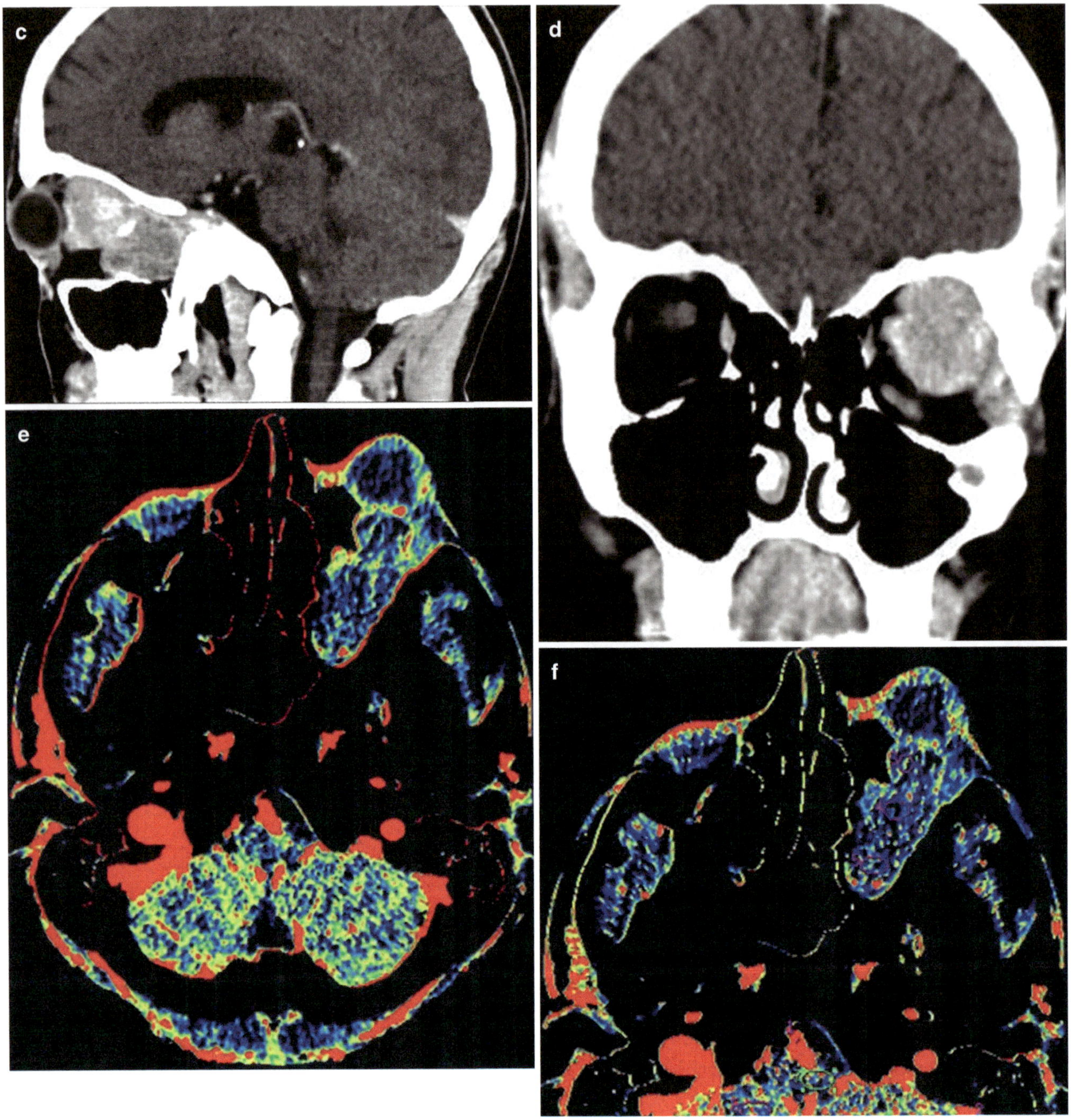

Fig. 2.21 (continued)

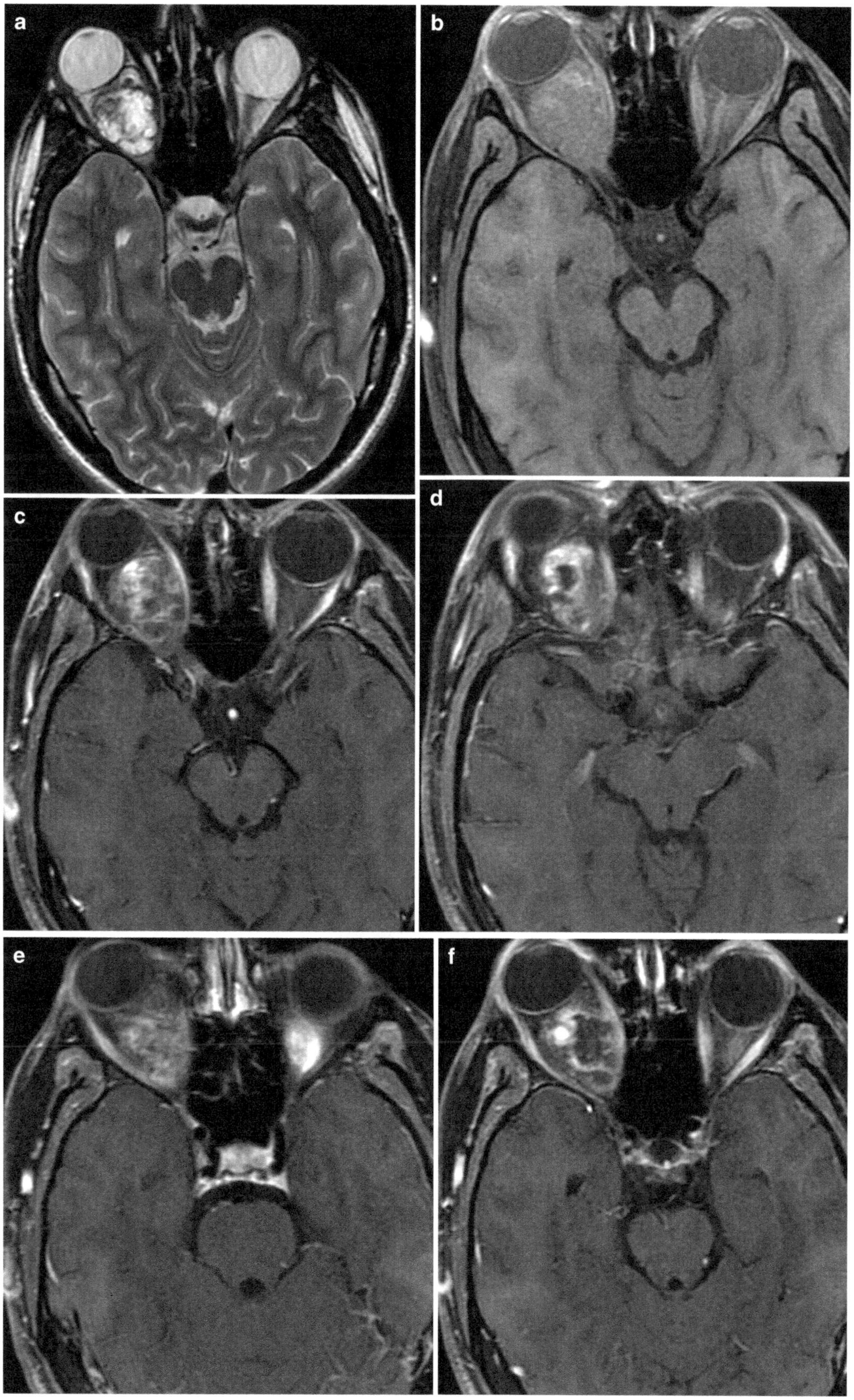

Fig. 2.22 Lymphangioma of the right orbit. Axial T2-WI (**a**), T1 + Fat-Sat without (**b**) and with (**c**–**f**) contrast enhancement MR scans on different levels detect polycystic tumor with inhomogeneous accumulation of the contrast medium

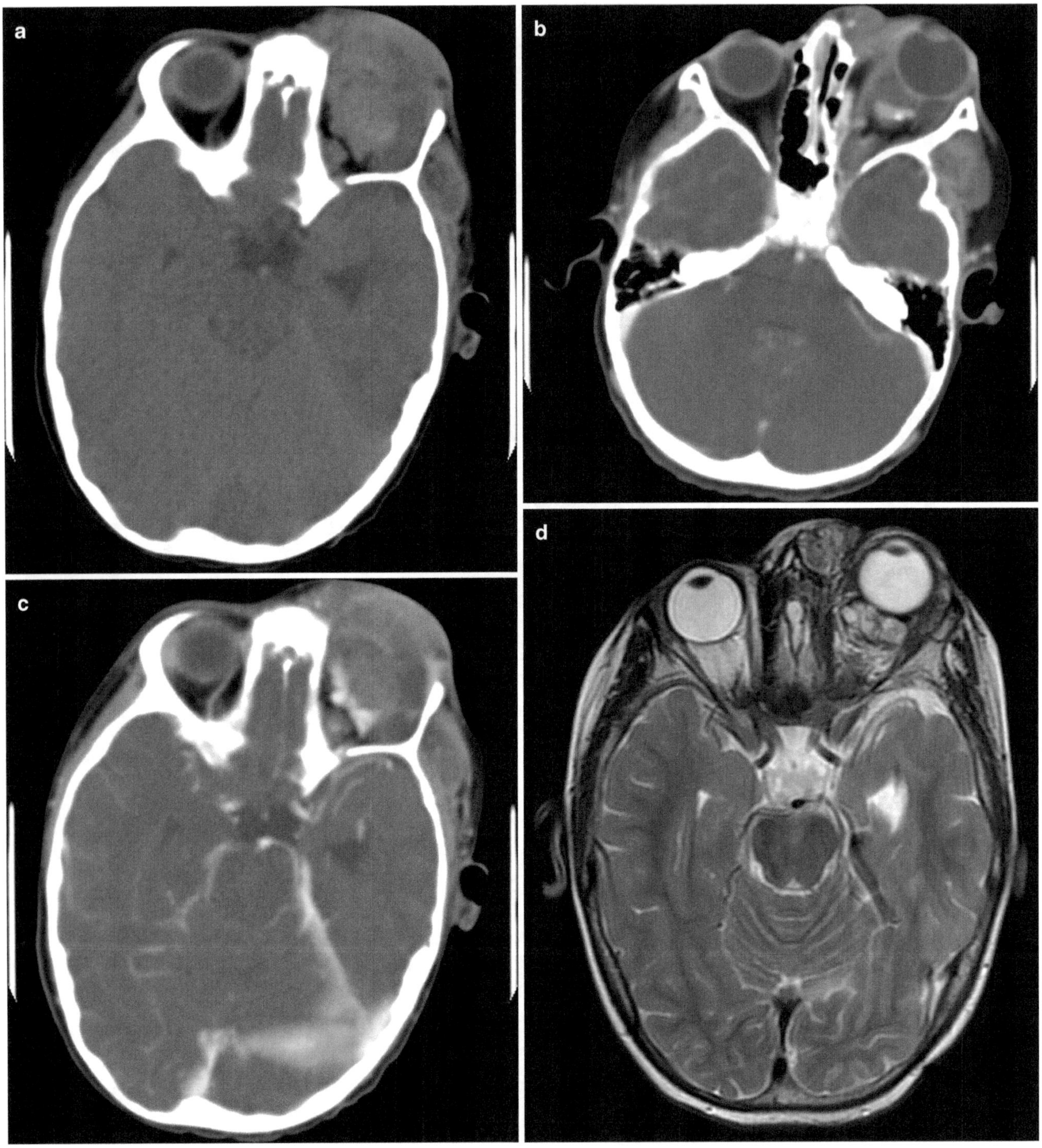

Fig. 2.23 Lymphangioma of the left orbit. Axial CT scans before (**a**) and after contrast enhancement (**b, c**) demonstrate tumor, which has intraorbital as well as extraorbital components and heterogeneously accumulates contrast medium. Lesion causes the proptosis. Axial T2-weighted (**d**), T1 + Fat-Sat without (**e**), DWI (**f**) scans demonstrate large intra-extraorbital lesion with hypo- iso-hyperintense MR-signal. Contrast-enhanced MR scans in the different projections better detect polycystic tumor with inhomogeneous accumulation of the contrast medium and wide spreading into the craniofacial region (**g–i**)

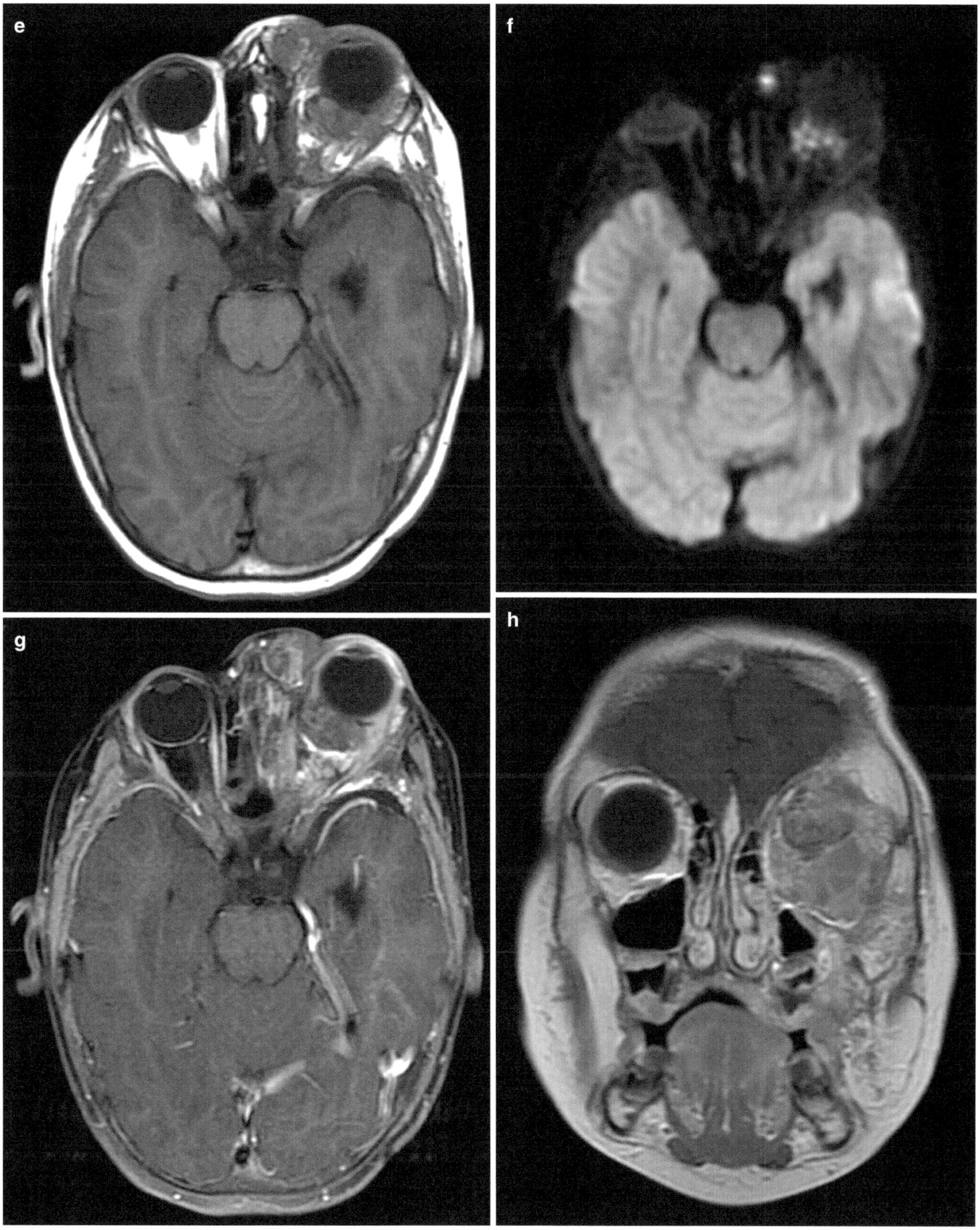

Fig. 2.23 (continued)

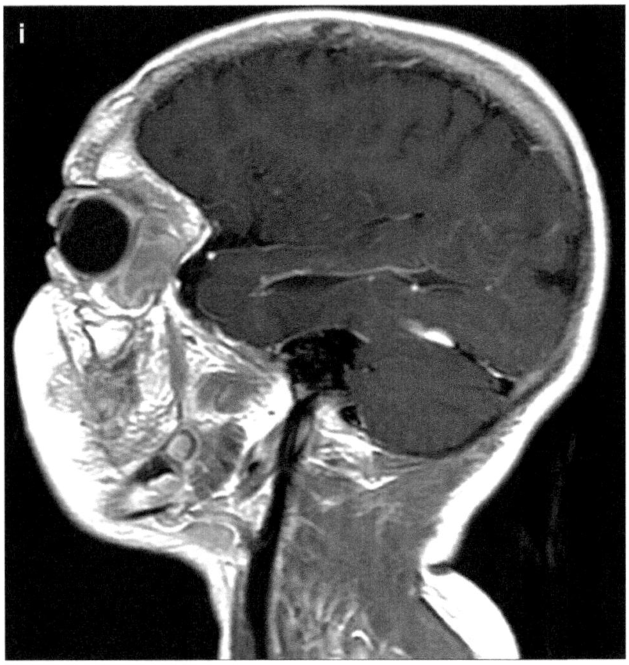

Fig. 2.23 (continued)

2.2.4.2 Diagnosis

The disease affects the retrobulbar fat, extraocular muscles, lacrimal gland, sometimes the optic nerve. If the lesion is located at the apex of the orbit, it may spread intracranially through the superior orbital fissure (Bencherif et al. 1993; Yan et al. 2000; Wasmeier et al. 2002). The pseudotumor can be both local and infiltrative process, in rare cases it may cause erosion of orbital bones (Tarasova and Drozdova 2005). On CT scan, it is distinguished as an isolated or generalized increase in the extraocular muscles (both unilateral or bilateral orbital involvement is possible), increased density of the retro-orbital fat. There is a moderately pronounced diffuse accumulation of the contrast agent in the abnormal tissue and low CT-perfusion parameters (Fig. 2.24). On MRI a pseudotumor is hypointense compared to normal orbital muscle on T1-weighted sequences and isointense or slightly hyperintense on T2-weighted (with fat suppression) and T2-STIR sequences. When using T2-STIR sequence, the neoplasm may also appear hypointense compared with the structures of the orbit due to pathologic cell infiltration and/or fibrosis. A hypointense MR-signal on MRI is indicative of the disease exacerbation. Following contrast enhancement, the contrast agent accumulation into the pseudotumor is diffuse and inhomogeneous (Fig. 2.25). Recommended MRI protocol: MR-sequences with fat saturation and contrast enhancement.

2.2.4.3 Differential Diagnosis

Thyroid-associated orbitopathy, sarcoidosis, Wegener's granulomatosis, lymphoproliferative disorders, primary lacrimal gland tumor, Sjögren syndrome (Gordon 2003).

2.2.5 Schwannoma and Neurofibroma

In addition to the optic nerve, there are cranial nerves III, IV, V, and VI and their branches, as well as the sympathetic and parasympathetic nerves in the orbit. Tumors of peripheral nerve sheaths accounts for 1–4% of orbital tumors (Carroll et al. 1999), and the most common are the tumors of sensory branches of the trigeminal nerve. These are mainly schwannomas, neurofibromas, or diffuse plexiform neurofibromas (Brovkina 2002).

Schwannoma is a benign, slow-growing tumor of the nerve sheaths, developing from the Schwann cells. It is well encapsulated and located eccentrically along the nerve. Schwannomas comprise 1/3 of all benign neurogenic orbital tumors. The age of patients ranges from 15 to 70 years, with women affected more often than men.

2.2.5.1 Clinical Manifestations

Orbital pain, swelling of the upper eyelid, partial ptosis, diplopia. Exophthalmos occurs in one third of cases. The eye repositioning is difficult. In 65–70% there is a papilledema, atrophy of the optic nerve occurs with long-term growth of the tumor (Brovkina 2008).

2.2.5.2 Diagnosis

There are two histological types of schwannomas: I—Antoni A, II—Antoni B. Tumors of type II are generally more vascularized and their characteristics MRI can vary greatly depending on the histological subtype. All schwannomas have an iso- to hypointense signal on T1-weighted images and their brightness varies from iso- to hyperintense signal on T2-weighted images, with an increase in hyperintensity in cases of cystic transformation. Type II tumors more prominently accumulate the contrast agent, heterogeneous contrast enhancement is not uncommon (Harnsberger et al. 2004b). On CT-perfusion imaging MTT prolongation and a moderate CBV elevation are typical for the most schwannomas. CBF values are close to those of the brain matter in the cerebellar hemisphere.

Schwannomas growing from sensory nerves inside the orbit, most often from branches of the trigeminal nerve, are usually located in the upper extraconal segment of the orbit. However, they can also be located in the muscle cone in the case of the schwannoma growth from nasociliary or motor branches of nerves III, IV, and VI (Figs. 2.26, 2.27, and 2.28). Schwannomas are often diagnosed as solitary lesions, unlike neurofibromas. Another difference is a tumor hemorrhage, which occurs in schwannomas and is well visualized on MRI in specialized sequences (SWI, SWAN, etc.).

Neurofibromas (NF) can be solitary, plexiform, and diffuse. Solitary NF usually develops in adults, while plexiform NF (typical for type I neurofibromatosis) develops within the first 5 years of life (Brovkina 2008). Plexiform (or reticular) neurofibromas are the most frequent in the orbit. Diffuse type is less common than plexiform and solitary ones, this

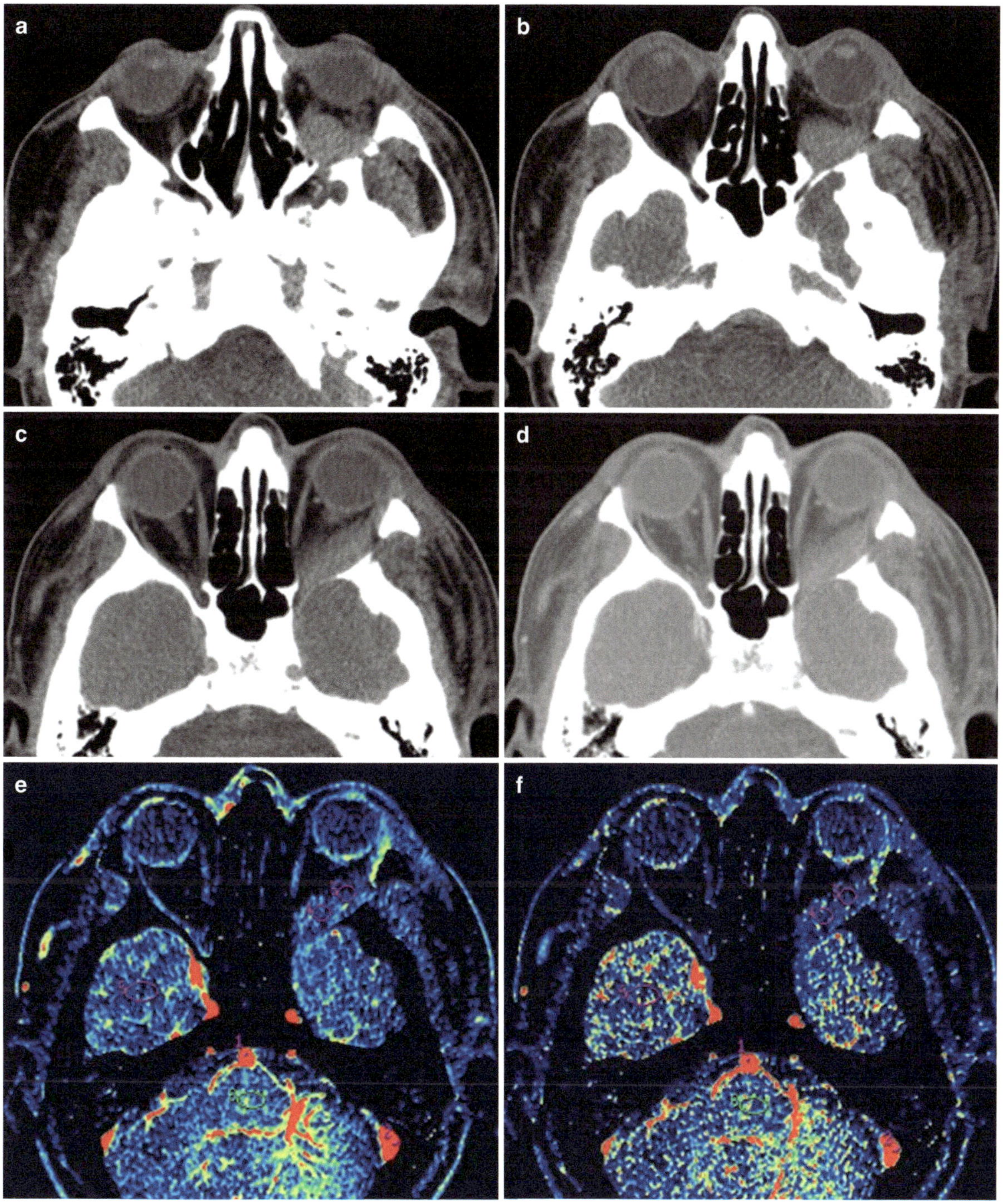

Fig. 2.24 Pseudotumor of the left orbit. Axial CT scans reveal infiltrative lesion with irregular shape, which is occupied the inferior and lateral parts of the orbit. The lesion leads to the lateral orbital wall thinning (**a**–**d**). Perfusion CT-maps demonstrate reduced hemodynamic parameters into the lesion (CBV—**e**, CBF—**f**)

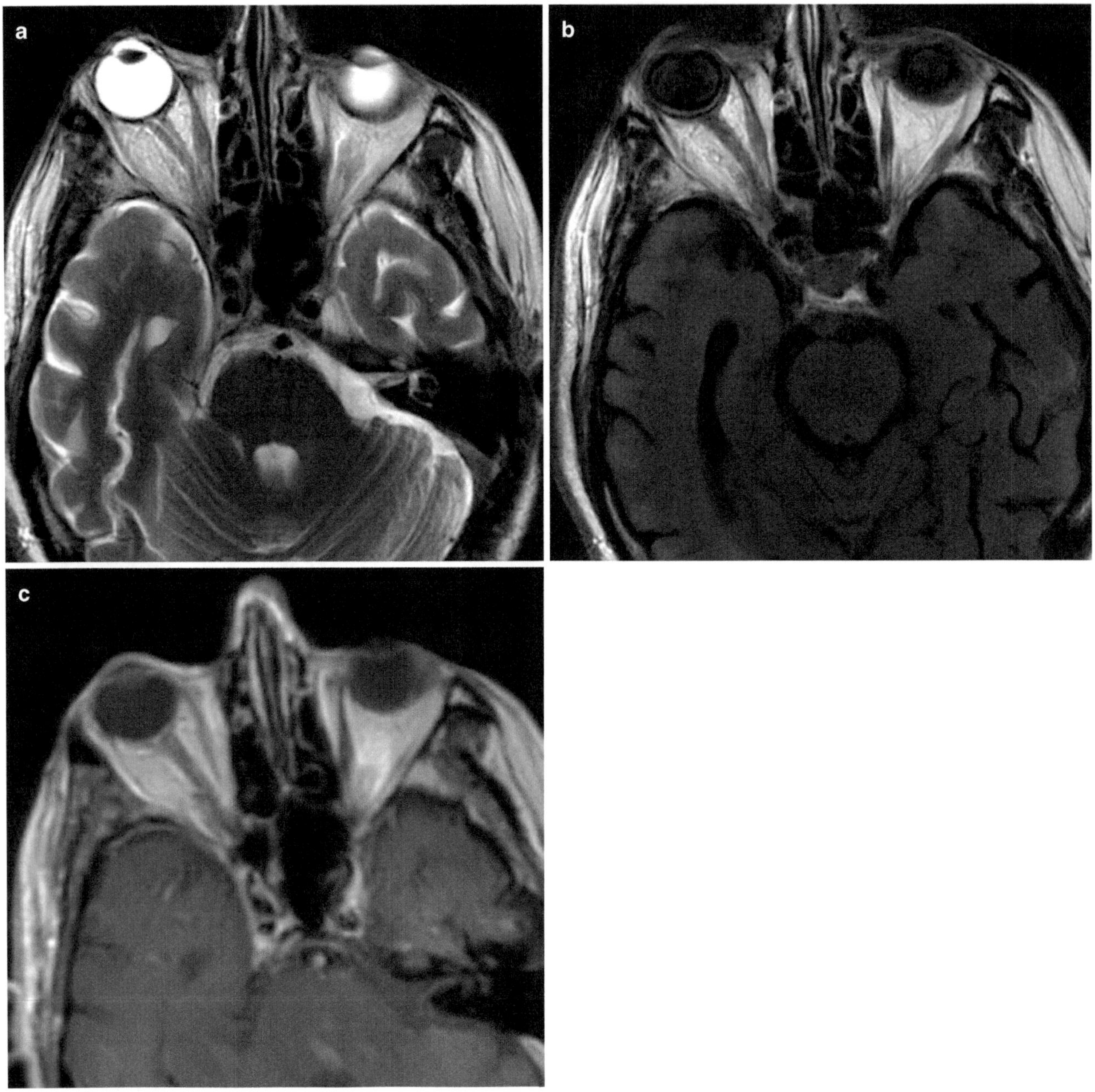

Fig. 2.25 Pseudotumor of the right orbit. Axial T2-weighed (**a**), T1-weighted before (**b**) and after (**c**) contrast enhancement MR-scans demonstrate retrobulbar infiltrative lesion, which is located between the lateral rectus muscle and intraorbital optic nerve. The optical nerve is shifted medially. Exophthalmos is rightwards

type is distinguished by its tendency to infiltrate the tissues located at some distance from the perineurium.

As a rule, solitary NF develops from the branches of the cranial nerve V. They can be single and multiple and are usually combined with neurofibromatosis. As with schwannomas, they are often located in the upper extraconal segment of the orbit. These tumors contain fibroblasts, Schwann cells, and myxoid material; they grow along the nerve bundles and have no capsule (Friedrich et al. 2010).

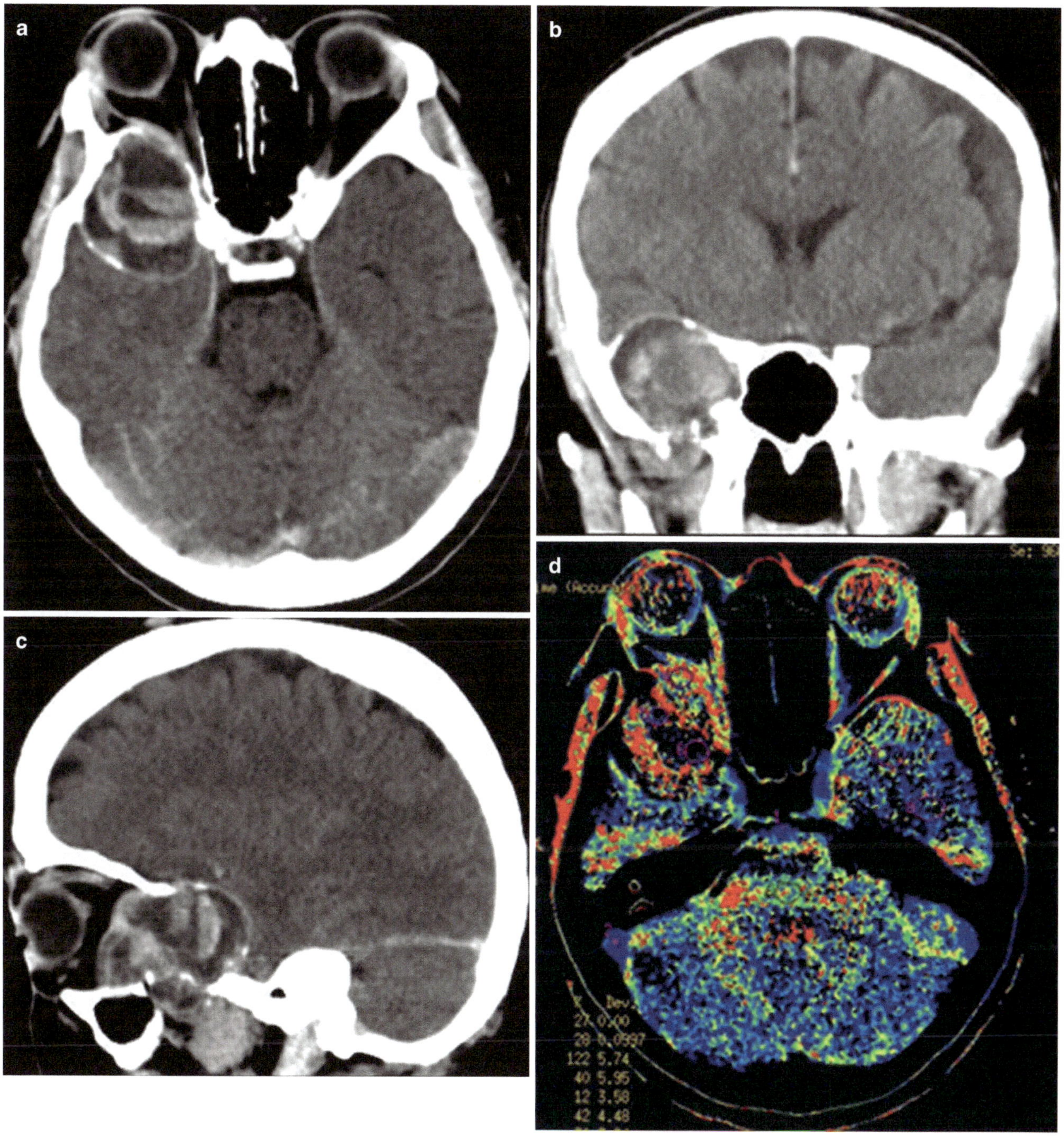

Fig. 2.26 Neurinoma of the right orbit with spreading into the middle cranial fossa. CT scans with contrast enhancement in axial (**a**), coronal (**b**), and sagittal (**c**) planes detect large tumor with heterogeneous structure and contrast agent accumulation. The tumor has apparent capsule. There are expansive bone changes with absence of lateral bone wall of the orbit. On perfusion CT CBF map (**d**) the slightly elevated tumor flow in peripheral parts of the lesion can be visualized. T2-weighed (**e**), T1-weighted without (**f**) and with (**g**, **h**) contrast enhancement MR-scans demonstrate heterogeneous structure of the tumor. Apparent diffusion coefficient is increased in solid and in cystic parts of the neurinoma (**i**)

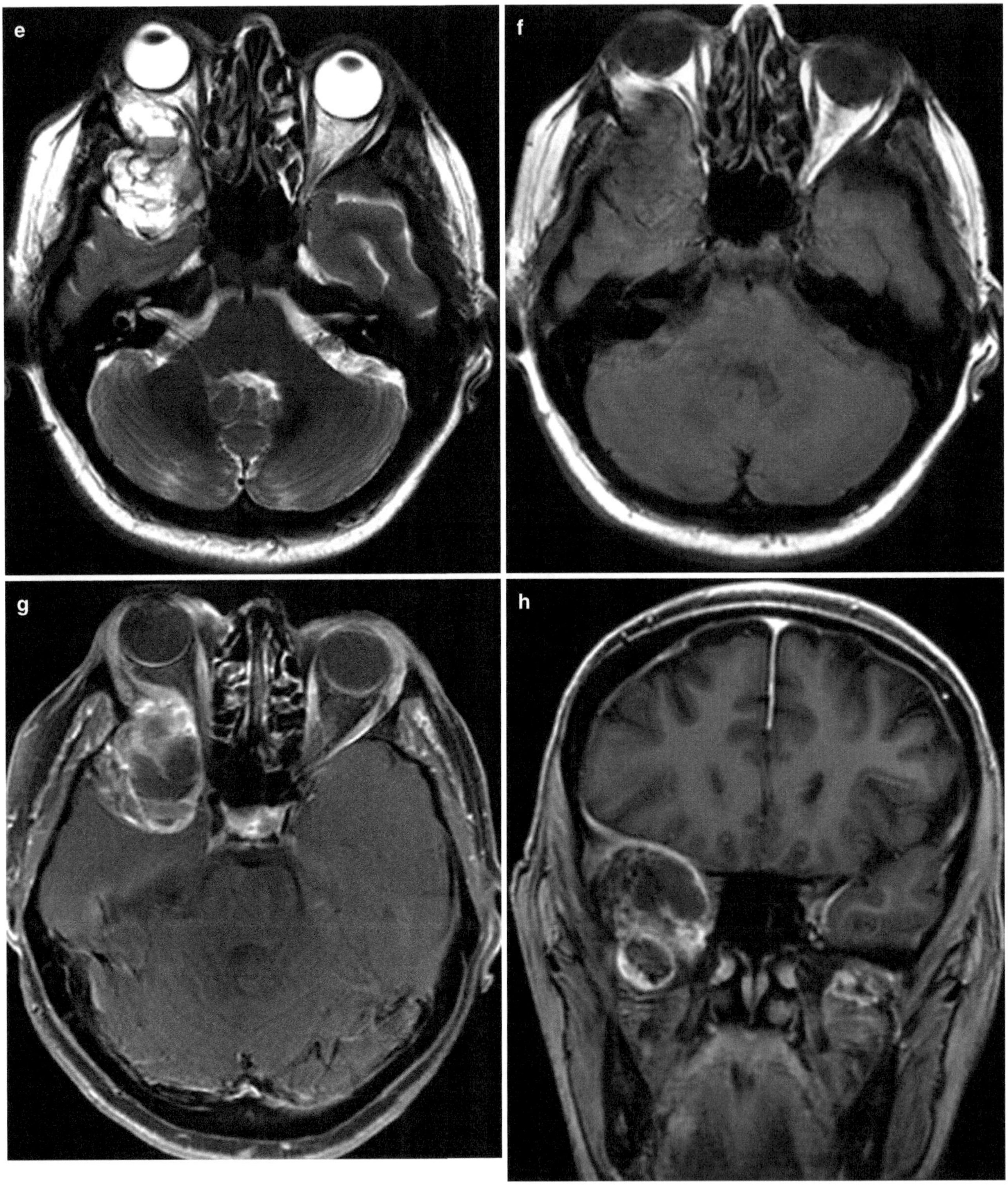

Fig. 2.26 (continued)

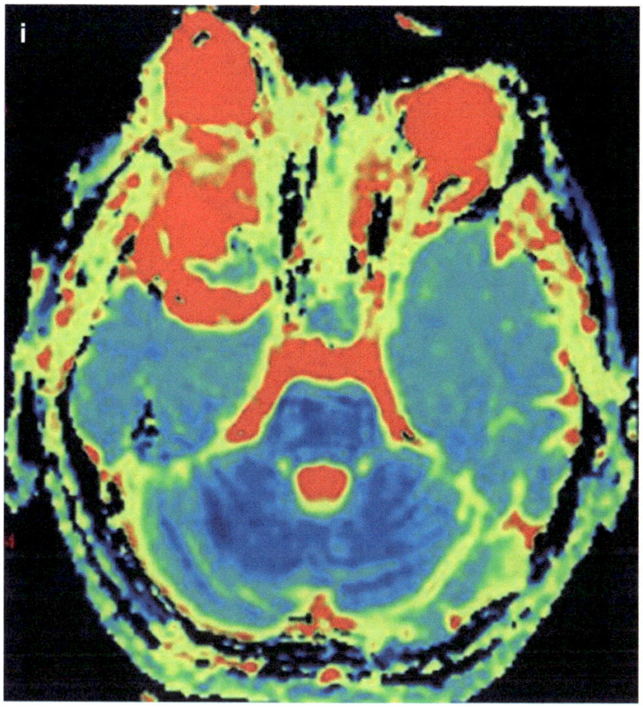

Fig. 2.26 (continued)

2.2.5.3 Clinical Manifestations

Swelling and elephantiasis of orbital tissues, ptosis of the upper eyelid, skin color changes, facial asymmetry due to the changes in its soft tissues.

2.2.5.4 Diagnosis

On CT, single NF looks like a rounded, oblong or oval encapsulated formation with a density close to that of the brain tissue; however, this pattern, in general, is nonspecific, it has a moderate degree of contrast enhancement. Sometimes the tumor pushes the orbital bone walls and causes an increase in orbit volume. Newborns may experience hyperplasia of the orbital bones, and, inversely, absence of the sphenoid bone wings or their dysplasia. On MR, NF has a homogeneous structure with irregular borders: the tumor is usually represented by infiltrative mass with irregular contours, which sometimes infiltrate the orbital adipose tissue. It is homogeneous and iso- or hypointense compared to the orbital muscle on T1-weighted images. On T2-weighted images, it can be homogeneously hyperintense or show a so-called "target sign"—a hypointense signal from the central area of the tumor, surrounded by a hyperintense rim. Contrast material is accumulated heterogeneously in NF, and their contrast enhancement pattern can be indistinguishable from that of schwannomas (Figs. 2.29, 2.30 and 2.31).

Plexiform neurofibromas are typical for neurofibromatosis type I. These are infiltrative lesions that develop in children, they contain nerve branches in its structure and are sometimes called "a bag of worms" (Castillo and Kaufman 2003; Harnsberger et al. 2004a). In the orbit, plexiform NF often grows into the eyelid and soft tissues, causing the sphenoid bone dysplasia (defects of the sphenoid bone greater wing, an enlargement of the middle cranial fossa, arachnoid cysts are often found). On MRI, plexiform NF has an iso- or hypointense signal relative to the orbital muscle on T1-weighted images and hyperintense on T2-weighted images. They heterogeneously accumulate contrast material (Figs. 2.32 and 2.33). According to our data with the use of CT-perfusion (four patients with plexiform NFs), this type of tumors had the highest MTT values among of all orbital tumors and a reduced CBF value in comparison to the white matter of the brain.

Malignization of neurofibroma is less frequent compared to the schwannomas. NF's malignization usually occurs in patients with neurofibromatosis type I. Most neurofibromas, as well as sarcomas, may be considered as malignant tumors of the nerve sheaths. In the case of malignization, they become more aggressive and may grow intracranially.

2.2.6 Metastases

Metastases to the orbit are frequently encountered in clinical practice. There is a difference in the origin of the primary tumor and the lesion sites in the orbit between children and adults, depending on age. In children, the eyeball is less frequently affected than in adults, with common primary tumors that metastasize to the orbit being neuroblastoma, leukemia, and Ewing's sarcoma. Metastases in children usually affect the orbital wall and grow into the subperiosteal space, thereby causing a mass effect in the intraorbital tissue.

In adults, the uvea, retrobulbar space, orbital bone walls (metastases of prostate cancer) are the most frequently affected. The most common primary tumors in adults are adenocarcinoma, breast cancer, prostate cancer, myeloma, lymphoma, and neuroblastoma (Lieb et al. 2010). Metastases to the paranasal sinuses can grow directly into the orbit. Malignant orbital tumors have metastatic origin in 34% or grow into the orbit from adjacent areas. Women are almost twofolds more likely to develop a tumor (Henderson 1994).

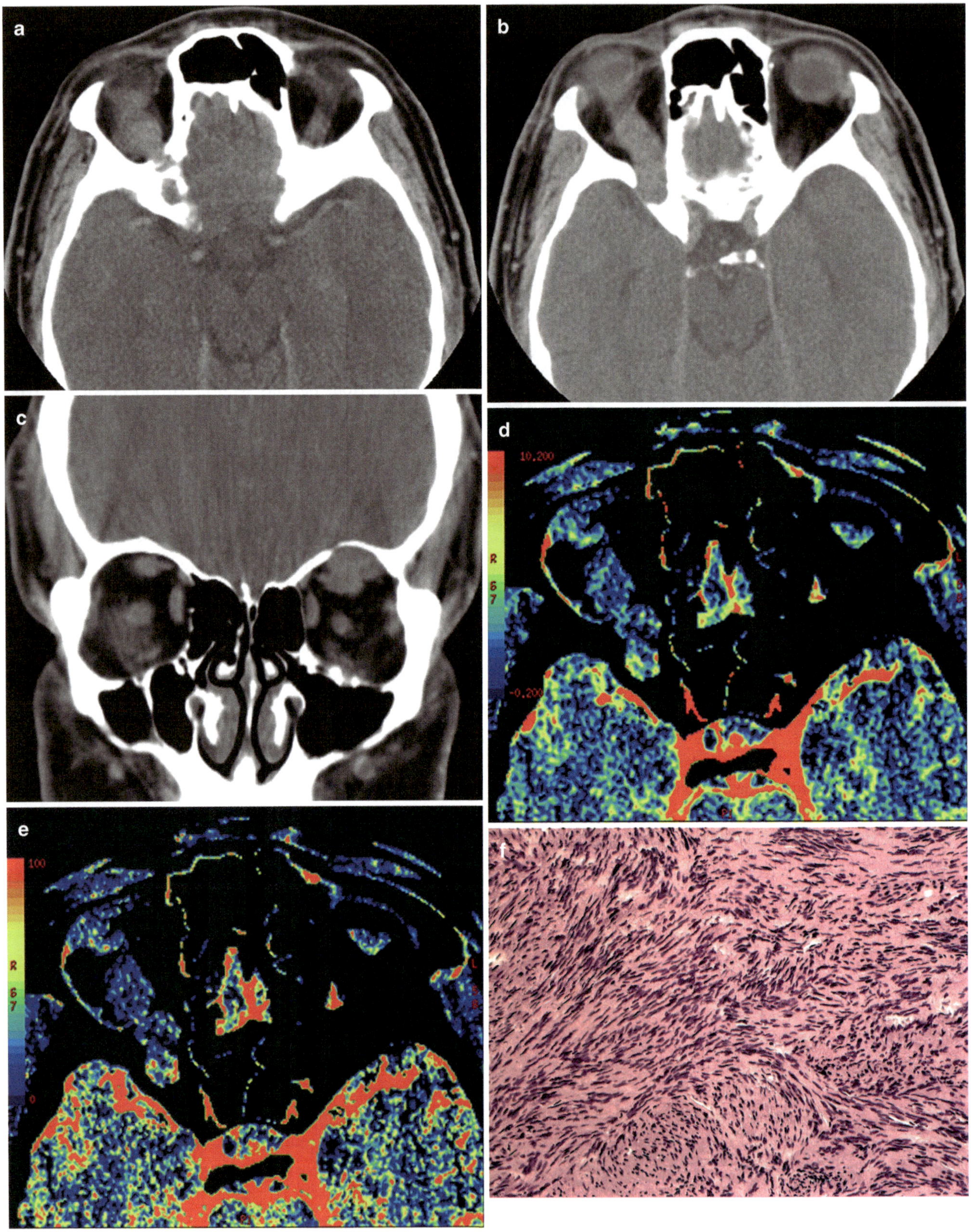

Fig. 2.27 Neurinoma of the right orbit. Axial (**a**, **b**) and coronal (**c**) CT scans on different levels demonstrate stretched tumor in the superior part of the orbit with the bone excavation of the lateral and superior orbital walls. On perfusion CT maps hemodynamic parameters (CBF—**d**, CBF—**e**) in the tumor are close to brain tissue. Histological specimen (**f**)

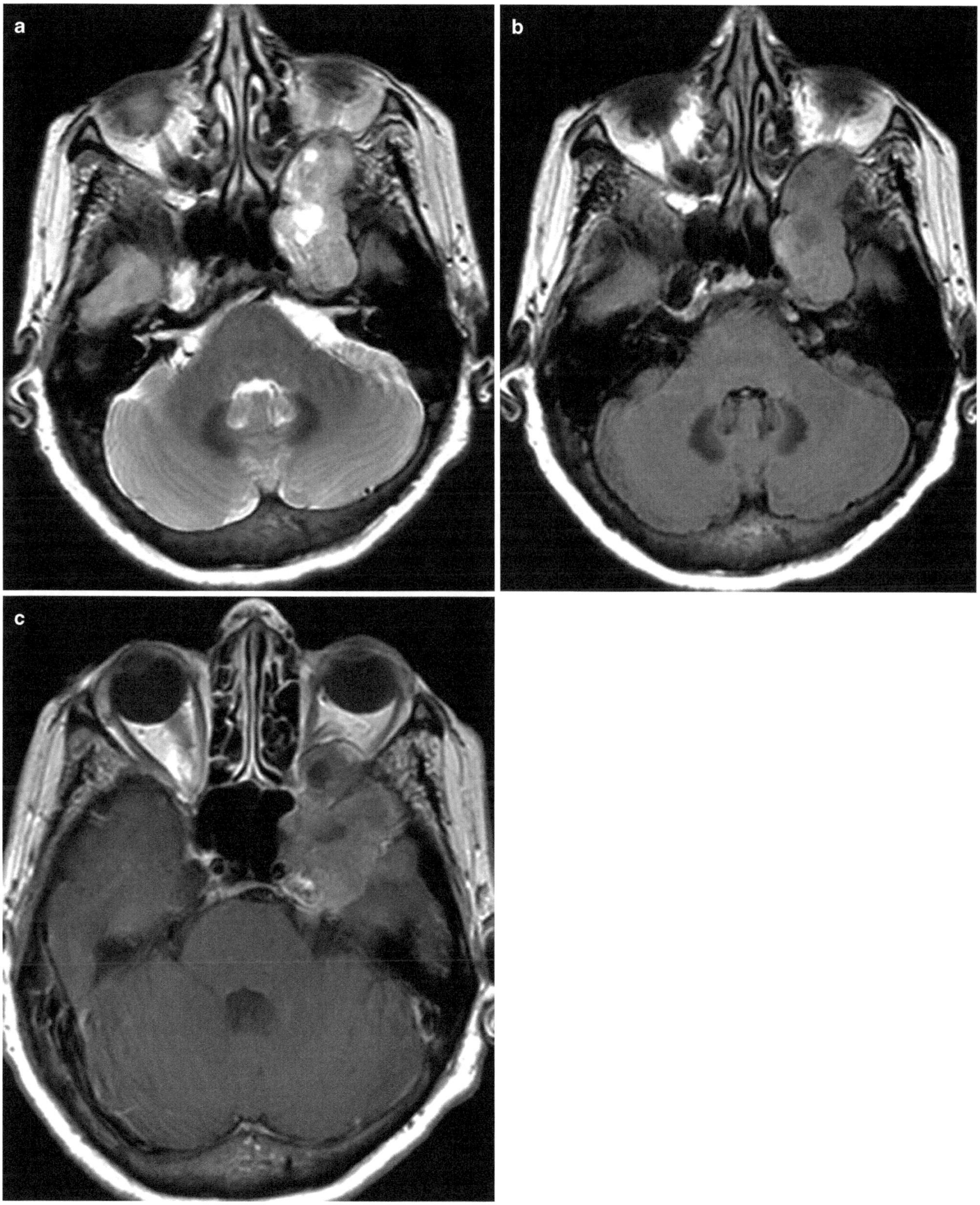

Fig. 2.28 Gasserian ganglion and the second branch of V-th nerve neurinoma of leftwards. T2 (**a**) and T2-FLAIR (**b**) MR images demonstrate tumor, which is placed at the base of the left middle cranial fossa. The tumor spreads forward and partial spreads through the lower orbital fissure into the cavity of the orbit. The neurinoma has sufficiently homogeneous contrast enhancement and there are small cysts in the tumor stroma (**c**)

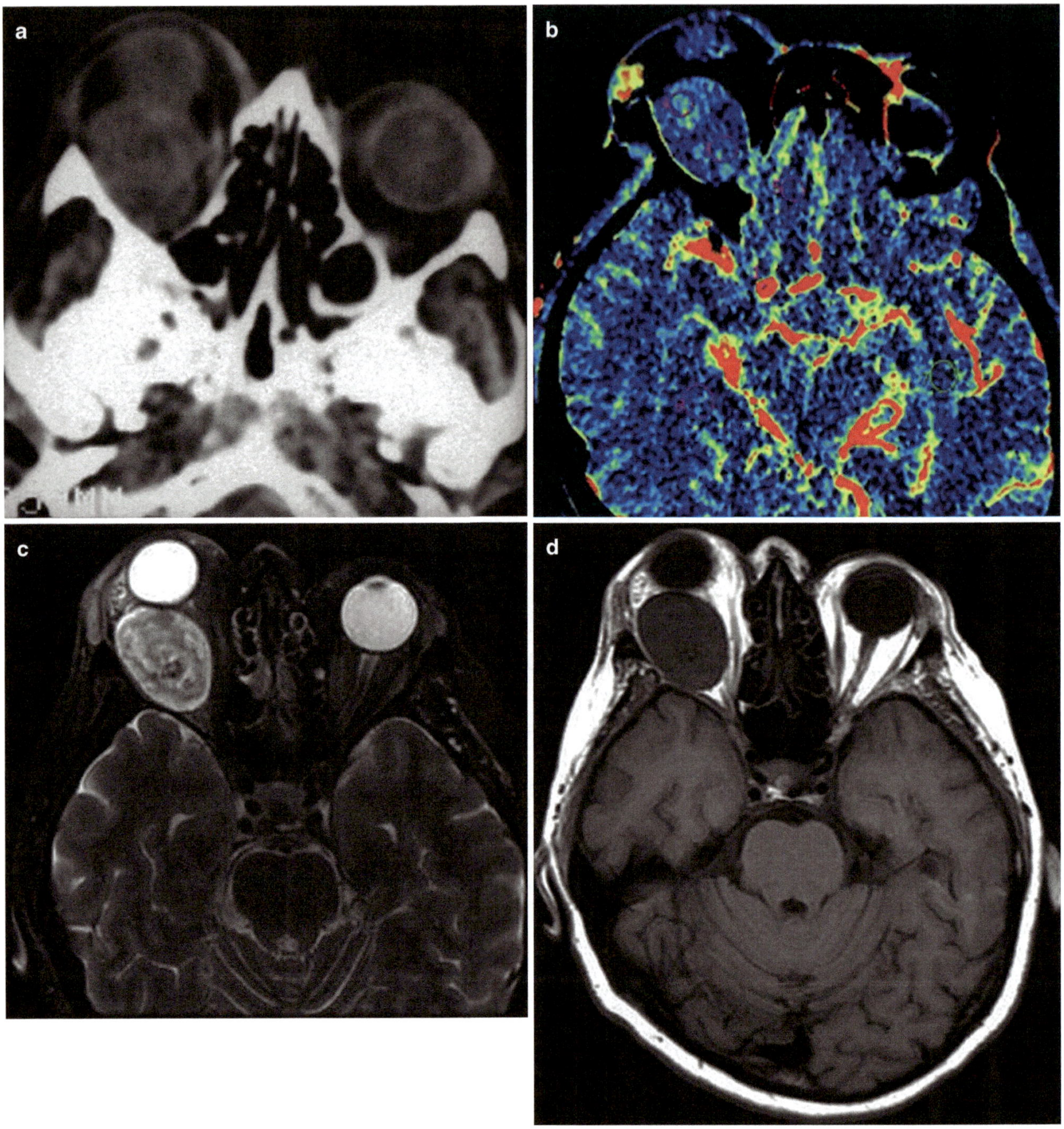

Fig. 2.29 Neurofibroma of the right orbit. CT scan (**a**) reveals large isodense retroorbital tumor, which leads to severe proptosis. On perfusion CT CBV-map (**b**) hemodynamic parameters in the tumor are slightly increased comparing to brain white matter. T2- (**c**, **f**) and T1-weighted (**d**) MR images demonstrate encapsulated tumor with heterogeneous MR-signal (hyperintense on T2-WI and hypointense on T1-WI) and with intensive inhomogeneous contrast enhancement (**e**)

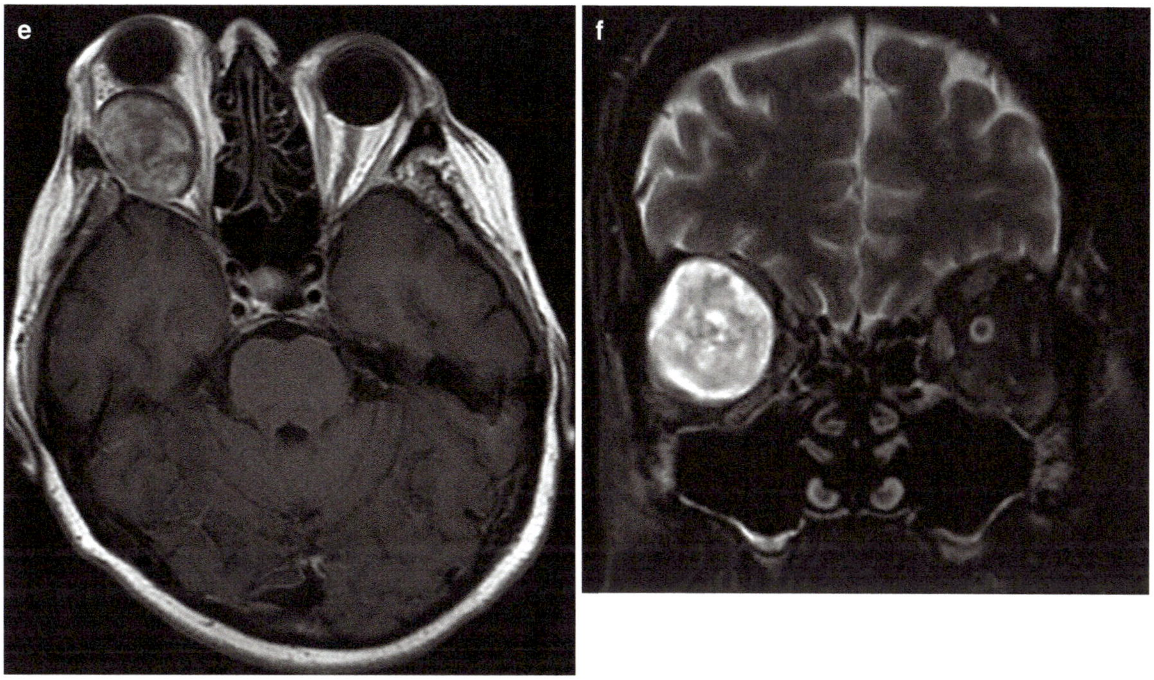

Fig. 2.29 (continued)

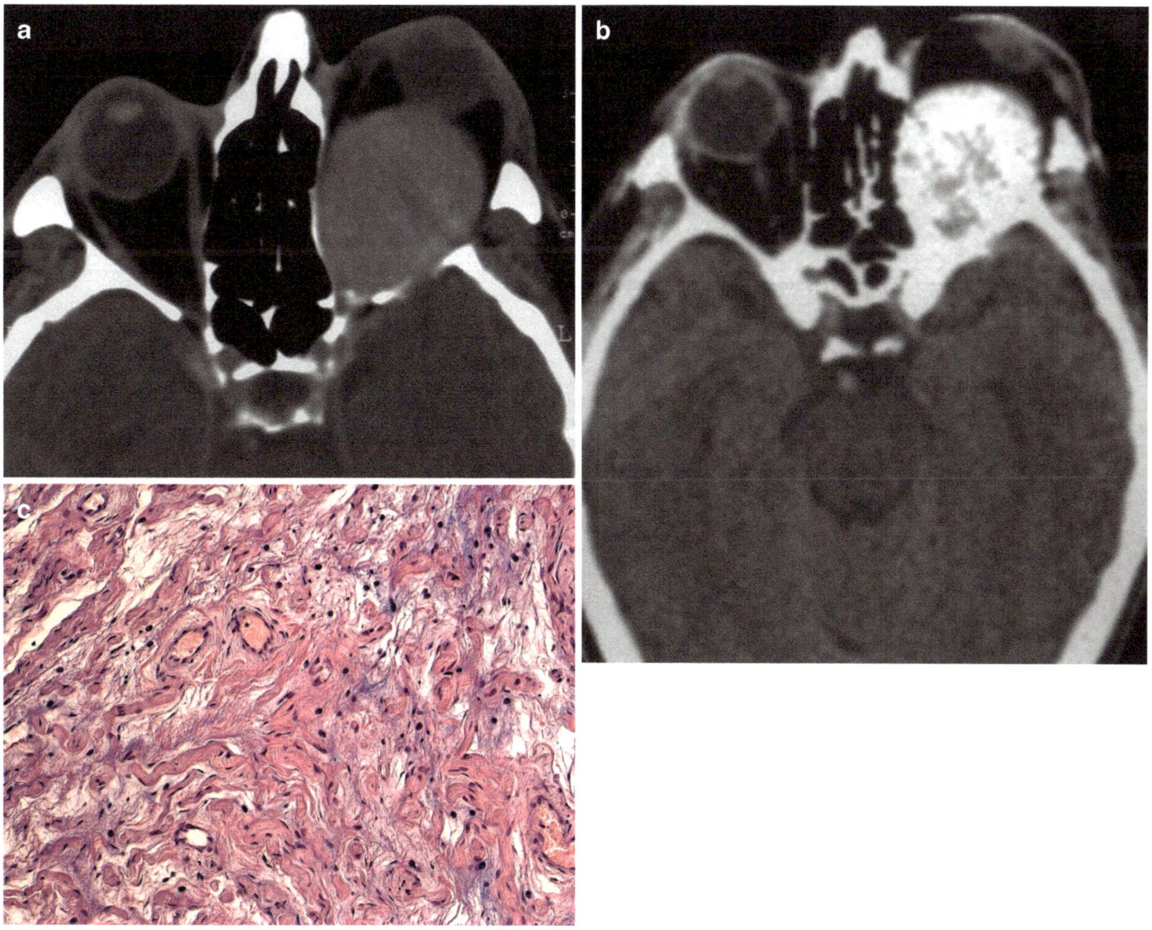

Fig. 2.30 Neurofibroma of the left orbit. Axial CT scans without (**a**) and with (**b**) contrast enhancement show large encapsulated retroorbital tumor, which is characterized by prominent contrast agent accumulation and leads to the bone changes of orbital walls. The orbit has increased size. Histological specimen of the neurofibroma (**c**)

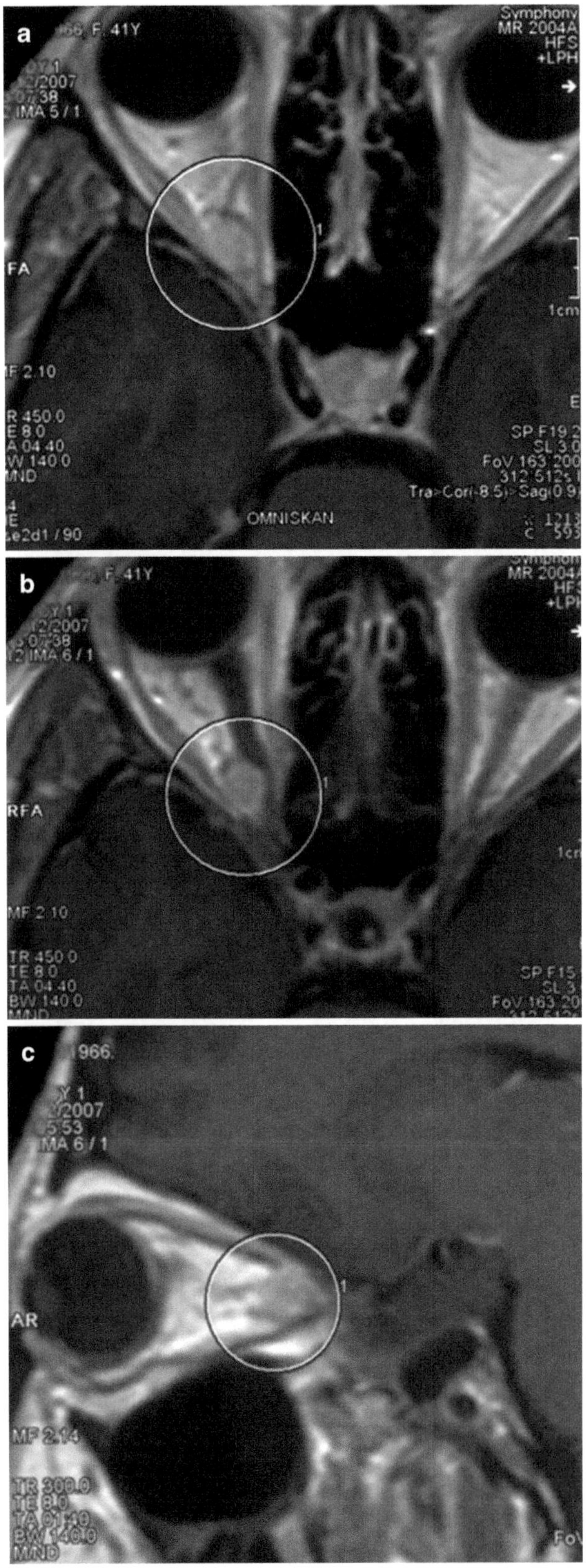

Fig. 2.31 Neurofibroma of the right orbit. T1-weighted MRI with contrast enhancement in axial (**a**, **b**) and sagittal projections (**c**) reveals small intraconal encapsulated tumor, which medially shifts optical nerve in the orbital apex. The tumor is characterized by moderate and homogeneous contrast agent accumulation

2.2.6.1 Clinical Manifestations

Exophthalmos, ophthalmoplegia, and tenderness in the affected orbit, possible strabismus, eyelid edema, red chemosis.

2.2.6.2 Diagnosis

The localization and the origin of the primary tumor strongly affect CT and MRI images of the pathological lesion. Thus, orbital metastases of breast cancer have a diffuse and heterogeneous growth, whereas metastases of carcinoid, renal cell carcinoma, and melanoma have clearly defined margins. Prostate cancer mts often involve the orbital bones and the greater wing of the sphenoid bone, significantly increasing the size of the orbit and causing a secondary sclerotic bone response. Changes in the bones are better diagnosed by CT. In the case of osteoplastic forms of the metastases, MRI shows abnormal hypointense lesions on T1- and T2-weighted images. All MTS accumulate contrast material, improving the visualization of the structure and lesion boundaries (Figs. 2.34, 2.35, 2.36, and 2.37). CT-perfusion helps to differentiate malignant tumor of the orbit with elevated hemodynamic parameters from benign lesions which are typically characterized low perfusion.

2.2.6.3 Differential Diagnosis

Lymphoma, pseudotumor, orbital cancer. In some cases, MRI is sufficient to differentiate between a pseudotumor and metastases. In general, they are more hyperintense in comparison with pseudotumors on T2-weighted images. However, metastases of some malignant tumors (myeloma, lymphoma, and neuroblastoma) are difficult to differentiate from a pseudotumor based on the MR signal intensity pattern.

2.2.7 Mesenchymoma

Stout (1948) first defined mesenchymoma as a tumor consisting of two or more elements of mesenchymal origin, where each separate element can be considered as a malignant neoplasm. The definition excludes malignant, fibroblast-like components that are common typical of all primitive sarcomas. Tissue elements that most often found in mesenchymomas include combinations of leiomyosarcoma/liposarcoma and rhabdomyosarcoma/liposarcoma. They are extremely rare in the orbit and are diagnosed in 0.37% (Brovkina 2008). This tumor can be located in any portion of the orbit and grows infiltratively.

2.2.7.1 Clinical Manifestations

Early signs of extraocular muscles dysfunction, compression of the superior ophthalmic vein, which manifests via the development of chemosis. There are no reports of tumor metastasizing in literature.

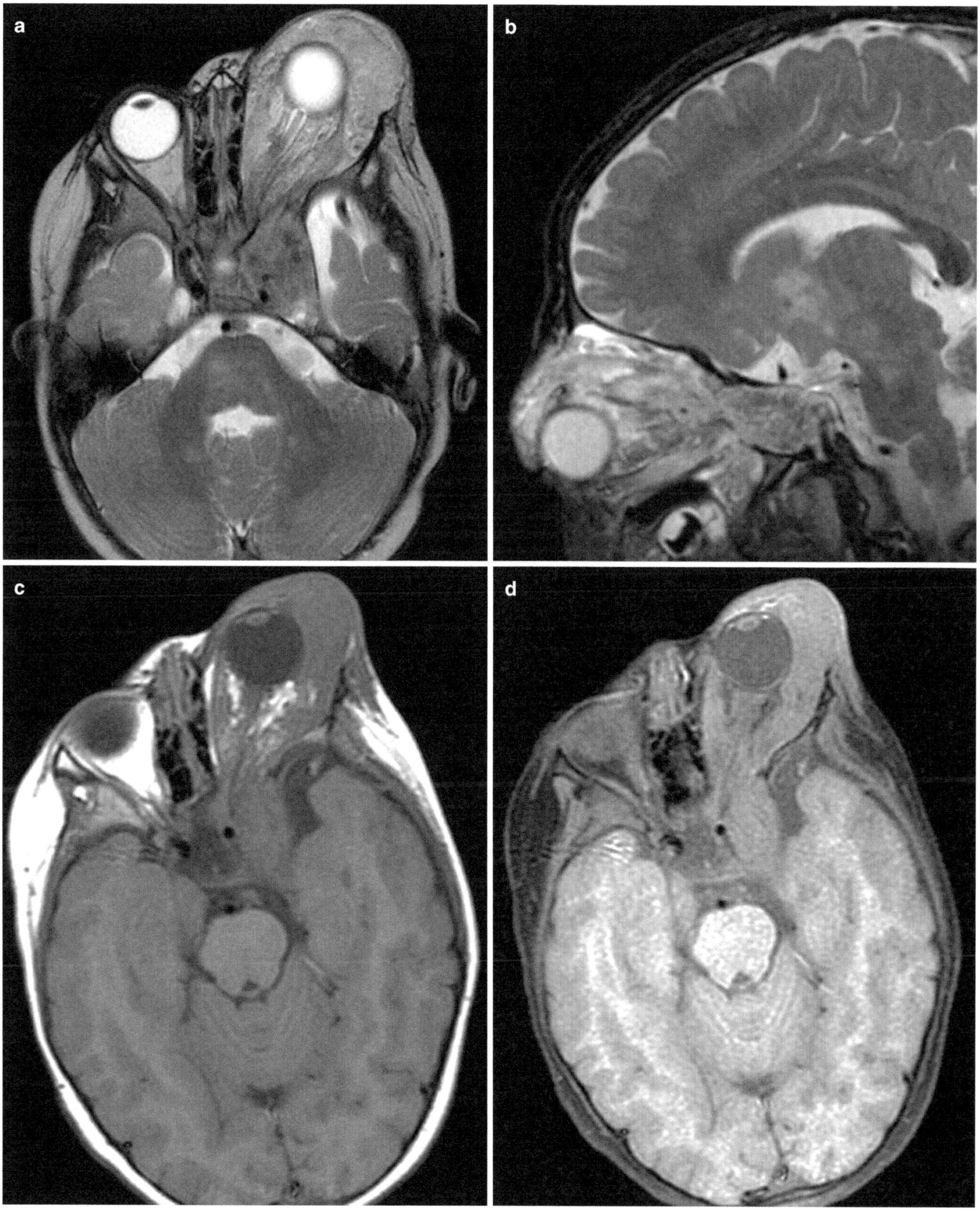

Fig. 2.32 Plexiform neurofibroma. T2-weighted (**a**, **b**), T1- (**c**) and T1 with Fat-Sat (**d**)-weighted MR images demonstrate large tumor of the left orbit, which infiltrates orbital structures. The tumor fills cavity orbit and grows into the eyelid and into the cavernous sinus leftwards. There is prominent proptosis. Axial (**e**) and sagittal (**f**) T1-weighted MRI with contrast enhancement reveals intensive contrast enhancement of the tumor tissue

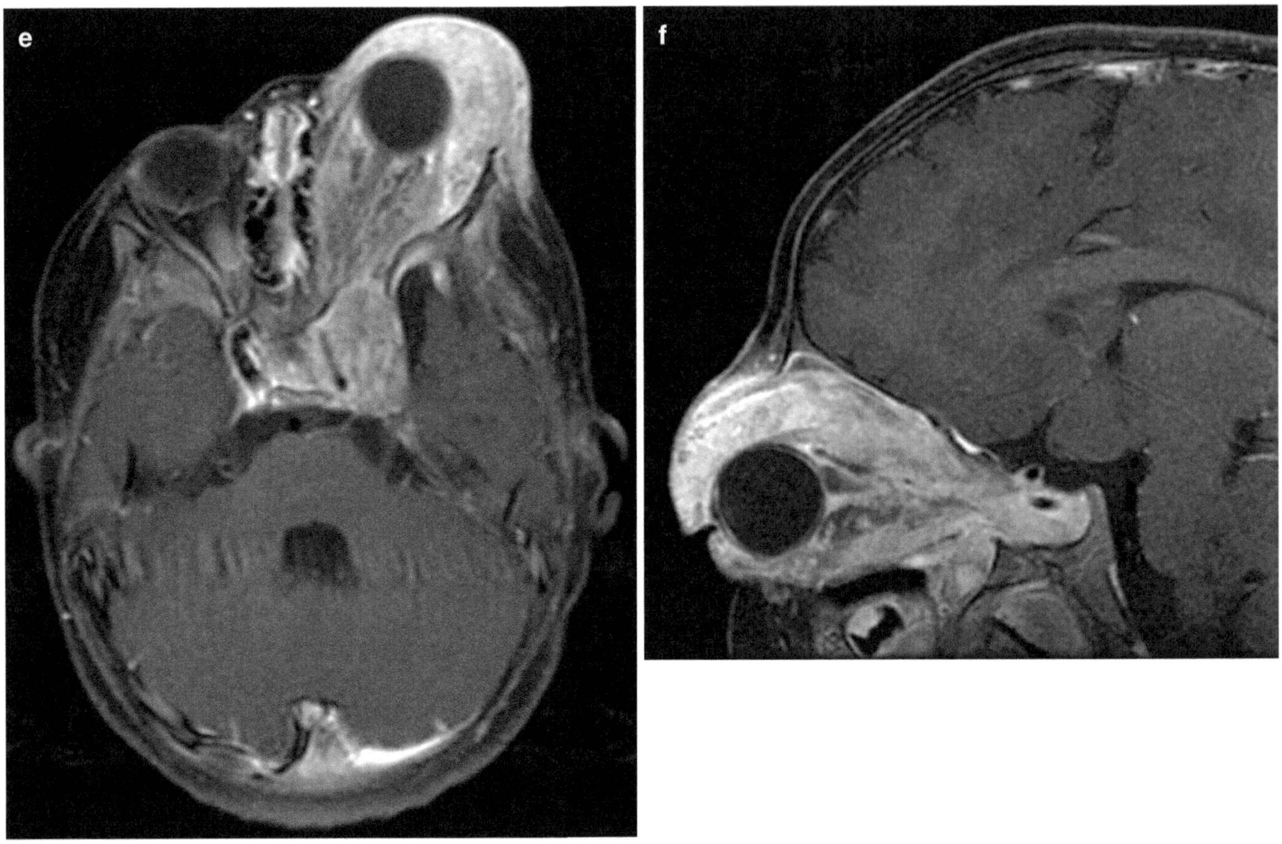

Fig. 2.32 (continued)

2.2.7.2 Diagnosis

We have a single case of patient with malignant orbital mesenchymoma. MRI showed the tumor as an infiltratively growing, isointense lesion on T1-weighted images and a hyperintense lesion on T2-weighted images (Fig. 2.38). The neoplasm caused partial destruction of the lateral orbital wall and marked exophthalmos.

2.2.8 Hemangioendothelioma

Hemangioendothelioma, also known as angiosarcoma, is a malignant tumor that develops from the vascular wall elements and has a tendency to metastasize. This tumor occurs predominantly at a young age, although is found in patients of 4–72 years of age (Brovkina 2008), mostly affecting men. It is usually localized in the upper internal quadrant of the orbit, has infiltrative distribution and affects the bones of the skull. In case of orbital involvement, the tumor spreads to the frontal bone. Angiosarcoma accounts for 1.5% of primary malignant bone tumors. The tumor size is usually 2–3 cm at the moment of primary diagnosis, but there are larger tumors. This tumor often grows from the orbit into the upper eyelid and the frontal bone.

2.2.8.1 Clinical Manifestations

Impaired function of the lacrimal glands, upper eyelid ptosis, exophthalmos, uneven skin pigmentation over the lesion.

2.2.8.2 Diagnosis

CT usually detects destruction of the adjacent bone and soft-tissue component. There may be calcifications present in the tumor. MRI detects a mottled pattern due to connective tissue trabeculae. Contrast enhancement is strong and heterogeneous (Figs. 2.39 and 2.40). CT-perfusion study demonstrates the heterogeneously prominent elevation of CBV and CBF parameters within the tumor structure, that is typical for majority of malignant orbital tumors.

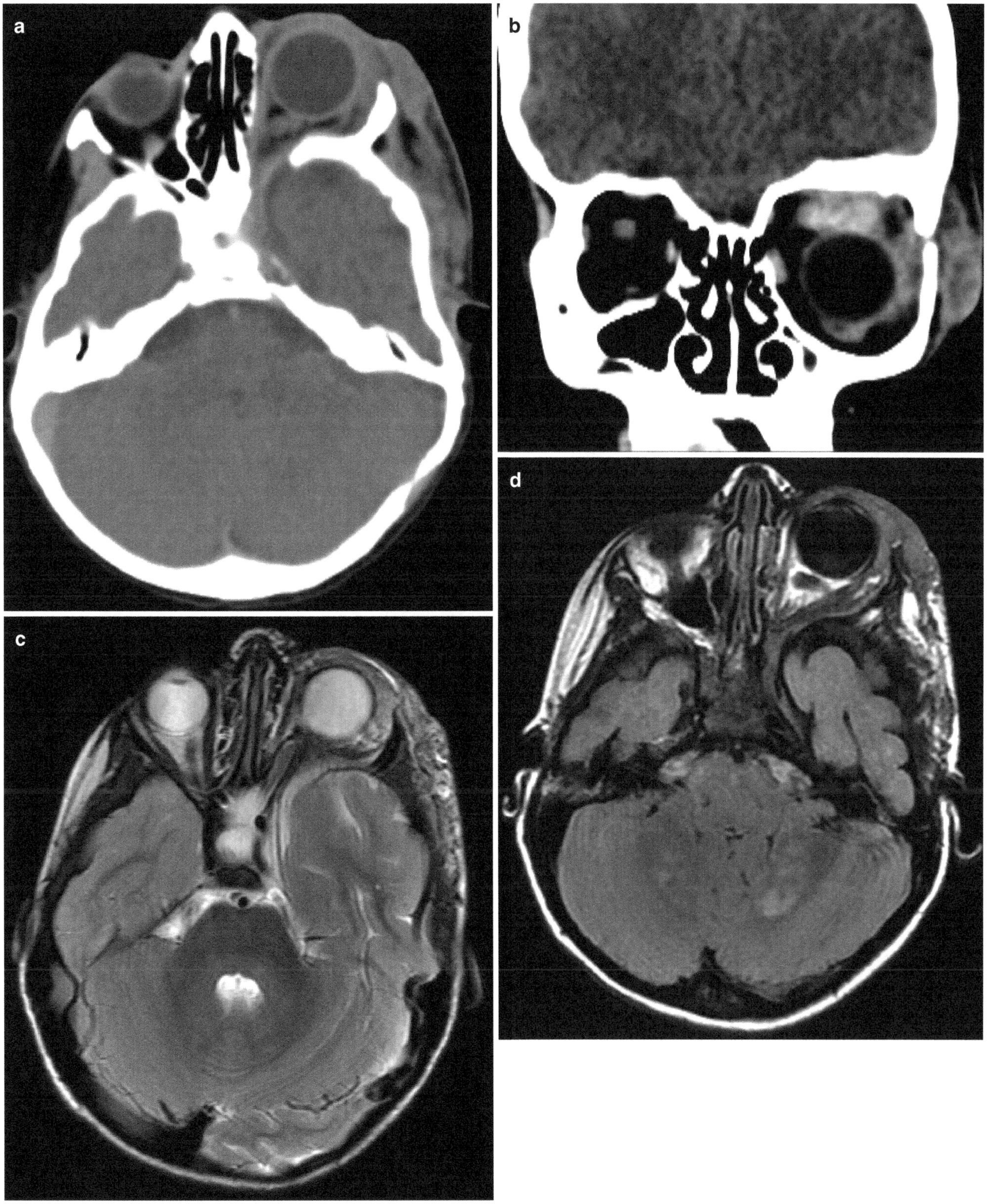

Fig. 2.33 Plexiform neurofibroma. Non-enhanced axial CT scan (**a**) and post-contrast coronal CT scan (**b**) detect diffuse infiltrative tumor of the left orbit. The tumor infiltrates the superior and lateral rectus muscles as well as the intraorbital fat. CT demonstrates the proptosis and deformation of left orbit and sphenoid wings leftwards. MRI with using T2- (**c**), T1-weighted scans before (**d**) and after (**e**) contrast enhancement demonstrates infiltrative nature of the tumor. It spreads to the optical nerve and chiasm. There is infiltration in extraorbital soft tissue of the left temporal region

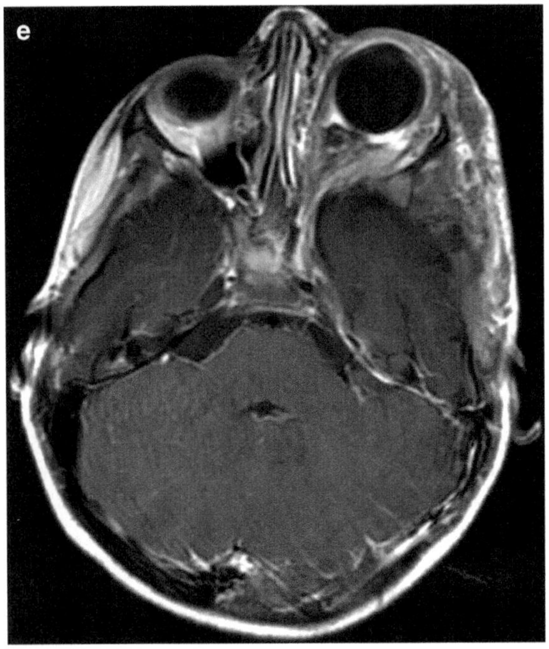

Fig. 2.33 (continued)

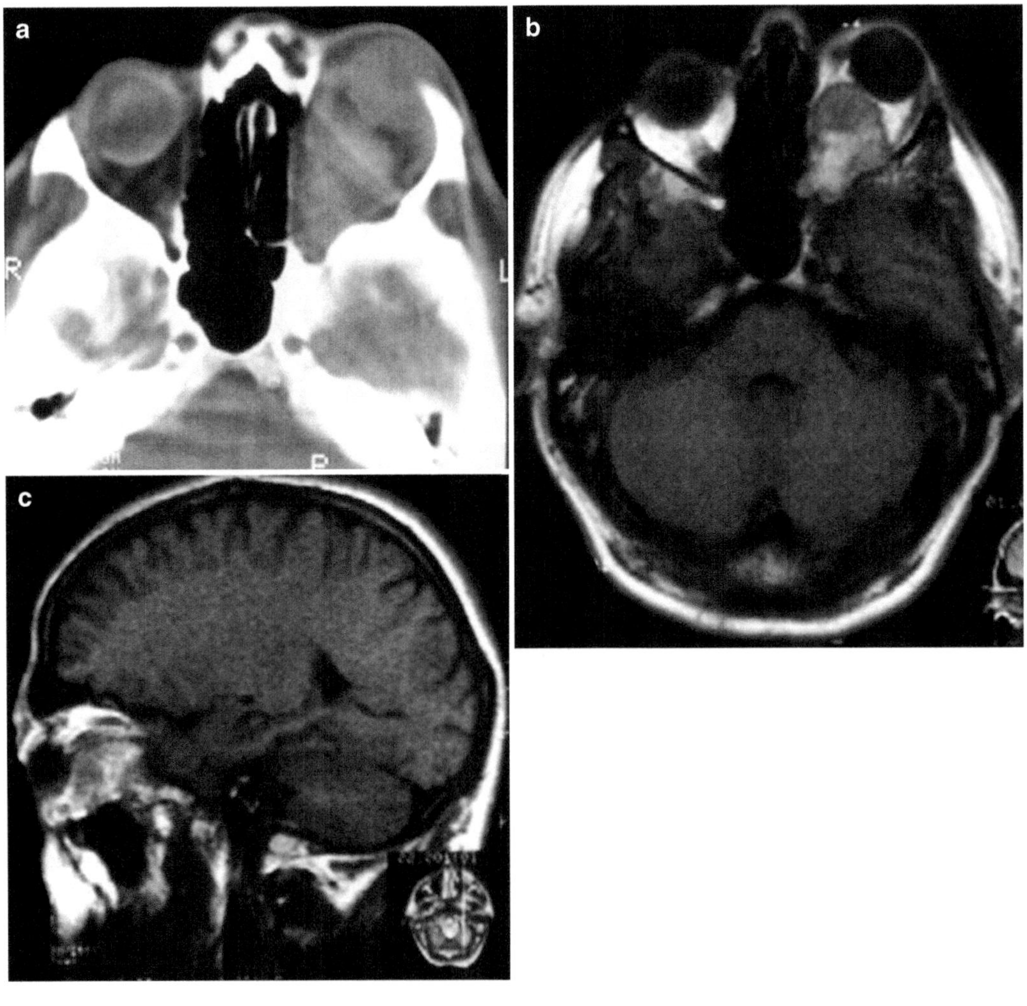

Fig. 2.34 Metastasis of melanoma to the left orbit. Axial CT scan (**a**) shows the soft-tissue tumor which has identical to the orbital muscles density and leads to the destruction of the medial orbital wall with exophthalmos. Axial (**b**) and sagittal (**c**) T1 -weighted post-contrast MR images demonstrate retrobulbar tumor with moderate heterogeneous contrast enhancement. Optical nerve is shifted upwards

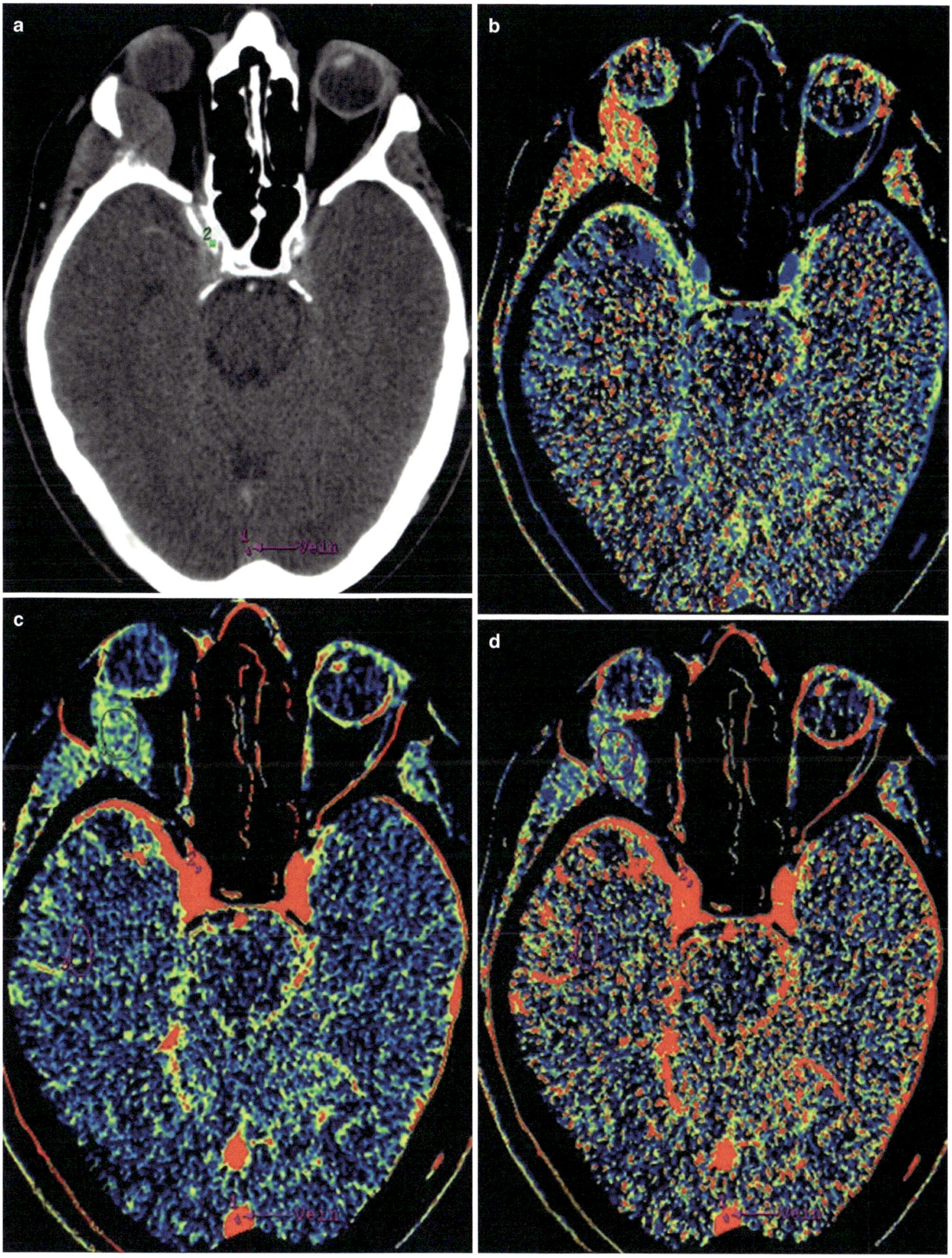

Fig. 2.35 Metastasis of adenocarcinoma into the right orbit. Axial CT scan (**a**) shows a mass, which is located in the lateral parts of the orbit. The tumor leads to local bone destruction. On perfusion CT an elevation of CBF (**d**), CBV (**c**) and MTT prolongation (**b**) can be detected. T1-weighted MRI (**e**, **f**) demonstrates tumor with homogeneous structure. Also, there are destruction of the lateral wall of the orbit and expansion of metastasis to the extraorbital soft tissue

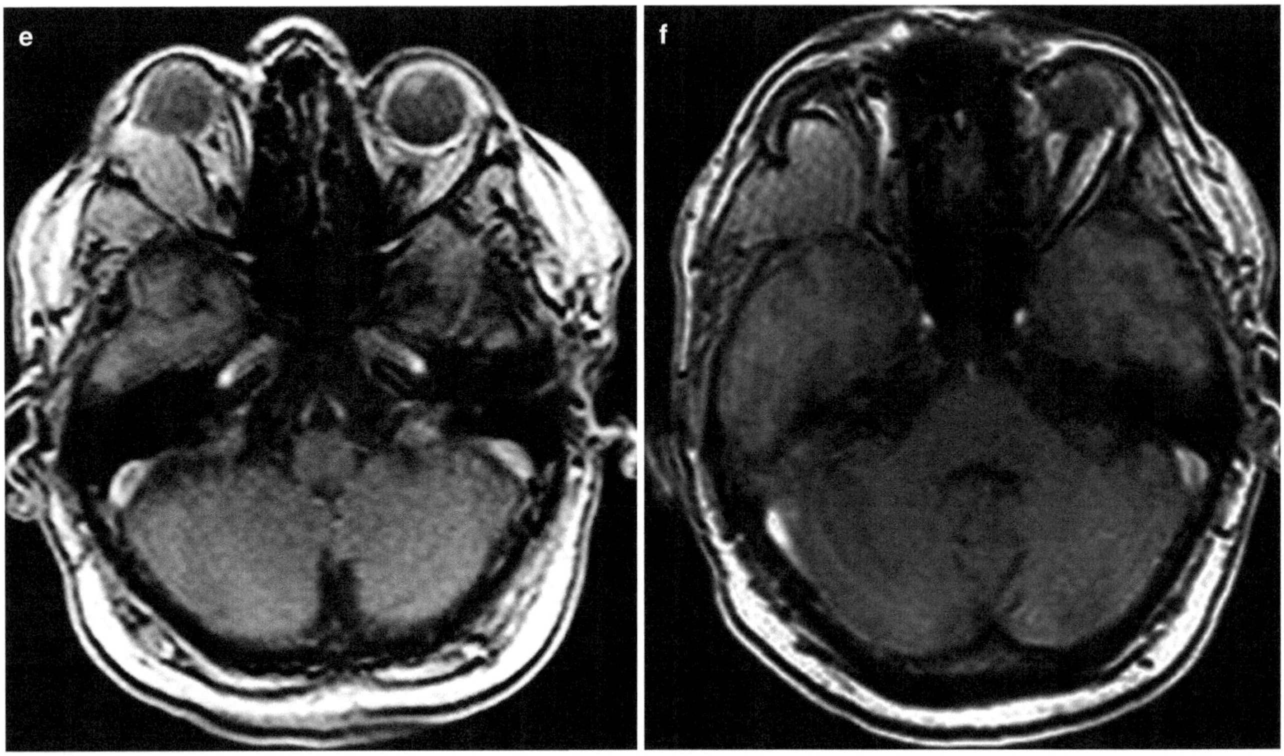

Fig. 2.35 (continued)

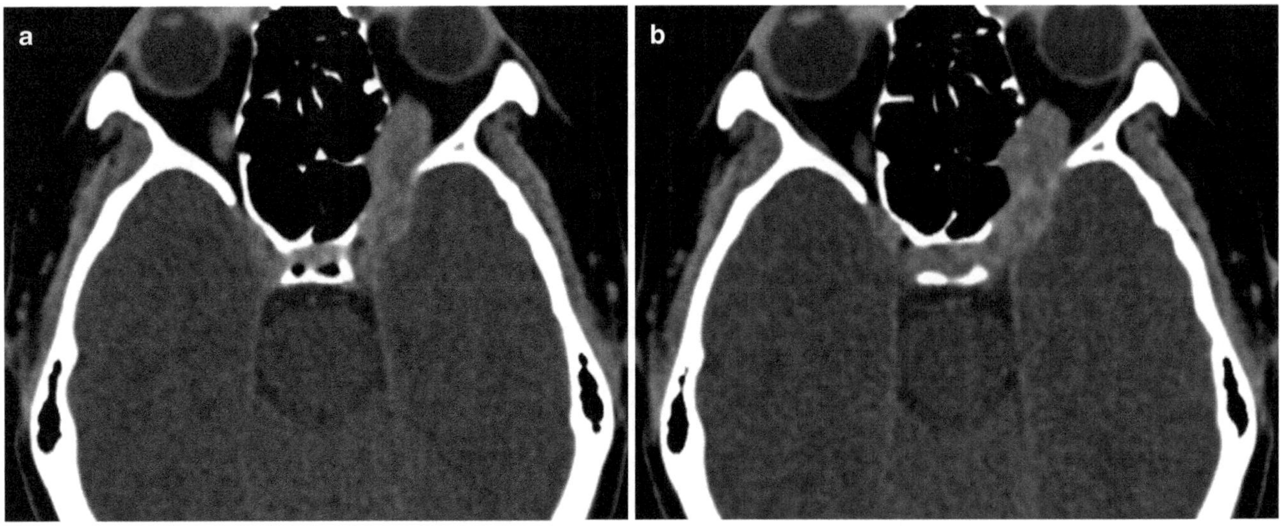

Fig. 2.36 Metastasis of the breast cancer into the left orbit. Axial CT images with contrast enhancement (**a**–**c**) demonstrate an enhancing tumor located in the orbital apex. There is destruction of adjacent bone structures. Perfusion CT study reveals the high hemodynamic values within the tumor tissue (CBF—**d**, CBV—**e**). MTT values are prolonged (**f**)

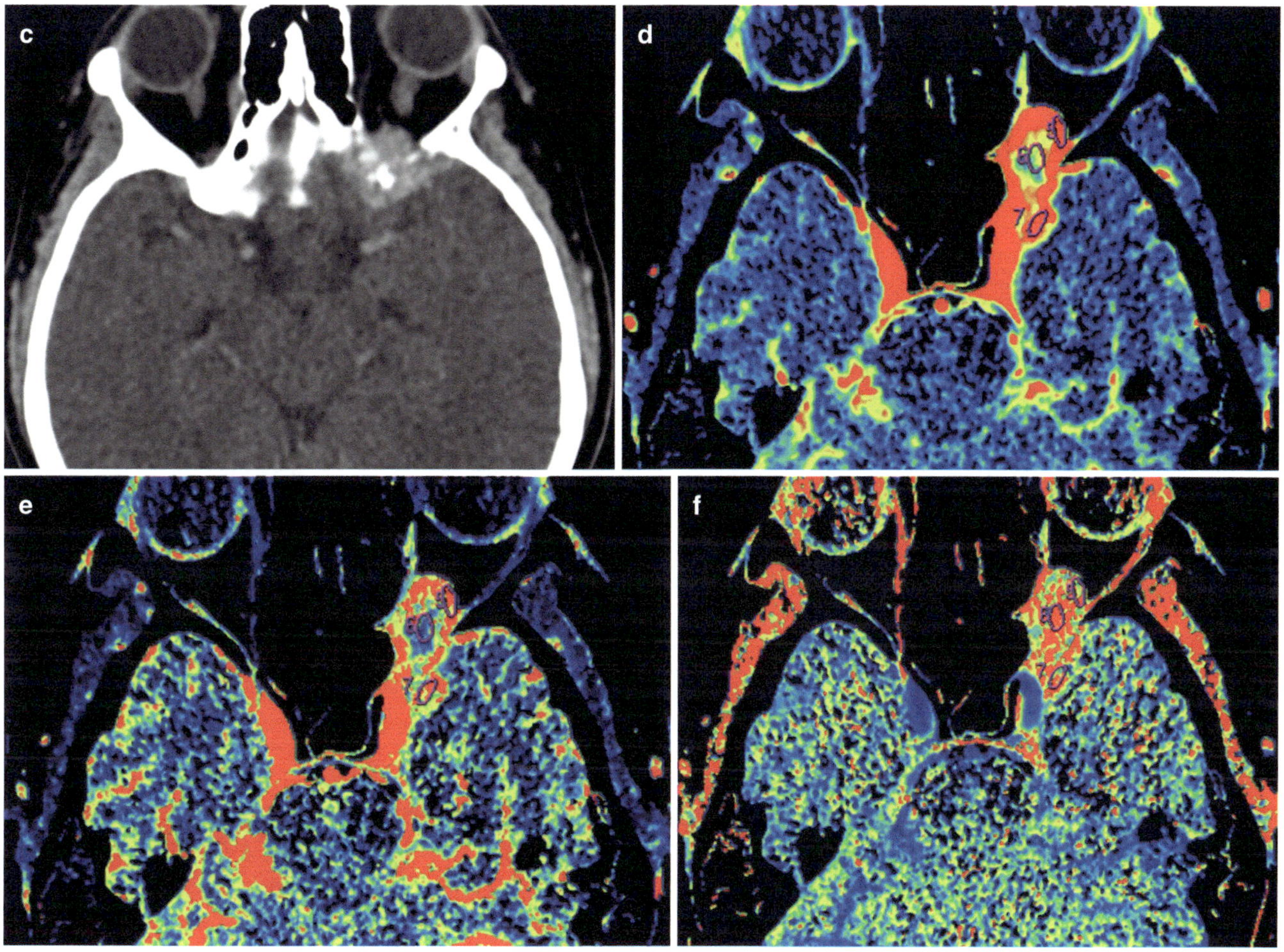

Fig. 2.36 (continued)

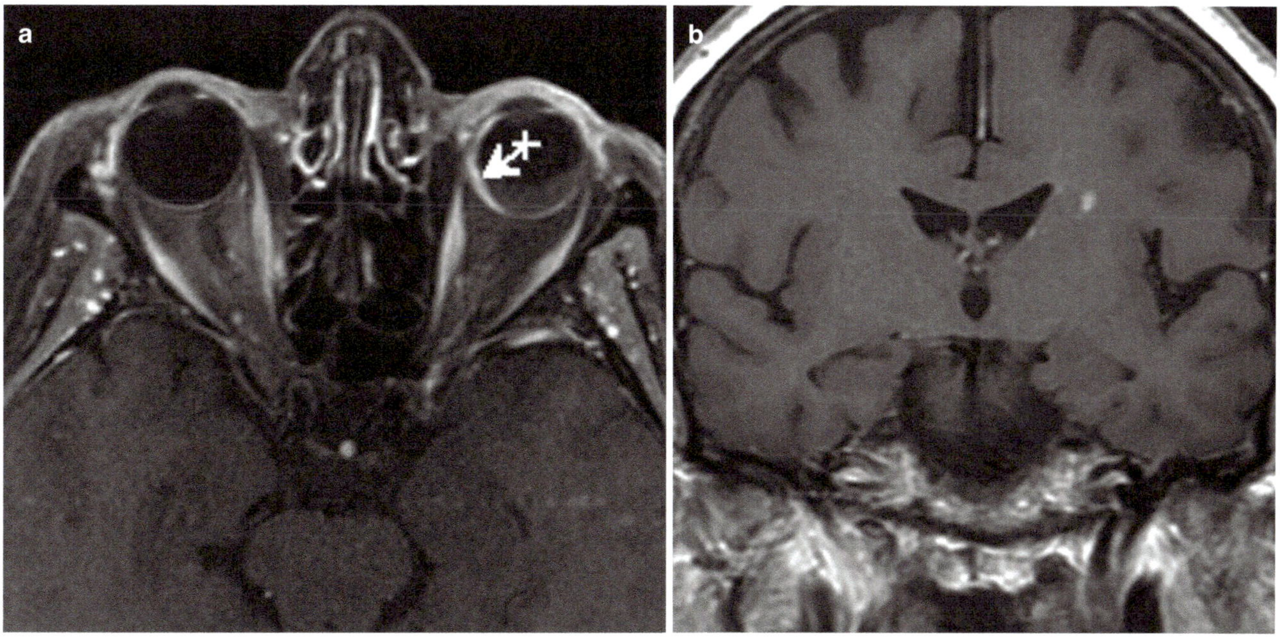

Fig. 2.37 Multiple metastases of lung cancer into the brain and eyeball leftwards. Axial T1 MRI with fat suppression technology (**a**) visualizes metastasis in the posterior medial wall of the eyeball leftwards (*arrow*). There is revealed related retinal detachment. Coronal post-contrast T1 MRI (**b**) reveals second (intraparenchymal) enhancing lesion in the left frontal paraventricular area. On whole-body DWI (**c**, **d**) multiple metastatic nodes in the spine, in the ribs, and also primary tumor node at the root of right lung were detected

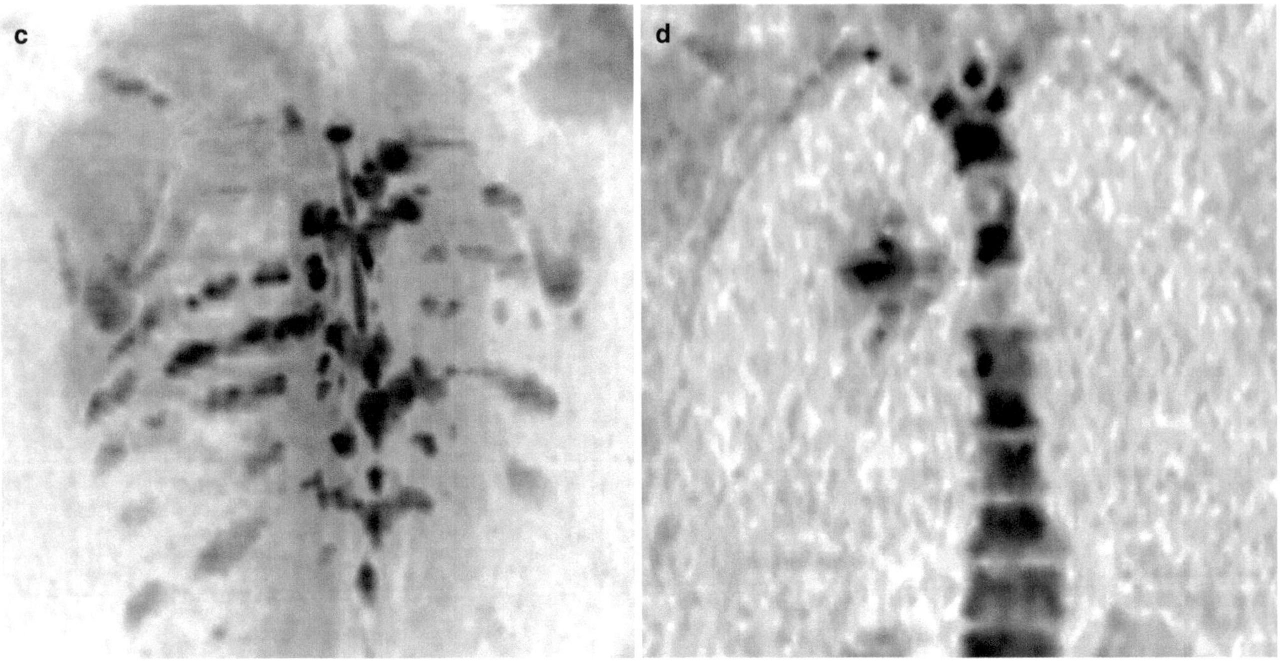

Fig. 2.37 (continued)

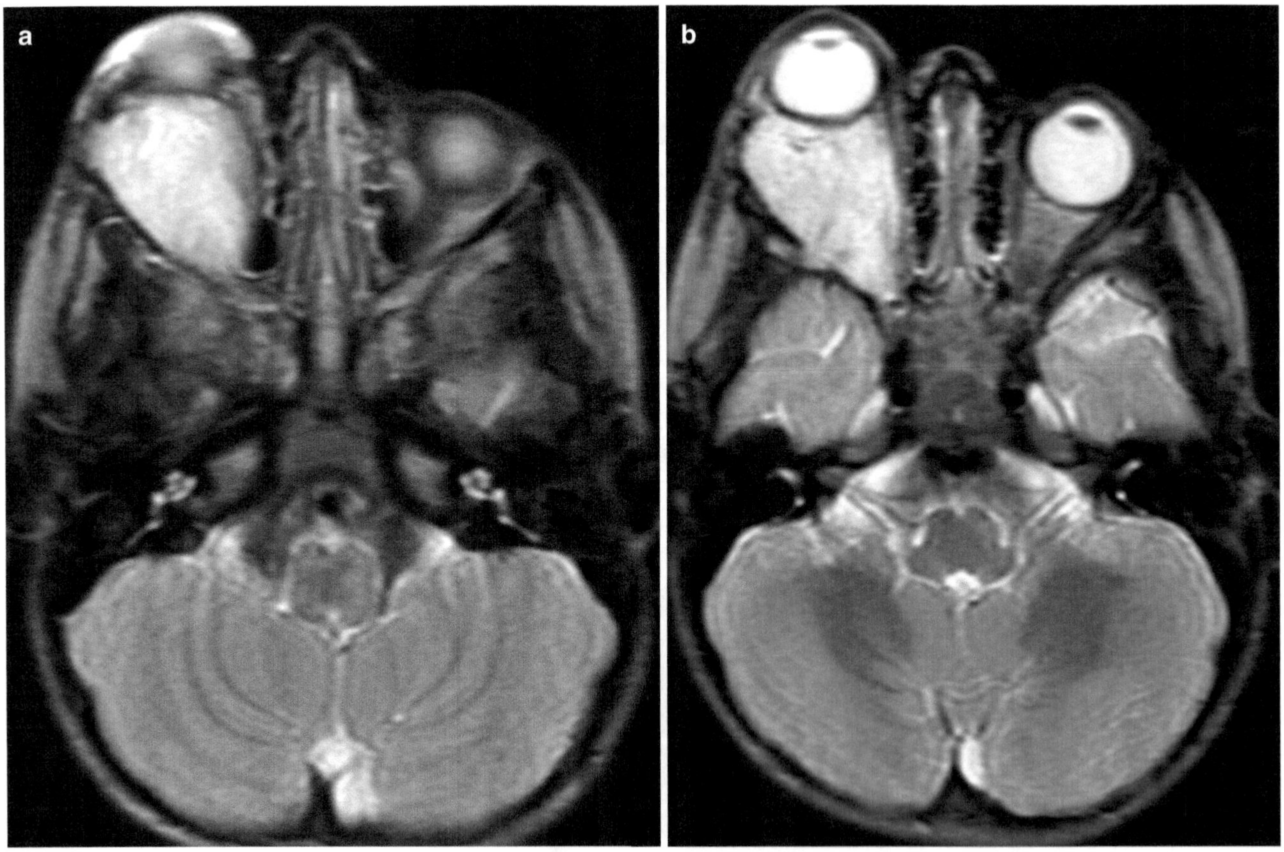

Fig. 2.38 Malignant mesenchymoma. Axial T2-weighted (**a**–**c**) and T1-weighted MRI (**d**–**f**) demonstrate homogeneous encapsulated tumor, which occupies a whole volume of the right orbit. There is prominent proptosis

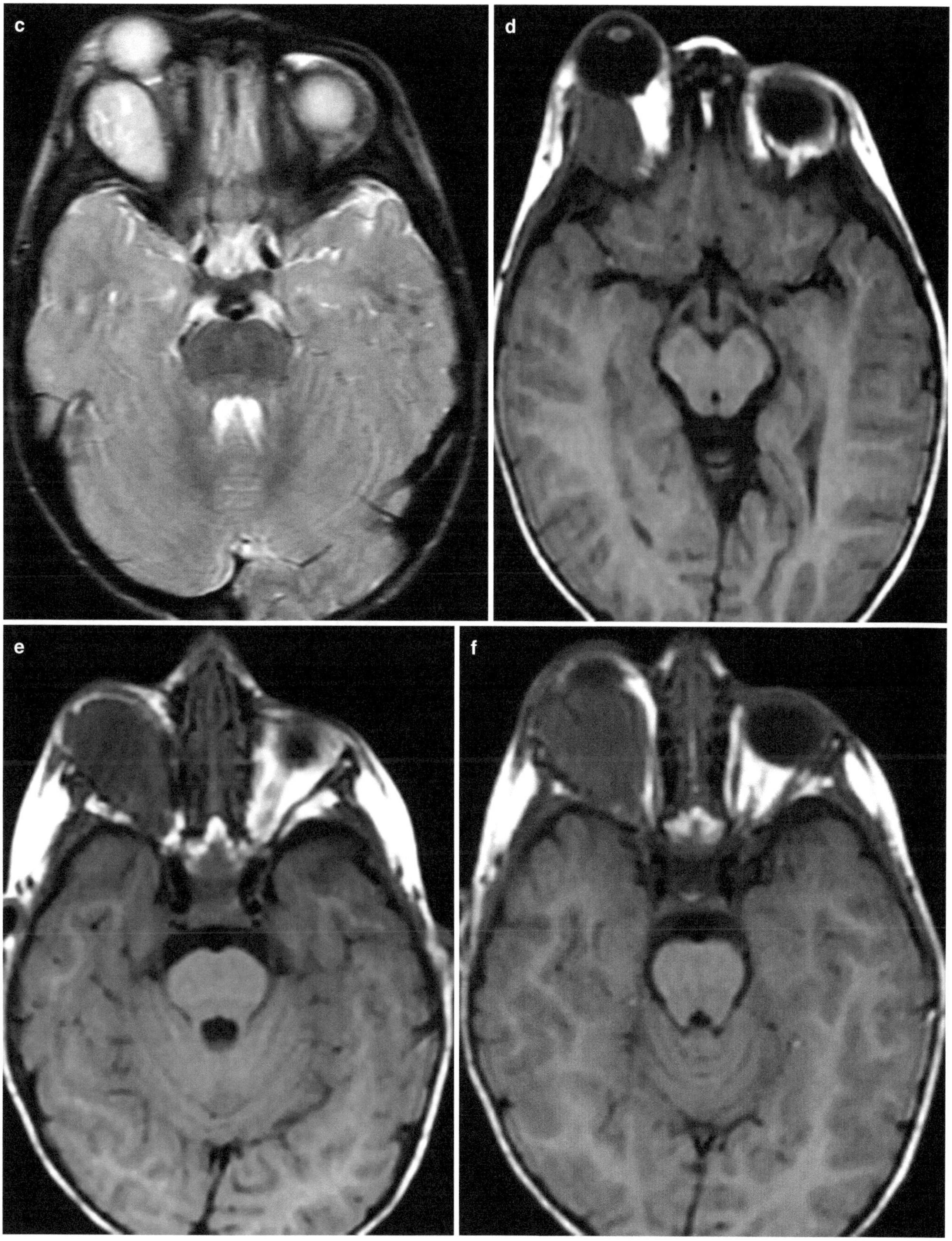

Fig. 2.38 (continued)

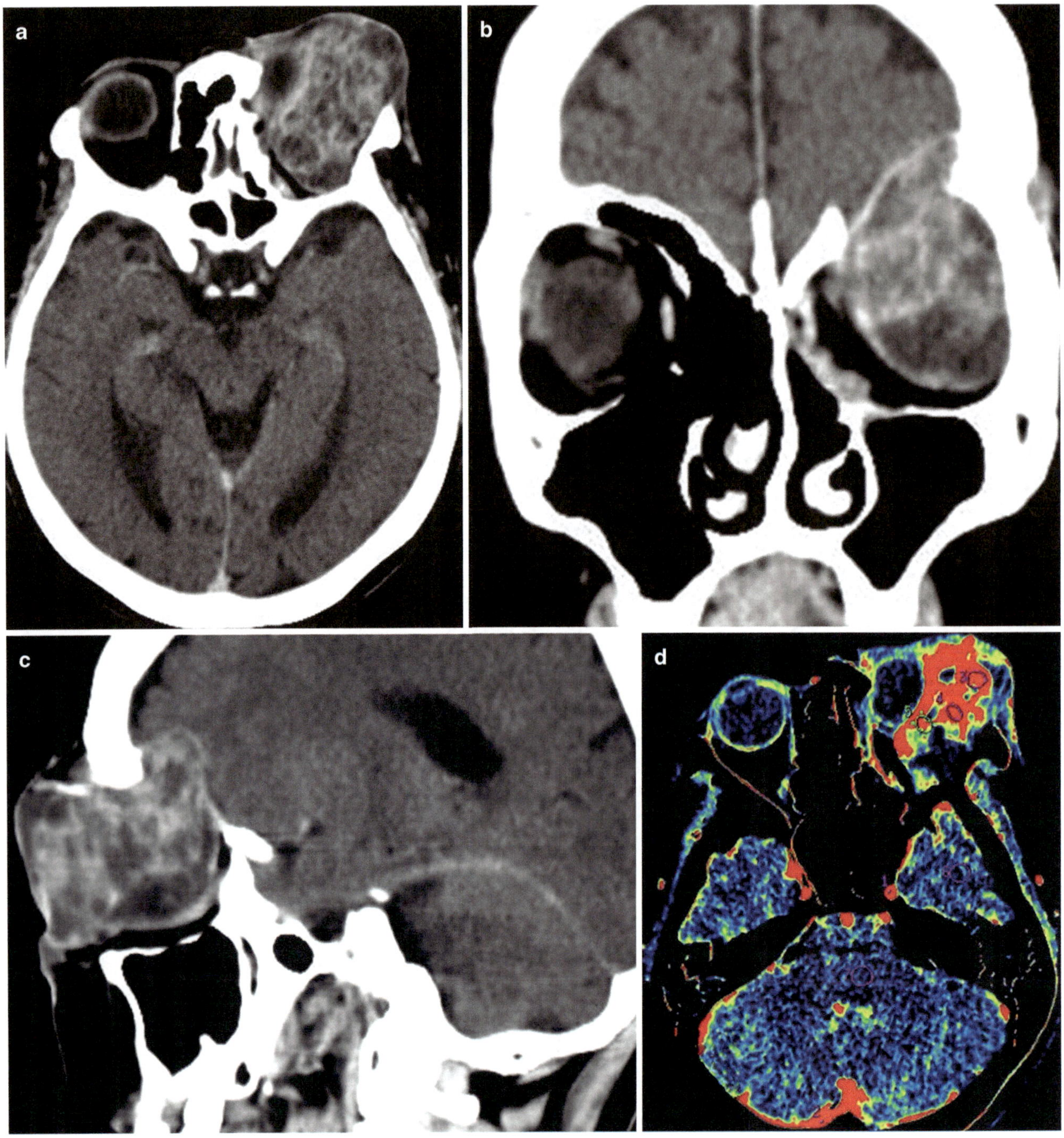

Fig. 2.39 Hemangioendothelioma. CT scans with contrast enhancement in axial (**a**), coronal (**b**), and sagittal (**c**) projections show a heterogeneously enhancing tumor of the left orbit which invades the superior orbital wall and frontal bone. Tumor contains many cystic cavities and septa, later are intensely enhanced. The tumor capsule is clearly visible. CT-perfusion maps reveal elevated blood flow and blood volume within the tumor (CBV–**d**, CBF–**e**). There is also moderate MTT prolongation (**f**)

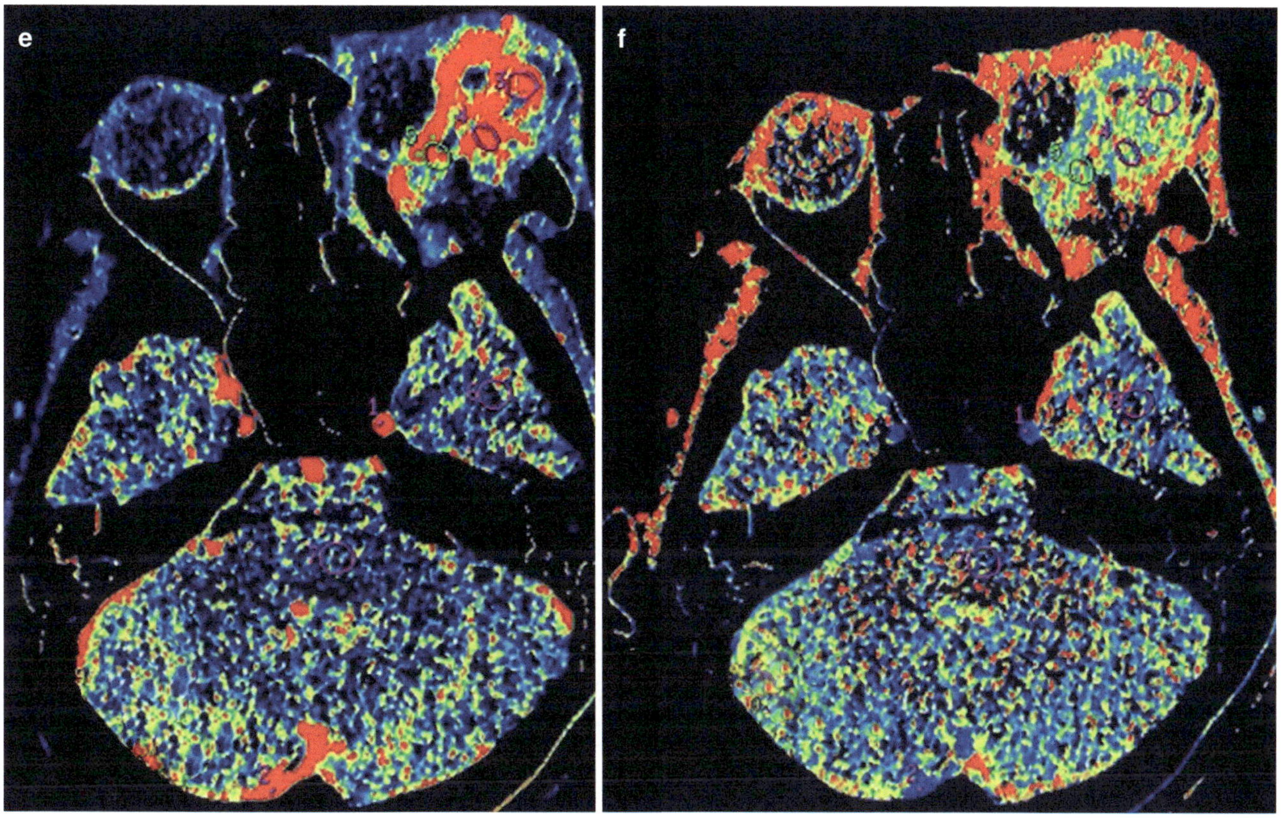

Fig. 2.39 (continued)

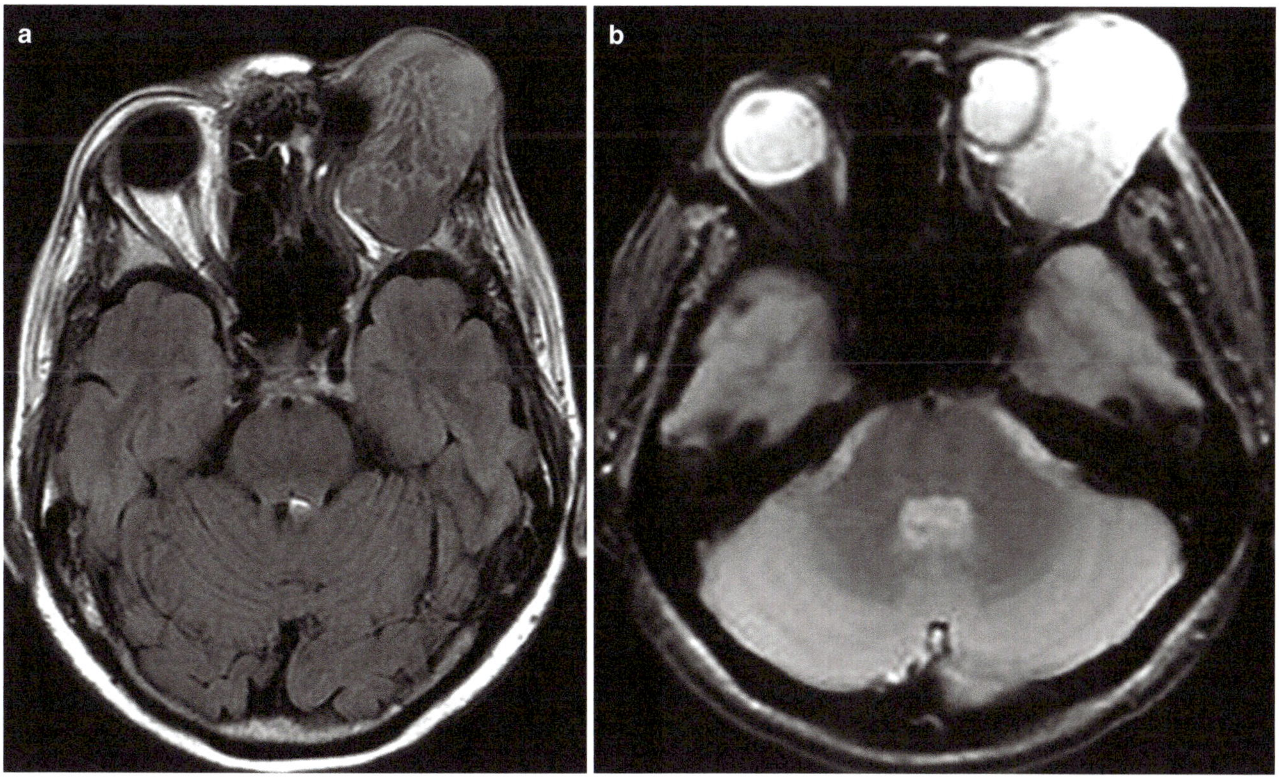

Fig. 2.40 Hemangioendothelioma (CT in Fig. 2.39). Axial T2-FLAIR (**a**) and T2* (**b**) weighted MRI demonstrate a large tumor of the lateral parts of the left orbit. The tumor has heterogeneous structure and multiple septa. There is high heterogeneous DWI signal (**c**) into the tumor probably due to hemorrhagic compounds. T1-weighted MR images in sagittal plane (**d**, **e**) and T2-WI in coronal projection (**f**) demonstrate the tumor, which has lobulated structure and infiltrates the upper layers of the eye globe with its deformation and shifting

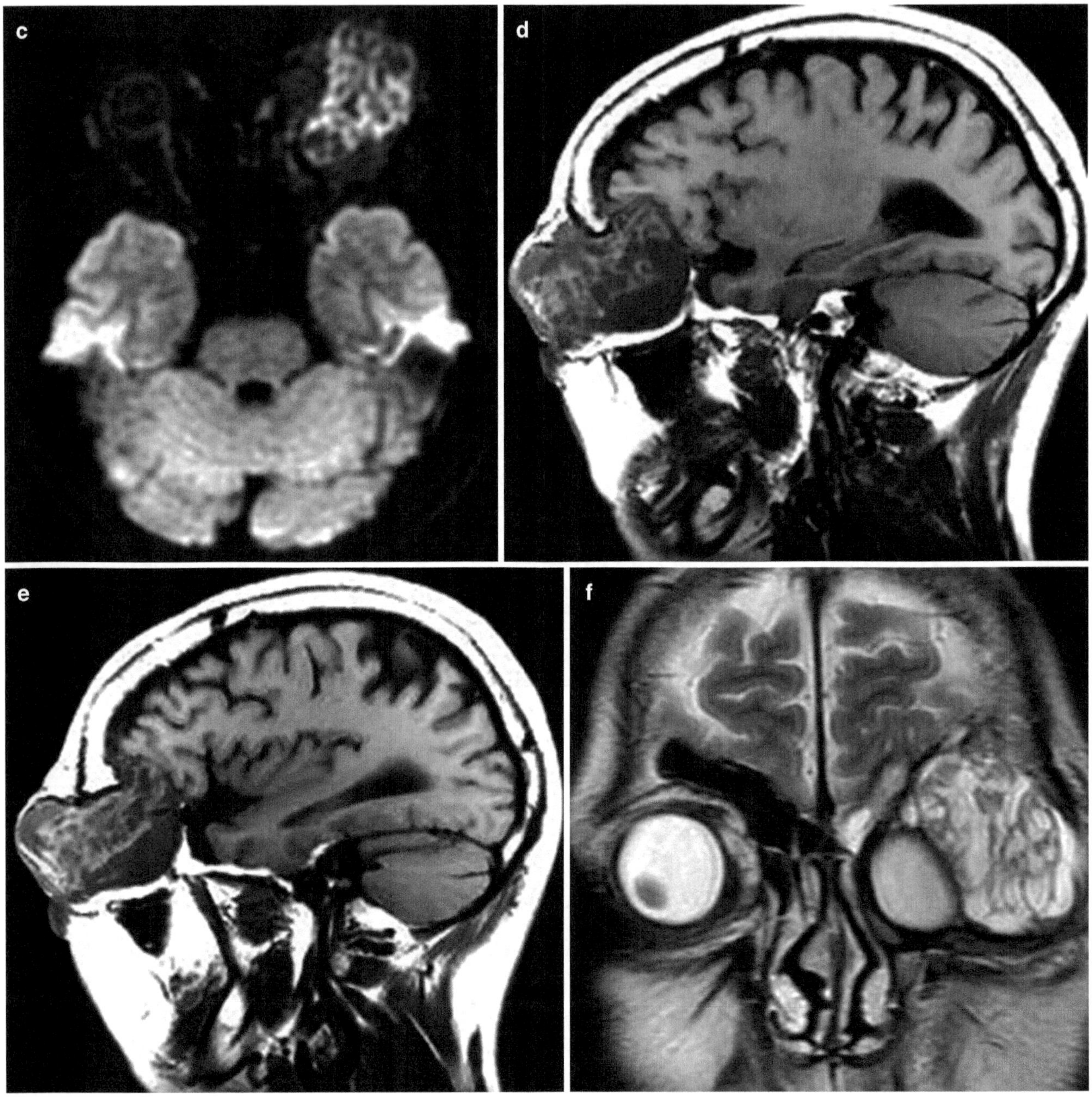

Fig. 2.40 (continued)

3 Intraconal Lesions with Involvement of the Optic Nerve

Contents

3.1 Tumors

Optic Nerve Gliomas differ by their course, types of treatment, histology, and prognosis, depending on their location along the nerve bundle. This is why more precise anatomical terms are introduced, such as glioma of the optic nerve, optic chiasm, and optic tract (a part of the optic pathway from the optic chiasm to the lateral geniculate nucleus). The term optic nerve glioma is used to designate gliomas of any portion of the anterior segment of the optic pathway. There are three tumor subtypes:

Tumor in children, associated with neurofibromatosis type I (NFI) (Thiagalingam et al. 2004);

Tumor in children, not associated with neurofibromatosis type I (NFI);

Tumor in adults, usually malignant—anaplastic astrocytoma, glioblastoma (Harnsberger et al. 2004a, b).

Optic nerve glioma is often a benign slow growing tumor, which accounts for 66% of all primary tumors of the optic nerve. In 65% of cases, glioma develops in the first decade of life, but only 5% of gliomas are detected until 2 years of age. According to Shields et al. (2004), gliomas account for 1–2% of all orbital tumors, and according to Baert and Sartor (2006), for 4%. Women are affected more often than men (3:2). 30–40% of patients with gliomas have manifestations of NF type I, and 15% of patients with NFI have an optic nerve glioma (Dutton 1994). The optic nerve involvement occurs in 1/3 of cases (Tow et al. 2003). 72% of patients have combined involvement of the optic nerve and chiasm (Cantore 2000; Brovkina 2008).

Clinical Manifestations A steadily progressive decrease in visual acuity is a typical sign of this disease. In young children, strabismus, nystagmus, axial or eccentric exophthalmos occur. Papilledema is found in the fundus as often as atrophy of the optic nerve (Balcer et al. 2001).

I. Pronin, V. Kornienko, *CT and MRI of Skull Base Lesions*, https://doi.org/10.1007/978-3-319-65957-2_3

Diagnosis On CT, glioma of the optic nerve is usually visualized as a spherical, spindle-shaped, or lobular space-occupying lesion growing along the optic nerve. Lobulation is caused by bends of the thickened optic nerve. The tumor spreading into the cranial cavity causes the expansion of the optic canal and is easily detected by CT. Typically, the density of optic nerve gliomas on CT ranges from 25 to 60 HU. Glioma is an isodense tumor as compared to the orbital rectus muscles. Following intravenous contrast enhancement, its density slightly increases (by 5–8 HU). There can be focal hypodense areas due to the presence of cysts. Glioma has clear contours, since it is located inside the nerve sheath. Calcifications in optic verve glioma occur extremely rare. A pathognomonic sign of glioma is considered to be an extension of the optic nerve bone canal (Brovkina 2008). Pilocytic astrocytomas, compared to other gliomas, are characterized by higher CBV and CBF values on CT-perfusion. Diffuse astrocytomas have all hemodynamic parameters similar to those of the brain white matter. In addition, an important diagnostic advantage of CT-perfusion over the standard procedure has become its ability to evaluate the structural tumor components with the possibility of differentiating pathologically hyperperfused foci (i.e., tumors) from cysts and other structures (Kornienko and Pronin 2009).

Based on MRI, the tumor has isointense or slightly hypointense MR-signal on T1-weighted images, as compared to the brain tissue, and a hyperintense signal in the peripheral regions on T2-weighted images (Cummings et al. 2000). There are hyperintense foci within the glioma structure due to small cysts. T2-weighted imaging successfully detects spreading of the tumor along the optic tract, even in cases where CT with contrast enhancement fails to visualize these changes. T1-weighted FAT-SAT sequence achieves a more accurate visualization of tumors, especially if they accumulate contrast agent. Contrast enhancement varies from low to intense; however, its use is mandatory in all cases (Figs. 3.1,

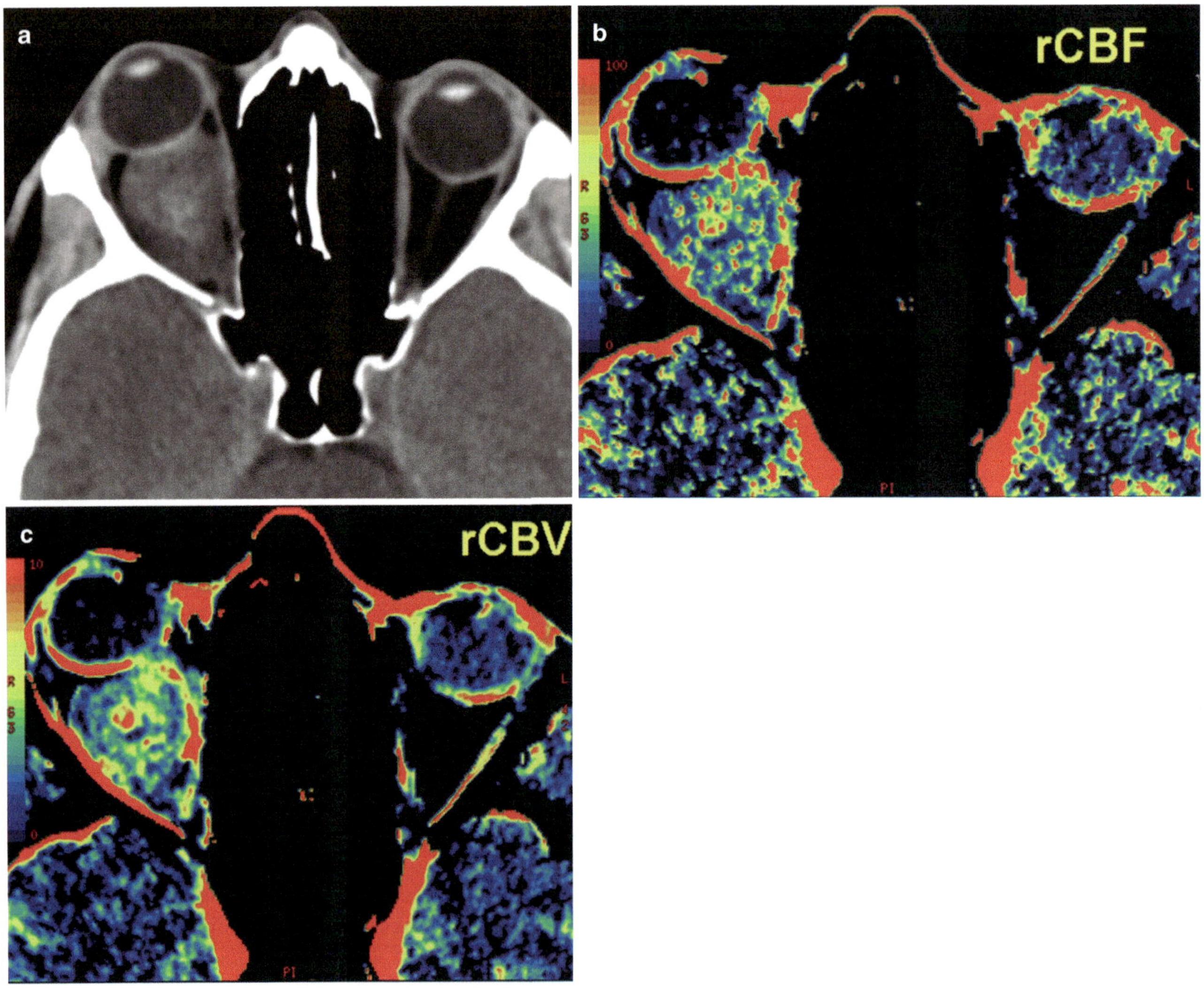

Fig. 3.1 Glioma of the right optic nerve. On CT scan in axial projection (**a**) a large heterogeneously enhancing (in the center) tumor is visualized. CT-perfusion study shows the heterogeneity of blood flow (**b**) and blood volume (**c**) values elevation within pathological tissue. Histological examination reveals pilocytic astrocytoma

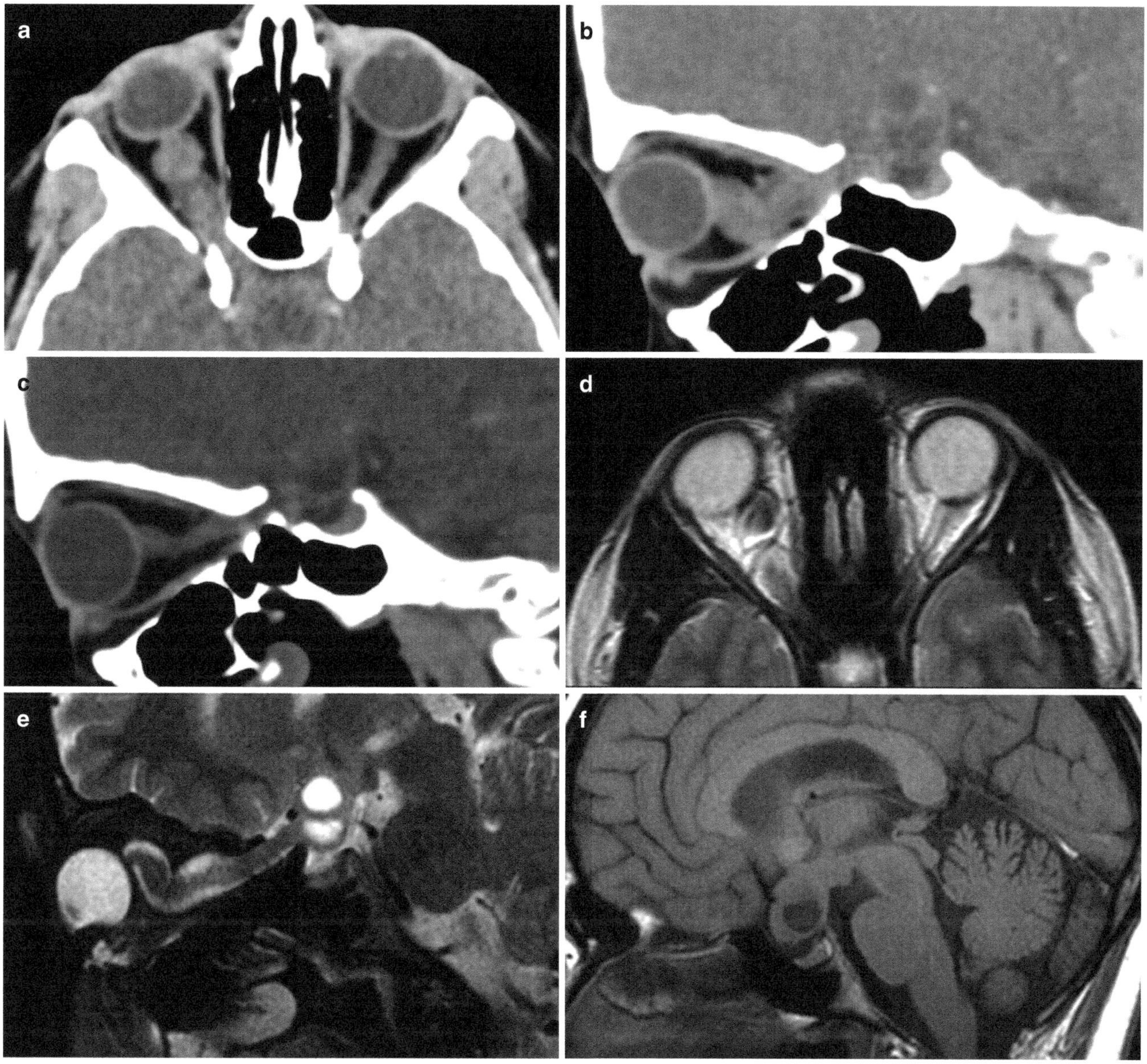

Fig. 3.2 Diffuse glioma (Grade I-II) of the right optical nerve and chiasm. CT scans in axial projection (**a**) and in sagittal reformats along the right (**b**) and left optical nerves (**c**) demonstrate a fusiform isodense tumor of the optical nerve, which is thickened and bended. On axial and sagittal T2-weighted (**d**, **e**) and sagittal T1-weighted (**f**) MR images (respectively) the tumor has heterogeneous "clutch-like" shape. There is MR-signal hyperintensity in peripheral area of the invaded nerve. Cystic changes are clearly visible in the chiasm projection

3.2, 3.3, and 3.4). For pilocytic astrocytomas from moderate to strong enhancement is typical. Majority of diffuse astrocytomas show the low degree of contrast enhancement (Fig. 3.5).

Differential Diagnosis Optic nerve sheath meningioma, optic neuritis, pseudotumor, sarcoidosis, etc. The main differences from the optic nerve sheath meningioma: expansion of the optic canal, rare calcifications, lack of hyperostosis of adjacent bones (Cabanis 1996). The presence of cystic degeneration, weak contrast enhancement or lack of it and low perfusion data can be highlighted among other characteristics of the optic nerve glioma (Kornienko and Pronin 2009).

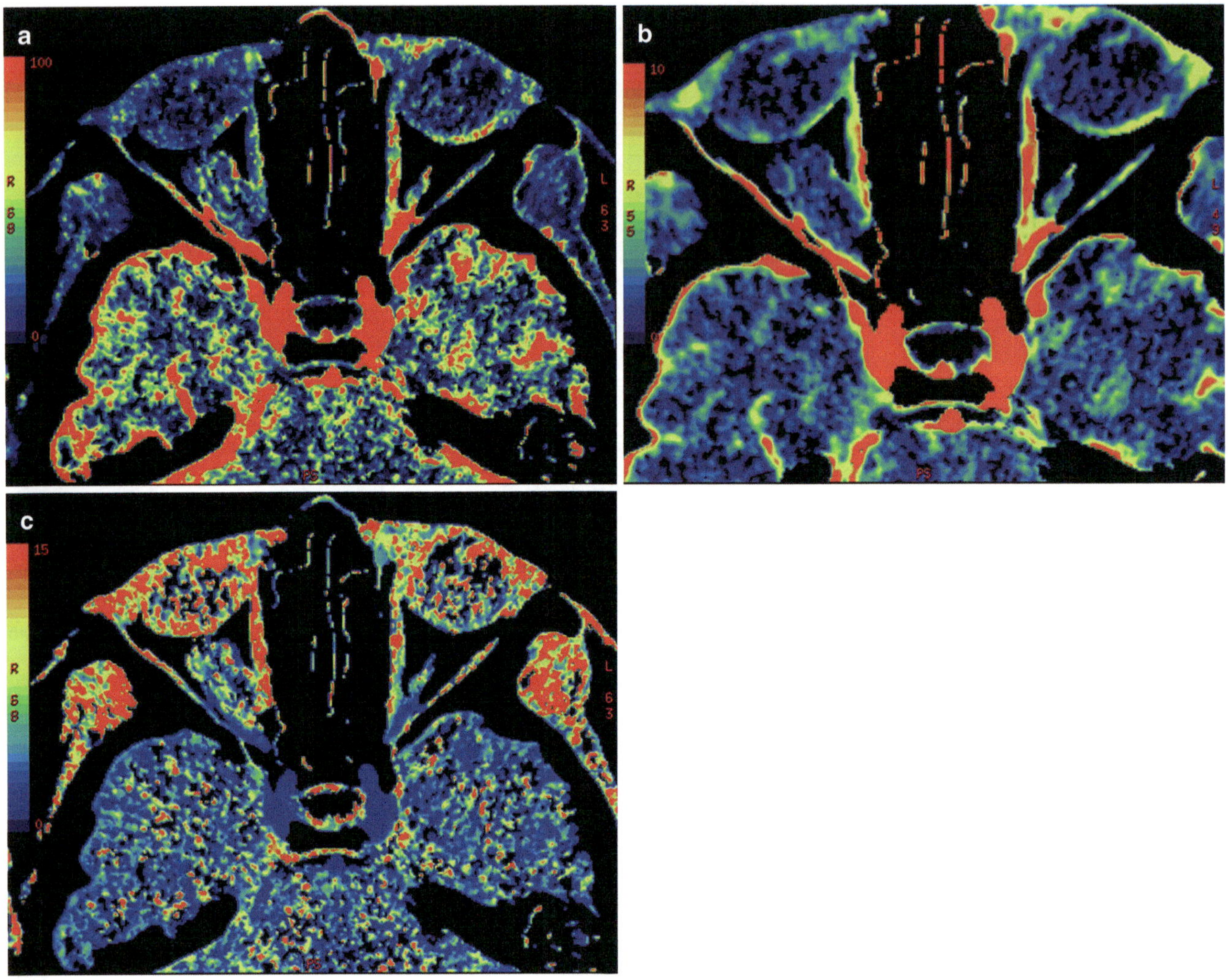

Fig. 3.3 The same patient as in Fig. 3.2. CT-perfusion study reveals minimal changes of blood flow (**a**) and volume (**b**) into the tumor tissue. Mean transit time of contrast agent (**c**) is lower in peripheral (hyperintense in T2-weighted MRI) lesion area

Optic Nerve Sheath Meningioma accounts for approximately 5% of primary orbital tumors, with about one third of primary tumors of the optic nerve (Turbin and Pokorny 2004; Taban and Perry 2007). The source of growth for meningiomas at this site are arachnoid villi between the dura and arachnoid membranes. Spreading via the intermeningeal space, the tumor can grow into the optic nerve sheath and infiltrate the orbital tissues. Orbital meningiomas are more common in women (80%) aged from 30 to 40 years old (Tailor et al. 2013). Meningiomas rarely occur in children, but they are characterized by aggressive growth in these cases.

Clinical Manifestations Pain in the orbit, progressive visual deterioration, asymmetric loss of visual fields, the eye repositioning is difficult, early development of the congestive optic disc (Egan and Lessell 2002).

Diagnosis CT shows a thickened optic nerve (a 4–6-fold increase in the diameter), eccentric tumor growth is possible with local thickening along the optic nerve. There may be both solitary and multiple calcifications. Intense contrast enhancement (up to 40–45 HU) of the tumor is a typical characteristic of meningiomas. Using helical CT scanning to obtain thin

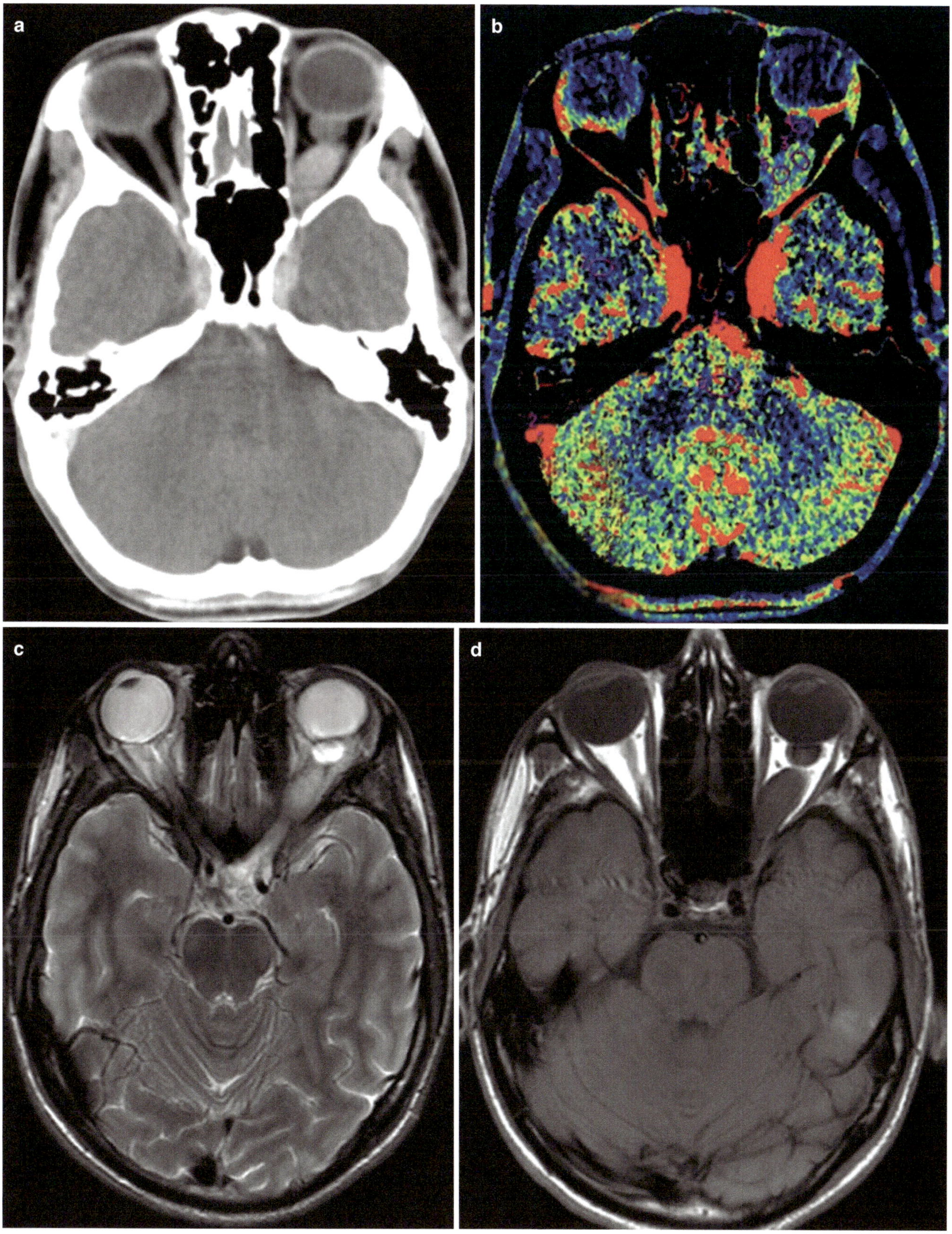

Fig. 3.4 Pilocytic astrocytoma of the left optic nerve. On axial CT scan with contrast enhancement (**a**) and CT-perfusion CBF map a mildly hyperdense tumor of the optical nerve without signs of blood flow elevation is revealed (**b**). T2-weighted image in axial plane (**c**) and T1-weighted MR images before (**d**) and after (**e**) contrast enhancement demonstrate well-defined fusiform tumor of the optical nerve. The tumor compresses the perineural CSF spaces and causes to local ampoule-shaped dilatation these spaces in the retrobulbar area. Post-contrast MRI demonstrates homogeneous and prominent contrast enhancement (**e**). (**f**)–histological specimen

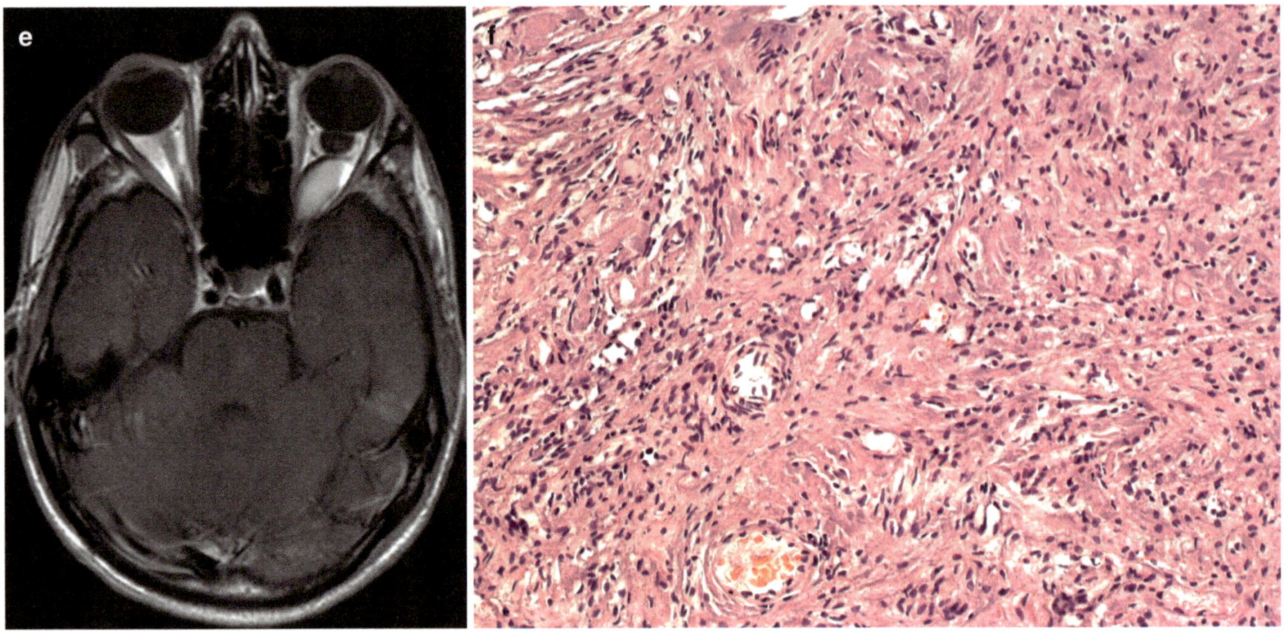

Fig. 3.4 (continued)

sections promotes better 2D reformation. The typical feature of this type of meningiomas is the visualization of optic nerve itself within the enhanced tumor tissue. A CT-perfusion study performed in our 18 patients with orbital meningiomas revealed the highest CBV values among other orbital neoplasms including malignant ones. CBF and MTT were higher than in the white matter of the brain but undistinguished from malignant tumors (Kornienko and Pronin 2009).

Nowadays 3.0 T MRI is considered as a more informative technology in the diagnosis of optic nerve sheath meningiomas due to high spatial resolution compared to 1.5 T MR scanners. The MR imaging pattern may vary depending on the histological subtype of the tumor. Meningioma may be isointense compared to the muscles on T1-weighted images and isointense or hyperintense on T2-weighted images (Mafee et al. 1999). The use of fat suppression techniques and contrast enhancement is most effective for detecting optic nerve meningiomas. In most cases meningiomas show strong contrast enhancement, and only in one quarter of cases contrast material accumulation is low. Optic nerve can be easily detected within the tumor tissue in majority of the cases (Figs. 3.6, 3.7, 3.8, 3.9, and 3.10).

Differential Diagnosis Optic nerve glioma, optic neuritis, pseudotumor, sarcoidosis, optic sheath schwannoma (Kim et al. 2002).

Fig. 3.5 Pilocytic astrocytoma of the right optic nerve. T2-weighted MR images in axial (**a**), coronal (**b**), and sagittal (**c**) planes show a optic nerve mass with hyperintense MR-signal surrounded by CSF (thin area of peripheral hyperintensity). Tumor shows isointense MR-signal on T1-weighted MRI (**d**) and prominent contrast enhancement on the post-contrast (**e**, **f**) MR image

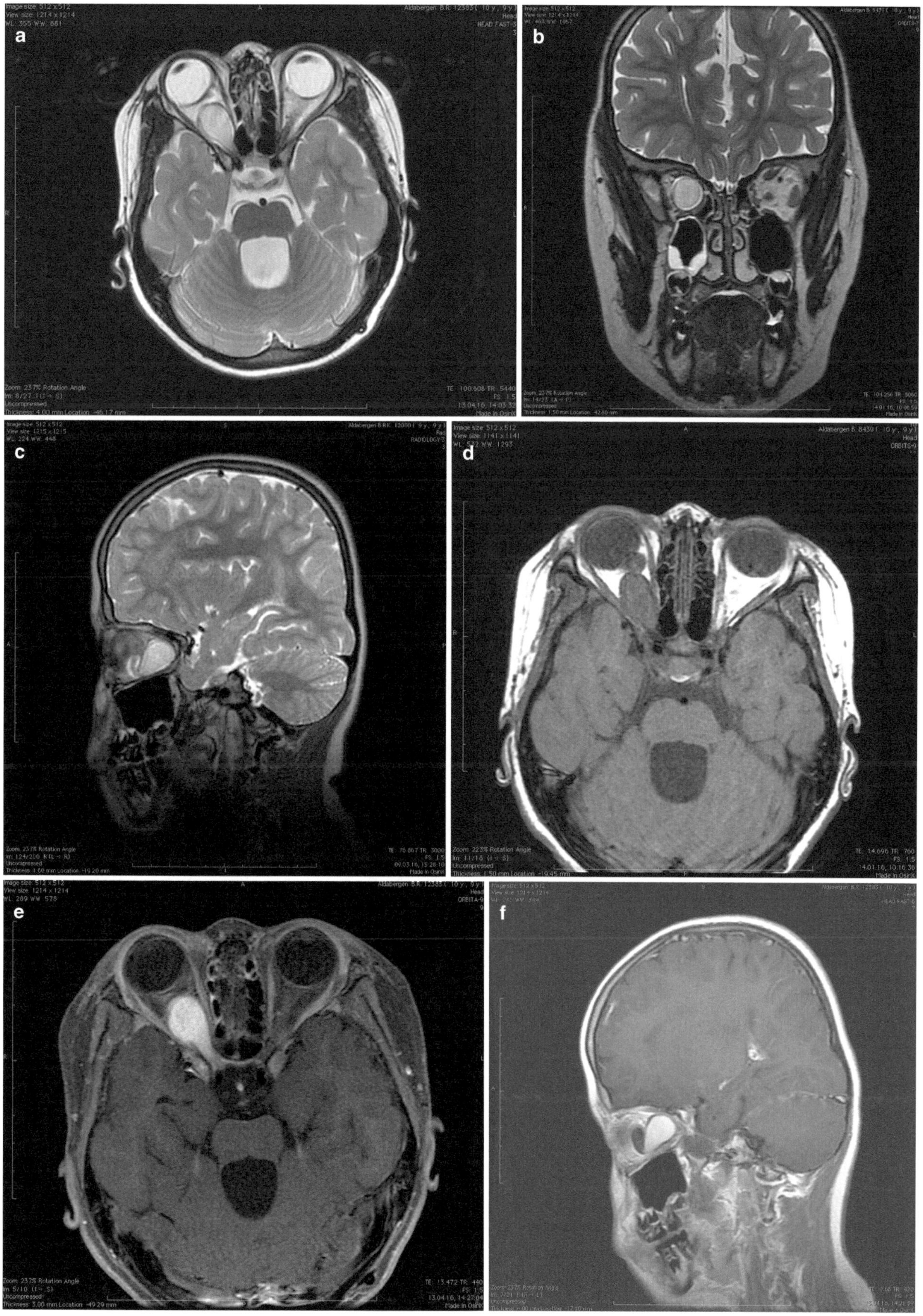
a
b
c
d
e
f

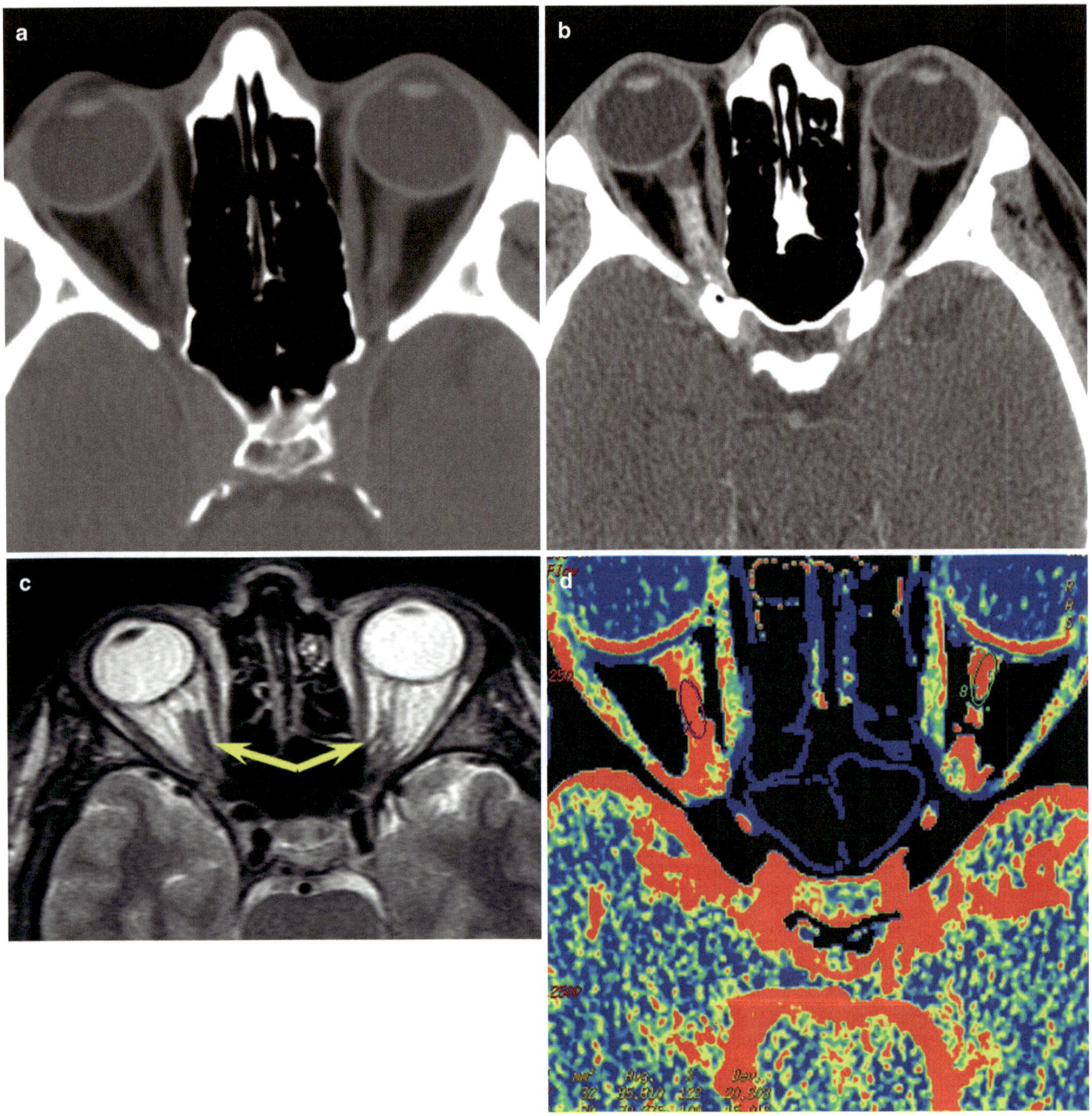

Fig. 3.6 Bilateral meningioma of the optical nerve sheaths. Axial noncontrast (**a**) and post-contrast (**b**) CT scans reveal an enhancing tumor of the middle and distal parts of the both optical nerves. The tumor leads to their thickening and deformation. T2-weighted MRI (**c**) demonstrates meningiomas that have hypointense MR-signal. On CT-perfusion CBF (**d**), CBV (**e**), and permeability (**f**) maps high values of these parameters within tumor tissue are visualized

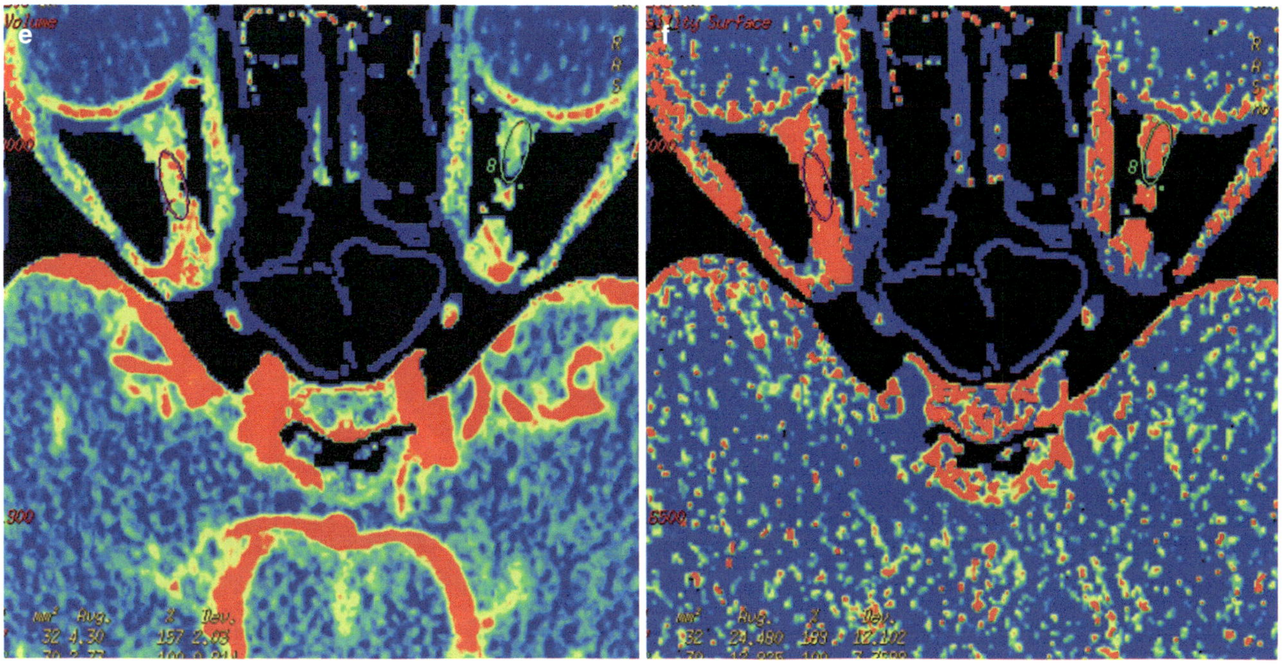

Fig. 3.6 (continued)

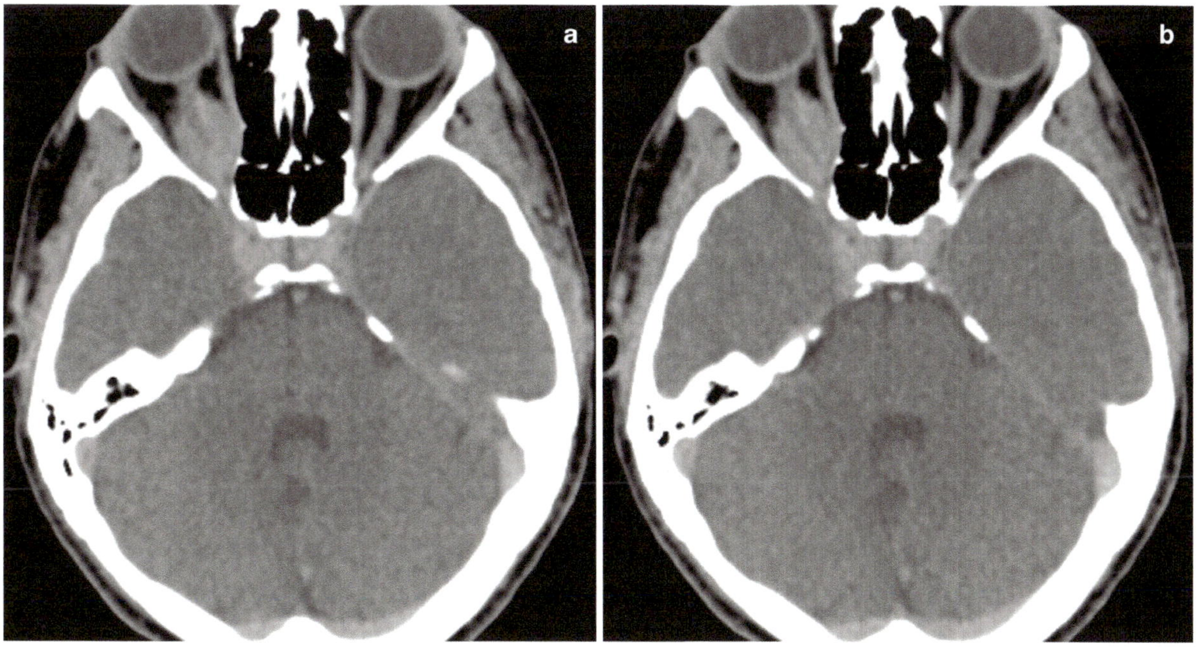

Fig. 3.7 Meningioma of the left optical nerve sheath. Postenhanced CT scans in axial plane (**a**, **b**) and with using coronal (**c**) and sagittal (**d**) reformations demonstrate "clutch-like" tumor, which wraps the optical nerve and grows from its sheath. The optic nerve itself can be visualized inside the tumor tissue. CT-perfusion CBV (**e**) and CBF (**f**) maps demonstrate significant blood flow elevation within the tumor

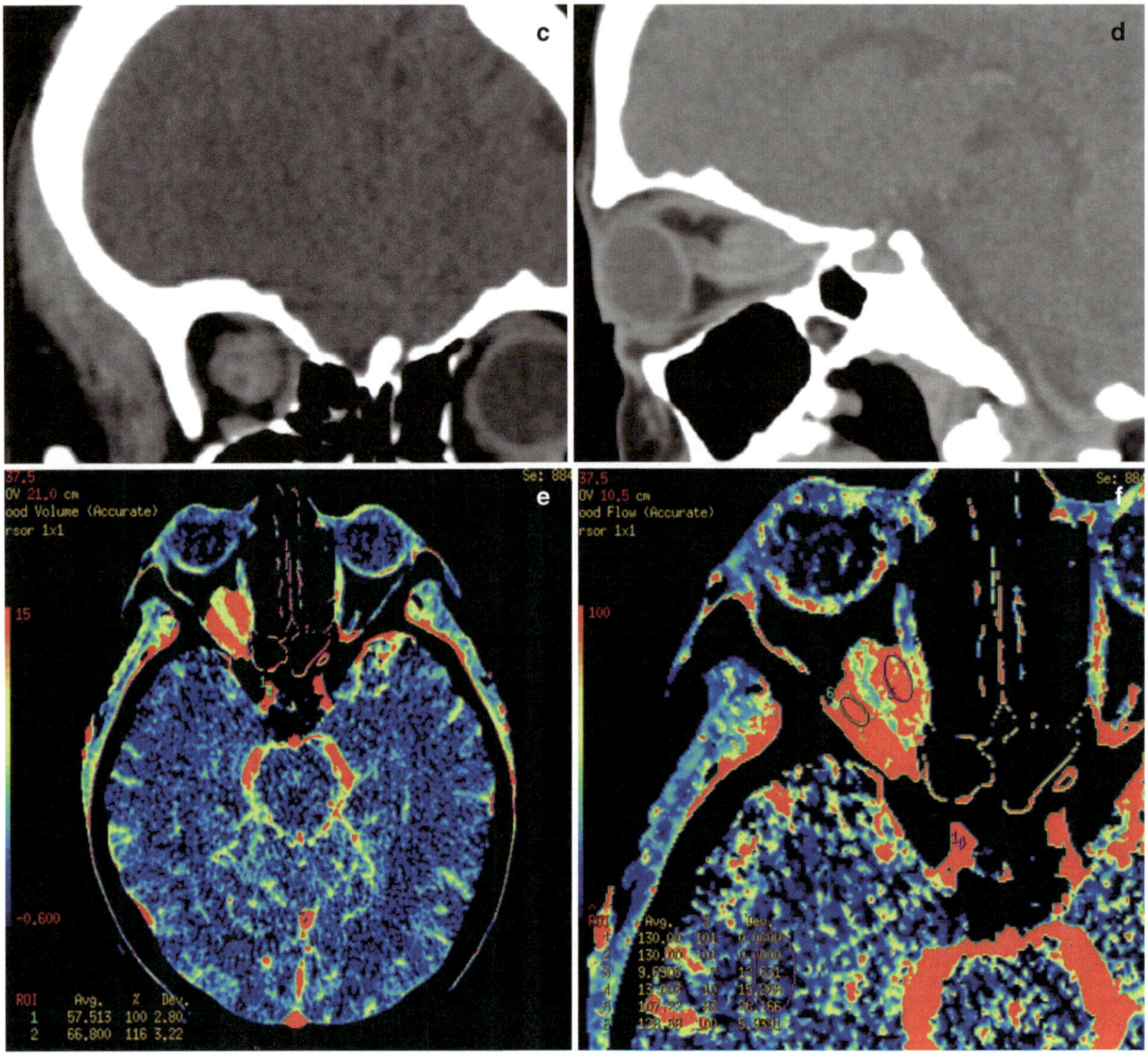

Fig. 3.7 (continued)

Fig. 3.8 Meningioma of the left optical nerve sheath. Axial non-contrast (**a**, **b**) and post-contrast (**c**, **d**) CT scans reveal an enhancing tumor of the retrobulbar location. The optic nerve can be visualized inside the tumor tissue. DSA (**e**, **f**) demonstrates prominent tumor blood supply from the ophthalmic artery

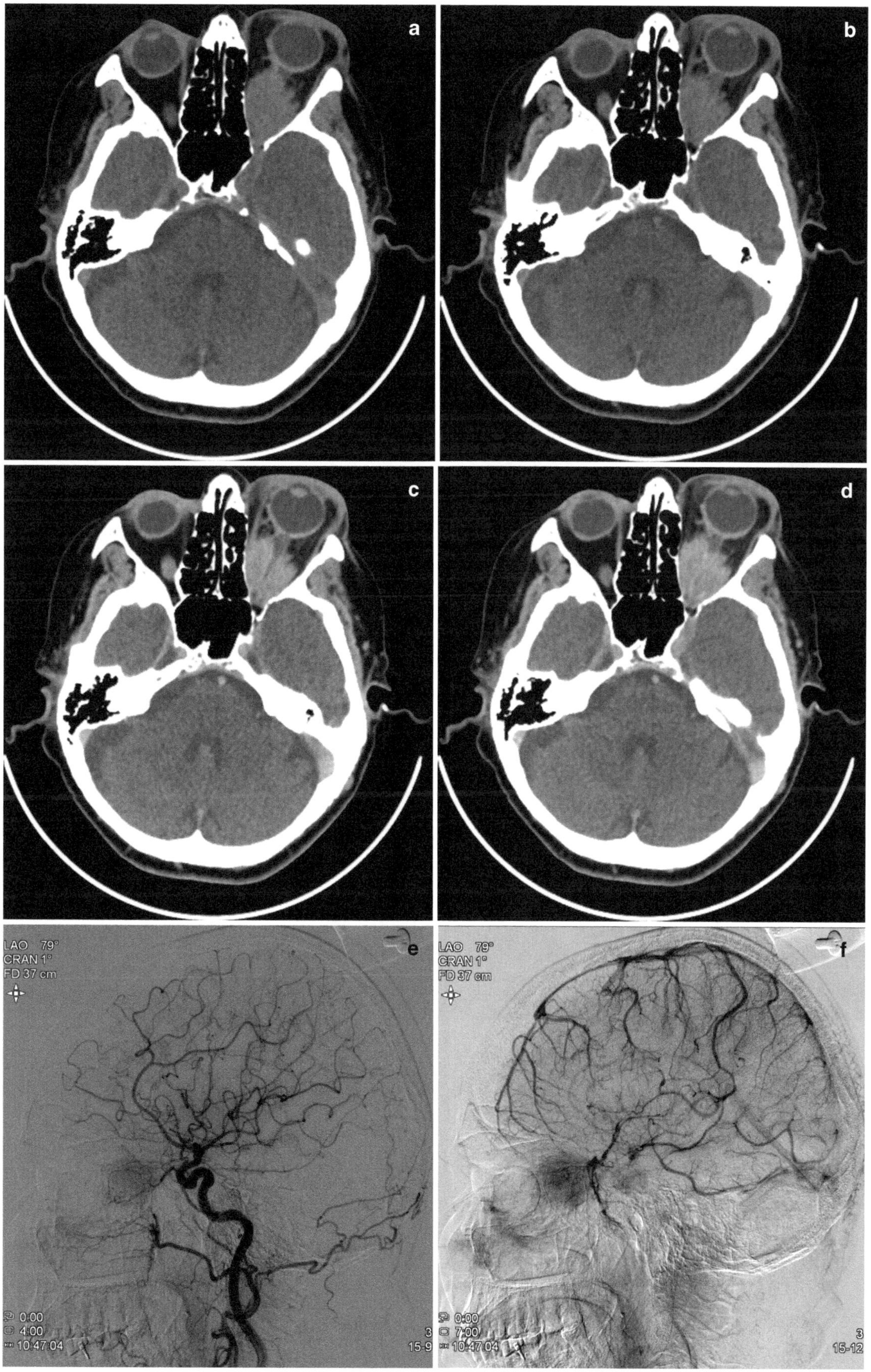
a
b
c
d
e
LAO 79°
CRAN 1°
FD 37 cm
0:00
4:00
10:47:04
3
15-9
f
LAO 79°
CRAN 1°
FD 37 cm
0:00
7:00
10:47:04
3
15-12

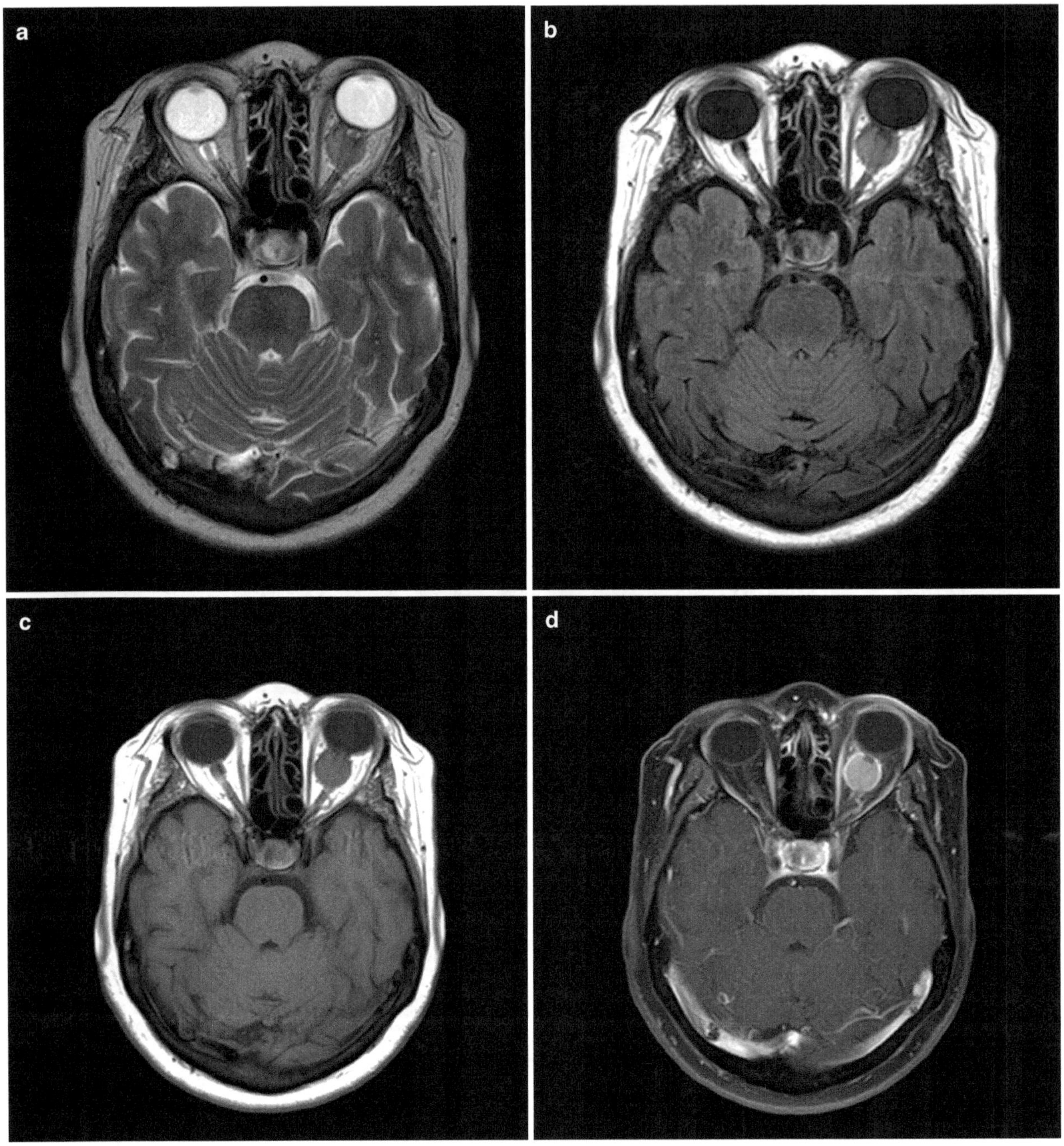

Fig. 3.9 Meningioma of the left optical nerve sheath. T2- (**a**), T2-FLAIR- (**b**), and T1- (**c**) weighted MR images demonstrate an isointense with white brain matter mass which wraps the optical nerve. The optic nerve can be visualized inside the tumor tissue. Enhanced axial T1-FatSat -weighted MR image shows marked enhancement of tumor (**d**). Postenhanced CT scans in axial plane (**e**) and with using coronal (**f**) reformation demonstrate enhanced "clutch-like" tumor of the left optic nerve. CT-perfusion CBF (**g**), CBV (**h**), and permeability (**i**) maps demonstrate significant elevation of these parameters within the tumor

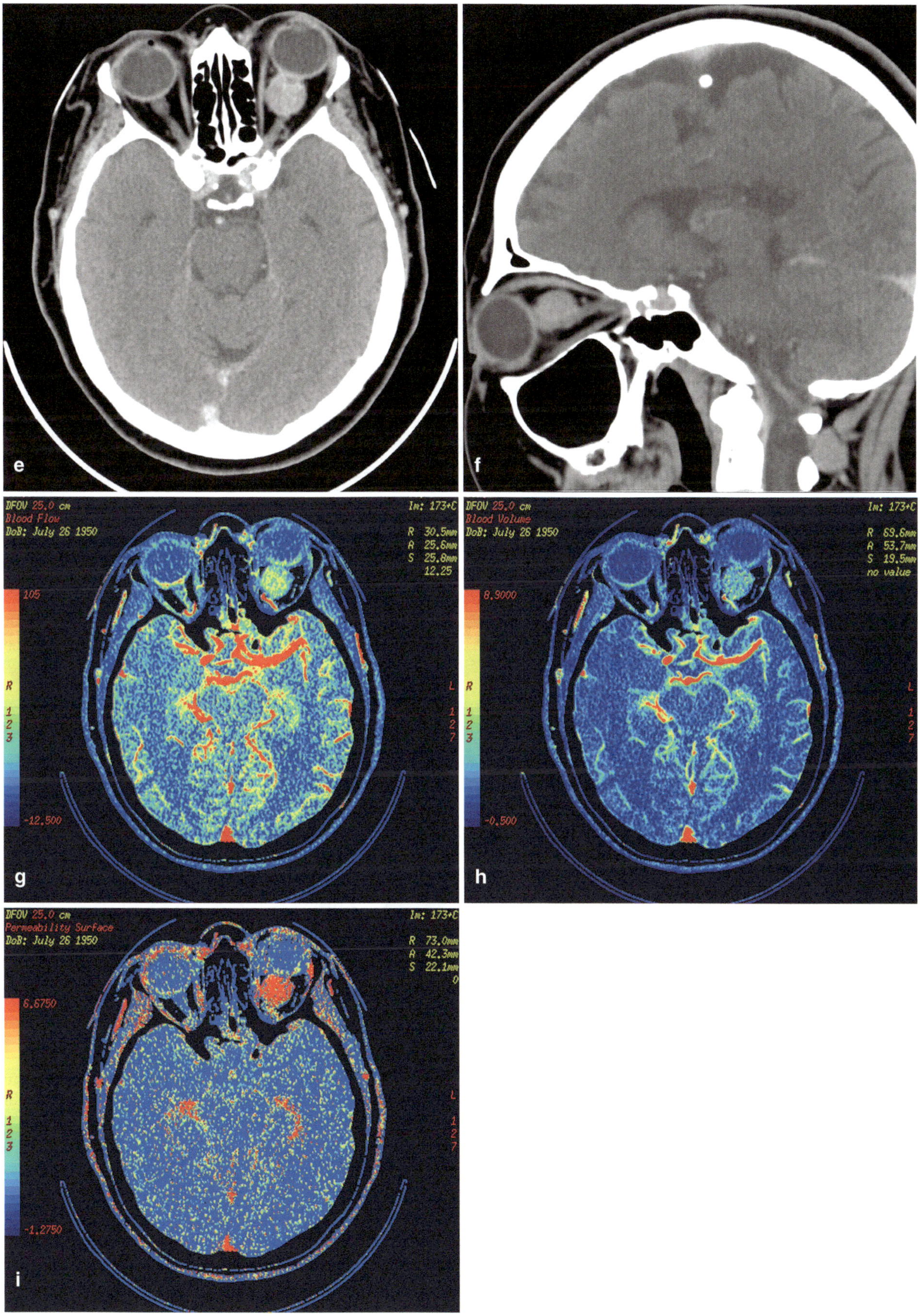

Fig. 3.9 (continued)

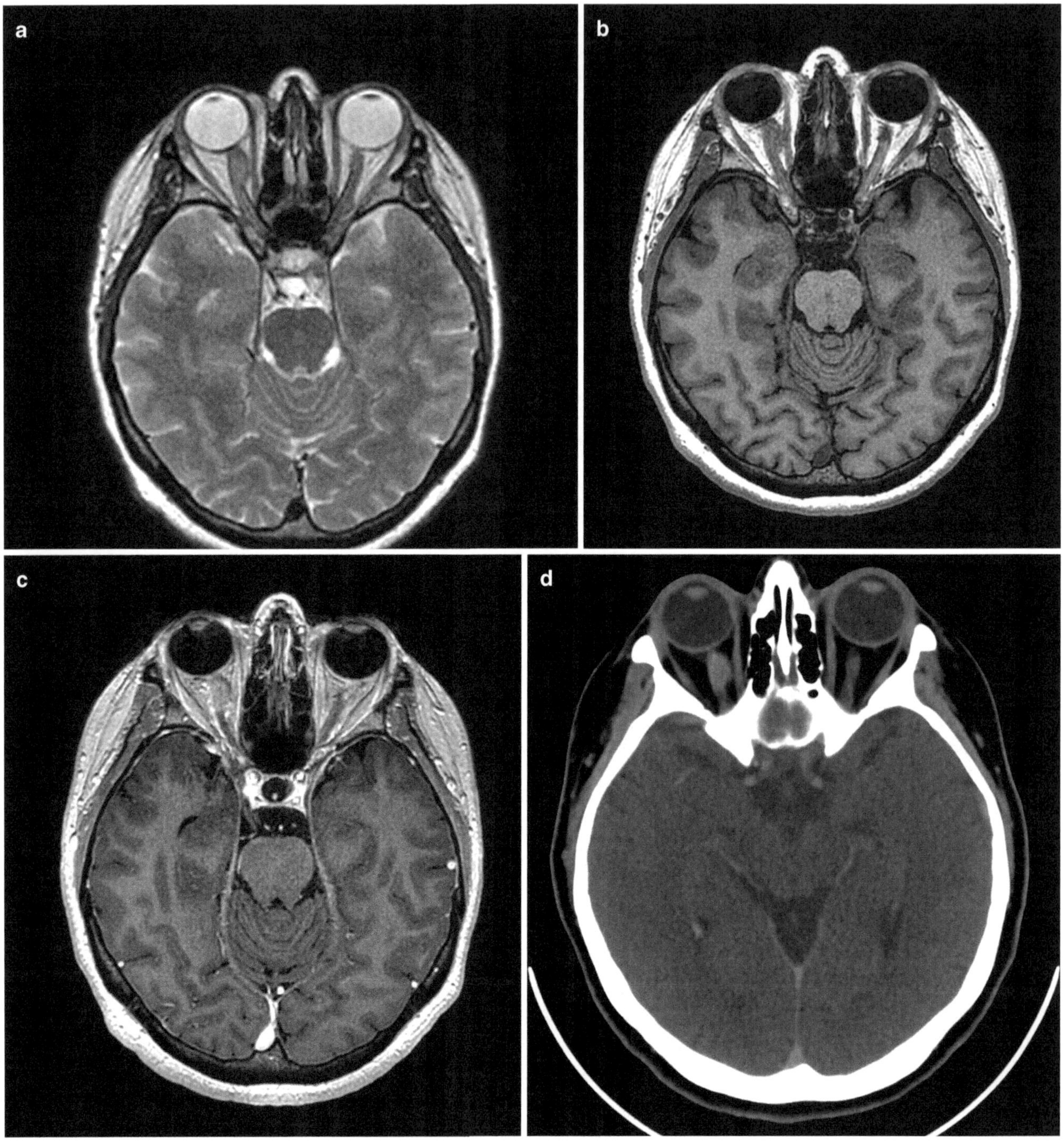

Fig. 3.10 Meningioma of the right optical nerve sheath. T2- (**a**), T1-before (**b**), and T1- after (**c**) contrast enhancement MR images demonstrate a small isointense with optic nerve mass which shows the marked enhancement and wraps the retrobulbar part of the optical nerve. Postenhanced CT scans in axial plane (**d**, **e**) and with using sagittal (**f**) reformation demonstrate marked enhancement of tumor. CT-perfusion CBF (**g**), CBV (**h**), and permeability (**i**) maps demonstrate significant elevation of these parameters within the tumor

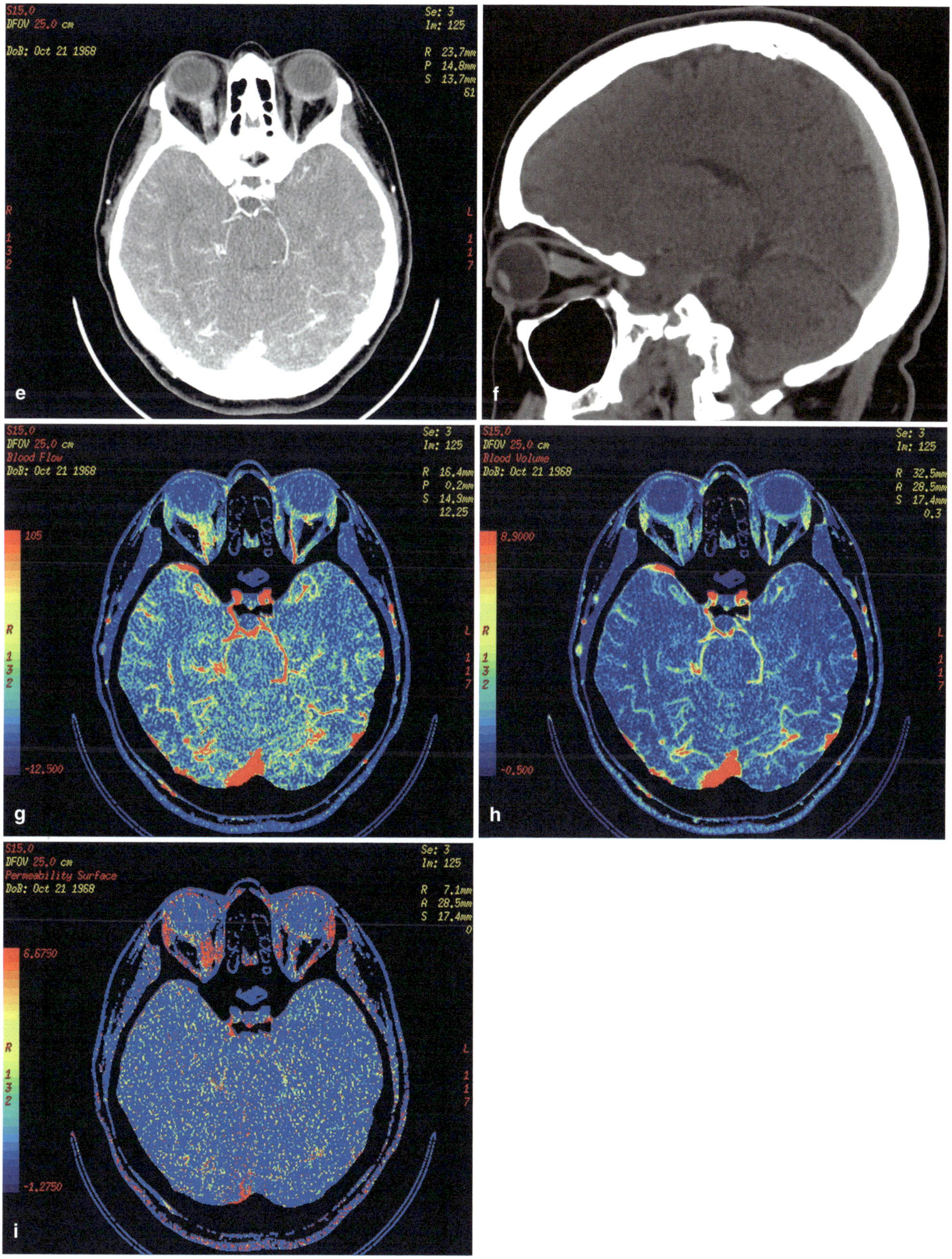

Fig. 3.10 (continued)

3.2 Inflammatory Diseases

Optic Neuritis Optic neuritis may be caused by multiple sclerosis, infection of the orbit, ischemia, meningitis. It is more common in young patients, with women being affected twice as often as men. Unilateral lesion occurs in 70%, the involvement of the anterior third of the optic nerve, middle part, intracranial part, and prechiasmal area occurs in 45%, 60%, 35%, and 7%, respectively. 50–60% of patients who suffered from optic neuritis may develop MS. In 15–20% of patients with MS, the disease starts with optic neuritis (Sorensen et al. 1999).

Clinical Manifestations Acute unilateral or bilateral loss of central visual acuity associated with central scotoma. Loss of contrast sensitivity and color vision, papillary defect often accompanied by pain in the postorbital region or during eye movements.

Diagnosis CT signs: the optic nerve is normal or slightly increased in diameter, can be poorly enhanced, mainly segmentally (in most cases not obviously). There are no signs of orbital destruction. Currently, CT is not used as a method of primary diagnosis.

On MRI, a marked thickening of the optic nerve can often be observed on T1-weighted images, as well as an increased MR signal on T2-weighted and T2-FLAIR images in most patients. Eighty one percent of patients have focal contrast enhancement that may be visualized both in the acute stage and in persistent disease. In order to visualize optic neuritis, thin coronary sections perpendicular to the optic nerve are used. It is recommended to use T1-weighted imaging with contrast enhancement and T2-weighted imaging with fat suppression technique, as well as STIR sequence due to the possibility of diminishing chemical shift artifacts and fat suppression (Harnsberger et al. 2004a, b). Using STIR with long TE is preferable because of the greater sensitivity in visualization of the optic nerve. Similar to their manifestations in the brain, demyelination lesions of the optic nerve and optic chiasm in MS are hyperintense on T2-STIR images. On diffusion-weighted MR images, the optic nerve lesions show the diffusion restriction. The combination of focal optic nerve lesions and the presence of lesions on T2-weighted images in the brain enhance the likelihood of a definite diagnosis of MS, in particular in young patients with primary complaints on a decrease in visual functions (Fig. 3.11). High-field MRI is more sensitive to detection of optic nerve lesion in patients with clinical manifestations of neuritis.

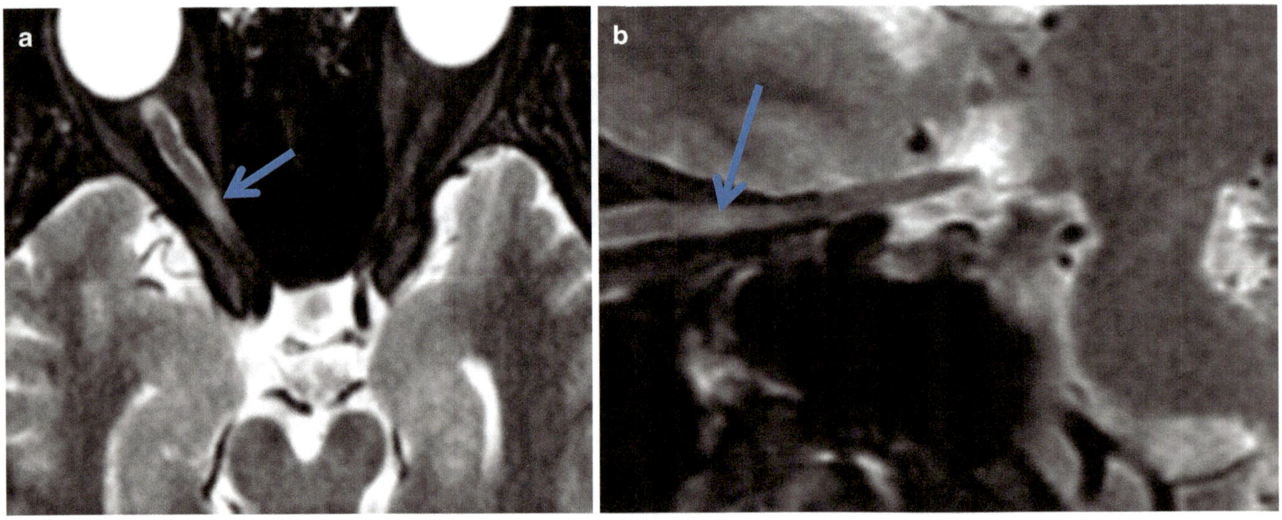

Fig. 3.11 Optical neuritis. Axial (**a**), sagittal (**b**), and coronal (**c**) T2-weighted MR images with Fat-Sat technology demonstrate a focal hyperintense lesion without sharp margins, which is located in the projection of the middle third of the right optic nerve (*arrow*)

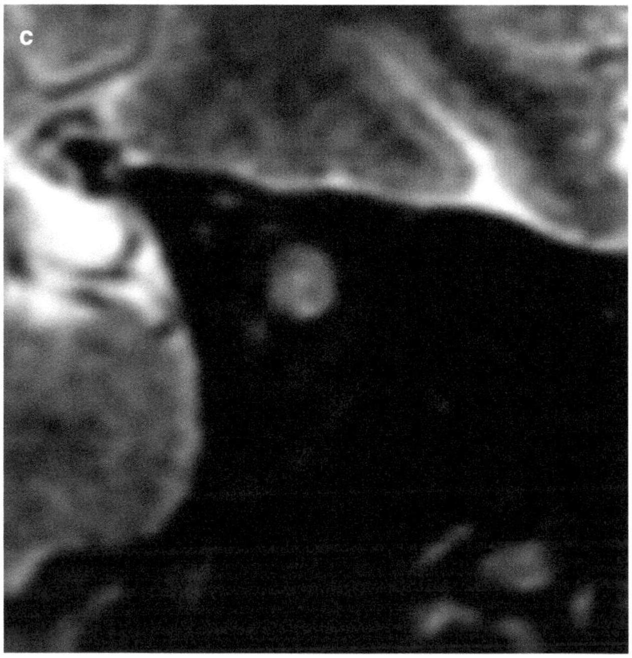

Fig. 3.11 (continued)

In typical cases with acute optic neuritis lesion can be enhanced after gadolinium-based contrast agent administration. In attempt to obtain better visualization of pathologic enhancement within involved optic nerve the increase of contrast agent dose can be recommended. Some authors believe that a triple dose of the contrast agent is most effective in 96% of cases of acute optic neuritis. Such contrast enhancement regimen revealed focal enhancement, as well as enhancement in the central part of the optic nerve in more than 90% of cases, which is most typical for this disease (Fig. 3.12).

Differential Diagnosis Ischemic neuropathy, infectious neuropathy, pseudotumor, optic nerve sheath meningioma, optic nerve glioma.

3.3 Intracranial Hypertension

Dilatation of the optic nerve subarachnoid space is a sign of intracranial hypertension. Modern literature emphasizes that pathogenesis of the optic disc edema and sheath dilatation is not completely clear. The frequency of these disorders in various brain diseases varies from 40% to 80% (Rohr et al. 2011). Severity of visual impairment varies from initial defects of visual fields to blindness. Processes that most often lead to an increased intracranial pressure include tumors, abscesses, arteriovenous malformations, hemorrhages, CSF circulation disorders, thromboses of sinuses and veins of the brain, congenital skull thickening and deformities. In addition, unexplained intracranial hypertension is detectable by MRI and CT. In order to diagnose intracranial hypertension, a direct measurement of cerebrospinal fluid pressure is required; however, since the method is invasive, its use is not always justified.

Clinical Manifestations Headache, nausea, vomiting, transient decrease in visual acuity, blurred vision mostly in the mornings, always bilateral.

Diagnosis CT and MRI studies of the optic nerves in intracranial hypertension are uncommon. MR-signal from the optic nerve is usually homogeneous, the nerve may look twisted with dilation of the subarachnoid space of the optic nerve throughout its length. Thus, an average diameter of the perineural space measured using MRI directly behind the eyeball is normally 5.52+/1.11 mm, while in case of a dilated sheath, it is 7.54+/1.05 mm. Marked flattening of the posterior sclera, the optic disc protrusion into the vitreous body are observed (Fig. 3.13). The optic disc protrusion is noted in 33% of patients with intracranial hypertension, swelling of the optic nerve and its thickening is found in 14% of cases and their combination occurs in 6% of cases (Rohr et al. 2011). Papilledema is always bilateral. Dilatation (up to 2.6 mm) of the superior ophthalmic vein is also noted (Donnet et al. 2008). The above signs do not necessarily subside following a decrease in the intracranial pressure, although it is described in literature as a pathognomonic sign of the effectiveness of treatment.

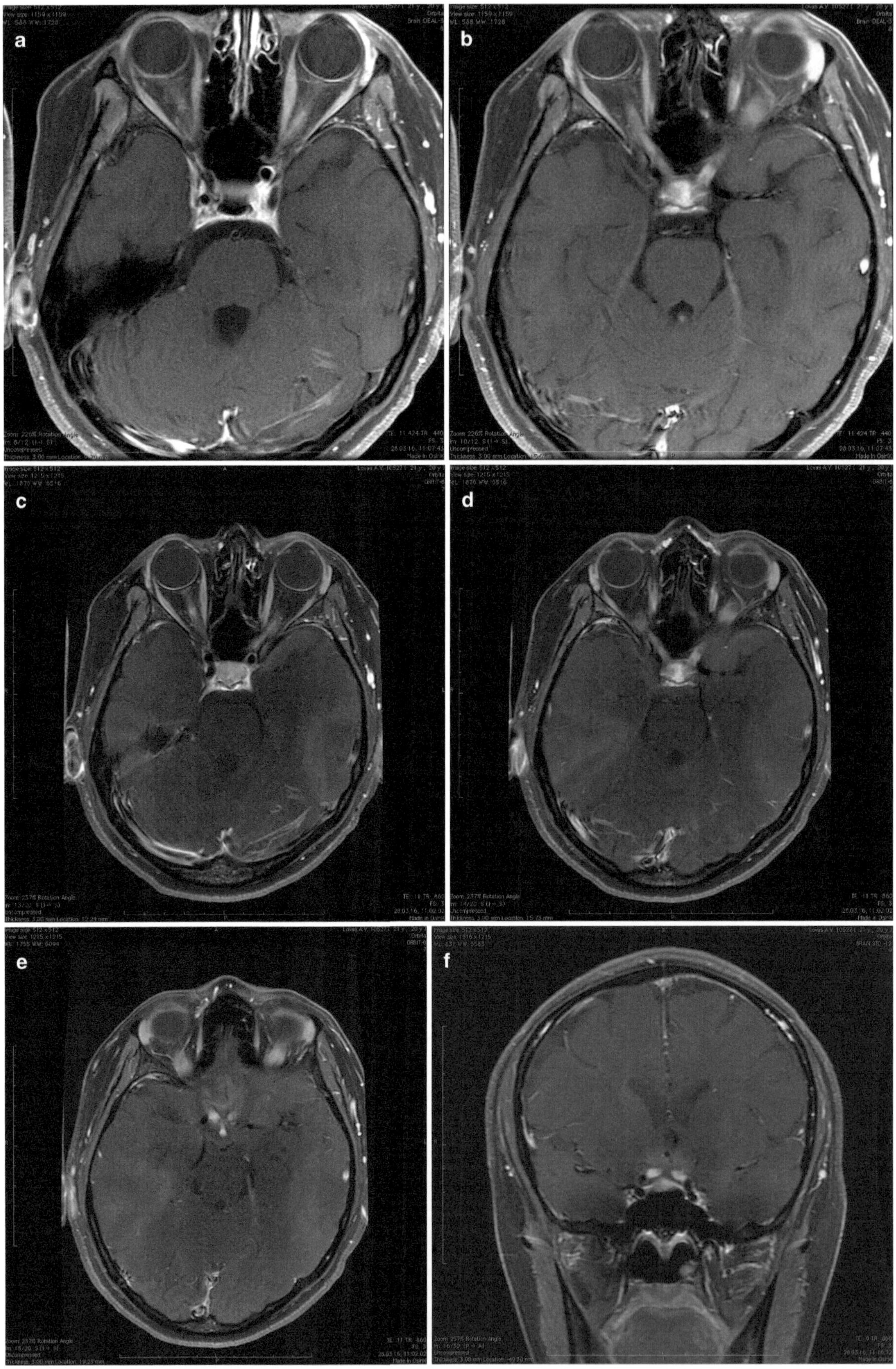

Fig. 3.12 Optical neuritis. Axial enhanced T1-weighted MR images with Fat-Sat technology (**a**–**e**) demonstrate a diffuse both sides lesion, which involves both optic nerves and chiasm. Both sides involvement is clearly depicted on coronal enhanced T1-weighted image (**f**). NMO IgG were seronegative in this case

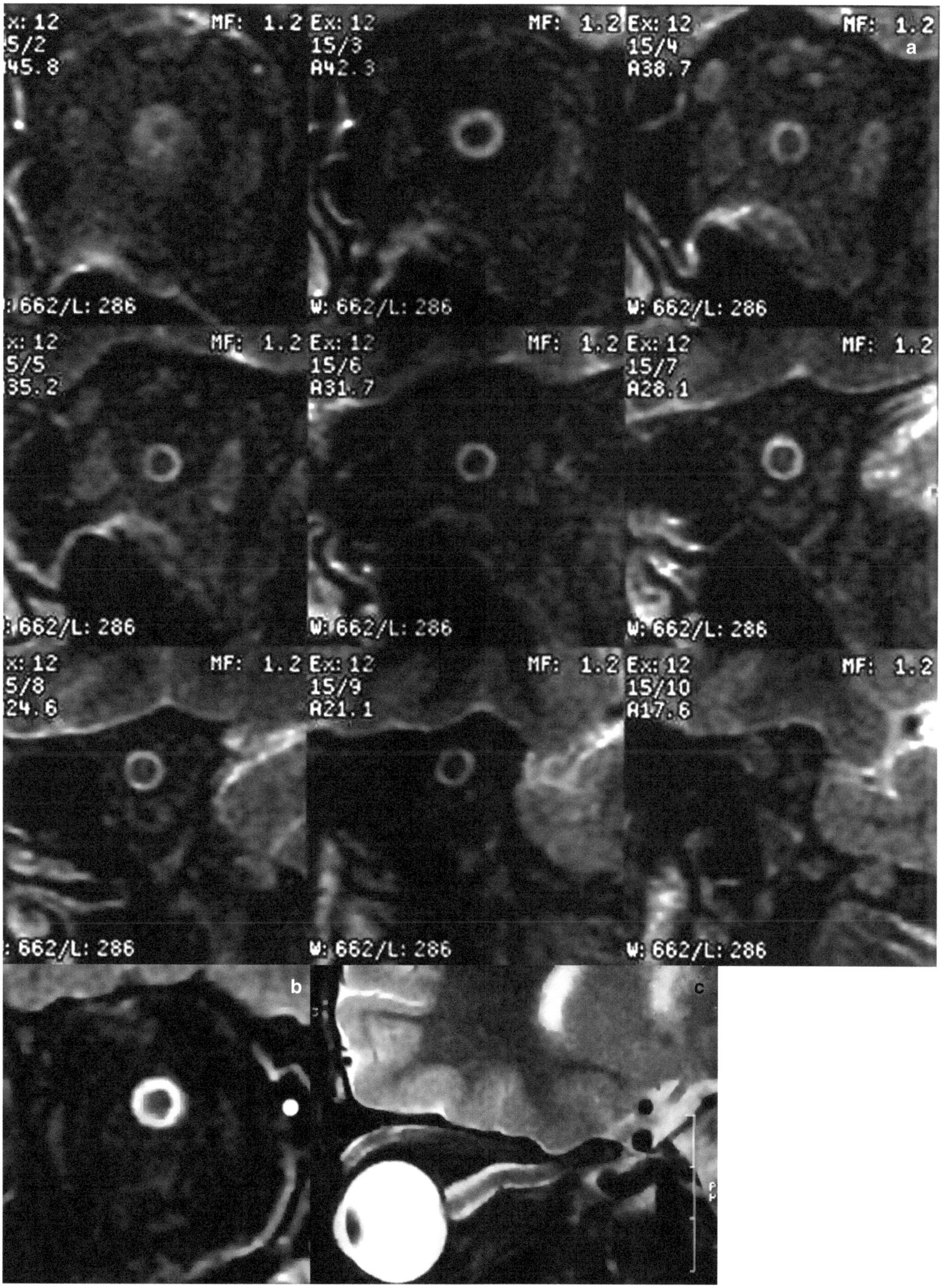

Fig. 3.13 Dilatation of optical nerve sheath in patient with intracranial hypertension due to intracranial tumor. Series T2-weighted MR images in coronal (**a**, **b**–zoom) and sagittal (**c**) projections demonstrate significant dilatation of perineural spaces around optical nerve

Muscle Cone Lesions

4

Contents

4.1 Endocrine Pathology

Thyroid ophthalmopathy (Grave's disease) is one of the most frequent reasons of orbital pathology, which develops in association with thyroid dysfunction. Autoimmune thyroid disease with its hyperfunction is called Basedow's disease in continental Europe, while it is called Grave's disease in English-speaking countries (Brovkina 2004).

The disease usually affects adults of young and middle age, most often aged 30–50 years, it is extremely rare in children, more common in women than men (4:1). Bilateral lesions are found in 90% of cases even if there are clinical signs of unilateral localization. Symmetrical changes are observed in 70%. Among patients with thyroid ophthalmopathy, 35–50% have orbital involvement with clinical manifestations (Kendler and Ozerova 1993). CT signs of the disease are detected in 70–90% of cases of this pathology (Lieb et al. 2010).

Clinical Manifestations Patients have exophthalmos, myopathy, retraction of the upper eyelid and diplopia, which are initially transient, later becoming permanent. Strabismus develops, usually downwards and inwards; limited mobility of the eye.

Diagnosis In case of typical clinical manifestations, CT is sufficient for diagnosis. The use of multislice spiral CT scanners with the ability of sagittal and frontal reformation is preferred. CT visualizes the extraocular muscles and the optic nerve in detail. An isodense thickening of the extraocular muscles with areas of decreased density is observed before using contrast enhancement. There can also be observed an enlargement in the orbital fat volume, which can compress the optic nerve. After contrast enhancement an abnormal increase in CT density of the affected muscles is

I. Pronin, V. Kornienko, *CT and MRI of Skull Base Lesions*, https://doi.org/10.1007/978-3-319-65957-2_4

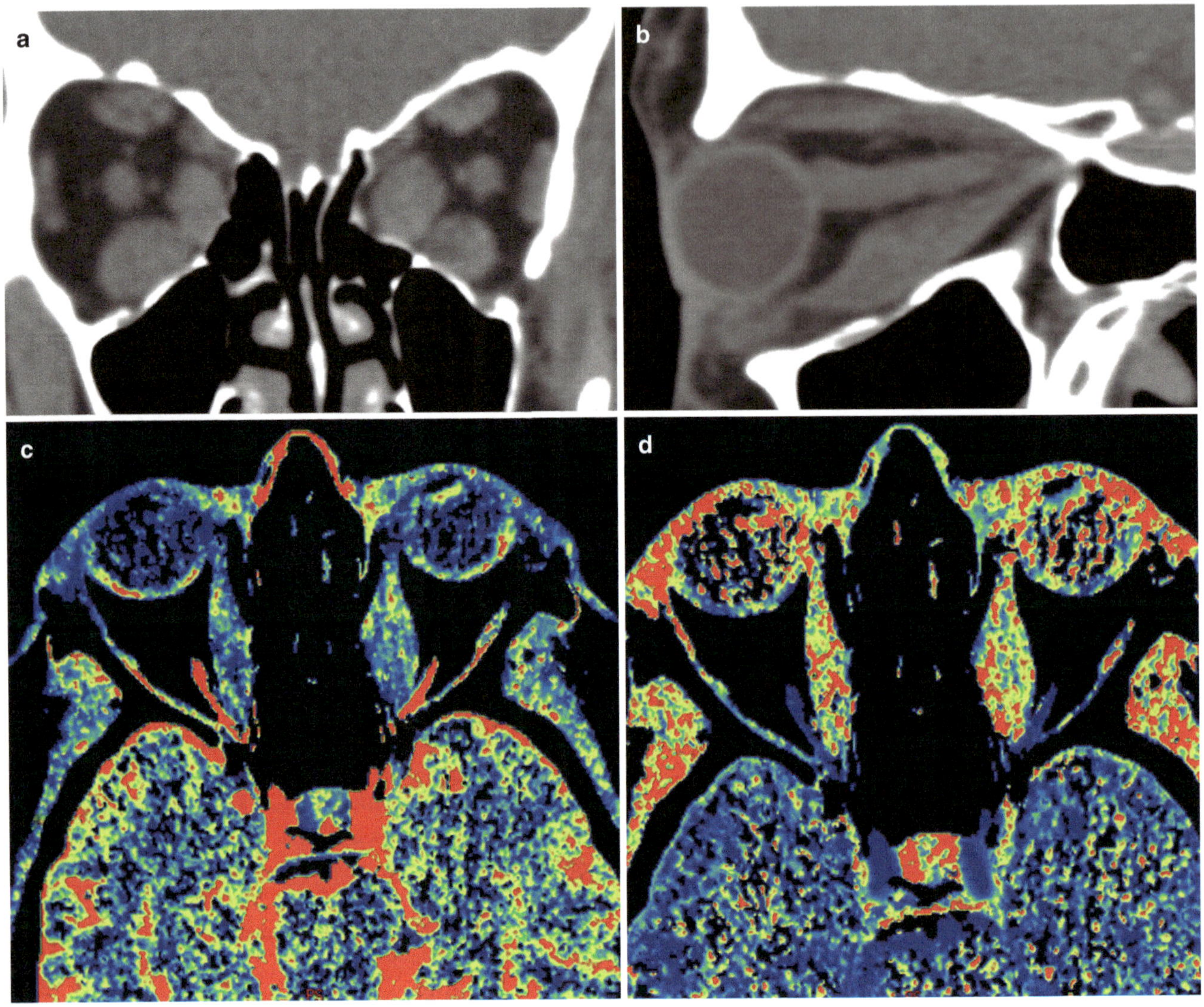

Fig. 4.1 Grave's ophthalmopathy. CT reformats in coronal (**a**) and (**b**) sagittal projections show bilateral asymmetric enlargement of medial and inferior rectus muscles. They have isodense density comparing to healthy muscles. On CT-perfusion CBF (**c**) and MTT (**d**) maps the moderate elevation of blood flow and prolongation in mean transit time is revealed

noted. CT-perfusion reveals the absence of XCBV and CBF elevation within muscular tissue with prolongation of mean transit time values (Fig. 4.1).

On MRI, T1-weighted sequences also revealed an increase in volume of the extraocular muscles with an isointense MR-signal. On T2-weighted images, edema (acute phase) of the affected rectus muscles with a diffuse hyperintensity of MR- signal can be observed, with a decreased signal in case of fibrosis (chronic phase). Changes in rectus muscles appearance on T2-STIR sequence can help in assessment of the disease activity, with an increased signal from the muscles being noted in the acute phase. Endocrine ophthalmopathy is characterized by prominent accumulation of the contrast material within involved muscles.

Coronal and axial MR-slices are needed in order to assess the muscle sizes and their location relative to the intraorbital structures. MRI is also more informative in differentiating acute edema and muscle fibrosis than CT scanning.

Differential Diagnosis Pseudotumor, infectious cellulitis/myositis, sarcoidosis, lymphoproliferative disease (most often non-Hodgkin's lymphoma), metastases.

4.2 Inflammatory Diseases of the Orbit

Cellulitis, Abscess, Cavernous Sinus Thrombosis Infectious diseases of the orbit usually have bacterial origin, however, viral and parasitic origin is also known (Kapur et al. 2009).

Nearly two-thirds of bacterial infections are caused by sinusitis, acute respiratory infections, traumatic injuries of orbital bone walls or postoperative infections. Spreading of inflammation from adjacent areas is possible in diseases of eyelids and lacrimal glands or in case of hematogenous transmission of infection in various purulent processes in the body (Tarasova and Drozdova 2005). Purulent process may also spread from the infratemporal and pterygopalatine fossae directly through the inferior orbital fissure or via venous anastomoses caused by vein thrombophlebitis of the pterygopalatine plexus.

The most common bacteria are *Staphylococcus, Streptococcus, Pneumococcus,* and *Pseudomonas*. Herpes simplex, herpes zoster, and cytomegalovirus are the main viral infections affecting the eye and the orbit. In immunocompromised and diabetes patients, fungal opportunistic infections may cause various sinonasal lesions of the orbit (Henderson 1994).

Bacterial infections of the orbit can be divided into five categories: preseptal cellulitis, orbital (postseptal) cellulitis, subperiosteal abscess, orbital abscess, and cavernous sinus thrombosis (Uehara and Ohba 2002). Preseptal cellulitis affects only the eyelid tissues located anteriorly to the orbital septum, without involvement of the orbital structure. Vision and pupillary reactions are not affected in this form of cellulitis. However, worsening of clinical symptoms in the form of exophthalmos, restriction of the eyeball mobility, chemosis, disorders of visual acuity indicate spreading of the inflammatory process into the orbital cavity. This type of orbital lesions (or postseptal cellulitis) is extremely dangerous, especially if fungal etiology is considered the most likely. Intracranial involvement is often detected with the development of the cavernous sinus thrombosis and even meningoencephalitis. Orbital abscess is a late stage of postseptal cellulitis, characterized by soft tissue infiltration along the orbital wall with dislocation of peripheral adipose tissue (Eustis et al. 1998).

Most cases of postseptal cellulitis are extraconal, most abscesses also have extraconal and subperiosteal localization. Infection can also spread via the venous blood flow in patients with lesions of the skin or sinuses. Orbital abscess is often a consequence of cellulitis or a traumatic injury of one of its walls. A subperiosteal abscess is localized between the periosteum and the orbital wall, while an orbital abscess is localized in the retrobulbar tissue.

Clinical Manifestations Orbital abscess is manifested by acute pulsating pain in the eye and general symptoms of inflammation (weakness, fever, nausea, vomiting). Local symptoms include swelling of the soft orbital tissues, exophthalmos, conjunctival edema, restriction of the eyeball mobility or complete ophthalmoplegia and displacement of the eyeball. These symptoms are caused by an acute increase in the intraorbital pressure (Harris 1999). There are no signs of venous stasis, papilledema in the fundus. In some cases, the process may involve the optic nerve and ciliary ganglion, which is accompanied by amblyopia or amaurosis, signs of neuroparalytic keratitis.

Although there is a significant response to conservative treatment in some cases, most patients need surgery to prevent deterioration and loss of vision.

Diagnosis The easiest and most affordable way to establish the correct diagnosis is spiral CT. Contrast-enhanced spiral CT scanning reveals a clearly defined focus, sometimes dislocating the corresponding rectus muscle, the lesion often has a characteristic capsule and there is marked concurrent edema of orbital tissues. Differentiation with subperiosteal hematoma, especially in case of chronic sinusitis, may be difficult (Griffeth et al. 1997).

A subperiosteal abscess is characterized by medium signal intensity on T1-weighted and proton MR images and hyperintense on T2-weighted images, with ring-shaped enhancement of the capsule after contrast agent administration. DW-MRI is also highly informative. Due to high viscosity of inflammatory detritus, abscesses have a high signal on DWI, characterized by a low diffusion rate, which allows for highly reliable differentiation from malignant gliomas that have similar signal characteristics in routine MRI and ring-shaped enhancement similar to that of abscesses (ring-like shape). In addition, the same characteristics of abscess visualization on DW-MRI allow differentiating it from other pathological processes with ring-shaped enhancement (fungal and parasitic diseases). Serious complications of orbital abscesses with mortality of approximately 21% are epidural or subdural abscesses, purulent meningitis, and cavernous sinus thrombosis (Fig. 4.2).

True orbital abscesses secondary to paranasal sinusitis or dental infection are extremely rare with timely treatment with antibiotics (Eustis et al. 1998).

Fungal orbital infections most frequently caused by Mucormycosis and Aspergillus are less common than bacterial infections. They are frequently found in patients with uncontrolled diabetes mellitus and in immunocompromised patients. The primary role of high-tech neuroimaging (CT and MRI) is to establish the relationship between the sinuses, orbit, and intracranial lesions (Eustis et al. 1998). On CT, nonspecific sinus mucosal thickening with bone erosion is observed in mucormycosis infection, which is not always distinguishable from sinusitis caused by Aspergillus. MR images demonstrate a hypointense T2-weighted signal from the source of fungal infection, with the presence of calcifications in the cavity of the sinuses on CT (Eustis et al. 1998).

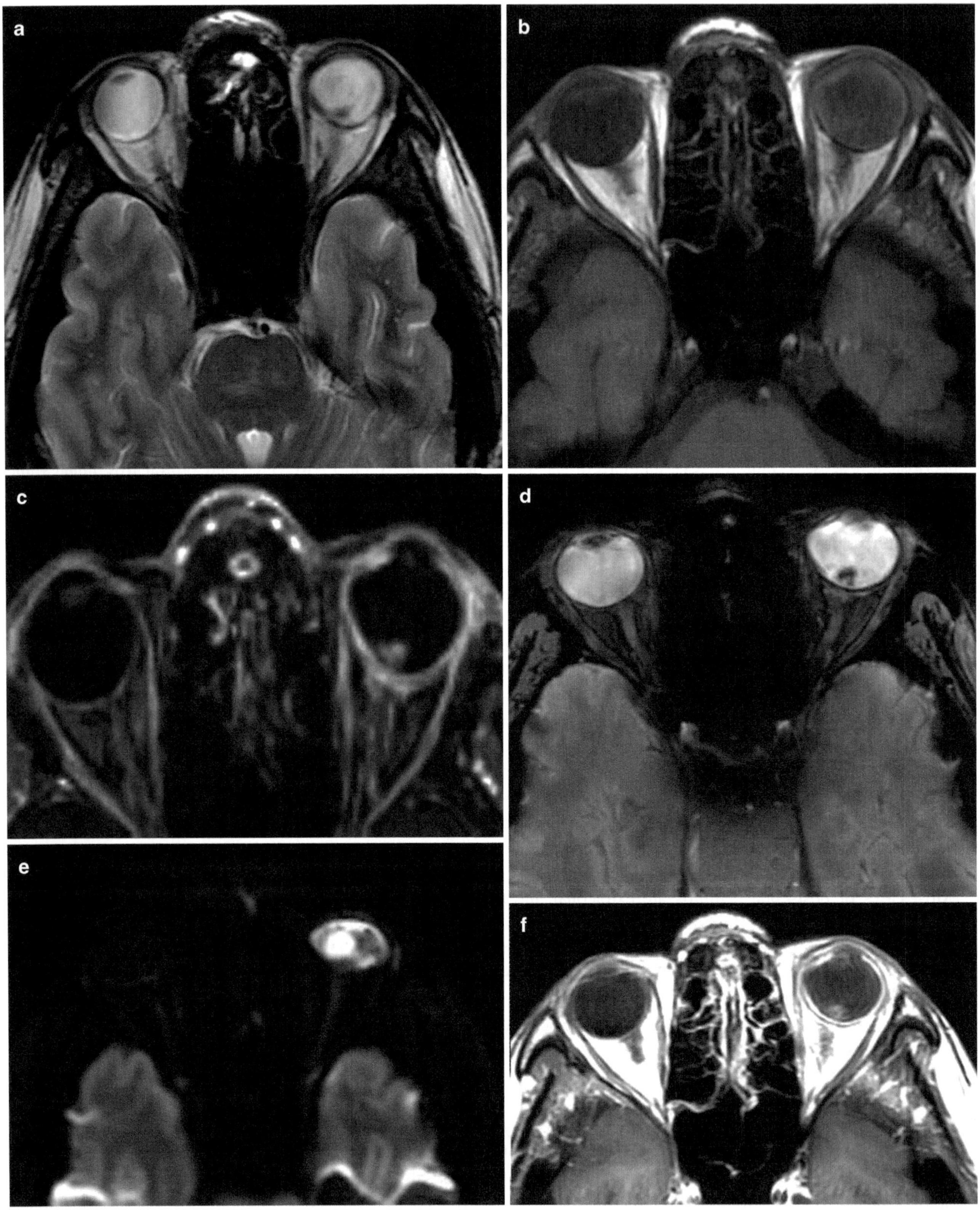

Fig. 4.2 Abscess of eyeball leftwards. Axial T2 (**a**)-, T2-FLAIR (**b**)-, and T1 (**c**) –weighted MRI reveal small lesion located inside left eyeball and attached to the internal surface. The lesion has hypointense signal on T2-WI MRI and SWAN (**d**). Diffusion MRI (**e**) shows an intraocular lesion with hyperintense MR-signal, which is typical for pus (surgically proved). T1-WI MRI with contrast enhancement (**f**) demonstrates local region, which slightly accumulates contrast medium. There is an intensive contrast enhancement of the choroid

4.3 Tumors

Cancer of the Orbit Among malignant orbital tumors, the most common are orbital sarcomas and lacrimal gland cancer, which constitute 13–16% of all tumors of the orbit. Primary orbital cancer also occurs. A tumor can be regarded as a result of transformation of dystopic epithelial cell during embryogenesis. The tumor grows without a capsule, has a stringy structure, and is dense and whitish. Primary orbital cancer is twice less likely to occur than sarcomas (Brovkina 2008). Sarcomas are located intra- and extraconally in 47% of cases. Most common types among sarcomas are rhabdomyosarcoma, fibrosarcoma, angiosarcoma, malignant fibrous histiocytoma, and others (Rao et al. 1999; Cunnane et al. 2011).

Clinical Picture Eyelid swelling, "bursting" sensation and pain, fast increasing exophthalmos, restriction of mobility and deformation of the eyeball, diplopia, optic nerve atrophy; regional and distant metastases.

Diagnosis Primary orbital cancer and sarcomas have unclear boundaries, irregular shape, bone destruction on CT. In general, sarcomas are isointense in relation to the muscles on T1-weighted MR images, while they are hypointense and rarely have a heterogeneous signal on T2-weighted images. The globe is often affected. Contrast enhancement is moderate, the recommended sequence being with fat suppression and contrast enhancement (Figs. 4.3, 4.4, and 4.5).

Differential Diagnosis Pseudotumor, abscess, neurofibromatosis, meningioma, lymphoma.

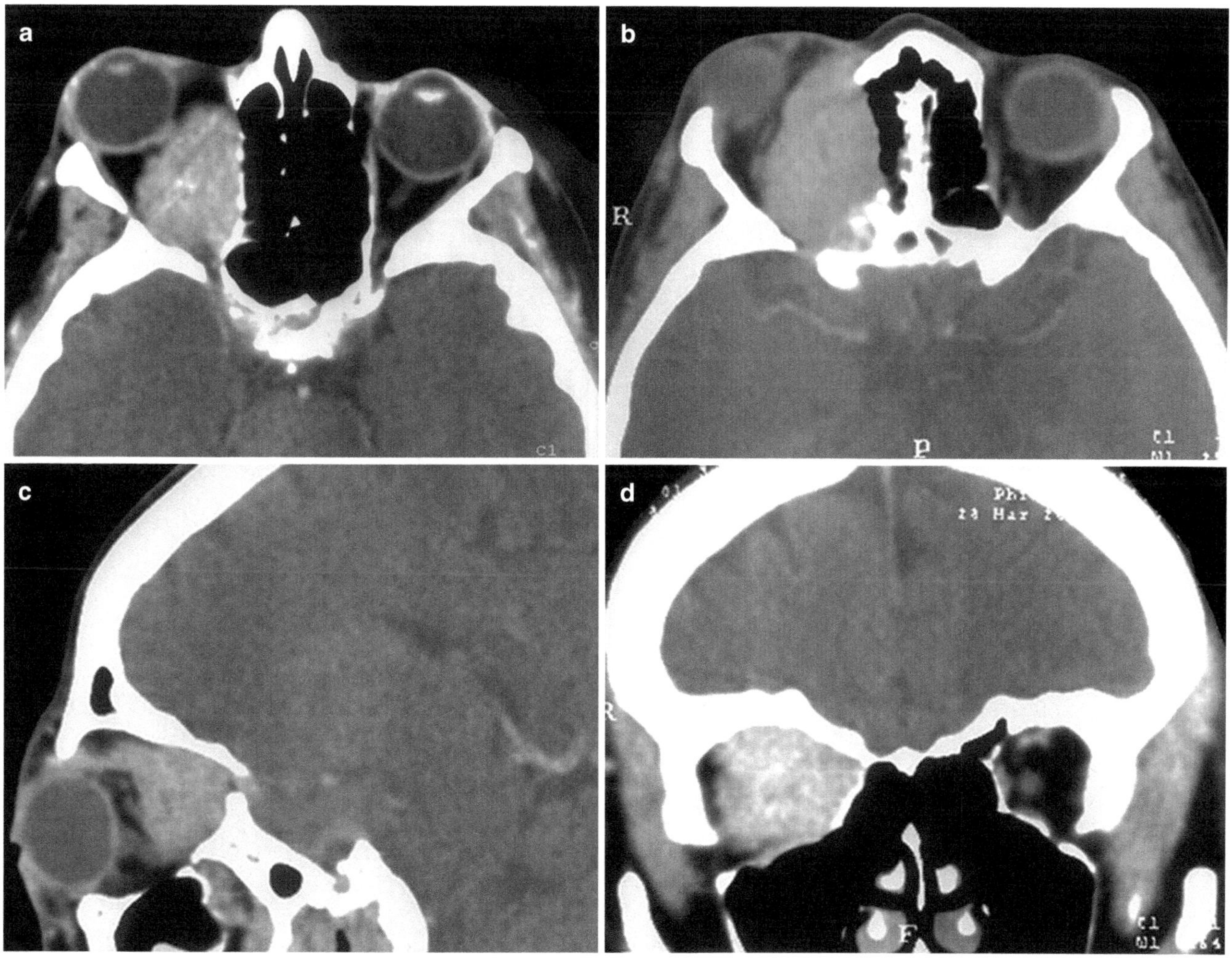

Fig. 4.3 Rhabdomyosarcoma. A large homogenous enhanced soft tissue tumor, which occupies retrobulbar space and produces the proptosis, is clearly visible on axial (**a**, **b**), sagittal (**c**), and coronal (**d**) CT scans after contrast enhancement. (**e**)–histological specimen

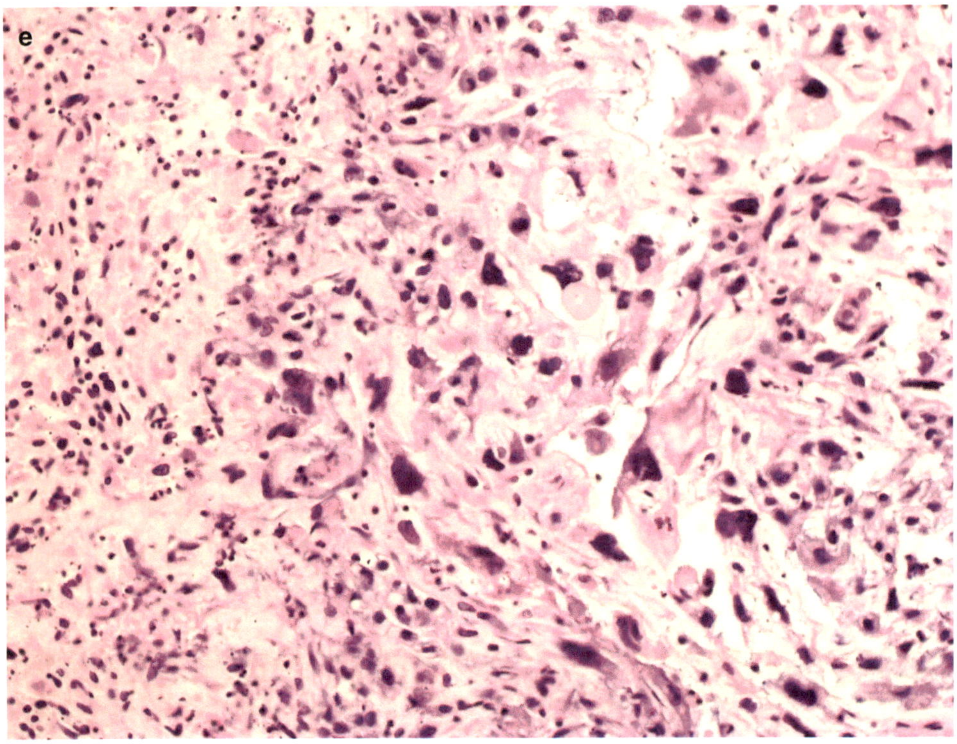

Fig. 4.3 (continued)

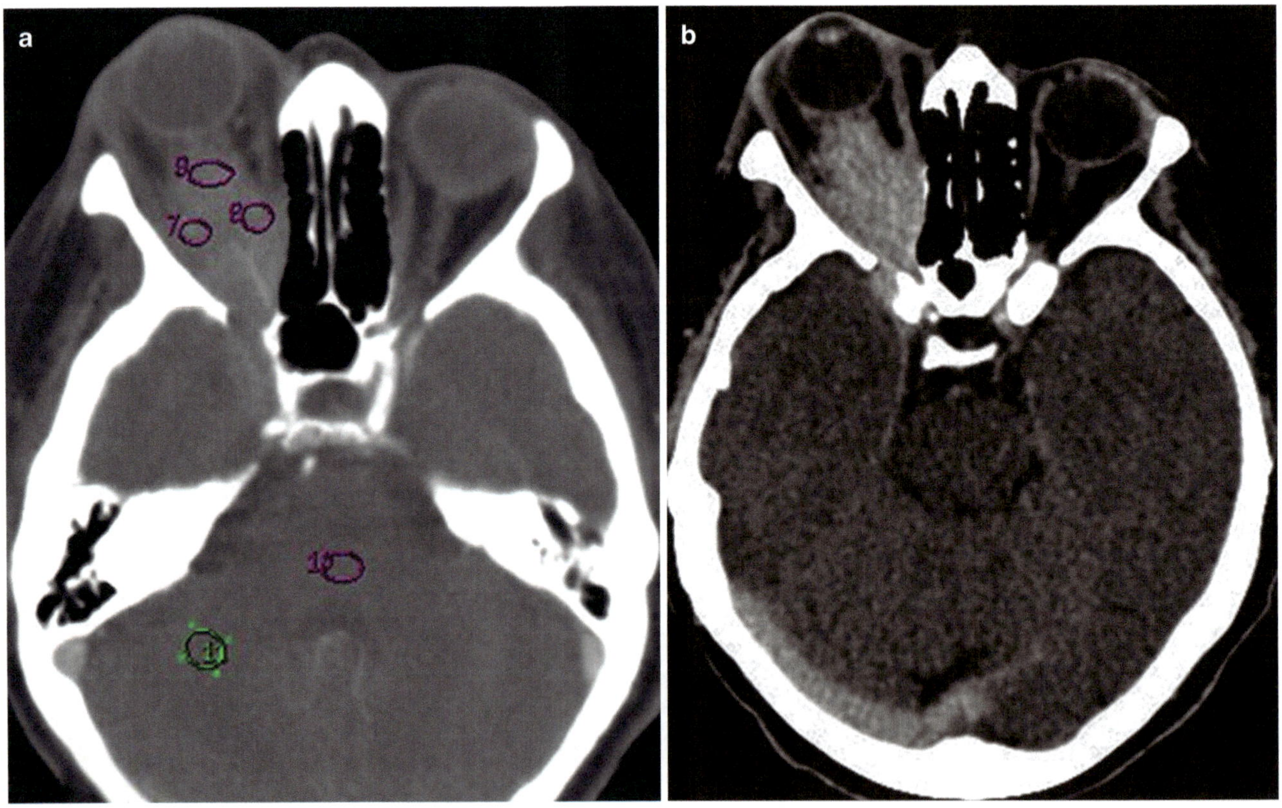

Fig. 4.4 Cancer of the right orbit. Post-contrast CT scans on the different levels (**a**–**c**) in axial projection demonstrate a large space occupied mass retroorbital location. The tumor demonstrates an intensive contrast enhancement and high values of perfusion parameters on CT- perfusion maps (CBF – **d**, CBV – **e**). There is prolongation of MTT in the tumor tissue (**f**)

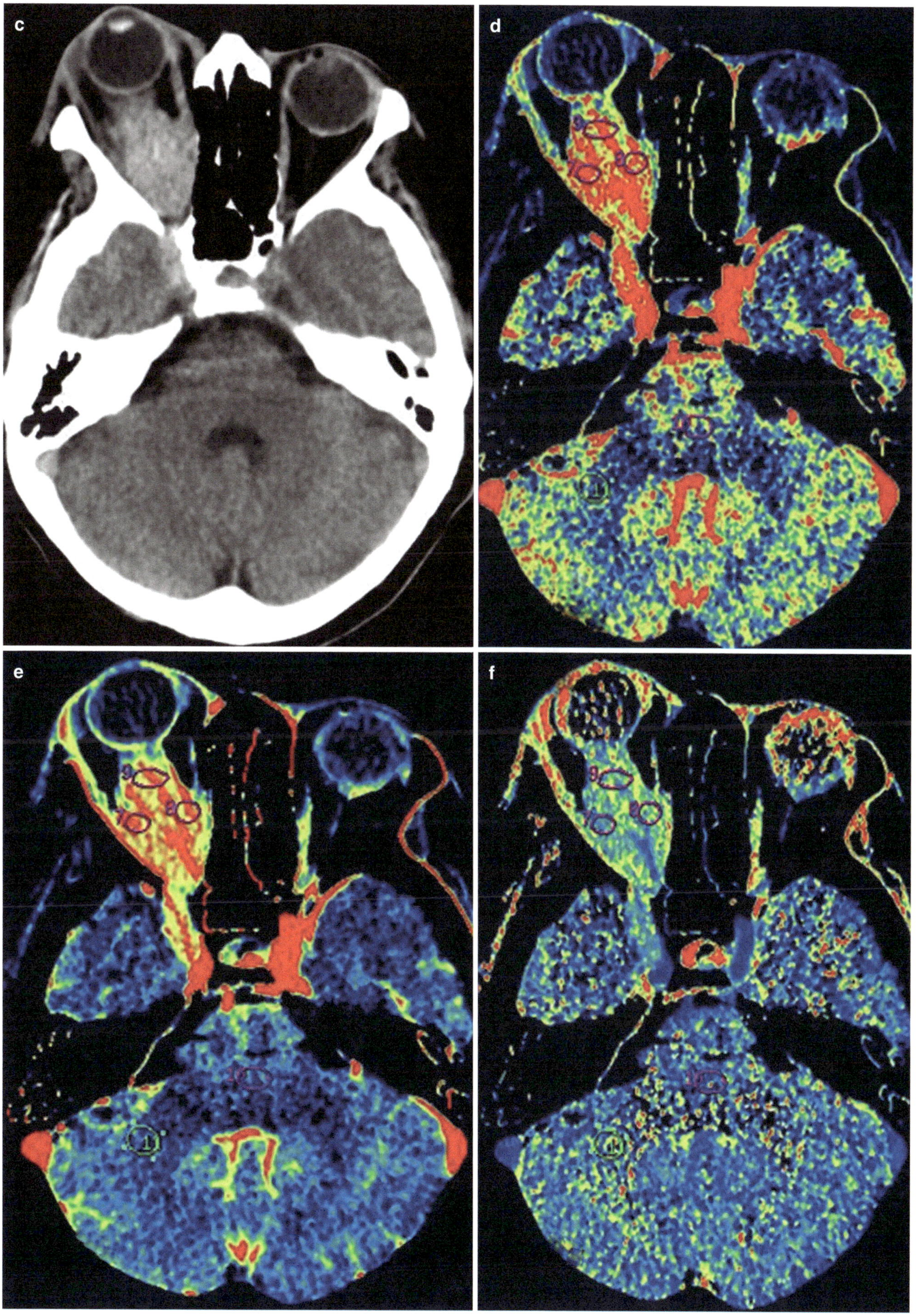

Fig. 4.4 (continued)

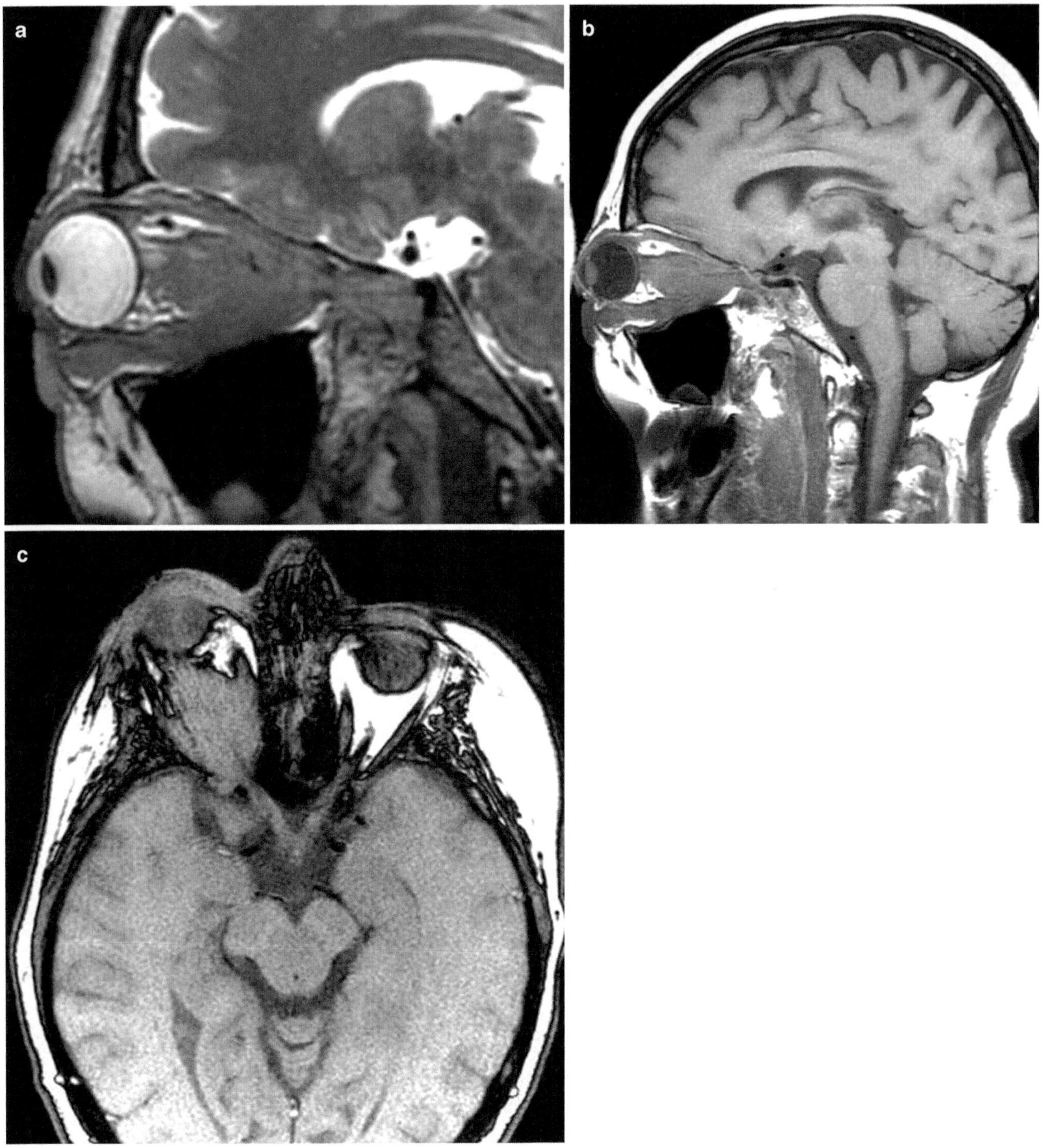

Fig. 4.5 Cancer of the right orbit. On sagittal T2-(**a**) and axial T1-weighted (**b, c**) MRI a large infitrative tumor, which envelops optical nerve and infiltrates the inferior rectus muscle of the right orbit is revealed. Tumor leads to prominent proptosis formation. The tumor has hypointense MR- signal on T2-weighted image

Lacrimal Fossa Lesions

5

Contents

Generally, 50% of the disorders affecting the lacrimal gland are inflammatory (acute or chronic), 25% of the lesions present lymphoma, and 25% of the lesions are primary lacrimal gland tumors (benign or malignant).

5.1 Tumors

adenocarcinoma, Wegener's granulomatosis, Sarcoidosis ACC is the second most common epithelial tumor of the lacrimal gland and the most common malignant epithelial tumor in this area, amounting to 50% of all malignant tumors and 25% of all tumors of the lacrimal gland (Henderson 1994). Lacrimal gland cancer occurs mainly at the age of 40–50 years. The average age is 45 years old, which is less than for other epithelial tumors. Its main morphological forms are adenoid cystic carcinoma (50–60%), malignant mixed tumor (34–48%), and adenocarcinoma (less than 20%).

The left eye orbit is affected almost twice as often as the right one.

Clinical Manifestations A rapid increase in symptoms is typical. As a rule, there is marked tenderness at the lesion area at palpation, pain with paresthesia occurs in 30–80%. Exophthalmos, ptosis, eyeball movement restriction are also noted.

Diagnosis The tumor is located outside the muscle cone, in the orbital portion of the lacrimal gland, sometimes grows into top of the orbit. These are isodense solid homogeneous masses without calcifications on CT. Lytic destruction is observed in the adjacent bone (unlike compression erosion), which is the only absolute sign that distinguishes a benign process from the malignant one. A sign atypical for ACC was noticed by Rootman (1988). The author believed that in young children invasive ACC manifestations are unobservable on CT due to the flexibility of bones in this age with followed expansion rather than invasion.

I. Pronin, V. Kornienko, *CT and MRI of Skull Base Lesions*, https://doi.org/10.1007/978-3-319-65957-2_5

On MRI, T1-weighted sequences reveal the tumor as solid homogeneous mass.

On T2-weighed images, ACCs have isointense characteristics, but occasionally they may be hypointense as well. After using intravenous contrast material administration diffuse contrast enhancement of the tumor is noted. The MR protocol must include T1-weighted imaging with contrast enhancement and fat suppression.

Adenocarcinoma differs from ACC by its histological characteristics, it affects more often men, rarely occurs in the orbit, metastasizes early compared to ACC. CT and MRI pictures of the tumor do not differ much (Fig. 5.1).

A short-term survival in these patients may be related to early tumor dissemination via the lymphatic system of the nasal cavity, paranasal sinuses, face, eyelids, and lacrimal glands.

Primary ACCs and adenocarcinomas have similar clinical and radiographic manifestations.

Differential Diagnosis Pseudotumor, Wegener's granulomatosis, sarcoidosis, myxoid adenoma, lymphoma, mucoepidermoid carcinoma.

Dermoid and epidermoid cysts belong to congenital lesions. These are slow-growing benign lesions. Histologically, a typical dermoid contains keratinized epithelium with inclusions of skin structures such as hair follicles and glandular cells. Epidermoid cysts contain only epithelial elements lying on the outer connective tissue layer. These are cystic, well-defined lesions including fat, fluid and myxoid components, usually adjacent to the periosteum, near bone sutures (Veselinovic et al. 2010). In most cases, they are localized extraconally in the superolateral portion of the orbit around frontomaxillary suture (65–75%). Their sizes are typically less than 1–2 cm. They are more common in children and adolescents with an average age of 15–20 years old. There is slight predominance in males.

Clinical Manifestations These are typically painful subcutaneous masses (85–90%). In 10–15% of cases, a cyst rupture occurs. Epidermoid cysts are characterized by slow growth, which takes years. In case of a rupture and inflammation, dramatic acceleration of its growth is observed.

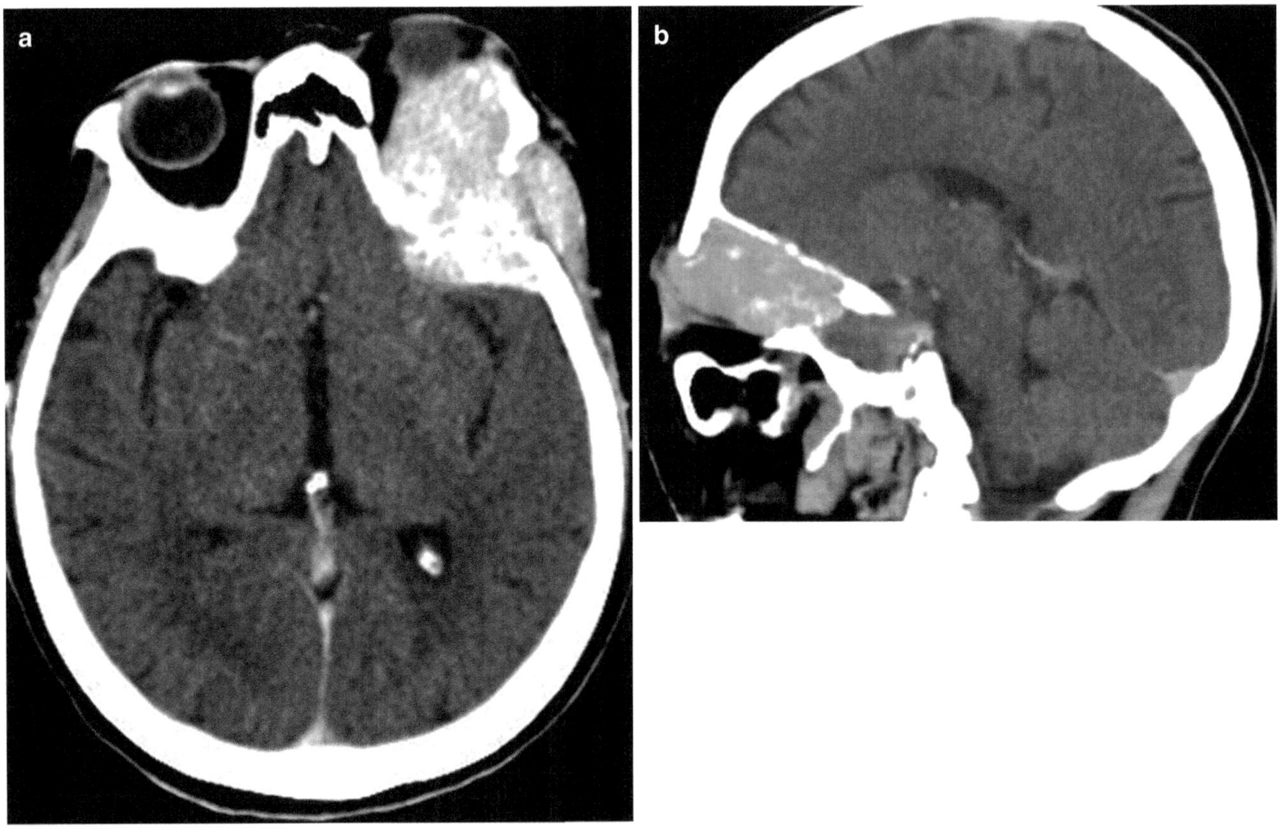

Fig. 5.1 Adenocarcinoma. CT scans in axial (**a**), sagittal (**b**), and coronal (**c**) planes with contrast enhancement demonstrate a large tumor in the left orbit, which spreads to supraorbital region and infratemporal fossa with intensive accumulation of contrast medium. Destruction of superior and lateral walls of the orbit is clearly visible. High values of CBF (**d**) and CBV (**e**) parameters are revealed on CT-perfusion. Transit time is shortened (**f**)

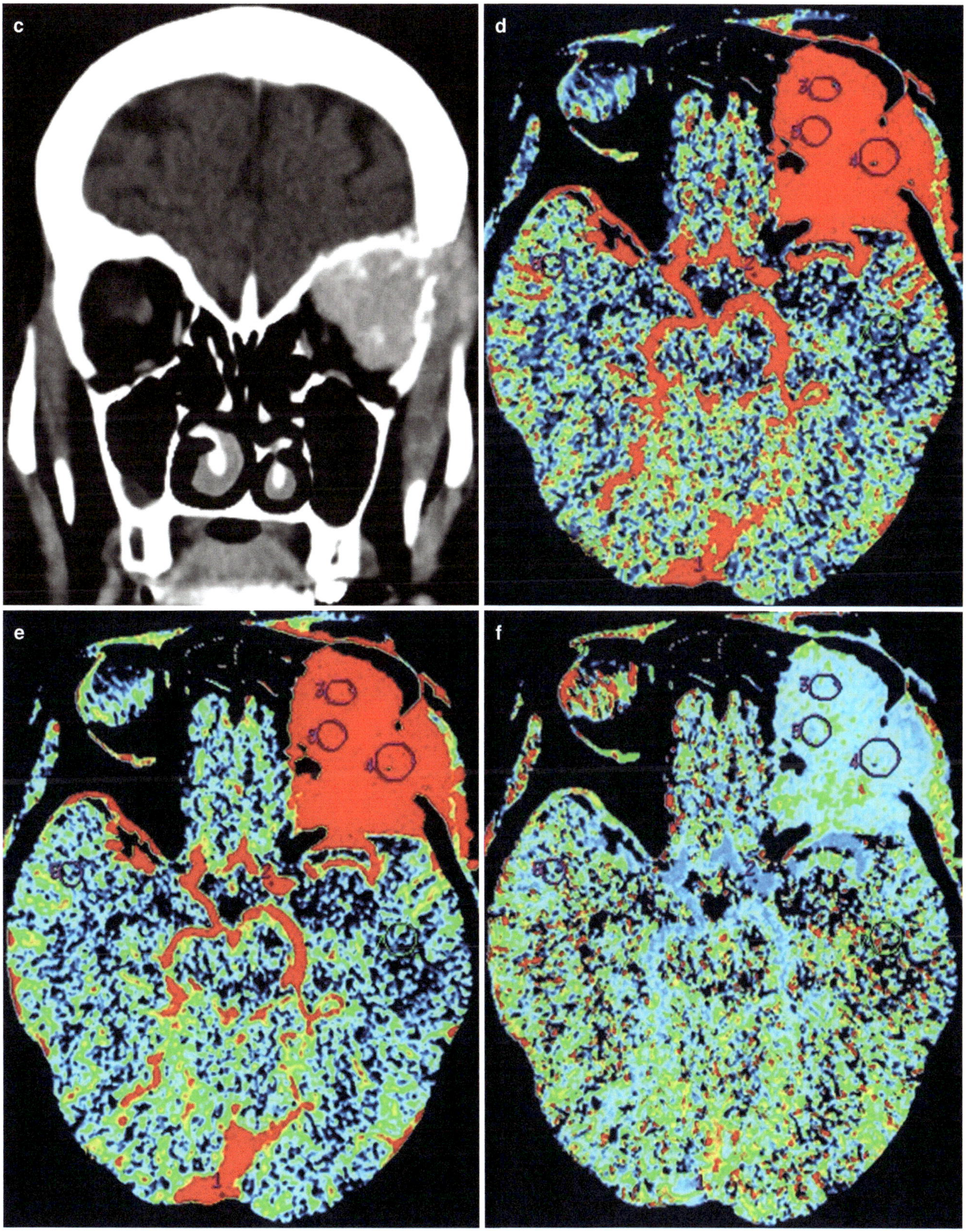

Fig. 5.1 (continued)

Diagnosis On CT, epidermoids are clearly defined hypodense cystic lesions located in the lateral portions of the eyebrows or in the middle of the upper eyelid. Contrast enhancement can be seen only in the capsule. The presence of calcifications helps distinguish them from mucoceles. Bone thinning caused by epidermoid cysts may lead to a local bone suture disruption. In case of the cyst rupture, there is a nonhomogeneous contrast enhancement of the lesion and perifocal inflammation (Cabanis et al. 1996).

On T1-weighted images, a hyperintense and isointense signals are observed from fat and the rest components, respectively. On T2-weighted images, an epidermoid cyst has a moderately hyperintense MR signal similar to that of the vitreous body. On diffusion and T2-Flair sequences, epidermoid cysts are usually hyperintense. On contrast-enhanced T1-weighted images, the contrast material accumulation is observed in the cyst capsule; in case of a rupture and inflammation, contrast enhancement becomes more diffuse. CT imaging without contrast enhancement is usually sufficient for a correct diagnosis; however, only DW-MRI sequence has high specificity.

Dermoid tumors are typically round-shaped on CT, with a pronounced capsule and inhomogeneously increased density (from 20 to 60 HU). Dermoids may have hypodense characteristics due to fat components. Tumors without any fat component may be encountered as well (Figs. 5.2 and 5.3).

There is often marked calcification of the capsule. An increase in the signal intensity is typical for dermoid tumors on T1-weighted MRI images. On T2-weighted MRI images, the tumor has a variable signal that ranges from hypo- to hyperintense nonhomogeneous. In the presence of hair in the tumor, threadlike portions of a reduced signal appear on MRI. In case of the tumor rupture, high-signal foci of fat-containing debris scattered throughout the intracranial space are detected (Fig. 5.4).

Differential Diagnosis Frontal mucocele, idiopathic orbital pseudotumor, vascular disorders, tumors of the lacrimal gland, lymphoma, rhabdomyosarcoma.

Myxoid Tumor This is a very rare tumor in the orbit, comprising less than 0.2% of all tumors. Although the fibrous

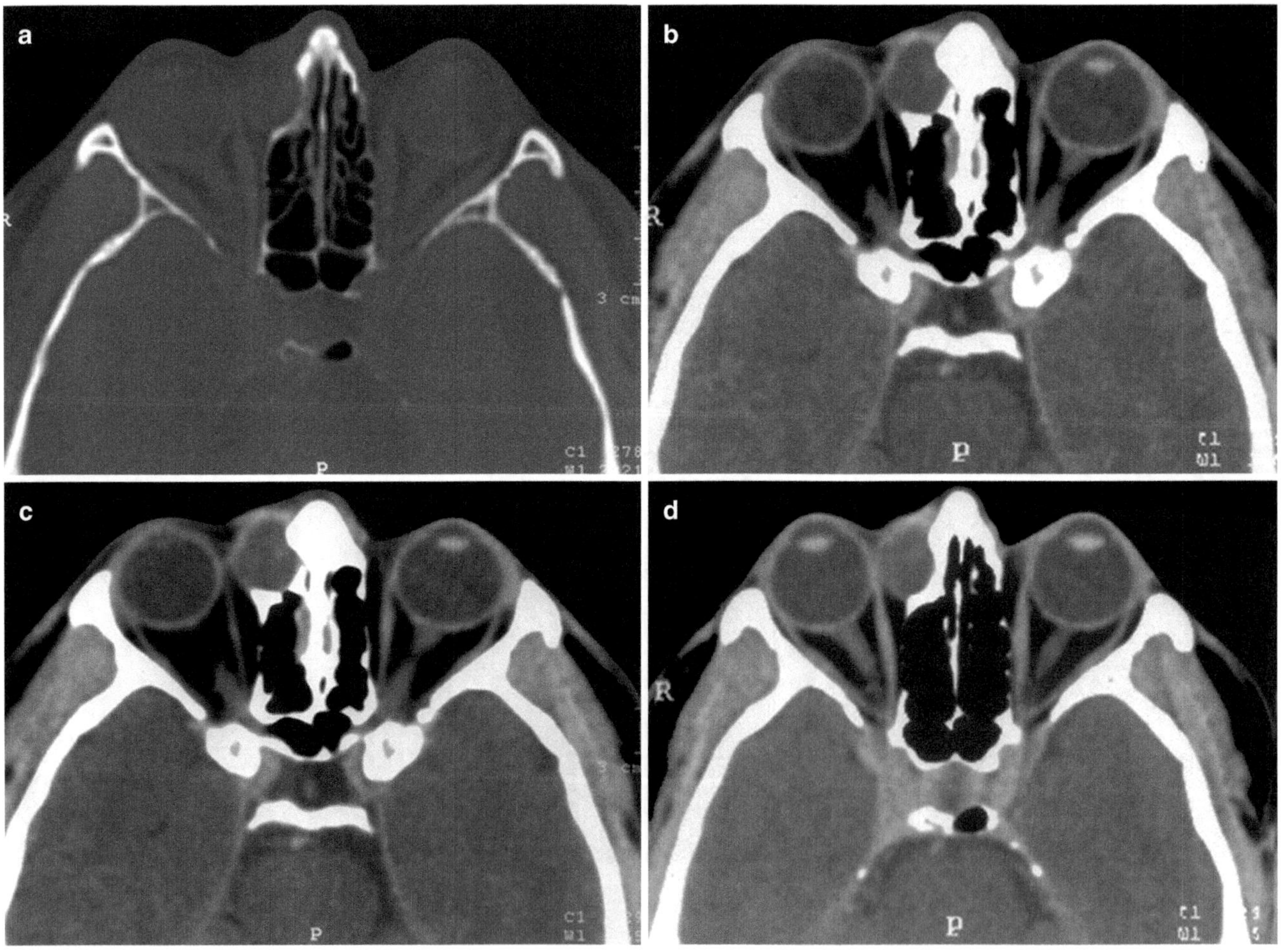

Fig. 5.2 Dermoid cyst of the right orbit. Axial CT series with contrast enhancement in bone (**a**) and regular (**b–d**) windows demonstrates a low density uniform lesion enhancing on the periphery, which located medially from eyeball. On sagittal (**e**) and frontal (**f**) CT reformats the excavation of the surrounding bone can be seen

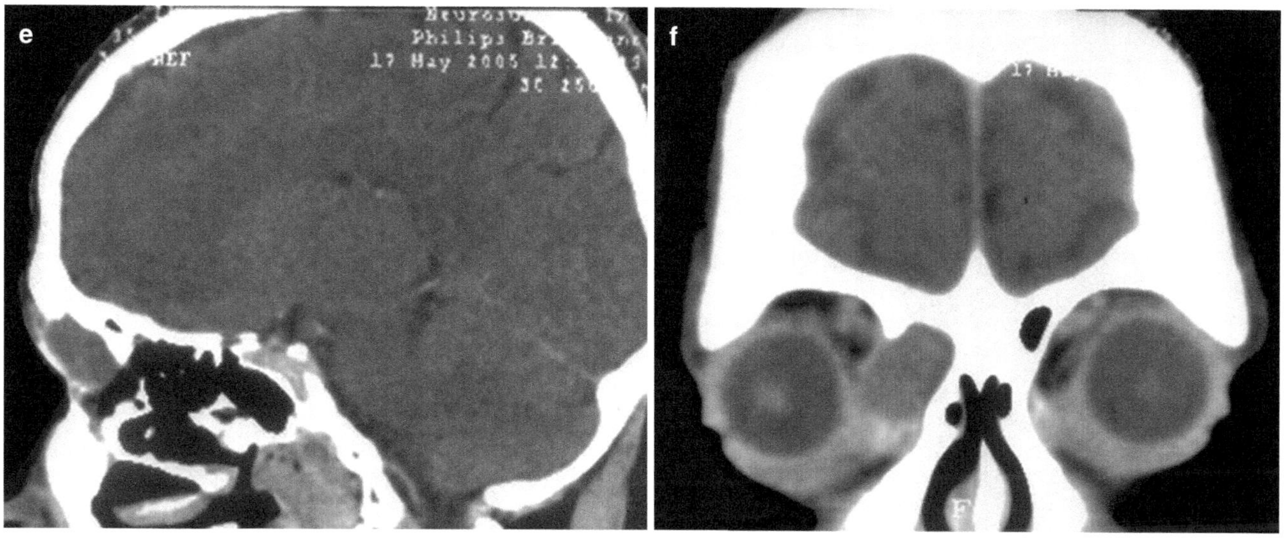

Fig. 5.2 (continued)

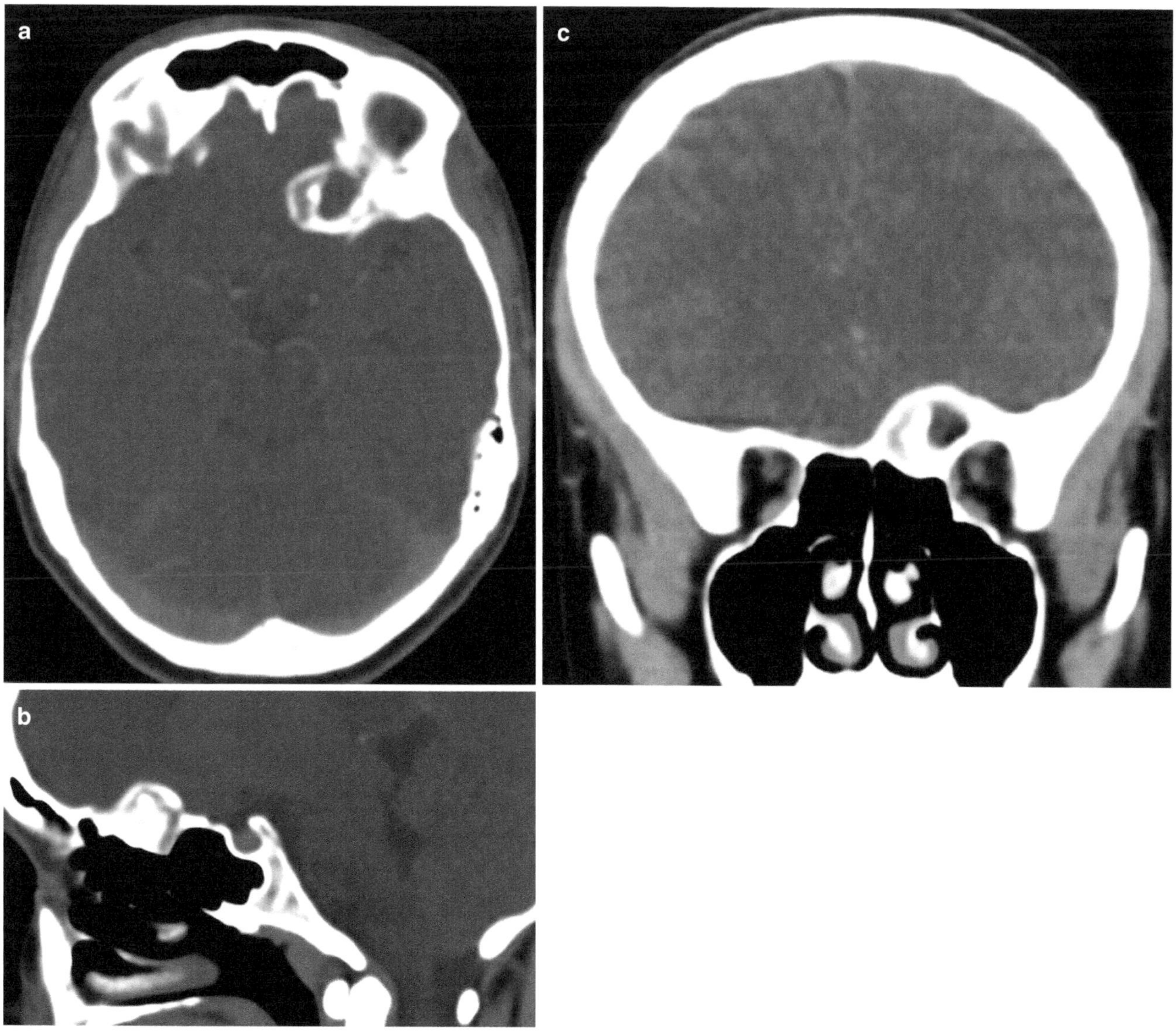

Fig. 5.3 Dermoid cyst of the left orbit roof. CT scans in axial (**a**), sagittal (**b**), and frontal (**c**) planes demonstrate a heterogeneous mass with irregular shape in the roof of the left orbit. The tumor contains calcifications in the center and causes of surrounding bone deformation

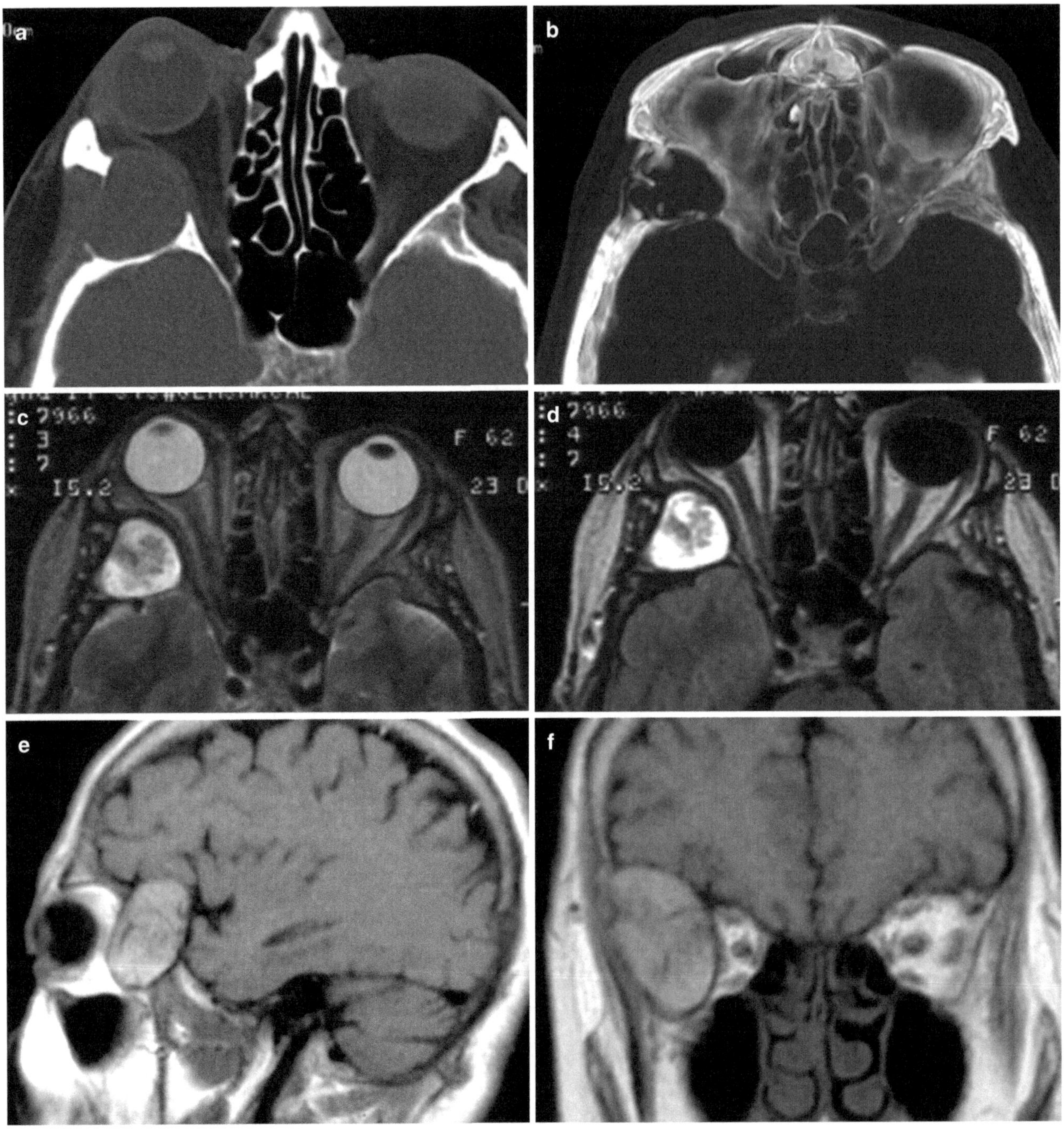

Fig. 5.4 Dermoid cyst of the pterional region. CT scans in axial projection (**a**, **b**) show an isodense mass in the lateral aspects of the right orbit, which leads to destruction of the lateral wall of the orbit. The tumor displaces an intraorbital lateral rectus muscle. Axial T2- (**c**) and T2-FLAIR-weighted (**d**) MR images demonstrate a lesion with hyperintense heterogeneous MR signal. The lesion shows the hyperintense MR-signal on T1-weighted images (**e**, **f**) and the absence of contrast enhancement

tissue and collagen are functional products of fibroblasts, they can also produce a mucoid substance. A benign myxoma might serve as an example. Enzinger (1965) stated that "it can be suggested that myxoma cells are modified fibroblasts that produce excessive amounts of mucopolysaccharides and are unable to form normal (mature) collagen fibers". In the orbit, the tumor grows as an isolated node.

Clinical Manifestations The majority of myxomas occur in the soft tissues of the extremities and pelvis. The palate is the most common site within the head and neck. Primary orbital myxomas are extremely rare. A noteworthy sign is a long duration of symptoms before the lesion is found in the orbit. This confirms its slow growth. Although patients develop exophthalmos or displacement of the eye, these are not always the initial symptoms of the disease. Blepharospasm, swelling of the upper eyelid, or diplopia may also be the initial symptoms of a slow-growing tumor. The tumor is usually isolated, lobular, and can be in any portion of the orbit.

5.2 Granulomatous Lesions

Wegener's granulomatosis is one of the most common diseases that can affect the orbit.

It is quite rare and nor fully clear disorder. Its underlying cause is an immune pathology characterized by necrotizing granulomatous lesions of the upper and lower respiratory tract, necrotizing glomerulonephritis and vasculitis of small vessels. The disease can occur in any body system: skin, eye, trachea, nervous system, heart, gums, prostate, stomach, vulva, neck (Leavitt et al. 1990). However, the orbital lesion is considered as a limited form of the disease and usually includes a small vessel soft-tissue component. The eye is involved in 42% of patients with Wegener's granulomatosis. Patients' age ranges from 13 to 77 years. The female to male ratio is 10:7. The right orbit is affected twice as often as the left one. Bilateral disease is less frequent.

Clinical Manifestations There are two groups of patients. The first group includes those who are already diagnosed with Wegener's granulomatosis at the time of orbital manifestations. These patients had necrotizing granulomatosis in the nasal cavities, paranasal sinuses, trachea, lungs, or mouth. In the second group of patients, the orbit was either a single anatomical site of the disease or one of the two. One third of patients with initial orbital manifestations have bilateral lesions. The duration of symptoms is from 1 to 14 years. Wegener's granulomatosis is more severe in patients from the first group. As a rule, the loss of vision, ophthalmoplegia, orbital wall erosion may occur.

Diagnosis CT findings in patients with Wegener's granulomatosis are varied and nonspecific. This space-occupying lesion may be located in any part of the orbit and be more local compared to the diffuse lesions in patients with extraorbital process. The local orbital lesion can accumulate contrast material to a varying degree, depending on the duration of the disease. "Younger" lesions are contrast-enhanced to a greater extent than those ones with more fibrotic tissue. Granulomas are generally homogenous and typically have irregular edges due to infiltration. This is what distinguishes Wegener's granulomatosis from non-vasculitis inflammatory tumors. When an orbital lesion is associated with diseases of the nasal cavities or adjacent paranasal sinuses, patients from the first group have osteitis, erosion, or destruction of the orbital wall adjacent to the affected sinus. Infiltration of the orbit is typical for these types of lesions.

T1-weighted MRI sequences show nodular masses with hypo- or isointense MR-signal comparing to rectus muscles. Abnormal masses have a reduced MR signal on T2-weighted images. A high signal due to the soft tissue edema is usually observed in the acute period. Pronounced and homogeneous contrast enhancement is typical (Fig. 5.5). MR techniques

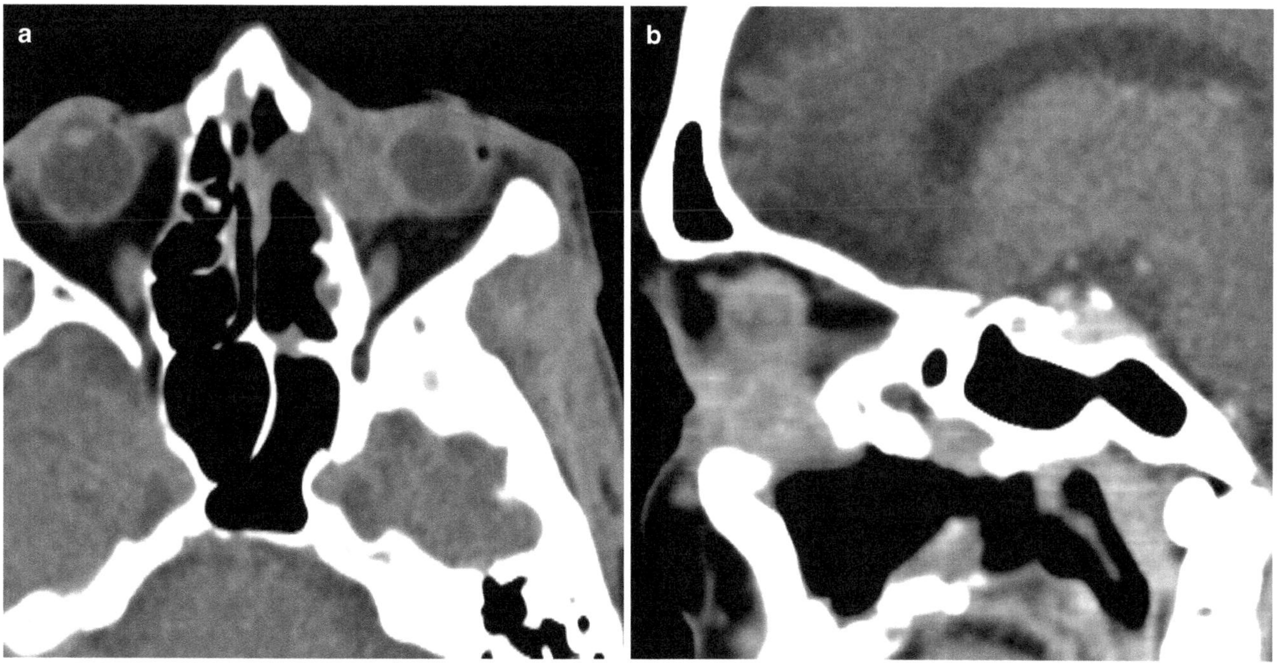

Fig. 5.5 Wegener's disease. Axial (**a**), sagittal (**b**), and coronal (**c**, **d**) CT scans with contrast enhancement demonstrate an infiltrative mass in the left infratemporal region, which spreads into the medial part of the left orbit. Local destruction of the medial orbital wall is revealed. The lesion shows an intensive contrast agent accumulation. On axial (**e**, **f**), coronal (**g**, **h**), and sagittal (**i**) MR images the widespread of the mass through skull base structures is clearly visible due to prominent contrast enhancement of the lesion

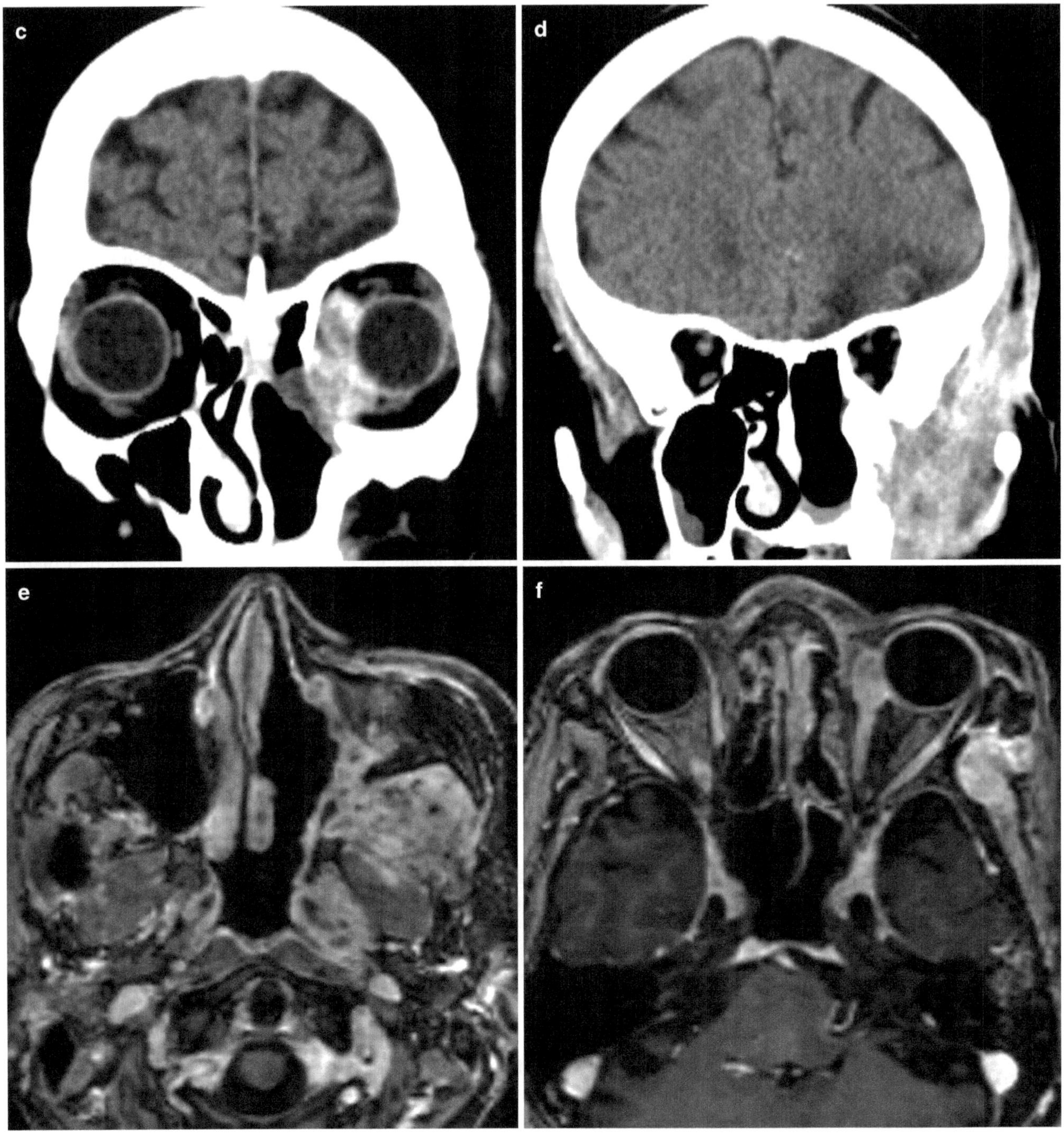

Fig. 5.5 (continued)

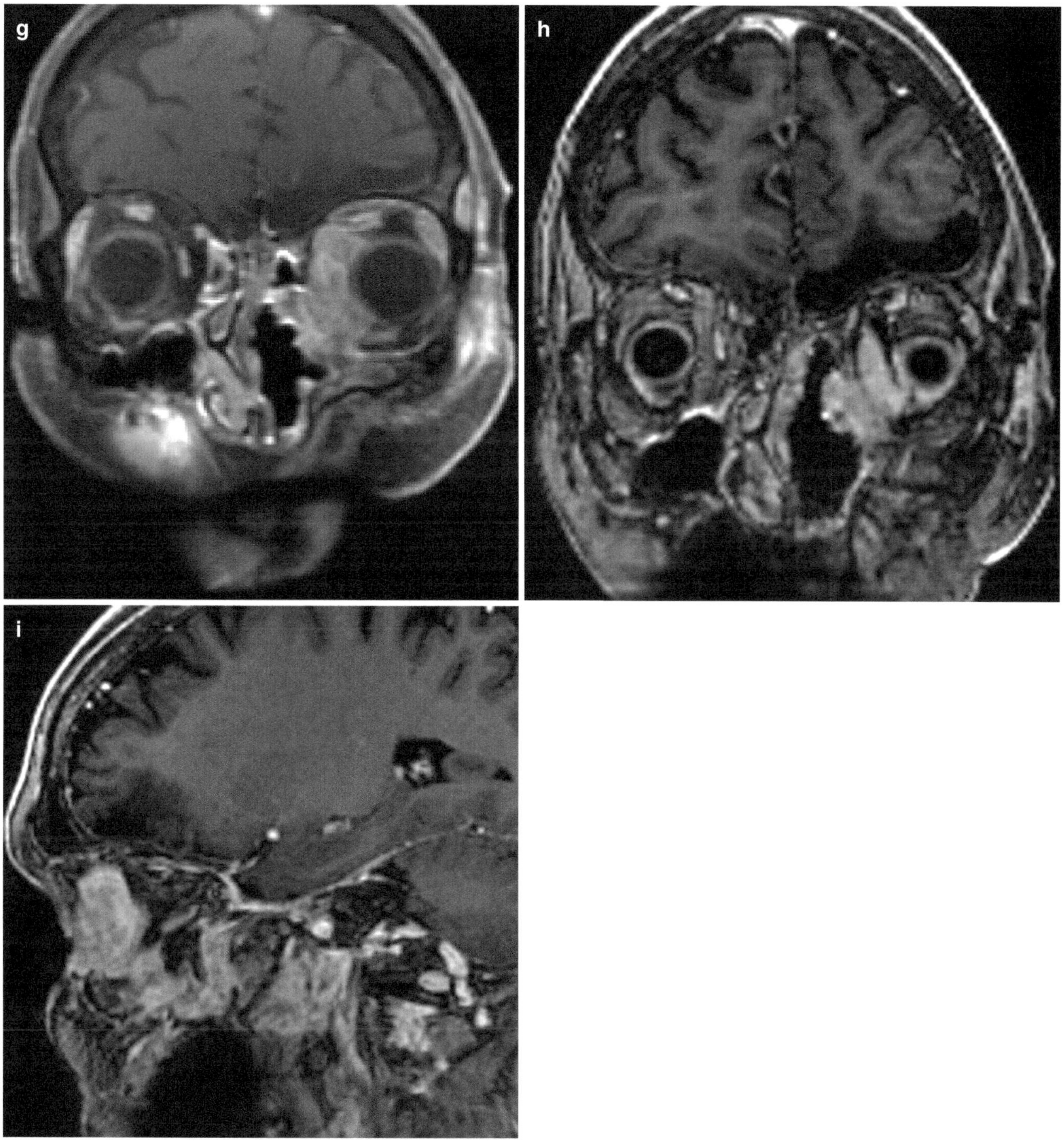

Fig. 5.5 (continued)

with suppression of fat signal should be considered principal in the diagnostic MR protocol.

Differential Diagnosis Sarcoidosis, idiopathic pseudotumor, thyroid ophthalmopathy.

Sarcoidosis is a chronic multi-system granulomatous disorder involving all body systems. In case of systemic involvement, clinical manifestations of sarcoidosis occur in CNS in 10% of cases (Mafee et al. 1999).

Clinical Findings In case of orbital involvement—acute uveitis, chronic dacryoadenitis, and enlargement of the lacrimal gland. Typical signs of the lacrimal gland lesions include: an increase in its size, painless at palpation, dry eyes. In case of involvement of the anterior chamber of the eye: soreness, conjunctivitis, and uveitis; posterior chamber: perivasculitis, infiltrates in the vitreous body and retinal changes, eyeball movement limitation and diplopia. Involvement of the optic nerve manifests by perineuritis, papillitis, and loss of vision. Sarcoidosis more often occurs in adults aged from 30 to 50 years old, predominantly in women. It is tenfolds more likely to be diagnosed among inhabitants of the African deserts. Also, the disease is common in Puerto Ricans, Irish, and Scandinavians (Brovkina 2008).

Diagnosis Sarcoidosis often mimics a pseudotumor and lymphoma.

An isodense enlargement in the nerve diameter is observed on CT scans before administration of contrast material. After contrast enhancement, abnormal accumulation of the contrast agent within the optic nerve and other intraorbital structures is identified. In addition, intravenous contrast enhancement shows an increase of the lacrimal gland, diffuse irregular thickening of the extraocular muscles. There are no erosions or compression changes in the bones of the orbital walls (Beardsley et al. 1984). However, none of these findings are specific for sarcoidosis.

T1-weighted MR-sequences reveal an isointense enlargement of the intraorbital structures. On T2-weighted images, hypointense (relative to normal muscle) or slightly hyperintense abnormal intraorbital masses can be visualized. T2-FLAIR sequence can demonstrate sarcoid parenchymal lesions in the brain. The optic nerve affected by granulomatous masses intensely accumulates contrast material. Contrast enhancement of the lacrimal gland and orbital muscles is also more pronounced than normally. In case of CNS involvement on MRI intracranial cisternal and parenchymal lesions can be detected (Camody et al. 1994; Ing et al. 1997). Optimal scanning sequences: a study with contrast enhancement and suppression of MR signal from the fat. Not only should the orbit be examined, but also the whole brain in order to identify other foci of sarcoidosis, as well as the lungs for histological confirmation of the diagnosis (Fig. 5.6).

Differential Diagnosis Idiopathic pseudotumor, thyroid ophthalmopathy, Wegener's granulomatosis.

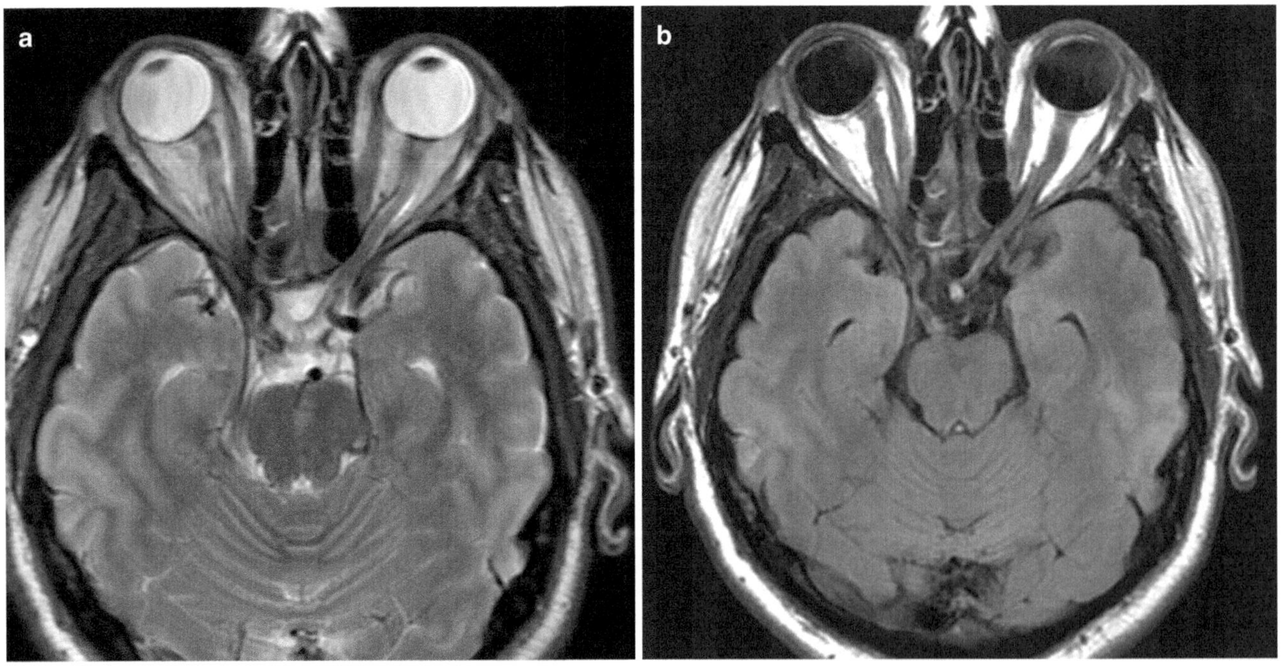

Fig. 5.6 Sarcoidosis. Axial T2 (**a**)-, T2-FLAIR (**b**)-, T2-FatSat (**c**), and T1 (**d**)- weighted images demonstrate irregular thickening of the lateral and medial rectus muscles of the right orbit. Enhanced T1-weighted MR images with FatSat technology in axial (**e, f**), coronal (**g**), and sagittal (**h**) projections show intensive contrast enhancement of right optic nerve sheath, lateral and medial rectus muscles. Infiltrative process involves the optic nerve sheath within optic canal with spreading intracranially. (**i**)—histological specimen

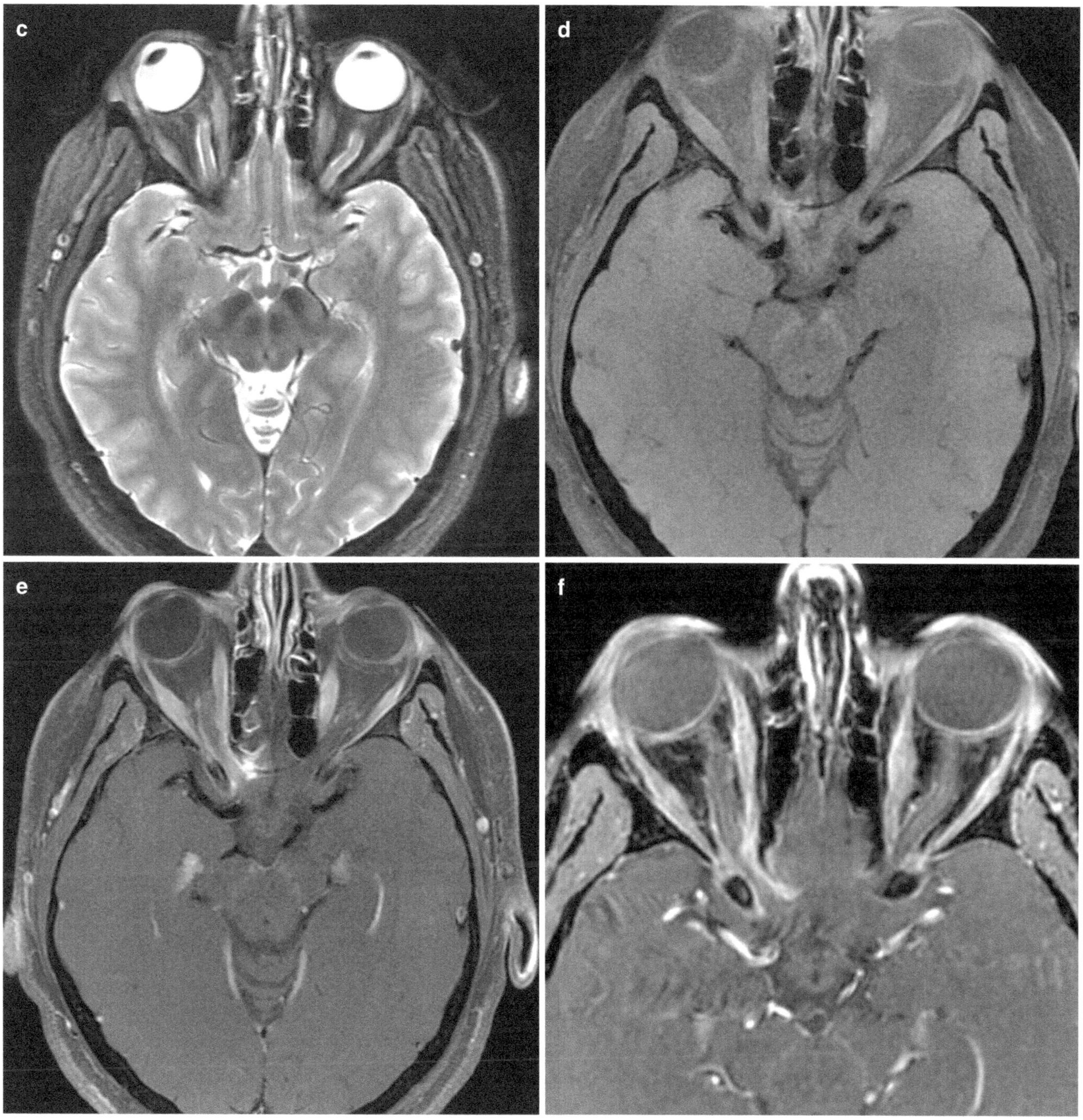

Fig. 5.6 (continued)

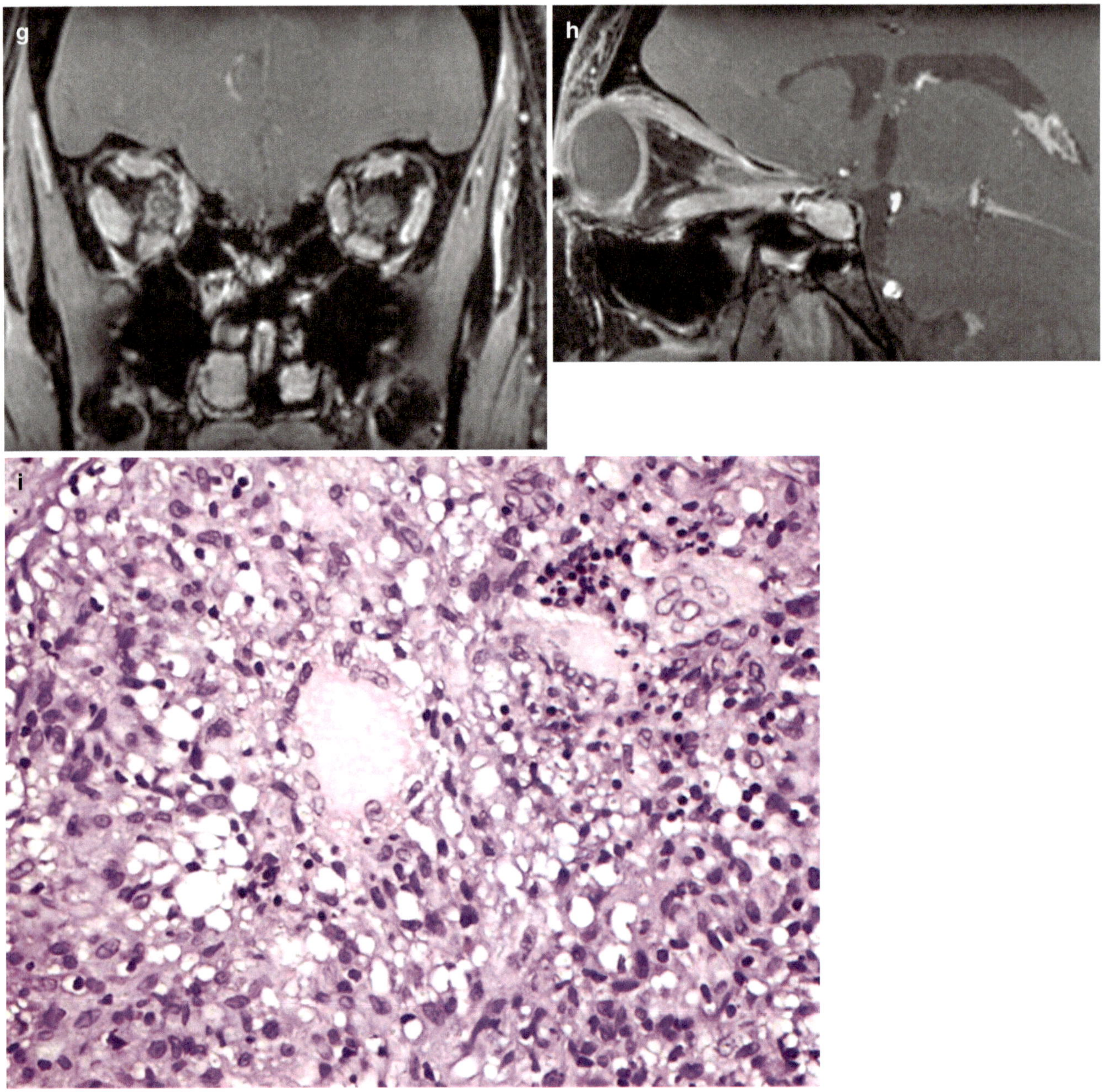

Fig. 5.6 (continued)

Eye Ball Lesions

6

Contents

6.1 Tumors

Melanoma Primary malignant melanomas of the ciliary body (10%), choroid (85%), and iris (5%) are rare. The majority of patients with secondary tumors underwent enucleation or evisceration of one eye. The tumor recurred within a year in 50% of cases. The prognosis is generally poor due to frequent metastases (Atlas et al. 1987).

Tumor development is possible from blue nevus, ectopic melanocytes, congenital peridermal melanosis (Brovkina 2008). According to Rice and Brawn (1990), the growth of primary melanoma is associated with periorbital pigmented lesions in 40% of cases. Melanoma can metastasize to the liver, lungs, kidneys, and brain. Elderly people suffer more often, the average age being 53 years old. The incidence of uveal melanoma increases with age. Less than 2% of tumors are seen in patients younger than 20 years age (Mafee 1998). The disease is diagnosed in men and women with an equal frequency. Northern Europeans are more prone to the disease, while in Africans the disease is extremely rare.

Clinical Manifestations Blurred vision, visual field defects, often no pain.

Diagnosis On CT scans melanoma is hyperdense and sharply demarcated in majority of the cases (Peyster and Augsburger 1985). Calcifications are rarely detected and occur more often after the treatment. The tumor diffusely accumulates contrast material (Fig. 6.1). High-resolution MRI is considered the gold standard in the diagnosis of orbital melanoma. The tumor is slightly to moderately hyperintense on T1-weighted images (comparing to the signal of the vitreous). The signal intensity increases together with an increase in the degree of pigmentation, which can be used to predict the treatment outcomes. Melanomas are hypointense on T2-weighted images (less MR-signal than in the vitreous). The tumor diffusely accumulates contrast material on T1-weighted images after intravenous injection (Motoyama et al. 2011) (Figs. 6.2 and 6.3).

I. Pronin, V. Kornienko, *CT and MRI of Skull Base Lesions*, https://doi.org/10.1007/978-3-319-65957-2_6

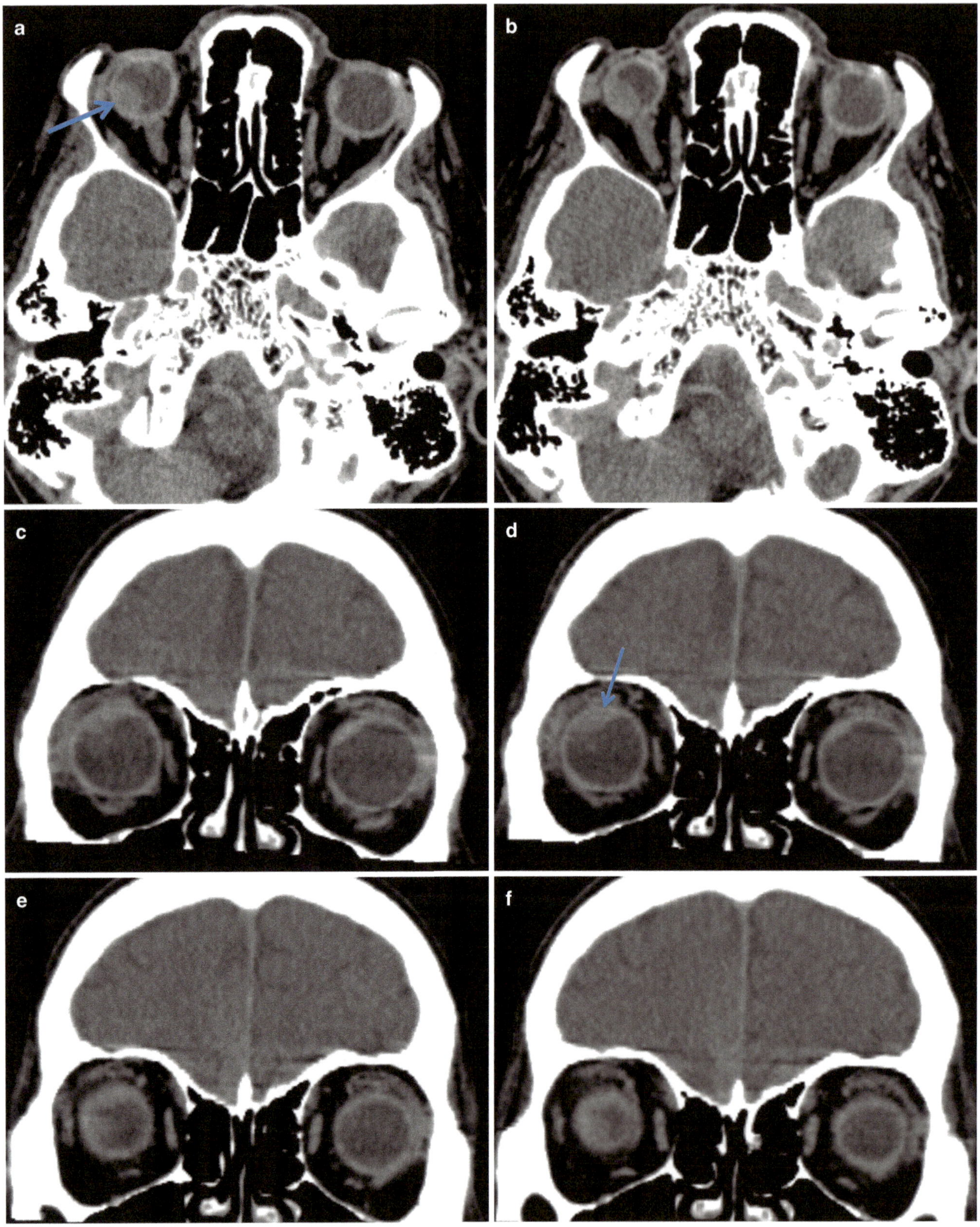

Fig. 6.1 Uveal melanoma. Lenticular hyperdense lesion with sharp edges is clearly visible on CT scans in axial (**a**, **b**) and coronal (**c**–**f**) planes (*arrows*). The tumor is located in supralateral segment of the right eyeball

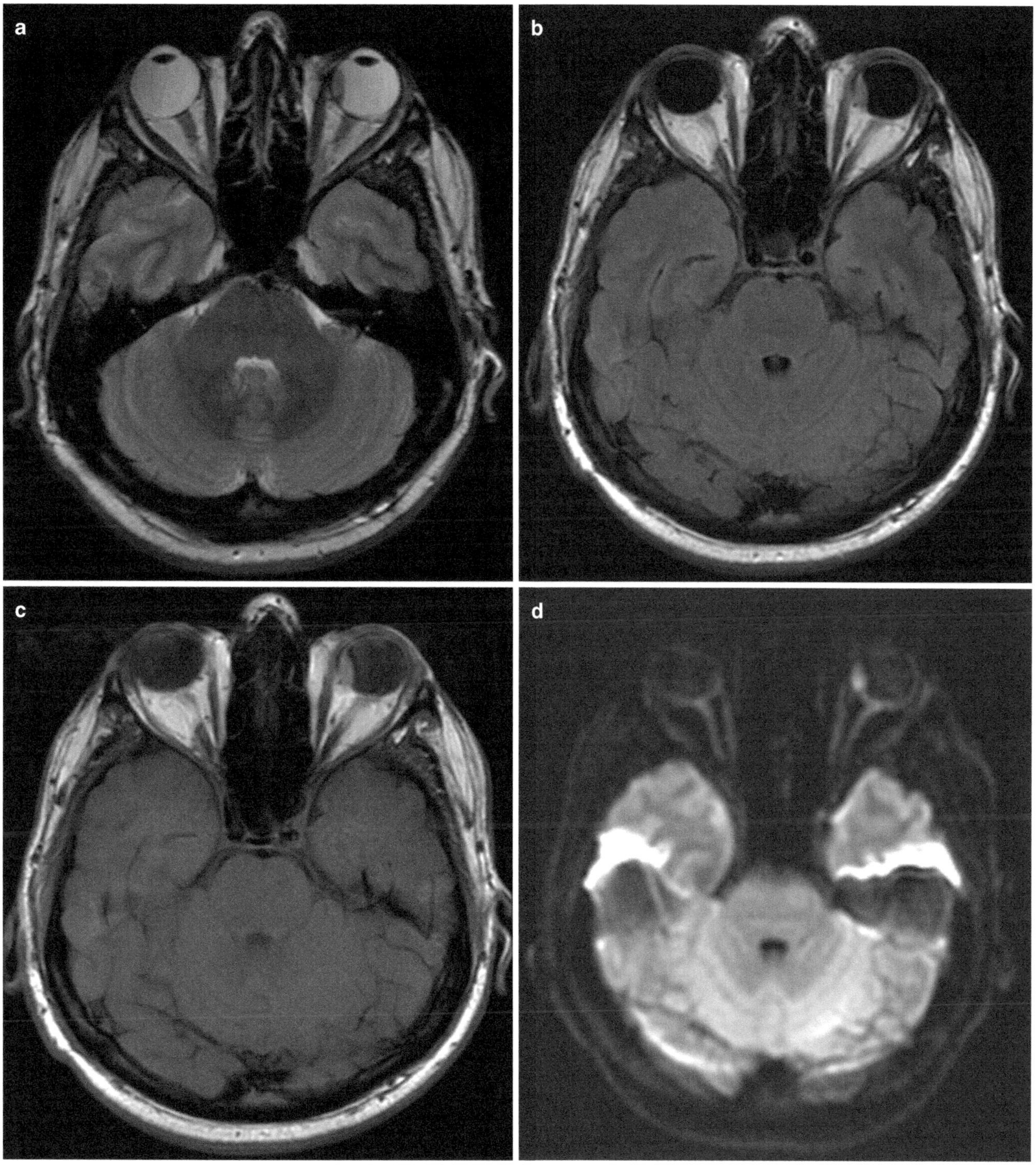

Fig. 6.2 Uveal melanoma. Axial T2-weighted MR image (**a**) shows a hypointense lesion of the medial aspect of left globe. Melanoma demonstrates a hyperintensity on T2-FLAIR (**b**), T1 (**c**) and diffusion-weighted (**d**) MR scans. Enhanced T1-FatSat MR images reveal a local mass on the medial wall of the left globe with intensive contrast enhancement (**e**, **f**)

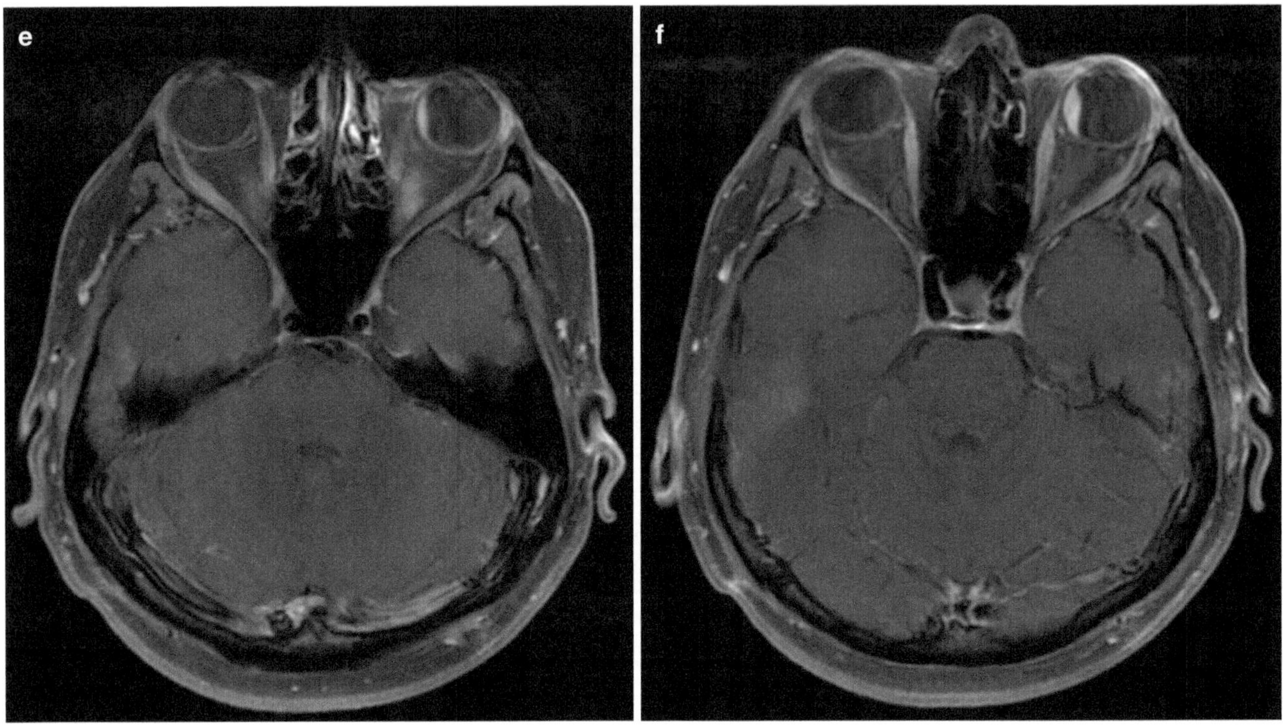

Fig. 6.2 (continued)

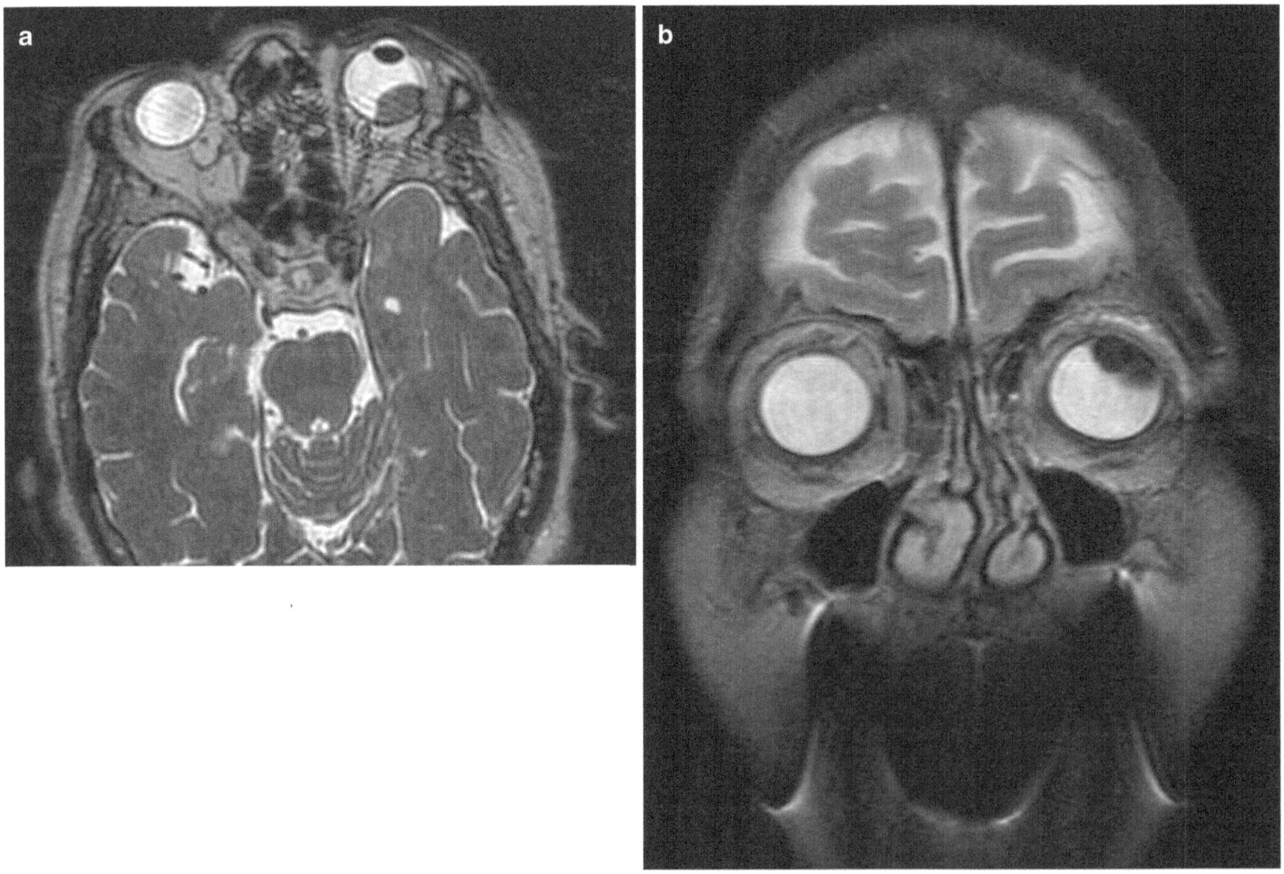

Fig. 6.3 Uveal melanoma. Axial (**a**) and coronal (**b**) T2-weighted MR images show a hypointense intraocular lesion. Melanoma demonstrates an intensive and homogeneous contrast enhancement (**c**—T1 before, **d**–**f**—post-contrast scans). There is involvement of optic disc region without extraocular extension

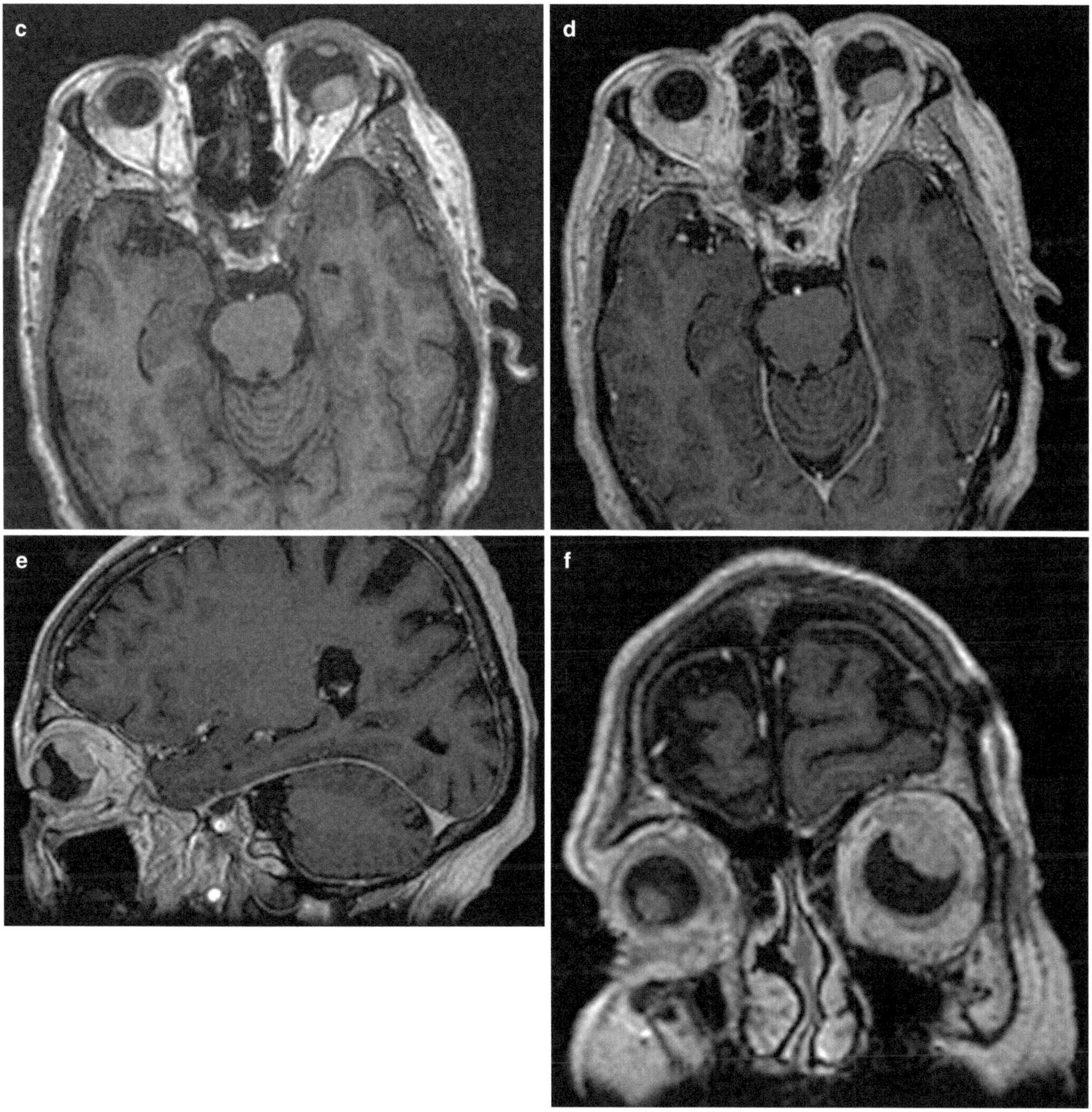

Fig. 6.3 (continued)

Differential Diagnosis Inflammation of the retina, metastases, retinoblastoma, and chorioretinal damage.

Retinoblastoma is a malignant tumor of the eye, most common in children. More than 90% of the identified cases of retinoblastomas are diagnosed in children younger than 5 years old with a uniform gender distribution (Castillo and Kaufman 2003; Balmer 2006; Cunnane et al. 2011). There are four types of retinoblastomas:

1. Non-hereditary, presumably caused by a postzygotic retinoblast mutation;
2. Retinoblastoma with autosomal dominant inheritance;
3. Retinoblastoma related to the RB1 gene mutation in the 13q14 chromosome;
4. Bilateral retinoblastoma in combination with a pineal tumor and suprasellar tumor (trilateral, tetralateral) (Johnson et al. 1985).

According to prognosis retinoblastoma can be classified as well into five groups (according to International Intraocular Retinoblastoma Classification from A to E). Group A differs from group E on the base of size (a small tumor that is away from the critical globe's structures (group A) and degree of anatomy and function of the eye destruction, and vitreous and subretinal dissemination as well (Murphree 2005).

The prognosis depends on the tumor stage. Retinoblastoma is a hereditary tumor occurring in 1:20,000 of newborns. About half of the cases are bilateral multifocal hereditary neoplasms. More than 15% of children have a unilateral retinoblastoma caused by abnormal development of the embryon (de Graaf et al. 2005). There are 200–300 newly diagnosed cases of retinoblastoma in the United States each year. Rootman (1988) established that the tumor occurs twofolds more often in the last 50 years. Prognosis: mortality <10% if the optic nerve is intact, and about 65% if the optic nerve is affected. Histological characteristics of retinoblastoma include small oval or round cells with a small amount of cytoplasm and enlarged nuclei, which may be poorly differentiated or have a high degree of differentiation. Formation of Flexner-Wintersteiner rosettes is possible. In case of rapid growth, retinoblastoma may contain foci of necrosis and calcifications. There are three types of retinoblastoma growth:

1. Endophytic—the tumor inhomogeneously grows anteriorly from the retina into the vitreous body, mimicking endophthalmitis;
2. Exophytic—retinoblastoma grows into the subretinal space, causing secondary retinal detachment, which leads to Coats' disease;
3. Diffuse—in this case, the tumor grows along the retina, forming a myxoid mass and mimicking inflammation or hemorrhage; this form is difficult to diagnose because of the lack of calcifications and due to occurrence outside the typical age group.

The most common clinical sign of retinoblastoma, which occurs in 60% of patients, is leukocoria, in 20% of cases strabismus is observed. Other clinical signs, such as eye pain, caused by secondary glaucoma occur much less frequently. More than 90% of retinoblastomas have calcifications both multiple and isolated, confluent or punctate (Essuman et al. 2010). CT for the diagnosis of retinoblastoma is considered preferable to MRI because of its greater sensitivity to calcifications. The most specific sign is the presence of calcifications in the eyeball (Fig. 6.4). Localization of the tumor can be either unilateral in 70–75% of cases or bilateral in 25–30% of cases. The optic nerve

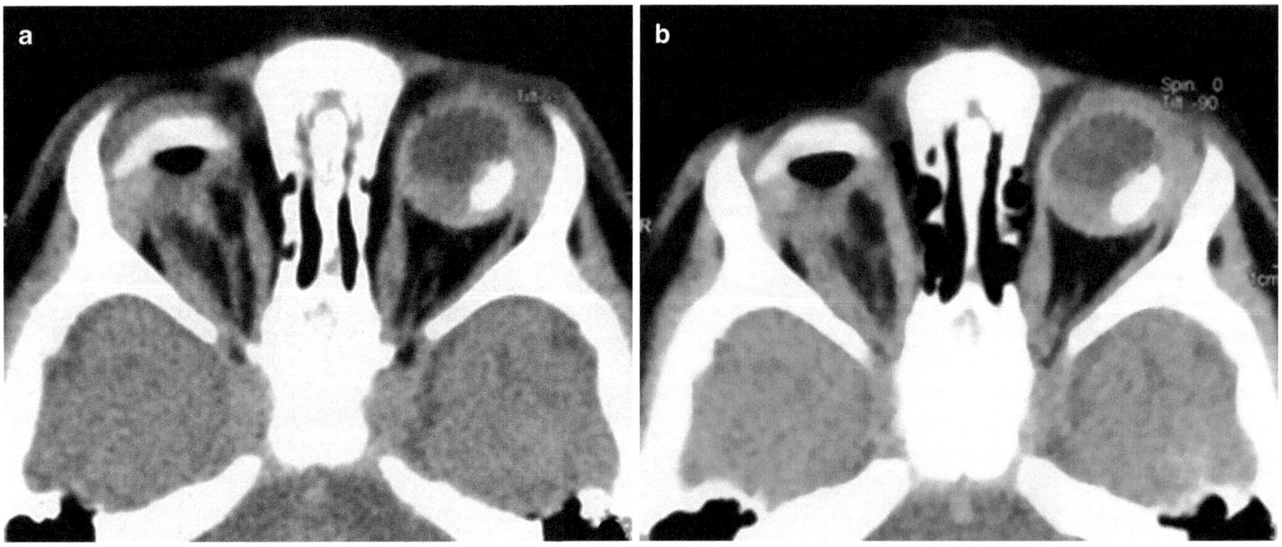

Fig. 6.4 Retinoblastoma, retinal detachment, right side enucleation due to retinoblastoma. CT scans in axial (**a**, **b**) and coronal (**c**) projections demonstrate an intraocular calcified lesion of leftwards. The left retinal detachment can be clearly visible. T2 (**d**)-, SWAN (**e**)-, T2-FLAIR (**f**, **g**)- weighted MR imaging reveals a tumor in the projection of the posterior *left* globe aspect, which visualized better on T2-weigthed and SWAN sequences as a hypointense focus. The tumor is clearly visible after intravenous contrast agent injection (**h**, **i**)

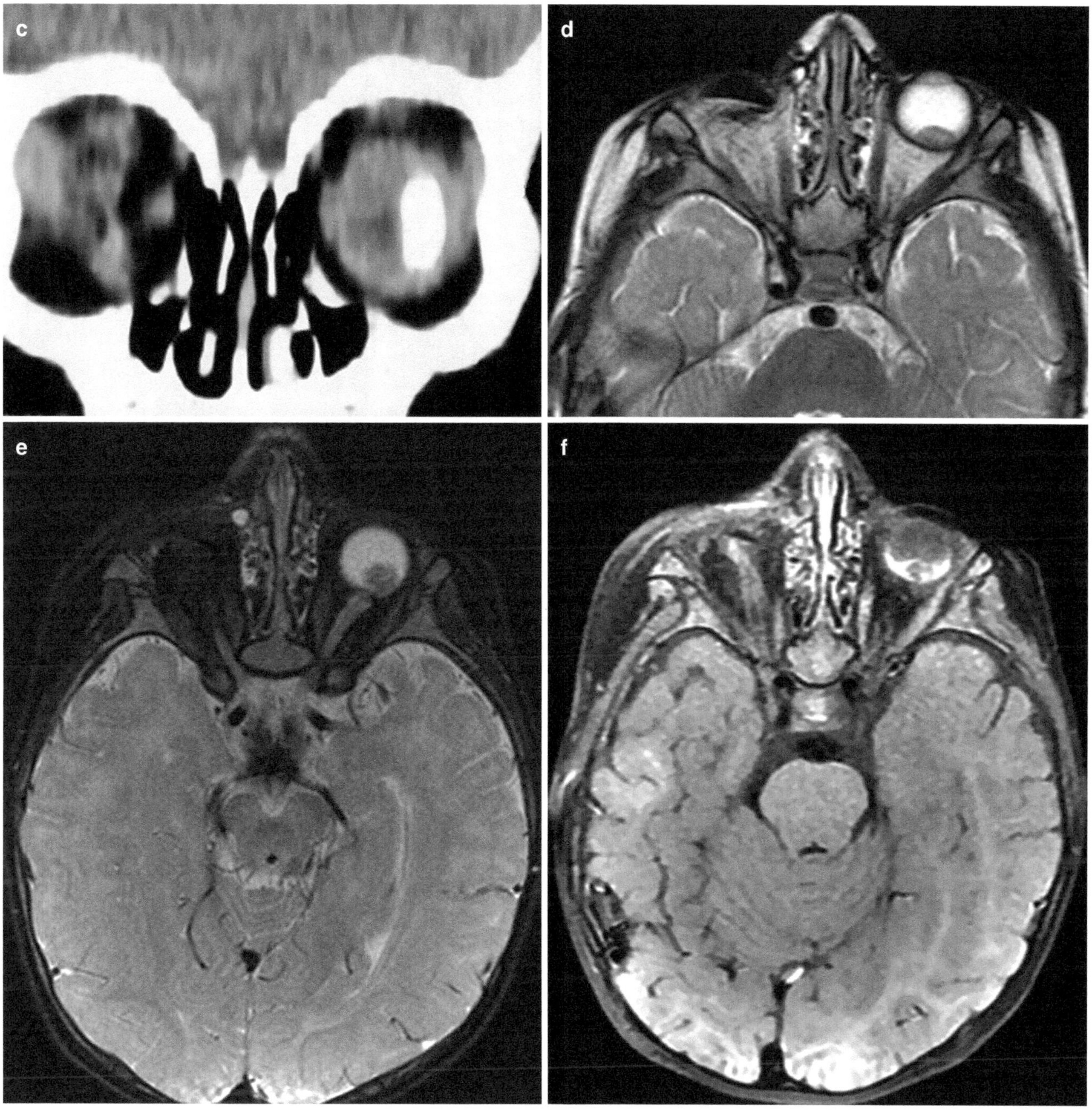

Fig. 6.4 (continued)

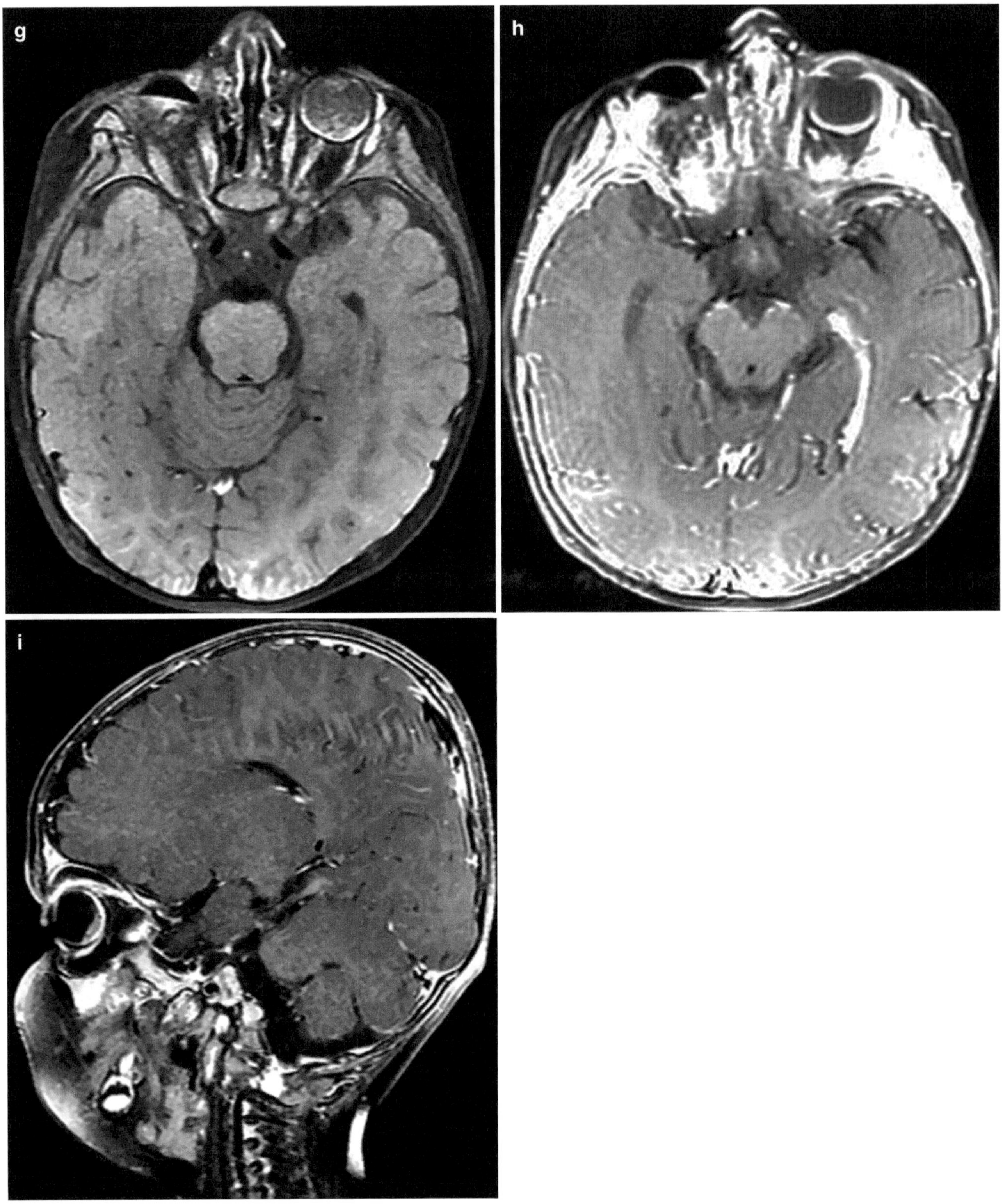

Fig. 6.4 (continued)

damage and intraorbital growth are infrequent events. Leptomeningeal metastases are rare.

Diagnosis CT scanning reveals a high-density lobular lesion with typical foci of calcification in 95% of cases (Baert and Santor 2006). The tumor intensely and heterogeneously accumulates the contrast agent.

A typical MRI picture includes a high or moderate signal hyperintensity on T1-weighted images and usually a hypointense signal on T2-weighted images. On the proton-density-weighted and T2-FLAIR images a demarcated tumor edge is visible. Growth into the distal optic nerve and into the vitreous body can be seen on the MRI. Contrast enhancement in the tumor is also quite pronounced on the MRI. For improvement of intraocular lesion visualization, the use of T2-heavy weighted sequences is recommended (Figs. 6.5 and 6.6).

Differential Diagnosis Coloboma, retinopathy, cat scratch eye disease, and other forms of leukocoria—retinal dysplasia, retinal hamartoma, hemangioma, retinal hemorrhage.

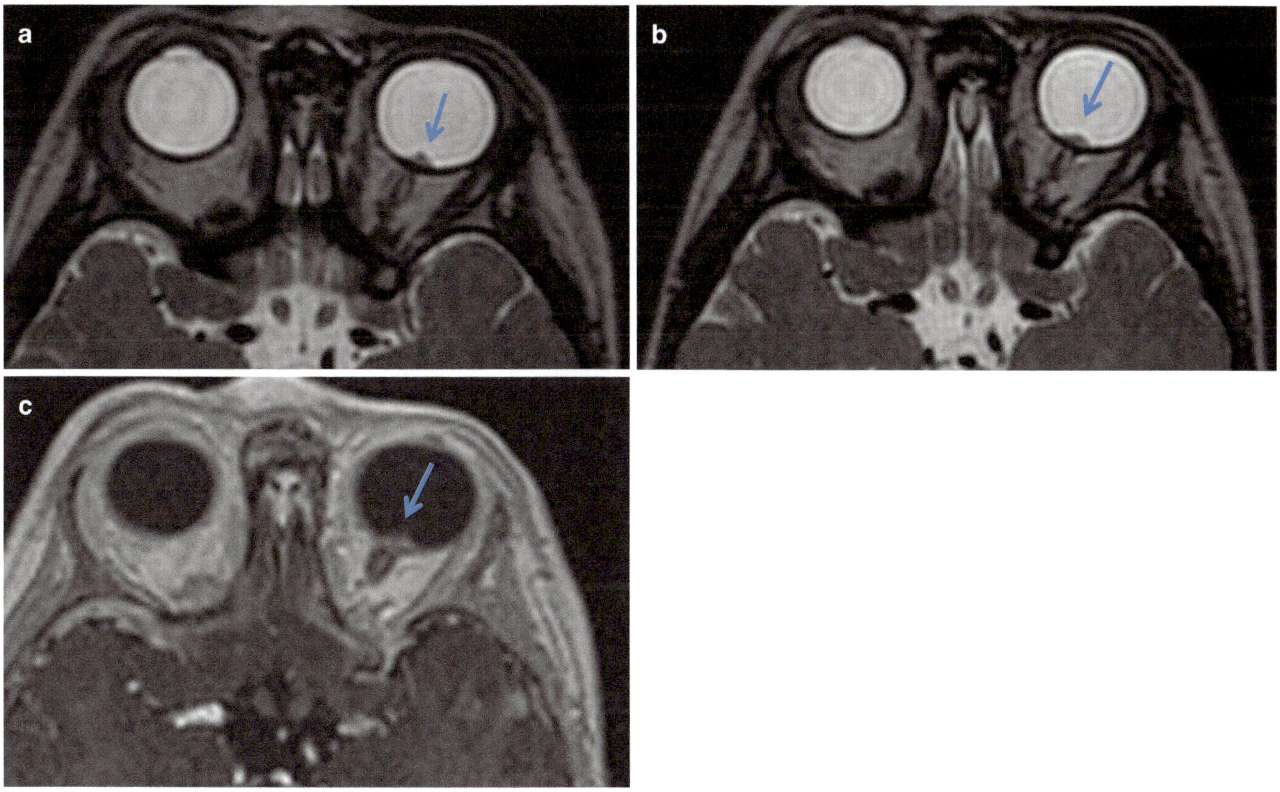

Fig. 6.5 Retinoblastoma of the left globe. Axial T2- heavy weighted MR images (**a**, **b**) demonstrate conical clearly delineated hypointense tumor in the optic disc projection. The tumor shows contrast enhancement on T1-weighted MR image (**c**). The lesion is less visible on T1 than T2-heavy weighted image (*arrows*)

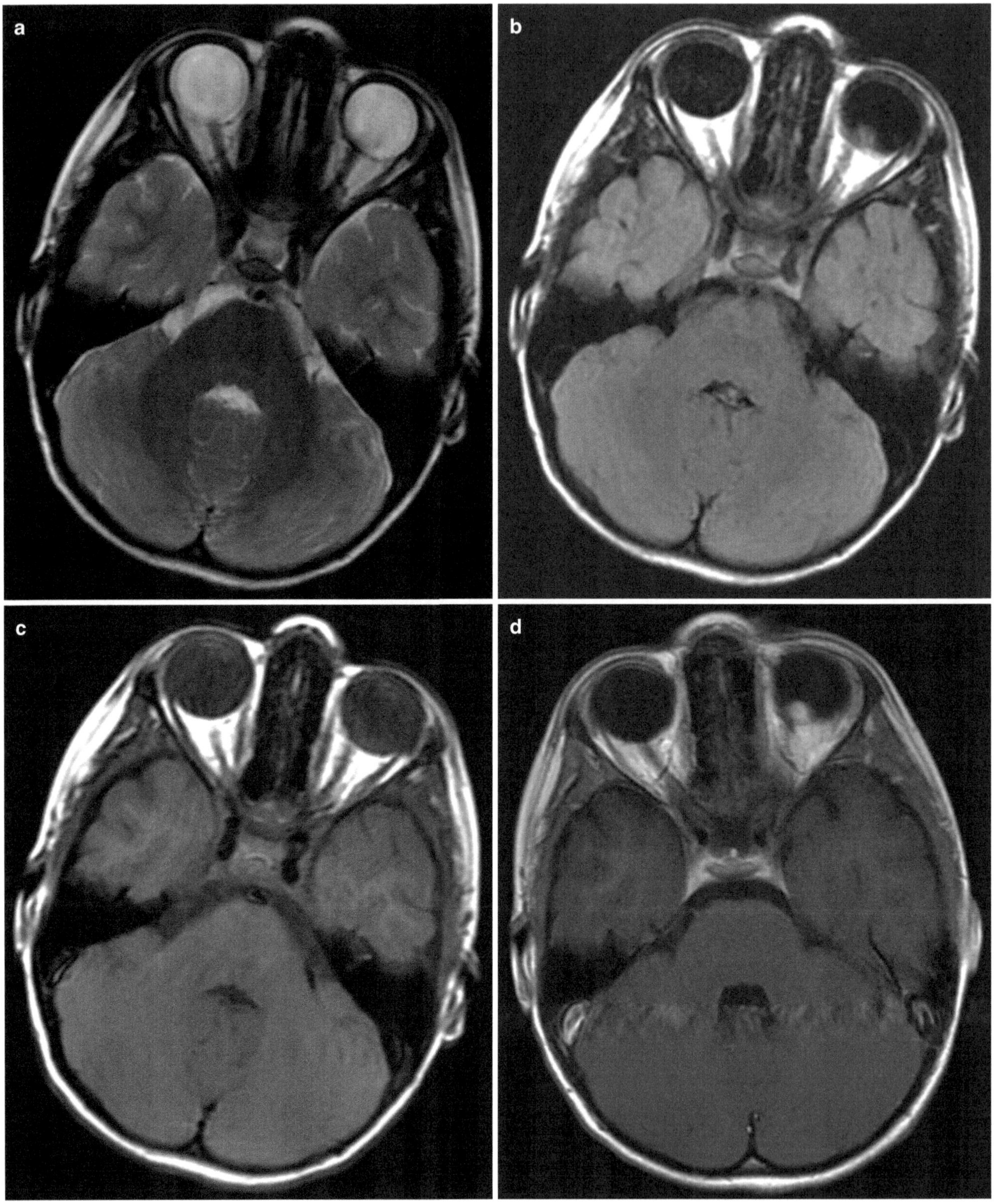

Fig. 6.6 Retinoblastoma. Axial T2- (**a**), T2-FLAIR—(**b**), and T1- (**c**) weighted MR images demonstrate an intraocular mass which is better visible on T2-FLAIR image due to hyperintense MR-signal. The tumor is characterized by prominent contrast agent accumulation (**d**–**f**). Enhanced T1-weighted MRI with Fat-Sat technology can improve the lesion delineation within the globe (**e**, **f**)

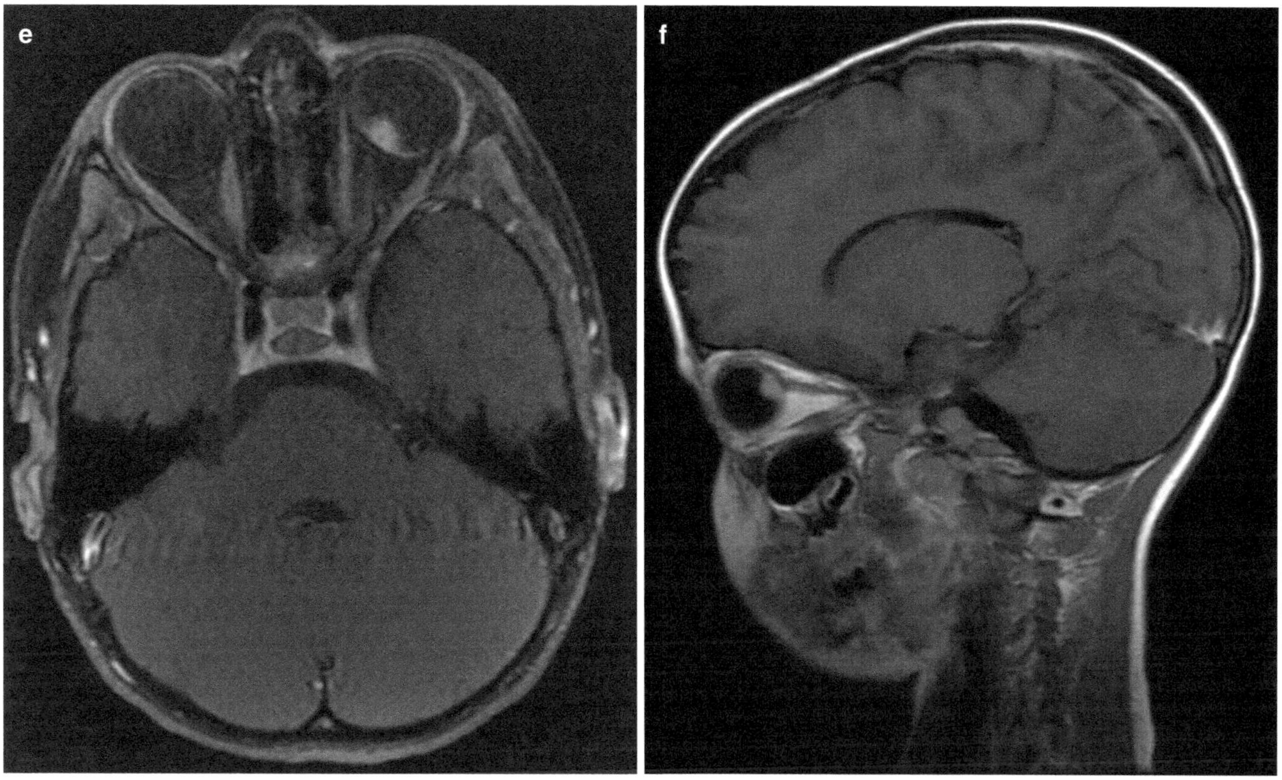

Fig. 6.6 (continued)

6.2 Congenital Disorders

Coloboma (from the Greek kolo-bos, meaning defect) is a defect in the eye membranes either acquired or congenital (genetic).

Coloboma occurs in all age groups, with equal frequency in men and women. This is a bilateral process in 60% of cases. The causes may include a traumatic brain injury or surgery, congenital or acquired defect of the orbital structures or it may develop as a result of incomplete closure of the choroidal fissure. Coloboma can occur in various systemic disorders, such as Joubert syndrome or Warburg syndrome.

There are two types of orbital coloboma: with excavation of the optic disc and without the optic nerve involvement. Congenital coloboma is a congenital abnormality occurring during organogenesis of the visual organs (Eagle 1999).

Diagnosis CT and MRI show a defect in the posterior wall of the eyeball with or without excavation of the optic disc. The defect typically is conical in shape and located in inferomedial sections of the eyeball. Sometimes there is a thickening of the optic nerve, as well as coloboma prolapse into the vitreous body.

CT reveals a cystic lesion that is isodense in relation to the vitreous body. Calcifications are rare, mostly at the edge of the lesion. Hyperdensity of the choroid is often caused by choroidal hemorrhage (Mafee et al. 1987).

Coloboma is isointense in relation to the vitreous body on T1- and T2-weighted MRI images (Fig. 6.7). In case of retinal hemorrhage, the MR signal depends on the stage of blood resorption. Any retroglobal cyst associated with microphthalmia should be regarded as a colobomatous cyst (Mafee et al. 1987).

Differential Diagnosis Peripapillary staphyloma, microphthalmic cyst, physiological myopia.

Unlike coloboma, staphyloma usually is not congenital, most cases develop secondary to severe myopia with dilation of the posterior segment of the eyeball. Another common cause of staphylomas is thinning of the sclera (Fig. 6.8).

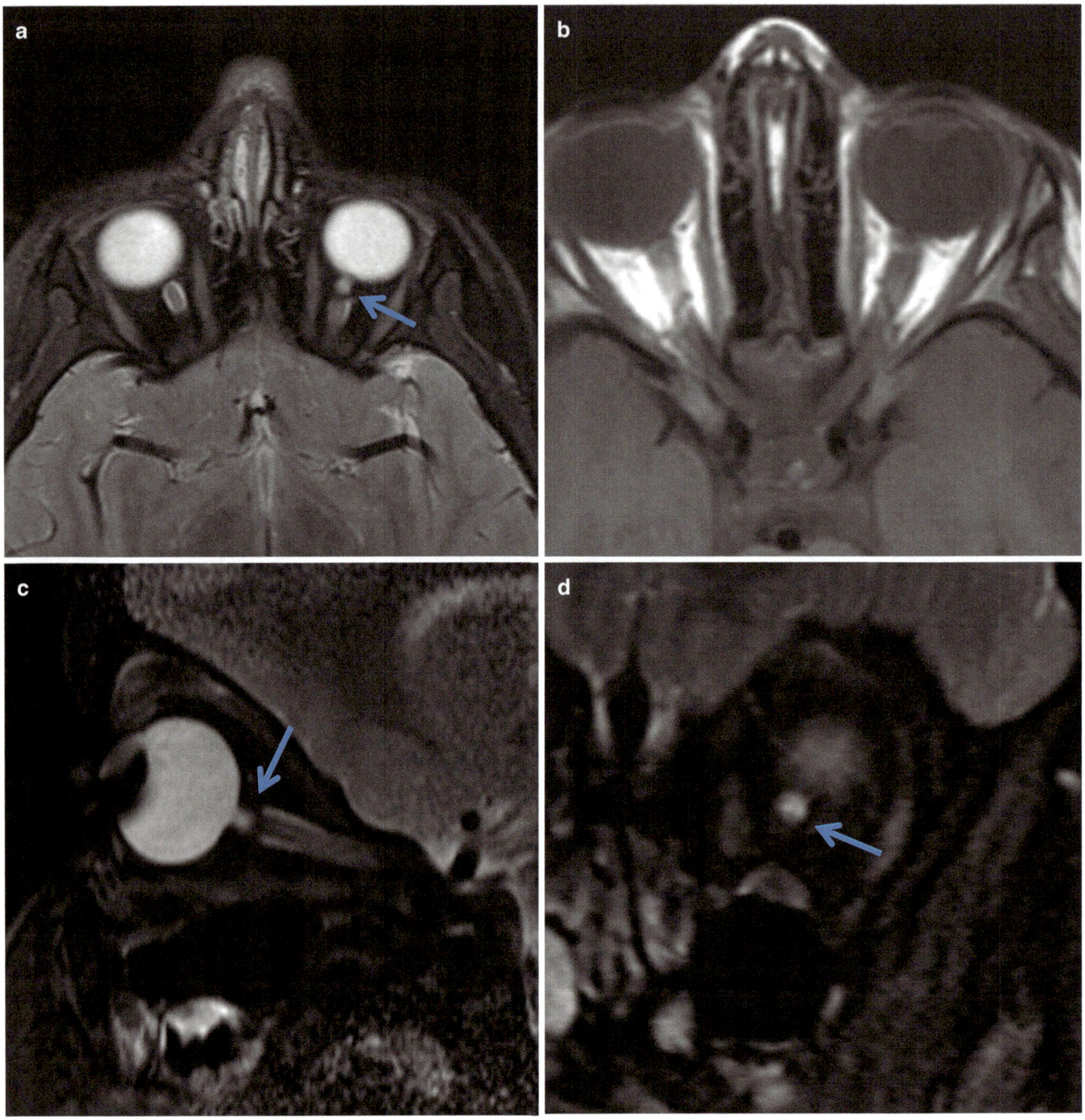

Fig. 6.7 Coloboma of the optic disc. T2-weighted (**a**) and T1-weighted (**b**) MR images demonstrate a defect of the posterior wall in the left globe in optic disc projection. The formation of a small cystic protrusion can be clearly visible on sagittal (**c**) and coronal T2 MRI (**d**) (*arrows*)

6.3 Vascular Disorders

Retinal detachment is the process of the retina separation from the choroid. They are closely adjacent in a normal eye. The retina consists of a sensitive layer and pigmented epithelium. A retinal tear is considered the main cause of retinal detachment. The retina does not move from its place if it is tight (retains its integrity) and has no tears. If there is a tear, then the vitreous fluid may seep under the retina, separating the retina from the choroid. Retinal tears can occur due to its dystrophy (thinning). Large tears often occur due to eye injuries. Other more rare causes of retinal detachment include already mentioned tractions (tension) by the modified vitreous body without retinal tears (this often happens in diabetic

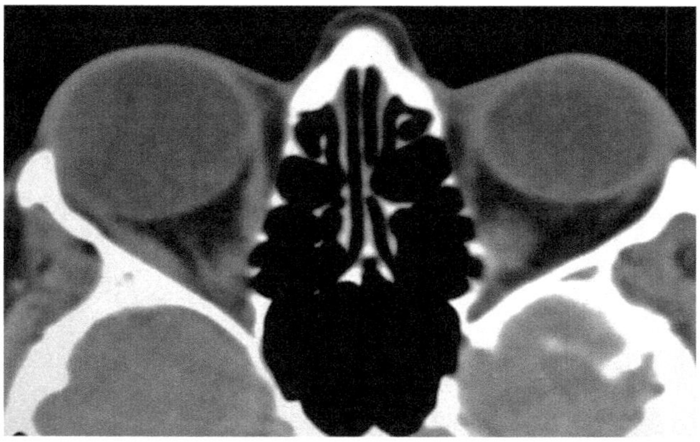

Fig. 6.8 Staphyloma. CT scan in axial plane shows thinning of the posterior wall of the globe. Also there is a right globe deformation and size increasing

retinopathy), as well as space-occupying lesions under the retina (tumors, fluid accumulation, etc.). The term "retinal detachment" includes detachment of the pigmented epithelium from the Bruch's membrane (Atlas 2009).

There are hemorrhagic (more common) and non-hemorrhagic retinal detachments, depending on the composition of the fluid. Non-hemorrhagic retinal detachment is caused by the penetration of the fluid of abnormally constricted retinal vessels. Non-hemorrhagic retinal detachment is often secondary to and occurs due to tumors (usually with melanoma, metastases, hemangiomas, or retinoblastomas). Also, non-hemorrhagic retinal detachment can occur due to inflammation and Coats's disease. Hemorrhagic retinal detachment occurs because of degeneration, retinal damage due to fibrosis or the eyeball hardening as a result of an injury. Spontaneous retinal detachment is extremely rare (0.00001%) (Atlas 2009).

Clinical Manifestations Partial loss of vision, occurrence of a veil before the eyes, turbid tears, low intraocular pressure. Flashes in the form of sparks and lightings also represent a typical sign of retinal detachment.

Distortion of letters, objects, loss of their separate parts from the visual field indicates that retinal detachment involves the retinal center.

Diagnosis On CT, hemorrhagic retinal detachment without contrast enhancement looks like a hyperdense lenticular area. MR studies require contrast enhancement. MR symptoms vary depending upon the composition of the fluid that caused the retinal detachment (the presence of hemorrhagic inclusions and proteins with different magnetic properties enhances the T1-weighted MR signal). Accumulation of the contrast agent in case of retinal detachment is V-shaped with a tip near the optic nerve on the inner surface of the fundus. Non-hemorrhagic retinal detachment presents as fluid with hypointense inclusions. In chronic retinal detachment, T1 and T2 shortening is observed due to an increased content of protein and blood in the fluid, which is accompanied by an MR signal reduction on T2-weighted sequences and an MR signal increase on T1-weighted sequences (Fig. 6.9).

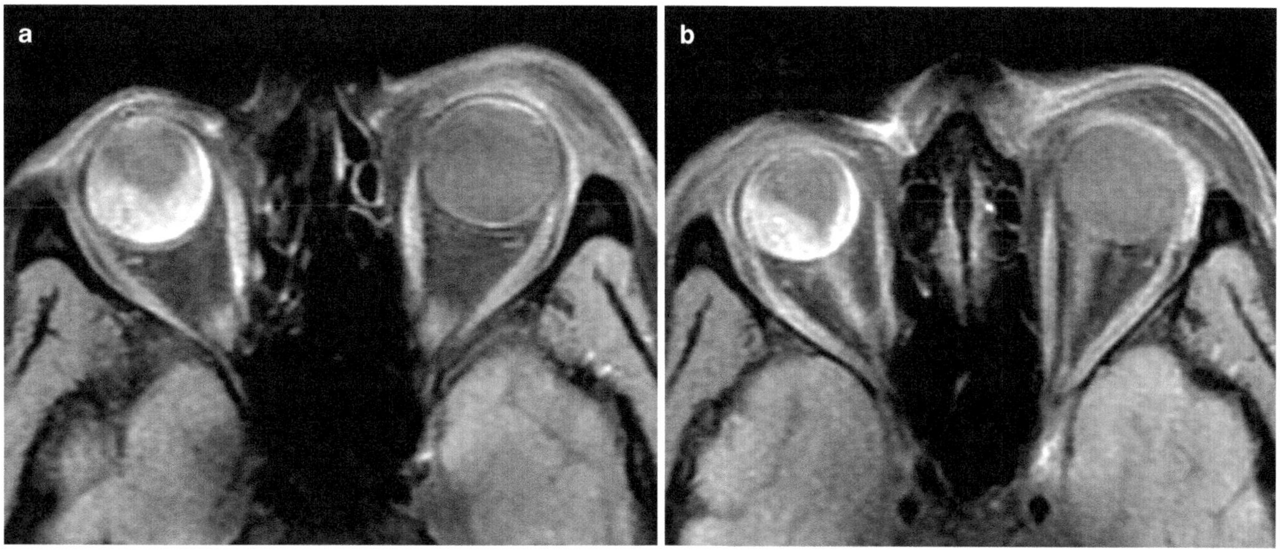

Fig. 6.9 Retinal detachment of rightwards. Series of T1-weighted MR images with Fat-Sat technology (**a**–**c**) as well as T2-FLAIR MR images (**d**–**f**) show a detached retina with typical V-shaped configuration and associated with presence of blood products (hyperintense MR-signal) in subretinal space

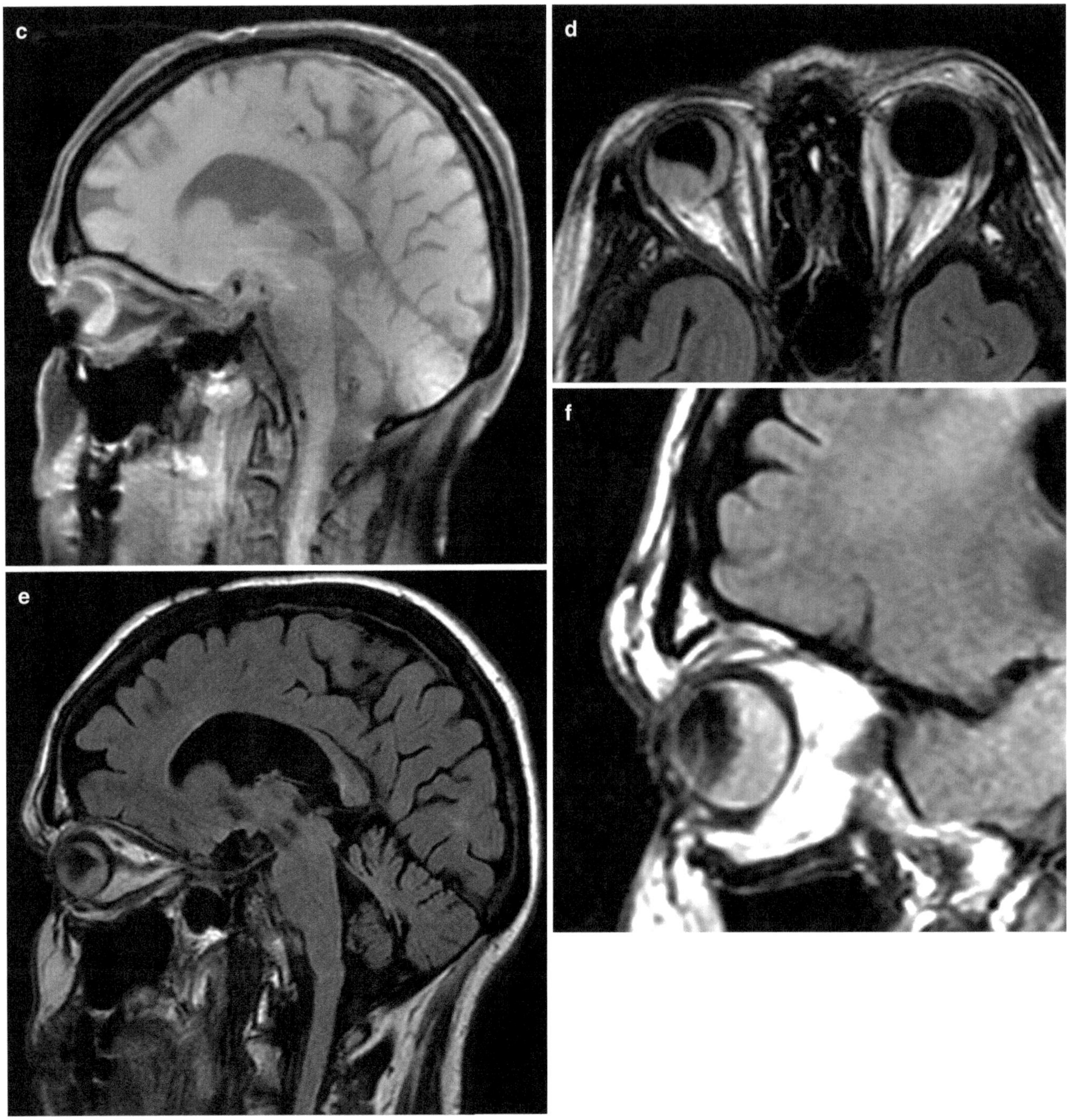

Fig. 6.9 (continued)

Tumors Involving the Orbit

7

Contents

7.1 Benign Tumors

Meningioma Primary orbital meningiomas are rare (Cherekayev et al. 1998; Ulivieri et al. 2001). Tumors penetrating into the orbit through the optic nerve channel from the cranial cavity or directly through the bone wall are diagnosed more frequently. As a rule, meningiomas of the sphenoid bone wing, cavernous sinus, sellar region grow into the orbit. Meningiomas are more common in middle aged and elderly women (2:1). Meningiomas generally constitute up to 26% of primary intracranial tumors. Among patients with unilateral exophthalmos, it is caused by meningiomas in 19% of cases (Ulivieri et al. 2001).

Clinical manifestations of the disease vary depending on the tumor expansion. The most typical are unilateral exophthalmos, decreased visual acuity, loss of visual fields predominantly of inferior halves. Occurrence of diplopia and restrictions of the eyeball movements due to lesions of nerves III, IV, VI indicate that the tumor spread to the area the superior orbital fissure or the cavernous sinus (Gabibov 1993).

Diagnosis In most cases (up to 75%), meningiomas have initially a varying degree of hyperdense characteristics on orbital CT. They are easily identified on the background of the orbital bone and fat structures, a dislocation of the extraocular muscles being quite clearly detected. The presence of calcifications is not an uncommon characteristic of the tumor. But most meningiomas growing into the orbital cavity cause hyperostotic changes to the bone structures (the greater wing of the sphenoid bone, the roof, and the medial wall of the orbit). Intravenous contrast enhancement facilitates a more precise differentiation of well-enhanced soft tissue component from the surrounding intra- and extraorbital structures. CT-perfusion imaging always reveals high CBV, CBF values. In most cases, MTT values are also increased in comparison with the white matter of the brain. Using a perfusion technique for meningiomas growing into the orbital cavity has become helpful in identifying the areas of invasion of the orbital walls and adjacent structures, such as muscles and the optic nerve (Fig. 7.1).

I. Pronin, V. Kornienko, *CT and MRI of Skull Base Lesions*, https://doi.org/10.1007/978-3-319-65957-2_7

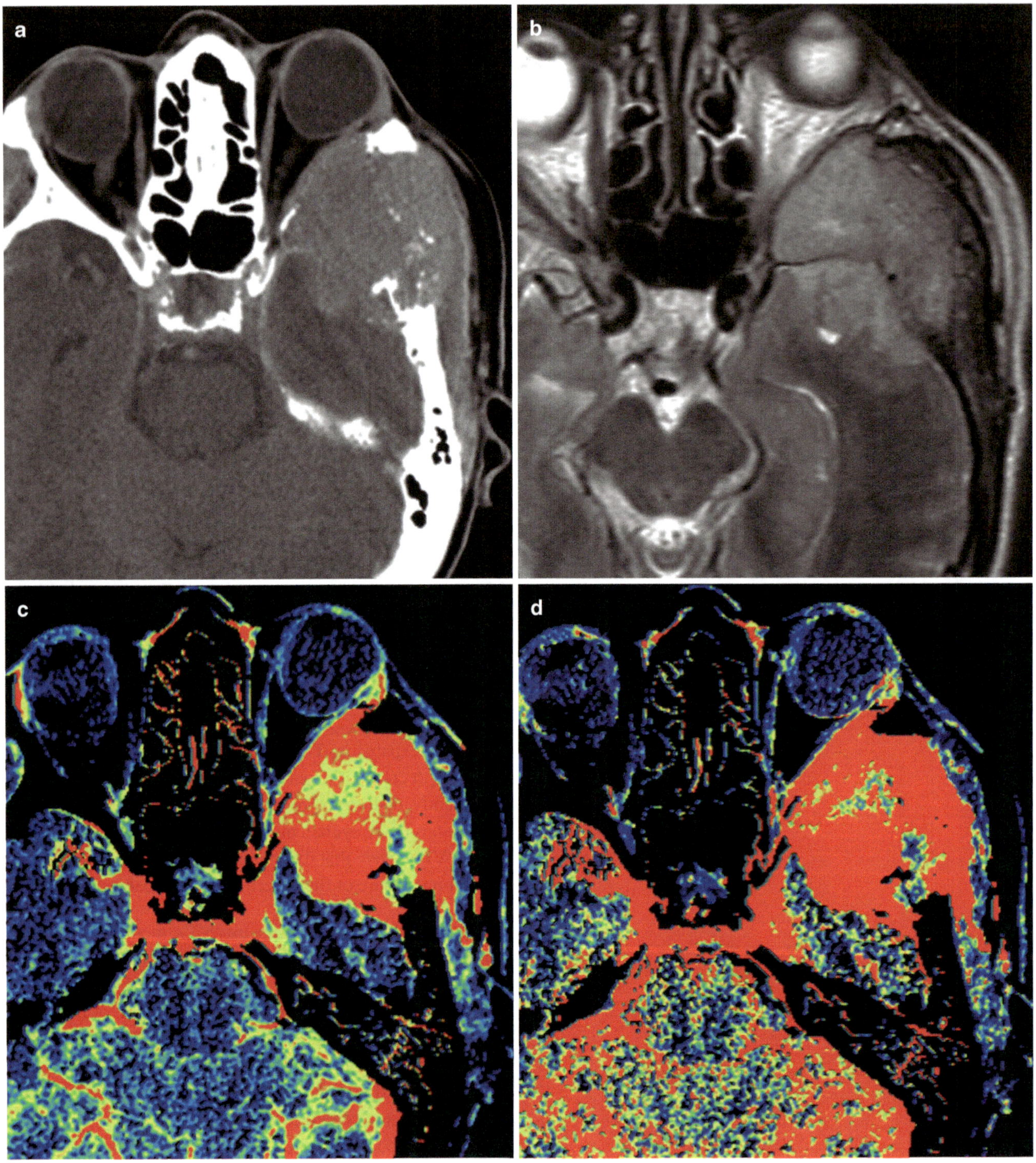

Fig. 7.1 Meningioma of the pterional region. Axial CT scan (**a**) demonstrates a large tumor of pterional region with lateral orbital bone wall destruction. On T2-weighted MRI (**b**) a mass shows hypointense MR-signal with spreading intracranially and into subtemporal fossa. There is left side proptosis due to tumor invasion of the orbit. CT-perfusion CBV (**c**) and CBF (**d**) maps demonstrate the high hemodynamic parameters of the tumor with MTT (**e**) prolongation as well. DSA revealed the prominent blood supply from (**a**) meningea media and other branches of external carotid artery (**f**)

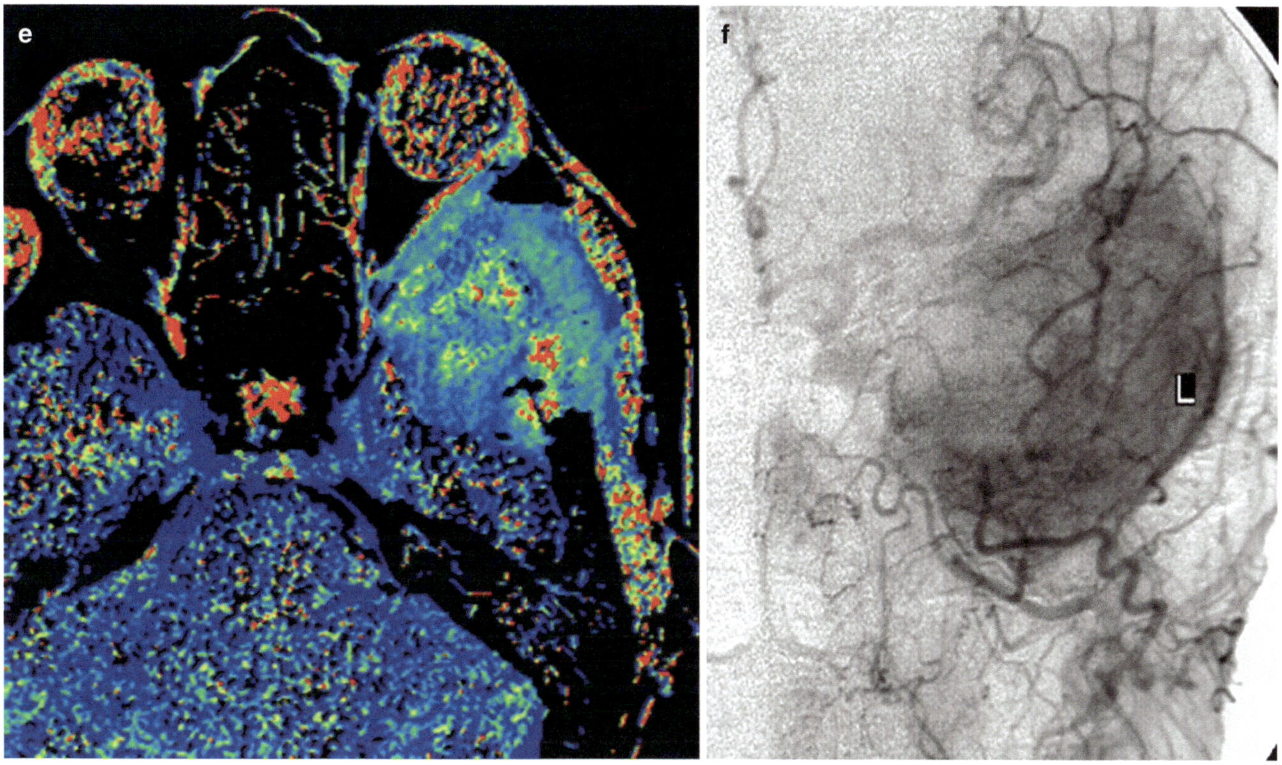

Fig. 7.1 (continued)

MR-characteristics of orbital meningioma are no different from those observed in meningiomas of the cranial cavity. On T1-weighted images, they usually are isointense to rectus muscle. MR-signal on T2-weighted images varies from iso- to slightly hyperintense. Hyperostosis is worse verifiable than on CT. However, the use of contrast enhancement with MR Fat-Sat techniques ranks MRI above CT, especially in imaging of the spreading of the lesion through the structures inside the orbit, penetration of the tumor into the cavernous sinus, and enclosing of the ICA siphon (Fig. 7.2). Selective direct angiography allows evaluating the degree of involvement of the major vessels, as well as the pattern of tumor vascularization, better than CT and MRI. However, the latter statement has been currently challenged in the study in the magnetic field of 3.0 T and application of new angiography protocols.

Differential diagnosis is carried out with fibrous osteodysplasia, osteoma, intraosseous hemangioma.

Orbital osteoma is a slowly growing benign primary bone tumor that predominantly affects the craniofacial area. It is quite specific for membranous bones (bones developing from the mesenchymal tissue) of the face and skull. The predominant lesion site in the orbit is the suture between the bones of the ethmoid and frontal sinuses in the anterior upper nasal portion of the orbit. These tumors are divided into three types: ivory, mature, and fibrous osteoma, depending on the histologic proportions of the bone. Osteoma pathogenesis is unknown.

Histologically, osteoma consists of misplaced bone plates, sometimes bordered by osteoblasts; intercostal spaces can be highly vascularized and consist of cellular or fibrous stroma, fibrovascular or adipose tissue, which may sometimes be interpreted as osteosarcoma (Wenig et al. 1988).

According to Atlas (2009), osteomas amount from up to 7% of the total number of orbital tumors. The age of patients ranges from 12 to 70 years old. Men are affected more often. According to most authors, both orbits are affected with the same frequency. Osteoma is usually asymptomatic and is discovered by chance, with patient noticing facial distortion, headache.

Diagnosis A solid, dense form of orbital osteoma contrasts well with the surrounding bone on standard craniograms and is more precisely demarcated by hypodense contents of the orbit on CT. The tumor has the bone density (Fig. 7.3). Tumor borders may be smooth in some cases and irregular and bulging in others, less frequently they have a pedicle or a mushroom shape. The latter is more common for tumors originating from the ethmoid and maxillary sinuses. A pronounced sclerotic type of fibrous dysplasia can mimic osteoma density on CT, but in such cases the CT bone mode may reveal slightly lower density, structural transparency in the inner part of fibrous dysplasia. On MRI, there is a marked hypointense (identical to the cortical bone) signal in all sequences.

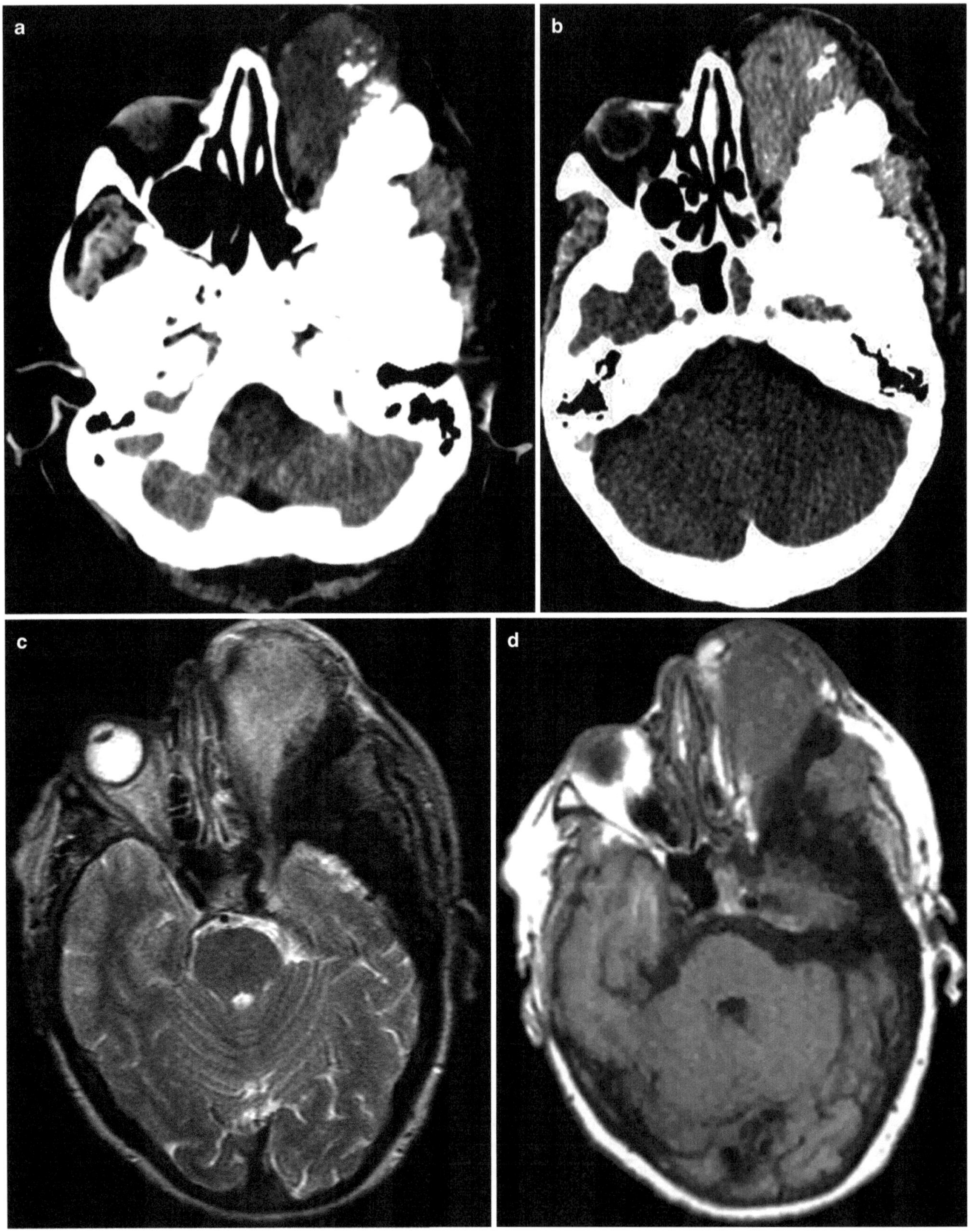

Fig. 7.2 Meningioma of the left orbit. Axial CT scans (**a**, **b**) demonstrate a large tumor with marked hyperostosis of the superior wing of sphenoid bone as well as temporal bone with soft tumor tissue within the left orbit cavity. The tumor intensively accumulates contrast agent. Soft tissue component of the meningioma is clearly visible on T2- (**c**), T1- (**d**) weighted images. The hyperostotic background changes have dark MR-signal. Widespreading of the meningioma can be seen better after intravenous contrast enhancement (**e**, **f**)

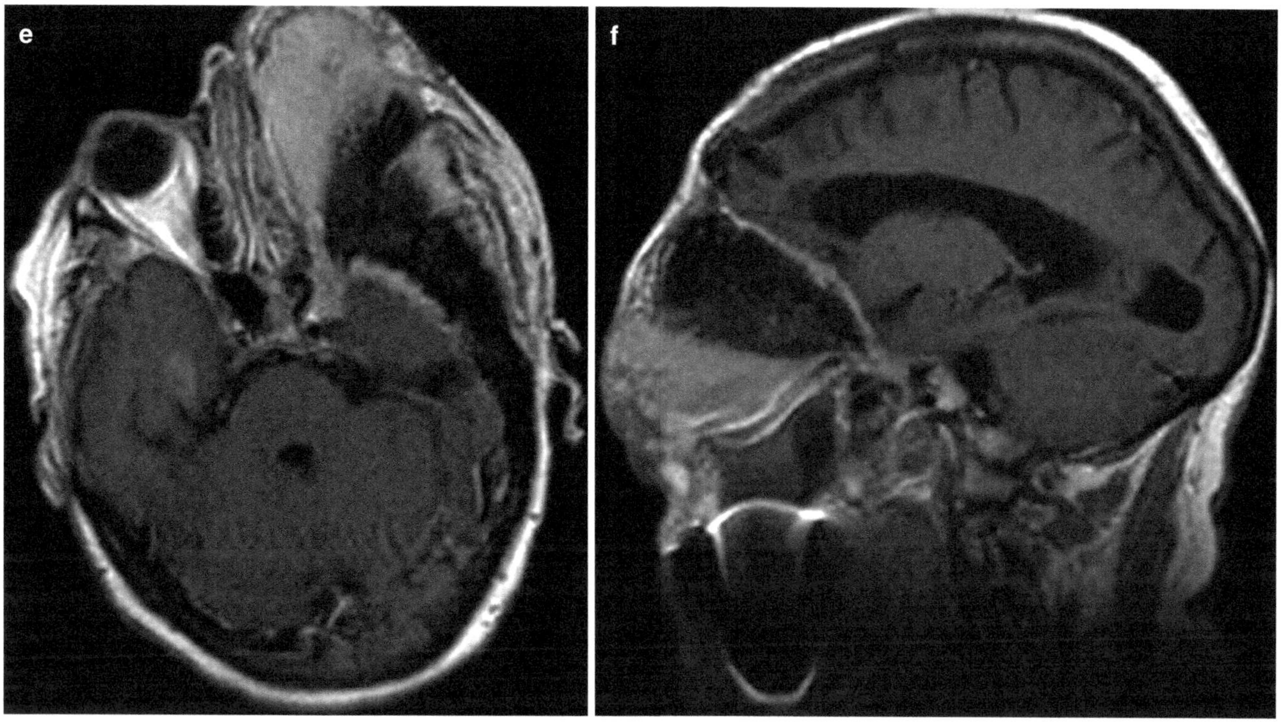

Fig. 7.2 (continued)

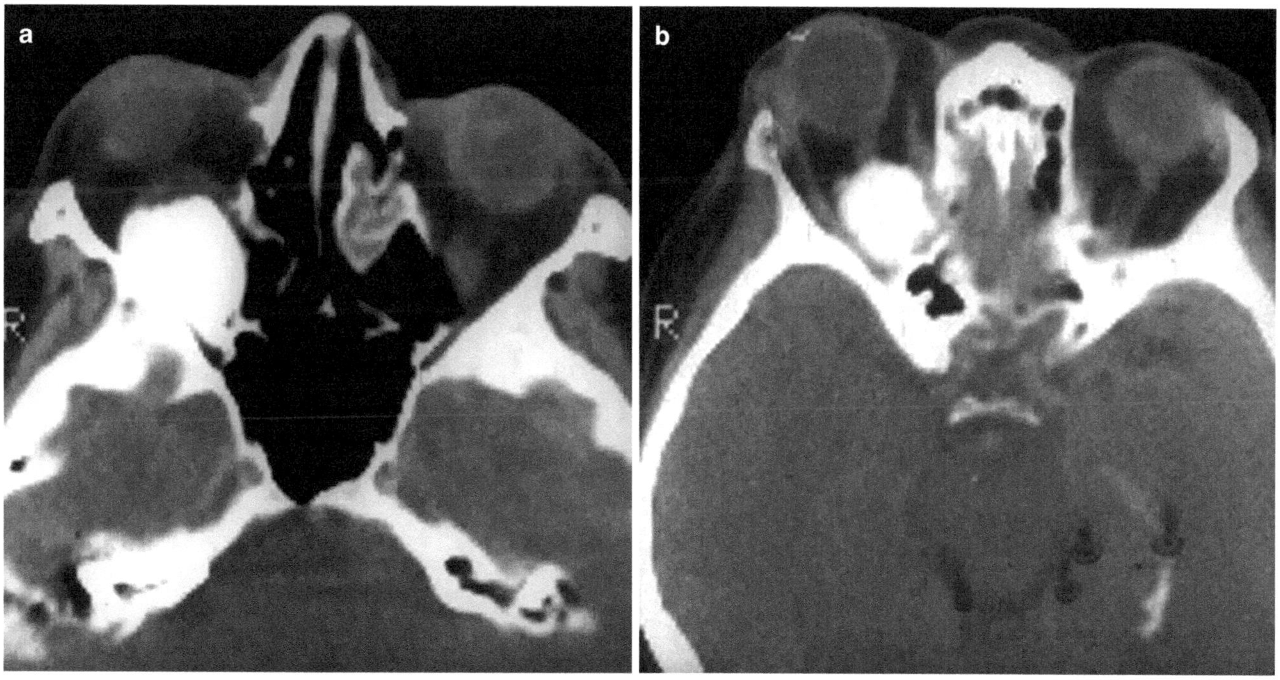

Fig. 7.3 Osteoma. CT scans in axial (**a**, **b**) and coronal planes (**c**, **d**) demonstrate hyperdense (which density is equal to bone) lesion within the right orbit without soft tissue component. There is a small right-side proptosis. T2 (**e**)- and T1 (**f**)- weighted MRI shows a hypointense mass in the apex of the right orbit

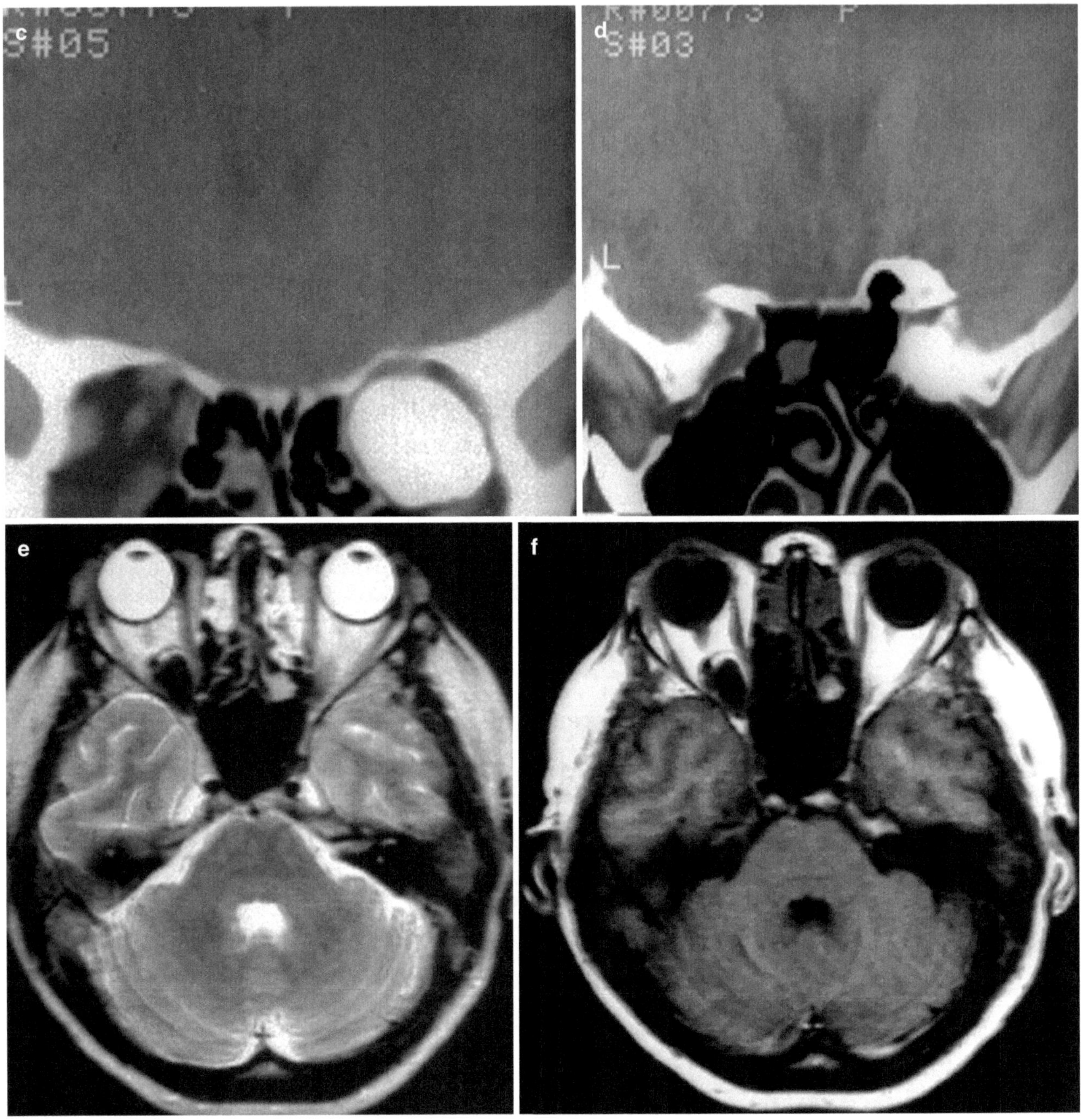

Fig. 7.3 (continued)

Differential diagnosis Ossifying fibromas, fibrous dysplasia, calcified meningioma.

7.2 Malignant Tumors

Cancer and Metastases Among malignant tumors growing into the orbit, the most common are primary cancer (squamous cell carcinoma and others) and metastases (Huh and Beverly 2006). Tumors can grow into the orbit from the adjacent areas: paranasal sinuses, wings of the sphenoid bone, chiasm-sellar area. They tend to cause destruction of the orbital walls, compression of its contents with further development of exophthalmos. Metastasis can affect the orbital muscles only (Gupta et al. 2011).

CT and MRI characteristics are nonspecific and not always depend on histology. Common diagnostic sings of these lesions include the presence of a solid soft tissue component, which is intensely enhanced after intravenous administration of the contrast agent, and extensive destruction of the bone structures (Demirci 2002). Helpful in the differential diagnosis is the use of CT-perfusion studies. Hemodynamic characteristics of tumors exhibit, in most cases, a varying degree of CBF, CBV elevation, as well as prolongation of mean transit time (MTT). The latter parameter has a certain dependence on the histological structure of the primary tumor (Figs. 7.4, 7.5, 7.6, 7.7, and 7.8).

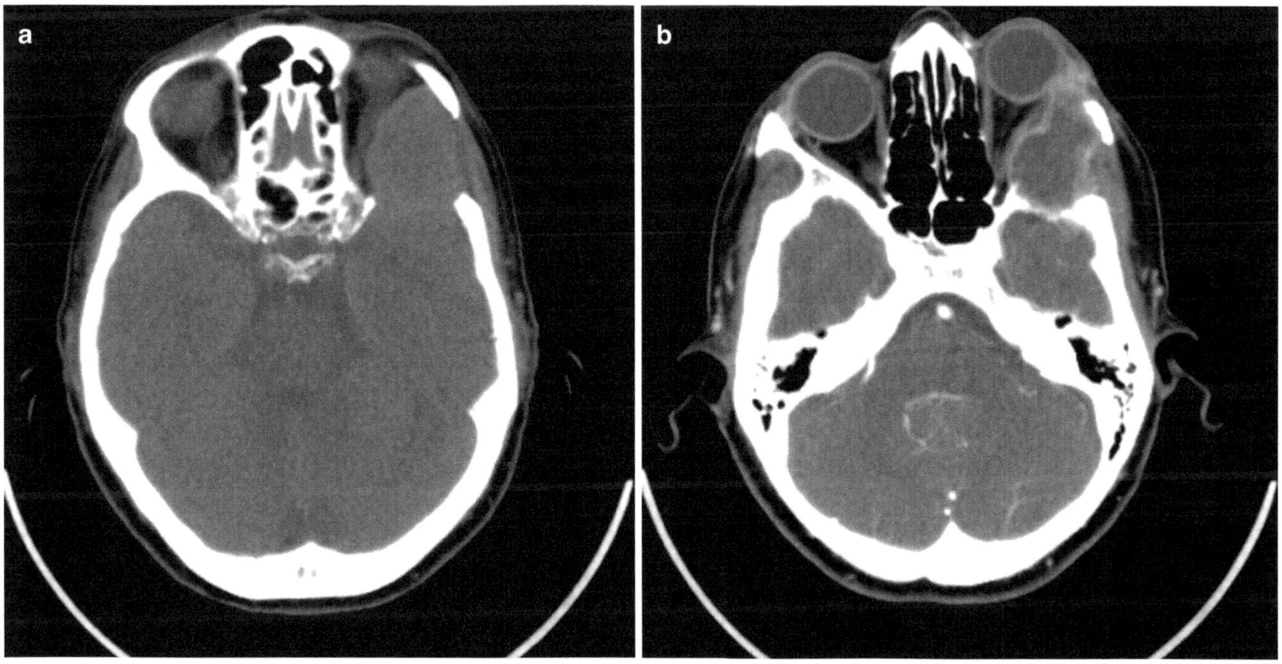

Fig. 7.4 Cancer of the left pterional region. Axial CT scans before (**a**) and after (**b**, **c**) contrast enhancement demonstrate a heterogeneous tumor of the left pterional region with lateral orbital wall destruction and lacrimal gland involvement. Post-contrast CT shows a peripheral pattern of contrast enhancement due to central part necrosis. There is a left-side proptosis. CT-perfusion CBV (**d**) and CBF (**e**) maps demonstrate an elevation of perfusion parameters in the peripheral parts of the tumor with MTT (**f**) prolongation through the whole cancer structure

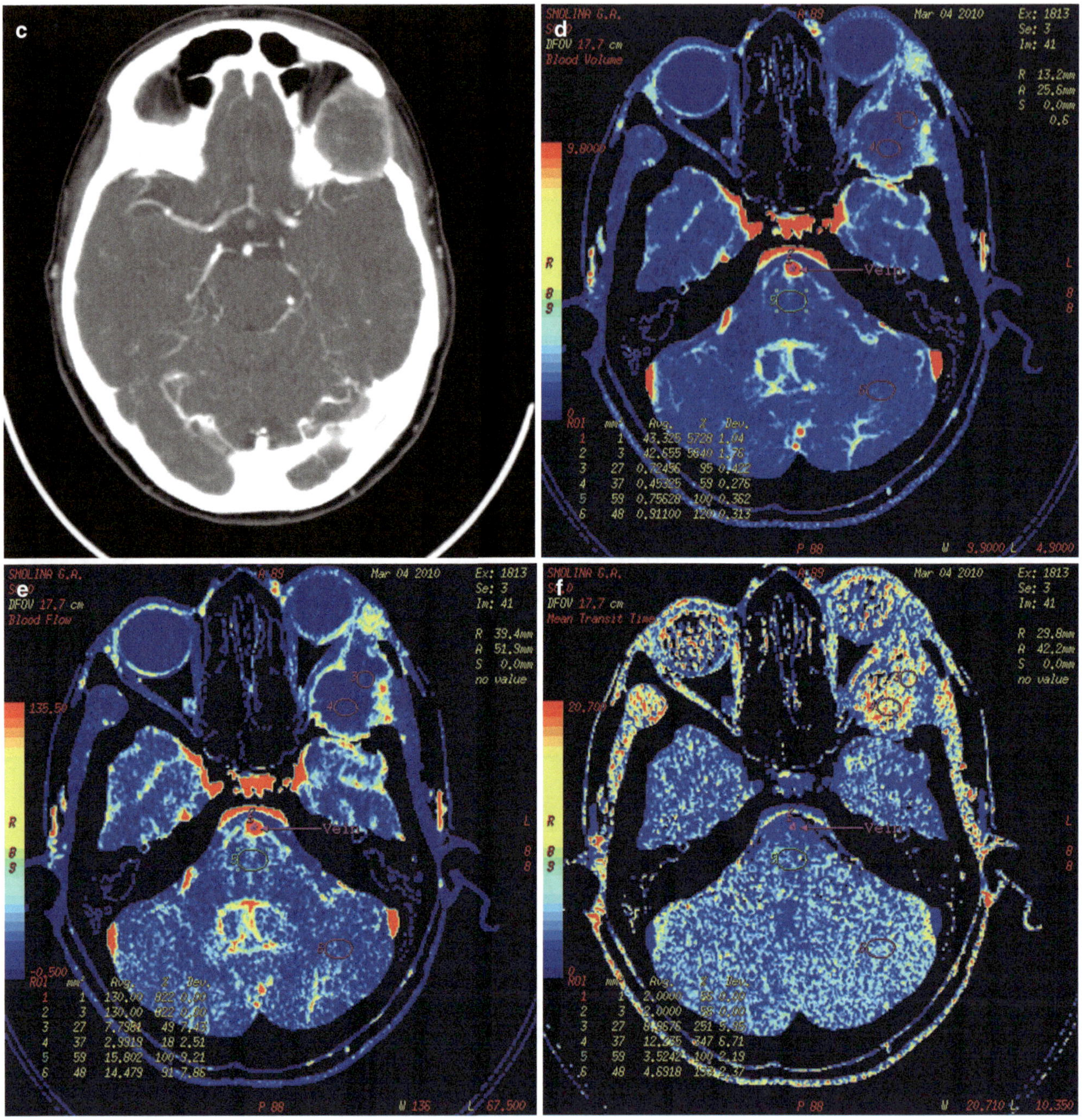

Fig. 7.4 (continued)

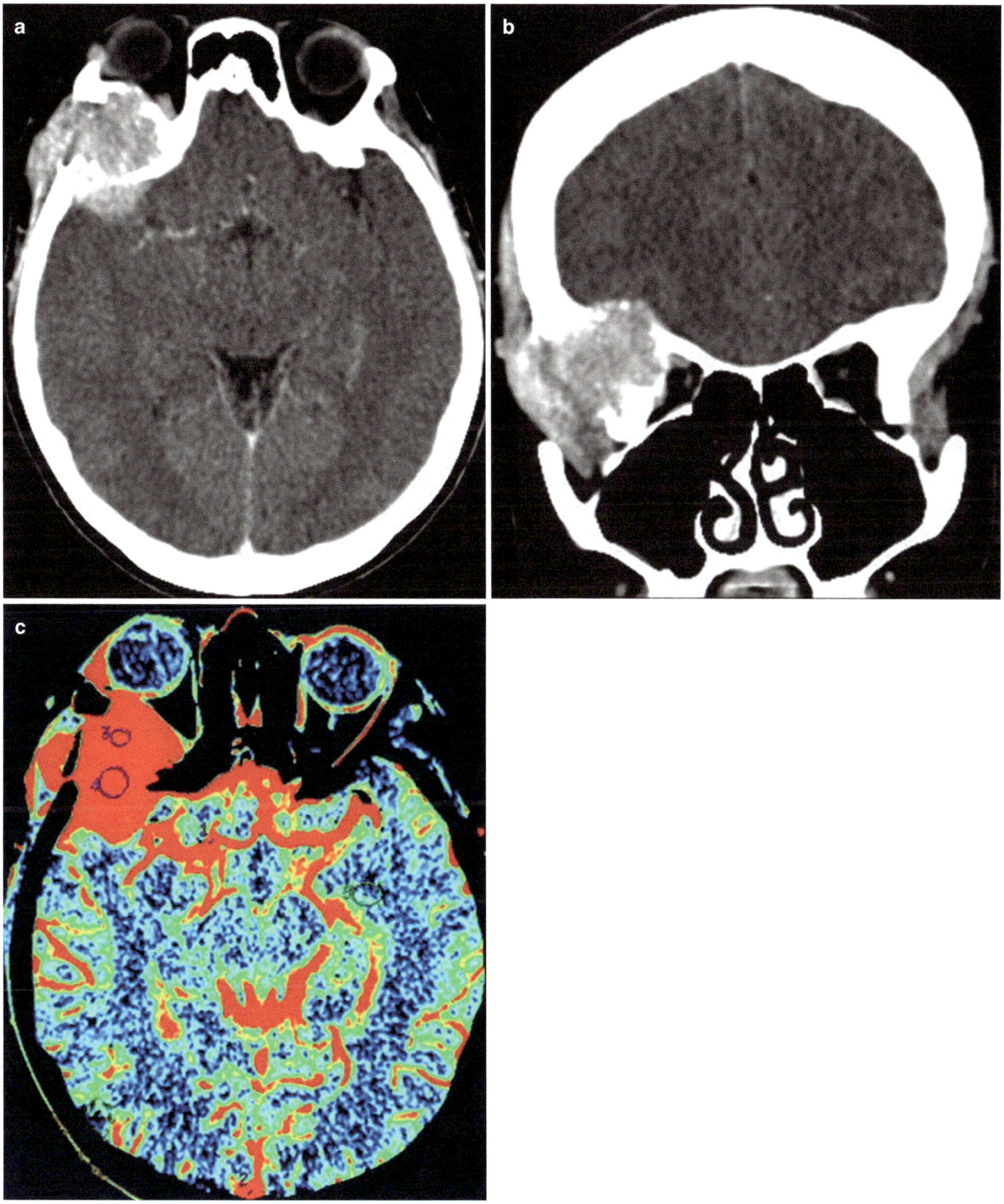

Fig. 7.5 Cancer of the right pterional region. Axial (**a**) and coronal (**b**) CT scans with contrast enhancement show a large enhanced mass with bone destruction and lateral aspects of the orbit involvement. The tumor is characterized by the high values of tumor blood flow on CT-perfusion CBF-map (**c**)

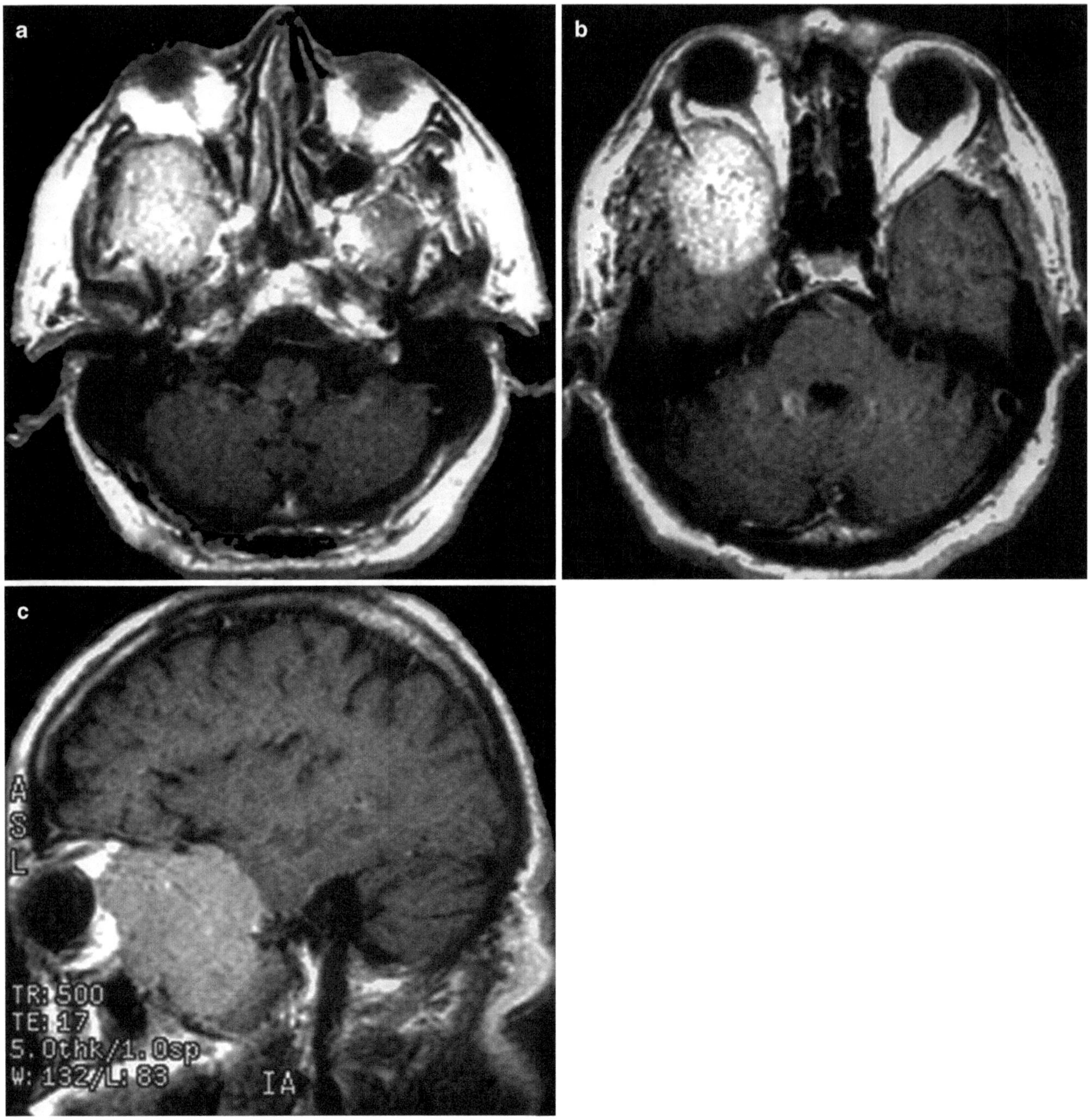

Fig. 7.6 Metastases of thyroid gland cancer. T1-weighted MR images with contrast enhancement in axial (**a**, **b**) and sagittal (**c**) planes demonstrate a space occupied enhanced lesion with involvement of right side skull base structures and spreading into the lateral part of the orbit

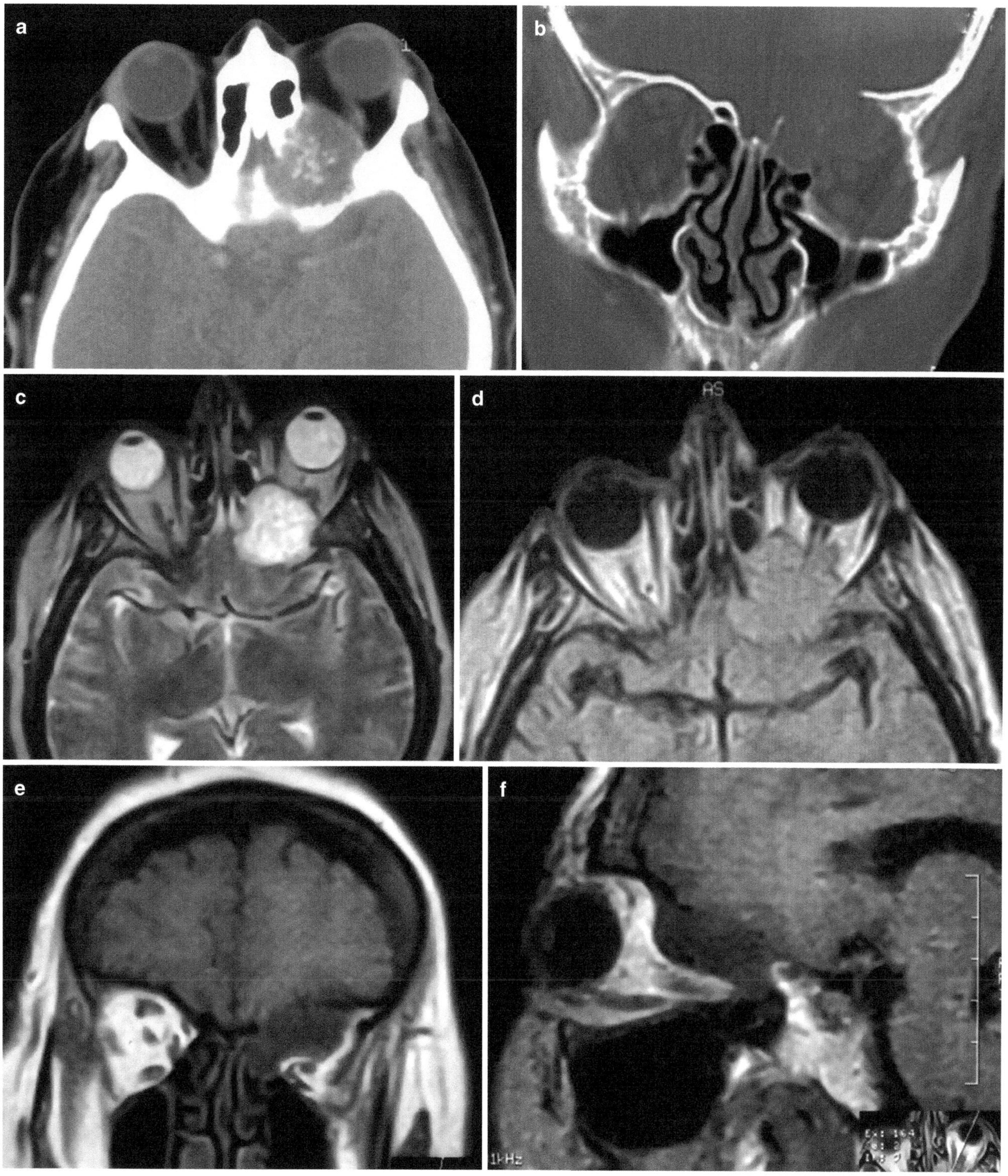

Fig. 7.7 Metastases of breast cancer. CT scans in axial (**a**) and coronal (**b**) planes detect a soft tissue tumor with calcifications in the central parts with wide destruction of the superior orbital wall. The tumor is visible better on T2- (**c**) than on T2-FLAIR- (**d**) weighted MR images due to hyperintense MR-signal. T1-weighted MR images in coronal (**e**) and sagittal (**f**) projections clearly delineate the tumor margins due to hypointense MR-signal from the tumor tissue on the background the high signal from the orbital fat

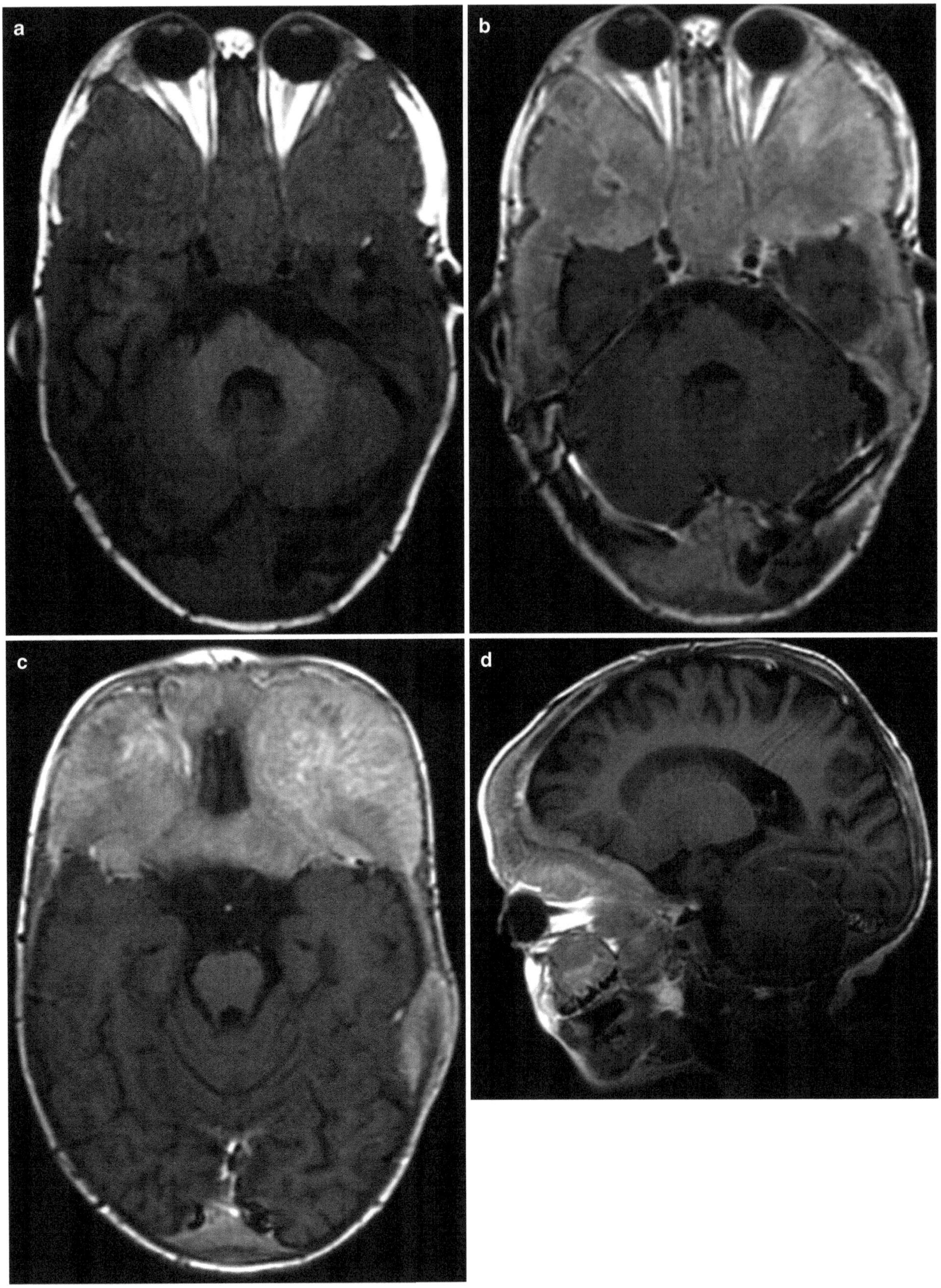

Fig. 7.8 Metastatic neuroblastoma. Bilateral soft tissue involvement of the calvaria, skull base, and craniofacial region is clearly visible on axial T1- before (**a**) and multiplanar post-contrast T1-weighted (**b**–**f**) MRI. There is an orbital structures compression. The pathologic tissue intensively accumulates contrast agent

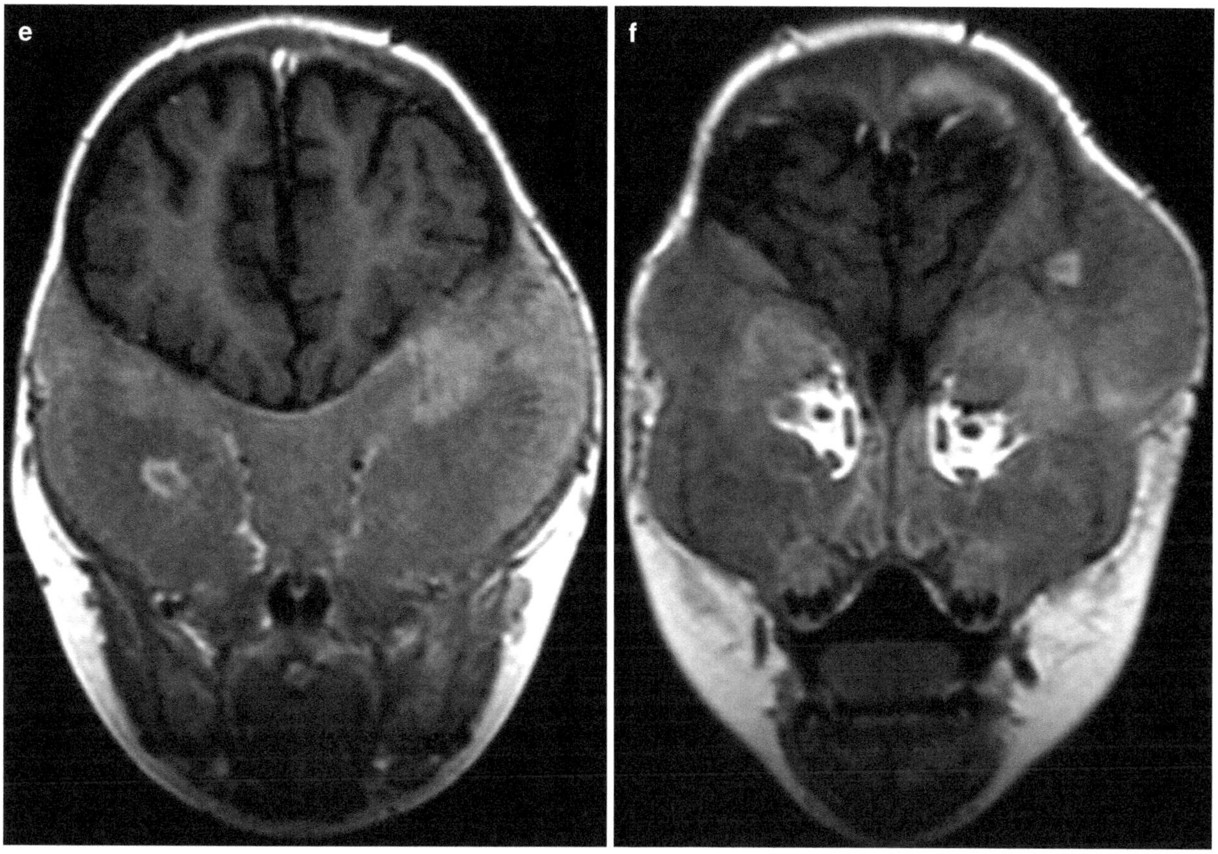

Fig. 7.8 (continued)

Presentation of Rare Cases of Orbital Disorders

8

Contents

I. Pronin, V. Kornienko, *CT and MRI of Skull Base Lesions*, https://doi.org/10.1007/978-3-319-65957-2_8

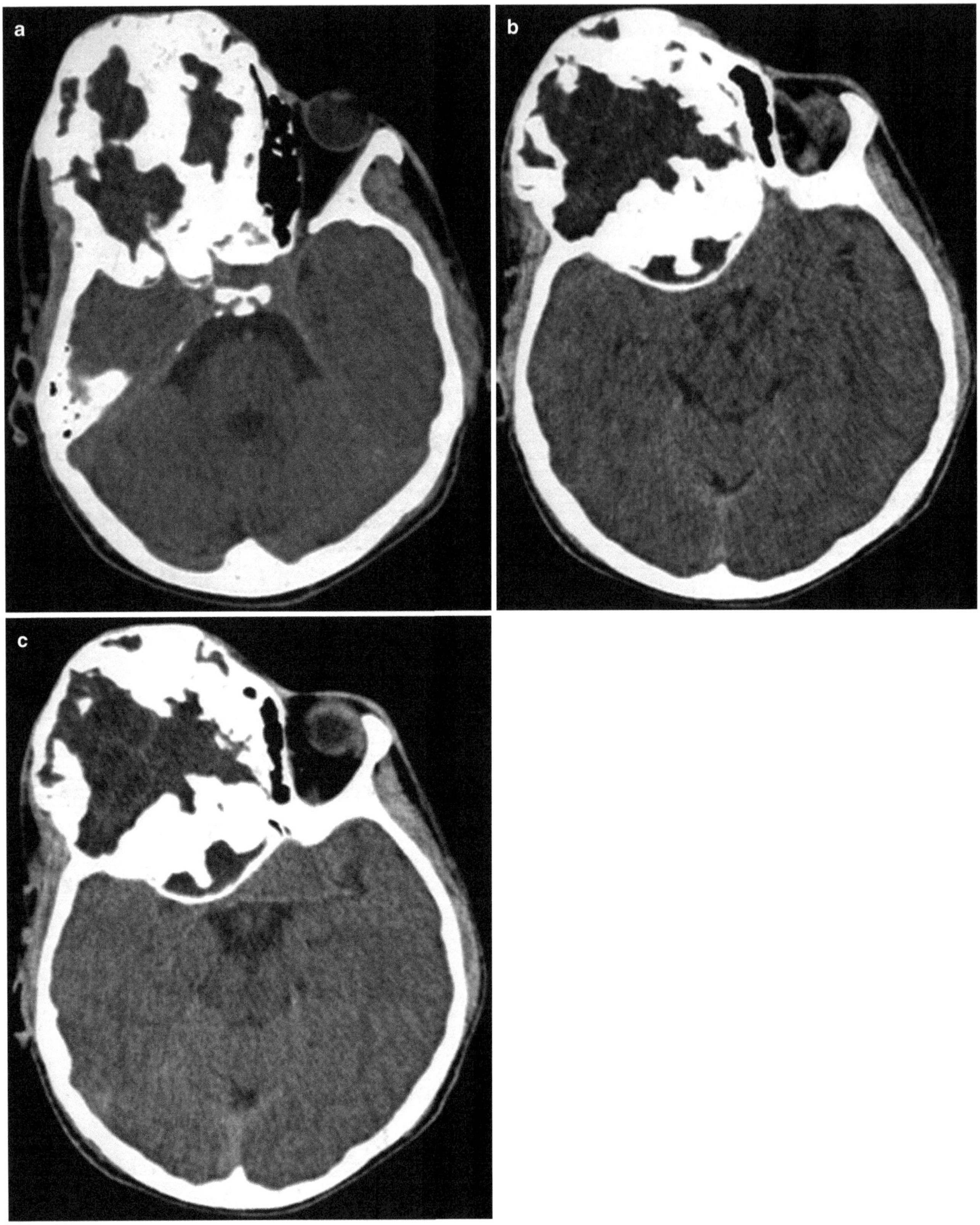

Fig. 8.1 Fibrous osteodysplasia. Axial CT scans (**a**–**c**) demonstrate a large mass of craniofacial region with the right orbit involvement, which contains as bone structures as soft tissue component. (**d**)—histological specimen with typical for fibrous osteodysplasia pattern

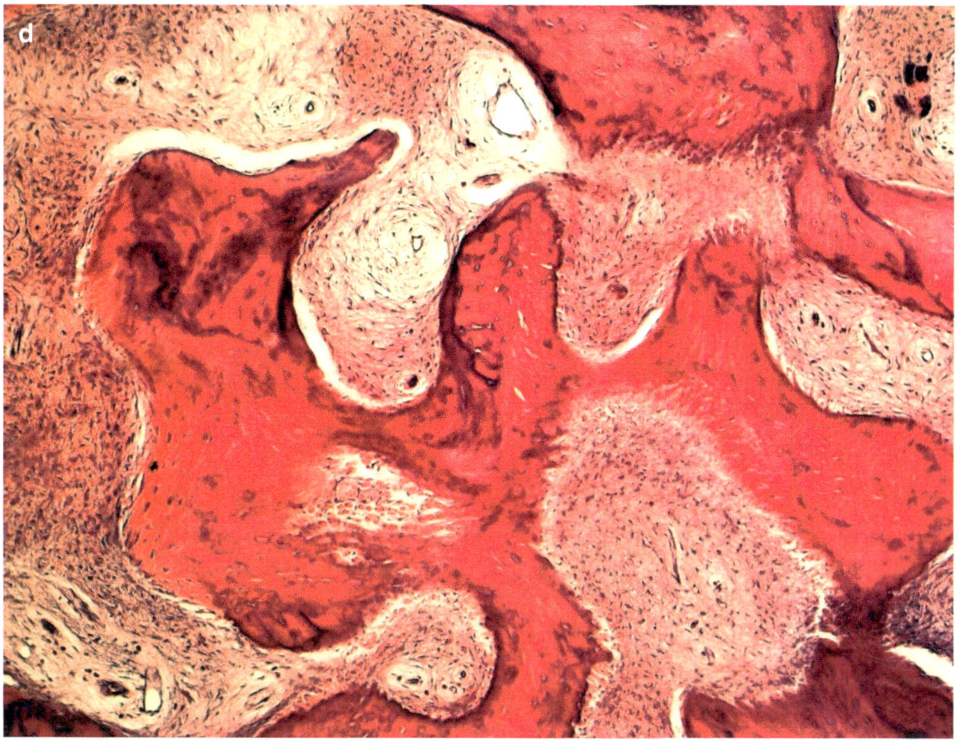

Fig. 8.1 (continued)

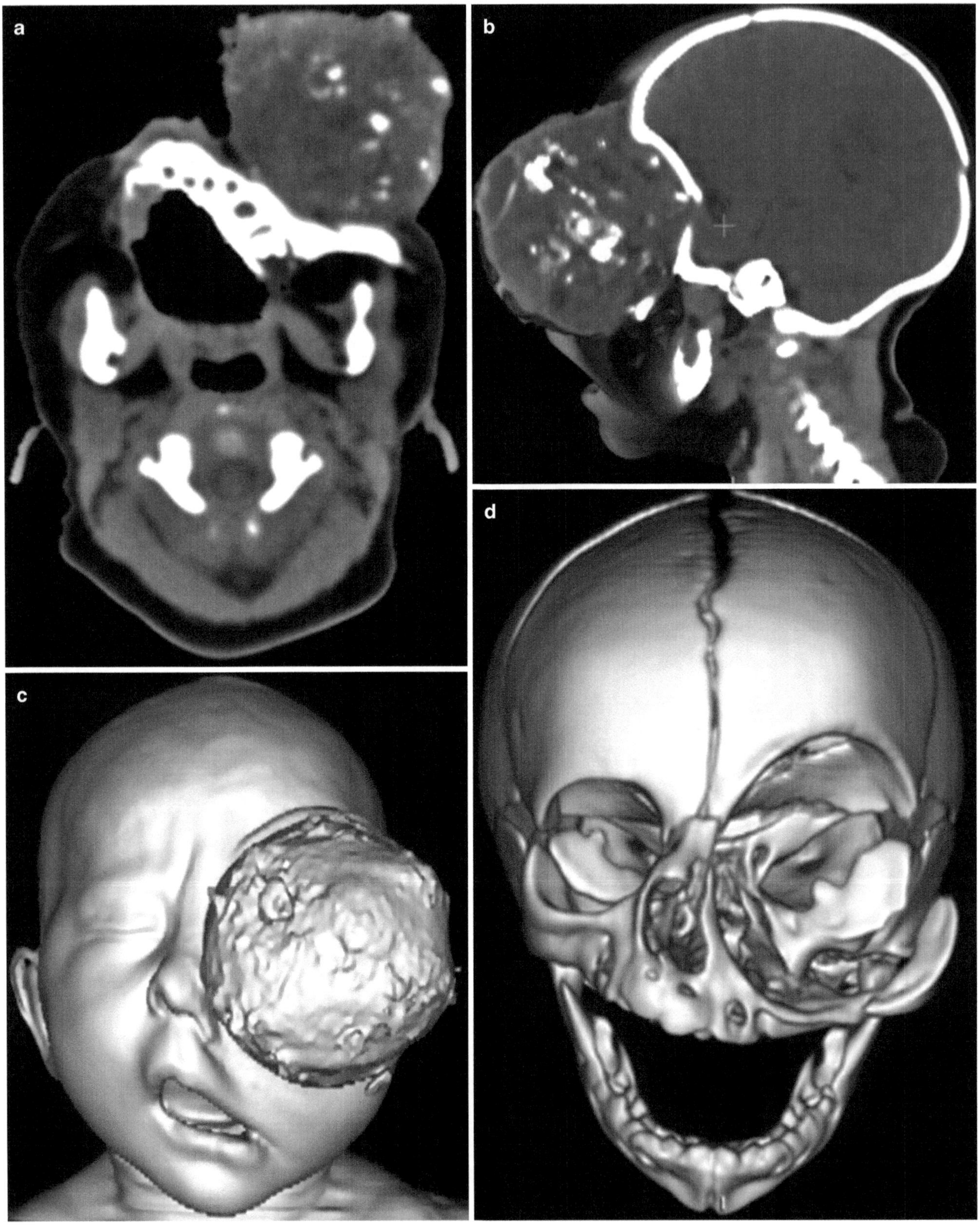

Fig. 8.2 Teratoma of the left orbit. CT scans in axial (**a**) and sagittal (**b**) planes and after 3D reconstruction (**c**, **d**) demonstrate a large intra-extraorbital tumor with multiple calcifications. There is a deformation of the orbital bones due to tumor. The tumor has heterogeneous structure and contrast enhancement. T2-weighted MR images in axial (**e**) and sagittal (**f**) planes show the predominantly hypointense mass with multiple cystic formations. Deformed globe can be clearly visible with its anterior displacement (**e**). The tumor demonstrates the heterogeneous contrast enhancement (**g**, **h**, **i**)

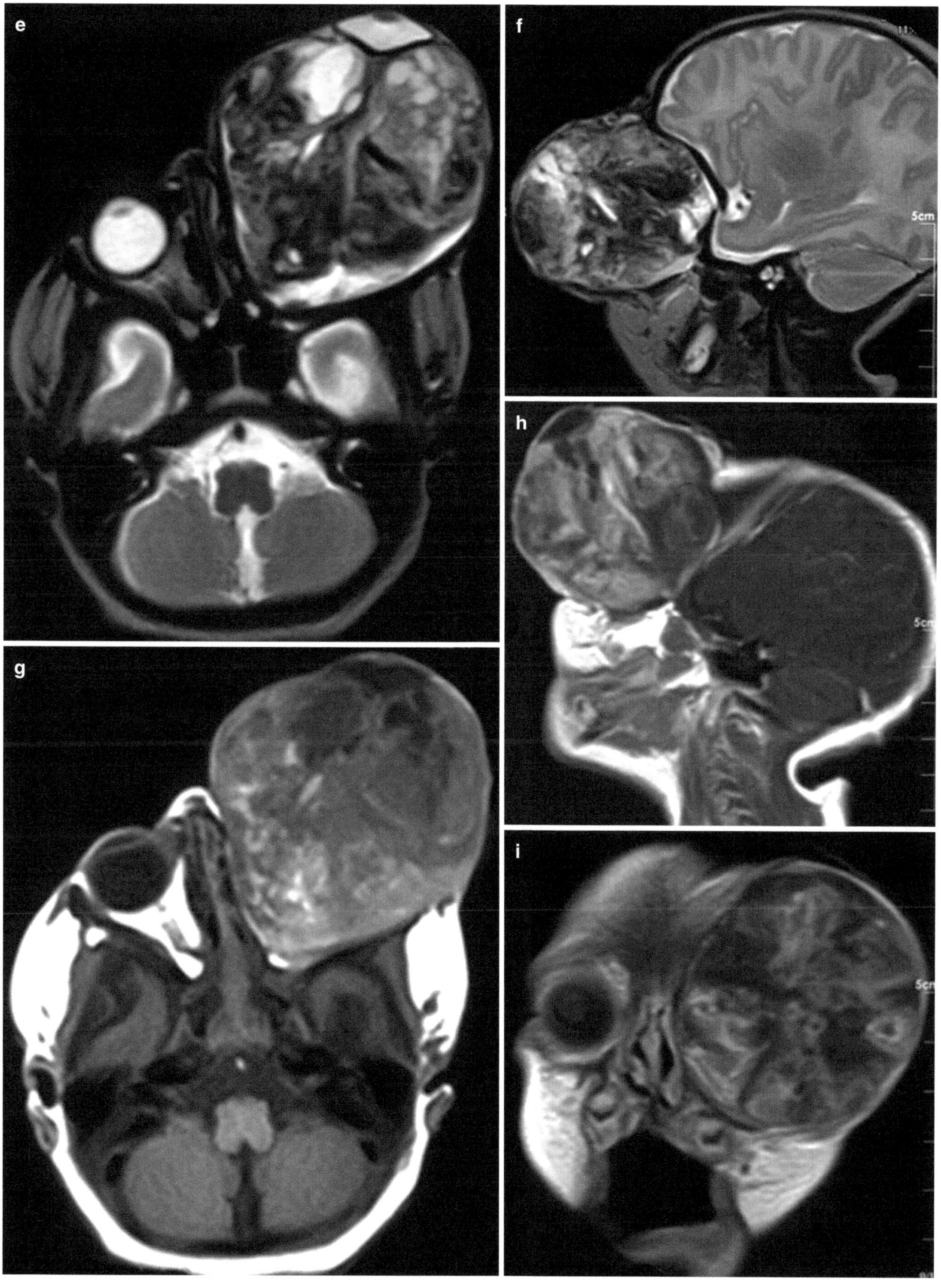

Fig. 8.2 (continued)

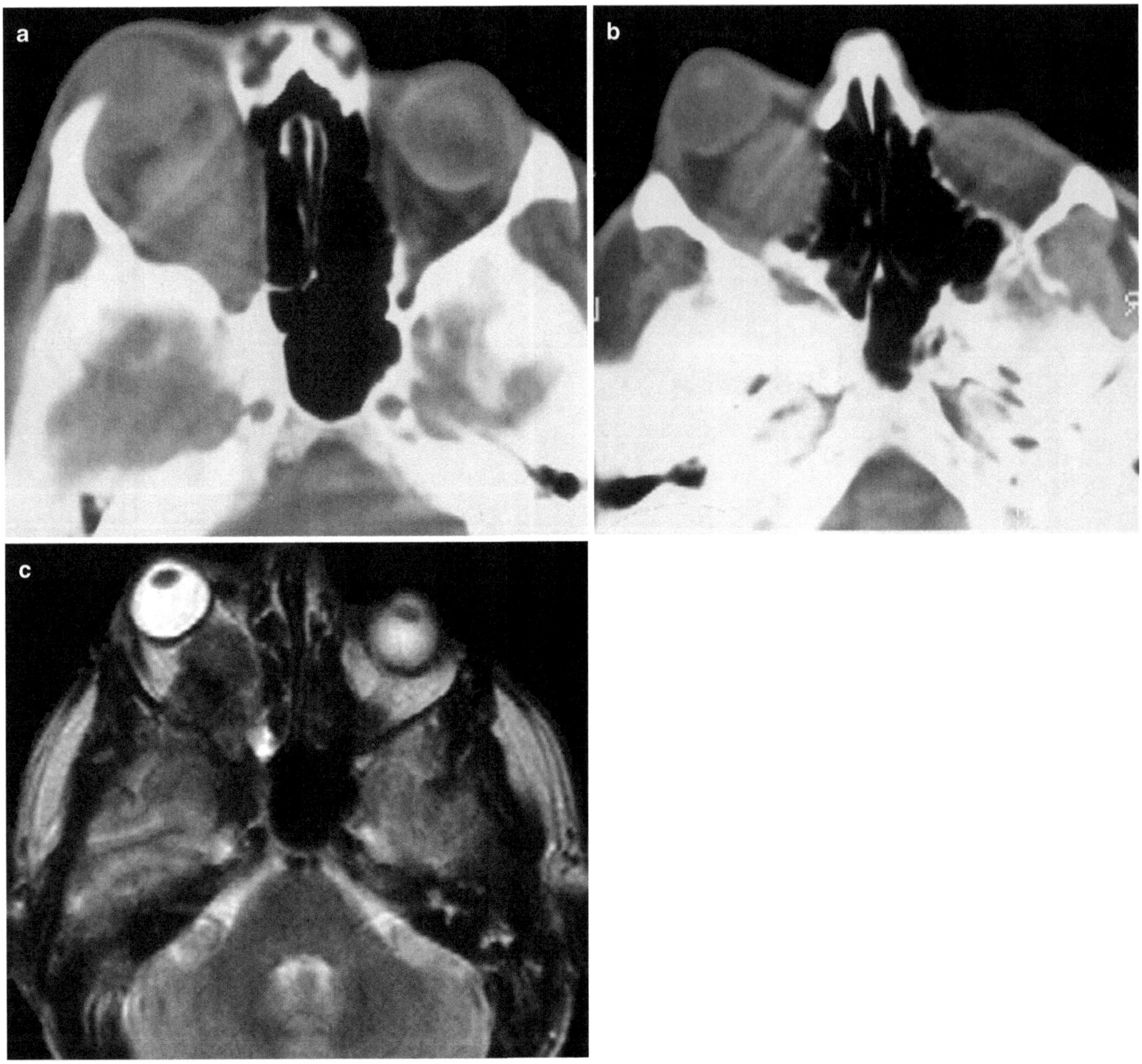

Fig. 8.3 Melanoma. Axial CT scans (**a**, **b**) demonstrate a retrobulbar mass with right side proptosis. On T2-weighted axial MRI (**c**) the dark MR-signal typical for blood products (or/and melanin) can be seen within the orbital tumor

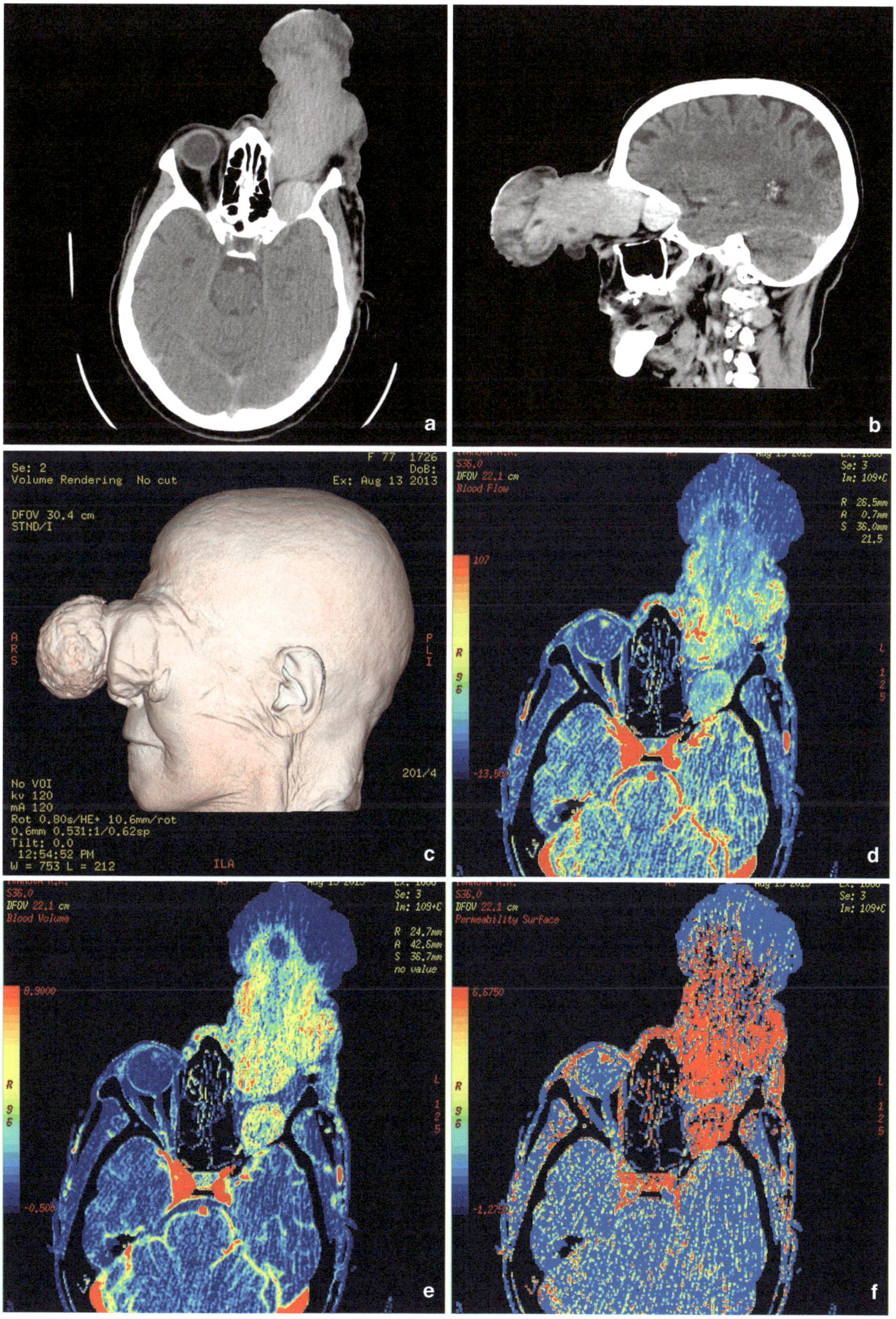

Fig. 8.4 Hemangiopericytoma of the left orbit. Axial CT scan (**a**) and sagittal reformat (**b**) as well as 3D reconstruction (**c**) show a huge intra-extraorbital mass with heterogeneous and intensive contrast enhancement. The tumor demonstrates the high values of CT-perfusion parameters with the use of CBF (**d**), CBV (**e**) and permeability (**f**) mapping

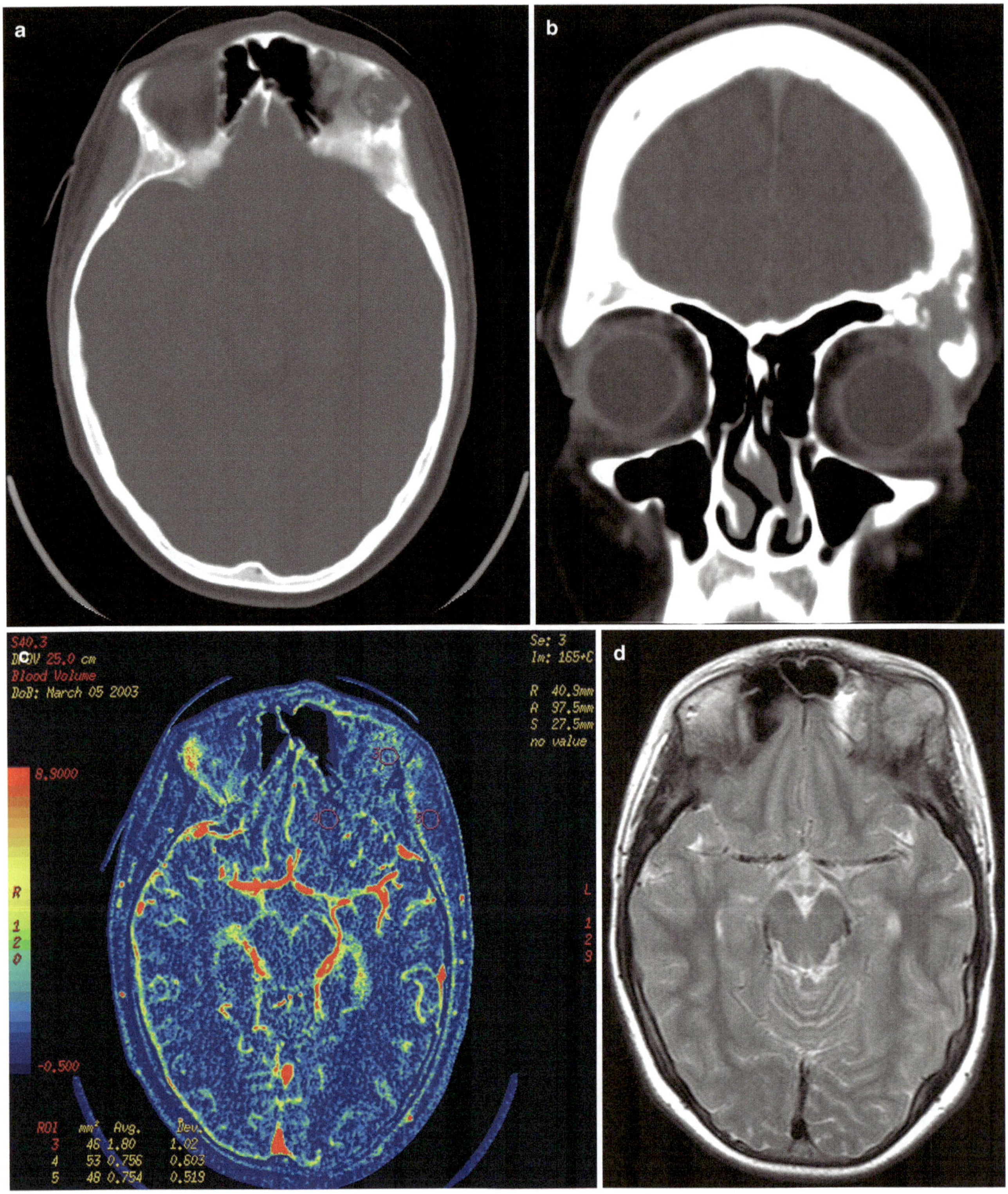

Fig. 8.5 Eosinophilic granuloma. CT scans in axial (**a**) plane and in coronal (**b**) reformat demonstrate a bone lytic lesion in projection of the left orbit roof. There is no lesion blood volume (CBV map-**c**) and blood flow elevation using CT-perfusion. T2- (**d**), T1- (**e**) weighted MR images show an isointense soft tissue mass in orbital roof with poor delineation. The lesion accumulates the contrast agent intensively and becomes more demarcated on enhanced T1-weighted MRI (**f**)

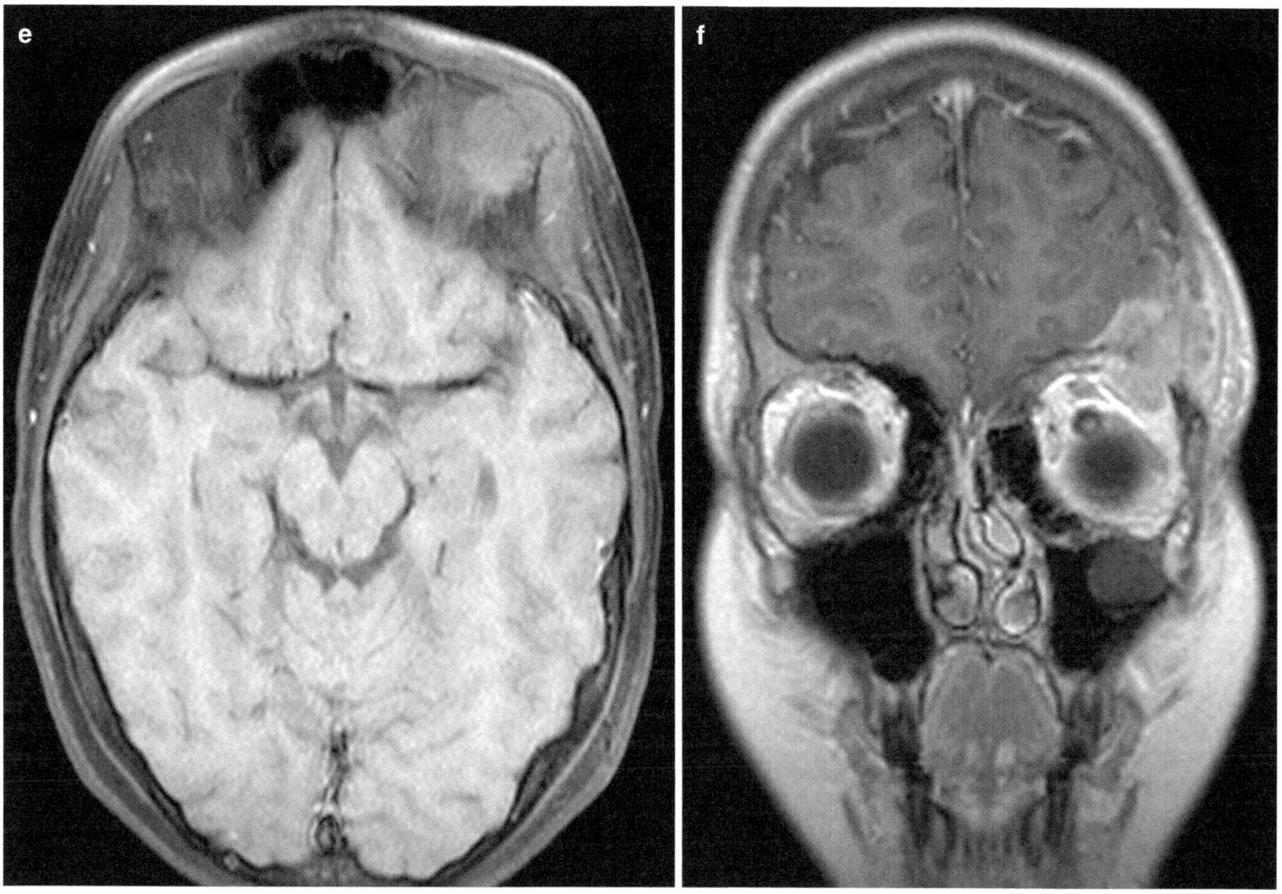

Fig. 8.5 (continued)

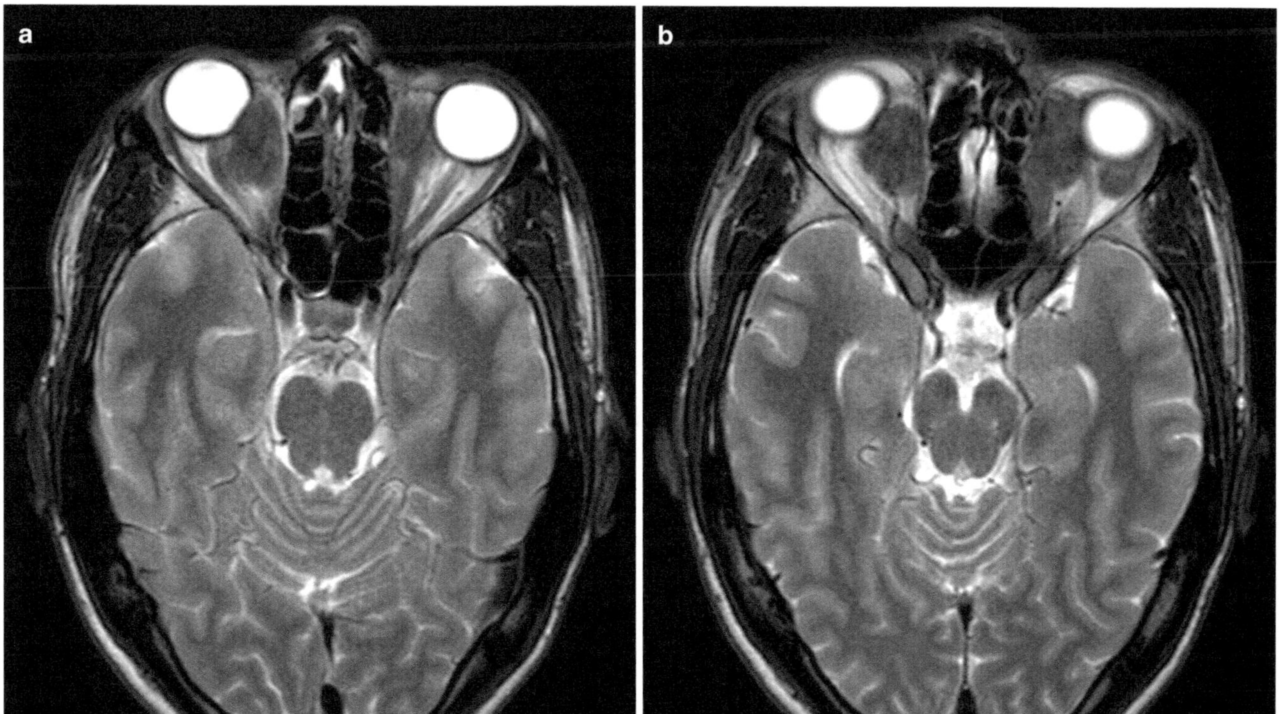

Fig. 8.6 Erdheim-Chester disease. MR imaging with using T2- (**a, b**) and T1- (**c–e**) weighted sequences reveals multiple infiltrative lesions with involvement of both orbits. Lesions show the dark MR-signal on T2-WI and hypointensity on T1-WI. After the intravenous contrast enhancement lesions demonstrate quite prominent and homogeneous accumulation of contrast material (**f**, **g**, **h**, **i**)

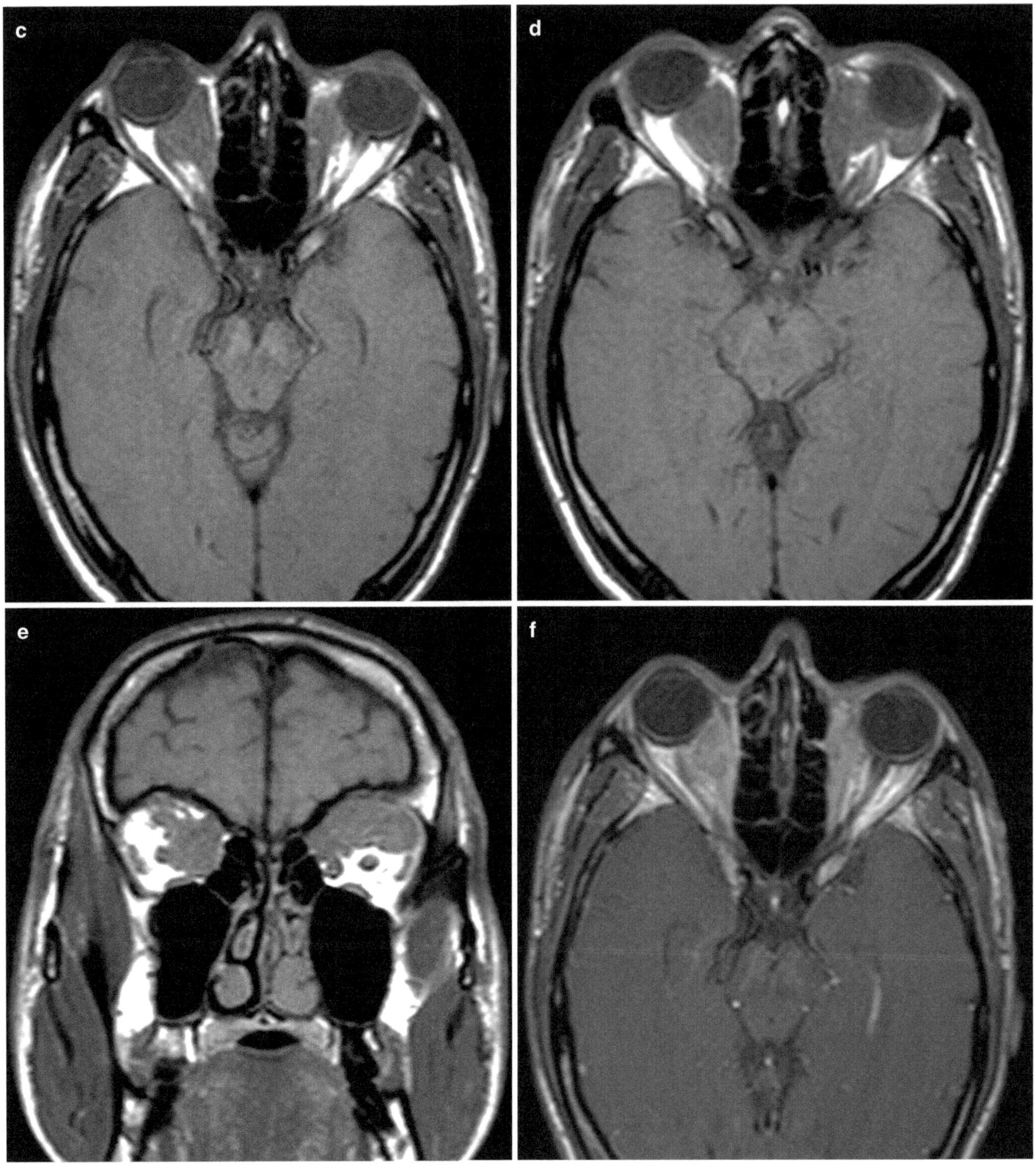

Fig. 8.6 (continued)

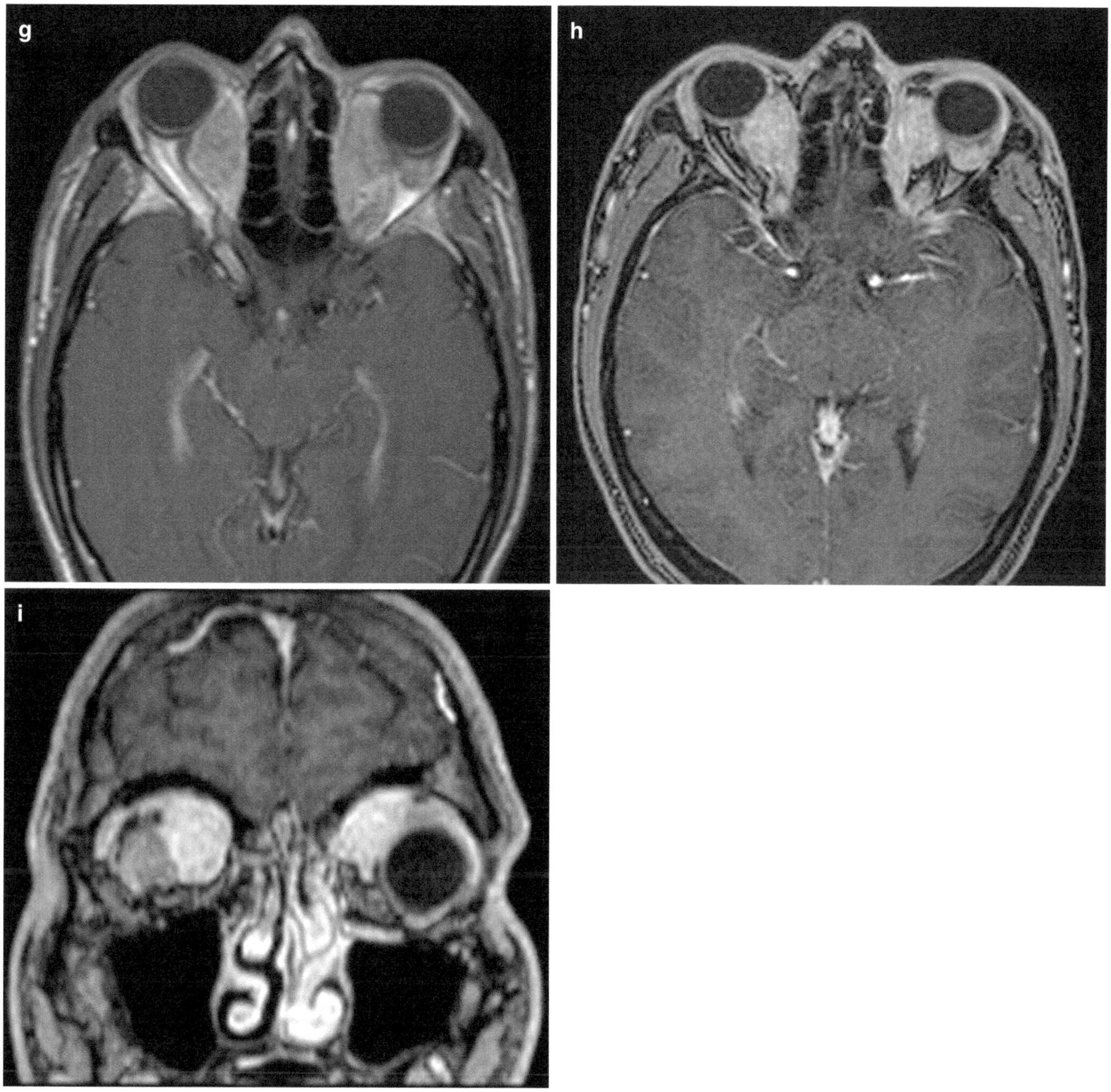

Fig. 8.6 (continued)

Part II

Anterior Cranial Fossa and Craniofacial Region Lesions

9 Introduction to Anterior Cranial Fossa and Craniofacial Region Lesions

The source of growth for the majority of tumors of the anterior cranial fossa (ACF) and craniofacial region (CFR) is a variety of structures and tissues in the specified area. These include: dura mater, olfactory nerves, mucosa of the upper nasal cavity and paranasal sinuses, orbital structures, tooth and the bones themselves. Neoplasms of this region of the head can be broadly classified from either epithelial or mesenchymal origin. Epithelial tumors may arise from mucosa (papillomas, squamous cell carcinomas, and adenocarcinomas), neuroendocrine tissue (sinonasal neuroendocrine carcinomas), minor salivary gland (from benign to malignant ones), and olfactory mucosa (olfactory neuroblastoma). Most often primary malignant tumors of this area are the squamous cell carcinoma, adenocarcinoma, and rarely occur melanoma and lymphoma. Metastases to this area are quite rare too. Among non-neoplastic lesions, inflammatory changes in the sinuses of the skull, different types of polyps, which, growing into the ACF region, can mimic neoplasms, are often encountered in radiological practice. Imaging of most ACF and CFR lesions is primarily aimed at determining the expansion of the lesion rather than determining its histological type, whether the tumor grows into ACF from the skull base, whether the brain substance is involved in the pathological process. What brain and vascular structures are involved in the affected area? In addition, there is a number of other issues in the evaluation of lesion expansion at the skull base, which radiologists have to resolve. For example, if the lesion spreads into the orbit. Tumors can often grow through the *lamina papyracea* and raise the periosteum of the orbit, not spreading into the orbital fat through this fibrous membrane. Extraconal fat in relation to the medial rectus muscle is a very important reference point: if the fat is intact and protrusion of the tumor into the orbital fat has a smooth edge, the lesion is limited by the periosteum.

If the tumor grows into the paranasal sinuses, a low MR-signal from the air is replaced by the signal representing the tumor. This is an important diagnostic symptom. However, inflammation or obstruction of the sinus cavity by inflammatory exudate also changes the signal in the sinus. Tumors themselves often cause a sinus cavity obstruction. In this case, both the tumor and inflammatory obstructive changes may be detected in the same sinus. The use of additional MR-sequences (inflammatory obstruction of the sinus has a high MR-signal on T2- and T2*-weighted images more often than tumors) or intravenous administration of contrast agents (most of skull base tumors enhance, while secretion into the sinus doesn't) is sometimes required in order to specify these issues.

The accuracy of topical lesion evaluation significantly increases when different MR-pulse sequences and modalities are used and the study is performed on multiple planes. In particular, a combination of orthogonal planes with oblique reformations better demonstrates expansion of the tumor into the skull base and CFR structures. The roof of the orbit and the cribriform plate are better visualized on the coronal images. Transition from the base of the ACF to the frontal bone wall is a smooth curve, along which neither axial nor coronal plane forms perpendicular slices, thus, cortical bone lines may be blurred. Sagittal images appear to be more informative in such cases. Routine diagnostic protocol of MR-studies of ACF and CFR has to include MR-sequences with fat signal suppression (both T2- and T1-weighted sequences), while post-contrast scanning is best to be obtained using spin echo T1-weighted sequences with fat signal suppression or new MR-technologies with Dixon method of fat saturation (T1-IDEAL (GE)) for better discrimination of the enhanced lesion from surrounding tissues (Curin and Cunnane 2009).

I. Pronin, V. Kornienko, *CT and MRI of Skull Base Lesions*, https://doi.org/10.1007/978-3-319-65957-2_9

Benign Tumors

10

Contents

About 25% of all nonepithelial tumors which are presented in CFR are osseous and fibroosseous lesions. In general, all these lesions can be classified as lesions of abnormal bone development (Paget's disease, fibrous dysplasia, cementoossifying dysplasia, giant cell granuloma), benign tumors (exostosis, osteoma, osteochondroma, osteoid osteoma, osteoblastoma, ossifying fibroma, chondroma, and giant cell tumor), and malignant tumors, such as osteogenic sarcoma and chondrosarcoma (Som et al. 2011).

Osteoma (Ost) is a benign, frequently solitary, well-circumscribed, slowly growing primary bone tumor, usually occurring in the paranasal sinuses. It arises from the sinus wall or the intersinus septum and typically extends into the sinus cavity. The tumor incidence is from 3 to 12% in general population. It is frequently detected in the craniofacial bones, most often in the frontal (80%), ethmoid (20%) sinuses, followed by the maxillary and sphenoid sinuses. It may also spread into the orbit and intracranial region. Other sites include bones of the external auditory canal, cranial vault, upper and lower jaws, sella turcica (Chen et al. 2008; Som et al. 2011).

The disease course is often asymptomatic. Only 5% of patients have clinical symptoms (sinusitis, headache, etc. depending on the process localization).

Imaging Osteoma is usually found during CT studies carried out for other reasons. On CT, osteomas visualize as a space-occupying lesion with homogeneous hyperdensity; however, it may include soft tissue areas (Figs. 10.1, 10.2 and 10.3). So the differentiation between the compact, cancellous, and fibrous types of osteoma can be based on CT-density. Large osteomas are also associated with a decrease in transparency of the sinus due to its obstruction. Mucocele formation as well as development of pneumocephalus, brain abscess, and subdural empyema as complications

I. Pronin, V. Kornienko, *CT and MRI of Skull Base Lesions*, https://doi.org/10.1007/978-3-319-65957-2_10

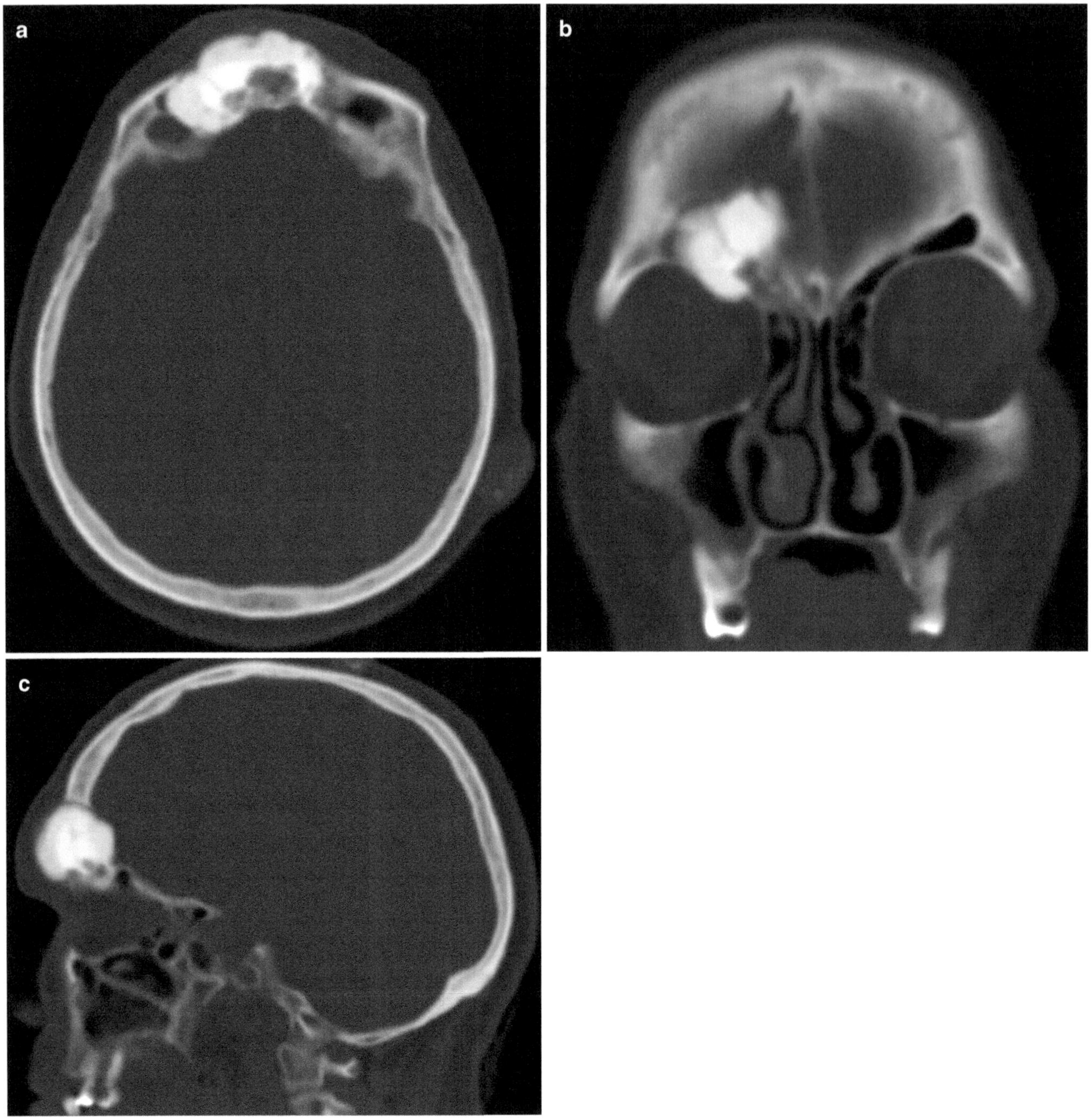

Fig. 10.1 Osteoma of the frontal sinus. CT scans in axial (**a**), coronal (**b**), and sagittal (**c**) projections show homogeneous hyperdense lesion with well-circumscribed margins. The lesion is located in the right part of the frontal sinus with bulging into the right orbit

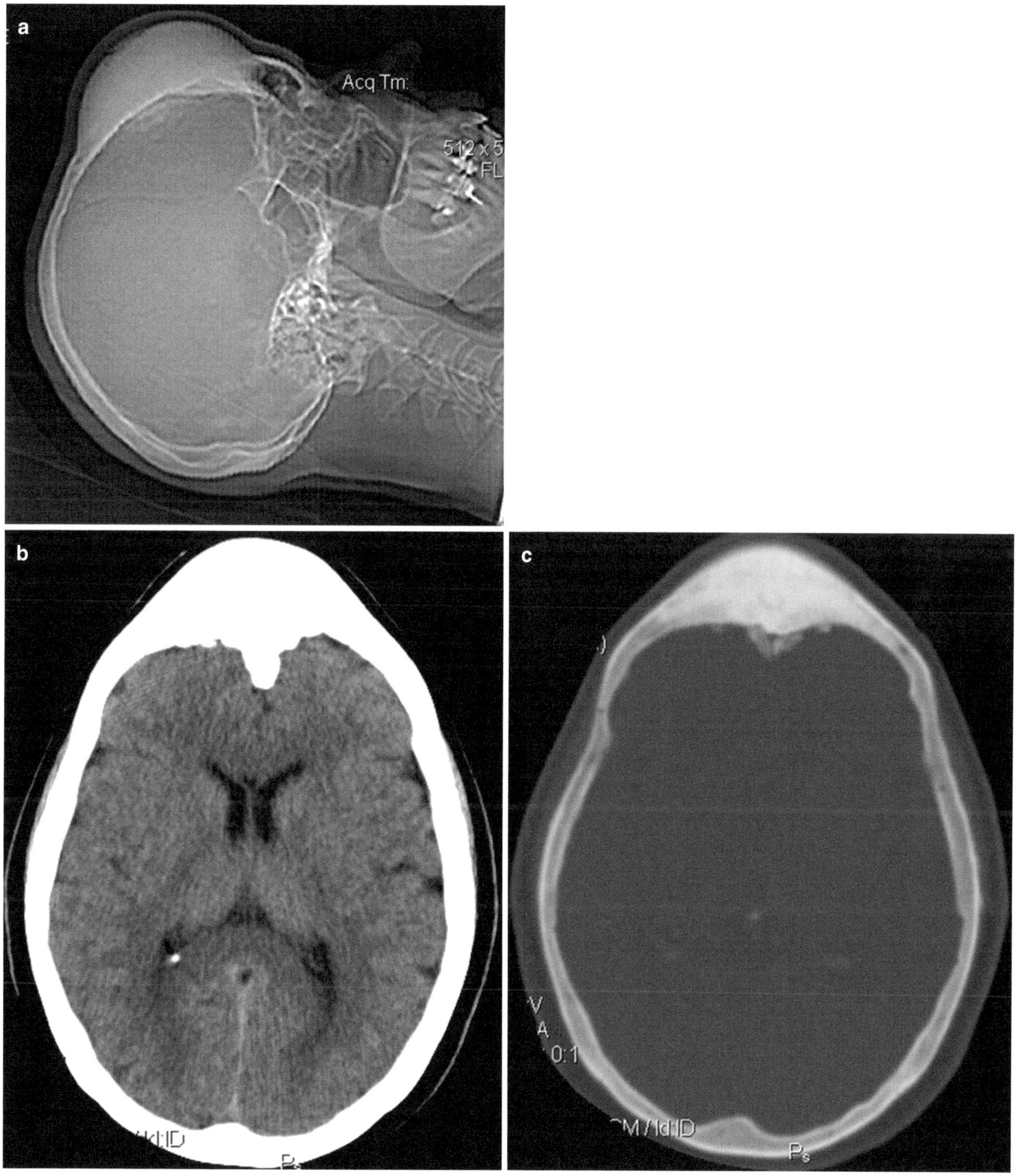

Fig. 10.2 Osteoma of the frontal bone and frontal sinus. Plan Rg (**a**) and axial CT scans in standard (**b**) and bone (**c**) windows reveal a large hyperdense lesion of the frontal bone with homogeneous structure

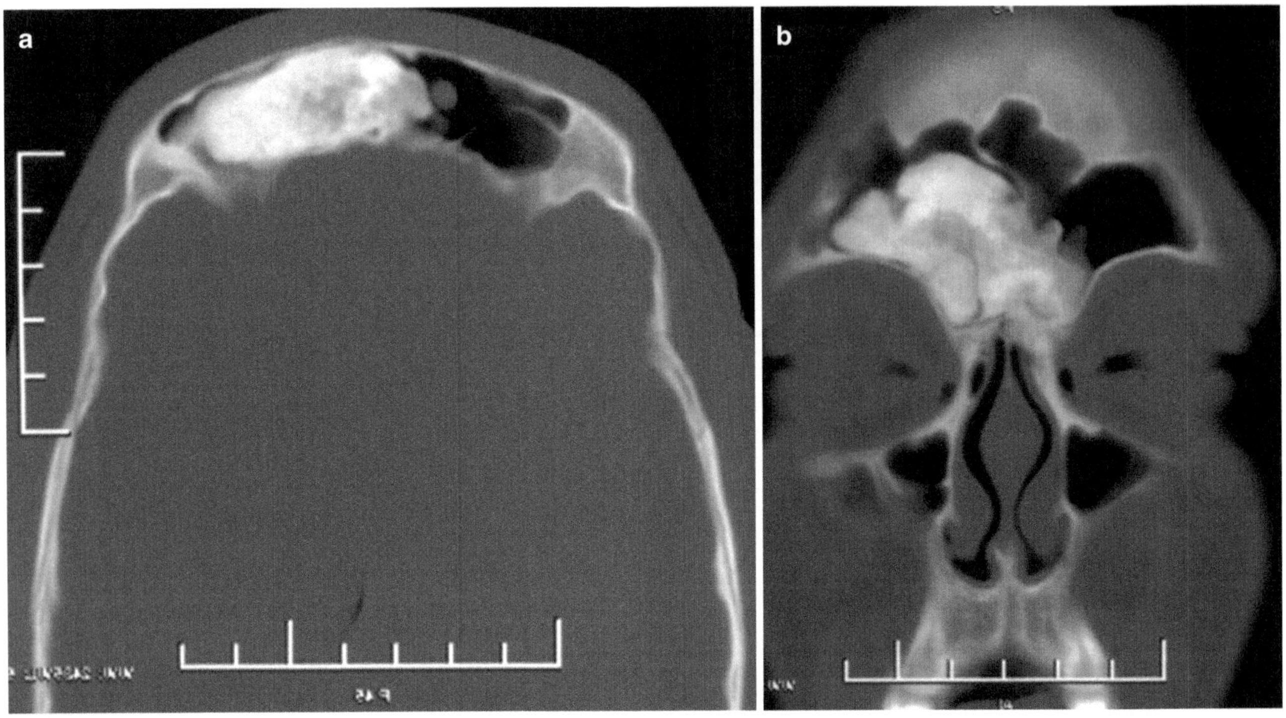

Fig. 10.3 Osteoma of the frontal sinus and upper ethmoids. CT scans in axial (**a**) and coronal (**b**) projections demonstrate a hyperdense and slightly heterogeneous mass, whose density is equal to the cortical bones. A lesion has a well-demarcated borders and doesn't extend beyond the sinus walls

of sinus obstruction is possible (Shady et al. 1994). Osteomas do not enhance after the contrast agent injection. Moreover, due to initially very high density of the neoplasm on CT the estimation of contrast enhancement degree can be masked (Earwaker 1993).

On T1-weighted MR images, osteoma has a low MR-signal, is poorly identified on scans and, therefore, and can be missed (can be confused with air), but its central portion may have a high MR-signal (bone marrow). Hypointense MR-signal on T2-weighted images is also typical for osteomas and varies from low to intermediate depending on the lesion matrix structure (Fig. 10.4).

MRI assesses the state of the sinuses (mucosal thickening, presence of effusion, etc.) better than CT.

Differential Diagnosis

1. Bone exostosis is a benign, expansile proliferation of mature bone that occurs on the surface of affected bone;
2. Fibrous dysplasia is a common bone disease with typical "ground glass" appearance; old lesions can mimic osteoma;
3. Ossifying fibroma is a primary nonossifying mass with a surrounding cortex, central part of the lesion often has a low density on CT;
4. Osteosarcoma is a malignant bone tumor; it is determined as tumor with osteoid matrix production. Enhanced soft-tissue component often being present.

Meningioma (M) is the most common extraaxial tumor in adults and consists of approximately 15–20% of all intracranial primary tumors (Graham and Lantoc 1997). It occurs most frequently in the falx and parasagittal area (50%), as well as in the base of ACF (up to 10% of all intracranial meningiomas). The neoplasm arises from the dura mater covering the intracranial surface of the skull or dural sheathes extending along some cranial nerves. Typical meningiomas are most frequent (80–85% of cases), atypical (10–12%) and malignant (3–5%) ones being less common. Bone hyperostosis is detected in about 5% of cases, however, the majority of patients are examined by MRI, and, therefore, many examinations do not clearly visualize and evaluate hyperostotic bone changes. Bone erosion can occur in all types of Ms, and they can also cause bone destruction, but still hyperostosis is more frequently observed. If meningioma is localized in the cribriform plate of the sphenoid bone or the planum sphenoidale, such a symptom as hyperpneumatization of the adjacent sinus can be observed (Castillo 2002).

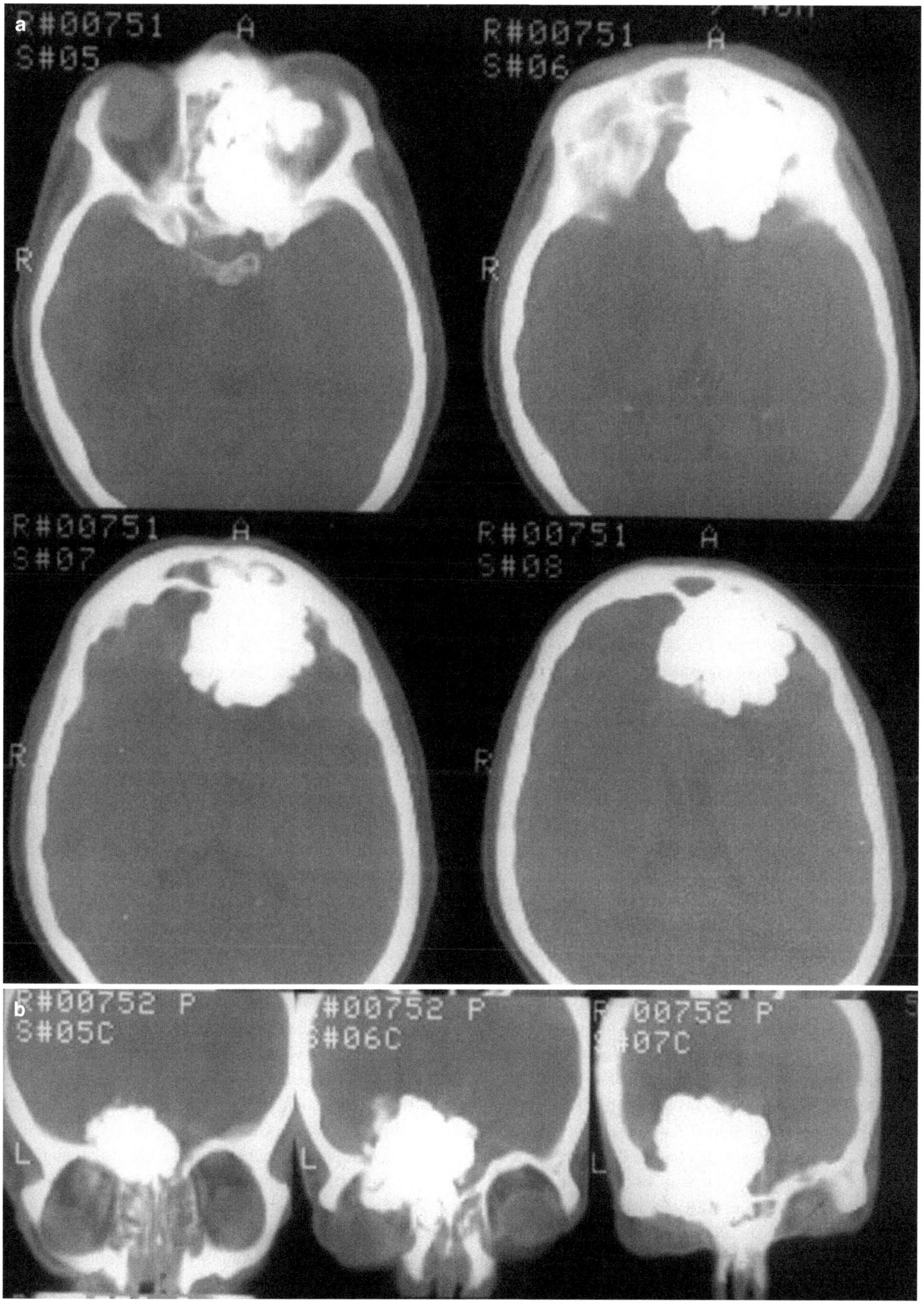

Fig. 10.4 Osteoma of the frontal sinus. Series of CT scans in axial (**a**) and coronal (**b**) projections show a hyperdense mass, which is located in the ethmoids, right part of the frontal sinus. The lesion spreads to the anterior cranial fossa with dislocation of frontal lobe and the anterior horn of the left lateral ventricle, and into the right orbit. Axial T2-weighted (**c**) and sagittal T1-weighted (**d**) MR images demonstrate low signal intensity from the osteoma. Surrounding cystic lesions as well as inflammatory changes within frontal sinus cavity with hyperintense MR-signal are visible on MRI

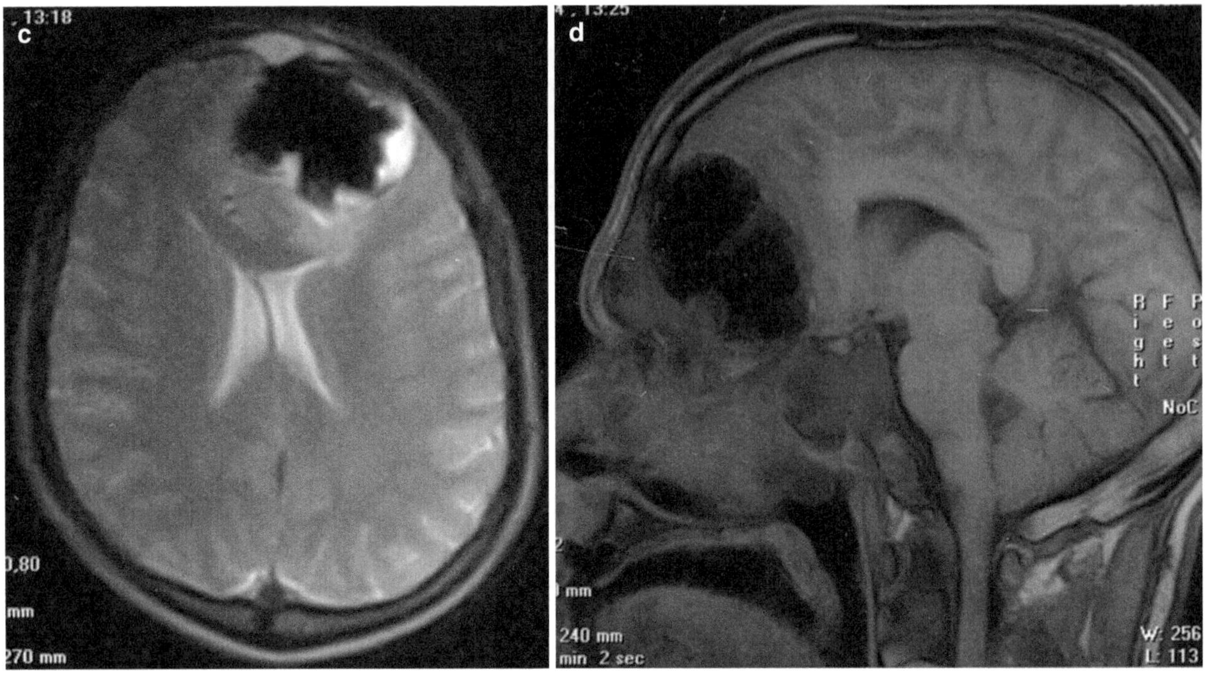

Fig. 10.4 (continued)

Imaging Since the most common site of Ms in the ACF is the cribriform plate (so-called olfactory meningiomas), this tumor has a typical form of one-sided convex lens on CT and MRI. Its contours are well defined and relatively rounded. Typical feature is a high degree of contrast enhancement with homogeneous distribution of the contrast agent within the M stroma (Fig. 10.5). Surrounding edema is present in almost 50% of all cases. Nodular forms of ACF Ms are more common, while a diffuse infiltrative growth pattern being rarer. The latter forms of meningiomas more often penetrate into CFR with extracranial components formation (Fig. 10.6). On CT-perfusion, most Ms are characterized by a marked elevation in the blood flow with an increase in CBF and CBV parameters. Various changes in mean transit time (MTT) from significant shortening to prominent prolongation can be found (Figs. 10.7, 10.8 and 10.9). Permeability of the contrast agent demonstrates the high values in majority of the meningiomas. 3D reconstructions are useful in hyperostotic forms of meningiomas assessment (Fig. 10.10).

Most Ms are isointense on T1-weighted MR images and strong enhancing tumor. On T2-weighted images, about 10% of Ms have a low signal compared to the brain, and MR-signal of intermediate intensity in 50% of cases and a hyperintense MR-signal in 40% of cases (Figs. 10.11 and 10.12). Lesions that are characterized by high (bright) MR-signal on T2-weighted images often have atypical histological picture. Contrast enhancement may extend beyond the main tumor nodule, with formation of the so-called dural "tails" or infiltrative changes in the dura mater on the periphery of a meningioma. This symptom occurs in 50% of all cases and only suggests the probable diagnosis of M, not being an absolute pathognomonic sign, and can occur with various tumors invading the dura matter such as metastasis, sarcomas, and others (Tokumaru et al. 1990). A dural "tail" sign can also occur in reactive changes of other origin in the brain meninges. There are disorders that affect the dura and cause its thickening similar to that in meningiomas. These are sarcoidosis, lymphoma, and various infections, in particular, tuberculosis and fungal infection. Contrast enhancement of the thickened dura may occur after lumbar puncture or intracranial hypotension syndrome.

Typical for olfactory fossa meningiomas is the visualization of the tumor vascular matrix that contains blood vessels running radially from the site of the primary M growth. Vessels are clearly visualized on sagittal T1- and T2-weighted MRI and can also be seen as hypointense structures after contrast enhancement on the background of enhanced tumor structure (Fig. 10.13). Current capabilities of high resolution MR-angiography practically superseded digital angiography from diagnostic preoperative algorithm of examining the patients with olfactory meningiomas, although it remains essential for neurosurgeons in case of large tumors in terms of preoperative embolization of the pathological tumor vessels (Fig. 10.14).

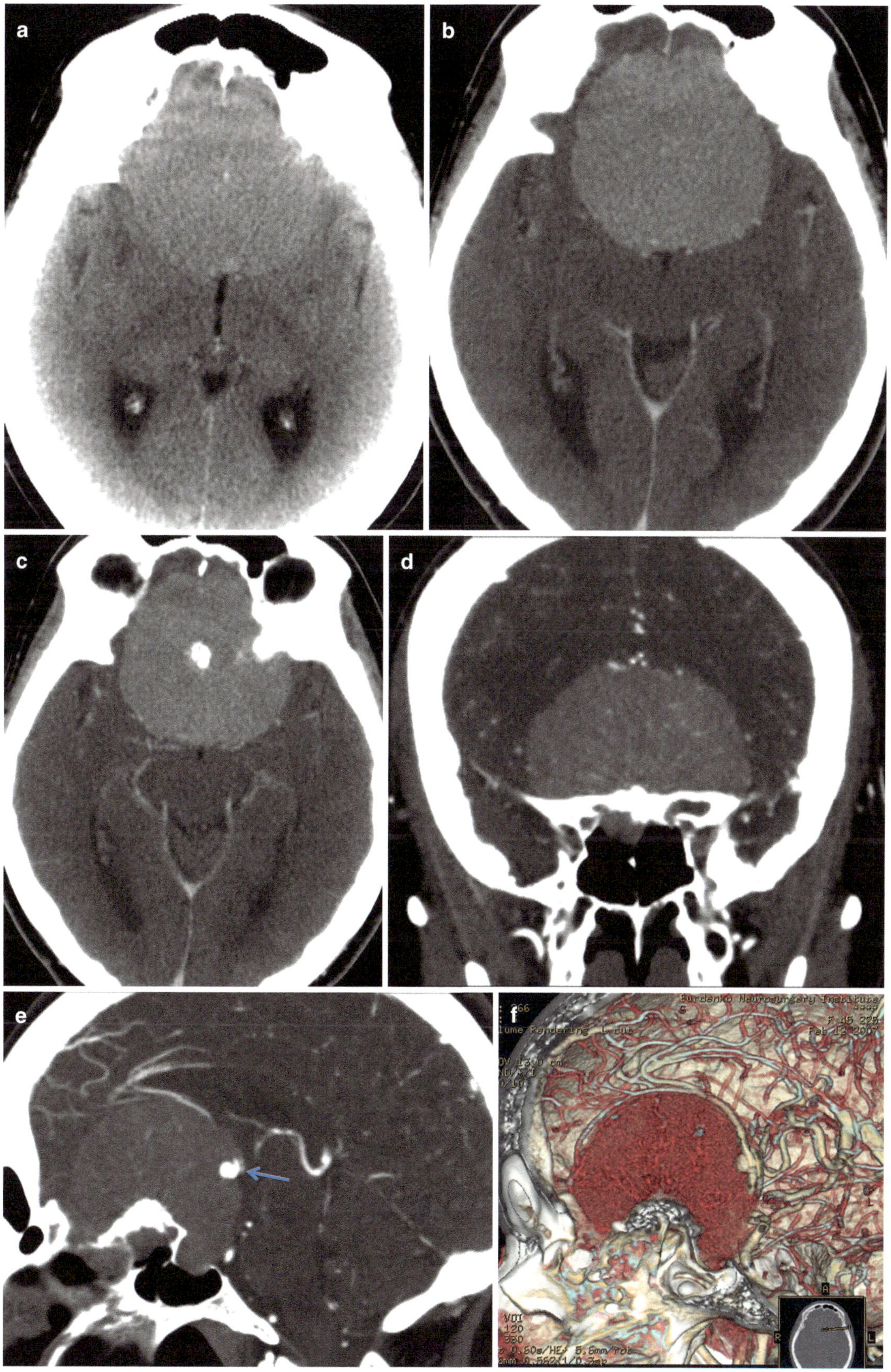

Fig. 10.5 Olfactory meningioma. Axial CT scans before (**a**) and after injection of contrast agent (**b**, **c**) as well as coronal (**d**) and sagittal (**e**) reformats reveal a large mass with homogeneous hyperdensity on non-contrast CT scan, located on the base of anterior cranial fossa. Tumor shows homogeneous and strong enhancement. The local hyperostosis of the planum sphenoidalis can be seen. On CT angiography (**e**, **f**), with the use of sagittal reformation and 3D-reconstruction all peculiarities of the meningioma are clearly visible. Additionally arterial aneurysm of the anterior cerebral artery is detected (*arrow*)

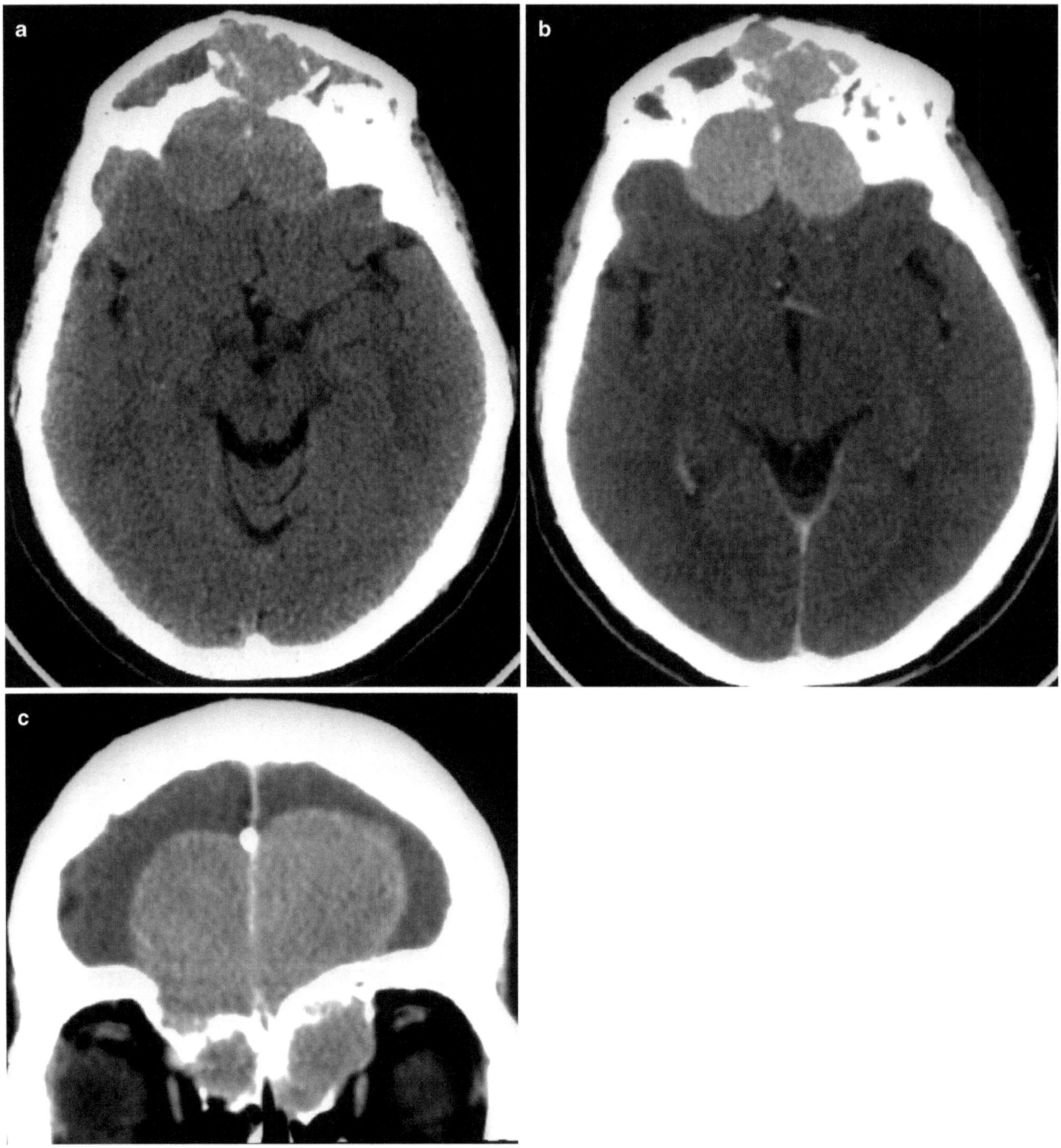

Fig. 10.6 Meningioma of anterior cranial fossa. On CT scans before (**a**) and after (**b**, **c**) contrast enhancement a large hyperdense and enhancing mass is visualized. The lesion spreads into the frontal sinuses due to the destruction of the internal wall. Coronal CT scan (**c**) demonstrates a tumor expanding into the ethmoids and both orbits

Fig. 10.7 Meningioma of planum sphenoidalis. On axial post-contrast CT scan (**a**) a small enhanced mass on the base of anterior cranial fossa can be visualized. Axial T2-weighted image (**b**) as well as axial (**c**) and sagittal (**d**) T1-weighted postenhanced images clearly demonstrates a tumor with homogeneous and strong enhancement. On CT-perfusion imaging (CBF (**e**), CBV (**f**)) a meningioma is detected as a lesion with elevation of blood flow and blood volume parameters. Moreover CT-perfusion maps show right-side located matrix of the tumor (*arrow*)

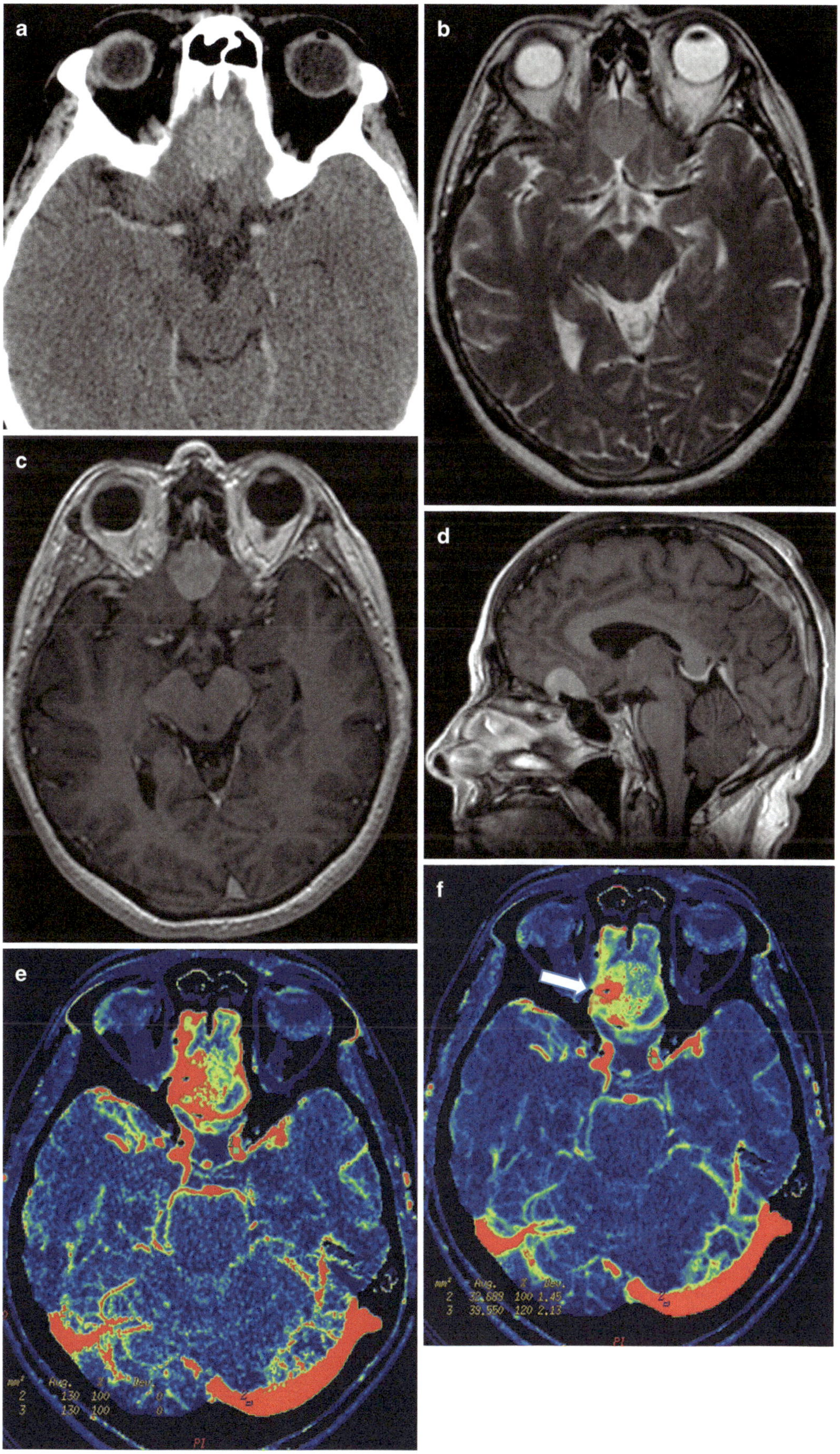
a
b
c
d
e
f

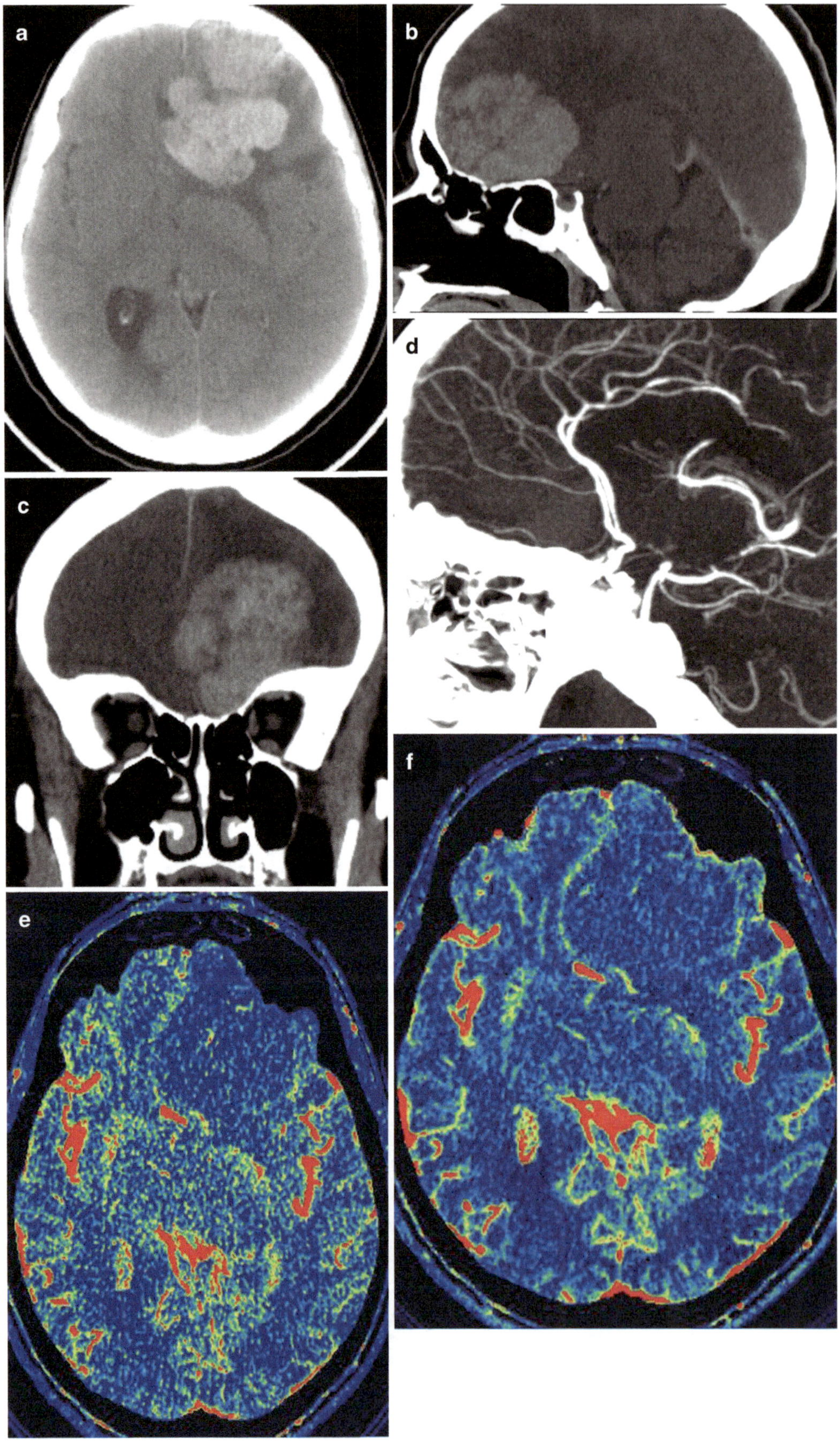

Fig. 10.8 Atypical chordoid meningioma of the anterior cranial fossa. Axial post-contrast CT scan (**a**) as well as sagittal (**b**) and coronal (**c**) reformats reveal a nonhomogeneous strongly enhancing mass with well-defined borders surrounded by edema. On CT-angiography (**d**) there is no tumor vascular network and only displacement of the anterior cerebral artery can be seen. CT-perfusion study (CBF-map (**e**) and CBV map (**f**)) demonstrates atypically low values of blood flow and blood volume within meningioma structure

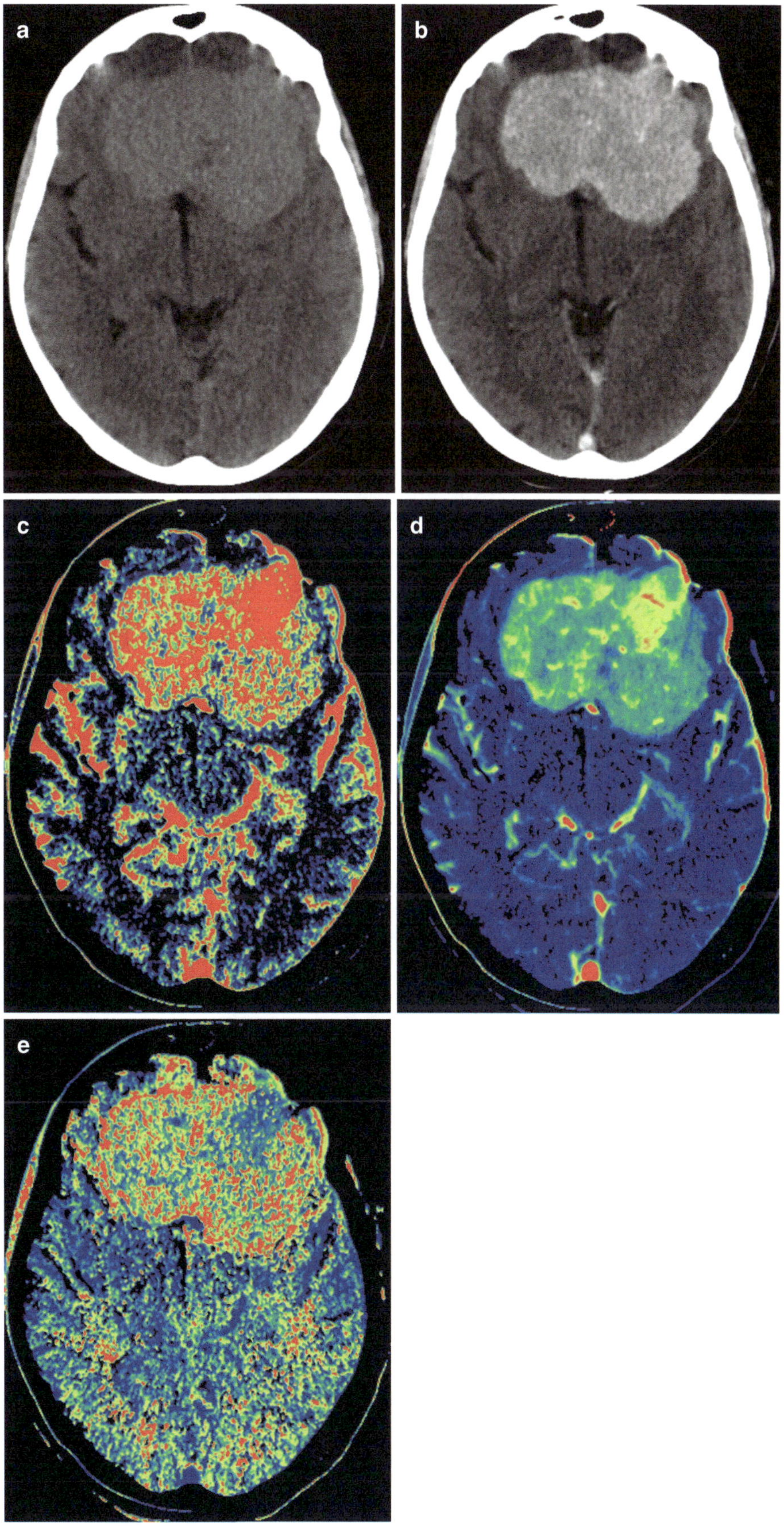

Fig. 10.9 Meningothelial olfactory meningioma. Axial CT scans before (**a**) and after (**b**) intravenous contrast enhancement show a large tumor in projection of anterior cranial fossa with strong and homogeneous enhancement. On CT-perfusion mapping (CBF (**c**), CBV (**d**), MTT (**e**)) the heterogeneous elevation of hemodynamics parameters can be seen

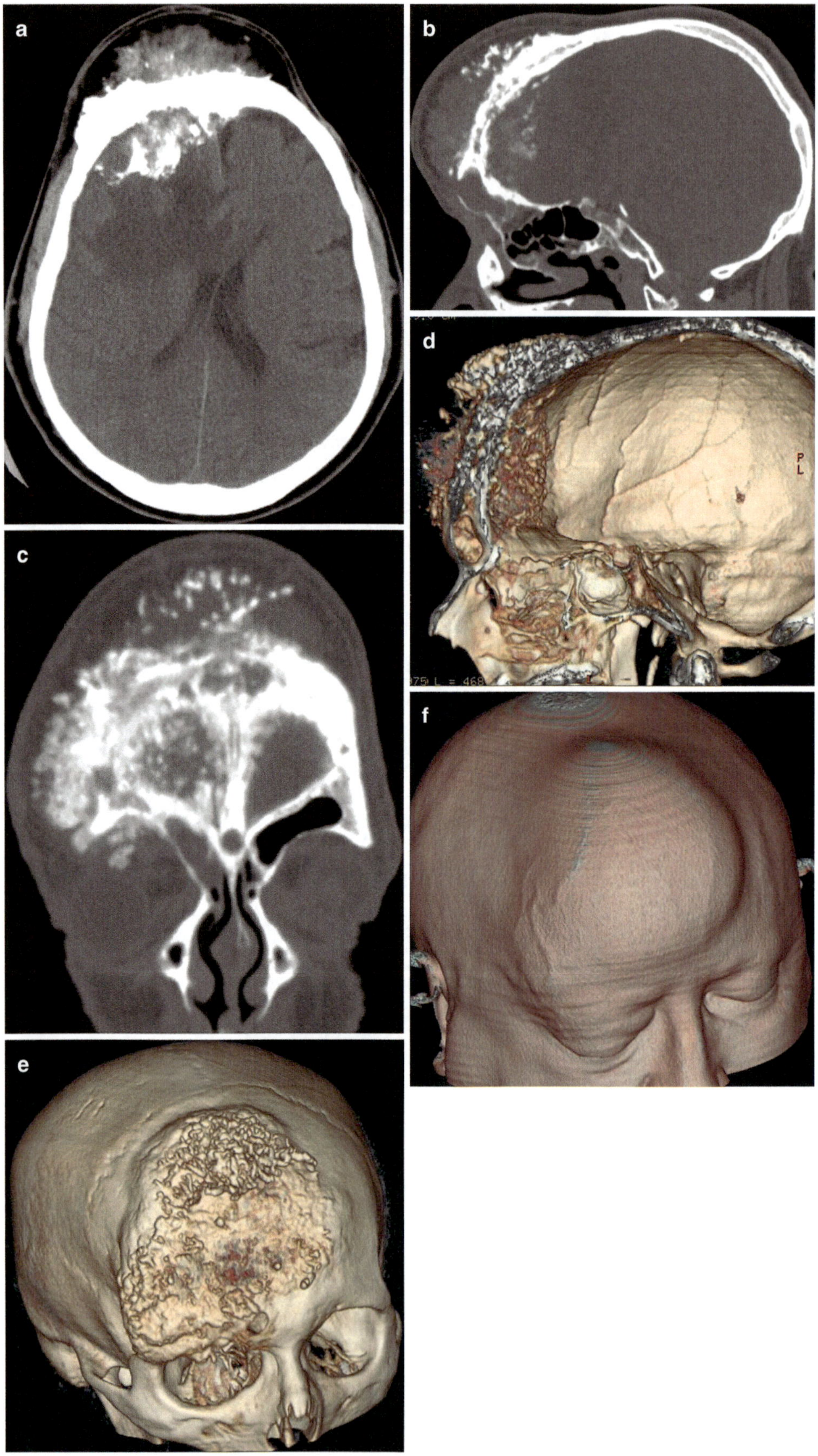
a
b
d
f
c
e

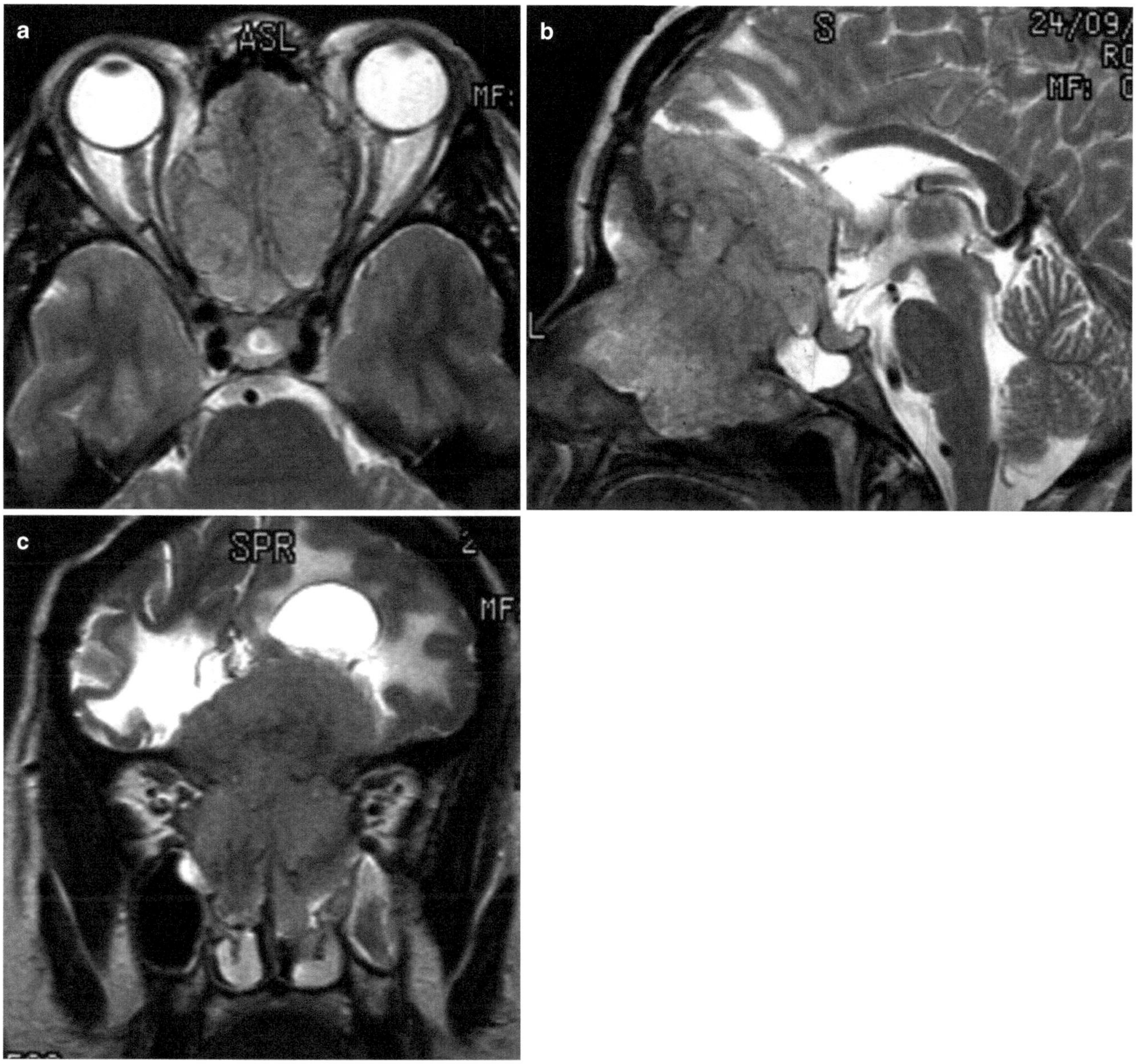

Fig. 10.11 Fibrous meningioma of the olfactory fossa. T2-weighted MR scans (**a**–**c**) demonstrate a large hypointense mass involving frontal sinus, ethmoids, upper part of nasal cavity and olfactory fossa. There is obstruction of sphenoid sinus. Intracranially, surrounded perifocal brain edema and cystic lesions can be seen

Fig. 10.10 Osseous meningioma of the right frontal bone. Axial CT (**a**) scan as well as sagittal (**b**) and coronal (**c**) reformats shows a large mixed density mass with calcification in fronto-orbital region. There is a frontal bone destruction and remodeling. Calcification in both intra- and extracranial (including left orbit) locations can be seen within soft-tissue meningioma portion. 3D reconstructions (**d**–**f**) add information about different aspects of bone involvement

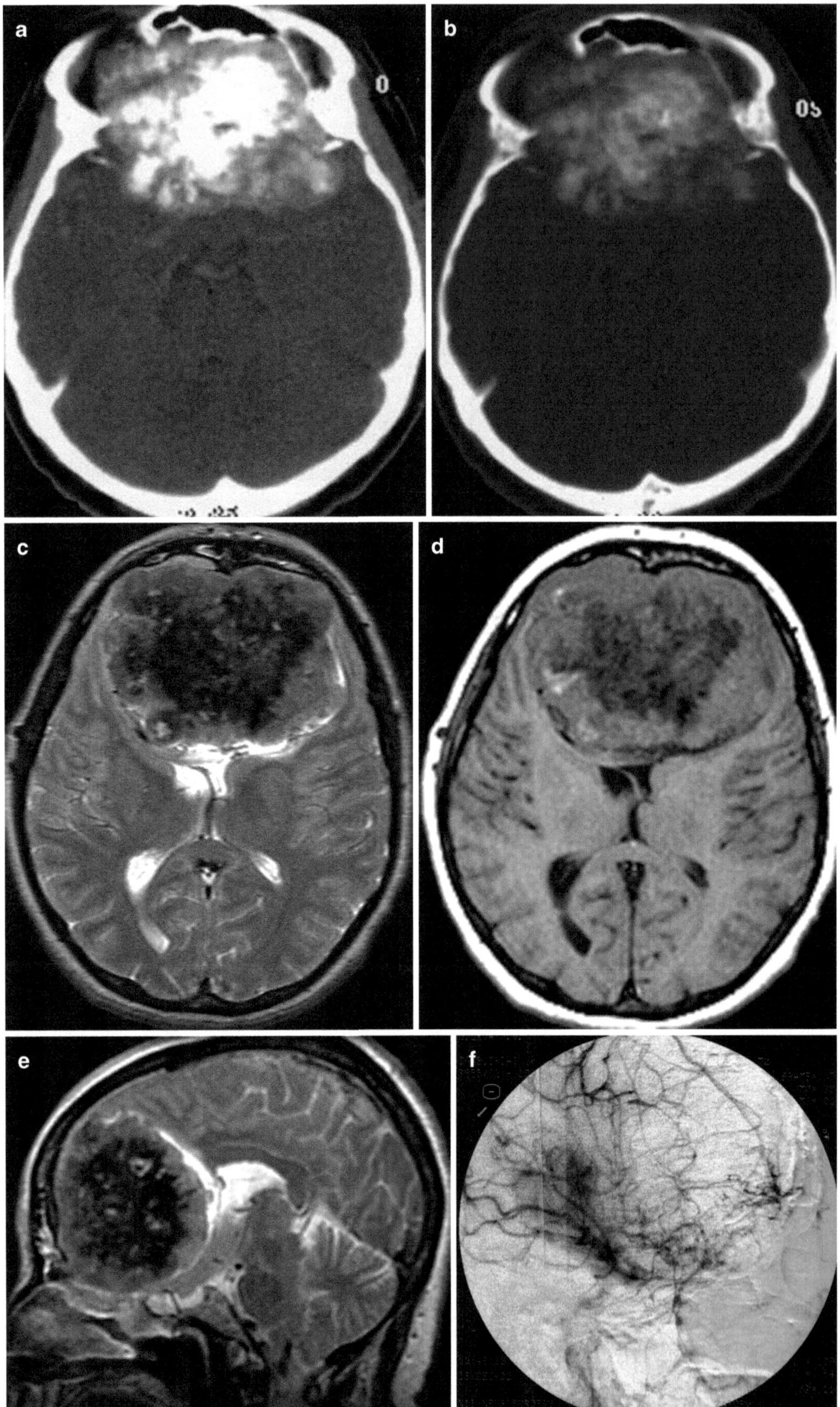

Fig. 10.12 Fibrous olfactory meningioma. Axial CT scans (**a**, **b**) with contrast enhancement show a huge size lesion located in the projection of anterior cranial fossa with massive calcifications. On T2-weighted (**c**, **e**) and T1-weighted (**d**) MR images a low MR-signal intensity from central calcified part of meningioma is visible. Soft-tissue portion of meningioma has isointense signal compare to the brain white matter. DSA (**f**) demonstrates pathologic vascular network of the tumor

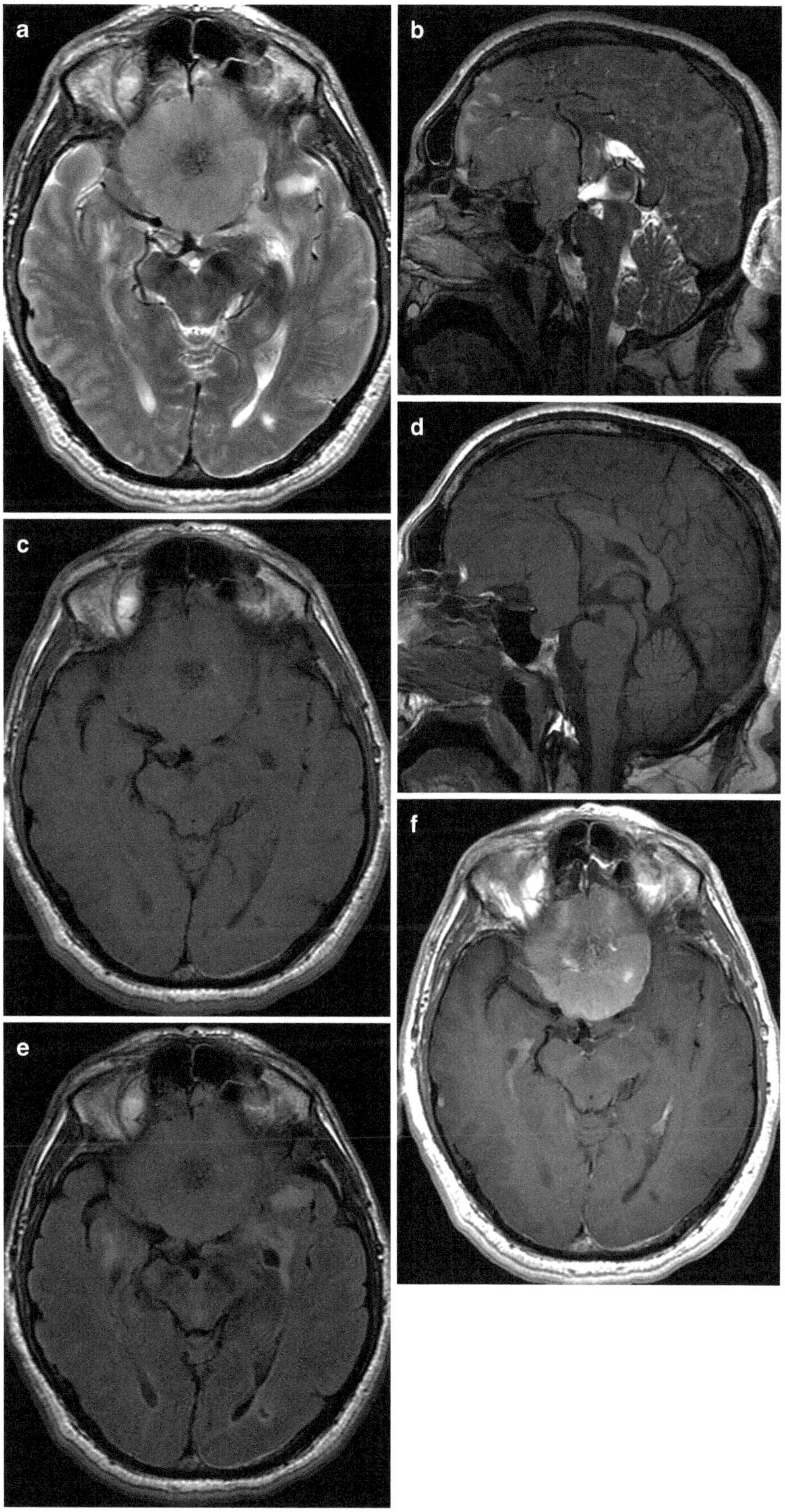

Fig. 10.13 Meningioma of the olfactory fossa. T2-weighted (axial (**a**), sagittal (**b**)), T1-weighted (axial (**c**), sagittal (**d**)), and T2-FLAIR (**e**) MR images show a huge size soft-tissue mass, which accumulates strongly contrast agent (**f**, **g**). Tumor has an isointense MR-signal in comparison to gray matter of the brain. Routine MRI as well as MR-angiography in sagittal (**h**) and axial (**i**) projections visualizes arcuate shift up (*short arrow*) of the anterior cerebral arteries, and arterial vessels of the tumor matrix (*long arrow*). Blood supply comes from a. ophthalmic, short branches of ICA, and A2 segment of anterior cerebral artery

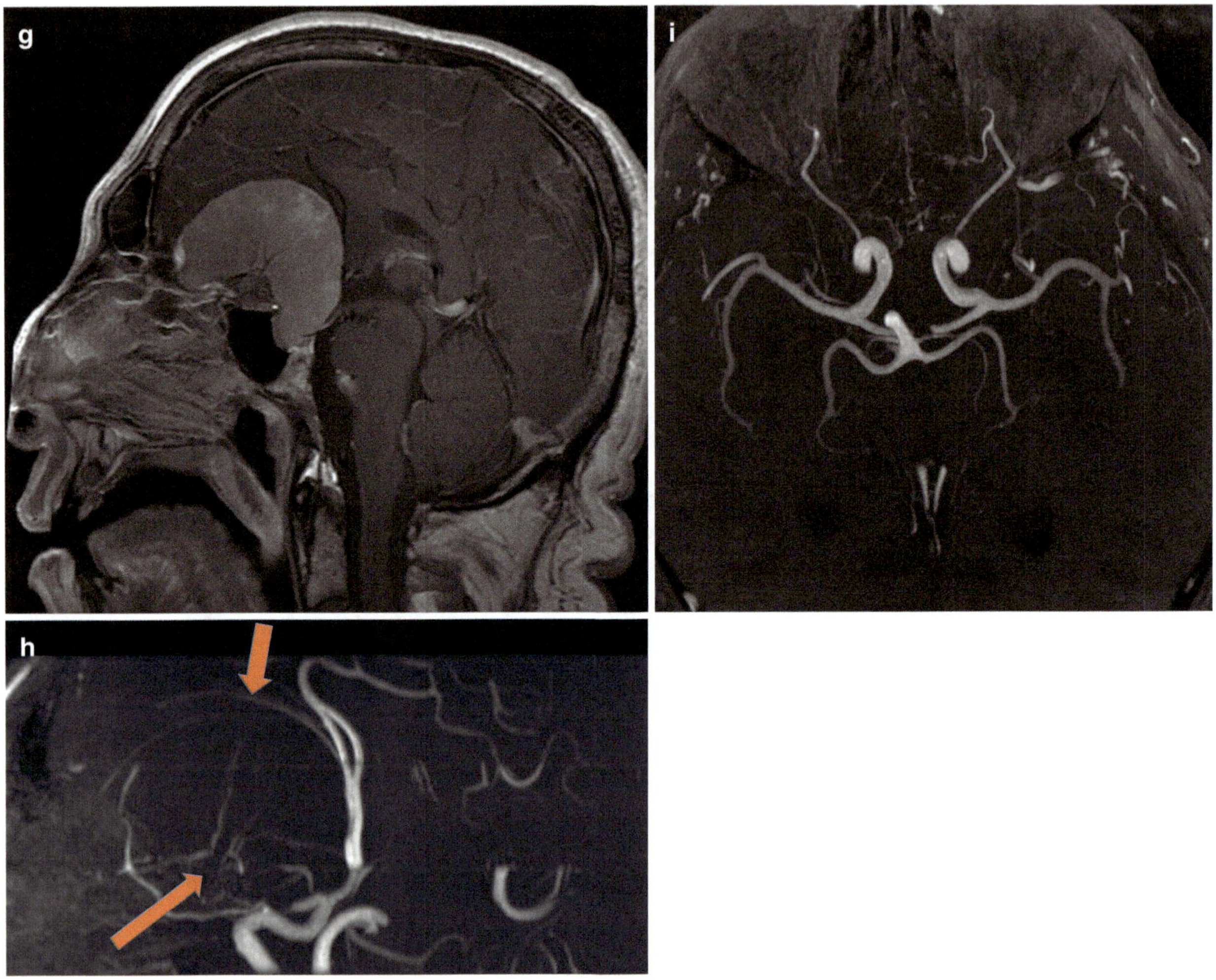

Fig. 10.13 (continued)

Differential Diagnosis

1. Olfactory neuroblastoma does not cause hyperostosis of the skull base, forms cysts on the border of the tumor and the brain;
2. Metastases cause the skull base bones destruction, they are often multiple with heterogeneous contrast enhancement;
3. Fibrous dysplasia (sclerotic form) may mimic osseous meningioma, but has no soft tissue enhancing component.

Ossifying fibroma (OF) (cementoossifying fibroma, central ossifying fibroma, central cementoossifying fibroma) is a benign fibroosseous space-occupying lesion consisting of an encapsulated mixture of the fibrous and immature bone tissue, well-circumscribed, with a heterogeneous soft tissue center (fibrosis) surrounded by a rim of ossification, which progressively ossifies starting from the periphery. OFs are most often detected in the mandible (75%); the incidence in the maxilla is about 10–20%, where it arises from periodontic ligament, most commonly in the molar and premolar regions (Som et al. 2011). OFs can also arise in the nasal cavity, usually from the lateral nasal wall or ethmoid bone. In cases with large size OF can involve the frontal, sphenoid, and maxillary sinuses.

The risk of malignancy is less than 0.5%. OFs can be combined with mucocele, lead to facial deformation, be complicated by pneumocephalus. This tumor most often occurs at the age of 20–40 years old and is five folds more common in women.

Imaging On CT, OF is a well-circumscribed, heterogeneous, soft-tissue density lesion with ossified walls. A classical CT

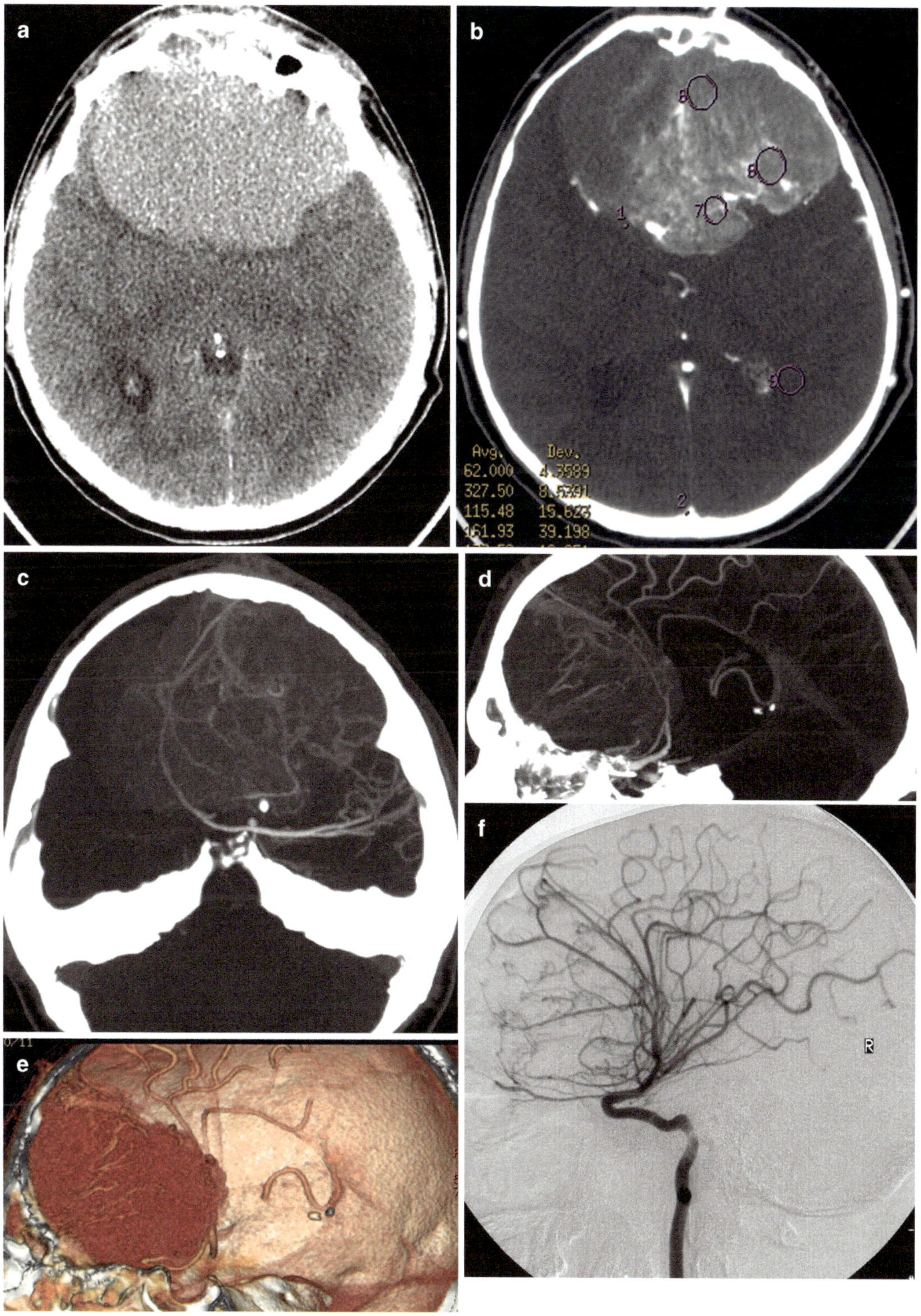

Fig. 10.14 Meningioma of the olfactory fossa. Axial CT scan (**a**) after contrast enhancement reveals a huge homogeneously enhancing tumor. On CT angiography (**b–d**) and 3D (**e**) reconstruction (from CT-Ag data) an intense pathologic vascular network within the tumor can be seen. Direct cerebral angiography (**f–i**) demonstrates an abundant arterial supply of the lesion from the distal branches of a. ophthalmic and arcuate shift up of the anterior cerebral arteries

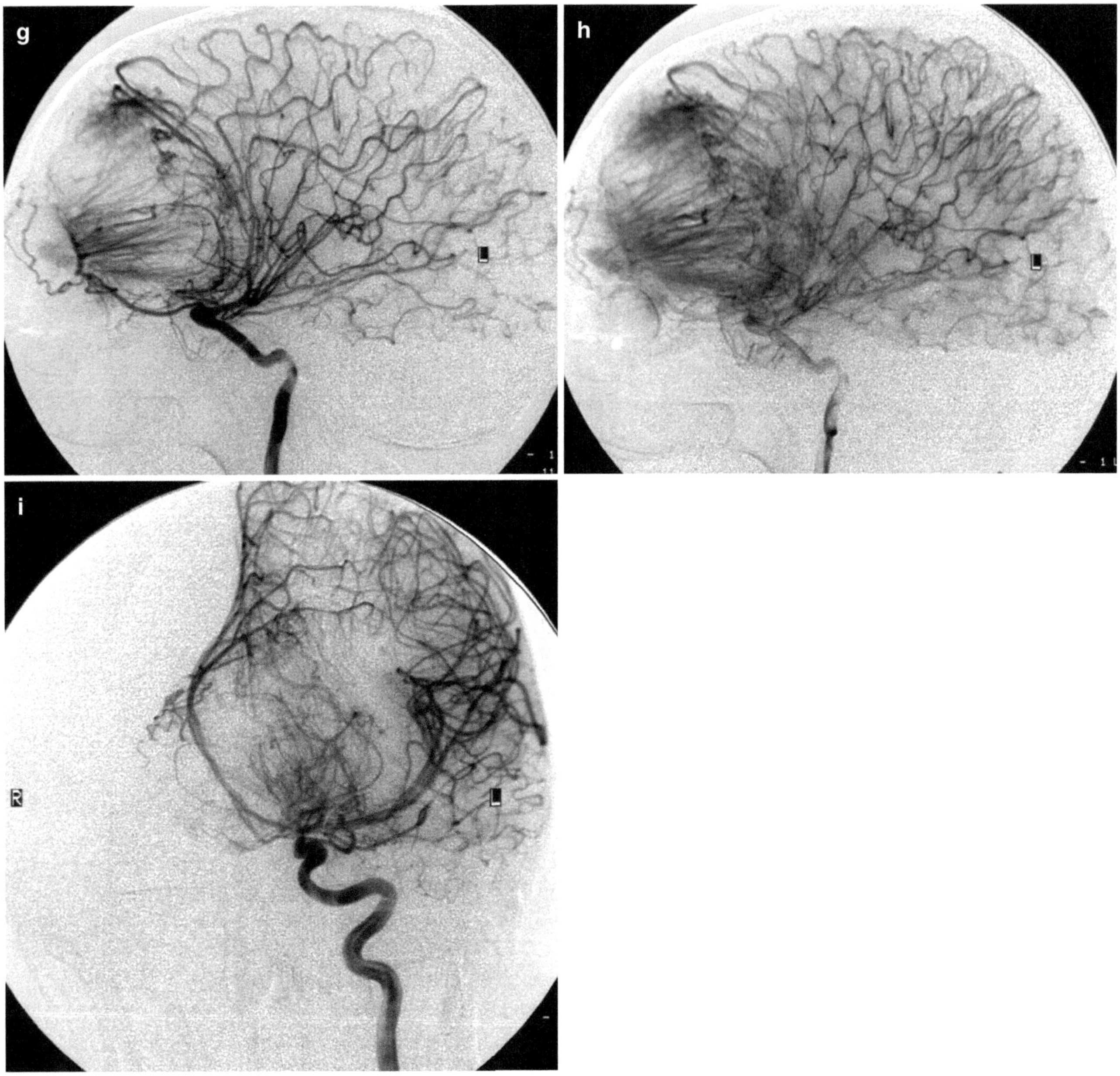

Fig. 10.14 (continued)

picture includes thick bony walls surrounding a fibrous center of low density (Fig. 10.15). The ossifying walls can be very thin. OF is sometimes difficult to differentiate from fibrous dysplasia. After intravenous administration of contrast agent, heterogeneous areas of enhancement can be detected (Engelbrecht et al. 1999).

On T1-weighted MR images, the intensity of MR-signal varies from medium to low; the fibrous center usually has MR-signal of intermediate intensity, while the ossified zone has hypointense MR-signal. On T2-weighted images, OF is presented by a heterogeneous signal: high signal from fibrotic areas (usually in the center) and hypointense ossified areas (on the periphery) (Kuta et al. 1995). The lesion may be accompanied by mucocele. MRI also detects heterogeneous accumulation of contrast agent by the fibrous portion of the tumor (Figs. 10.16 and 10.17) (Khoury et al. 2002).

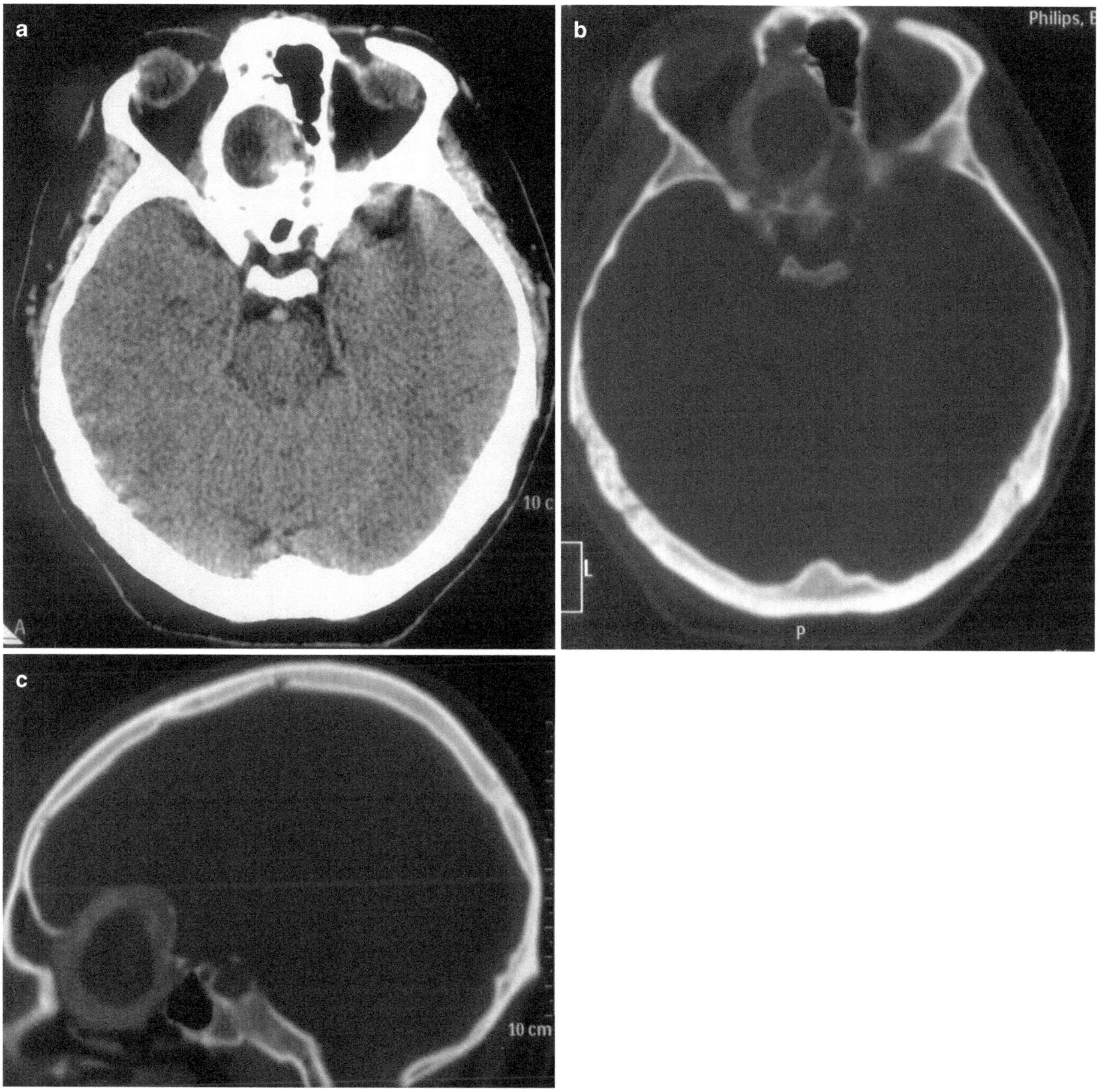

Fig. 10.15 Ossifying fibroma of the ethmoid sinus. On CT in axial (**a**, **b**) and sagittal (**c**) projections a lesion has typical hyperdense ossifying contour with (hypodense) fibrous center

Differential Diagnosis

1. Fibrous dysplasia is a lesion without well-defined contours, which is characterized by an enlargement of the facial bones, the skull base region and the cranial vault with a classic "ground glass" sign (in cases with multiostotic involvement), possible cystic areas formation;
2. Osteoma is a solid with high-density on CT lesion, often localizes in the frontal sinus;
3. Cementoma (cementoblastoma) is a benign cementum-producing lesion of the mesodermal periodontal ligament in young males (Mehhlisch et al. 1972);
4. Osteosarcoma is most frequently diagnosed in adolescent boys, an aggressive malignant tumor of craniofacial bones; periosteal response is observed.

Juvenile angiofibroma (JNAF) (juvenile nasopharyngeal angiofibroma) is a benign, slowly growing, highly vascular,

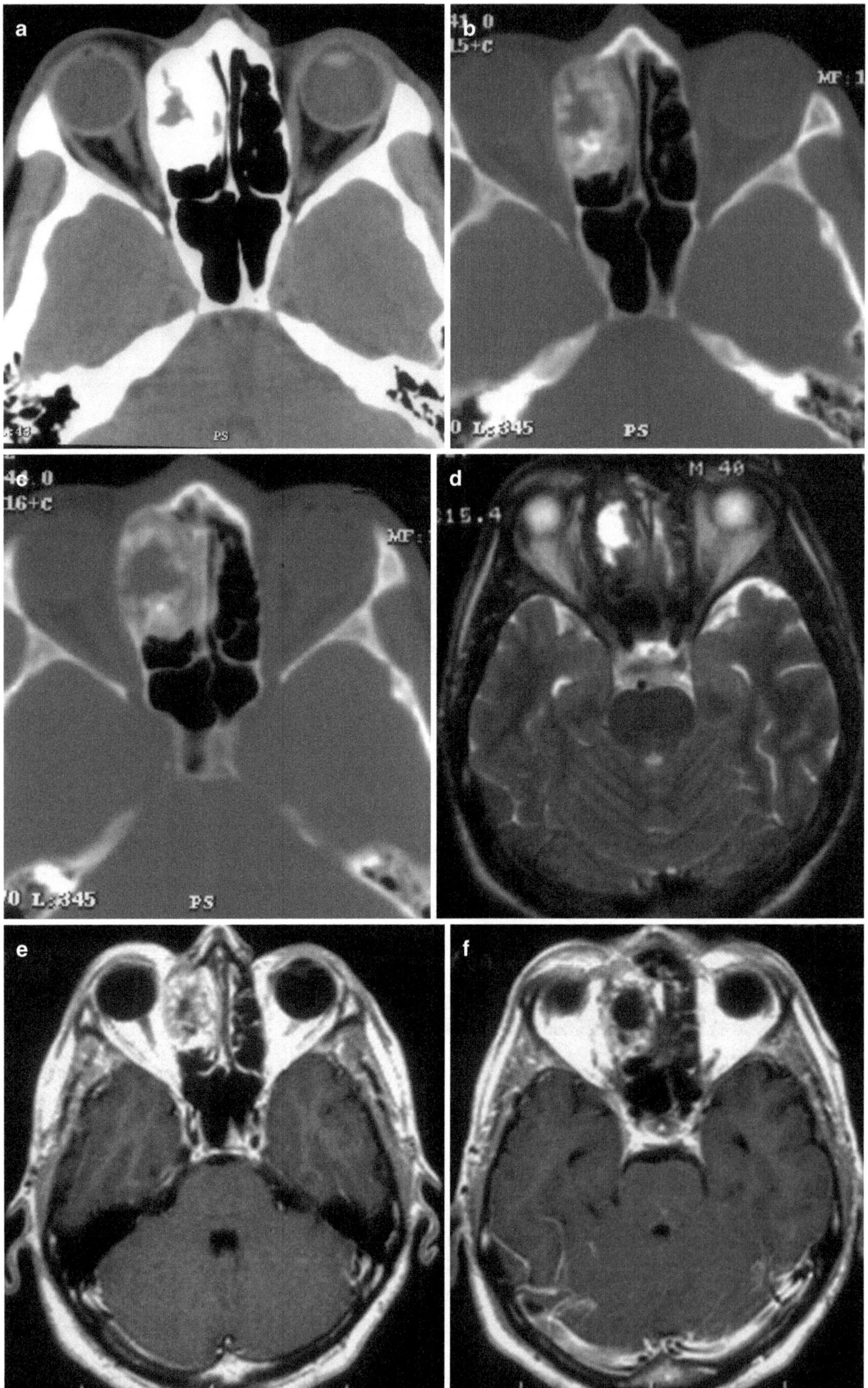

Fig. 10.16 Ossifying fibroma of the anterior ethmoids. Axial CT scans (**a**–**c**) reveal a lesion with dense ossifying periphery and soft tissue central part. T2-weighted (**d**) and T1-weighted (**e**, **f**) MR images after contrast enhancement demonstrate a mass with heterogeneous structure (low MR-signal from the periphery and high MR-signal from the central part), which is characterized by intermediate contrast enhancement by its fibrous part

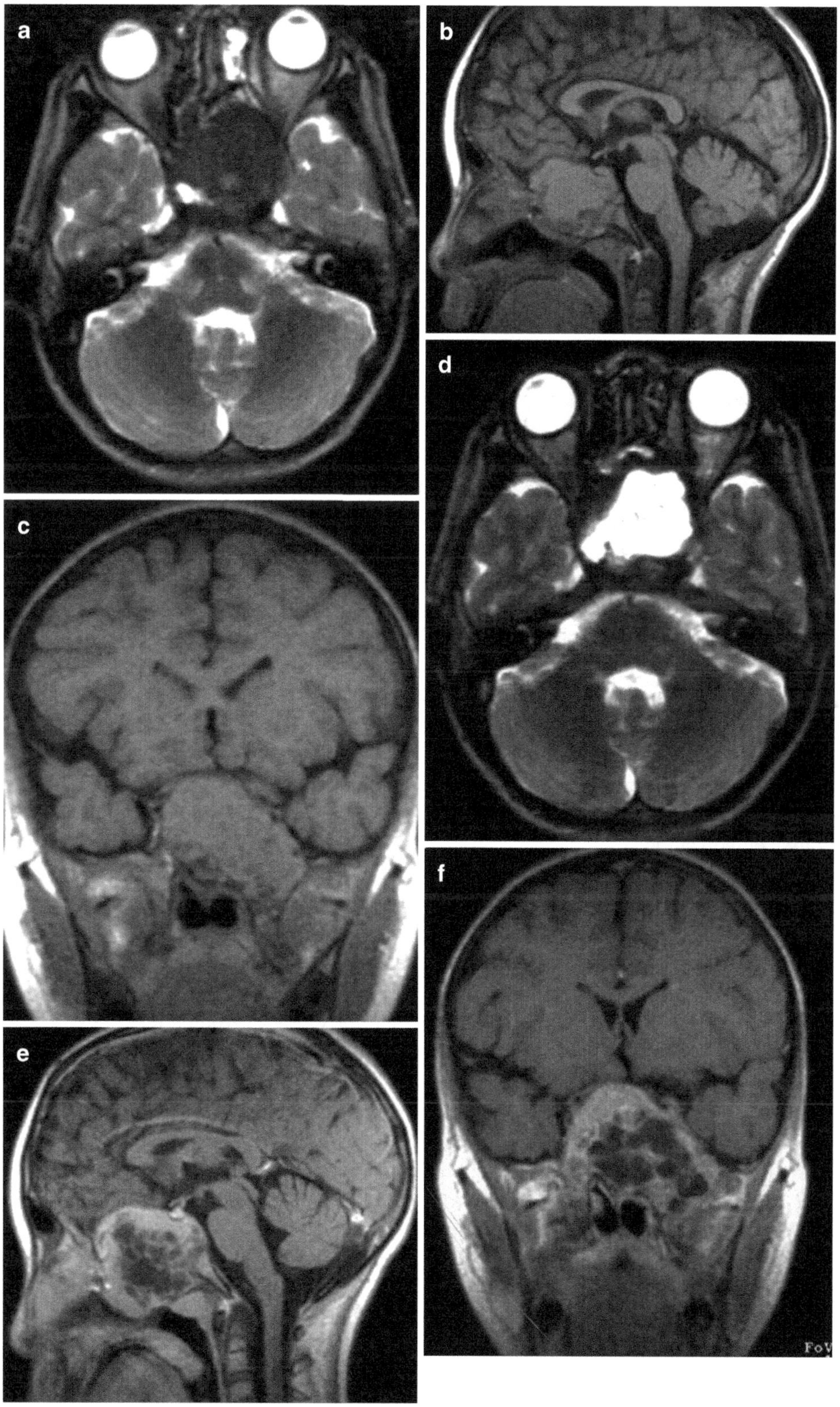

Fig. 10.17 Ossifying fibroma of the sphenoid sinus. On axial T2-weighted (**a**) and T1-weighted MR images in sagittal (**b**) and coronal (**c**) planes a hypointense (on T2) and isointense (on T1) lesion is visualized. A lesion has heterogeneous structure. MRI, performed 1 year later after partial resection, reveals a mass with high MR-signal from the central part of the tumor on T2-weighted image (**d**). Sagittal (**e**) and coronal (**f**) post-contrast T1-weighted MR images show an intense contrast enhancement in peripheral parts of the fibroma with cystic central transformation

nonencapsulated polypoid and locally invasive tumor found only in males during adolescence (Lopez et al. 2017). JNAF accounts for about 0.05% of all head and neck tumors. The tumor affects only males from 10 to 25 years old. Juvenile angiofibroma of the skull base is histologically benign but a clinically aggressive tumor with a significantly high rate of relapses and rapid prolonged growth (Yadav et al. 2002). The complexity of the topographic anatomy of the nose, paranasal sinuses, edematous hypertrophic mucosa after the surgical treatment are the causes of errors and late diagnosis of tumor relapses. Local relapses after the treatment are observed in 6–24% of cases (Petruson et al. 2002; Mann et al. 2004).

JNAF of the posterior parts of the nasal cavity usually grows into the anterior nasal cavity, nasopharynx, pterygopalatine fossa (one of the earliest pathways of growth) (90%). It spreads into the sphenoid sinus in 60% of cases through the roof of the nasopharynx, can grow into the maxilla (43%) and ethmoid sinuses (35%), the infratemporal fossa and the clivus. Finger-like pattern of growth can affect the orbit, middle cranial fossa (parasellar region) and compress the cavernous sinus (Harnsberger et al. 2004a, b).

Common presenting symptoms include nasal obstruction and epistaxis. More advanced tumors may present with facial swelling and visual or neurological disturbances. The evaluation of patients with juvenile angiofibroma relies on diagnostic imaging. Preoperative biopsy is not recommended. The mainstay of treatment is resection combined with preoperative embolization.

Imaging On CT, the tumor is visualized as a soft-tissue lesion at the nasal cavity and nasopharynx with extensive expansion throughout this area. There is a significant reorganization and destruction of surrounding bones, the rear wall of the maxillary sinus is usually pushed out anteriorly. An enlargement of the nasal cavity and pterygopalatine fossa is observed (Lloyd and Phelps 1986). There are no calcifications within the tumor. JNAF is a diffusely and strong enhancing lesion. CT-perfusion study is an important minimally invasive diagnostic method for angiofibromas vasculature assessment. According to our data these tumors are characterized by quite homogeneous and extremely high perfusion (Fig. 10.18), which allows not only visualizing, but also quantifying the tumor tissue hemodynamics itself as well as the pathways of tumor growth. CT-perfusion is a highly effective method in identifying a residual tumor both in the early period after surgery, accompanied by edematous mucosa in the sinuses and nasal cavities, and in the long term angiofibroma recurrence (Figs. 10.19 and 10.20). Differences between BV and BF values from the tumor tissue, and edematous and thickened mucosa of the paranasal sinuses obtained in our 14 patients were so significant that they allowed to differentiate precisely angiofibroma remnants or recurrence, and mucosal hyperplasia, which is often almost impossible to obtain with standard CT or MRI According to CT-perfusion data, JNAF is characterized by sufficiently uniform elevation in hemodynamic parameters: BV (21.78 ± 13.35 ml/100 g), BF (104.7 ± 35.22 ml/100 g/min) for the tumor tissue were significantly elevated in all 14 patients compared with those for the white matter of the brain (CBV (2.09 ± 1.62 ml/100 g), CBF (23.60 ± 13.07 ml/100 g/min)), mucosa of the sinonasal cavities (BV (6.84 ± 8.03 ml/100 g), CBF (42.79 ± 35.26 ml/100 g/min)), and temporal muscle (CBV (2.28 ± 1.58 ml/100 g), CBF (13.61 ± 11.6 ml/100 g/min) (Fig. 10.18).

On T1-weighted MR images, the tumor has a heterogeneous, intermediate intensity MR-signal with small foci of signal intensity loss (flow-void phenomena) from large tumor vessels. On T2-weighted images, the lesion is also heterogeneous; MR-signal intensity varies from moderate to high. Local microfoci of loss MR-signal from the blood vessels are also visualized. For contrast-enhanced MRI, it is appropriate to use Fat-Sat techniques better at the coronal plane in order to exclude or confirm JNAF's growth into the cavernous sinuses, sphenoid sinus, and skull base region (Lloyd et al. 2000a, b). However the main problem with MRI is the difficulties of distinguishing the marginal tumor areas from the altered and usually inflamed and thickened mucosa that, similar to the tumor on routine MR imaging, intensively accumulates contrast material as well (Fig. 10.21).

MR angiography detects hypertrophy of the external carotid artery branches, in particular, the maxillary artery on the affected side. DSA typically reveals intense capillary network of the tumor with supplying from the external carotid artery branches (maxillary and ascending pharyngeal arteries are frequent supplying vessels). If the tumor spreads into the cavernous sinus, it may be supplied by the branches of the internal carotid artery (Fig. 10.22).

Differential Diagnosis

1. Encephalocele is a lesion connecting with the intracranial subarachnoid space, contains the brain parenchyma and/or meninges, does not accumulate the contrast material;

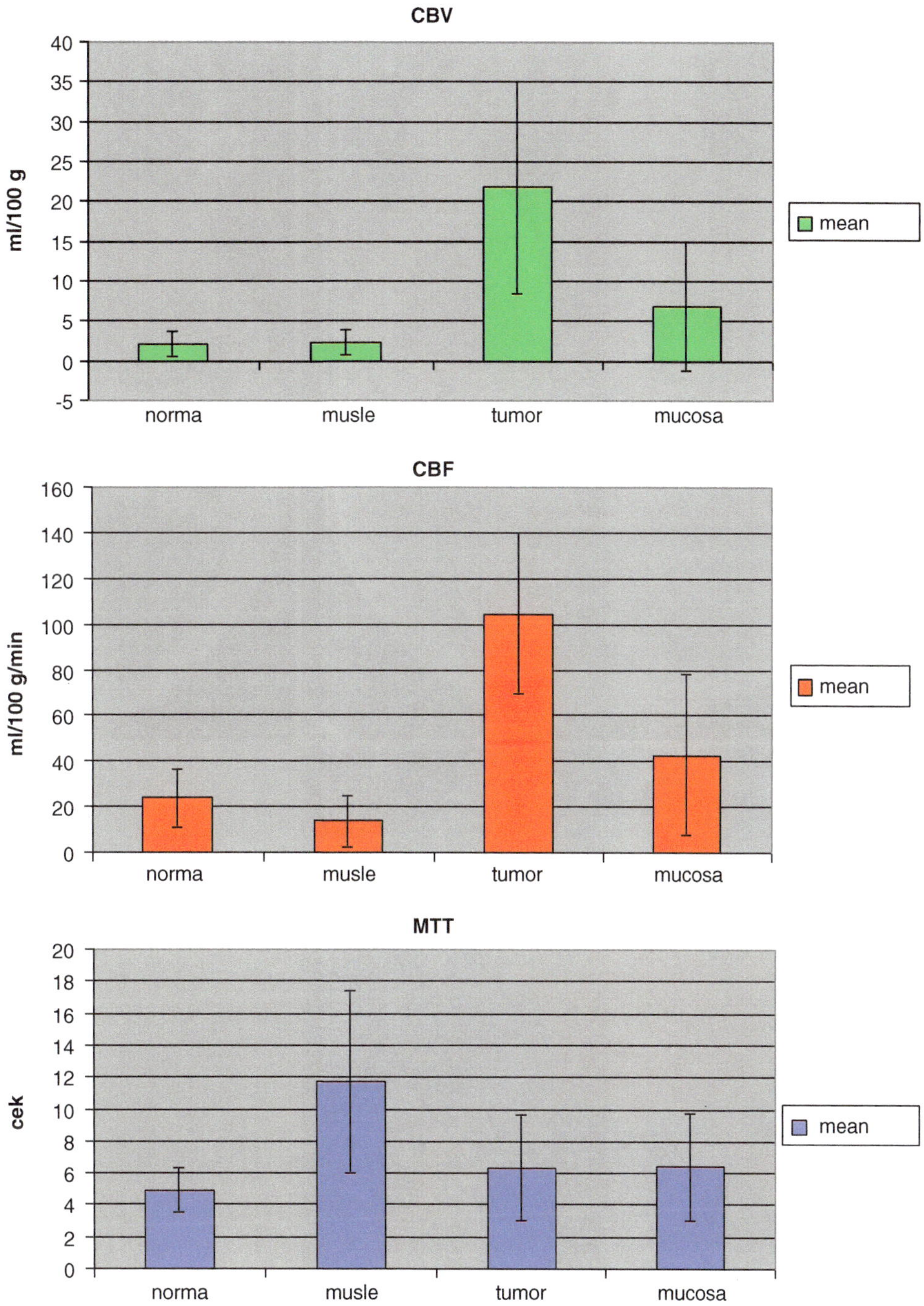

Fig. 10.18 CT-perfusion data of the patients with juvenile angiofibromas compared to white matter, temporal muscle, mucous of sinuses. (**a**) CBV, (**b**) CBF, (**c**) MTT

2. Polyps in the nasal cavity and maxillary sinuses—masses that fill the sinuses cavity; pterygopalatine fossa is usually not involved; the lesion prolapses into the anterior nasal cavity, then into the nasopharynx;
3. Hemangioma is usually localized in the nasal cavity; there are no areas of MR-signal loss from the blood vessels; occurs not only in young males;
4. Rhabdomyosarcoma is a soft-tissue mass with bone destruction, occurring not only in the posterior portion of the nasal cavity, usually does not spread into the pterygopalatine fossa; rapid invasive and destructive growth are the main characteristic features.

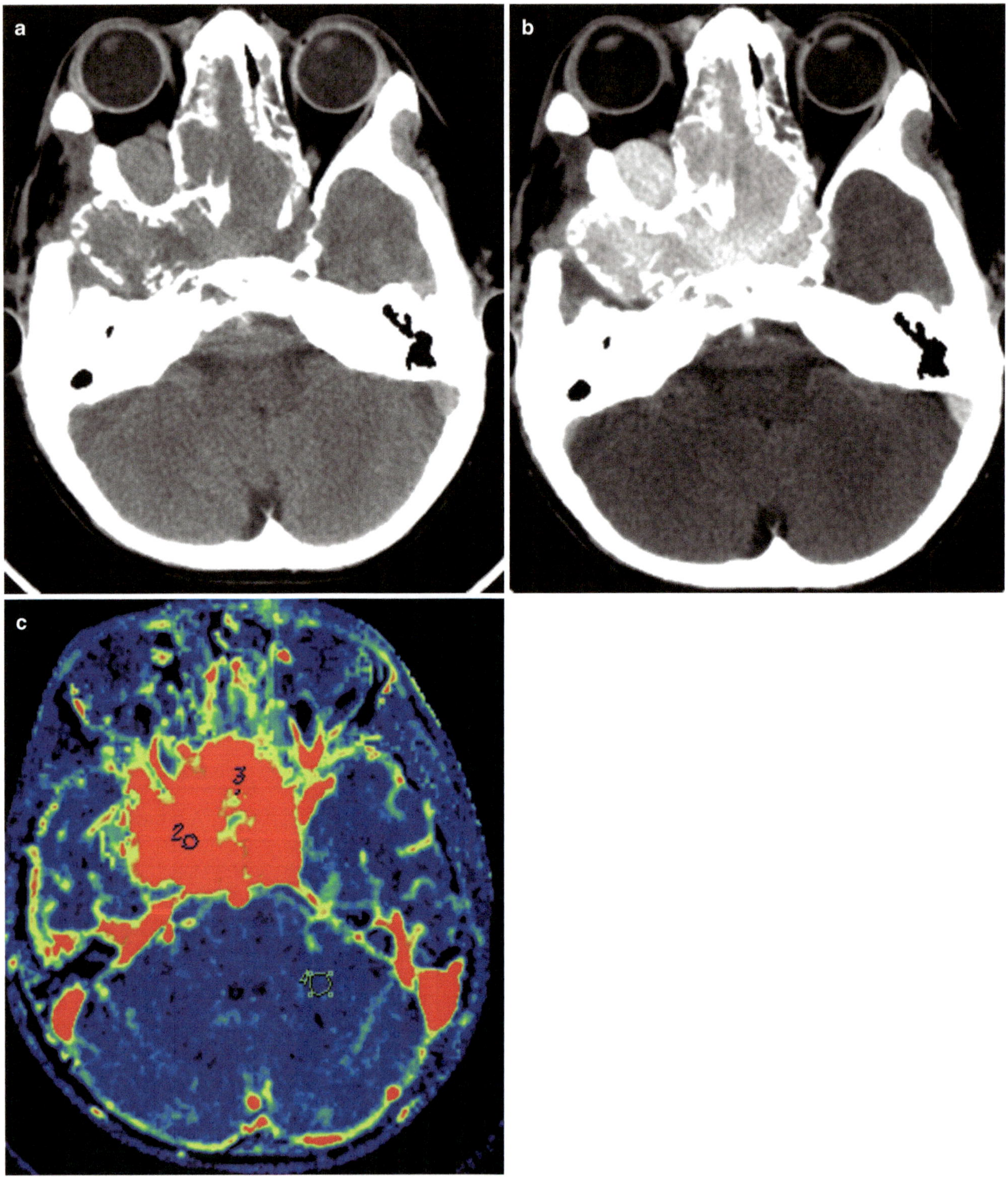

Fig. 10.19 Juvenile nasopharyngeal angiofibroma. Axial CT scans before (**a**) and after (**b**) contrast enhancement demonstrate a large tumor extending to the nasal cavity, ethmoids, sphenoid sinus, the right orbit, and temporal region. The tumor is characterized by a homogeneous contrast enhancement. There is a bone destruction and remodeling. CT-perfusion study reveals a very high tumor blood flow values (CBF (**c**))

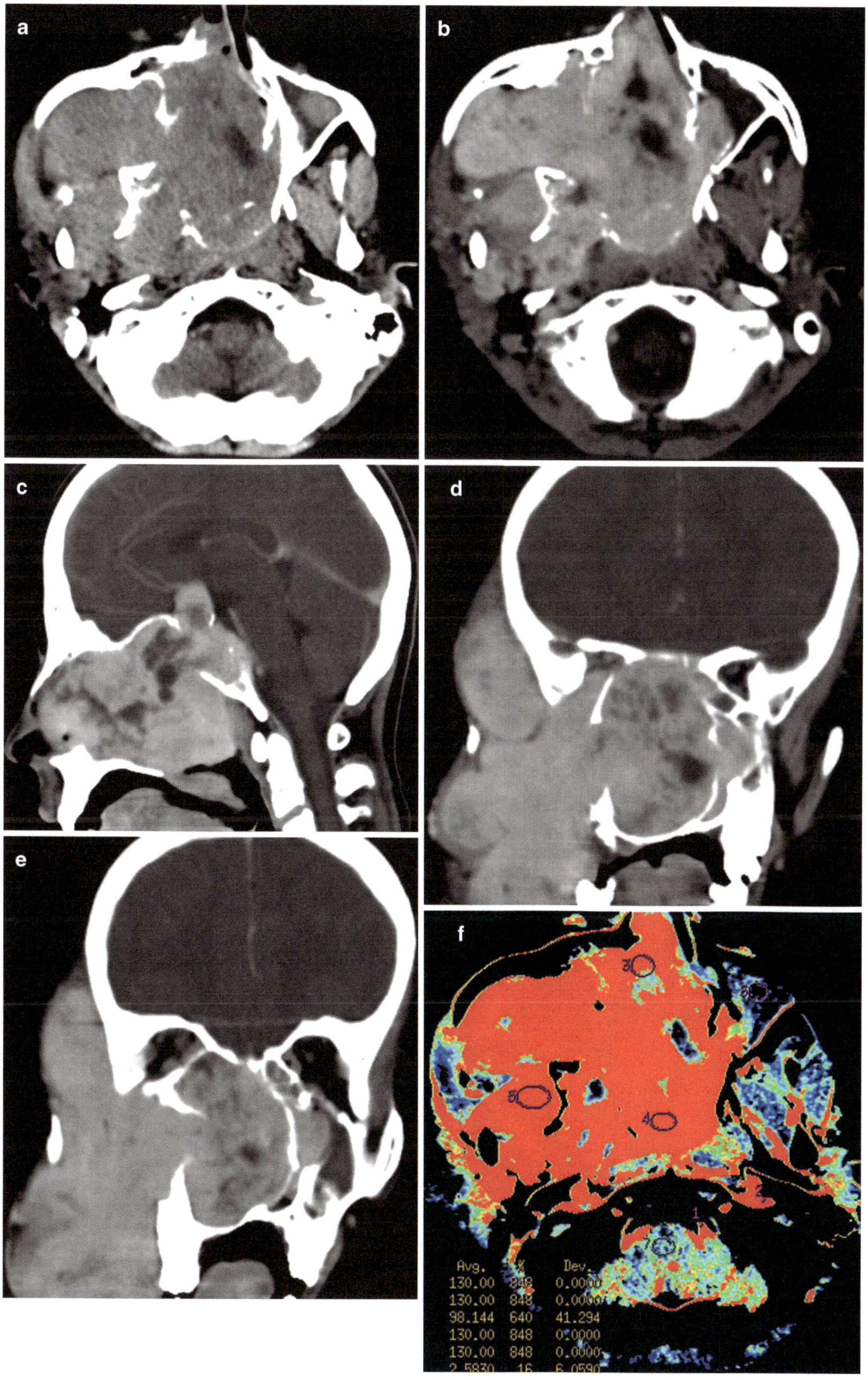

Fig. 10.20 Juvenile angiofibroma. Axial CT scans before (**a**) and after contrast enhancement (axial (**b**), sagittal (**c**), coronal reformats (**d**, **e**)) show a huge strongly enhancing mass with involvement of the nasal cavity and paranasal sinuses. The tumor spreads into nasopharynx and pterygopalatine fossa, and leads to bones destruction in the craniofacial area. CT-perfusion study demonstrates extremely high values of cerebral blood flow within the tumor (CBF (**f**))

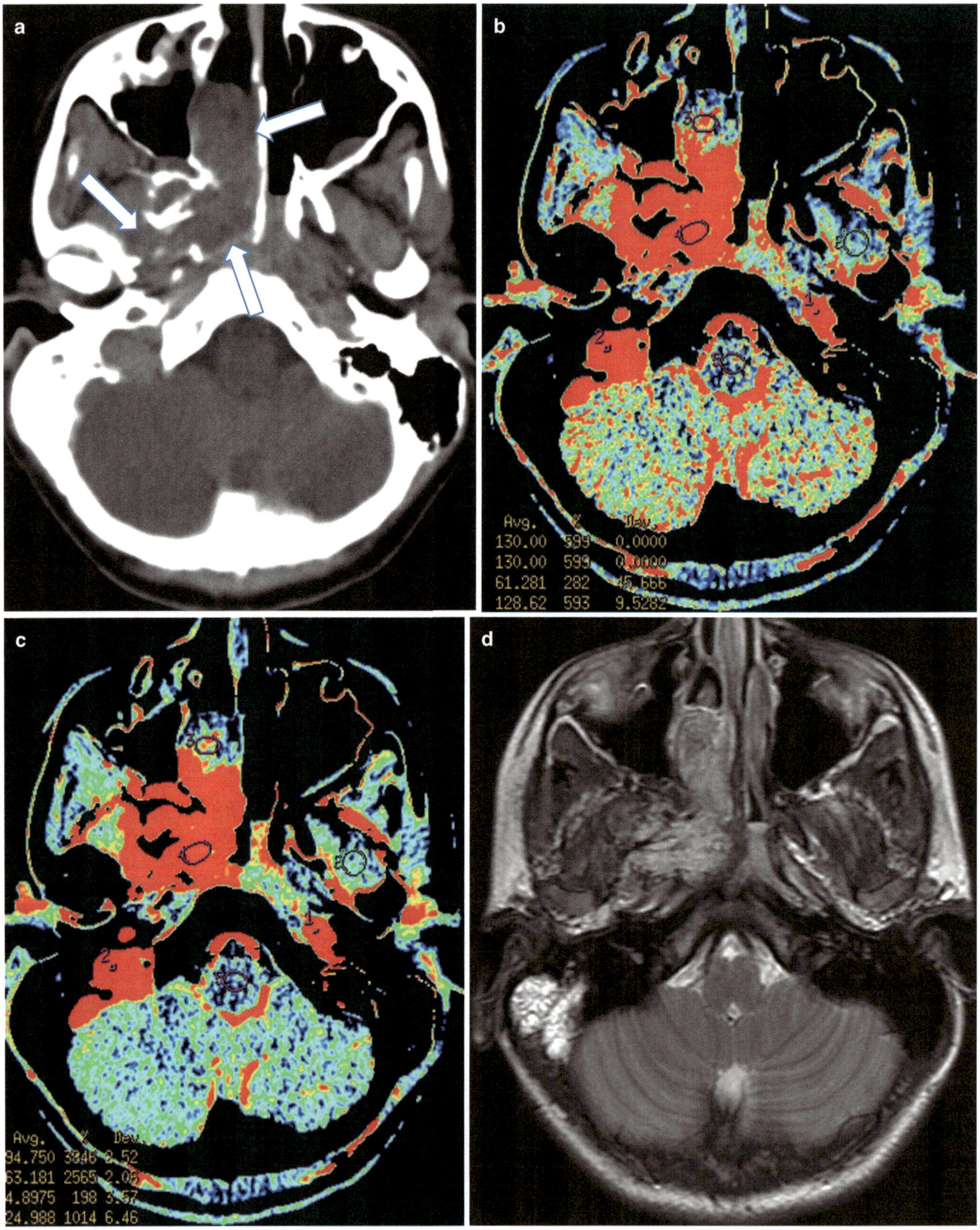

Fig. 10.21 Juvenile nasopharyngeal angiofibroma of a 14-year-old boy. Axial CT scan (**a**) shows a slightly hypodense with muscles soft-tissue tumor in the right pterygopalatine fossa and nasopharynx (*arrows*). CT-perfusion study (CBF (**b**), CBV (**c**)) demonstrates high values of blood flow and blood volume for the tumor. On T2-weighted MRI (**d**) the angiofibroma has hyperintense MR-signal, on T1 (**e**) it has isointense to muscle MR-signal. On T1-WI with contrast enhancement (**f**) and on T1 + fat suppression (**g**–**i**) the angiofibroma enhances homogeneously and intensely (*arrows*). Pathologic vascular network (areas of MR-signal loss of tortuous shape) in the projection of pterygopalatine fossa can be seen on T1-Fat-Sat MR image (**g**) (*short arrows*)

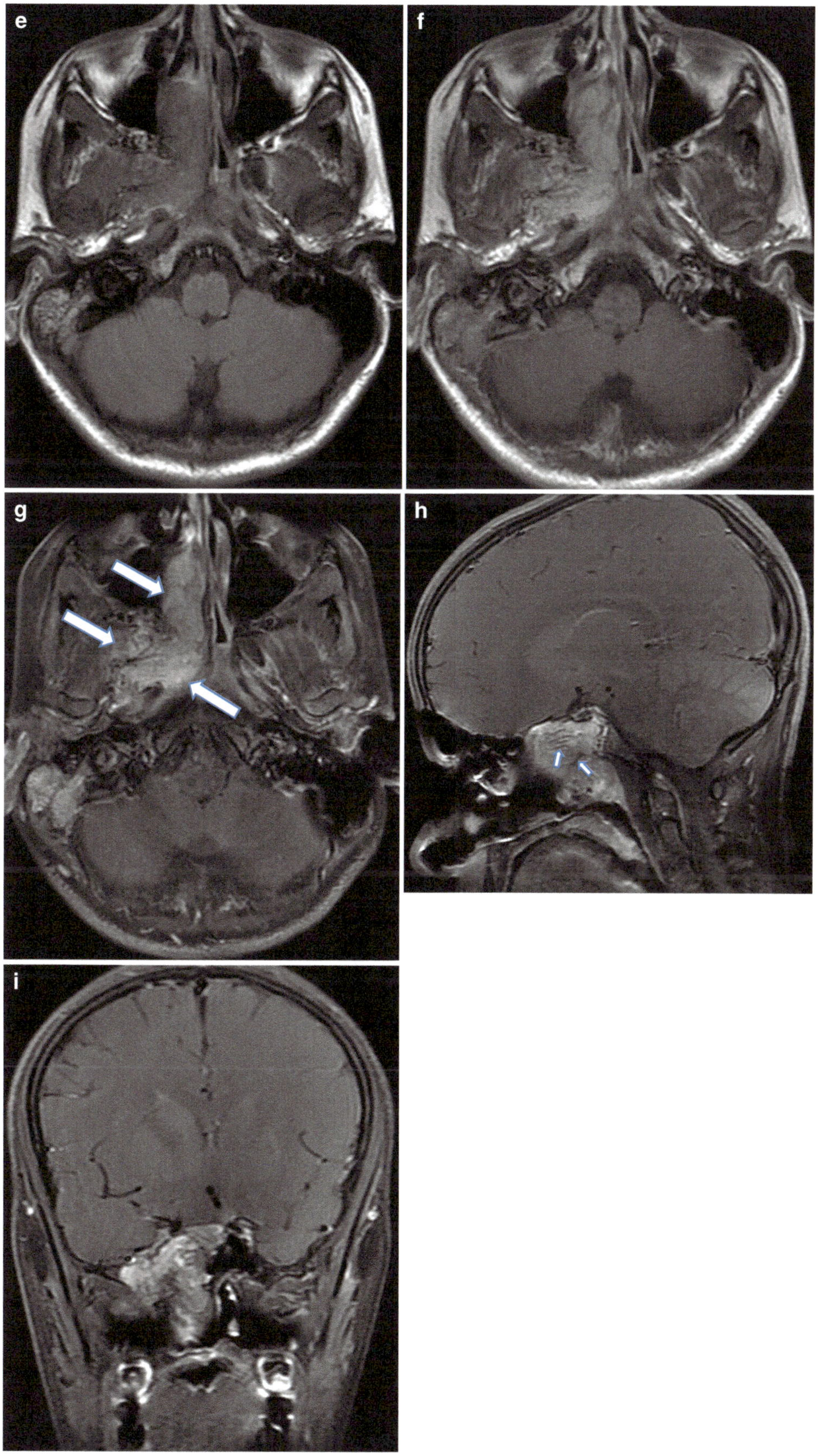

Fig. 10.21 (continued)

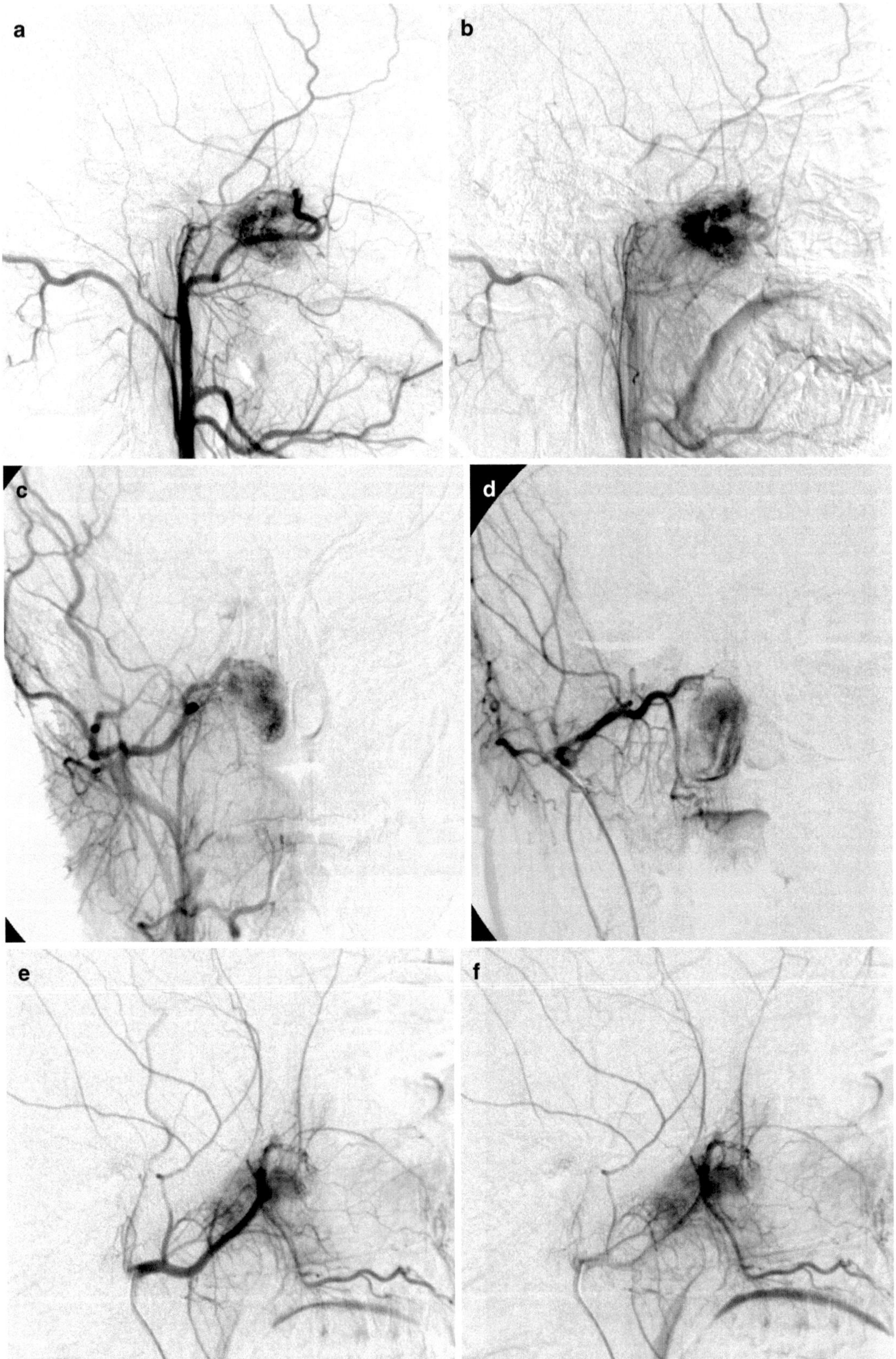

Fig. 10.22 Juvenile angiofibromas of a 14-year-old patient (**a–c**) and of a 20-year-old patient (**d–f**). Direct superselective angiography demonstrates an abundant blood supply from branches of the maxillary artery in both cases

10.1 Hemangioma

Hemangiomas of the nasal cavity occur most commonly in area of the nasal septum (65%), then lateral wall (18%), and vestibule (16%) (Som et al. 2011). According to the literature the lesions arising in the anterior septum are typically of the capillary type. In area of lateral wall the lesions have usually the cavernous structure. Epistaxis and nasal obstruction are the most common clinical presentation of the lesion. Even a small size hemangiomas can lead to severe epistaxis. Sometimes the spontaneous regression can be observed. In craniofacial region the hemangiomas that primarily involve the bone structure can also occur. These lesions account for 0.7% of all primary bone tumors and can arise in area of skull base, mandible, nasal bone (Barnes 1985).

Imaging Hemangiomas which are located within nasal cavities have isodense structure on NECT and strong contrast enhancement. On MRI this lesion is characterized by intermediate MR-signal in all sequences and, as on CT, demonstrates prominent contrast enhancement (Fig. 10.23). Sometimes on T2-weighted images the tortuous areas of MR-signal loss can be visualized within the lesion—pathologic vascular net. Hemangiomas that predominantly grow inside the facial and skull base bones can have different appearance—a"sunray," "honeycomb," and "soap bubble." They have low or intermediate signal intensity on T1 MRI and hyperintensity on T2-weighted images. Hemangiomas both enhance on CT and MRI. For better demarcation of lesion borders it is recommended to use Fat-Sat technology on MR studies, especially after contrast enhancement.

10.2 Giant Cell Tumor (GCT)

Giant cell tumor of bone (old name was osteoblastoclastoma or osteoclastoma) is a benign, expansile lesion with potentially local aggressiveness. This lesion accounts up to 5% of all primary bone tumors (Kujas et al. 1999; Som et al. 2011) and the epiphysis of long bones is the most common primary site of the GCT. The location in craniofacial region is extremely rare for this tumor (Kujas et al. 1999).

Imaging CT imaging is a very good modality for early detection of the bone destruction and bone remodel that can be demonstrated in cases with GCT. Initially GCT is a hyperdense lesion. Contrast enhancement is mandatory in all cases because GCT is prominent enhanced lesion. MR-appearance of GCT is dependent on tumor structure. With cystic formation MR-signal on T2-weighted images becomes higher than that in the soft-tissue component which is usually has dark MR-signal on T2 (Fig. 10.24). Contrast enhancement is prominent, and more obvious with Fat-Sat technology MRI. In out perfusion studies with using MRI and CT GCTs demonstrate from low to intermediate increase of BF and BV parameters.

10.3 Aneurysmal Bone Cyst (ABC)

Aneurysmal bone cyst—80–90% of primary aneurysmal bone cysts are detected in patients younger than 20 years old. It is not a pure tumor, but rather an increasing cystic lesion (not a true cyst) of an unknown origin, which accounts up to 2% of primary bone tumors (Som et al. 1991; Kaffe et al. 1999). The lesion is covered by intact periosteum, under which there is a thin calcified layer. ABC appears as a network of cavities with different sizes, filled with non-coagulated blood or protein contents. Sometimes ABC can be presented as a unilocular lesion. The walls of cameras have no vascular endothelium and are covered with fibrous tissue and often contain bone-like tissue (Pawha 2009). ABC can be primary or secondary, i.e. be associated with other bone lesions (giant cell tumor, chondroblastoma, fibrous dysplasia, osteosarcoma, etc.). Between 3 and 12% of all ABC occur in the head-neck area, and they also have been reported in the maxilla, orbit, ethmoid, and frontal bone (Citardi et al. 1996).

Imaging Expansion and thinning of the cortical bone is one of the main radiological characteristics. ABC appears as a lytic expansile lesion limited by a thin peripheral cortical bone (an "eggshell" sign), which may be intermittent, sometimes there are barely distinguishable trabeculae. On CT and MRI, ABC may be unilocular or may demonstrate multilocular pattern. On CT scans ABC may appear as "soap-bubble" or "honeycomb" radiological pattern (Kaffe et al. 1999). CT successfully distinguishes between the bone and soft tissue structures that can accumulate contrast material.

MR-signal of the lesion may vary and, depending on the contents of the cysts (non-coagulated blood or blood-containing fluids), have a high signal on T1- and T2-weighted sequences, whereas in the absence or low protein content, the intensity of MR-signal can be low on T1-weighted, and high on T2-weighted images. The lesion is usually surrounded by a low-intensity rim. The fluid–fluid levels or the sedimentation effect are one of the principal ABC characteristics (Beltran et al. 1986; Zimmer et al. 1984). However, sedimentation can also be observed in more aggressive lesions, such as telangioectatic osteosarcoma. These lesions can be differentiated only via biopsy. Also, ABC is often confused with giant cell tumors. The utility of contrast enhancement demonstrates quite pronounced, but heterogeneous contrast enhancement of the soft tissue components of ABC (Figs. 10.25 and 10.26).

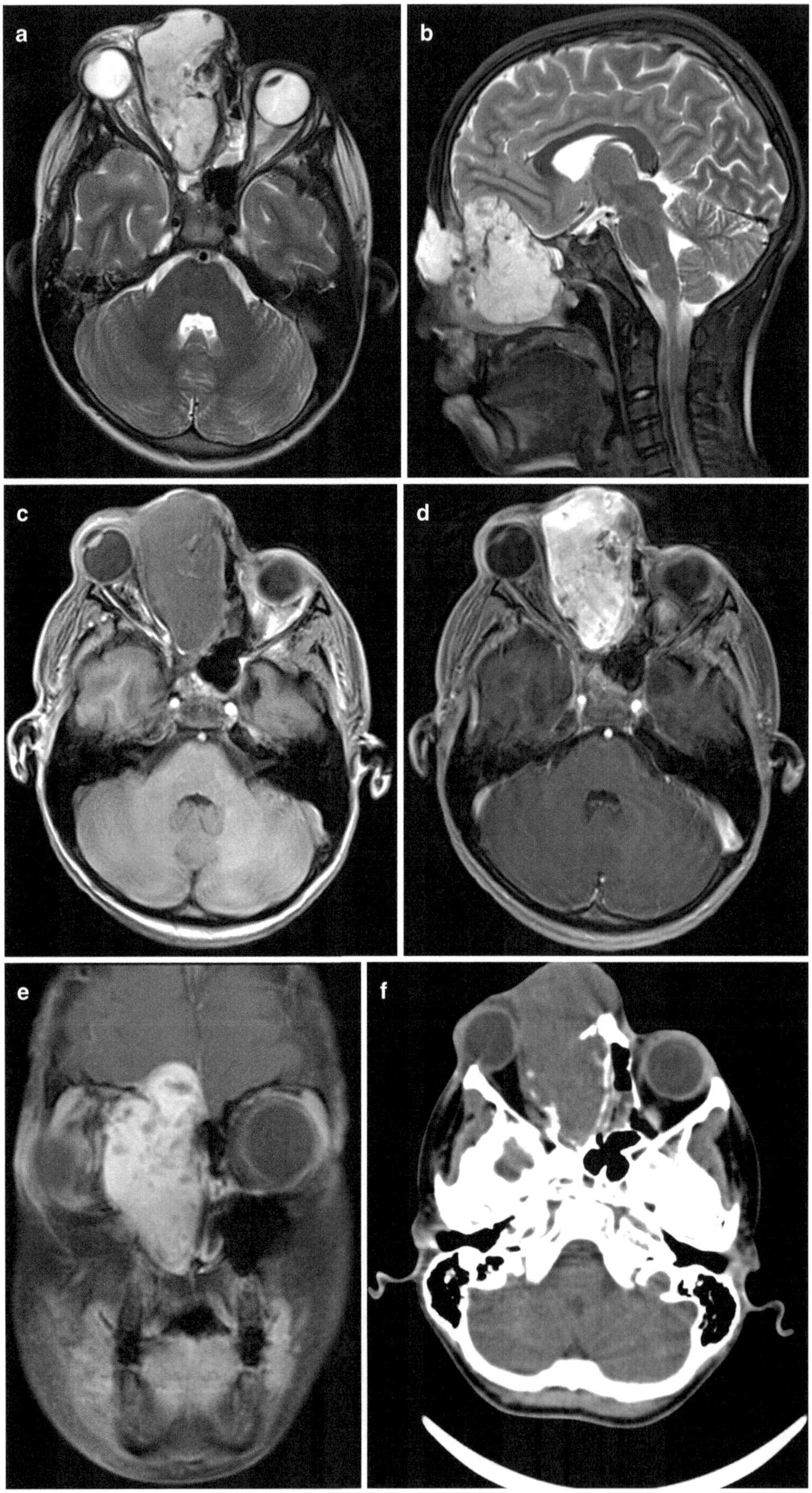

Fig. 10.23 Hemangioma (capillary type). T2- (**a**, **b**) and T1- (**c**) weighted MR images show an expansile large mass in the projection of right ethmiod complex extending into nasal cavities, intracranially as well as extracranially in area of dorsum nose. Right globe is dislocated laterally. A lesion has hyperintense on T2 and hypointense on T1-weighted images, and strongly and homogeneously enhances (**d**, **e**). CT scans before (**f**) and after (**g**) contrast enhancement demonstrate a soft tissue tumor with prominent enhancement and bone remodel rather than destruction (**h**, **i**)

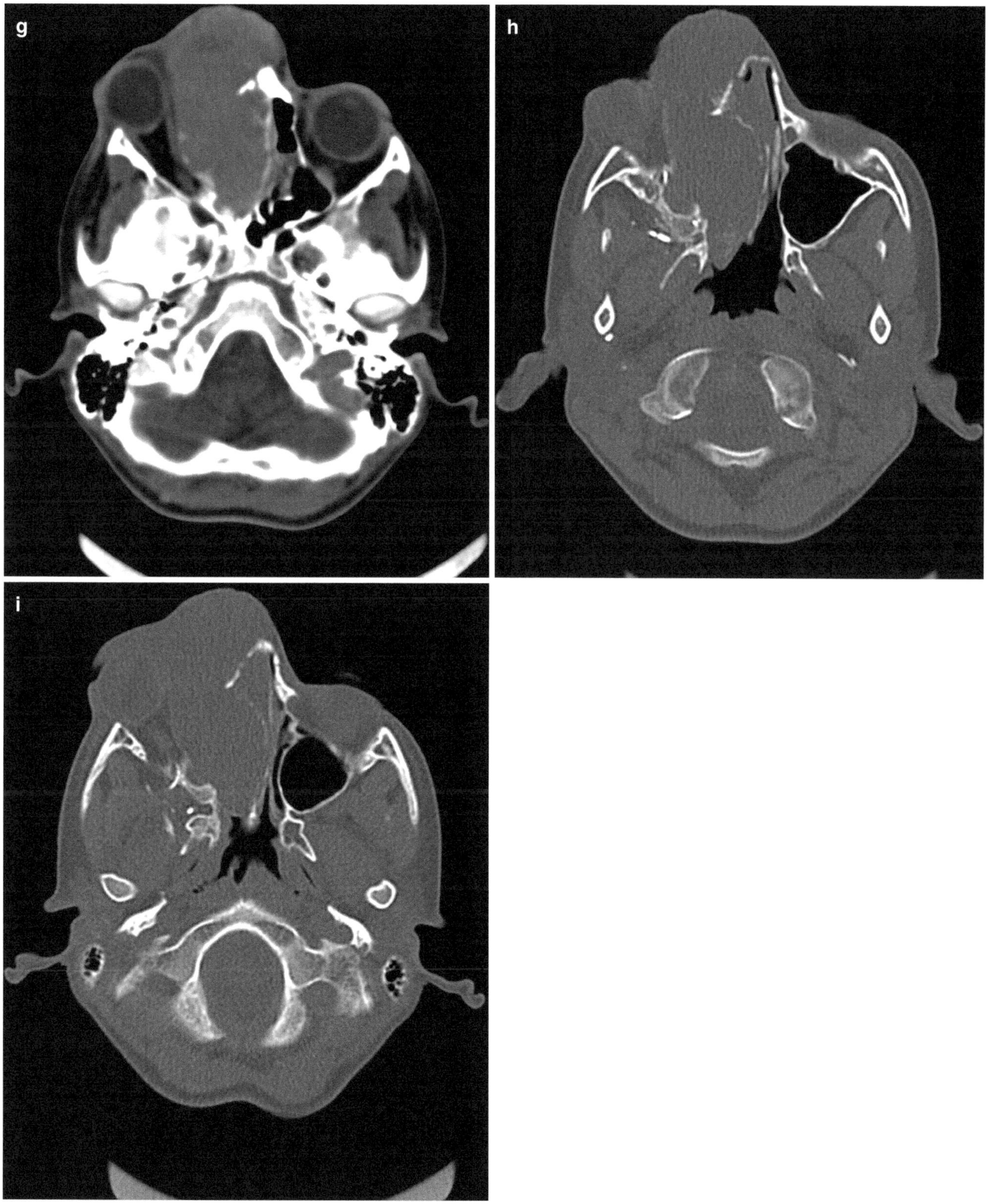

Fig. 10.23 (continued)

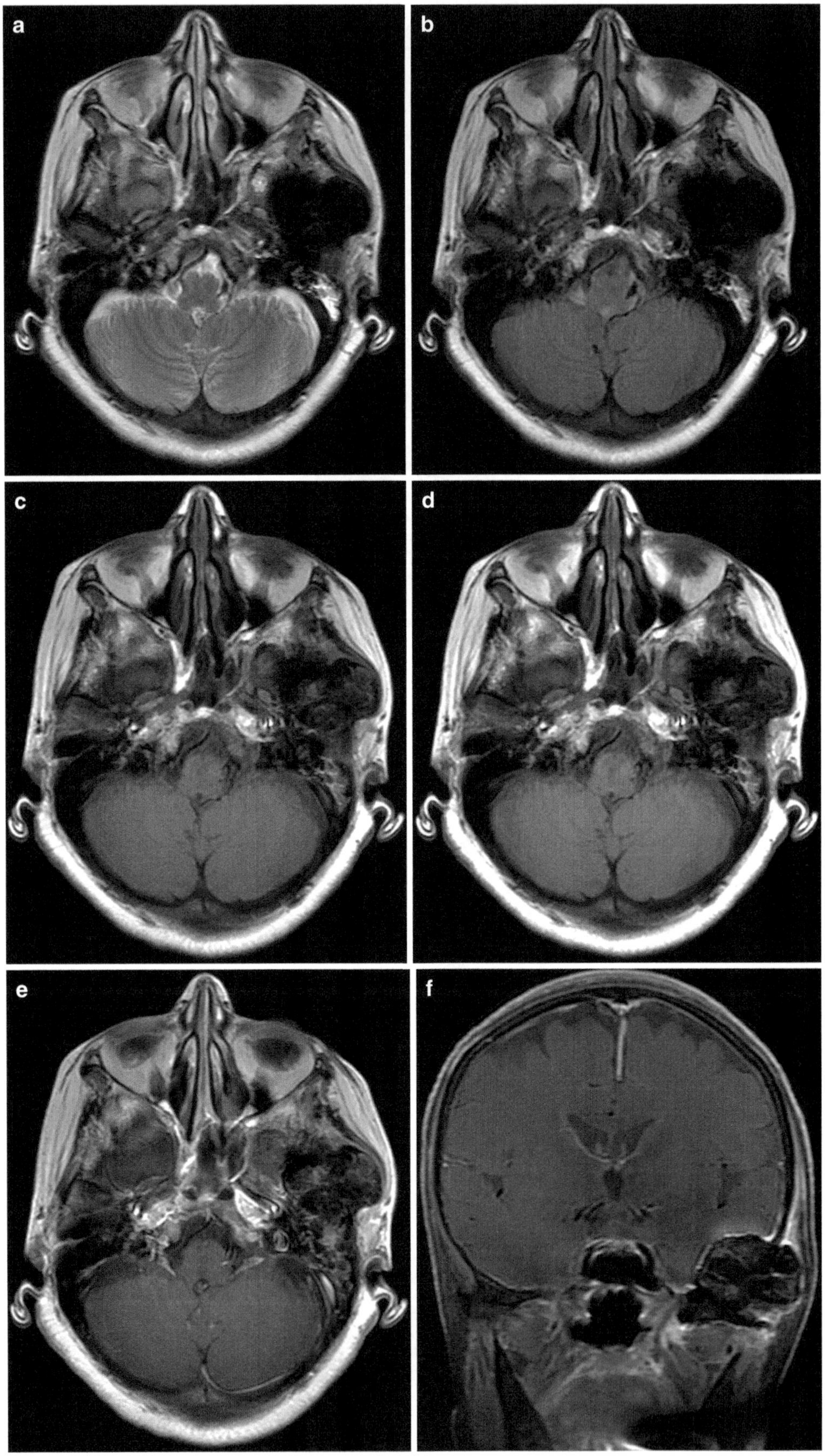

Fig. 10.24 Giant cell tumor of the temporal area. Axial T2- (**a**), T2-FLAIR- (**b**) and T1- (**c, d**) weighted MR images show a hypointense in all sequences mass with MR-signal which is comparable to bone. Soft tissue septa can be seen inside the lesion. Contrast enhancement has low degree and is not so obvious (**e**) even using Fat-Sat technology (**f**). CECT imaging (**g–i**) better than MRI showed extent of bone destruction as well as bone remodel

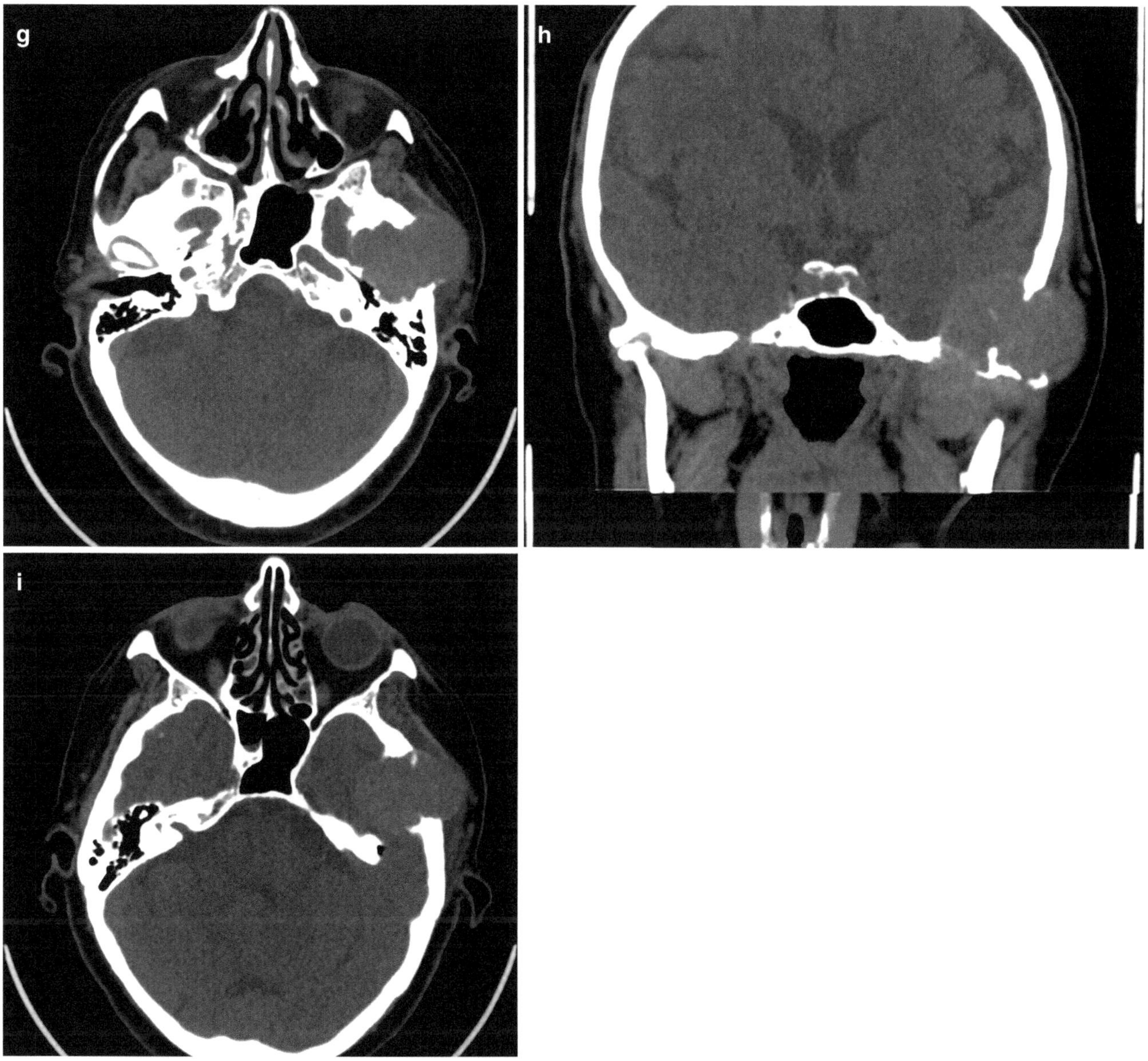

Fig. 10.24 (continued)

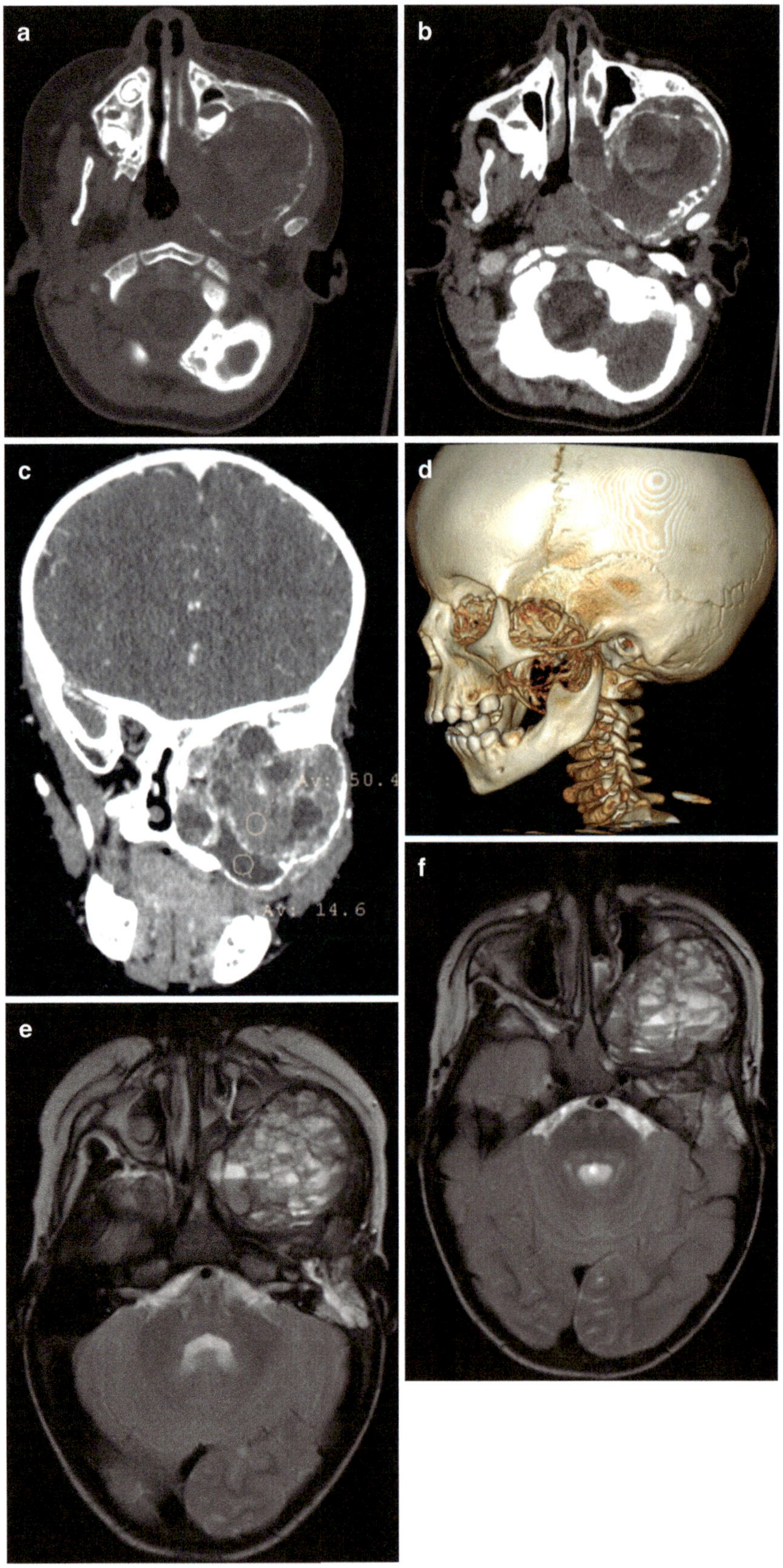

Fig. 10.25 Aneurysmal bone cyst in the craniofacial region (child, 2 years old). CT scans before (**a**) and after (**b**, **c**) contrast enhancement demonstrate a large expansile mass, growing in the left craniofacial area. A lesion leads to surrounding bone remodeling (3D-reconstruction (**d**)). A mass has heterogeneous structure with multicystic formation and prominent contrast enhancement of soft tissue components. T2-weighted MR images (**e**, **f**) show a multilocular cystic mass with different hyperintense MR-signal into them and the effect of sedimentation (fluid-fluid level) within cystic lesions.T1-weighted MR images before (**g**) and after (**h**) contrast enhancement show intense contrast agent accumulation within soft tissue portion of the lesion. MR-angiography (**i**) doesn't show pathologic vascular net of the lesion

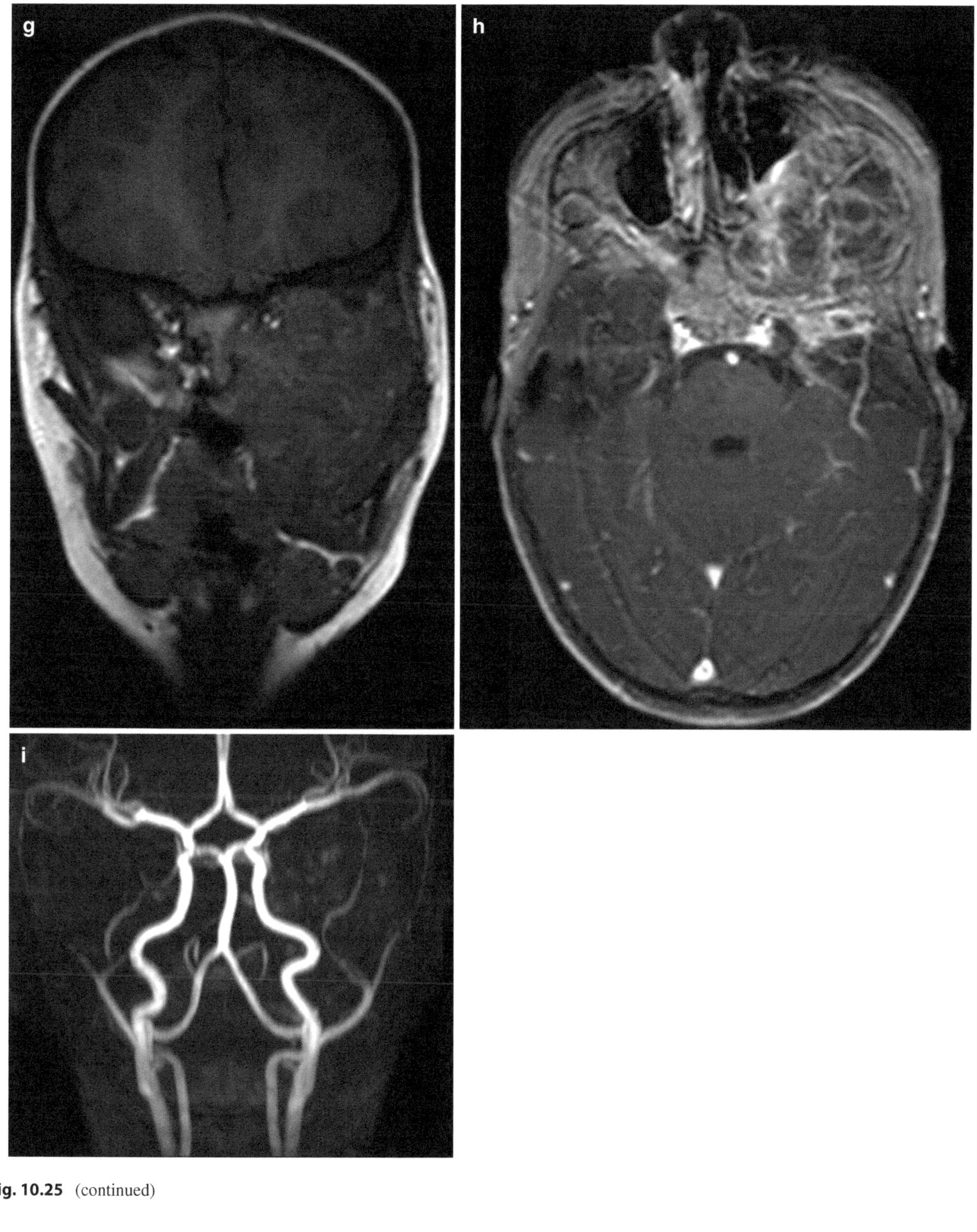

Fig. 10.25 (continued)

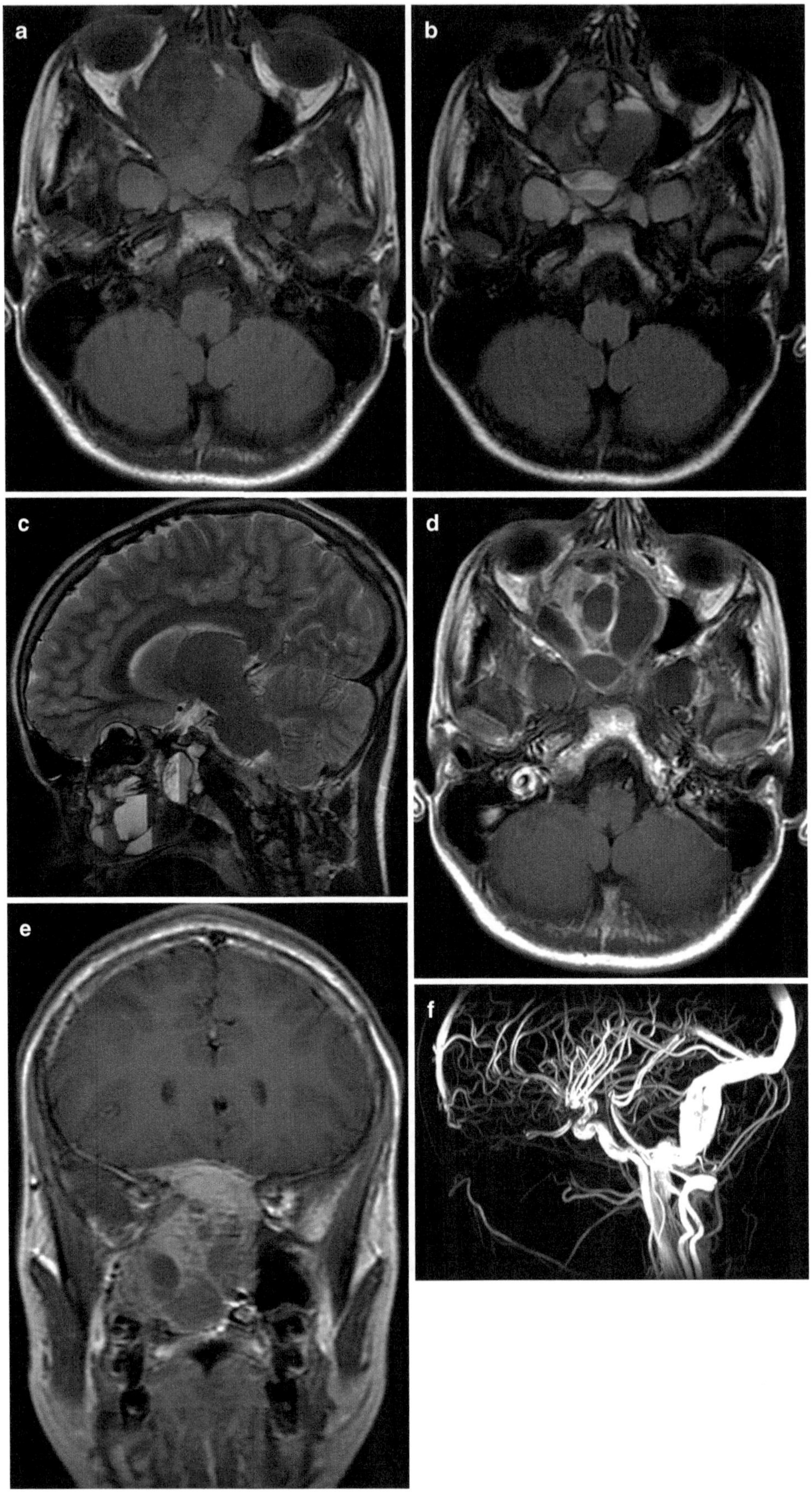

Fig. 10.26 Aneurysmal bone cyst of the nasopharynx. T1- (**a**), T2-FLAIR- (**b**), and T2- (**c**) weighted MR images demonstrate an expansile lesion, which consists of multiple cavities with fluid components. In some of the cavities the effect of sedimentation is clearly visible. Soft-tissue part of the lesion intensely enhances (**d**, **e**). MR-angiography (3D PC) reveals avascular region in projection of the tumor location (**f**)

Differential Diagnosis Chondrosarcoma, fibrous dysplasia, malignant fibrous histiocytoma, telangioectatic osteosarcoma, and giant cell tumor.

10.4 Ameloblastoma

Ameloblastoma is a benign tumor originating from odontogenic epithelium of the mandible or maxilla, which accounts from 10 to 18% of all odontogenic tumors and only 1% of all lesions of the jaw (Scholl et al. 1999). In general, this is a mixed-density, cystic, and solid lesion. The posterior mandible is the most common site of the tumor origin. In the upper jaw, it is often localized in the area of the first molars and premolars.

Imaging On CT, this is a single-chamber lesion in 20% of cases and a multi-chamber lesion with wavy edges, a "bubble" symptom, resorption of surrounding teeth in 80% of cases. There is also thinning of cortical layers of the mandible or maxilla, which would remain intact in case of a small lesion. The lesion has a low density (osteolytic changes) with nonhomogeneous structure and doesn't enhance on CT. If the lesion extends beyond the boundaries of the bone tissue, accumulation by the soft tissue component can be intense. However, spreading outside the bone tissue is a rare feature of the tumor. On T1- and T2-weighted MR images, a lesion has heterogeneous structure (Hughes et al. 1999; Asaumi et al. 2002). A tumor shows strong but inhomogeneous contrast enhancement with a multilocular pattern created by small cystic lesions that don't enhance and separate from enhancing tumor (Weissman 1993; Asaumi et al. 2002). This last feature is considered as importing radiologic pattern in the distinguishing ameloblastoma from others, especially malignant tumors of craniofacial region (such as squamous cell carcinoma) (Weissman 1993) (Fig. 10.27).

Differential Diagnosis

1. Periapical cyst (abscess)—severe pain;
2. Follicular cyst is a single-chamber cystic lesion, may be similar to ameloblastoma;
3. Odontogenic keratocyst is often indistinguishable from ameloblastoma;
4. Fibrous dysplasia—"ground glass" sign, even if the cysts are present, there are always matrix calcifications;
5. Aneurysmal bone cyst is more common in children, a rounded, multi-chamber lesion with fluid–fluid levels.
6. Squamous cell carcinomas of the nasal sinuses are generally homogeneous, multilocular and cystic structure is not typical. Marked hyperintensity on T2-weighted images on ameloblastomas as well as the degree of contrast enhancement would be unusual for squamous cell carcinomas.

10.5 Chondroma

According to the WHO classification, chondromas belong to benign cartilaginous tumors. It is characterized by slow growth. Spine is usual chondroma localization. The tumor is extremely rare, occurs in craniofacial region. Nevertheless, the majority of head and neck chondromas have been reported in the nasal cavity and ethmoids (70% of all cases). There is no gender predilection. Approximately 60% tumors occur in patients younger than 50 years old (Barnes 1985).

Imaging Chondromas are typically well-circumscribed, sometimes encapsulated lesions.

On CT, these tumors tend to be expansile, remodel bone, and appear as a hypodense lesion compared to muscle. Typical CT-feature is the calcification within the tumor matrix, but in some cases they are not visible. On MR imaging, they usually are characterized by hypointense MR-signal on T1-weighted images and high MR-signal on T2-weighted images with foci of low intensity due to intratumor calcifications. In most cases the contrast enhancement is prominent but heterogeneous. CT-perfusion demonstrates low values of tumor blood flow and blood volume (Figs. 10.28 and 10.29).

10.6 Neurofibroma

Neurofibroma (NF) is a benign, well-circumscribed, but nonencapsulated tumor arising from the nerve sheath. Together with schwannomas and referred to as peripheral nerve sheath tumors they are very common for the head and neck area. Craniofacial and sinonasal cavity involvement is considered as rare primary site of these types of the tumors (less than 4% (Hillstrom et al. 1990). Histologically, this tumor composes of fibroblastic cells and neuronal elements within a collagenized matrix. It can be a solitary tumor or be multifocal, especially in patients with neurofibromatosis (NF Type I). In some cases these tumors can have malignant degeneration (5–15%) (Oberman and Sullenger 1967).

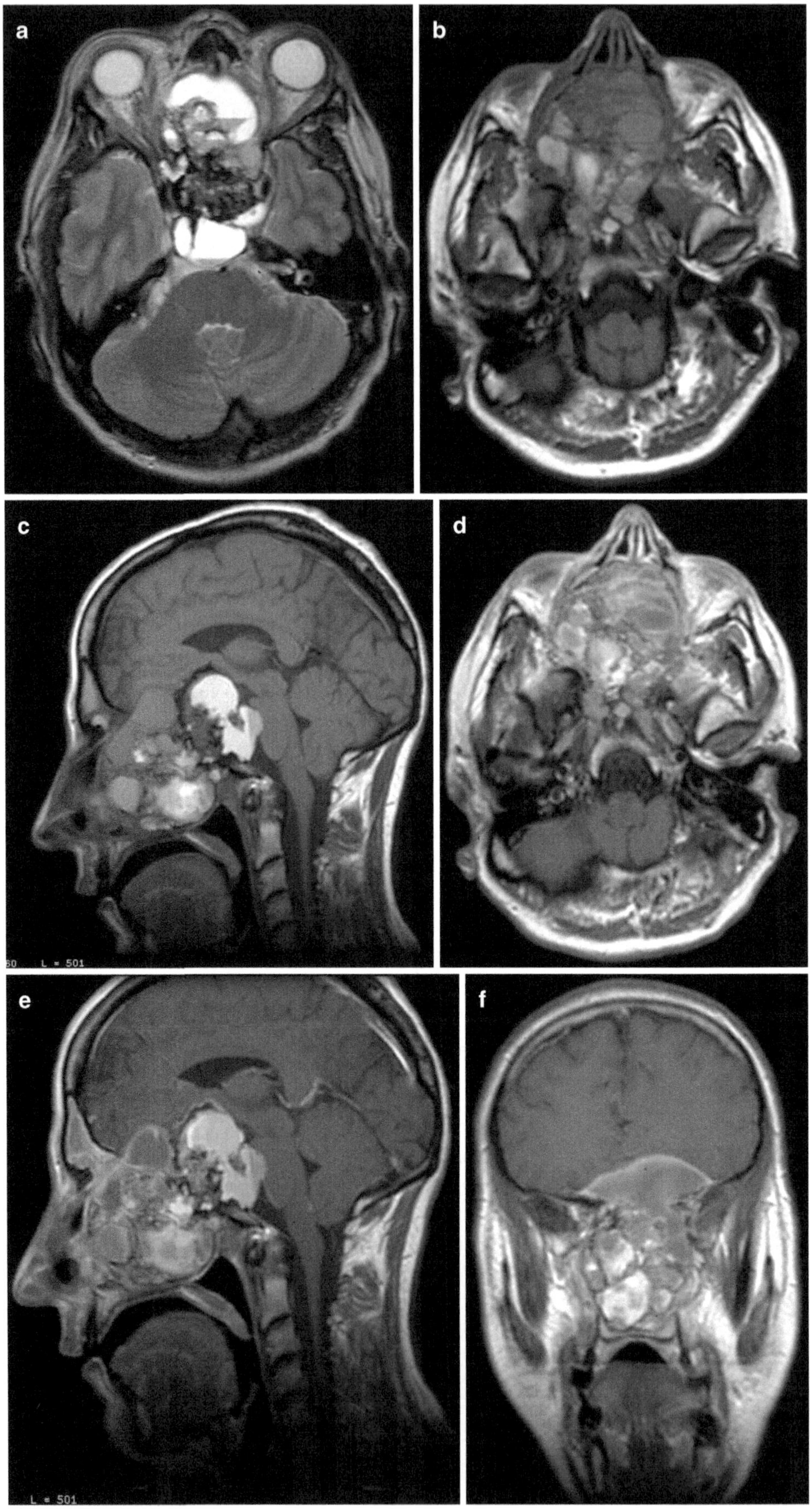

Fig. 10.27 Ameloblastoma of the anterior cranial fossae with intracranial spreading. T2- (**a**) and T1 (**b**, **c**) MR images show an expansile multicystic mass with wide involvement of nasal cavity, nasopharinx, sphenoid bone, and sphenoid sinus. In some of the cavities the effect of sedimentation is clearly visible. Dark T2 MR-signal in central part of the lesion represents the intralesional calcifications. There is a difference in signal intensity between cystic lesions with the most bright signal from the cysts located into intracranial part of the tumor. The obstruction of the frontal sinus can be seen. Post-contrast T1-weighted images (**d**–**f**) demonstrate the contrast enhancement of the solid components and in the septa between the cystic lesions (**d**–**f**)

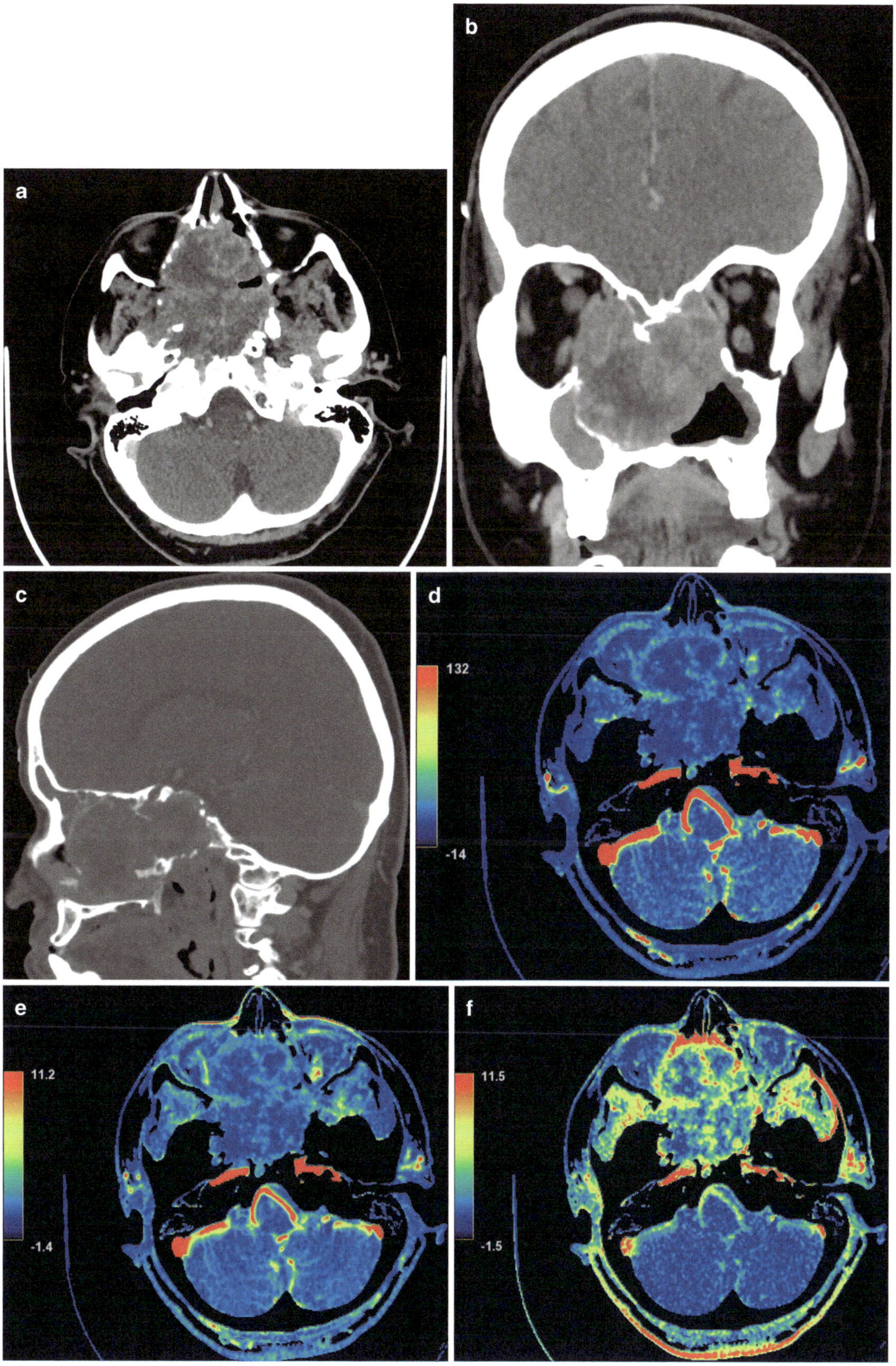

Fig. 10.28 Chondroma of the nasal cavities and ethmoid bone. Axial contrast-enhanced CT scan (**a**) and coronal (**b**), and sagittal (**c**) reformats demonstrate a heterogeneous expansile mass with involvement of the nasal cavities and ethmoid bone, extending in both orbits and sphenoid sinus. A lesion has intermediate contrast enhancement underlying the cystic portions of the mass. There is expansive bones destruction and remodeling. CT-perfusion study demonstrates low values of tumor blood flow (**d**) and blood volume (**e**). Capillary permeability parameter is heterogeneously elevated (**f**)

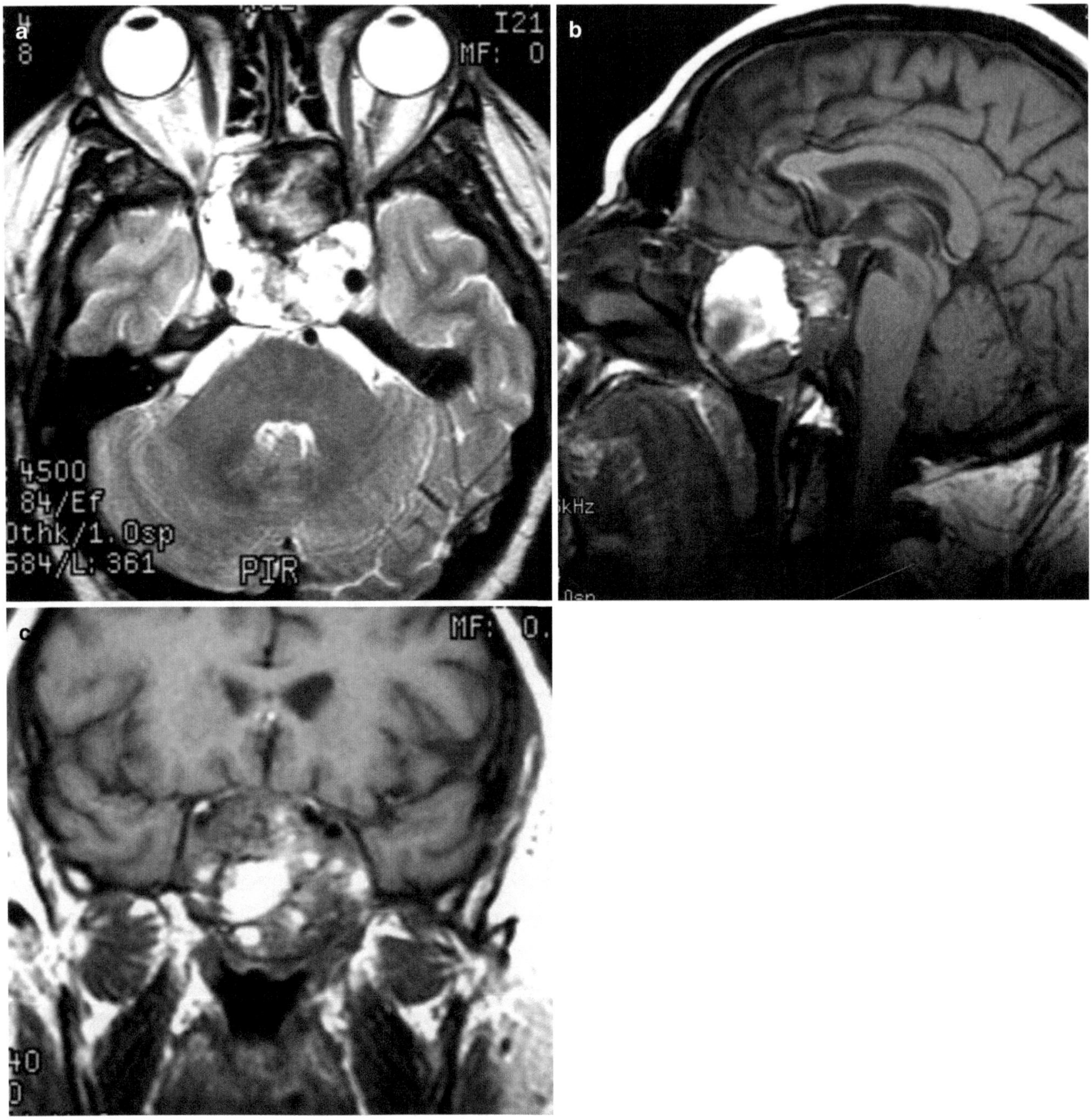

Fig. 10.29 Chondroma of the sphenoid bone and sphenoid sinus. T2-weighted (**a**) and T1-weighted MR images in axial, sagittal, and coronal planes (**b**, **c**) show an expansile mass in the sphenoid bone with expansion into posterior ethmoids. Lesion has a heterogeneous MR-signal with areas of hypo- (calcifications) and hyperintensity. The hyperintensive MR-signal on T1-weighted images is caused by blood products presence within the cystic portion of the lesion. Tumor displaces the hypophysis upwards and internal carotid artery siphons laterally

Imaging Due to mixture structure these tumors can have a variable CT and MRI appearance. On NECT lesion reveals usually as isodense to the muscle mass. Cystic part of the lesion shows a hypodensity. Contrast enhancement within a solid component of the lesion is moderate, cystic parts don't enhance and look as hypodense areas inside the tumors. But in most cases NFs is a soft-tissue and predominantly solid mass with oval shape and well-defined margins, which doesn't show bone destruction. CT clearly demonstrates the bone excavation and bone remodel causes by NF. Bone destruction due to NF growth is suspected for malignant transformation of the lesion. On MR imaging they have an inhomogeneous intermediate signal intensity on T1-weighted and variable signal intensity (from hypo- (common) to hyper (rare) on T2-weighted images. The plexiform type of Nf commonly has a high MR-signal on T2-weighted images with so-called a "bag of worms" pattern (Fig. 10.30).

10.7 Myxoma and Fibromyxoma

Myxoma and fibromyxoma are tumors that develop from pluripotential mesenchymal cells, and have been related with fibroosseous tumors, however they have no odontogenic or osseous structure. These lesions occur commonly during 2–3 dozen of life.

Imaging On CT and MRI this tumor appears as soft-tissue, space-occupying mass with filling nasal cavities. CT can reveal thin strands of calcification that dispersed within tumor's tissue. Sometimes bone destruction and cystic transformation can be observed (Som et al. 2011). MR imaging demonstrates a heterogeneous hyperintense on T2-weighted sequences mass with septas within the tumor with low MR-signal. In our case in spite of hyperintense MR-signal on T2-WI diffusion-weighted imaging showed a low signal from the lesion. Contrast enhancement was prominent and helps better characterize the lesion structure (Fig. 10.31).

10.8 Leiomyoma

Leiomyoma is a benign, smooth-muscle tumor, rarely occurs in the craniofacial region, which arises from perivascular smooth-muscle tissue that is abundant in the sinonasal tract. Leiomyoma and leiomyosarcoma are very rare lesions within sinonasal cavities. In literature less than 100 clinical cases with these tumors located in sinonasal area have been reported (Huang et al. 2000; Lippert et al. 1996; Strasser et al. 1998; Harcourt and Gallimore 1993; Kuruvilla et al. 1990). In compiled series described by Barnes et al. (2000) from 257 head and neck leiomyomas, the most common sites of occurrence were the cervical esophagus (36%), subcutis (23%), and oral cavity (20%). The nasal cavity and sinuses were involved in eight (3%) cases only.

Imaging CT and MRI studies demonstrate in majority of cases a soft-tissue, homogeneous mass with prominent contrast enhancement. Bone destruction is not typical for leiomyoma rather than for leiomyosarcoma. On MRI, lesions show hypoisointensity on T1-weighted and hyperintensity on T2-weighted images. CT-perfusion and ASL–MR study demonstrate low values of blood flow and slightly elevated blood volume within the tumor (Figs. 10.32 and 10.33).

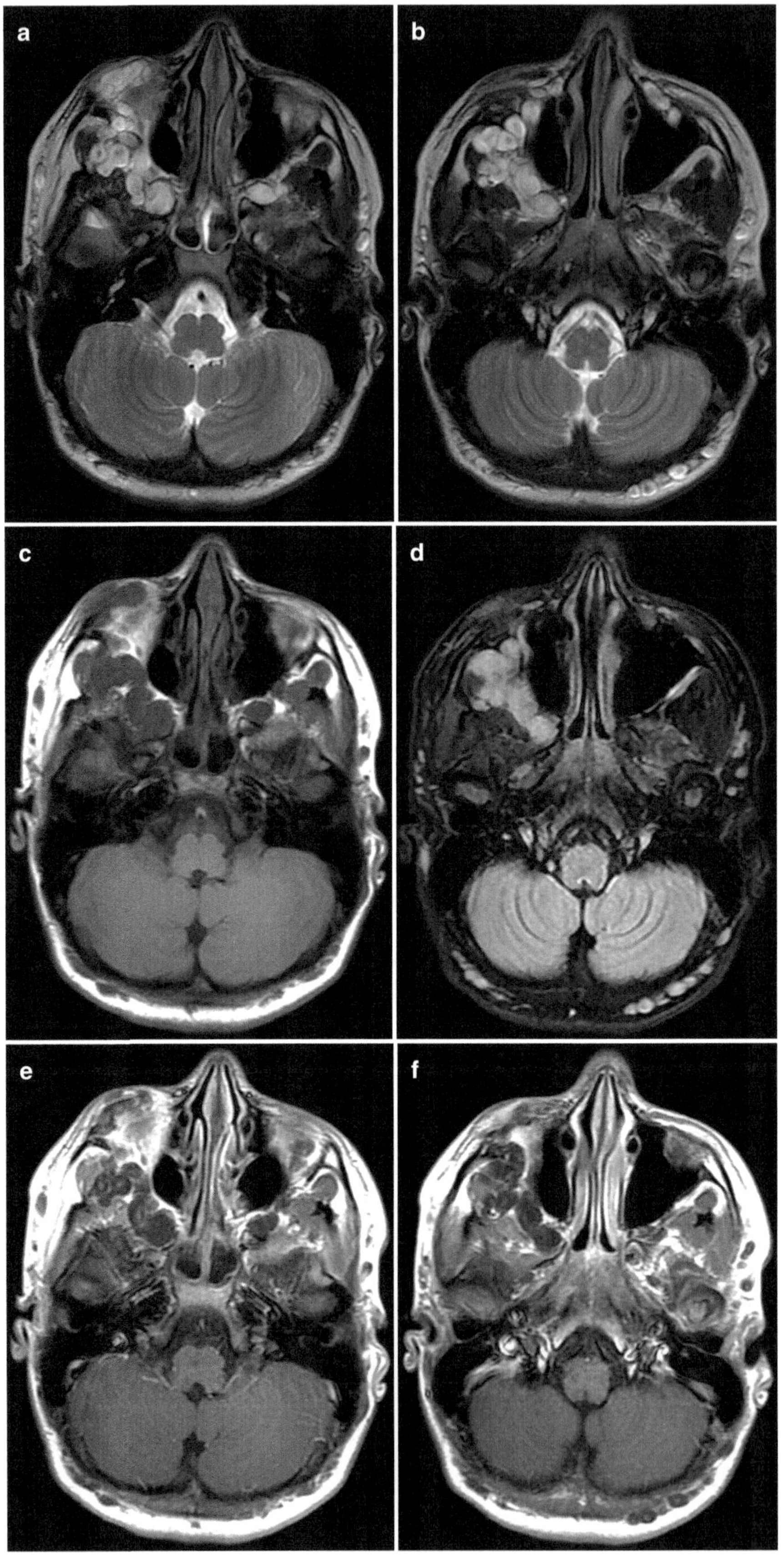

Fig. 10.30 Multiple neurofibromas in patient with NF I type. Axial T2- (**a**, **b**), T1- (**c**), and T2-FLAIR- (**d**) weighted MR images show a conglomerate of multiple oval lesions with hyperintense MR-signal (on T2 and T2-FLAIR images) located in projection of right maxilla involving lateral wall of maxillary cavity and spread into infraorbital area ("bag of worms" pattern). There are plenty other small round lesions on the left side, especially in occipital regions under the skin of both sides. Contrast enhancement demonstrates the hererogeneous predominantly central accumulation of contrast agent—"target-sign" within the lesions (**e**, **f**)

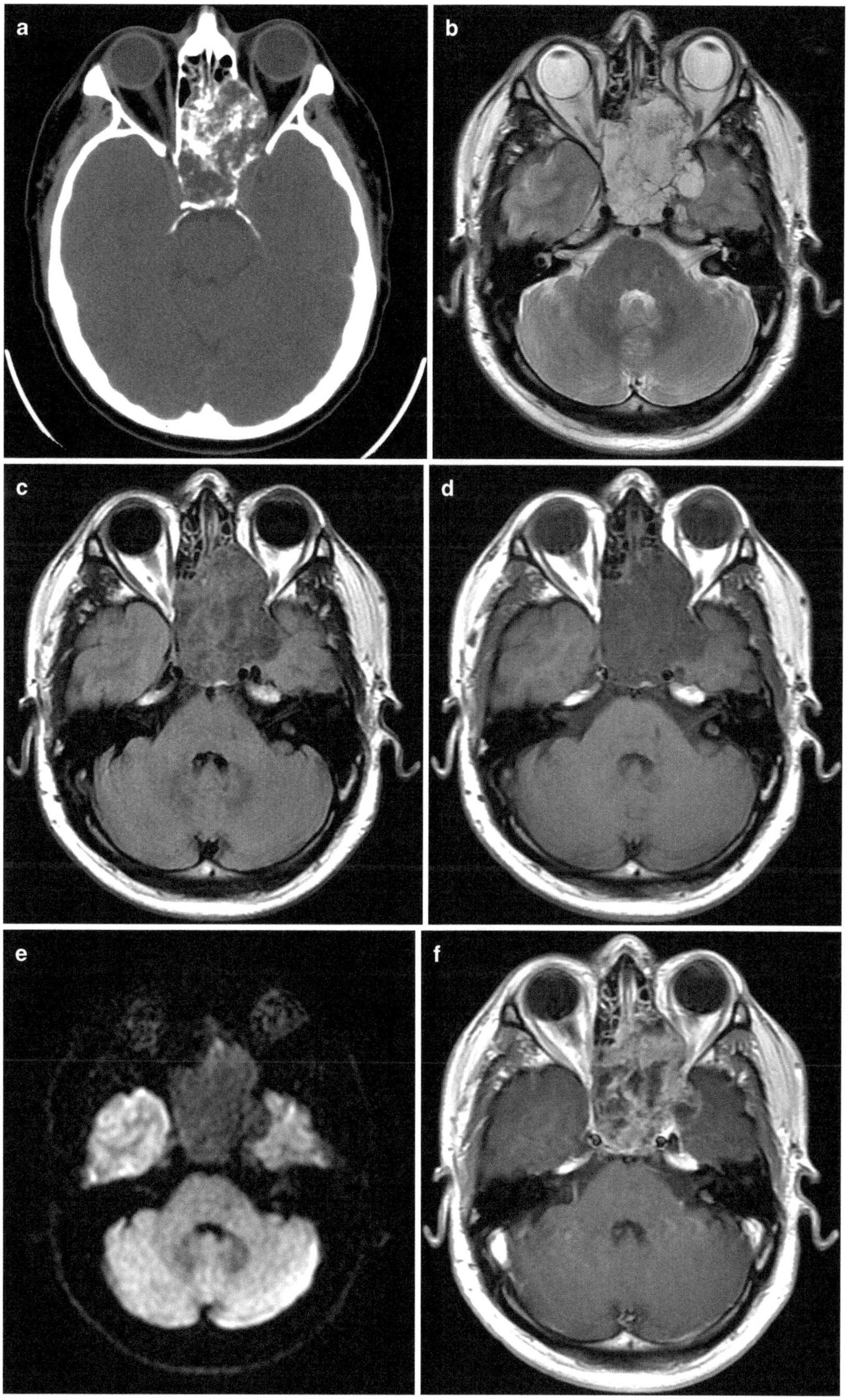

Fig. 10.31 Myxoma of ethmiod and sphenoid bones. Axial CT scan (**a**) and MR imaging with using T2- (**b**), T2-FLAIR- (**c**), and T1- (**d**) weighted images show an expansile heterogeneous mass with hyperintense MR-signal on T2-WI extending intracranially. A lesion has a slightly hypointense signal on T2-FLAIR (cystic formation) and T1-WI. DWI (**e**) demonstrates hypointense compared to brain MR-signal as well. Calcifications are diffusely dispersed within the lesion (**a**). Contrast enhancement study helps better to characterize the tumor structure with presence as solid as cystic portions (**f–h**). FIESTA sequence is very useful in demarcating the lesion from surrounding tissues including brain (**i**)

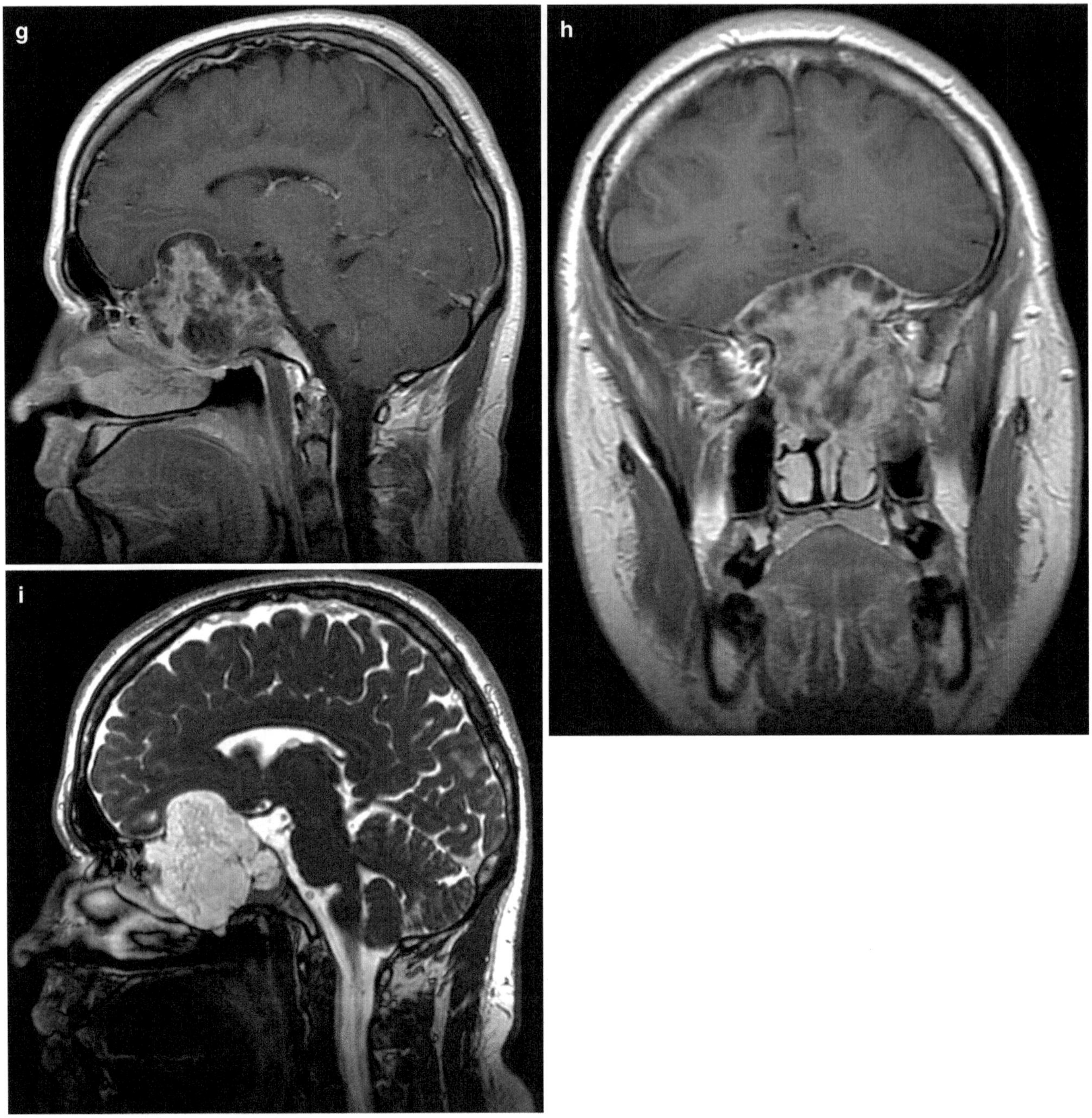

Fig. 10.31 (continued)

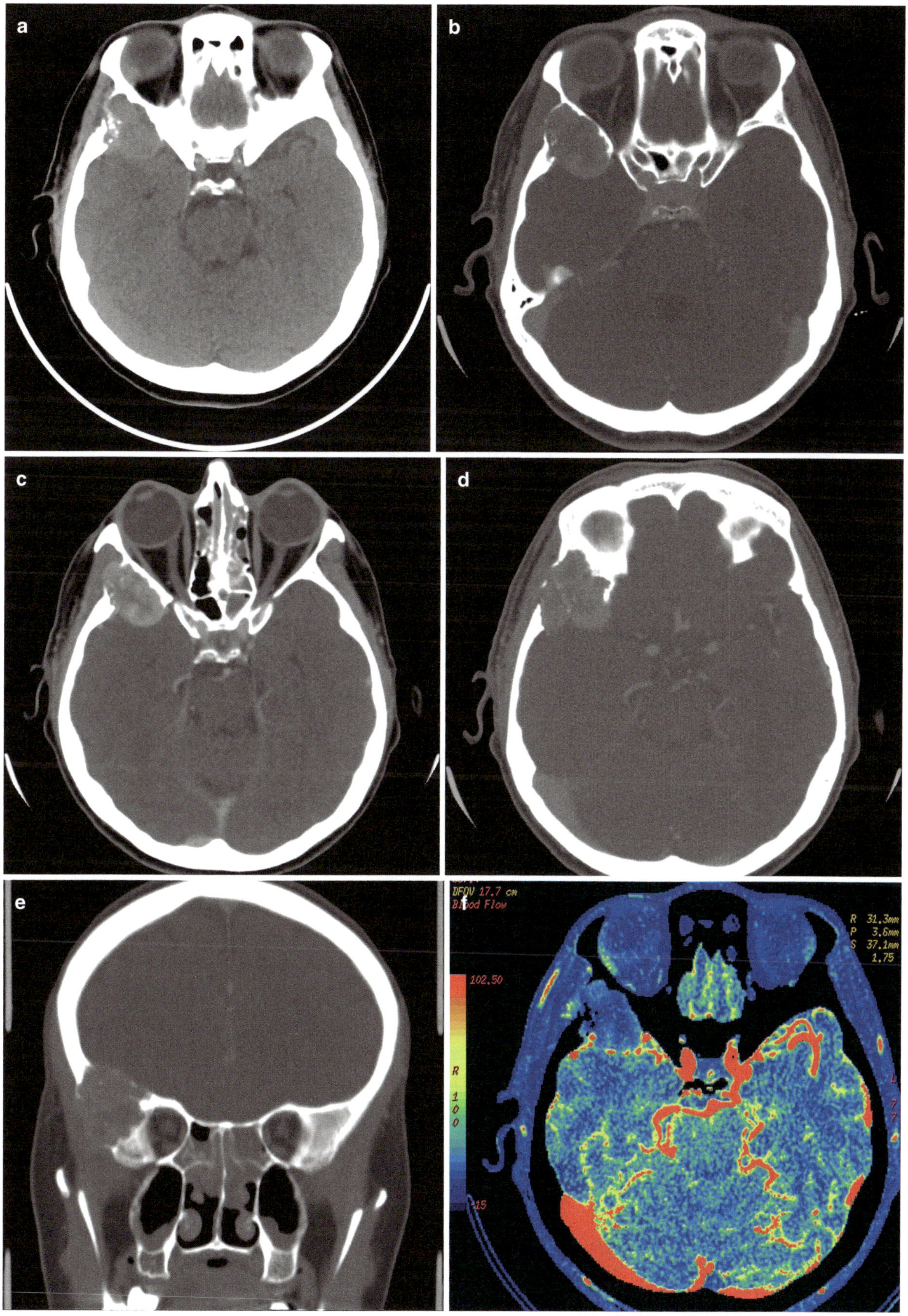

Fig. 10.32 Leiomyoma of the right pterional region. Axial CT scans before (**a**) and after (**b**–**e**) contrast enhancement demonstrate a isodense and enhancing mass with destruction of the temporal bone and partially lateral orbital wall. Small calcifications in lateral part of the lesion can be seen. Contrast enhancement is prominent and homogeneous. CT-perfusion study shows low values of blood flow within the lesion (**f**)

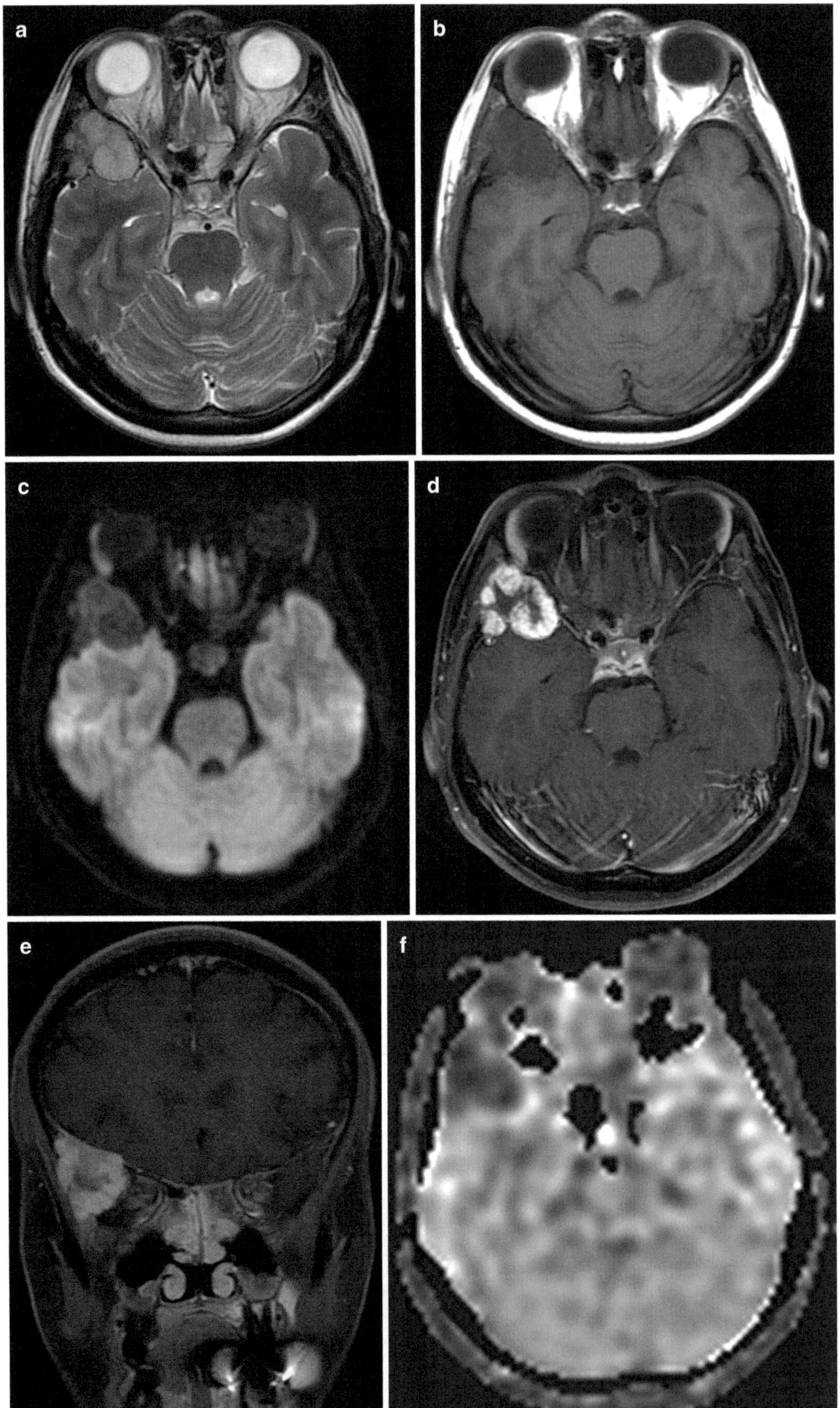

Fig. 10.33 Leiomyoma of the right pterional region (CT study is presented in Fig. 10.32). T2- (**a**) and T1- (**b**) weighted MR images demonstrate a slightly hyperintense on T2 and slightly hypointense (on T1) mass with partial destruction of the temporal bone base and lateral orbital wall. On DWI (**c**) a lesion has a hypointense MR-signal. Contrast enhancement is prominent but heterogeneous with nonenhanced central area (**d–e**). ASL study shows low values of blood flow within the lesion (**f**)

Malignant Tumors

11

Contents

11.1 Chordoma (Ch)

Chordoma develops from the embryronic remnants of the notochord and occurs most common in the sacrococcygeal area (50%), clivus (30–35%), along the cervical and thoracic spine (15–19%). Chordomas are malignant neoplasms (account about 1% of all primary malignant bone tumors), which is characterized by aggressive and locally invasive growth with a high metastatic rate (10–40% of all patients) (Barnes 1985). At the ACF and CFR, primary chordomas are revealed extremely rarely, being usually characterized by antegrade tumor growth from the clivus. Bone destruction and expanding into the nasal cavity are typical features of tumors located at this area. In that cases where chordomas arise in ethmoid, maxilla, frontal sinuses, and mandible as a primary site, it is considered that these tumors presumably arise in notochordal remnants that separated from the main notochord during the extreme mesodermal movement of the face that take place in early period of embryogenesis (Shugar et al. 1980; Miro et al. 1998; Som et al. 2011). Chordomas don't have a capsule and grow expansively with tumor "finger-like" outgrowths formation. If histologically tumors have cartilaginous inclusions, they are referred to as chondroid-chordomas. The latter is characterized by an earlier patients age and better prognosis, as compared with typical chordomas (Heffelfinger et al. 1973).

Imaging On CT, from 30 to 70% of chordomas contain calcifications and bone fragments. The extent of bone destruction is clearly visualized. Intravenous contrast enhancement is mandatory in preoperative CT diagnosis. CT-perfusion imaging Ch pattern is characterized by low blood volume and blood flow parameters.

MRI reflects the heterogeneous structure of Ch. In most cases, the tumor has an isointense MR-signal on T1-weighted images and a relatively high MR-signal on T2-weighted images (Yuh et al. 1985). Chondroid type may exhibit a moderately hyperintense MR-signal on T2-weighted images. All chordomas are contrast enhancing lesions with various

I. Pronin, V. Kornienko, *CT and MRI of Skull Base Lesions*, https://doi.org/10.1007/978-3-319-65957-2_11

degree of contrast agent accumulation, varies from low to high. Intratumor soft-tissue trabeculae are better detected with contrast enhancement, which is considered as a very specific characteristic in Ch visualization (Fig. 11.1).

Differential Diagnosis Metastases, plasmocytoma, primary sarcoma and other secondary lesions spreading into CFR from the clivus area (nasopharyngeal cancer, meningioma).

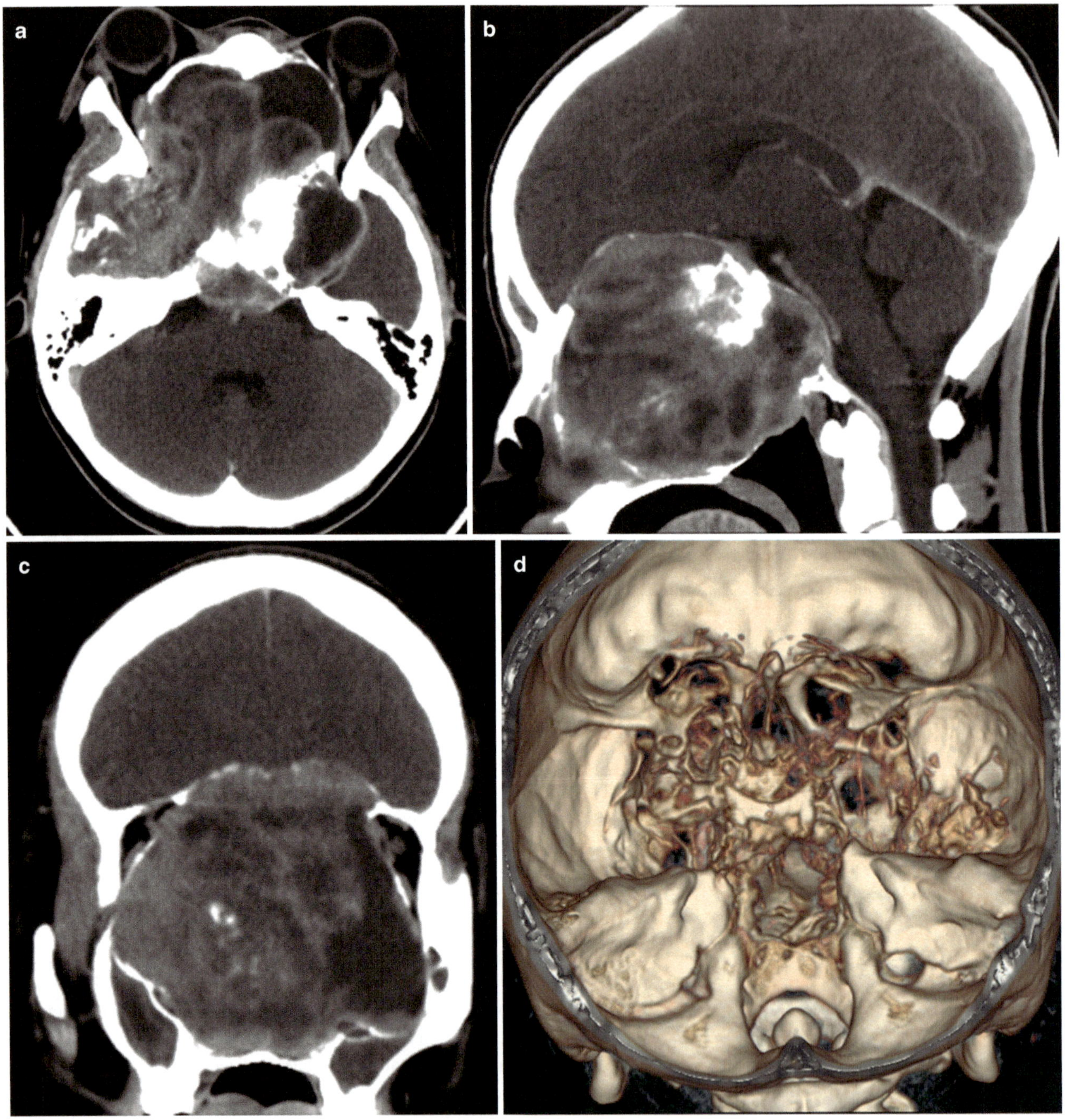

Fig. 11.1 Chondroid-chordoma of the craniofacial region. Contrast-enhanced axial CT (**a**) image and sagittal, and coronal reformats (**b**, **c**) demonstrate a huge tumor with heterogeneous structure, spreading into nasal cavities, ethmoids, sphenoid bone, and sinus as well as in both orbits and right middle cranial fossa. The involvement of both cavernous sinuses can be seen. The tumor has a moderate and inhomogeneous contrast enhancement, and leads to extensive bone destruction (3D reconstruction (**d**). CT-perfusion study (row data scan (**e**), CBF (**f**)) shows low values of blood flow in the tumor. On digital cerebral angiography (**g**–**i**) an avascular area at the skull base with displacement of internal carotid artery is visible (*arrows*)

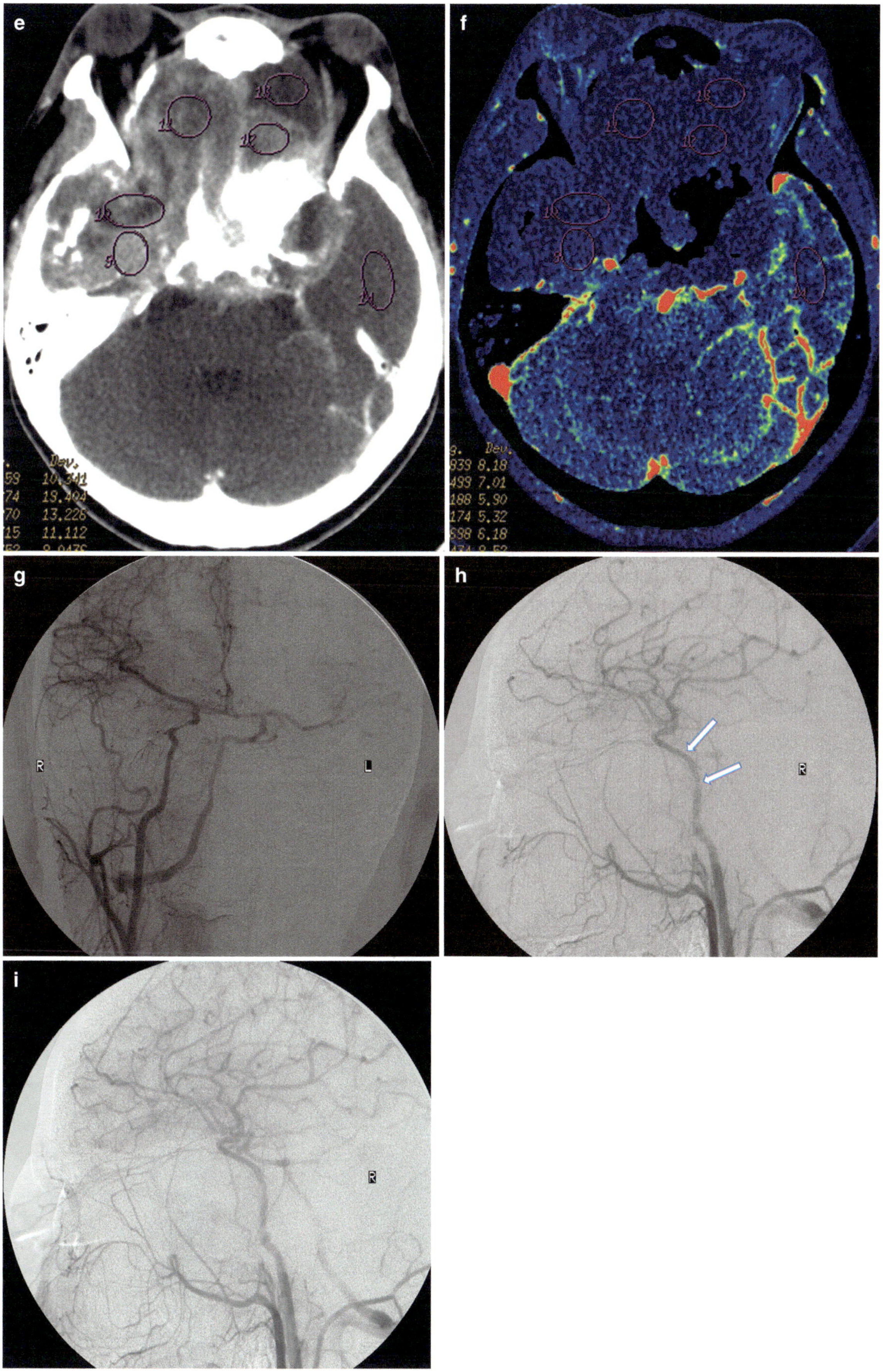

Fig. 11.1 (continued)

11.2 Chondrosarcoma (COS)

Chodrosarcoma is a rare tumor arising from the skull base, its pathogenesis remains unclear. COS is characterized by the abnormal production of a specific cartilage matrix. Although COS can manifest in any bone, this cancer preferentially develops in the pelvis, humerus, femur, scapula, and ribs and can present at any age (Leddy and Holmes 2014). Based on the histological profile, four different subtypes of COS have been identified: (a) conventional COS, which is the most common (approximately 90% of diagnosed cases); (b) dedifferentiated COS (approximately 10% of diagnosed cases); (c) mesenchymal COS, the most rare but also the most aggressive; and (d) clear cell chondrosarcoma, a rare variant. COS has been shown to be resistant to the chemotherapy and radiotherapy. Consequently, an improved prognosis for patients is based on an extremely precise surgery, but unfortunately, patients with COS usually relapse and inevitably have a poor prognosis (Frezza et al. 2015). At the skull base they are suggested to develop from chondrocytes within the endochondral cartilage. Unlike the calvarium bones, where the latter develops to form intramembranous ossification, the skull base bones, including the larger part of the petrous portion of the temporal bone, areas of petro-occipital, spheno-occipital, spheno-petrosal synchondroses, mature predominantly by endochondral ossification. The preferred site of the skull base chondrosarcoma is the area of the petro-occipital synchondrosis, therefore, they are located mainly asymmetrically with respect to the midline. Chondrosarcoma is detected in 6% of skull base tumors and 0.15% of intracranial tumors. In estimation by Som et al. (2011) on the base of experience of 500 cases with chondrosarcomas from Memorial Sloan-Kettering Cancer Center, only 5% (25 cases) occurred in the head and neck area. Most often localization of chondrosarcomas of the CFR are maxilla sinus (about 45%), nasal septum, ethmoid, and sphenoid (41%), then followed mandible (10–11%) and nasal tip (3–4%) (Saito et al. 1995; Rassekh et al. 1996; Gadwal et al. 2000).

Imaging On CT, this is an invasive tumor causing bone destruction at the site of its growth. Lesion has a heterogeneous structure with variable degree of calcifications (Grossman and Davis 1981; Meyers et al. 1992; Cherekaev et al. 2001) and with the presence of soft tissue enhanced component. Calcifications are always much more pronounced than in chordomas. On CT-perfusion imaging, this tumor is distinguished from chordomas by a higher degree this perfusion with heterogeneous and elevated blood flow and volume values (Fig. 11.2).

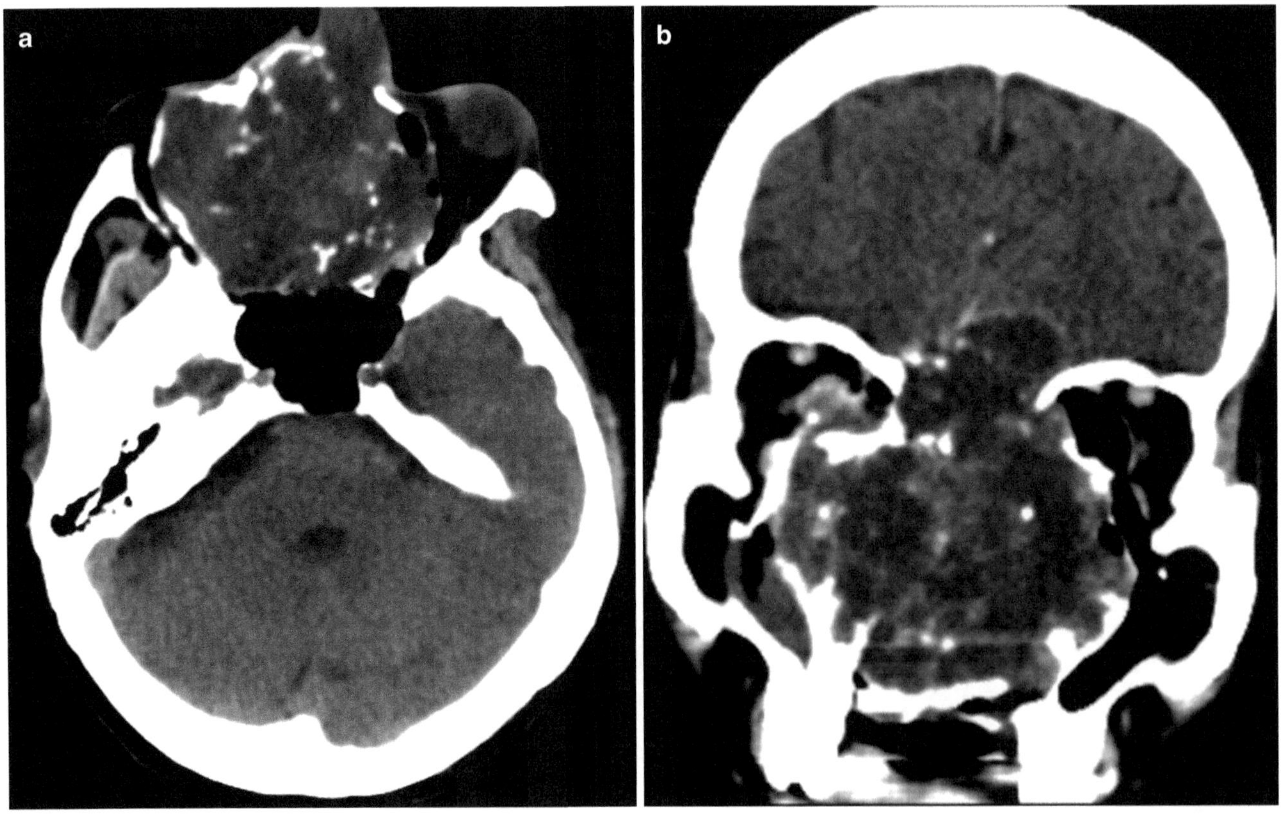

Fig. 11.2 Chondrosarcoma of the nasal cavities and ethmoid bone. CT scans in axial plane (**a**) and contrast-enhanced CT scans with reformations in coronal and sagittal planes (**b**, **c**) visualize a heterogeneous tumor with plenty calcifications in it. The tumor has intermediate and inhomogeneous contrast enhancement, and leads to wide destruction of surrounding bones, including floor of anterior cranial fossa with intracranial spreading. CT-perfusion study (CBF (**d**), CBV (**e**), MTT (**f**)) demonstrates atypically low values of blood flow and blood volume parameters in the tumor with foci of hyperperfusion (on CBV map). MTT-values are prolonged

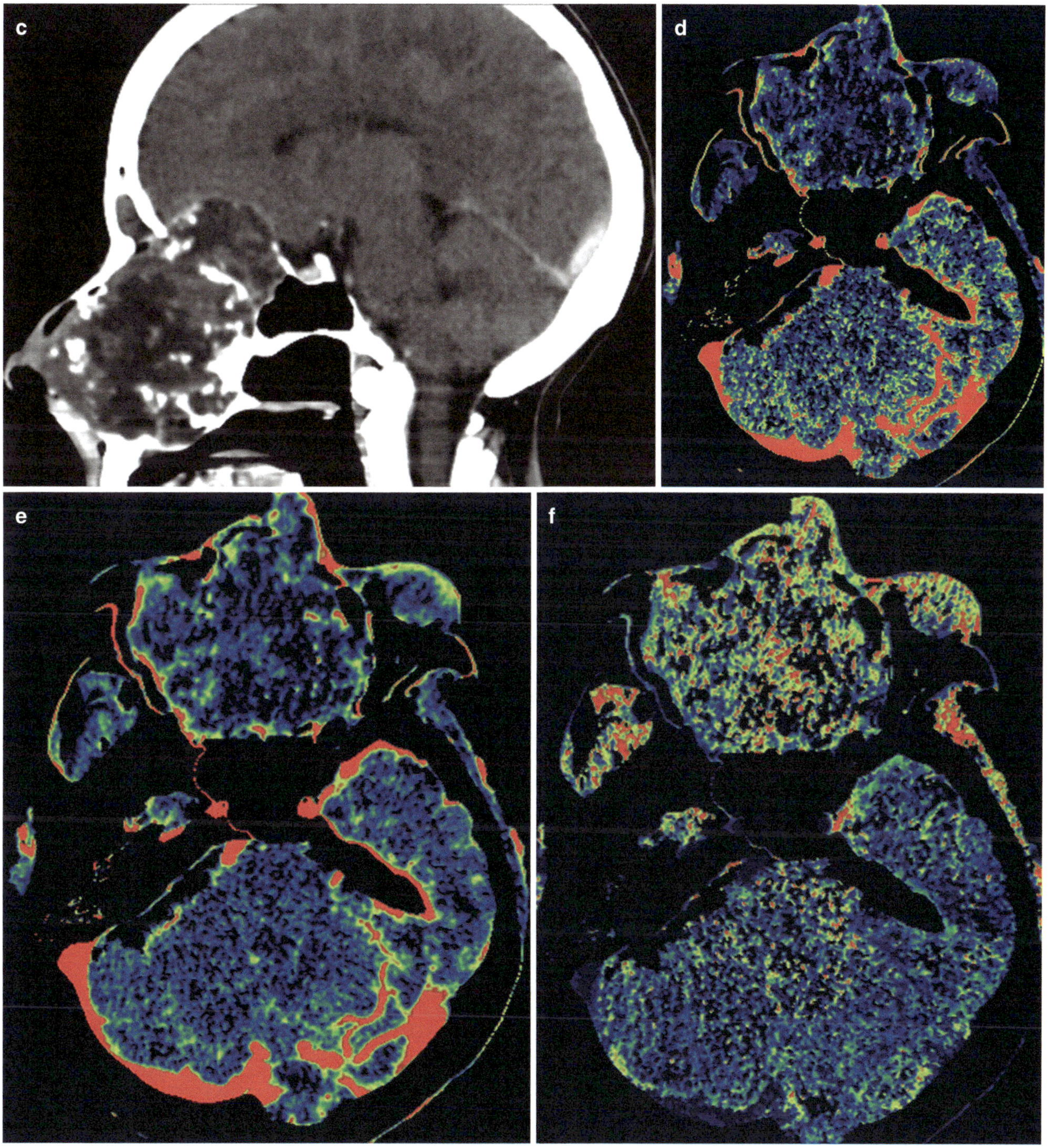

Fig. 11.2 (continued)

Heterogeneity of the tumor structure due to calcifications is reflected on MR imaging. On T1-weighted sequences, the tumor has a heterogeneous MR-signal, while on T2-weighted images it is hypointense in regions with calcifications and hyperintense in the soft tissue areas. Accumulation of the contrast agent is observed mainly within a soft-tissue portion of chondrosarcoma. MR-imaging demonstrates the tumor invasion extent into the bones of the skull base and intracranially (typically extradural) better than CT, especially when using simultaneously techniques with fat-saturation and contrast enhancement (Fig. 11.3).

Differential Diagnosis All malignant tumors of the skull base, which cause bone destruction and calcification. Unlike most chondrosarcomas, clivus chordomas are commonly localized at the midline and have a lower degree of perfusion. The majority of studies show that no reliable signs have been identified allowing to distinguish between chondrosarcomas and chordomas on the routine images (Brown et al. 1990; Meyers et al. 1992). In our opinion CT-perfusion can help to resolve with differential dilemma due to different perfusion patterns these two entities. Primary bone cancer of the skull base causes the destructive changes in the bone, rarely generates calcifications in its stroma.

11.3 Olfactory Neuroblastoma (ONB)

Olfactory neuroblastoma (referred to as well as esthesioneuroblastoma) belongs to the group of malignant tumors arising from the olfactory mucosa of the superior parts of the nasal cavity, growing primary from the olfactory neuroepithelium. A lesion commonly becomes calcified. It occurs in 3–6% of all cancers of the nasal cavity and in 20–40% of cases gives metastases into the regional lymph nodes, lungs, and bones (Jethanamest et al. 2007; Howell et al. 2011). Olfactory neuroblastoma looks like a "dumbbell" lesion of ACF and nasal cavity with a "waist" at the

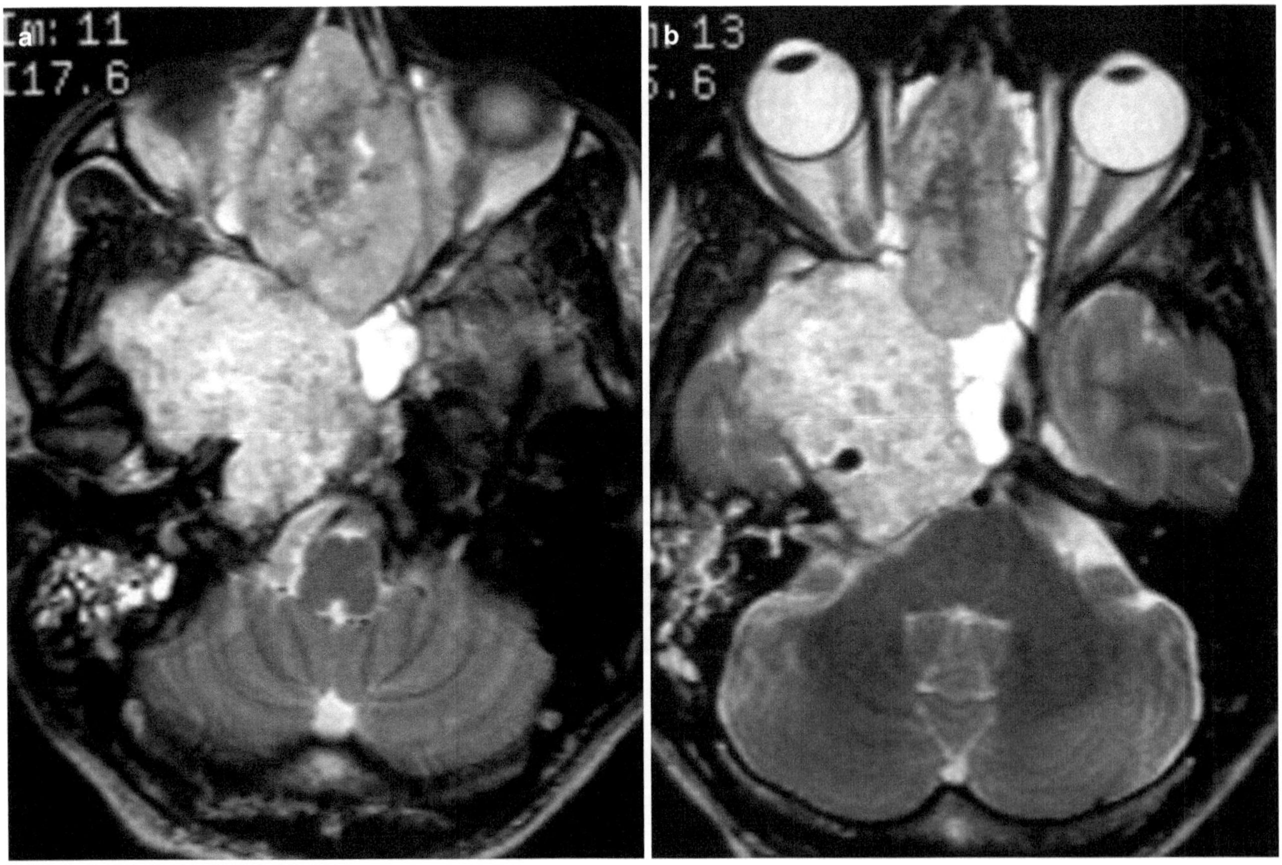

Fig. 11.3 Chondrosarcoma. Axial T2-weighted MR images (**a**, **b**), T1-(**c**), and T1-weighted images after contrast enhancement (**d**–**f**) demonstrate a large expansile heterogeneous mass with involvement of nasal cavity, ethmoids, sphenoid bone and sinus, extending into base of middle cranial fossa. The tumor has hyperintense MR-signal on T2-weighted images. There is no intraorbital invasion but the local intracranial invasion in retrosellar and retroclivus area can be seen. The lesion strongly accumulates the contrast agent and becomes hyperintense on T1-weighted images

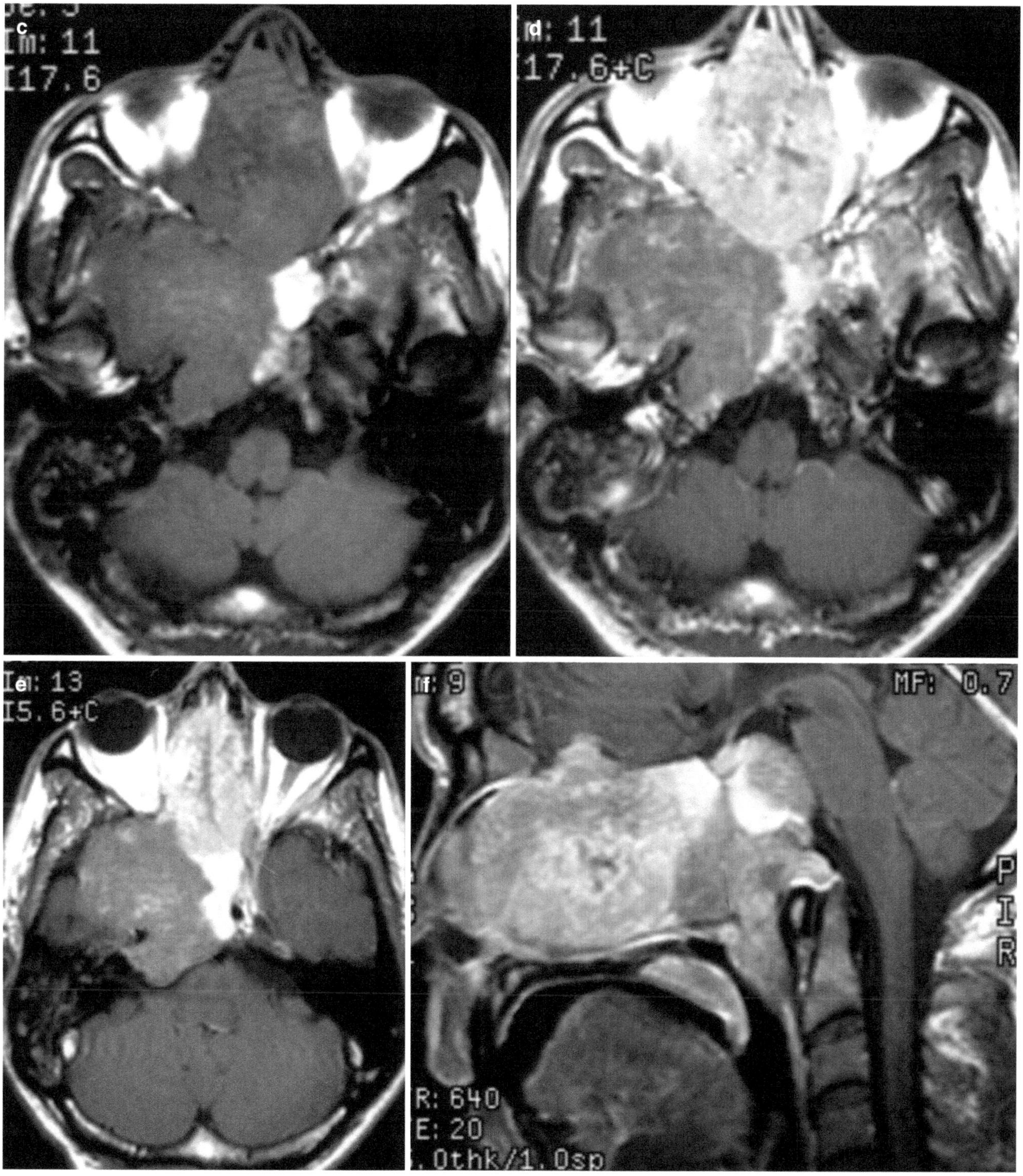

Fig. 11.3 (continued)

cribriform plate level. There may be cysts visualized at the margins of the intracranial mass. These specific features of the tumor shape and structure suggest its histological type with a high level of accuracy. Small size lesions are usually localized at the arch of the nasal cavity, while large ones are localized in the anterior cranial fossa, ethmoid bone, maxillary sinuses and can later spread even into the orbit.

Common symptoms include: obstruction of the sinuses, epistaxis, anosmia, rhinorrhea, headache and pain in projection of the orbit. In case of a successful total removal of the tumor, 8-year survival reaches in 80% cases.

Imaging On CT, a tumor is visualized as a soft-tissue space-occupying lesion localized at the ethmoidal bones and the base of ACF (Rao et al. 2001). Sagittal CT reformations clearly visualize the dumbbell shape of the tumor and the extent of bone changes, especially in the area of cribriform plate. Destructive bone changes are typical, but local hyperostosis can also be observed (Regenbogen et al. 1988). Olfactory neuroblastomas homogeneously enhance with contrast agent administration (Figs. 11.4 and 11.5).

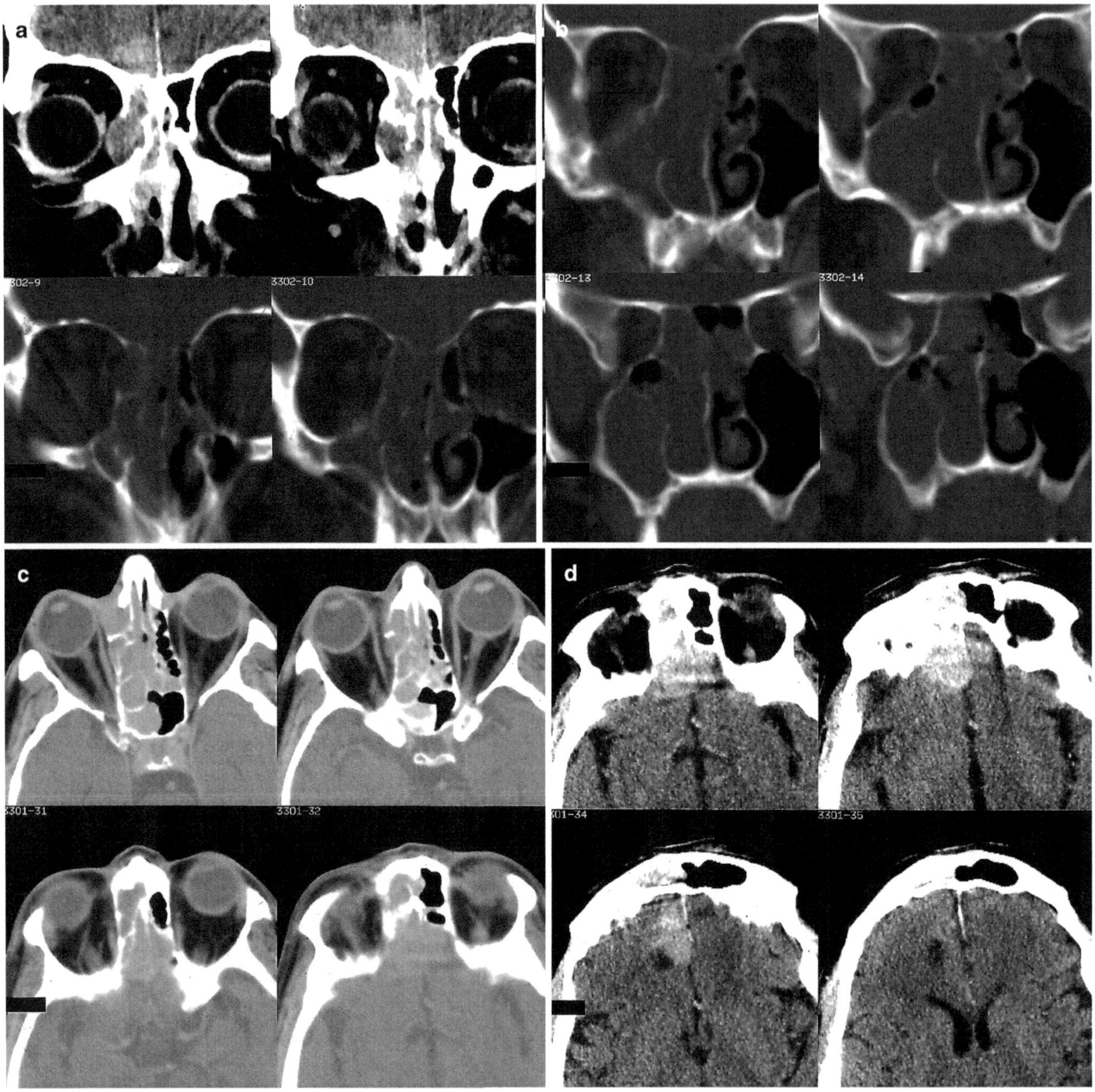

Fig. 11.4 Olfactory neuroblastoma (esthesioneuroblastoma) of right nasal cavity. Series of coronal (**a**, **b**) and axial (**c**, **d**) CT scans demonstrate a soft tissue intranasal mass, which spreads to the anterior cranial fossa and partially into the right orbit. The tumor causes of obstruction of the right maxillary sinus. The lesion has intensive and inhomogeneous contrast enhancement (**c**, **d**). The tumor also has area of cystic transformation in the upper pole. On the digital angiography (**e**, **f**) the tumor capillary network is visible. Its blood supply comes from the ophthalmic and maxillary arteries (*arrows*)

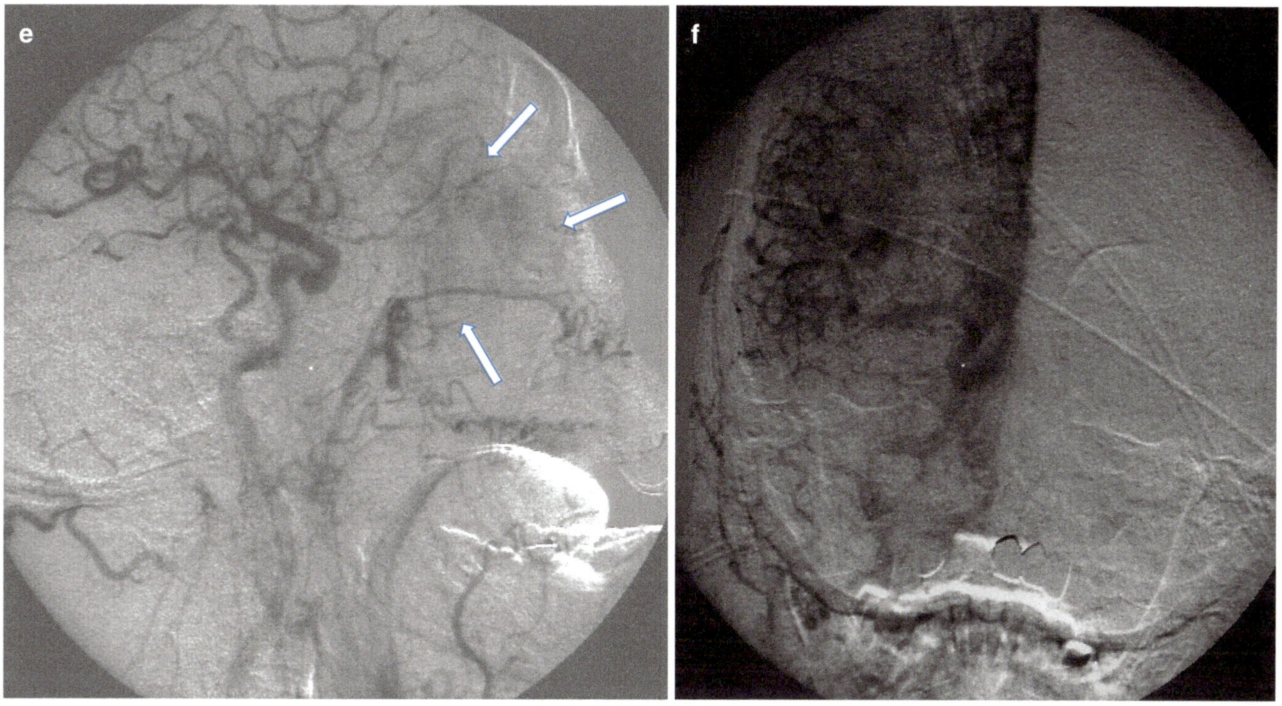

Fig. 11.4 (continued)

On T1-weighted MR images, the tumor has a hypo- or isointense MR-signal compared to the brain. Foci of hemorrhage are detected as areas with high signal intensity. On T2-weighted MR images, signal intensity of tumor tissue varies from moderate to high, commonly the areas of cystic degeneration are identified, adjacent sinuses may be obstructed by the presence of thickened and inflamed mucosa and effusion into the sinus cavity (Som et al. 1994). T2-weighted images better differentiate the tumor and mucosal contents of the obstructed sinuses. Contrast agent accumulation on MRI is often pronounced and rather homogeneous (Fig. 11.6), but can also be heterogeneous, when there are necrotic areas in the tumor (Li et al. 1993; Dulguerov et al. 2001; Bradly et al. 2003; Constantinidis et al. 2004). CT- and MR-perfusion study typically demonstrates the elevation on TBF and TBV even in cases with small tumor size (Figs. 11.7 and 11.8) which is usually associated with an abundant vascular network of ONB (Fig. 11.9).

Differential Diagnosis

1. Olfactory meningiomas with extracranial growth: hyperostosis of the skull base is frequently revealed, tumor structure being dense, no cystic changes, distinct vascular tumor matrix;
2. Squamous cell carcinoma is extremely difficult to distinguish from olfactory neuroblastoma, if it is diagnosed in the nasal cavity; its more common accounts in the maxillary sinuses, contrast agent accumulation isn't so intensive and strong.
3. Non-Hodgkin's lymphoma of the nasal cavity appears as a dense mass on non-enhanced CT, more homogeneously accumulate contrast material compare to olfactory neuroblastoma and typically doesn't destroy skull base bones;
4. Sinonasal undifferentiated carcinoma is difficult to distinguish from olfactory neuroblastoma, this tumor is more common in elderly patients, there are no reliable differential radiologic features.

Squamous cell carcinoma (SCC) is a malignant epithelial tumor growing from the epithelium of the sinus or nasal cavity mucosa. A tendency to aggressive spread into surrounding structures is clearly pronounced. Representing 3% of all malignant tumors of the head and neck, SCC most commonly affects the sinonasal area (80%), in 15% of cases dissemination into the regional lymph nodes can be seen in early stage.

A tumor is more frequently observed at the age range of 50–70 years, and is more common in men. Arising within the sinonasal area SCC appears as an aggressive soft-tissue lesion

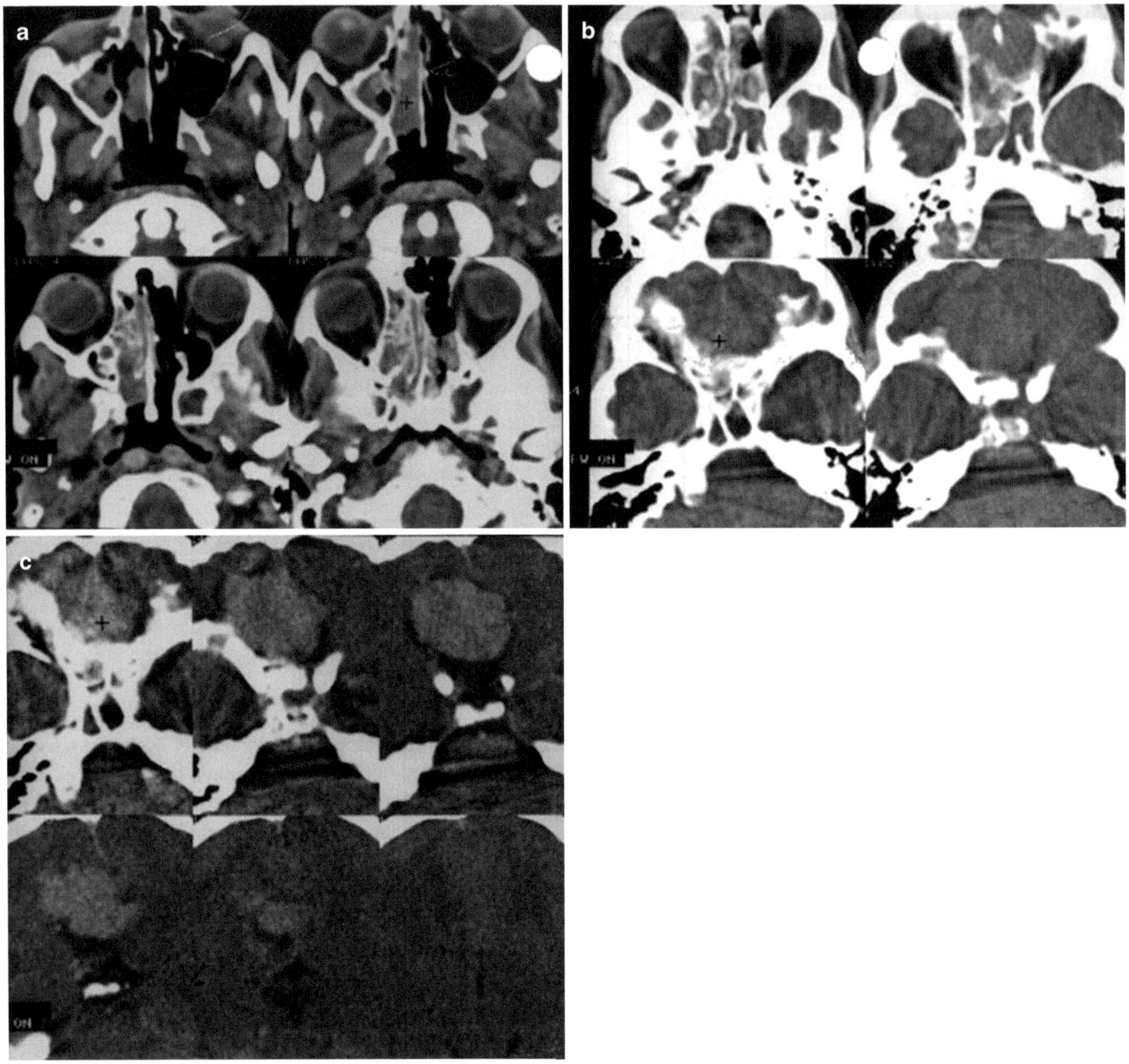

Fig. 11.5 Olfactory neuroblastoma (esthesioneuroblastoma) of right nasal cavity. Series of axial CT scans without (**a**, **b**) and after (**c**) contrast enhancement show a soft tissue mass within the upper part of right nasal cavity. The tumor extends intracranially into anterior cranial fossa and strongly enhances. There is an obstruction of the right maxillary sinus

with bone destruction of the sinus walls, common has a unilateral localization, involving the nasal cavity, the maxillary sinus, or the ethmoid bone. The growth initially begins in the sinus (75%) and in the nasal cavity (about 30%). Secondary extension to maxillary sinus is common, occurring in 80% of patients with sinonasal carcinoma (Som et al. 2011).

Imaging As nearly 80% of sinonasal malignancies are squamous cell carcinomas, CT and MR imaging studies are not expected to establish the pathologic diagnosis. On CT, this is a soft tissue tumor with irregular margins and isodense to the neck muscles, which leads to bone destruction in majority of the cases. Usually on CT SCC has a solid structure with slight and heterogeneous contrast enhancement (Fig. 11.10).

On T1-weighted MR sequences, the tumor has intermediate MR-signal intensity; areas of subacute hemorrhages can be visualized (foci with high MR-signal). On T2-weighted images, the MR-signal from the tumor varies from intermediate to high as compared to the muscles. However, as noted by most authors, MR-signal with this sequence is lower than that

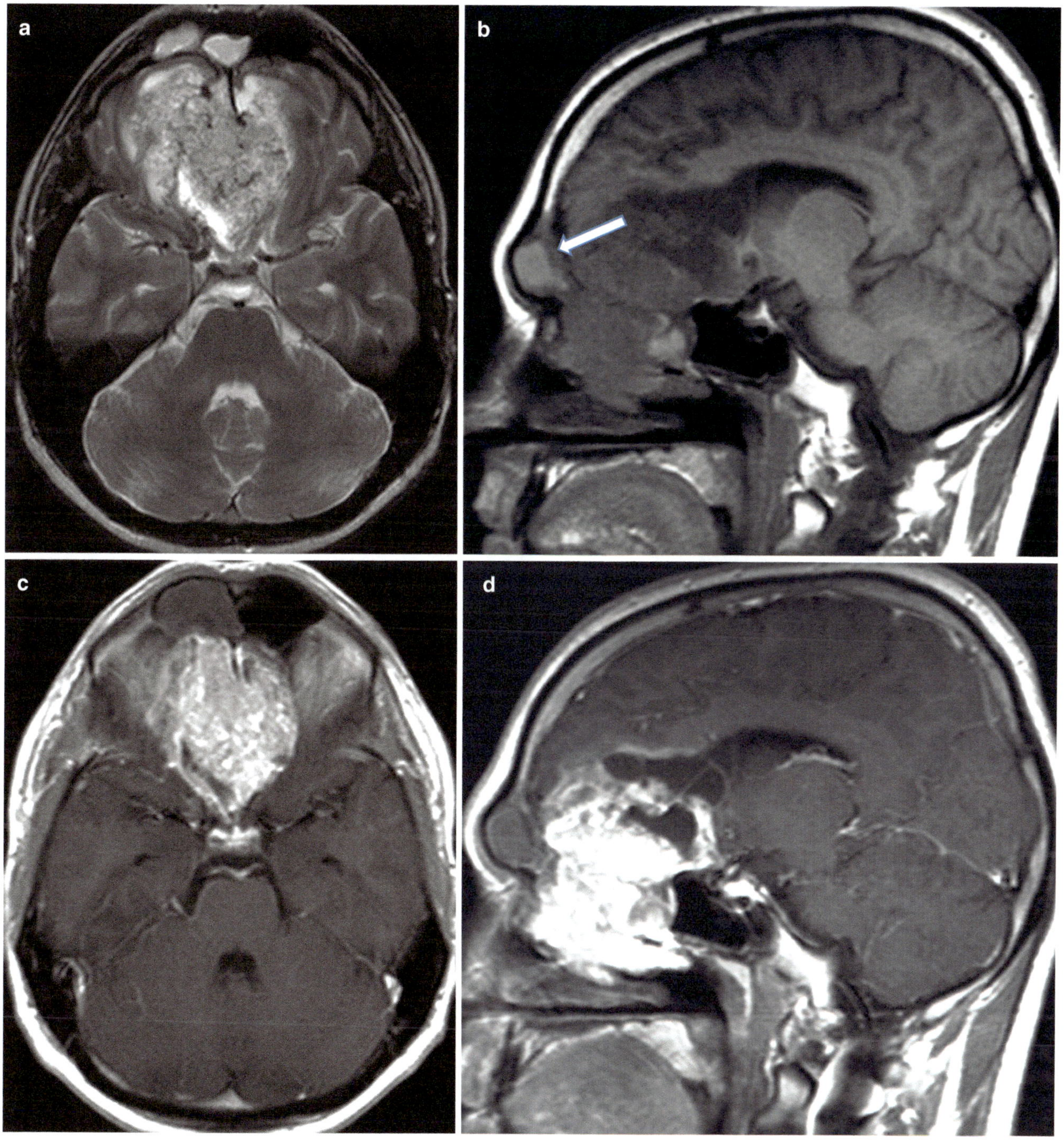

Fig. 11.6 Olfactory neuroblastoma (esthesioneuroblastoma) of right nasal cavity, which extends into anterior cranial fossa. Axial T2-weighted (**a**) and T1-weighted (**b**) MR images show a soft tissue mass with heterogeneous increased intensity of MR-signal on T2. On T1-WI the tumor has slightly hypointense to the brain tissue MR-signal. There are cysts in area of the intracranial extension. Intravenous injection of contrast agent produces intensive and inhomogeneous contrast enhancement (**c**–**e**). MR-angiography (**f**) on the background of contrast enhancement demonstrates the dislocation of intracranial vessels only. The tumor leads to obstruction of the frontal sinus and formation of mucocele there (**b**) (*arrow*)

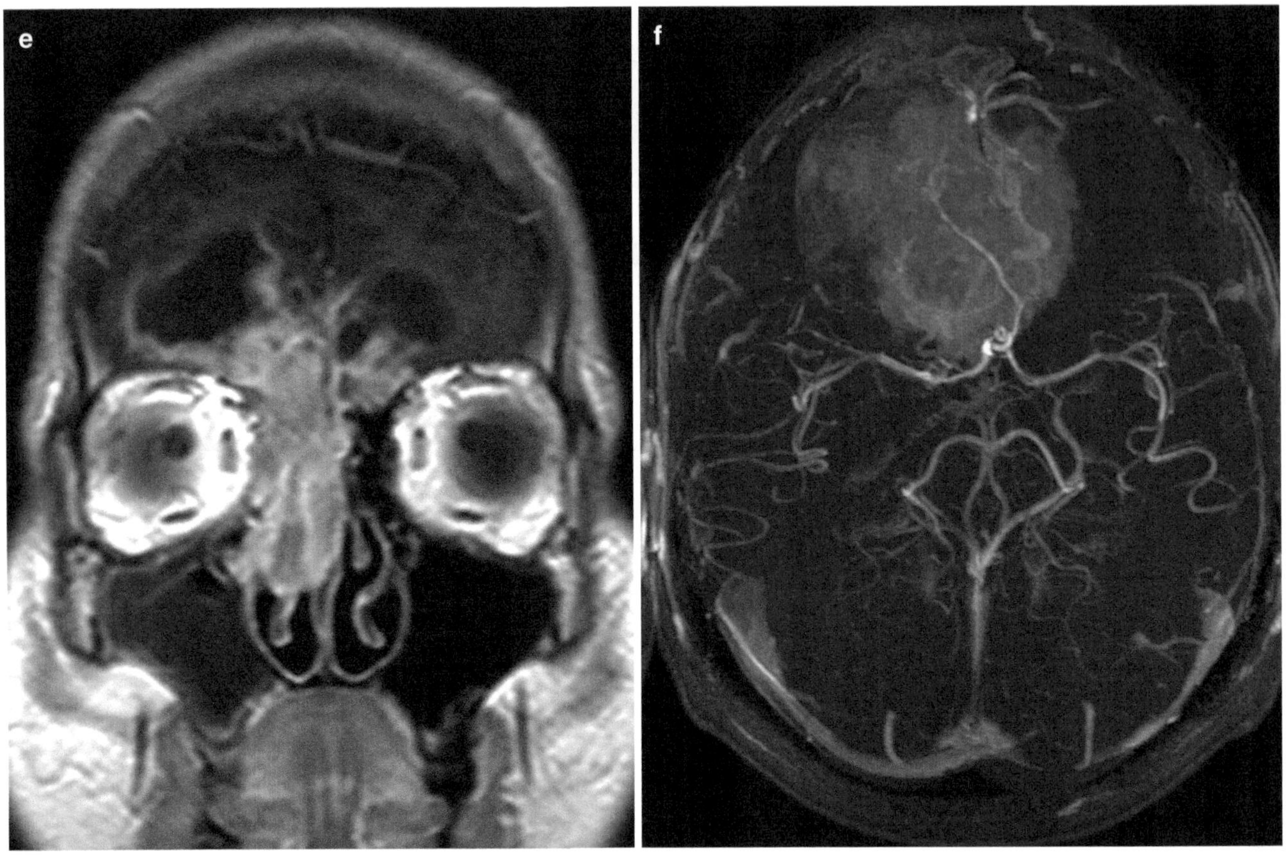

Fig. 11.6 (continued)

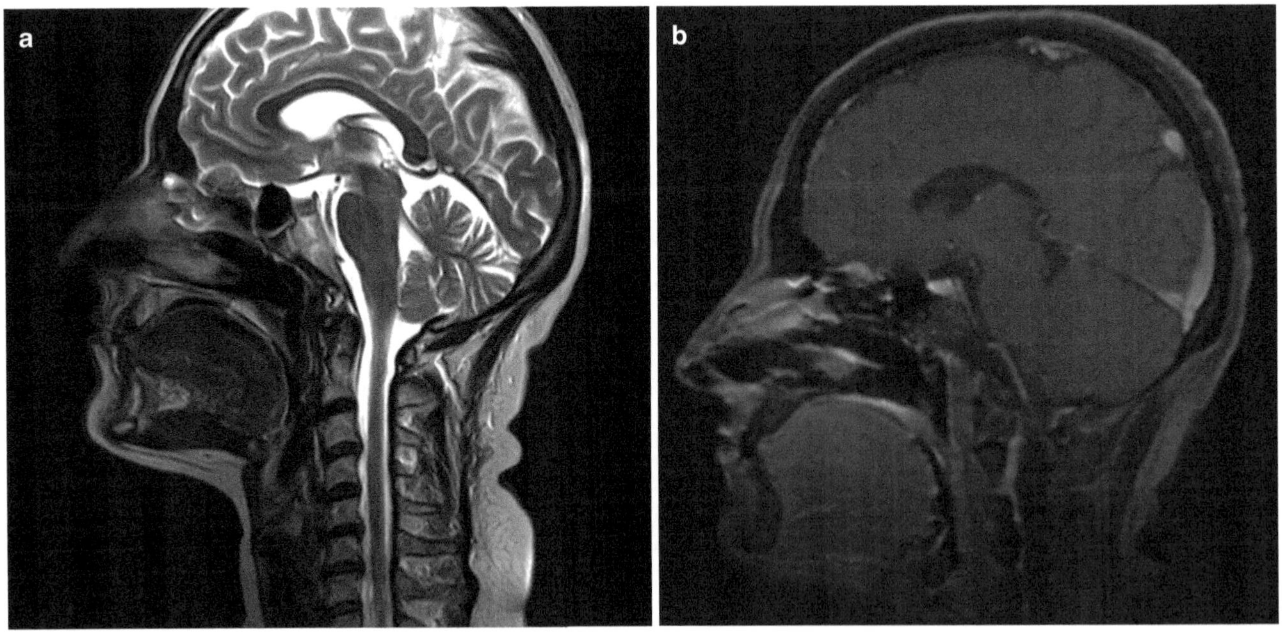

Fig. 11.7 Olfactory neuroblastoma (esthesioneuroblastoma). Sagittal MR images using T2-(**a**) and post-contrast T1-(**b**) weighted sequences demonstrate a small soft tissue lesion that is located in projection of anterior cranial fossa floor. The lesion has prominent contrast enhancement and mimics olfactory meningioma. CT-perfusion study (CBV map (**c**)) shows a high blood volume values within the tumor (*arrows*)

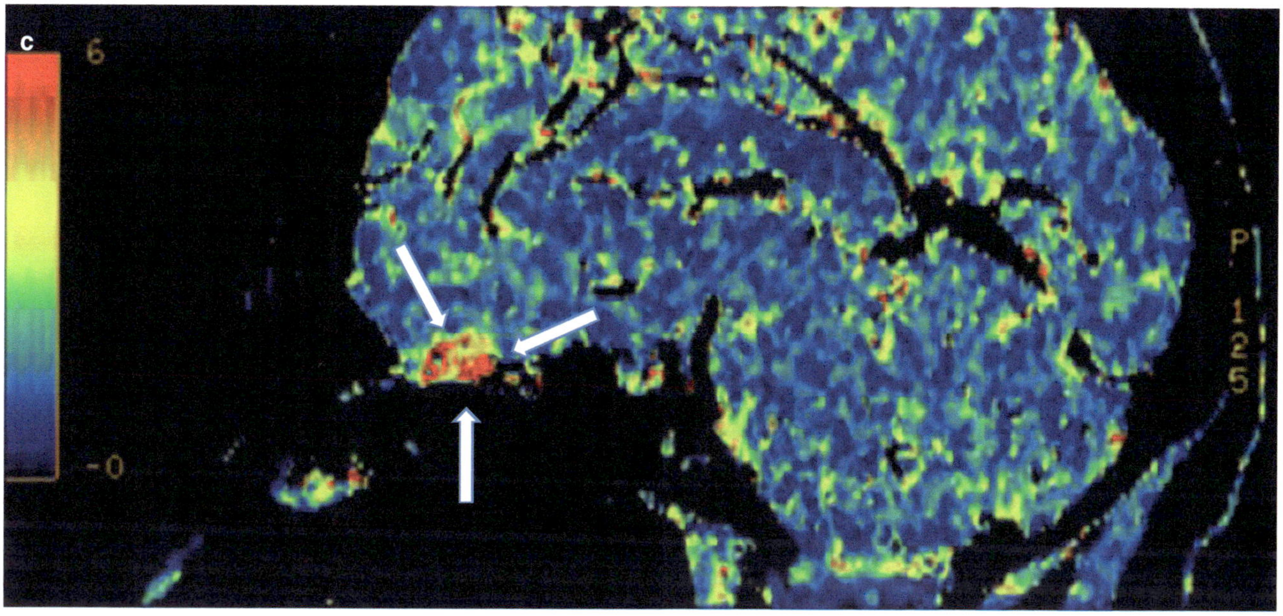

Fig. 11.7 (continued)

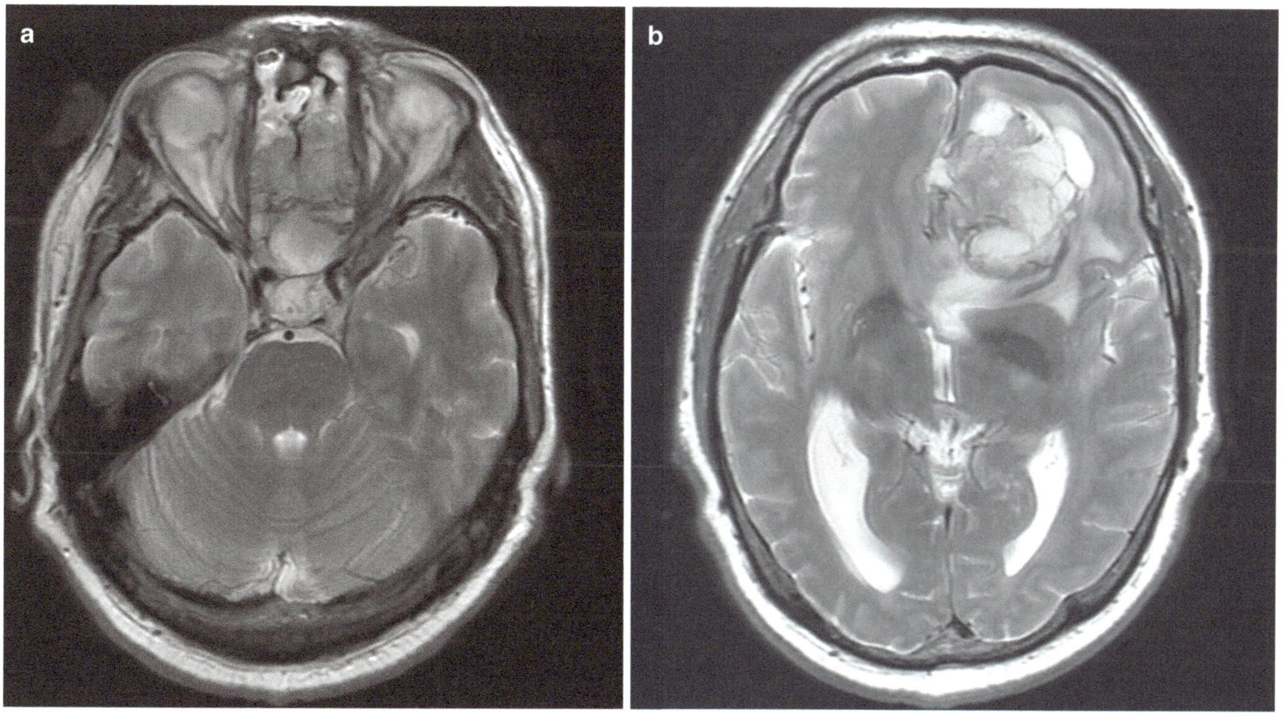

Fig. 11.8 Olfactory neuroblastoma (esthesioneuroblastoma). Axial T2-weighted (**a**, **b**) MR images show a mixed expansile mass with heterogeneous intensity of MR-signal expanding ethmoid complex and nasal cavities with spreading intracranially (isointense to brain from soft tissue portion and hyperintense MR-signal from cystic parts). DWI demonstrates a restriction of diffusion with hyperintense MR-signal from the lesion (**c**). Intravenous contrast enhancement produces intensive and inhomogeneous accumulation of contrast agent with better demarcation of cystic components on the border with brain (**d**–**f**). On ASL MR imaging a lesion is characterized by prominent increase of tumor blood flow (**g**). 3D TOF MR-angiography (**h**, **i**) demonstrates the abundant blood supply from different sources—branches of a. maxillary and anterior cerebral artery

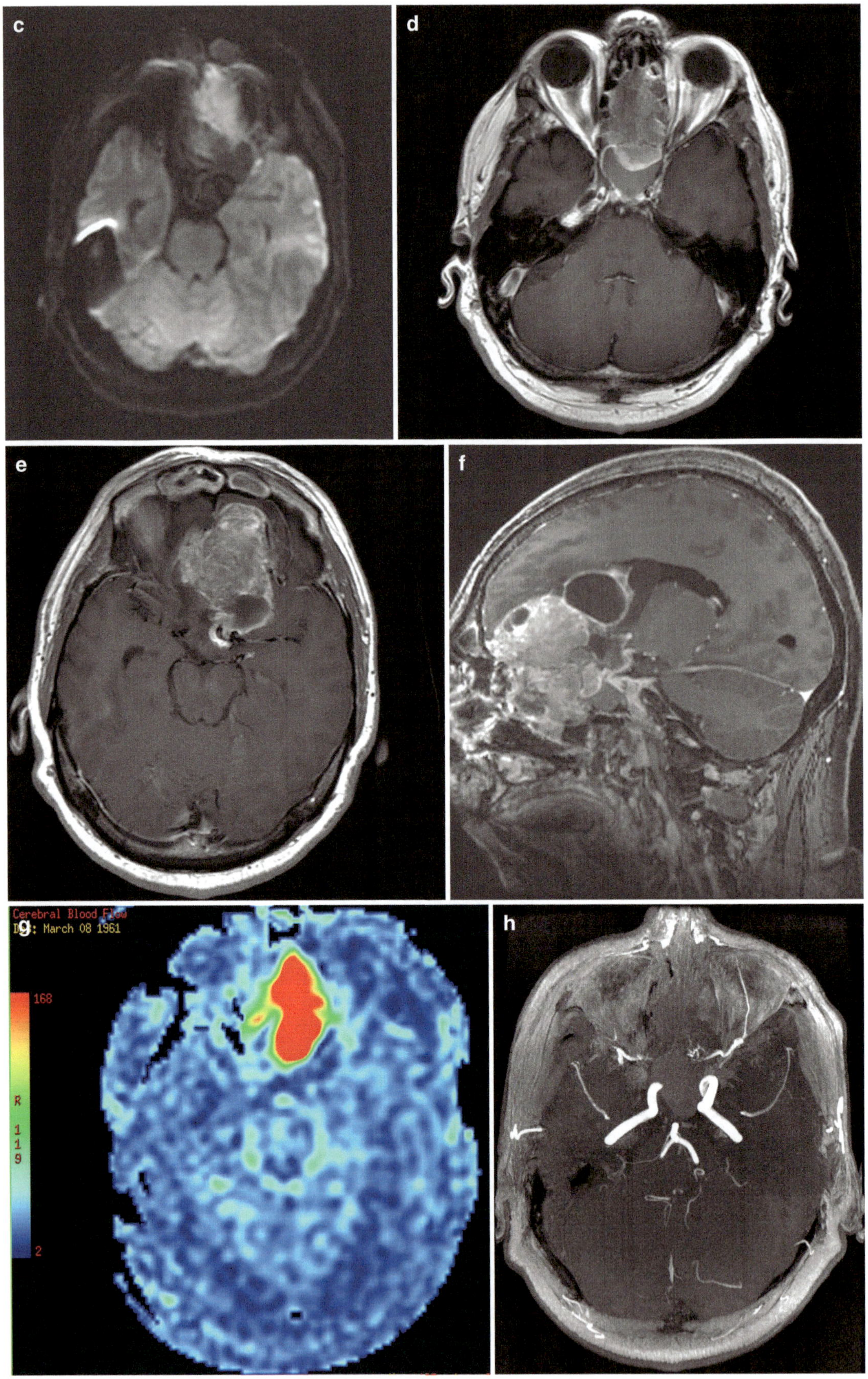

Fig. 11.8 (continued)

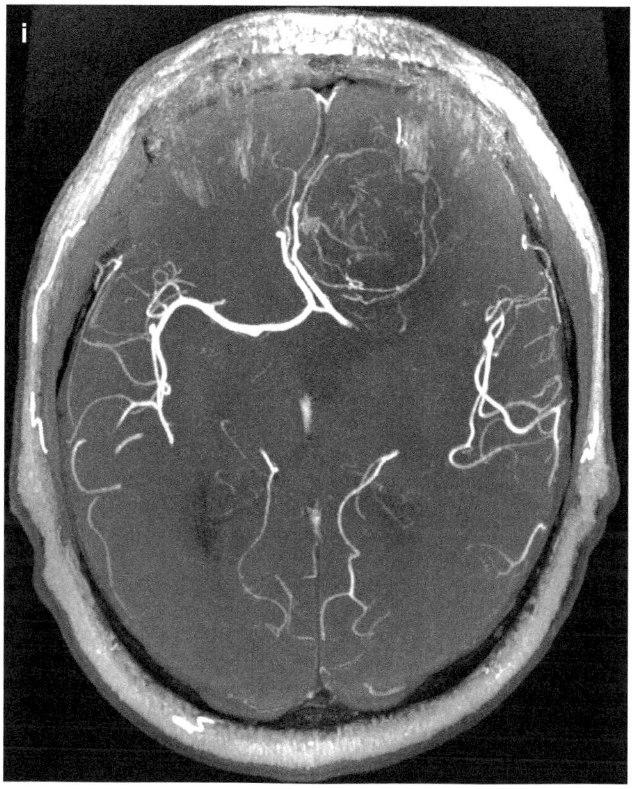

Fig. 11.8 (continued)

in other malignant tumors of the skull base (Som et al. 2011). A low MR-signal on T2-weighted images is due to high cellularity (a large amount of small cells) with a high nuclear-cytoplasmic ratio. Accumulation of MR contrast agents also varies widely from moderate to high, from homogeneous to heterogeneous patterns. The degree of contrast enhancement is lower than in adenocarcinoma, melanoma, and olfactory neuroblastoma. Using post-contrast T1-weighted sequence with Fat-Sat technology is mandatory in assessment of the tumor growth within the skull base bones (Figs. 11.11, 11.12, and 11.13). PET reveals a high degree of 18F-FDG accumulation into the SCC due to their hypermetabolism (Hermans et al. 1999) and helps better demarcate the lesion from surrounding tissues as well as better than CT and MRI demonstrates the dissemination of tumor to the regional lymph nodules.

Because of their proximity to the skull base, SCCs often spread into the base of the anterior and middle cranial fossa. The extradural and/or intradural extension can often be seen.

Differential Diagnosis

1. Fungal sinusitis is a rapidly progressive destructive disease, may cause invasion of the internal carotid artery and its thrombosis; more common in immunocompromised patients;

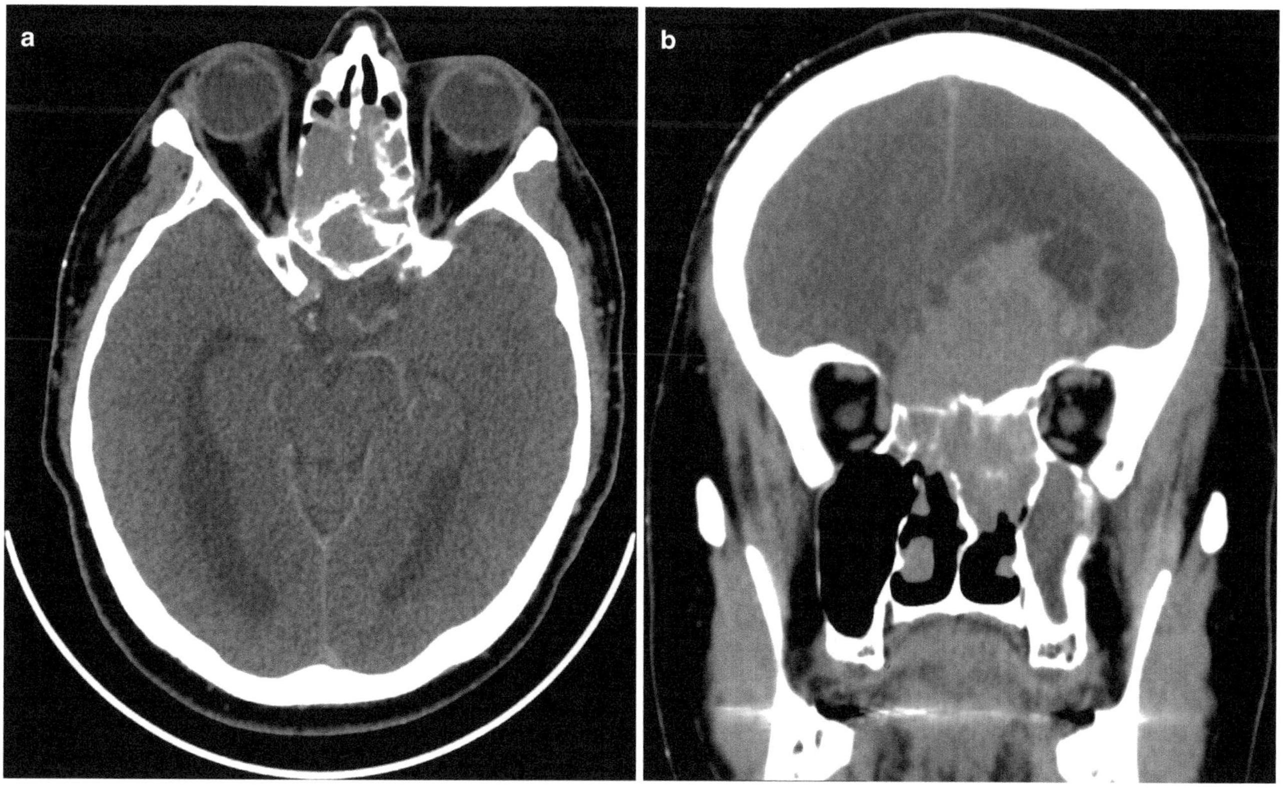

Fig. 11.9 Olfactory neuroblastoma (MRI is presented in Fig. 11.8). Post-contrast CT scans in axial (**a**) plane and with coronal (**b**, **c**) and sagittal (**d**) reformats show a soft tissue enhancing expansile mass with involvement of ethmoid complex, nasal cavities and sphenoid bone and sinus. A lesion locally invades in right orbital cavity and spreads intracranially. There are as bone remodel as destruction. CT-perfusion study ((**e**) TBF, (**f**) TBV) demonstrates an elevation of blood flow and blood volume parameters from the tumor. DSA revealed an abundant blood supply from a. maxillary, a. ophthalmic and anterior cerebral artery (**g**–**i**)

Fig. 11.9 (continued)

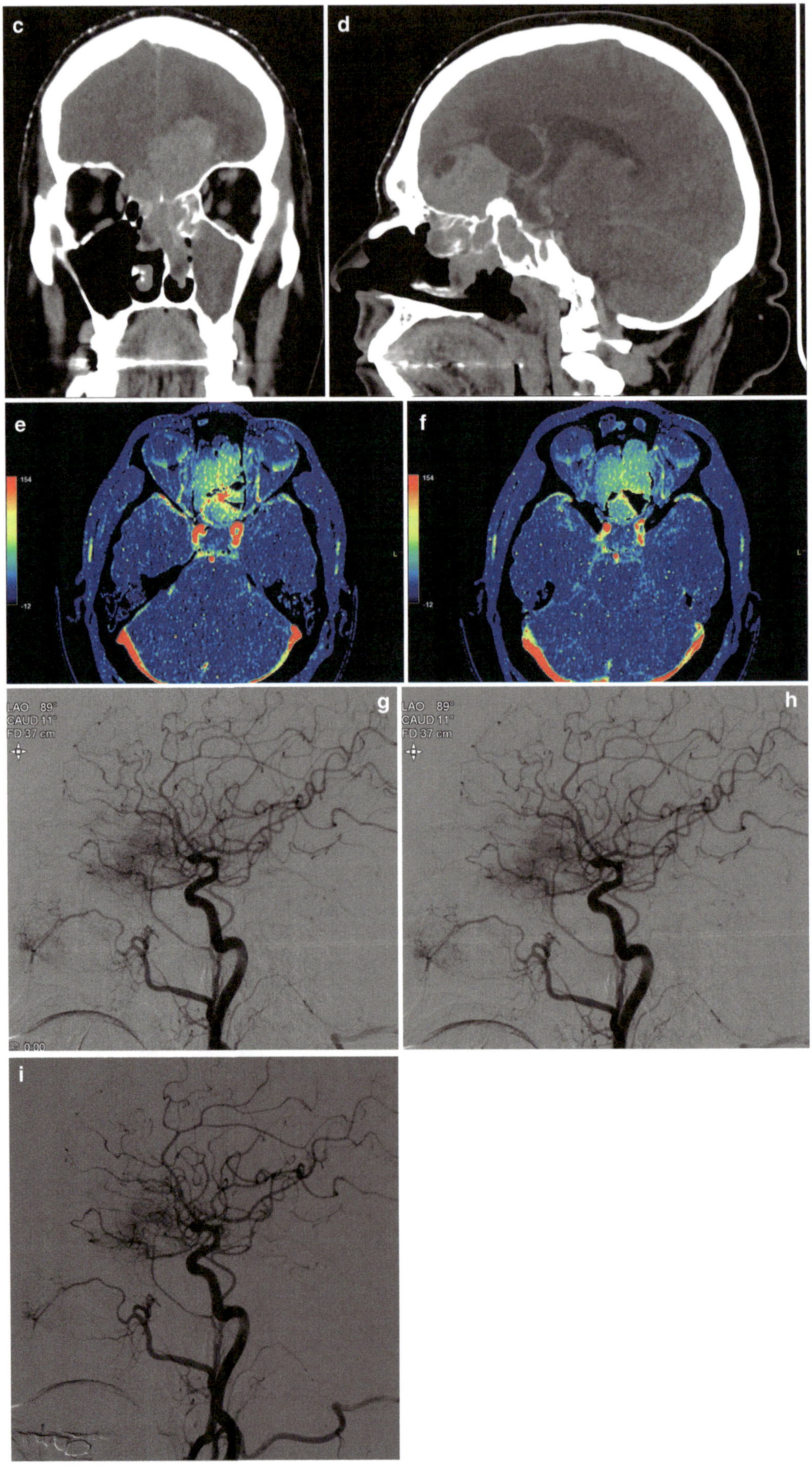

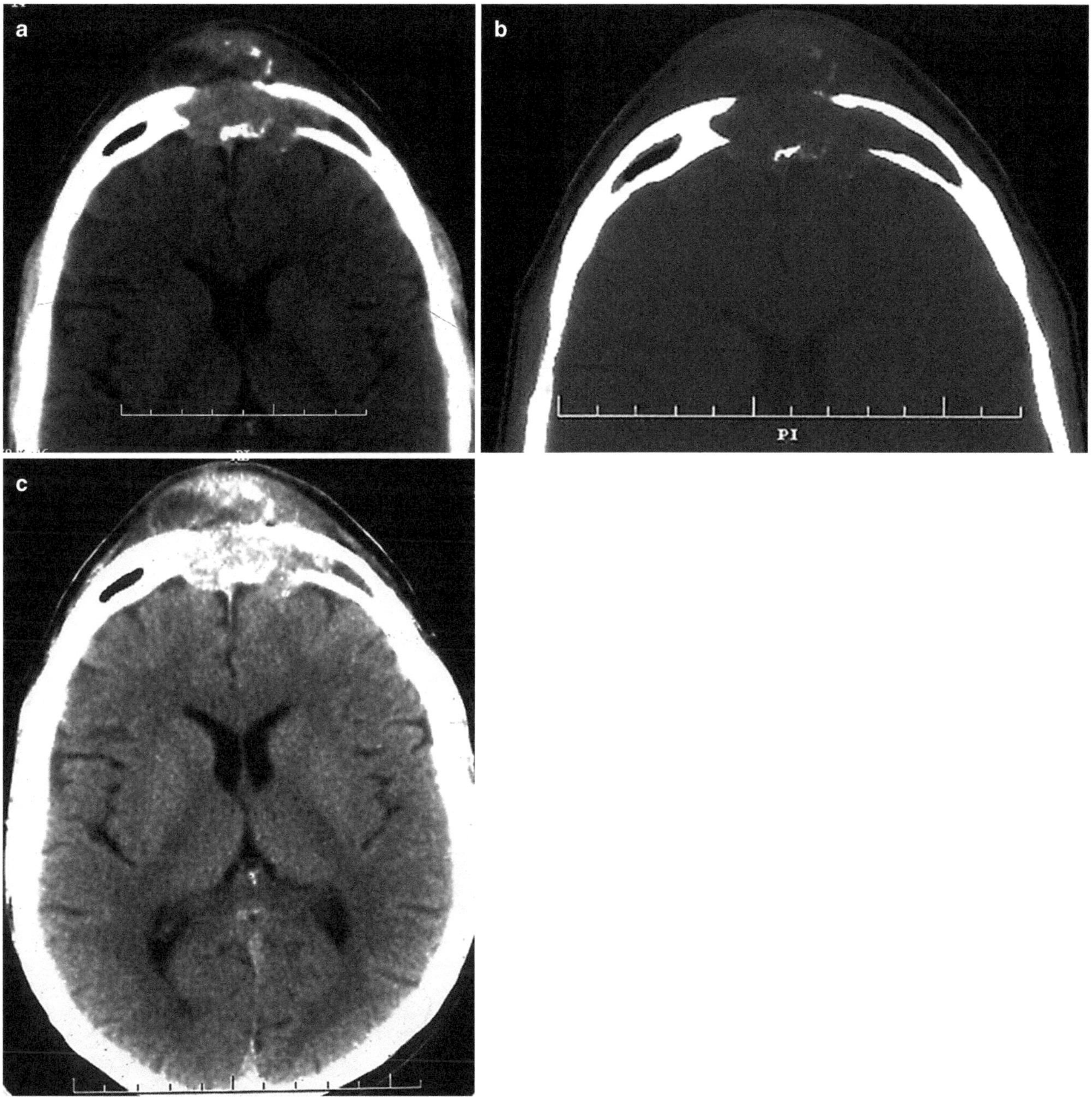

Fig. 11.10 Squamous cell carcinoma of the frontal bone and sinus. Axial CT scans (**a–c**) demonstrate a soft tissue mass with calcifications and wide bone destruction. After contrast enhancement (**c**) the solid part of the tumor heterogeneously accumulates the contrast agent and becomes hyperdense. Extra- and intracranial extension can be clearly seen

2. Granulomatosis typically causes destruction of the nasal bones, chronic sinusitis, a combination with tracheobronchial or kidney disorders;
3. Non-Hodgkin's lymphoma—a high degree of homogeneity of contrast enhancement and high signal on diffusion-weighted MRI are typical radiological characteristics;
4. Sinonasal undifferentiated carcinoma is difficult to distinguish from squamous cell cancer, typically is characterized by rapid growth.

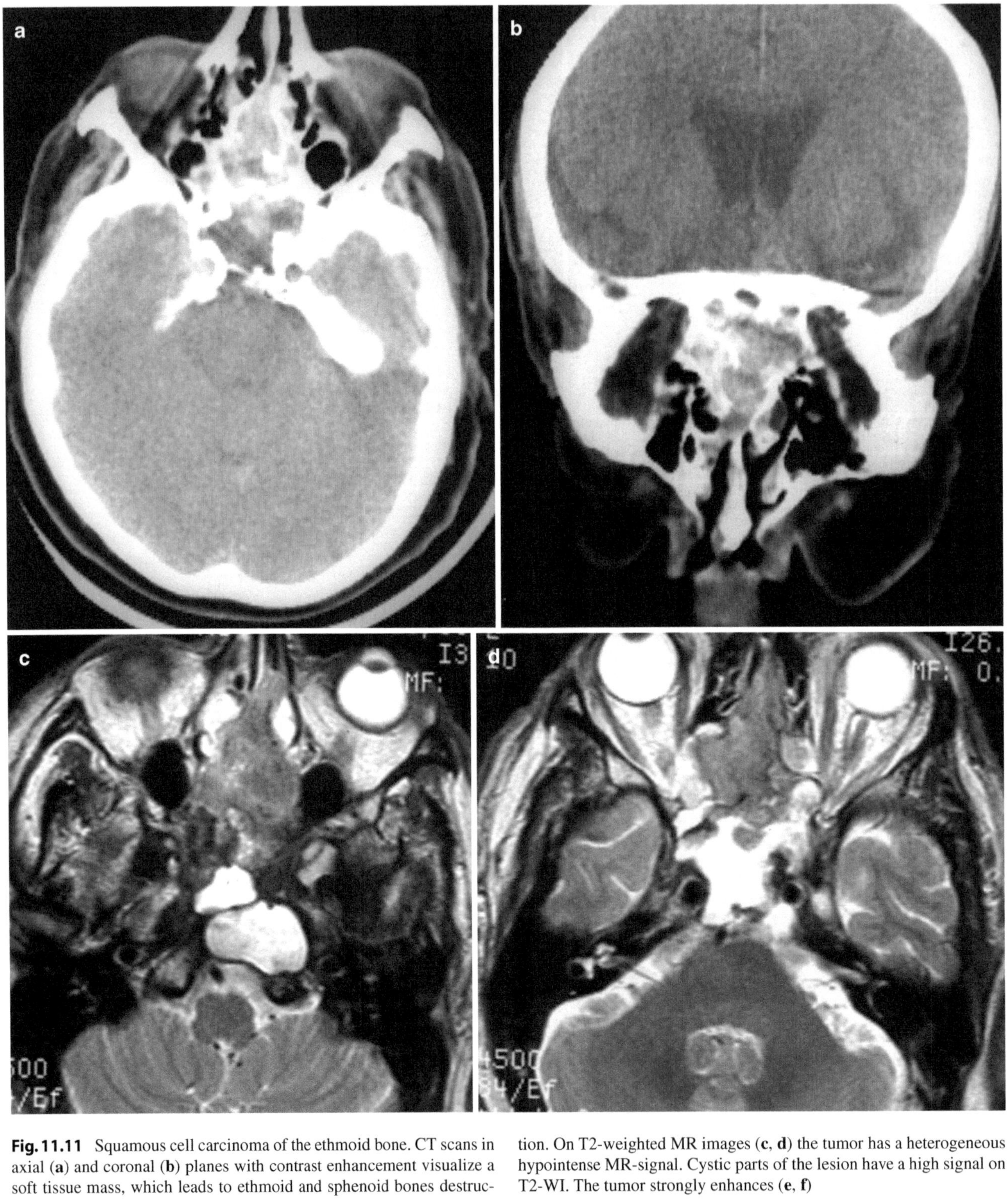

Fig. 11.11 Squamous cell carcinoma of the ethmoid bone. CT scans in axial (**a**) and coronal (**b**) planes with contrast enhancement visualize a soft tissue mass, which leads to ethmoid and sphenoid bones destruction. On T2-weighted MR images (**c**, **d**) the tumor has a heterogeneous hypointense MR-signal. Cystic parts of the lesion have a high signal on T2-WI. The tumor strongly enhances (**e**, **f**)

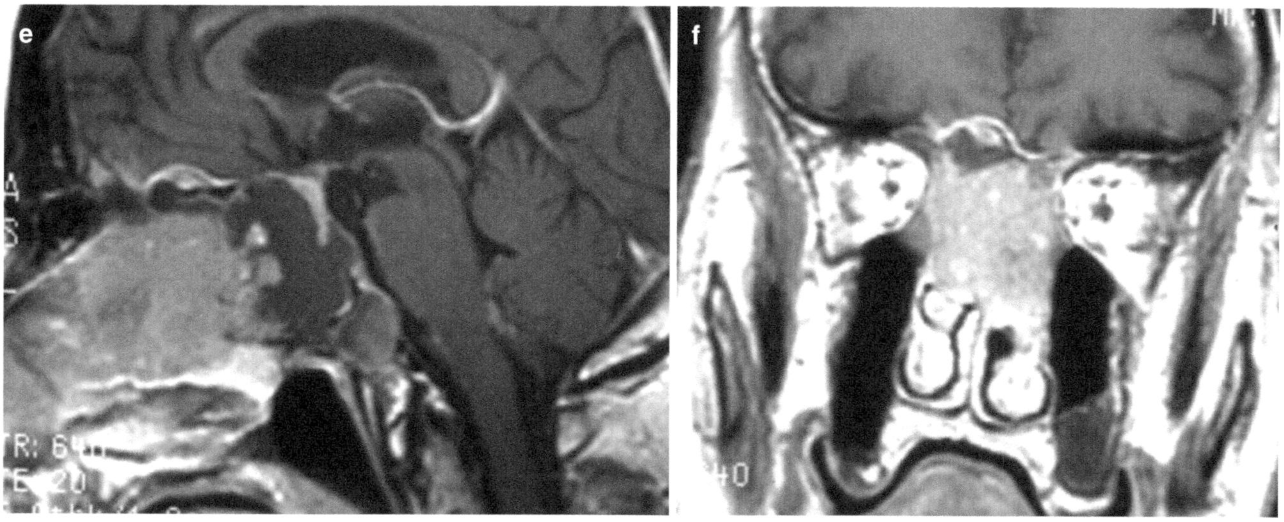

Fig. 11.11 (continued)

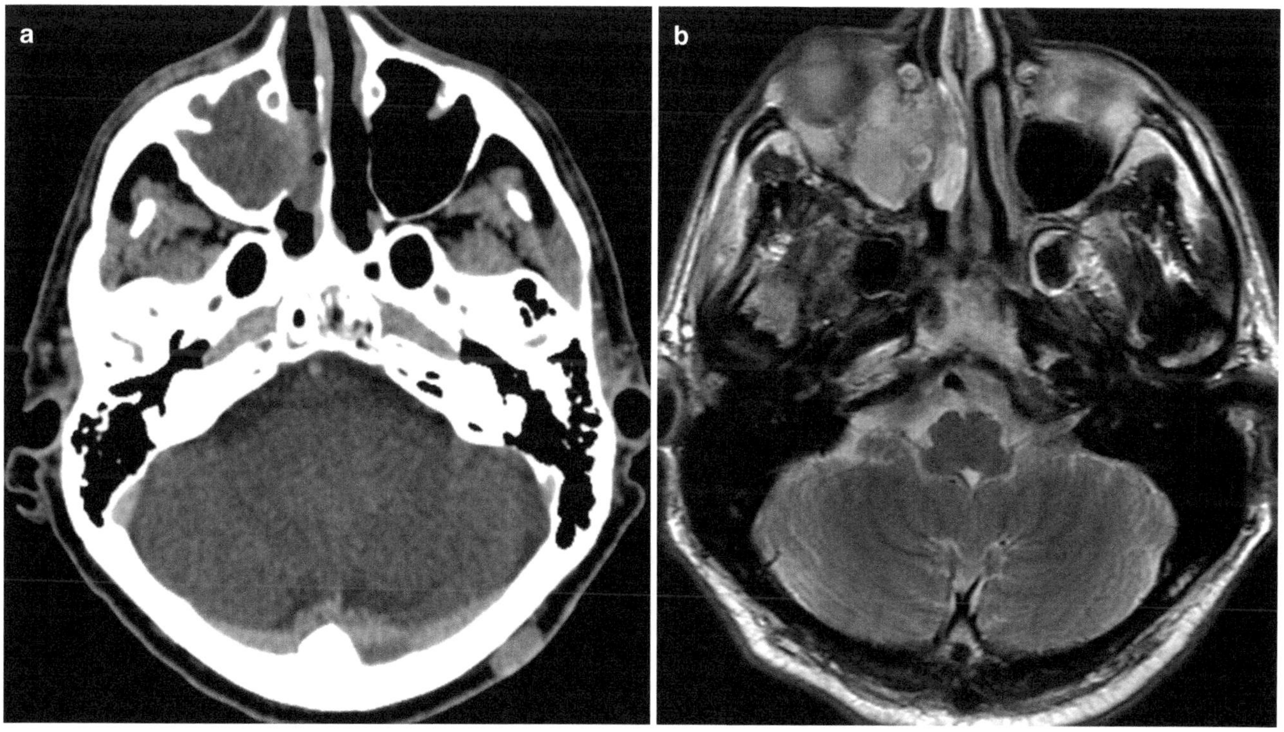

Fig. 11.12 Squamous cell carcinoma of the right nasal cavity. CT scan (**a**) and T2-weighted MR images (**b**, **c**), and T1-weighted image (**d**) demonstrate a soft tissue mass located in the right parts of nasal cavity. The tumor accumulates intensively contrast agent (T1 + fat sat (**e**)) and leads to obstruction of the right maxillary sinus with presence of pus in it (high MR-signal on DWI (**f**))

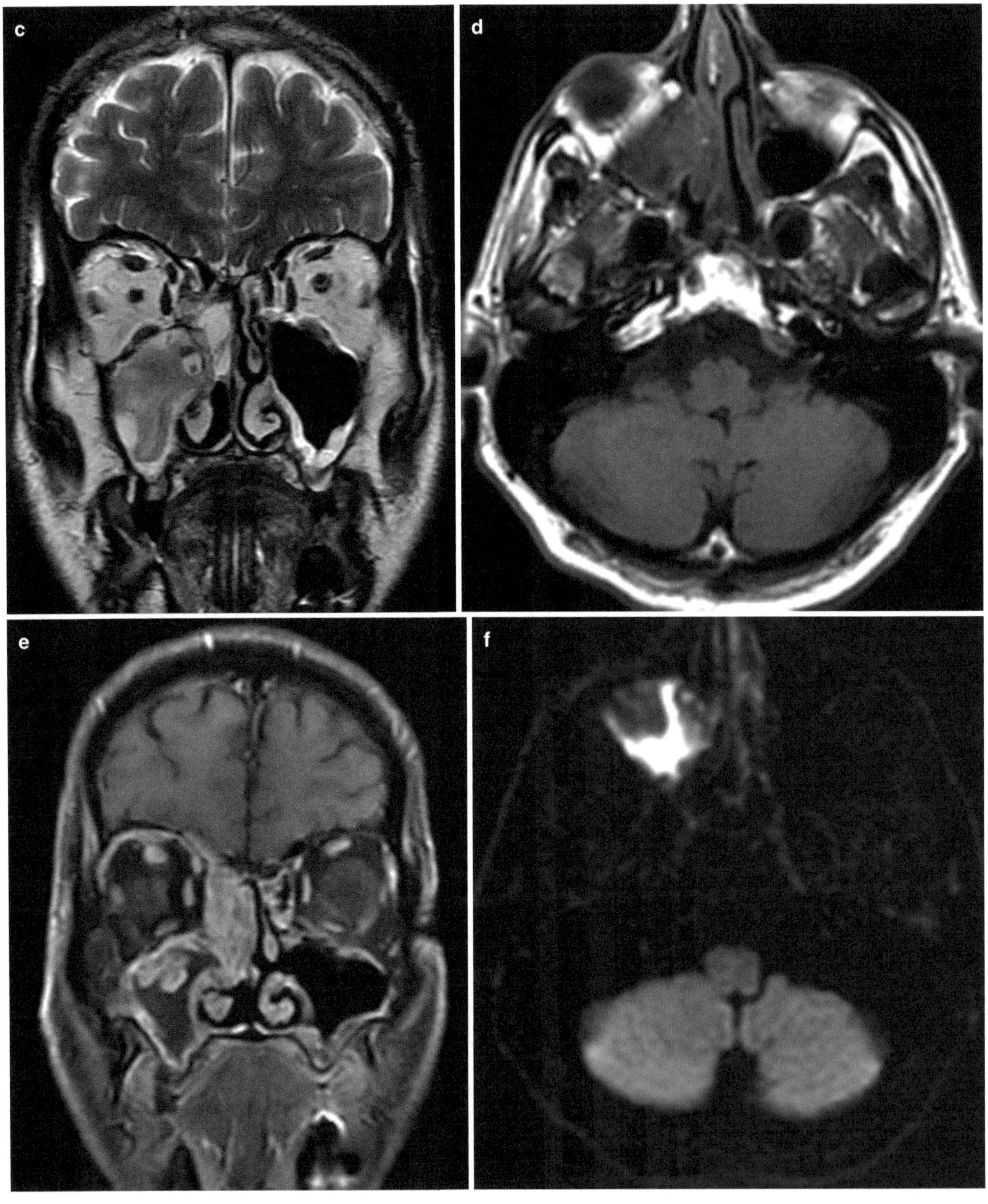

Fig. 11.12 (continued)

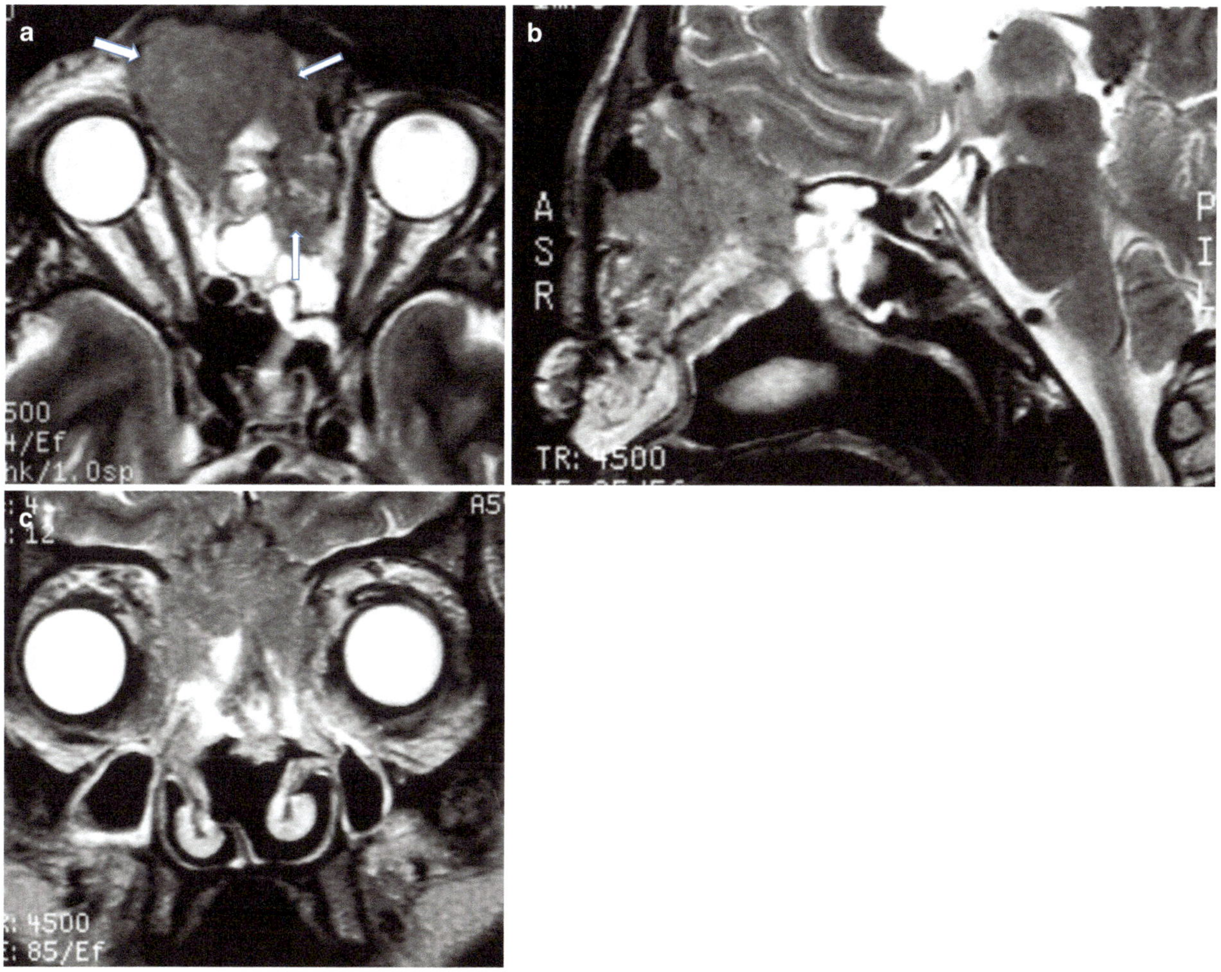

Fig. 11.13 Recurrence of squamous cell carcinoma of the frontal sinus and ethmoid bone. On T2-weighted MRI (**a**–**c**) on the background of post-surgical changes an isointense mass with involvement of ethmoids, frontal sinus, upper part of nasal cavity is detected. The tumor has a heterogeneous structure, a solid part has isointense to brain MR-signal (*arrows*)

11.4 Undifferentiated Carcinoma (UDC)

Undifferentiated carcinoma (undifferentiated malignant tumor)—this tumor as a separate entity was described by Frierson et al. (1986) and then Levine et al. (1987). These tumors have no obvious differentiation and are characterized by aggressive growth, extensive destruction of tissue in most cases, involvement of the orbital structures and the anterior cranial fossa, petrous portion of the temporal bone; it commonly forms an intracranially located part of the lesion very rapidly (Robertson and Hugh 2000). There is often a need in morphological differentiation of UDC from melanoma, lymphoma, rhabdomyosarcoma, and lymphoepithelioma. The prognosis for this type of cancer is unfavorable, especially in case of intracranial localization and infiltration of the brain matter. There are only a few cases of survival for 18–52 months reported (Levine et al. 1987).

Imaging On CT, undifferentiated craniofacial cancer looks like a space-occupying lesion, with a wide skull base extension into intracranial area, as well as into the sinuses, orbits, causing destruction of the bone structures, obstruction of the paranasal sinuses, with inhomogeneous contrast enhancement. On T2-weighted MRI, the tumor is characterized by a hypo- and isointense MR-signal relative to the brain matter. The structure of the tumor is typically heterogeneous. On T1-weighted images, the larger part of the tumor has an isointense and more homogeneous MR-signal. Areas of hemorrhages appear as bright foci in the stroma and on the periphery of the lesion on T1-WI. When the tumor grows into the sinuses, it causes their obstruction and secretion accumulation within the sinus cavity, which can be seen on MRI as high MR-signal both T1- and T2-weighted images with different brightness. When the tumor grows into the cranial cavity, it elevates the dura (dura remains intact for a long time) and may deform the frontal lobes. Poorly differentiated cancer is characterized by pronounced heterogeneous contrast enhancement. Using the contrast enhancement improves differentiation of the tumor mass from the surrounding structures of the facial skeleton especially with using Fat-Sat technology (Figs. 11.14, 11.15, 11.16, and 11.17). CT-perfusion study demonstrates intermediate elevation of tumor blood flow and blood volume, and high elevation of permeability (Fig. 11.18).

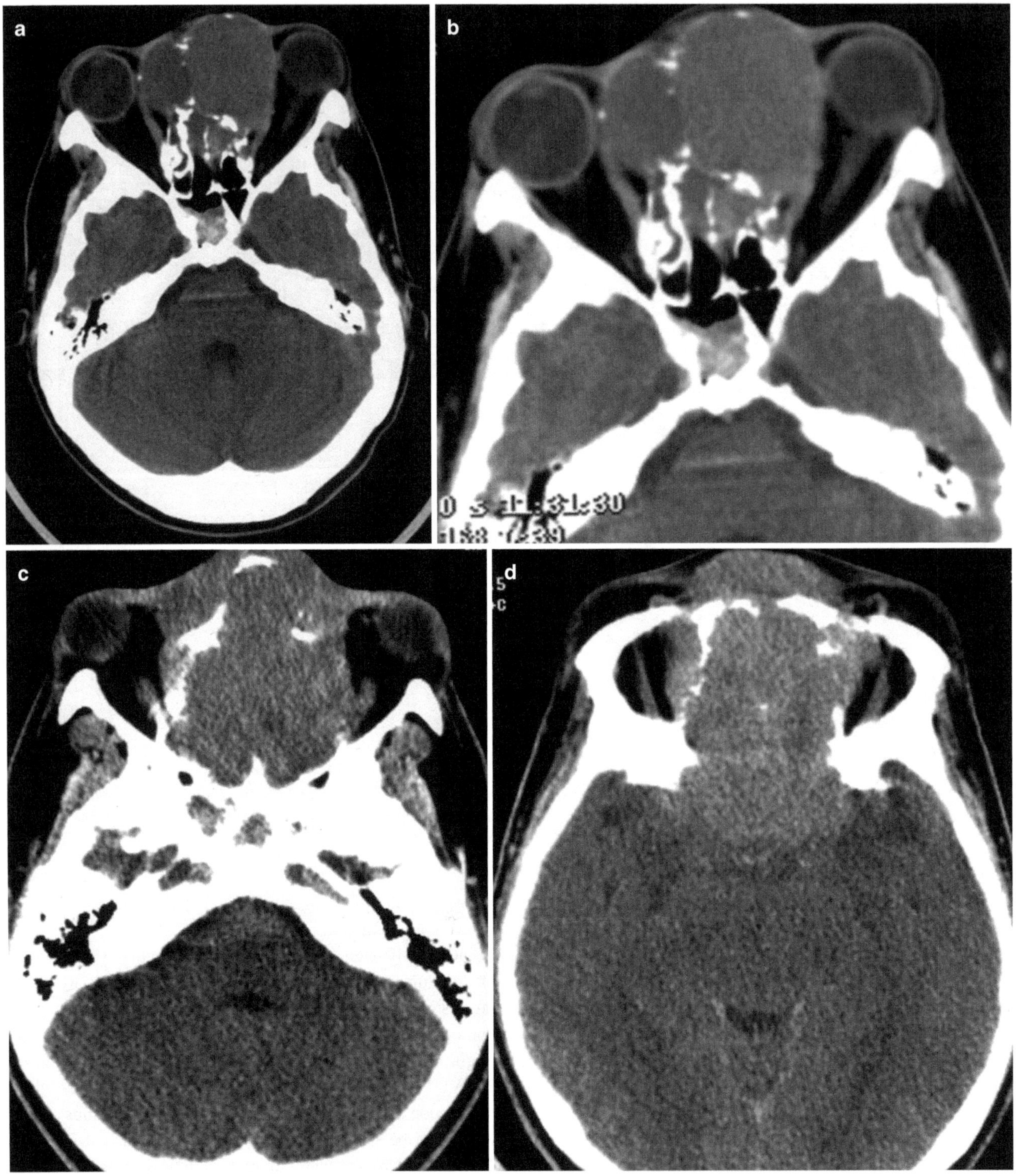

Fig. 11.14 Undifferentiated cancer. Axial CT scans before (**a**) and after injection of contrast medium (**b–f**) demonstrate a large and heterogeneous mass in area of ethmoids and frontal bone, and sinus, which extends intracranially to frontal region with brain edema as well as into the orbits with globes displacement. The tumor leads to wide destruction of the bones. Contrast enhancement is inhomogeneous and intensive

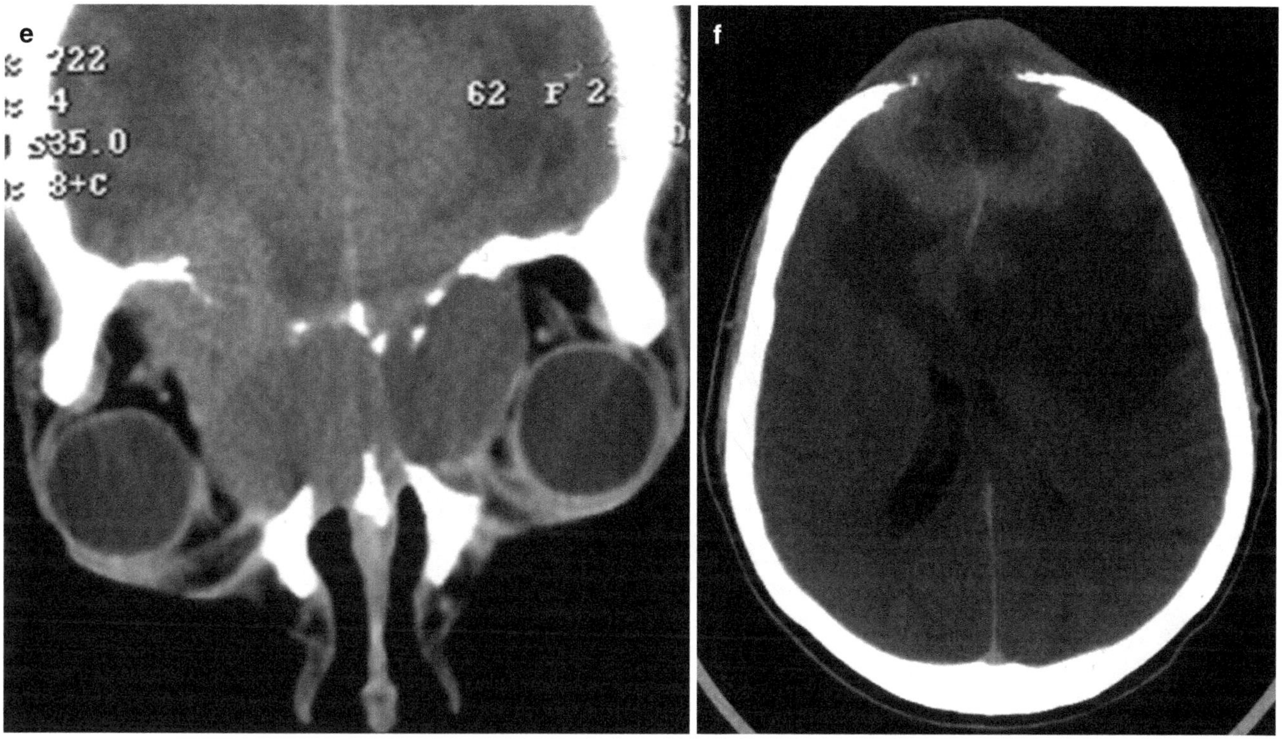

Fig. 11.14 (continued)

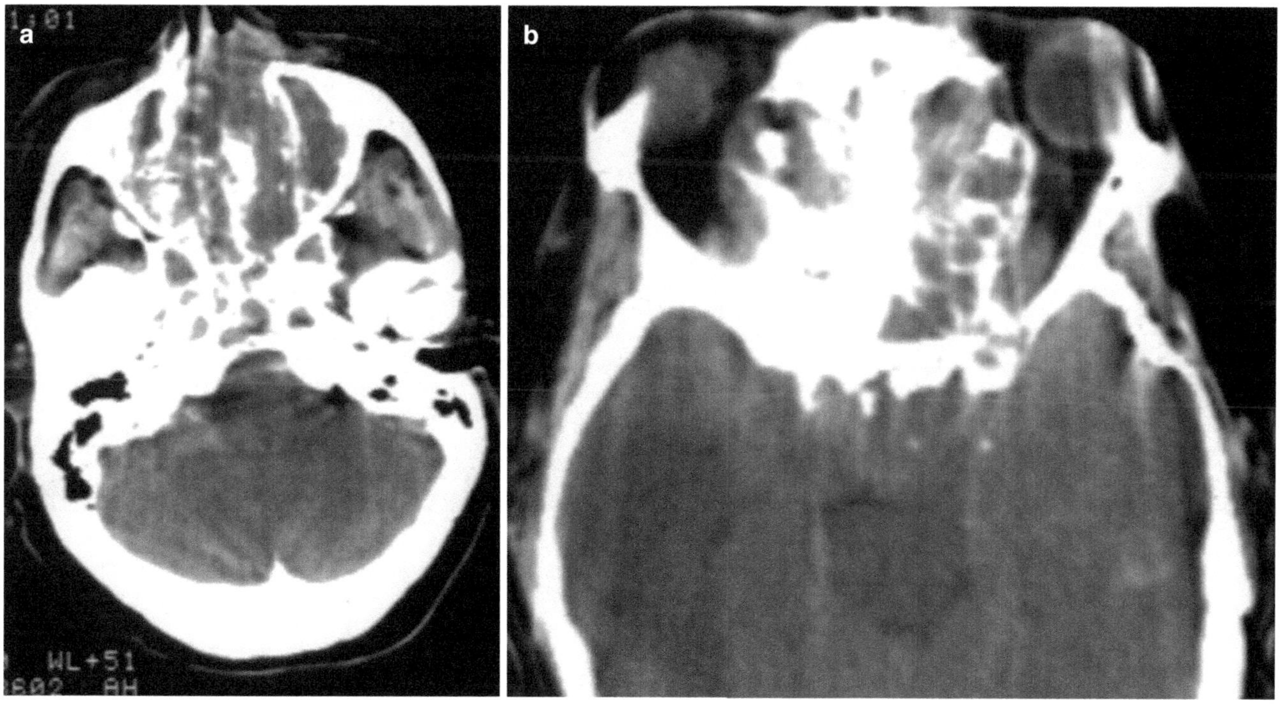

Fig. 11.15 Undifferentiated cancer of the nasal cavity, frontal and sphenoid bones and sinuses, and ethmoid bone. Axial (**a**, **b**) and coronal (**c**) CT scans reveal an expansile mass with calcification that leads to wide destruction of the bone structure. Also, the tumor leads to obstruction of the maxillary sinuses. There is a gross intracranial invasion causes of extensive brain edema. On T2-weighted (**d**, **e**) and T1-weighted (**f**) MR images the tumor has a heterogeneous structure with presence as solid as cystic components. On T2-weighted MRI the tumor has an isointense with brain MR-signal but slightly hypointense on T1-WI

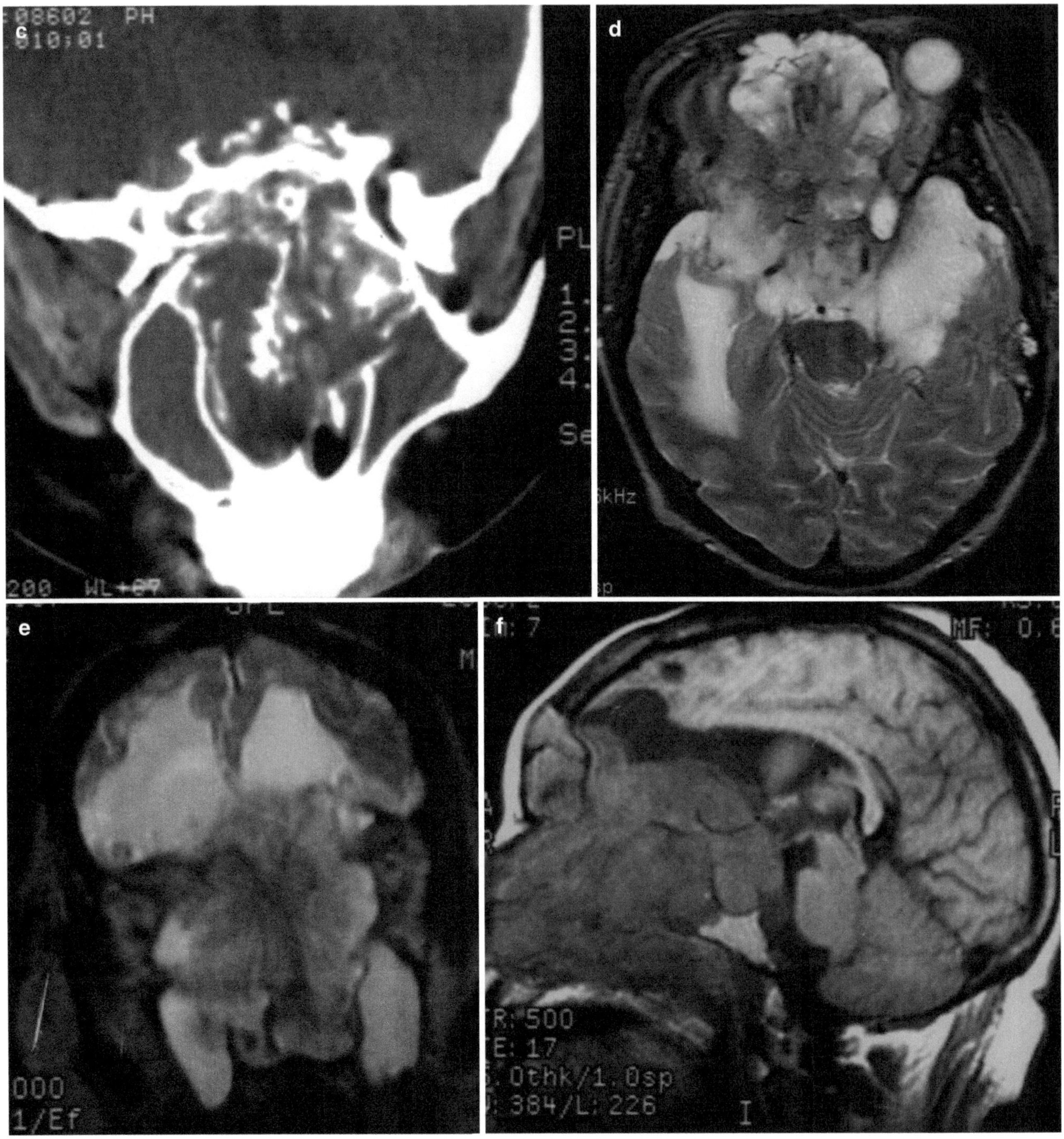

Fig. 11.15 (continued)

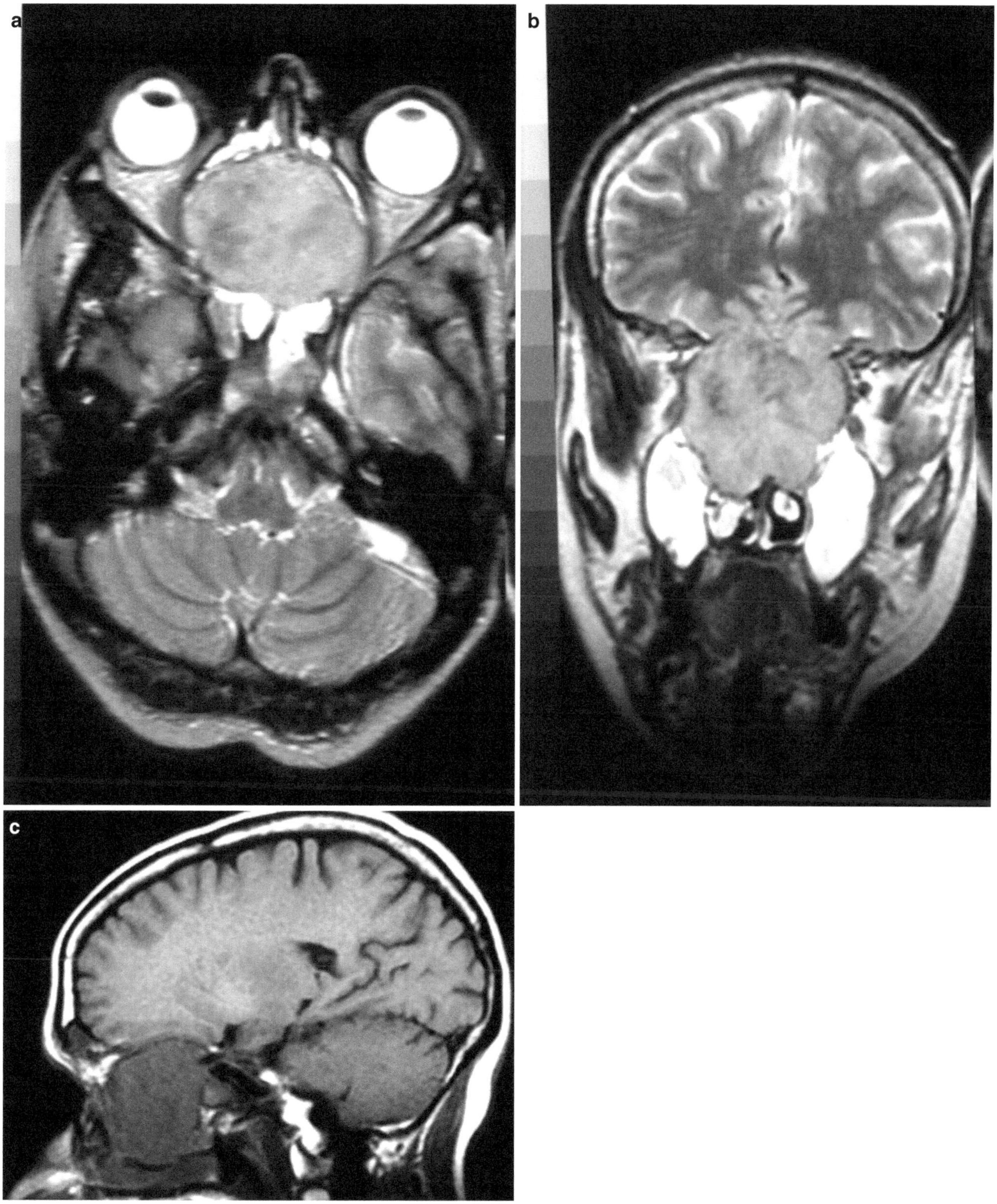

Fig. 11.16 Undifferentiated cancer of nasal cavity and ethmoid bone. T2-weighted (**a**, **b**) and T1-weighted (**c**) MR images visualize a soft tissue solid mass with slightly inhomogeneous structure, which leads to obstruction of the maxillary sinuses. Tumor destroys the ethmoid bones and extends into both orbits

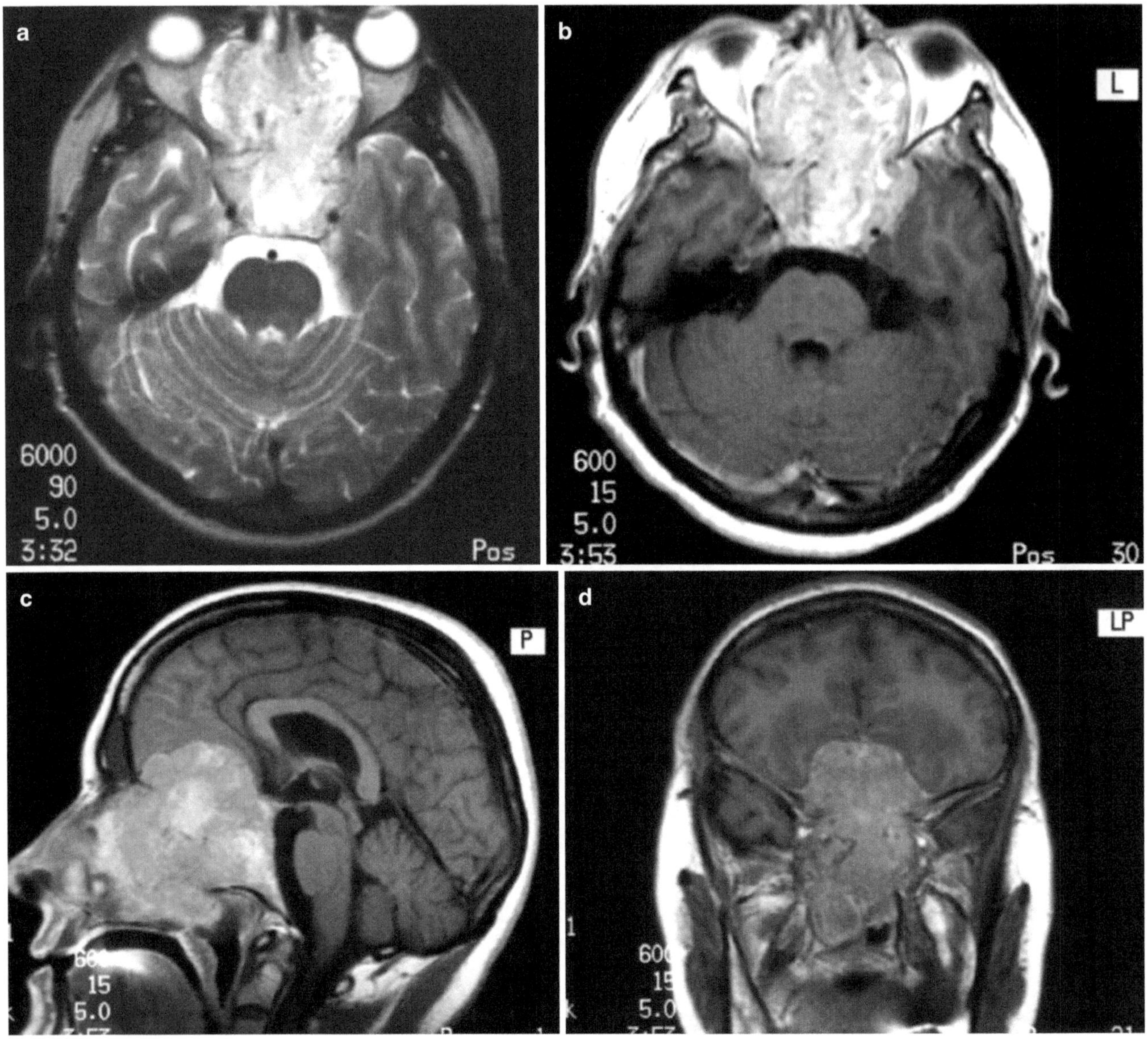

Fig. 11.17 Undifferentiated cancer of nasal cavities and ethmoid bone. T2-weighted (**a**) and T1-weighted MR images with contrast enhancement (**b**–**d**) show a large expansile soft tissue mass, which extends intracranially and strongly enhances. The tumor also has extended into both orbits and cavernous sinuses

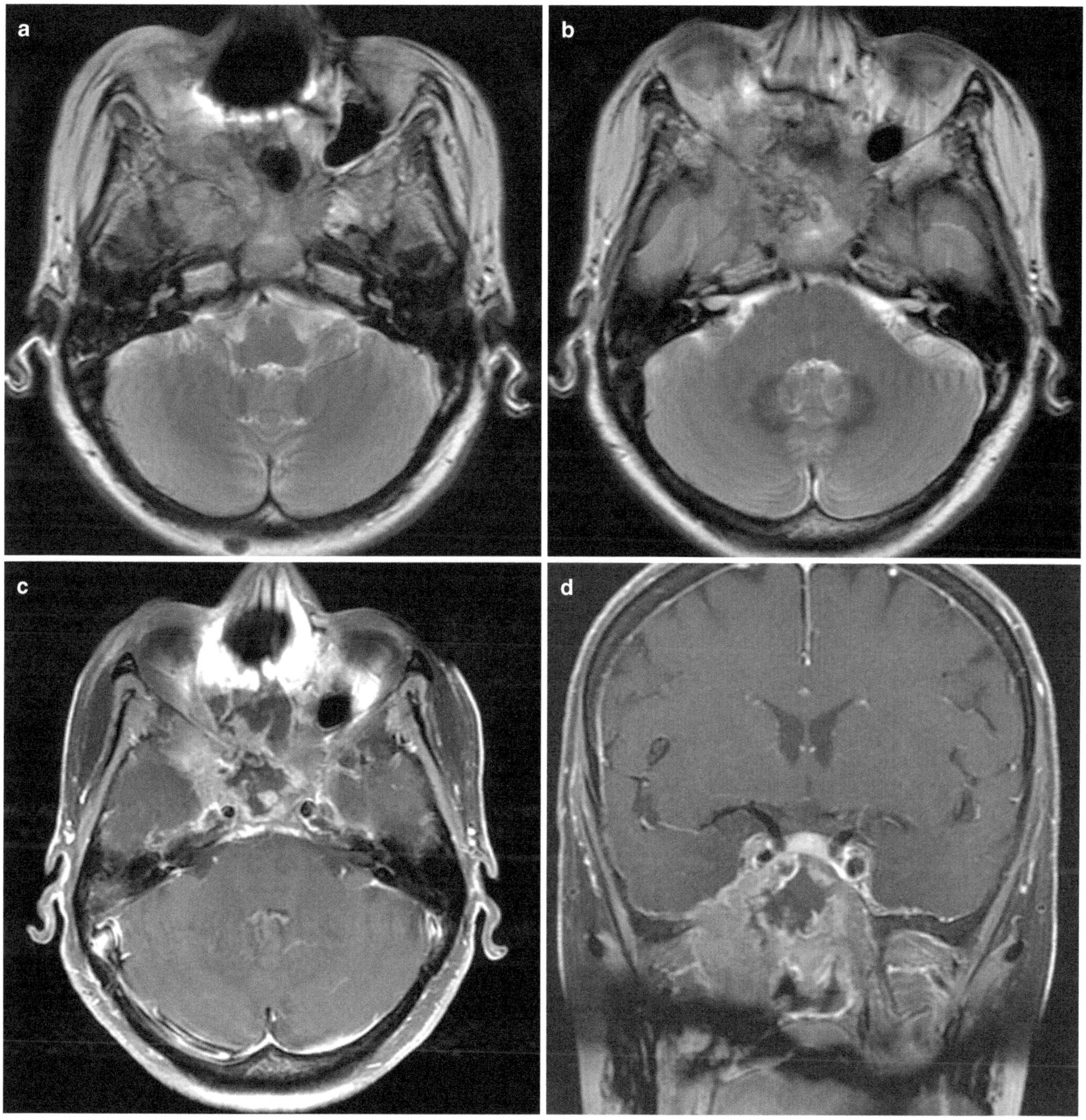

Fig. 11.18 Undifferentiated cancer. Axial T2-weighted (**a**, **b**) and contrast enhanced T1-weighted (**c**–**e**) MR images in axial and coronal planes demonstrate a hypointense on T2 and strongly enhancing mass with involvement of the nasopharynx, sphenoid bone, ethmoids, and right maxillary sinus. This tumor has intracranial extension in the right middle cranial fossa and cavernous sinus. CT scans (**f**–**h**) demonstrate a wide area of skull base bone destruction. CT-perfusion study (TBF map (**i**)) shows a heterogeneous elevation of perfusion parameters in solid part of the tumor (*arrows*)

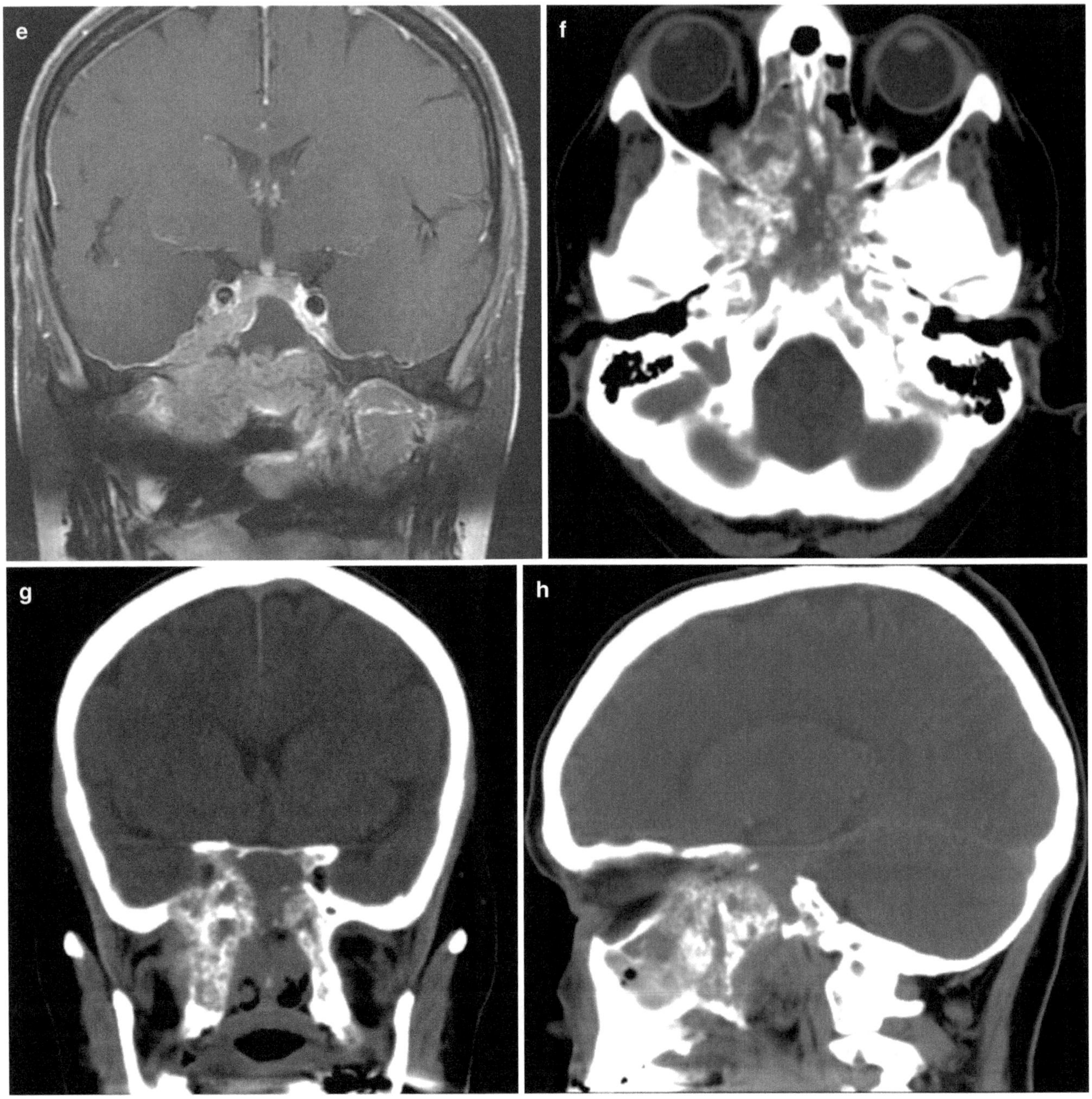

Fig. 11.18 (continued)

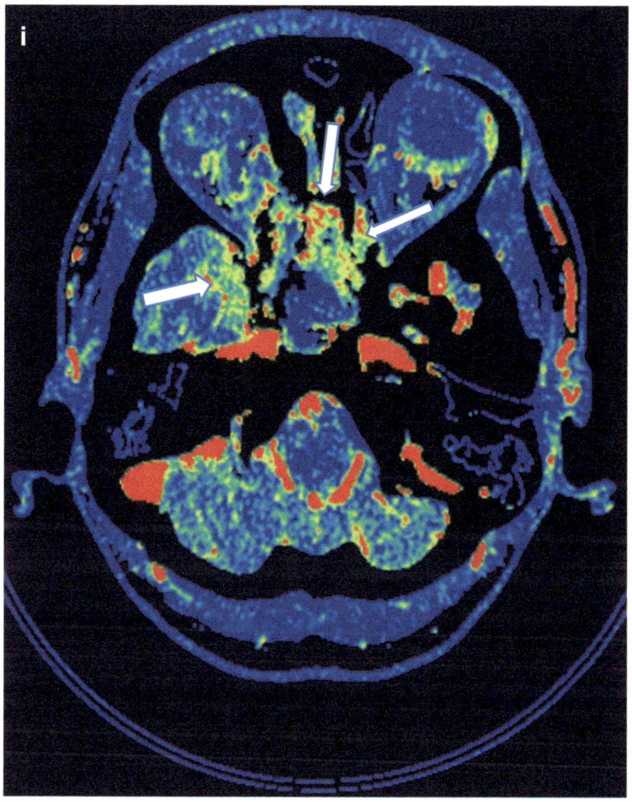

Fig. 11.18 (continued)

11.5 Sinonasal Adenocarcinoma (SA)

Sinonasal adenocarcinoma is a malignant neoplasm which typically has grandular origin and occurs in 10% of all sinonasal tumors (Barnes 1985). This is a solid, poorly defined lesion in the sinuses and nasal cavity with involvement of the ethmoid and skull base bone; it may grow from the hard palate (Sklar and Pizarro 2003). SA commonly causes an obstruction of paranasal sinuses, which mimics sinusitis, delaying the correct diagnosis. A clinical presentation of the disease is frequently characterized by epistaxis, pain, and facial asymmetry. The tumor is more common in men. Sinonasal adenocarcinomas can be subclassified as salivary type, intestinal type, neuroendocrine, and "other" (Som et al. 2011).

Imaging On CT, this is a soft tissue lesion without well-defined borders, causing wide bone destruction and heterogeneously enhancing.

On T1-weighted MRI, the tumor has intermediate MR-signal intensity, there may be areas of hemorrhages within the tumor; on T2-weighted images, MR-signal varies from intermediate to relatively high. Contrast agent accumulation is diffuse and heterogeneous. As with other skull base lesions, a combination of contrast-enhanced series with Fat-Sat technique is mandatory (Fig. 11.19). Nevertheless the imaging features of these tumors are non-specific and are indistinguishable from those of SCC.

Differential Diagnosis All malignant craniofacial tumors, such as squamous cell carcinoma, esthesioneuroblastoma, sinonasal undifferentiated carcinoma, etc.

11.6 Adenoid Cystic Carcinoma (ACC)

Adenoid cystic carcinoma (sometimes referred to as adenocyst, malignant cylindroma, adenocystic, adenoid cystic carcinoma) is a rare malignancy of exocrine glands defined by the presence of a dual population of cells (epithelial and myoepithelial cells) organized in varying combinations of cribriform, tubular, and solid patterns (Fusco et al. 2015). This neoplasm most frequently originates in the salivary glands; however, it can also occur in other anatomical sites, including the breast, lacrimal gland, lung, brain, Bartholin gland, trachea, and the paranasal sinuses (Marchio et al. 2010). It is the third most common malignant salivary gland tumor overall (after mucoepidermoid carcinoma and polymorphous low grade adenocarcinoma). It represents 28% of malignant submandibular gland tumors, making it the single most common malignant salivary gland tumor in this region. Patients may survive for years with metastases because this tumor is generally well-differentiated and slow growing.

ACC most commonly arises in the palate and then extends into nasal fossae and paranasal sinuses. These type of tumors usually arise in whites between 30 and 60 years of age.

Imaging Very common sinonasal salivary tumors form spherical masses rather than the more typical polypoid, or diffuse lesions (Som et al. 2011). On CT, ACCs may appear nonhomogeneous because of a mesenchymal component, cystic degeneration, necrosis, or serous and mucous collections can be presented (Klintenberg et al. 1984).

On MRI, these tumors tend to have an intermediate MR-signal intensity depending on the cellularity of the lesion. Tumors with low-cellularity index usually have high MR-signal on T2-weighted images (Sigal et al. 1992). On T1-weighted images a lesion has typically isointense with muscles MR-signal and shows the intermediate contrast enhancement. CT-perfusion study demonstrates the elevation of blood flow and blood volume in the tumor tissue (Fig. 11.20).

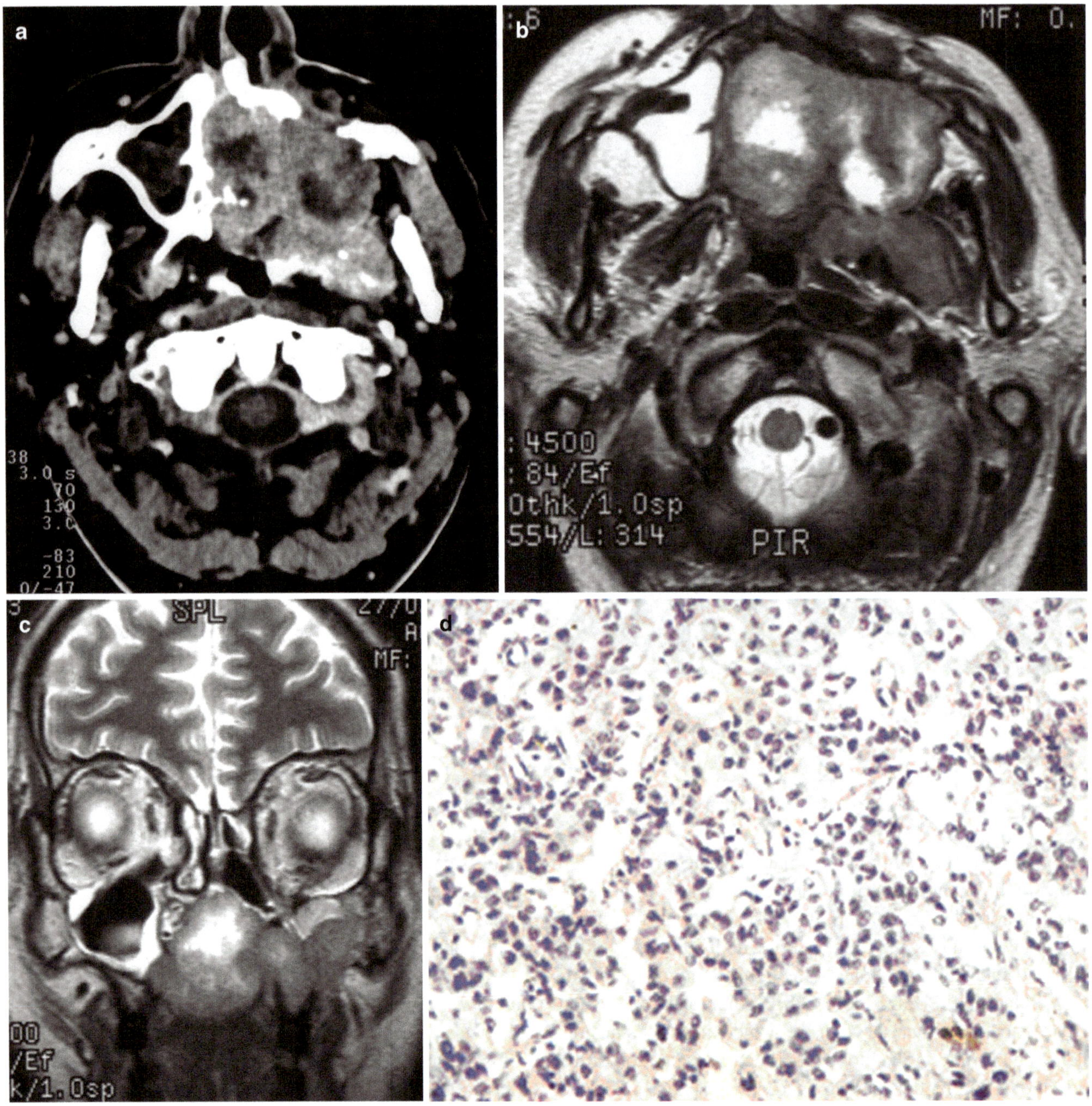

Fig. 11.19 Recurrence of sinonasal adenocarcinoma. Axial CT scan (**a**) with contrast enhancement and T2-weighted MR images (**b**, **c**) in axial and coronal planes demonstrate a heterogeneous expansile soft tissue mass, extending into the left maxillary sinus. These is a wide bone destruction of the maxilla and the hard palate. (**d**) histological specimen

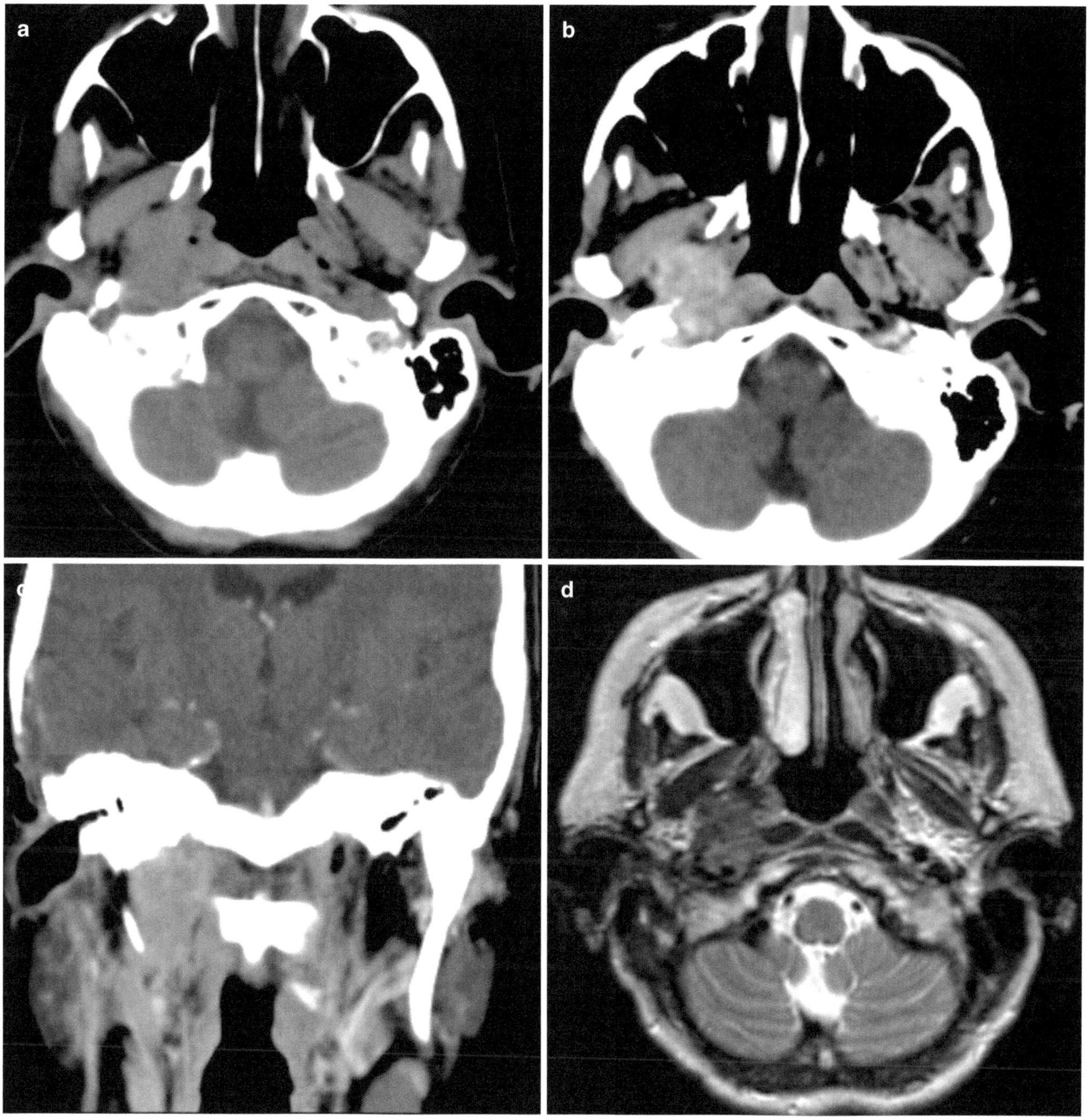

Fig. 11.20 Adenoid cystic carcinoma (cylindroma). Axial CT scans before (**a**) and after (**b**, **c**) contrast enhancement show a soft tissue enhancing mass that occupies the right parapharyngeal space. Internal carotid artery is dislocated backwards. On T2-weighted MR image (**d**) a tumor has hypointense MR-signal compared to fat tissue. On T1-weighted image (**e**) a lesion is characterized by isointense MR-signal to muscles and intermediate degree of contrast enhancement (**f**). CT-perfusion study demonstrates an elevation of tumor blood flow (TBF map (**g**)) and blood volume (TBV map (**h**)) as well as capillary permeability values (PS map (**i**))

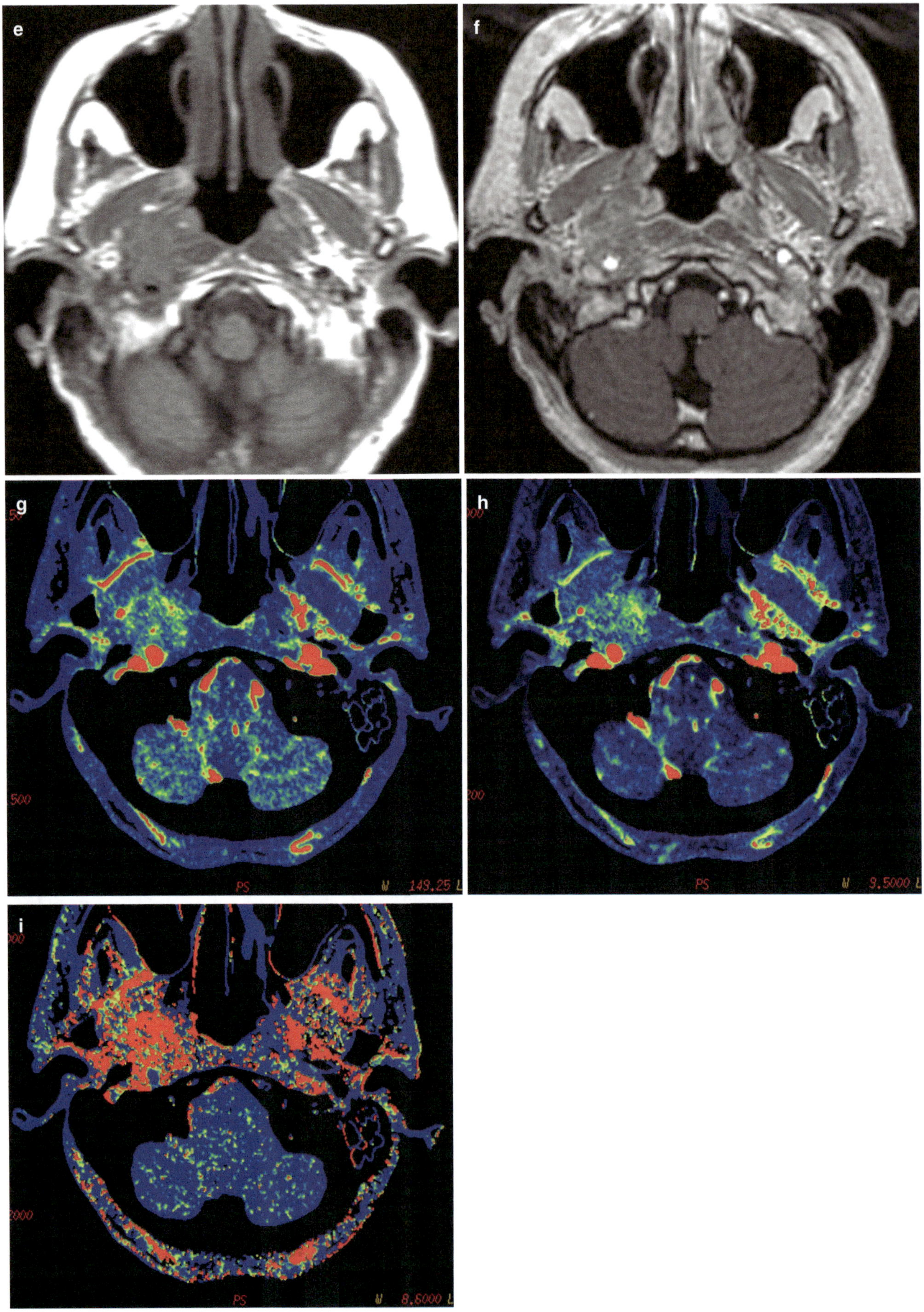

Fig. 11.20 (continued)

11.7 Plasmacytoma and Multiple Myeloma

Plasmacytoma is a tumor that is characterized by a malignant proliferation of plasma cells. This plasma cells proliferation leads to the bone marrow involvement with the following bone destructive process. Multiple myeloma is more common disorder among all plasma cell dyscrasias and usually affects patients over the age of 40 years. In patients with multiple myeloma multiple skeletal lytic lesions are found in 85% cases. Osteoporosis and pathologic bone fractures are typical clinical and radiologic features in majority of cases, even in beginning of the disease. Some authors consider the solitary plasmacytoma is a first stage of multiple myeloma (Barnes 1985). In general, solitary plasmacytoma is a rare plasma cells proliferation lesion, nevertheless extramedullary plasmacytoma represents 3–4% of all sinonasal cavity tumors (Som et al. 2011). The head and neck area is a common primary site for this lesion. Next locations are nasal cavity and paranasal sinuses.

Imaging On CT, head and neck plasmacytoma is a homogenous, strongly enhancing polypoid (if located in sinonasal cavity) lesion. Surrounding bone remodel is a typical radiologic feature (Kondo et al. 1986). On MRI, these tumors have intermediate MR-signal intensity on all sequences, typically strongly enhances and demonstrates the bone destruction. These lesions are characterized by a high vasculature, flow-void phenomena within the lesion can be seen on T2-weighted MR images and it is associated with elevation of perfusion parameters on CT- and MR-perfusion studies. The main radiologic feature of this tumor is a very discrete bone destruction area, which is different from that in cases with metastatic lesions where margins bone infiltration is a most typical sign (Fig. 11.21).

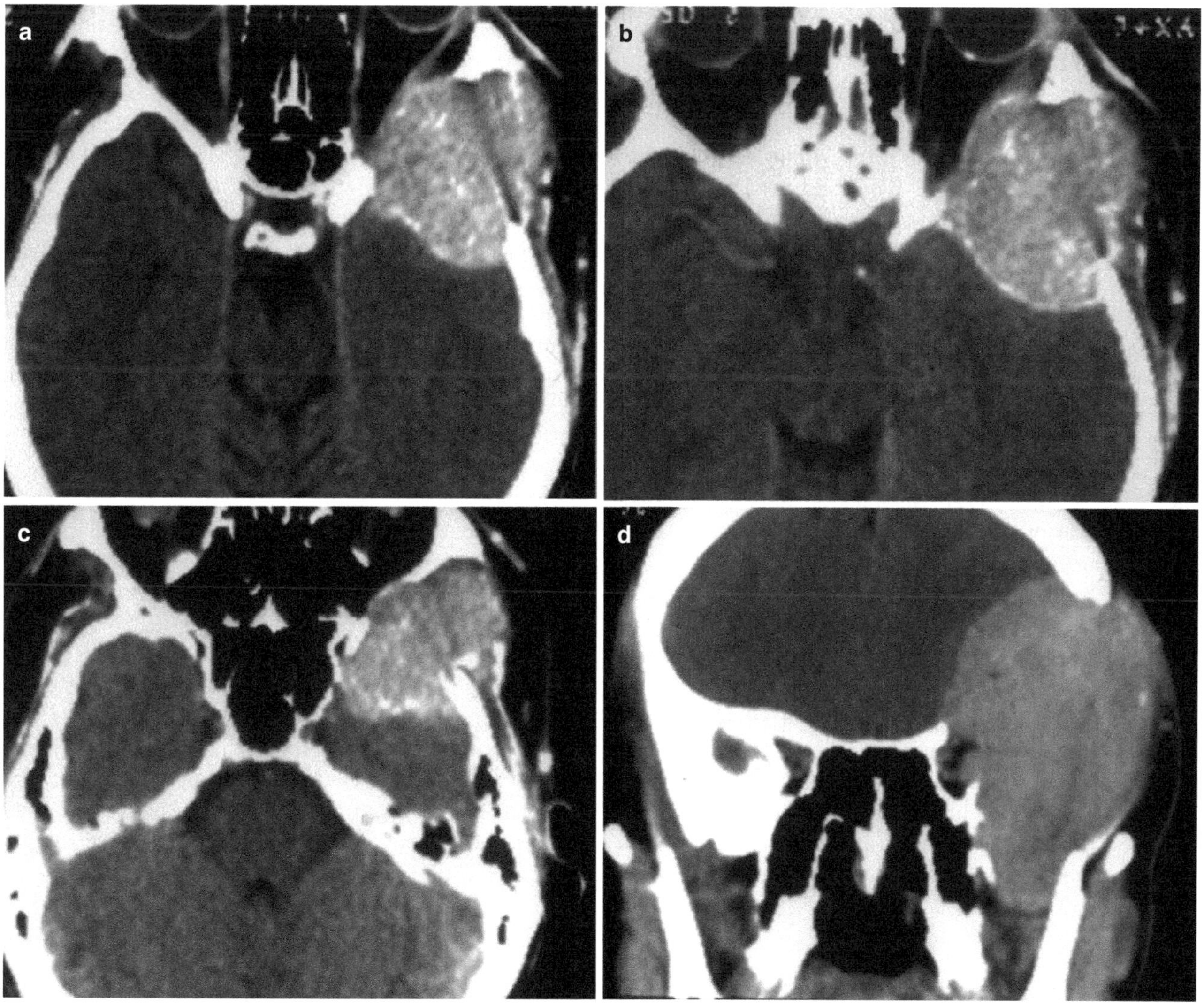

Fig. 11.21 Plasmacytoma. CT scans in axial (**a**, **b**, **c**) and coronal (**d**, **e**) planes demonstrate a large soft tissue mass in left pterional region. A lesion leads to wide bone destruction and extends into middle cranial fossa and left orbit. Contrast enhancement is strong and homogeneous. Axial CT scan in bone window mode shows an extent of bone destruction (**f**)

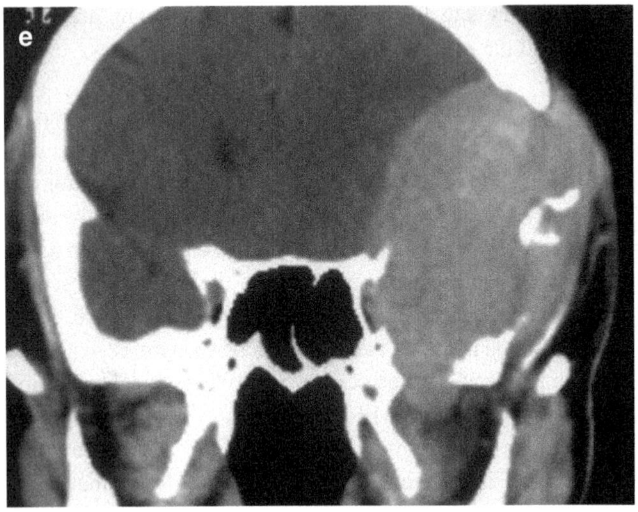

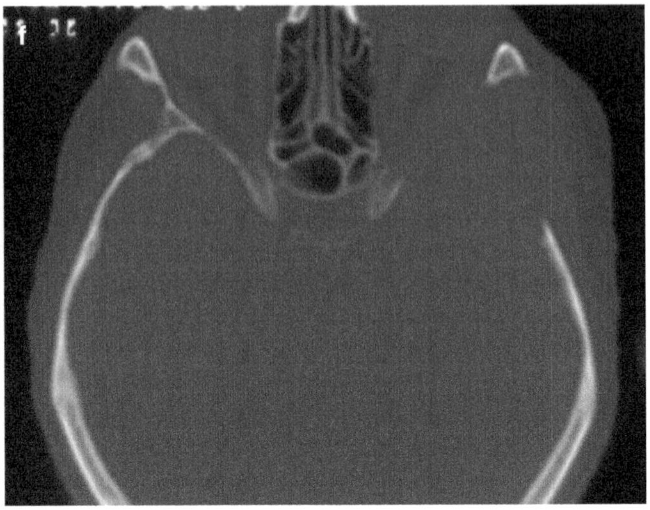

Fig. 11.21 (continued)

11.8 Malignant Fibrous Histiocytoma (MFH)

Malignant fibrous histiocytoma is regarded as a type of soft tissue sarcomas in adult patients with revealing both fibroblastic and histiocytic phenotypes. The incidence of this tumor in the head and neck is rare and considered about 3–10% (Barnes and Kanbour 1988; Som et al. 2011). The most common sites of initial growth of these tumors in head and neck area are paranasal sinuses; also, MFH can grow from the craniofacial skeleton, pharynx, soft tissues of the neck and mouth, pure sinonasal malignant fibrous histiocytomas are extremely rare. Neoplasms developing from the sinonasal cavities and craniofacial bones are characterized by highly aggressive growth, high recurrence rate, and distant metastases (25–30%). Metastases to the regional lymph nodes are rarely detected. 2-year survival for all MFH is up to 60% (Barnes 1985; Barnes and Kanbour 1988; Som et al. 2011).

Imaging MFH of the craniofacial region on CT appears as a mass with heterogeneous structure, causing bone destruction and spreading both intra- and extracranially: into the orbits, paranasal sinuses and other craniofacial structures. But CT-characteristics are nonspecific.

Contrast enhancement is moderate and inhomogeneous (Fig. 11.22). On MRI, fibrous histiocytoma usually has intermediate MR-signal intensities using T2- and T1-weighted imaging, contrast enhancement is typically heterogeneous.

11.9 Fibrosarcoma (FS)

Fibrosarcoma is one of the most common malignant soft tissue tumors, which is formed from immature fibrous connective tissue. This lesion is referred to as desmoid tumor or aggressive fibromatosis (Som et al. 2011). It often occurs in the muscles of the extremities (hip, shoulder) or torso. Involvement of the craniofacial area is considered extremely rare. There are infantile fibrosarcoma (usually occurs in children under 10 years of age) and adult fibrosarcoma (common in children older than 10 years of age and in adults, more often at the age of 40–55 years old) (Toro et al. 2006). The division of FS into grades (from I to III) is existed as well.

Diagnosis CT and MRI manifestations of craniofacial FS are generally indistinguishable from those of other malignant tumors growing in this area. By the time of primary diagnosis, the tumor is usually has wide extension. On CT, this is a soft-tissue space-occupying lesion, causing the destruction of bone structures in the anterior cranial fossa and craniofacial region (Fig. 11.23). Presence of calcifications in the tumor stroma is untypical. MRI pattern depends on the predominant histological structure. On T1-weighted images, this is usually an isointense lesion as compared to the brain, while on T2-weighted images, MR-signal is variable from hypo- to slightly hyperintense.

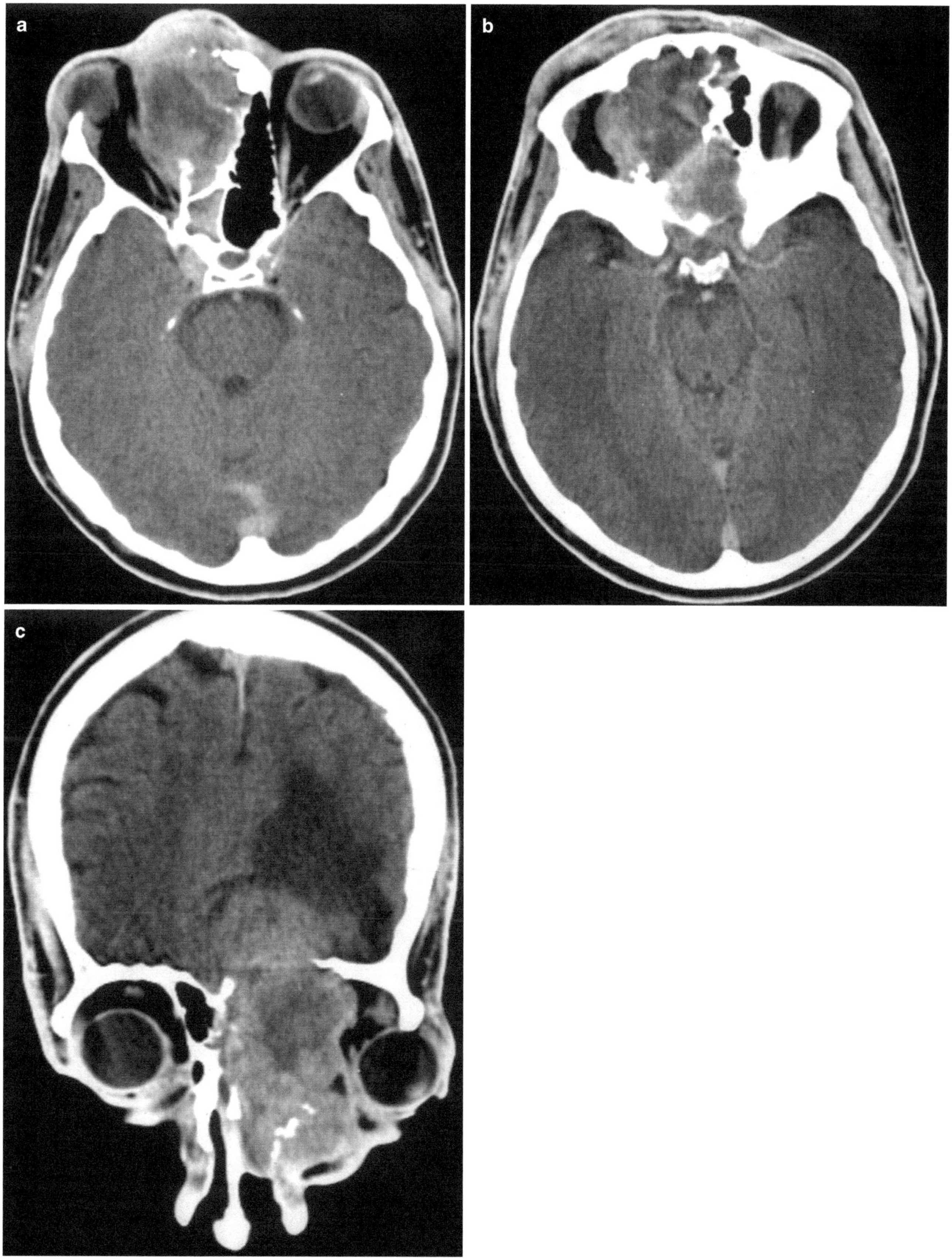

Fig. 11.22 Malignant fibrous histiocytoma of craniofacial area. CT scans (**a–c**) with contrast enhancement show a bone destructive mass with heterogeneous structure that involves the right nasal cavity and ethmoid complex with intracranial extension due to destruction of right orbital roof. The tumor contains area with cystic transformation. Solid component of the tumor is characterized by prominent contrast enhancement

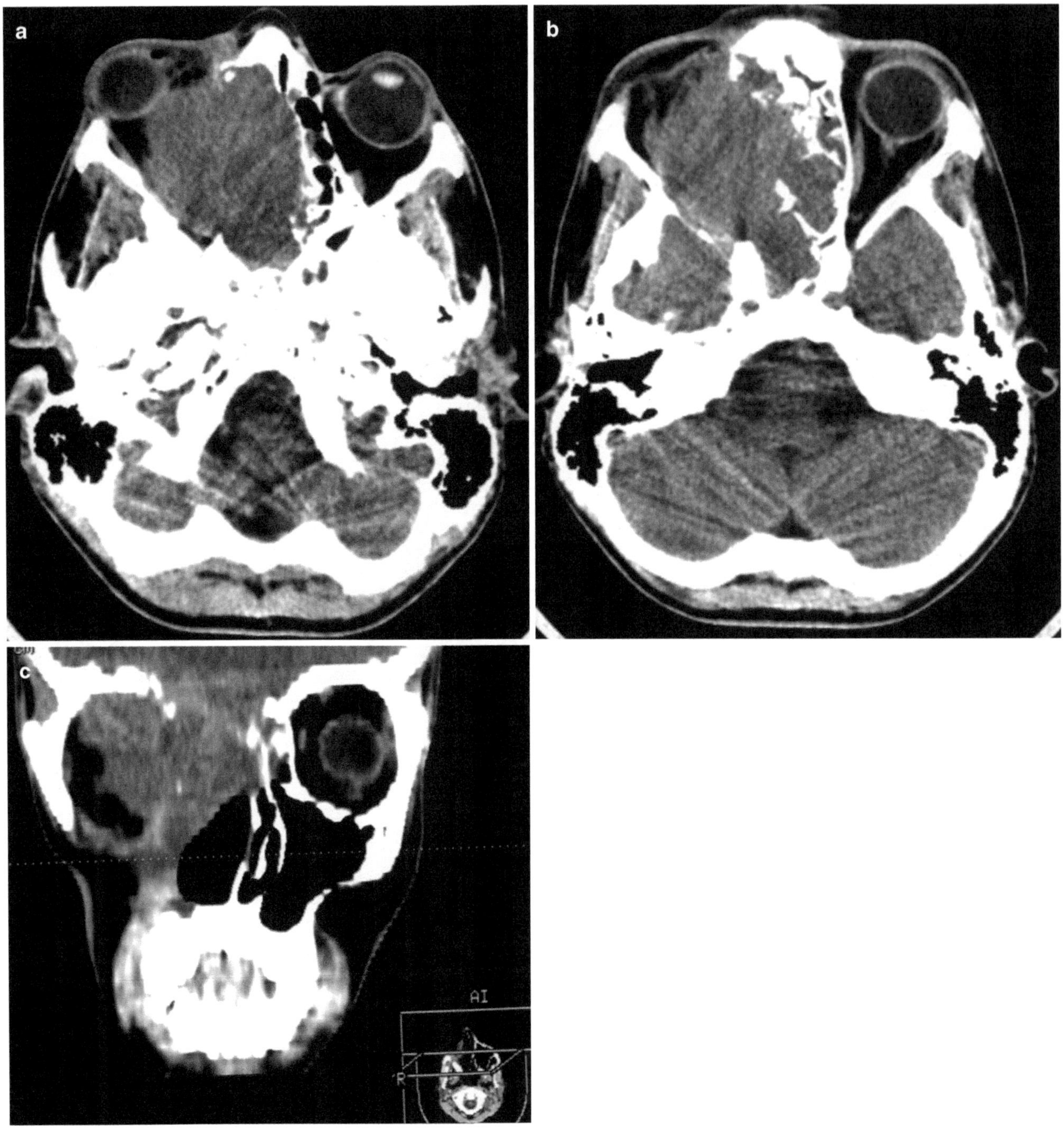

Fig. 11.23 Fibrosarcoma of craniofacial area. Axial (**a**, **b**) and coronal (**c**) CT scans reveal a soft tissue expansile mass, which leads to wide destruction of bones in the anterior cranial fossa, ethmoid complex, and right orbit. The tumor spreads to the right orbit and right maxillary sinus

11.10 Rhabdomyosarcoma (RMC)

Rhabdomyosarcoma is the most common soft tissue sarcoma of skeletal muscle derivation, especially in children; but it can appear in any part of the body. Majority of patients with RMS are younger than 12 years (up to 78% of all cases) and it accounts for 4–8% of all malignancies in patients under the age of 15 years (Soule et al. 1968; Sutow et al. 1970). The head and neck is the principal location for childhood rhabdomyosarcoma, especially the orbit; however, this anatomic region is rare in adults RMS (Feldman 1982; Nayar et al. 1993). The ethmoidal sinus is the most common site of origin of head and neck rhabdomyosarcomas in adults (Nayar et al. 1993). Its biological behavior varies widely, and despite the absence of specific clinical or radiological characteristics, rhabdomyosarcoma should be taken into account in the differential diagnosis of solid tumors in children. Histologically, rhabdomyosarcomas are classified into four types: embryonal, botryoid, alveolar, and pleomorphic (Enzinger and Weiss 1988; Feldman 1982). The embryonal type is the most common and accounts for 70–80% of all rhabdomyosarcomas. It affects mainly but not exclusively children between birth and 15 years of age and occurs predominantly about the head and neck, the genitourinary tract, and the retroperitoneum. The botryoid type is a variant of the embryonal type. Alveolar rhabdomyosarcoma is less frequent; it accounts for 10–20% of all RMSs and affects mainly children and young adults between 10 and 25 years of age. Pleomorphic rhabdomyosarcoma is actually the least common type in general, but the predominate type in adults. Embryonic and alveolar types are more common for RMC head and neck area (Som et al. 2011). In the head and neck region RMSs can involve different areas, the most common sites are orbit (36%), nasopharynx (15.4%), middle ear and mastoid (13.8%), sinonasal cavities (8.1%), face (4.5%), neck (4.1%), larynx (4.1%), and oral cavity (Jee et al. 1996; Som et al. 2011).

Imaging On CT, the head and neck rhabdomyosarcomas can be described as a poorly defined, inhomogeneous soft tissue masses destroying adjacent bone (Latack et al. 1987; Ng et al. 1990; Jee et al. 1996). After intravenous injection of contrast material, the masses enhance generally to the same degree as muscle. CT-perfusion demonstrates an elevated TBF and TBV within the tumor. Capillary permeability is increased as well indicating high level vascularity of the tumor which usually is associated with high degree of malignancy (Fig. 11.24).

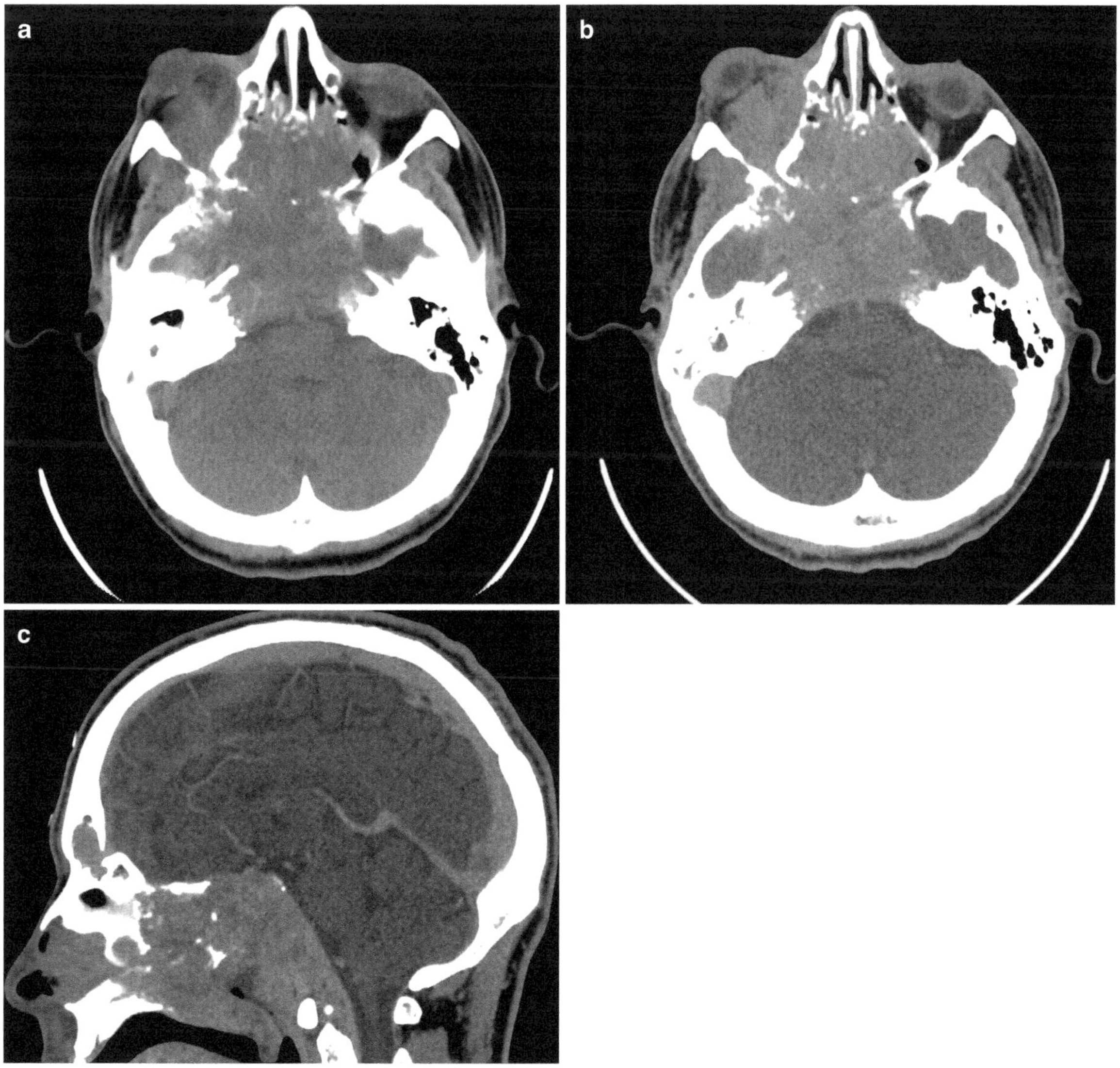

Fig. 11.24 Rhabdomyosarcoma. Axial and sagittal CT scans before (**a**) and after (**b**, **c**) contrast enhancement show a widespreading soft tissue enhancing mass with involvement of skull base bones. A tumor leads to wide bone destruction including nasal, ethmoid, and sphenoid bones, petrous bones both sides, clivus, right maxillary bone and extends into nasal cavities and maxillary sinuses. Tumor has a homogeneous and strong contrast enhancement. CT-perfusion study demonstrates an elevation of blood flow (**d**), blood volume (**e**), and capillary permeability (**f**) indicating high degree of malignancy of the tumor

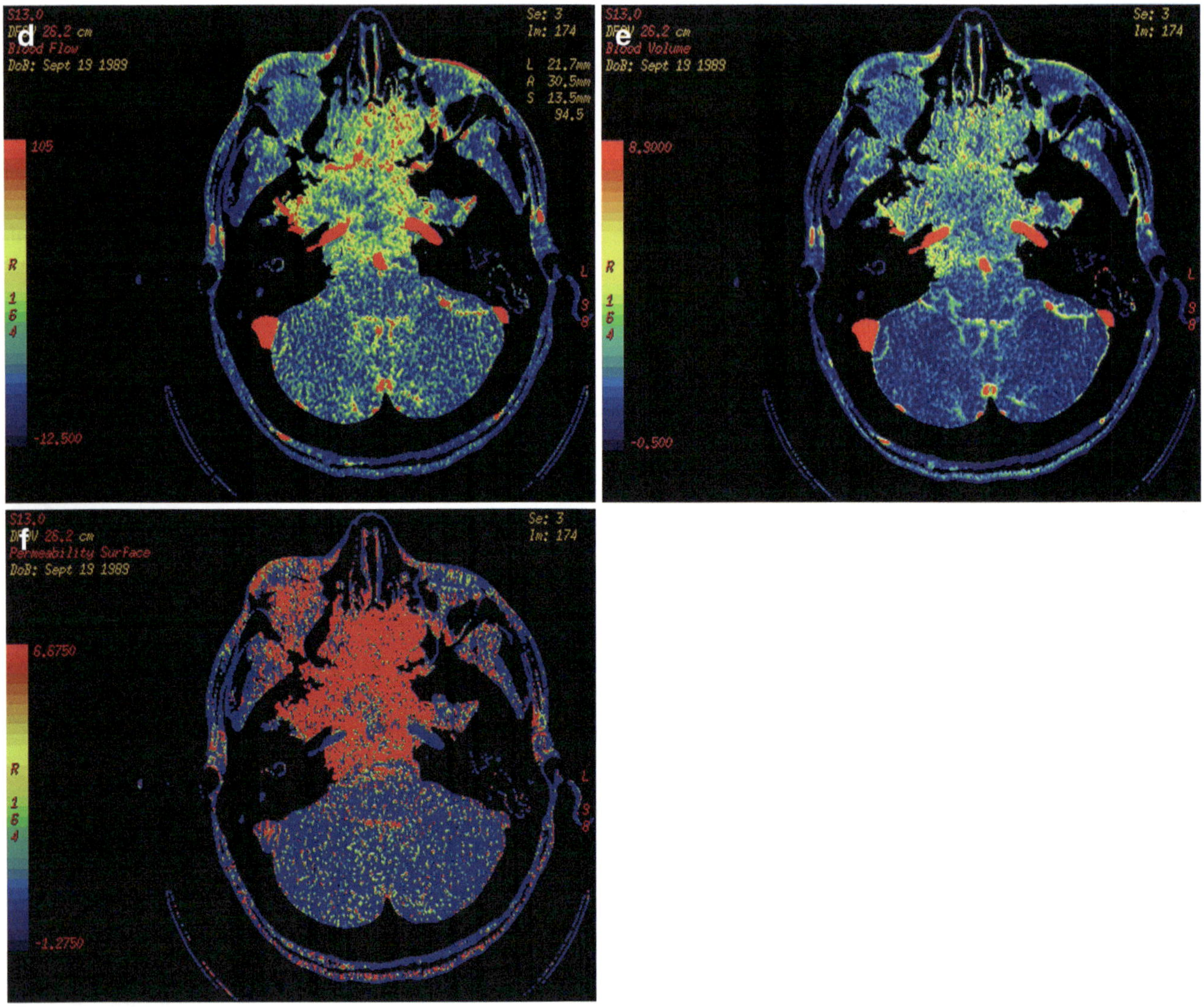

Fig. 11.24 (continued)

The most commonly reported MR imaging appearance of rhabdomyosarcoma in the head and neck is that of a homogeneous mass, isointense or minimally hyperintense relative to muscle on T1-weighted images and hyperintense relative to both muscle and fat on T2-weighted images, with postcontrast images showing enhancement of the tumor (Yousem et al. 1990; Jee et al. 1996; Som et al. 2011). RMSs of the head and neck in adults are different from those of childhood in their site of origin (Nayar et al. 1993), but they produce similar imaging findings.

MR imaging seems to be better than CT for initial and follow-up examination of rhabdomyosarcomas because of its multiplanar capability and ability to precisely define the extent of tumor, especially with using high-resolution T2-weighted images and Fat-Sat technology on T1-weighted imaging after contrast agent injection. ASL technology can be used as additional method in prediction of tumor vasculature severity (Figs. 11.25 and 11.26).

Differential Diagnosis Malignant tumors in the head and neck in children and in adults demonstrate very similar imaging findings. But some clinical and imaging characteristics can be very helpful in differential diagnosis.

- Liposarcomas usually have components of fat density on CT and signal intensity on MRI—lymphomas can be differentiated from rhabdomyosarcomas in its multifocal involvement and is less often associated with invasion and destruction of adjacent bony structures.
- Chordoma and chondrosarcoma typically have areas of calcification,
- Osteosarcoma on CT has "sunburst" pattern of periosteal reaction.
- Other malignant tumors of the head and neck, such as squamous cell carcinomas, usually have imaging findings similar to those of rhabdomyosarcoma, but age at diagnosis of RMS is younger than that for squamous cell carcinoma.

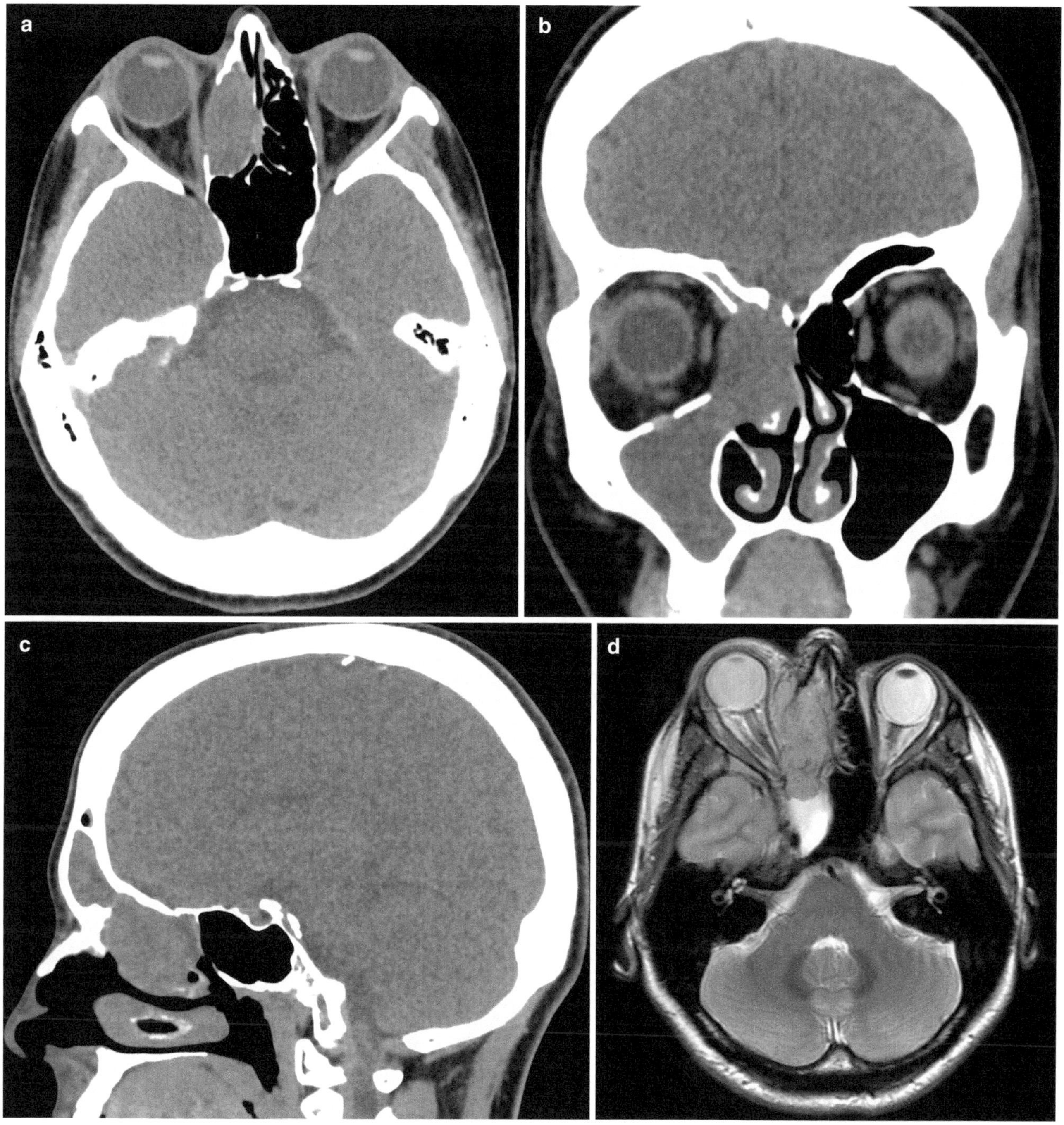

Fig. 11.25 Rhabdomyosarcoma. Post-contrast CT scans in axial plane (**a**) and using coronal (**b**) and sagittal (**c**) reformations show a small size soft tissue enhancing mass located into right ethmoid sinus and nasal cavity. A lesion causes the obstruction of frontal and maxillary sinuses. There is a destruction of medial orbital wall. On MR imaging (performed 1 month later) a mass demonstrates an intensive growth with invading the right orbit and spreads even intracranially along sphenoid bone wing. Tumor has an isointense brain MR-signal on T2- (**d**), T2-FLAIR- (**e**) and T1- (**f**) weighted MR images. Extension and borders of the tumor can be better estimated on post-enhanced T1 (**g**, **h**) and T1 with Fat-Sat (**i**) images

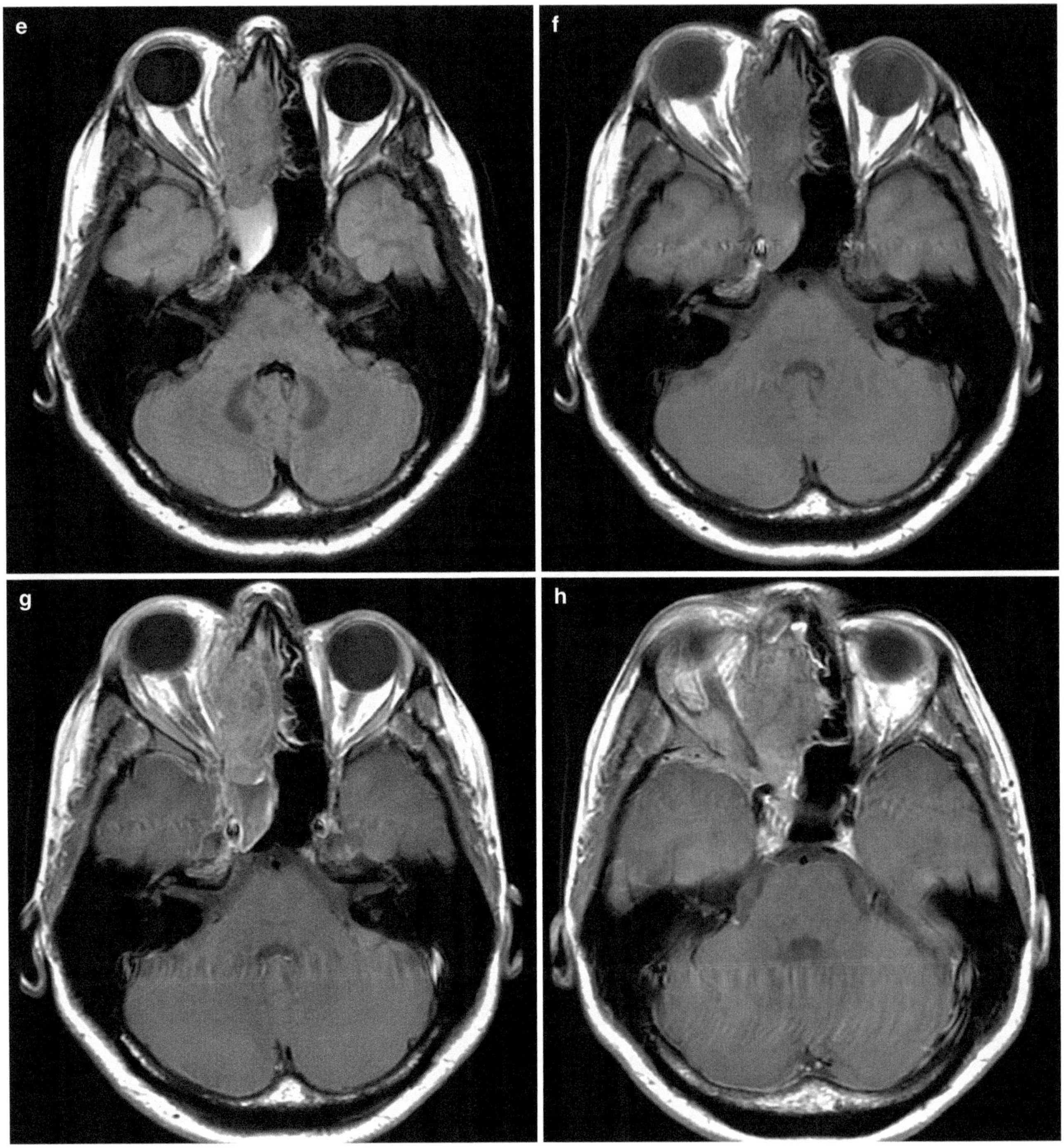

Fig. 11.25 (continued)

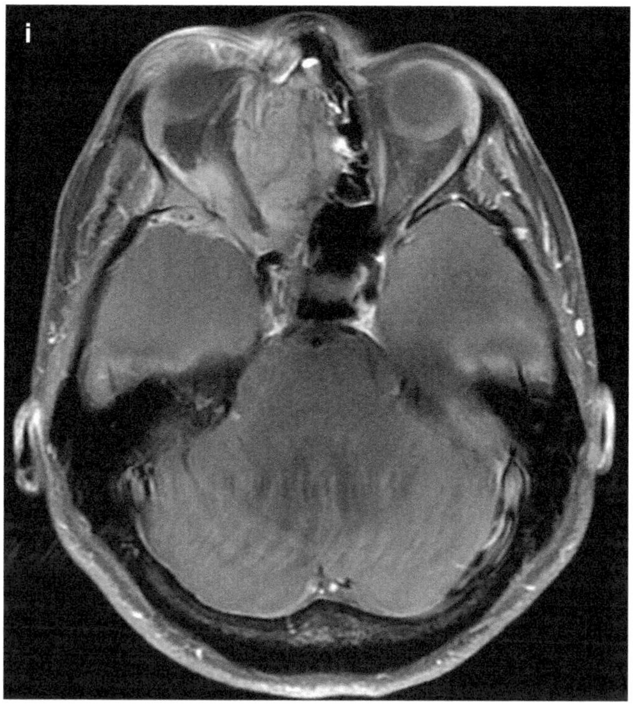

Fig. 11.25 (continued)

11.11 Osteogenic Sarcoma (OS)

Osteogenic sarcoma is another primary bone tumor, commonly occurs in children and adolescents (Ottaviani and Jaffe 2009). This type of sarcoma is the most common primary bone tumor. Based on the histological analysis, it has been observed that several subtypes of OS (including chondrosarcoma) exist. Among them, the most commonly diagnosed is conventional OS, which can be osteoblastic, chondroblastic or fibroblastic depending on the histology. In general, OS is a tumor in which the malignant cells produce an osteoid matrix. In head and neck area these neoplasms account very rare. According to the presented data by Som et al. (2011) in series of more than 1000 cases of OS, only 7% arose in the head and neck, usually in the jaws. Maxillary OS is more common than mandibular OS.

Imaging On CT, with common cases of OS a "sunburst" pattern of periosteal reaction is typical (Figs. 11.27 and 11.28). Focal areas of bone destruction usually can be seen. In some cases the sclerotic bone may be present, especially in the maxilla alveolus. Soft tissue component is also pres-

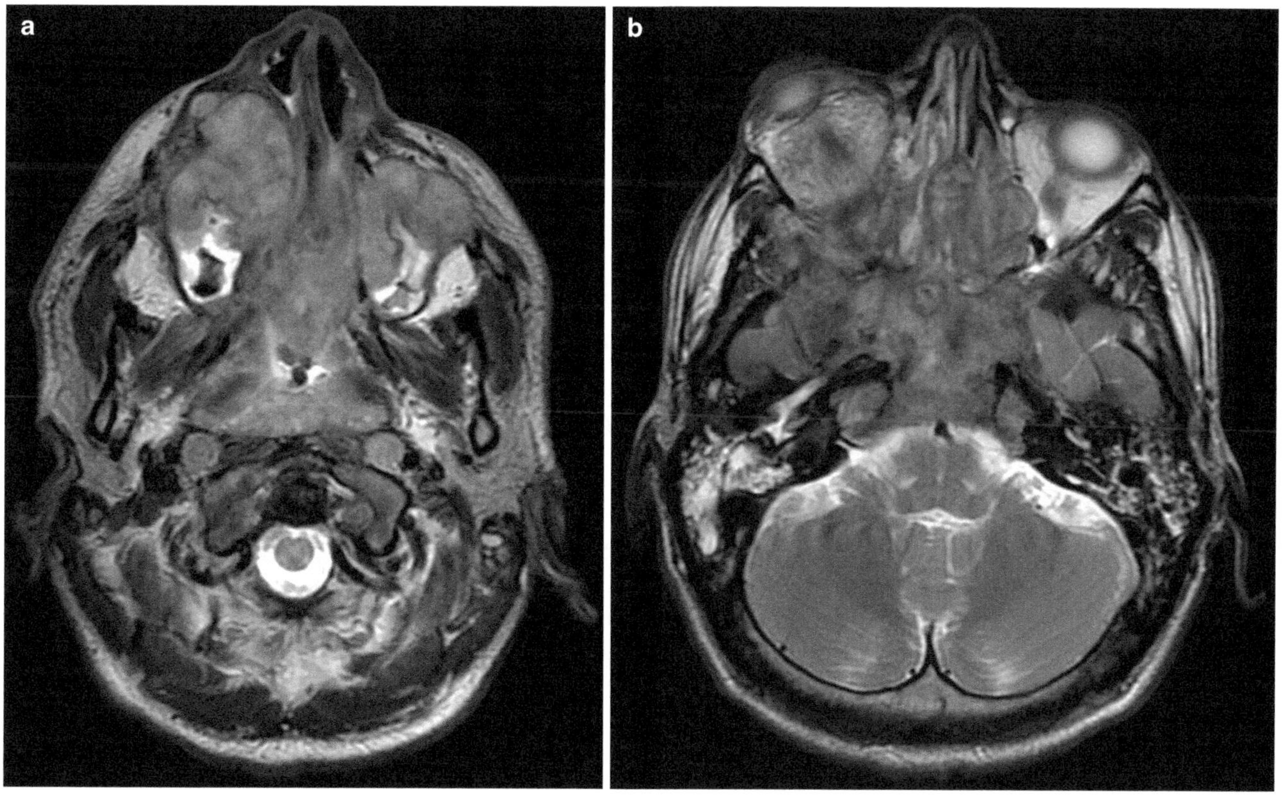

Fig. 11.26 Rhabdomyosarcoma of the craniofacial area. MR imaging using T2- (**a**, **b**) and T1- (**c**) weighted images demonstrates a widespreading through skull base structures soft tissue mass. Tumor has a slightly hyperintense MR-signal compared to muscles on T2-weighted images and isointense signal on T1. DWI demonstrates a restriction of diffusion in tumor tissue (high signal on DWI (**d**)). On ASL MRI perfusion (**e**) a lesion is characterized by focally increased blood flow within the tumor masses. The contrast enhancement and multiplanar imaging improves the assessment of tumor structure and extension (**f–i**)

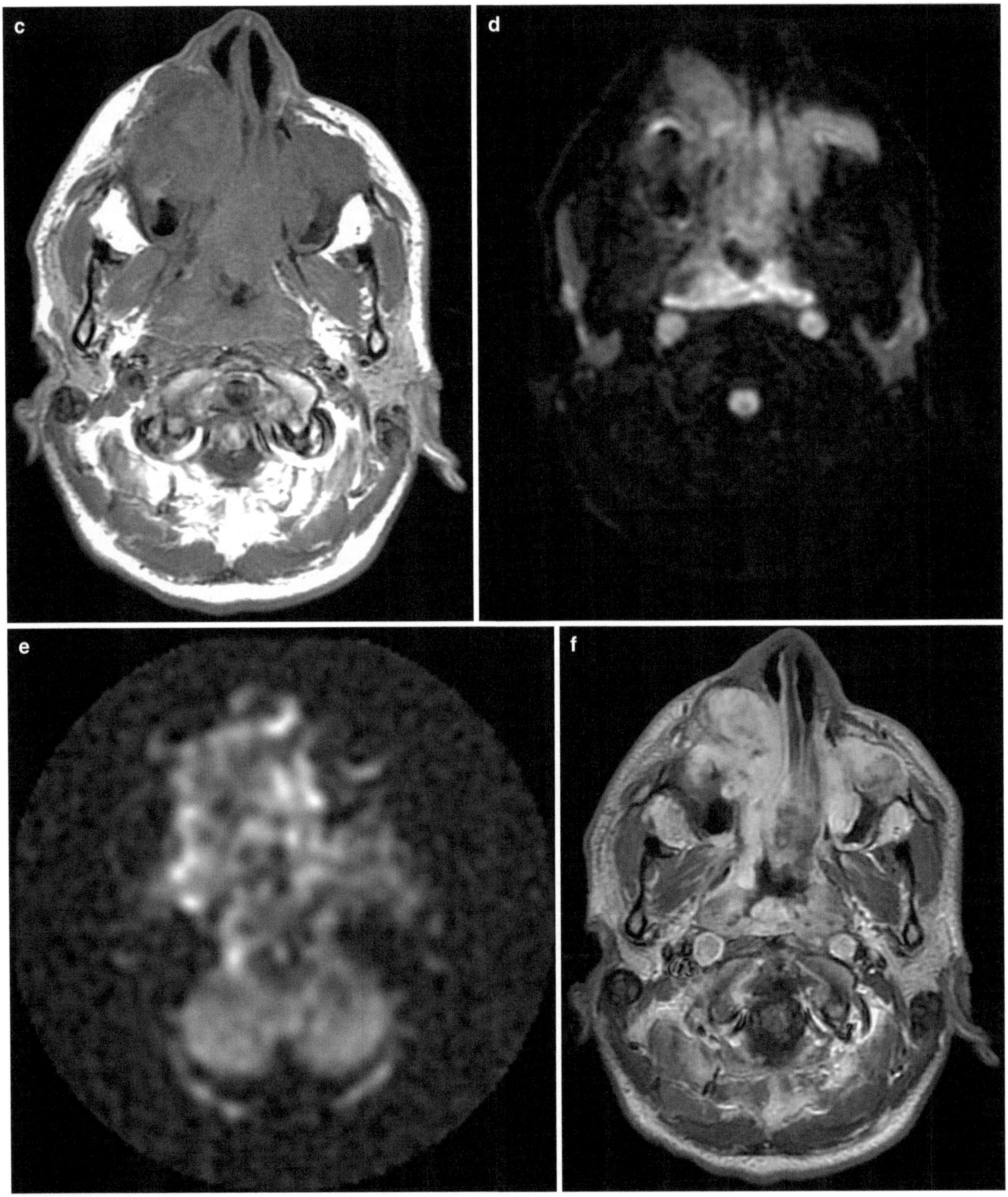

Fig. 11.26 (continued)

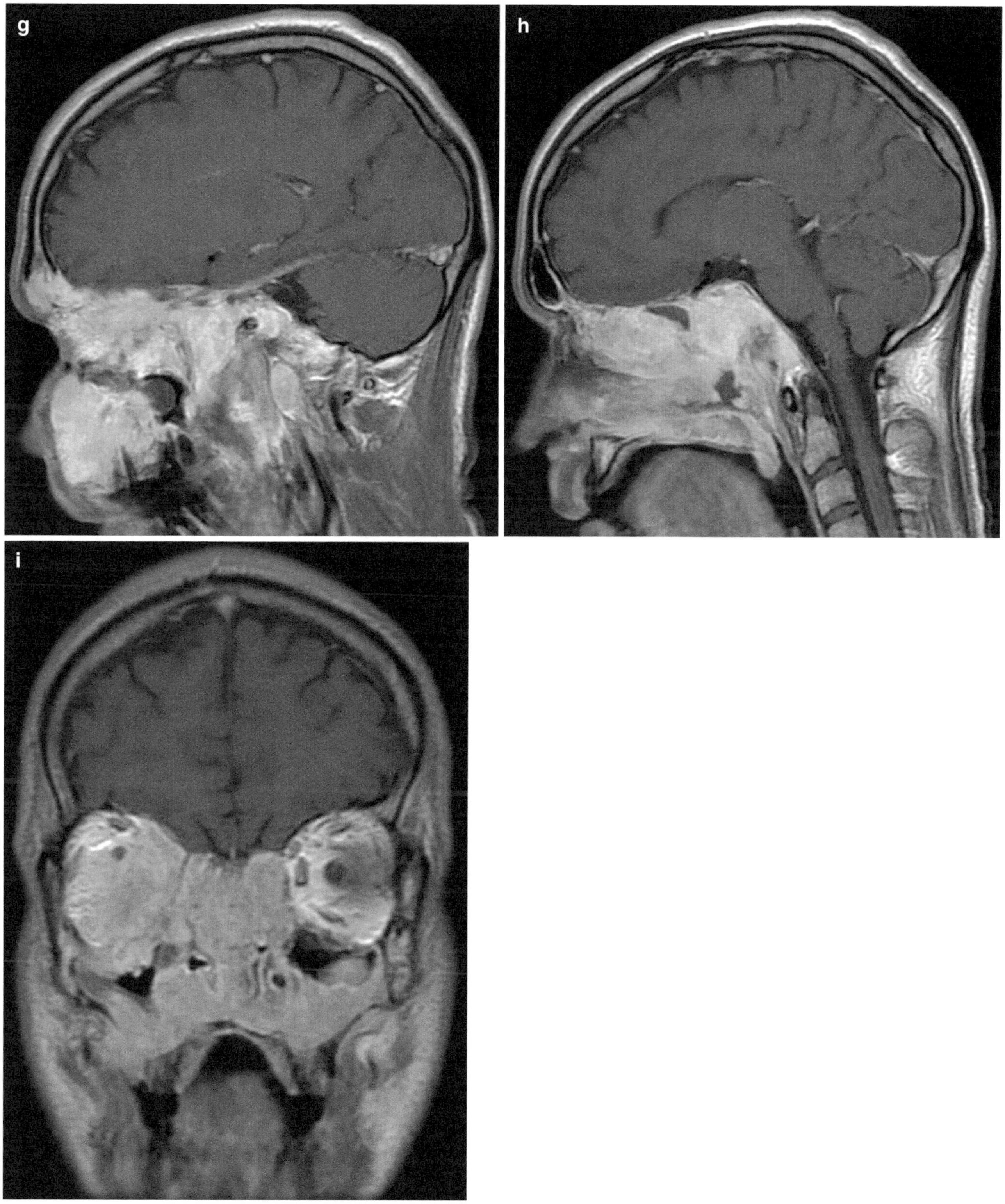

Fig. 11.26 (continued)

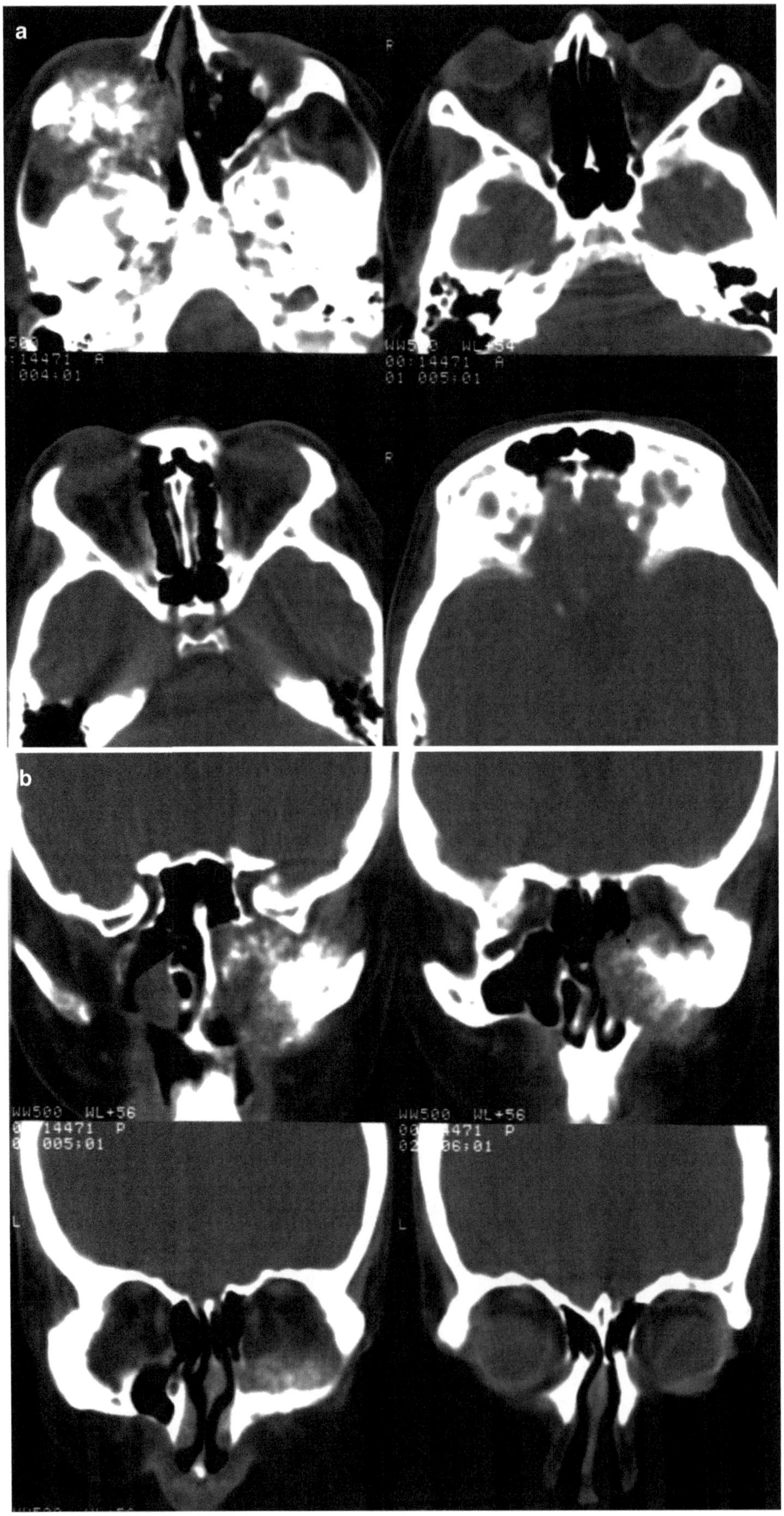

Fig. 11.27 Osteogenic sarcoma of maxilla. Series of axial (**a**) and coronal CT (**b**) scans demonstrate a bone destructive mass in right maxilla with a typical "sunburst"-type periosteal reaction. Within the tumor irregular areas of calcification or ossification can be seen

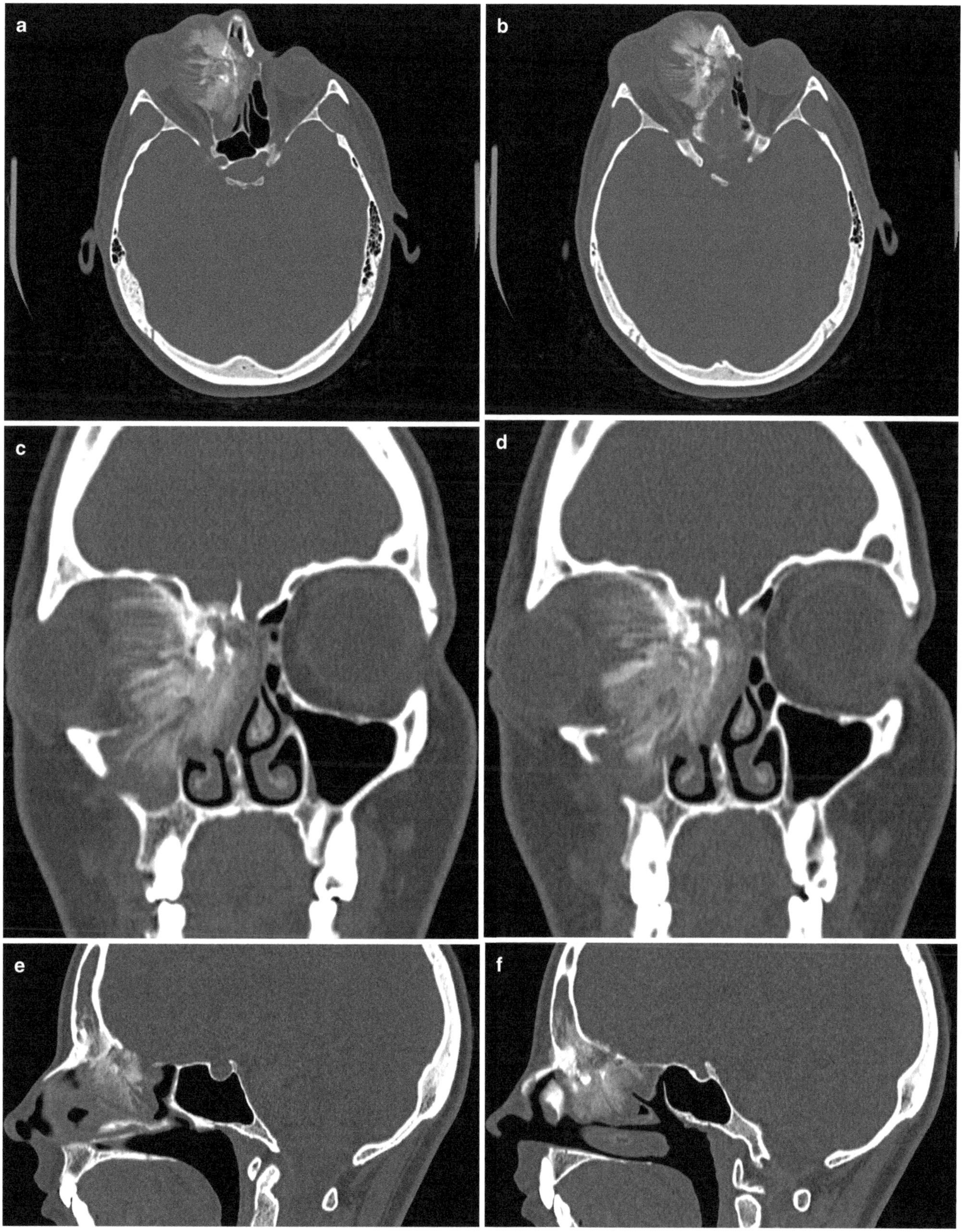

Fig. 11.28 Osteogenic sarcoma of ethmoid complex and nasal cavity. Series of non-contrast axial CT scans (**a**, **b**), as well as coronal (**c**, **d**) and sagittal reformats (**e**, **f**) show a predominantly hyperdense mass in the projection of right ethmoids and right part of nasal cavities with spreading into maxillary cavity. There are bone remodel and bone destruction. CT imaging clearly visualizes the "sunburst" pattern of periosteal reaction

ent, but its contrast enhancement is not so obvious due to dense sclerotic bone tissue. On MR imaging the appearance of the OS depends on the ratio between sclerotic and soft tissue components. On T1-weighted images OS usually demonstrates a low MR-signal from bone part and isointensity with muscle from soft tissue portion. MR-signal on T2-weighted images can vary, usually being from hypo- (from sclerotic bone) to intermediate (from soft tissue part) (Yamaguchi et al. 2004). Contrast enhancement also varies from intermediate to strong. For improvement the tumor margin identification the Fat-Sat MR-technology should be used. In our case with OS of craniofacial area where CT-perfusion was used soft tissue component of the tumor showed the moderate elevation of BV and BF as well as capillary permeability on the background low perfusion parameters from the sclerotic central part of the lesion (Fig. 11.29).

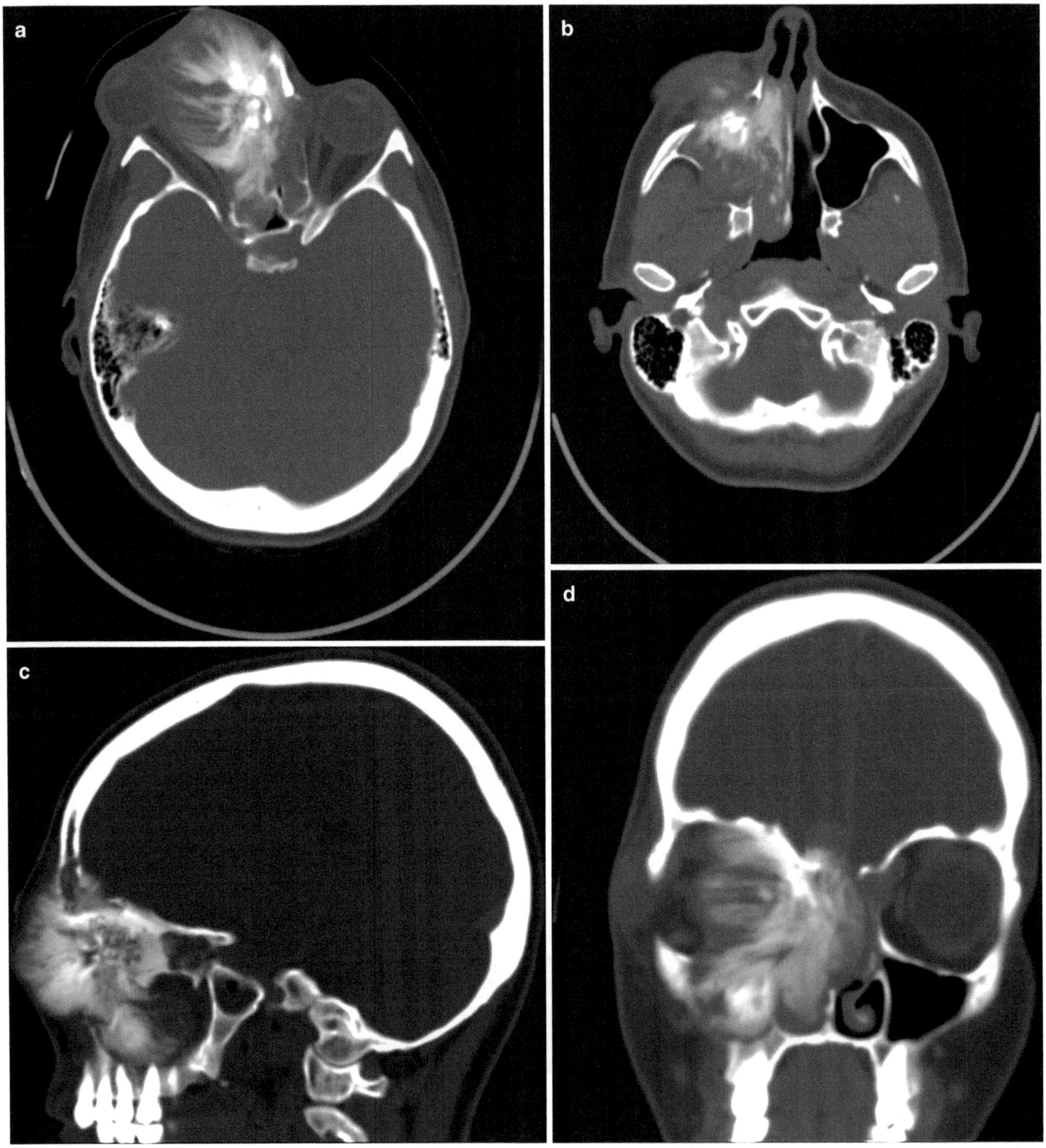

Fig. 11.29 Osteogenic sarcoma of ethmoid complex and nasal cavity. Series of contrast enhanced axial CT scans (**a**, **b**), as well as sagittal (**c**) and coronal (**d**) reformats show a mixed mainly hyperdense mass in the projection of right ethmoids and right part of nasal cavities with spreading into maxillary and frontal cavities. The "sunburst" pattern of periosteal reaction can be clearly seen. CT-perfusion study demonstrates an intermediate elevation of blood volume (**e**) and blood flow (**f**) within the soft-tissue portion of the tumor (*arrows*)

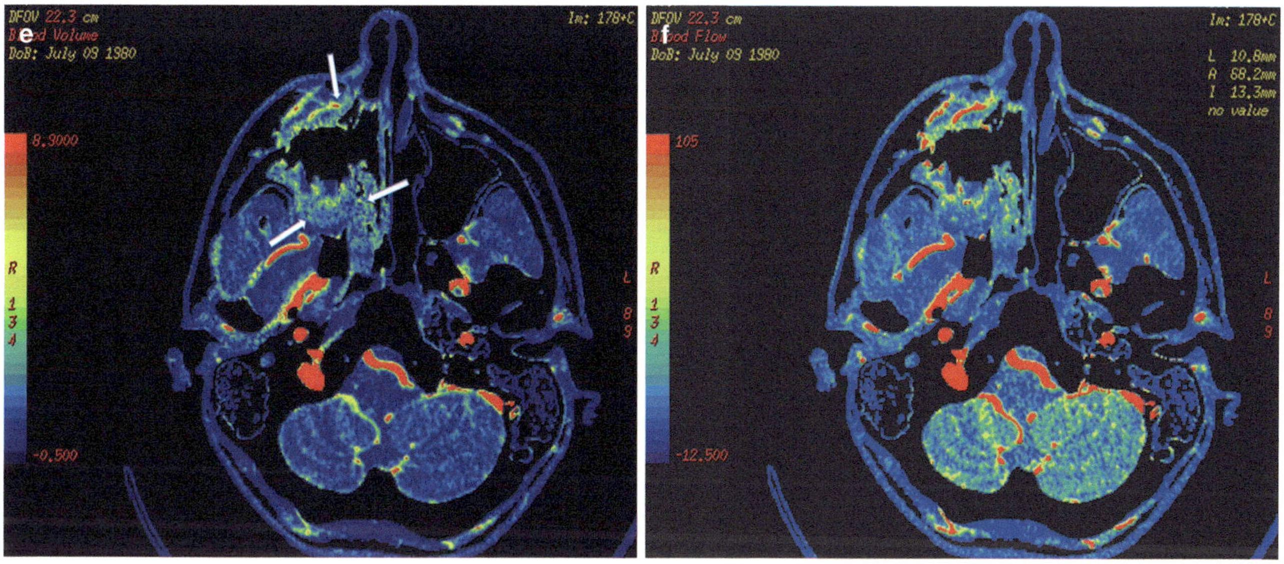

Fig. 11.29 (continued)

Differential Diagnosis

1. Osteomyelitis causes of bone destruction without formation of new bone-like tissue;
2. Metastasis—aggressive bone destruction, no periosteal reaction and calcification.

11.12 Lymphoma

In general, lymphomas of the head and neck are very common malignancy of this area with involvement of cervical lymph nodes but only in 10% of cases these lesions have extranodal origin, usually involving tonsils, sinonasal tract and thyroid (Fellbaum et al. 1989). Most often the lesion is located in the nasal fossae and maxillary sinuses. Less common, tumors can be found in projection of ethmoid sinuses and more rare in frontal and sphenoid sinuses (Vidal et al. 1999).

According to Som et al. (2011) sinonasal lymphoma is the second most frequent group of extranodal lymphomas after gastrointestinal form of lesions. Sinonasal lymphomas can be categorized as either B-cell or T-cell phenotypes with some differences regarding histology. B-cell lymphomas more often involve paranasal sinuses while T-cell lymphomas more commonly affect the nasal cavities and have more aggressive, and invasive behavior with necrotic cavities formation and bone destruction.

Imaging On CT and MR imaging, lymphomas of craniofacial and sinonasal areas look like homogeneous soft tissue masses that is characterized by from moderate to strong enhancement. CT is a more accurate method in assessment of surrounding bone remodel (common) or destruction (rare). MR-imaging better than CT demonstrates the tumor extension through craniofacial region, especially with using contrast enhancement and Fat-sat technology. DWI is also very useful in lymphoma visualization within sinonasal cavities due to high MR-signal, indicating the restriction of diffusion (Fig. 11.30).

Metastases—the central nervous system is more frequently affected by lung, breast, kidney cancers, melanoma and less frequently by cancers of the gastrointestinal tract, bladder, prostate, ovaries. Metastases can be found in the skull bones and the dura mater, in the vertebrae and epidural space, in the pia-mater with its diffuse extensive involvement, as well as in the brain tissue (Figs. 11.31 and 11.32). Metastatic involvement of paranasal sinuses is a very rare disorder and more common in patients with renal cancer (Grossman and Yousem 1994). CT-perfusion study is a reliable method for hypervascular metastatic lesion discrimination from tumors with low vasculature (Fig. 11.33).

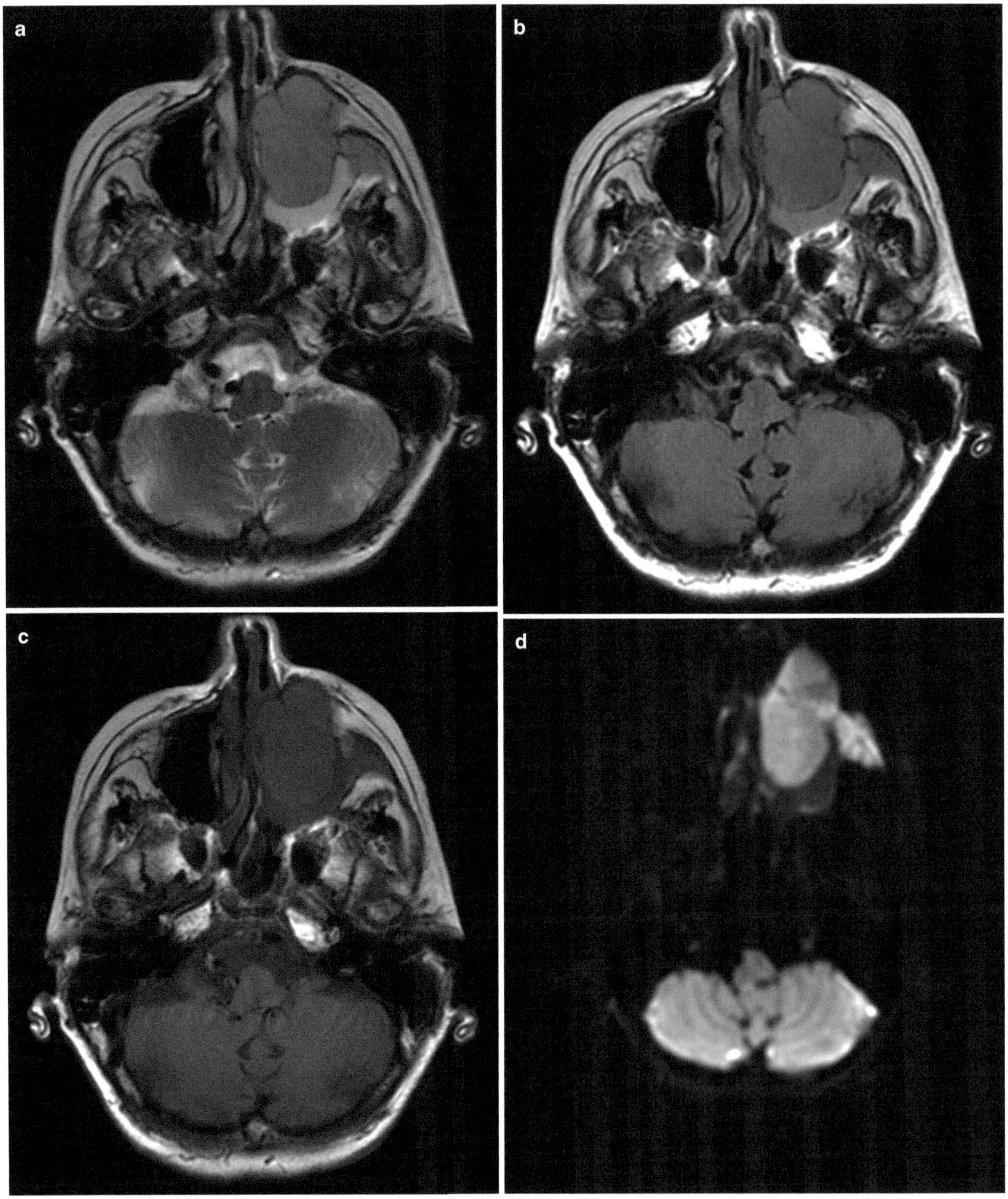

Fig. 11.30 Lymphoma of craniofacial area. Axial T2- (**a**), T2-FLAIR- (**b**), and T1- (**c**) weighted MR images show an expansile soft tissue mass with homogeneous structure into projection of maxillary sinus, expanding into nasal cavity. There is obstruction of the remnants of maxillary sinus. On DWI (**d**) and ADC map (**e**) tumor demonstrates the restriction of water diffusion (high MR-signal on DWI and low values of ADC on ADC-map). Row-data scan of 3D TOF MR-angiography doesn't show pathologic vessels within the lesion (**f**). A tumor is characterized prominent and homogeneous contrast enhancement on T1 fat-sat weighted images (**g–i**)

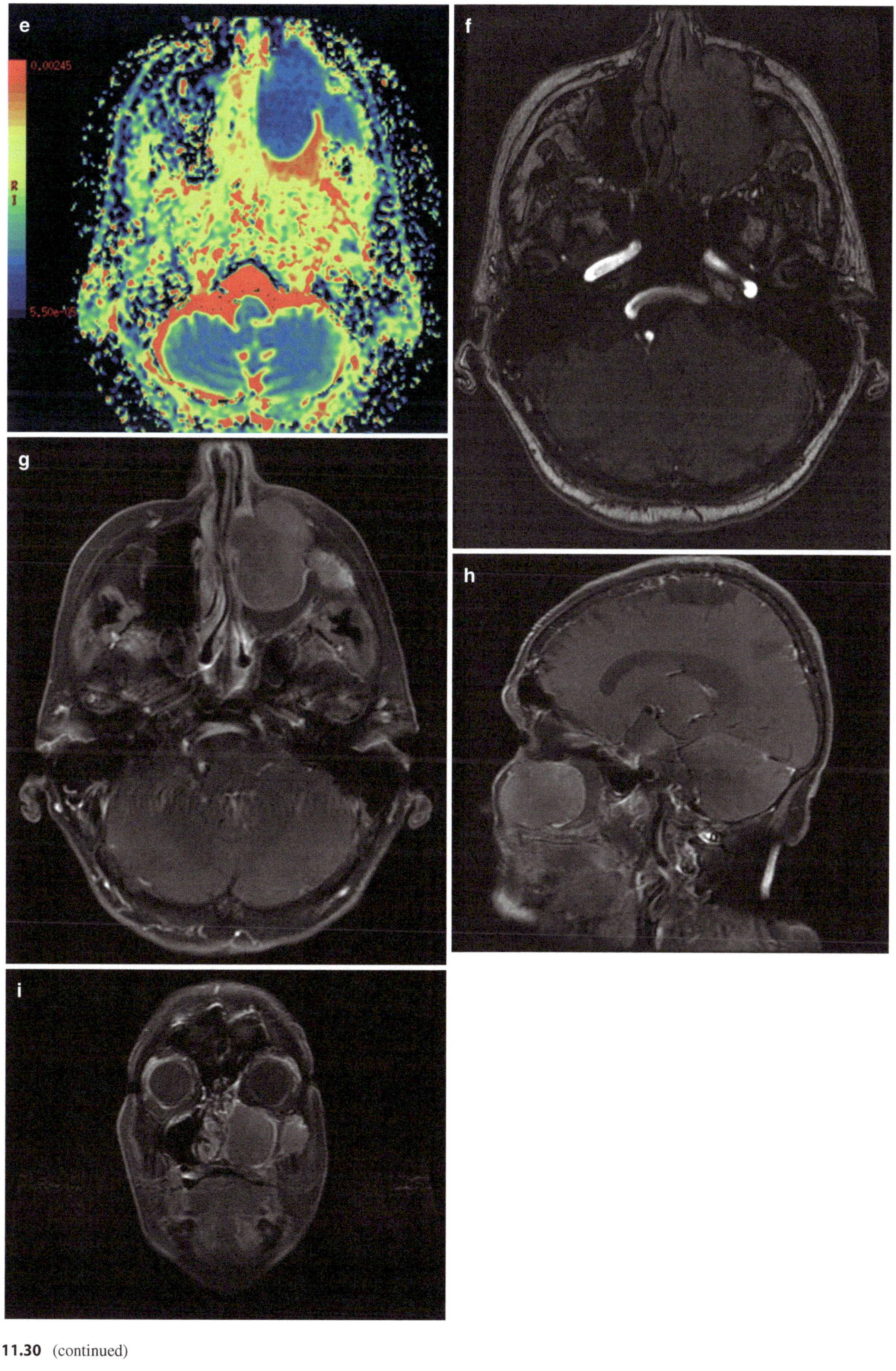

Fig. 11.30 (continued)

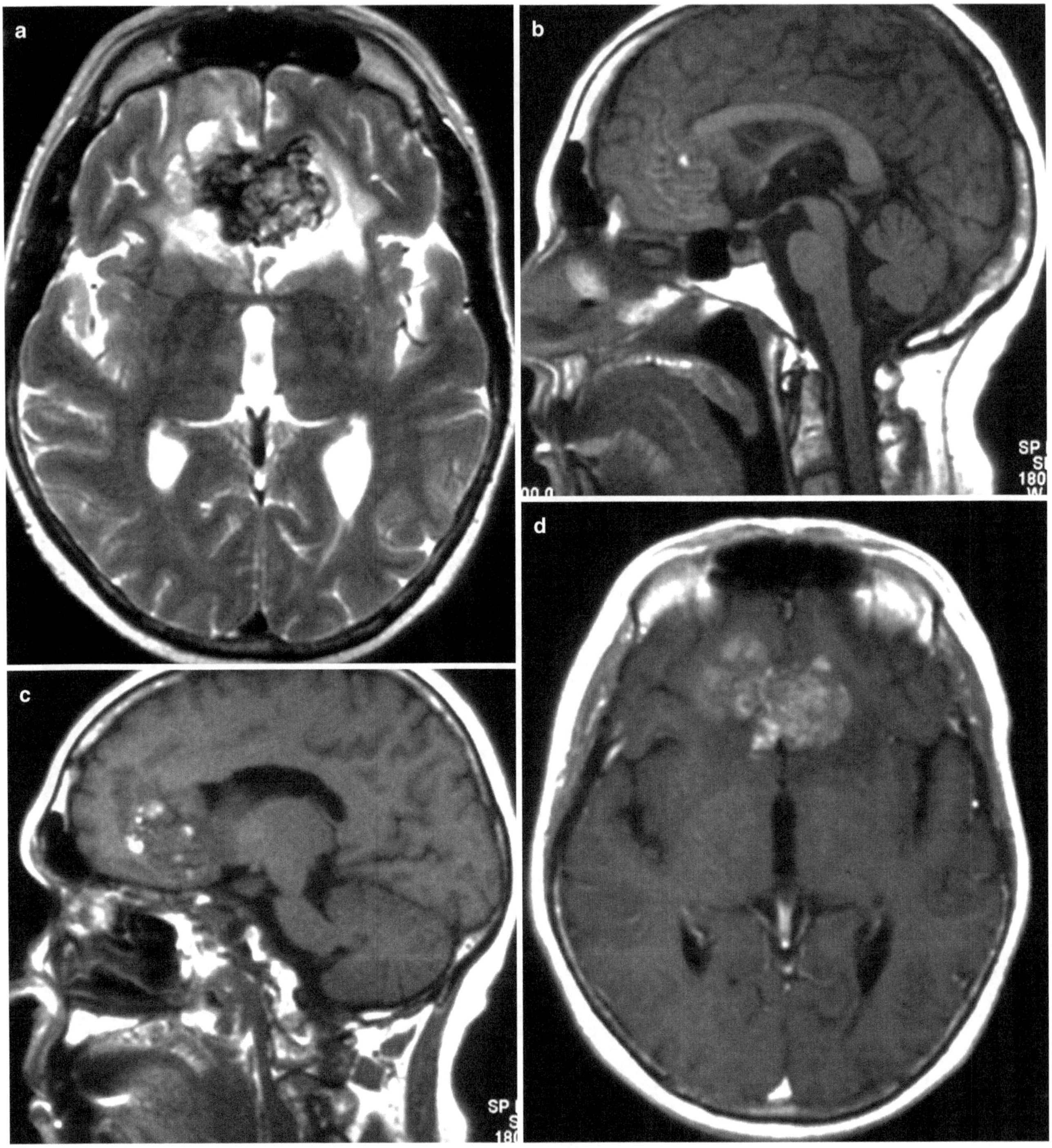

Fig. 11.31 Metastasis of cancer in the anterior cranial fossa. Axial T2-weighted (**a**) and sagittal T1-weighted (**b**, **c**) MR images reveal a heterogeneous in structure, dark on T2, with bright foci on T1 (hemorrhages), mass surrounded with perifocal edema. There is intensive inhomogeneous accumulation of contrast agent (T1 + Gd (**d**, **e**, **f**)). Digital angiography shows abnormal vascular network (**g**–**i**) of the tumor

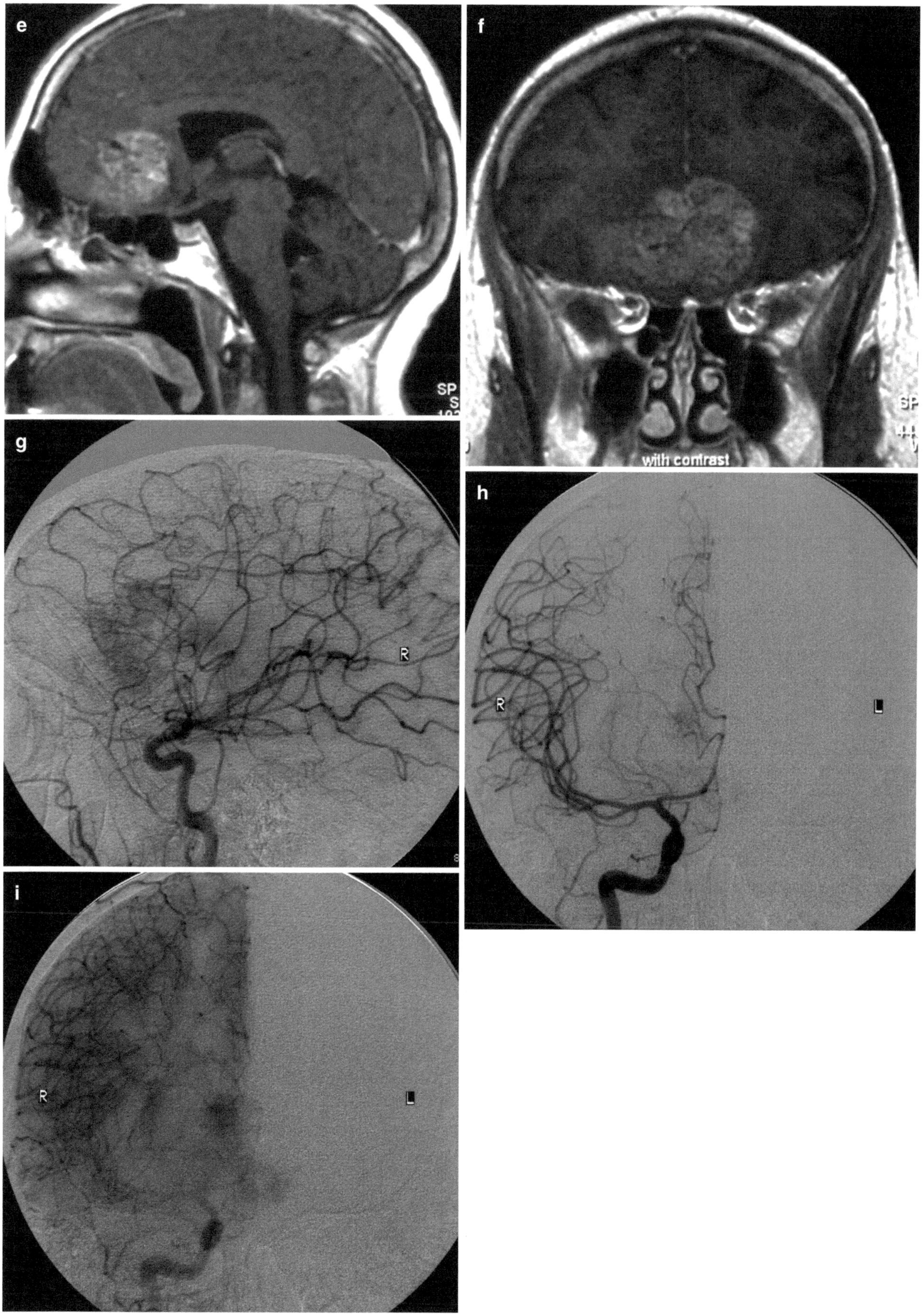

Fig. 11.31 (continued)

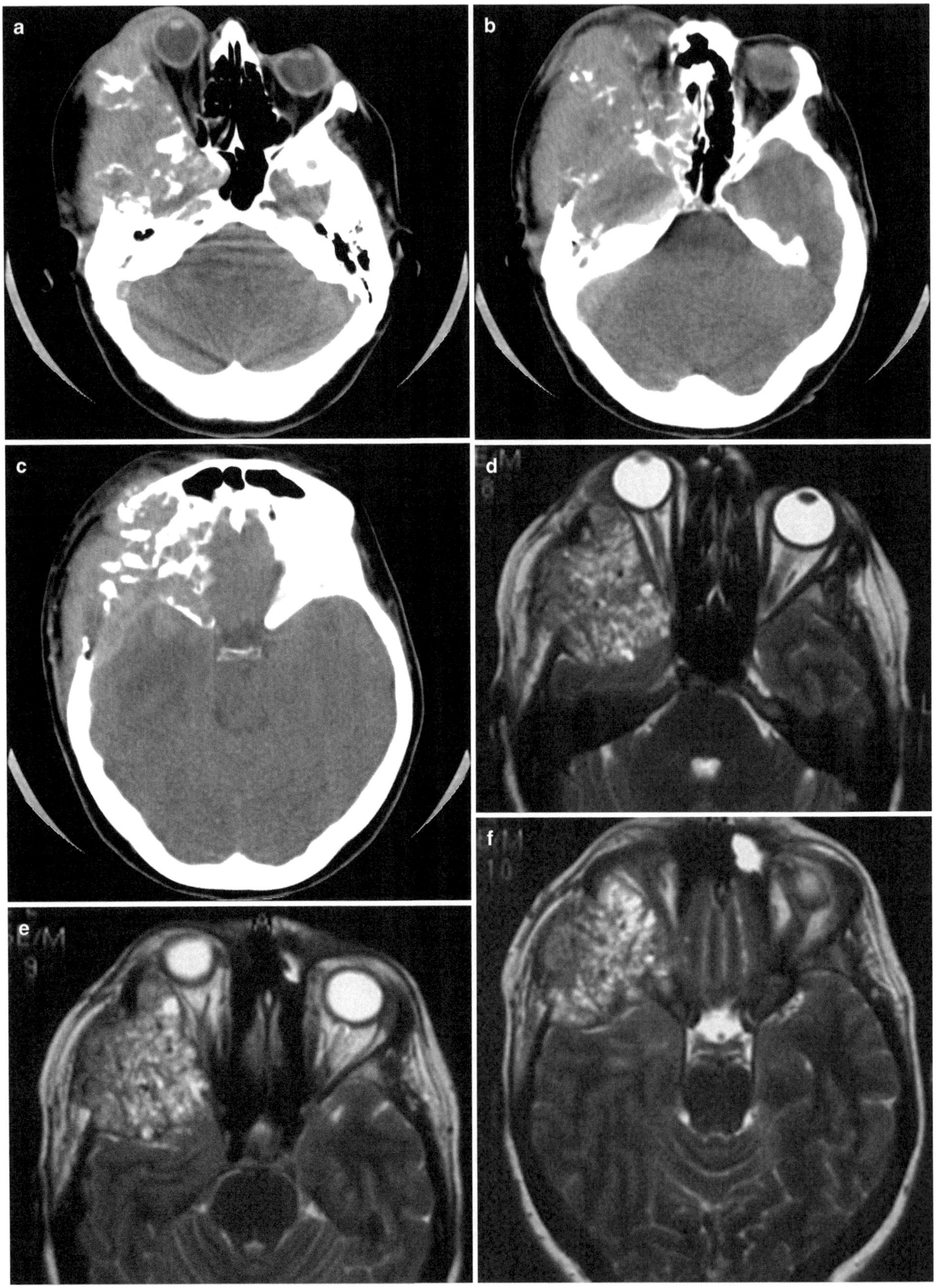

Fig. 11.32 Metastasis of cancer in right craniofacial region. Axial CT scans after (**a**–**c**) contrast enhancement demonstrate a large soft tissue mass with calcifications and wide bone destruction, strongly enhancing and involving right temporal frontal region. There is a invasion of lateral aspects of right orbit with dislocation of the globe. On axial T2-weighted images (**d**–**f**) a lesion has heterogeneous MR-signal due to multiple intratumor microcystic formations

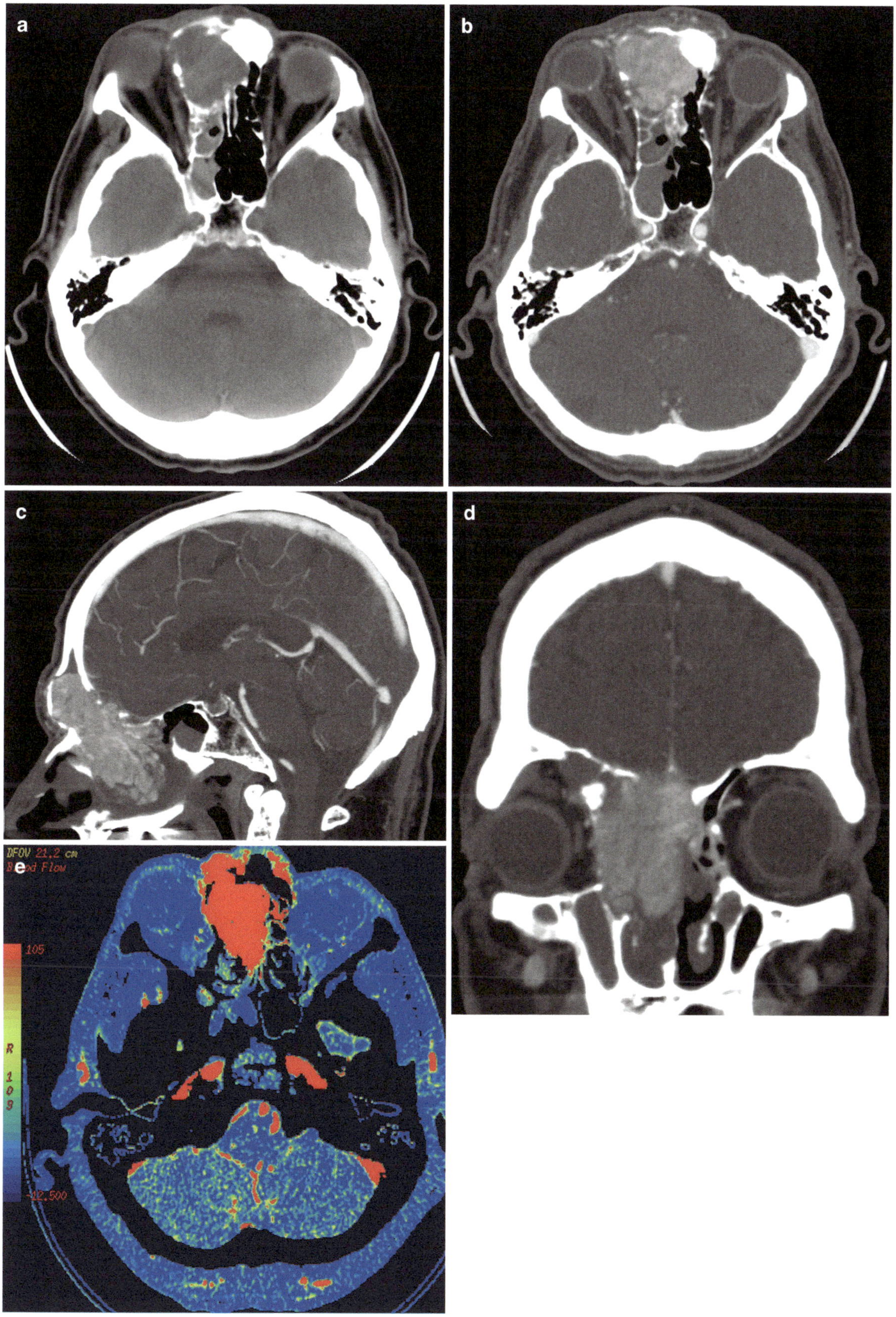

Fig. 11.33 Metastasis of kidney cancer in the ethmoid bone. CT scans before (**a**) and after (**b–d**) contrast enhancement demonstrate a large soft tissue mass, strongly enhancing and involving ethmoid and frontal sinuses as well as right nasal cavity. There is surrounding bone destruction including nasal septa and lamina papyracea on the right. CT-perfusion study ((**e**) TBF map, (**f**) TBV map) shows a very high values of blood flow and blood volume in the tumor, that were associated with presence of abundant vascular network of the tumor on performed DSA (**g–i**)

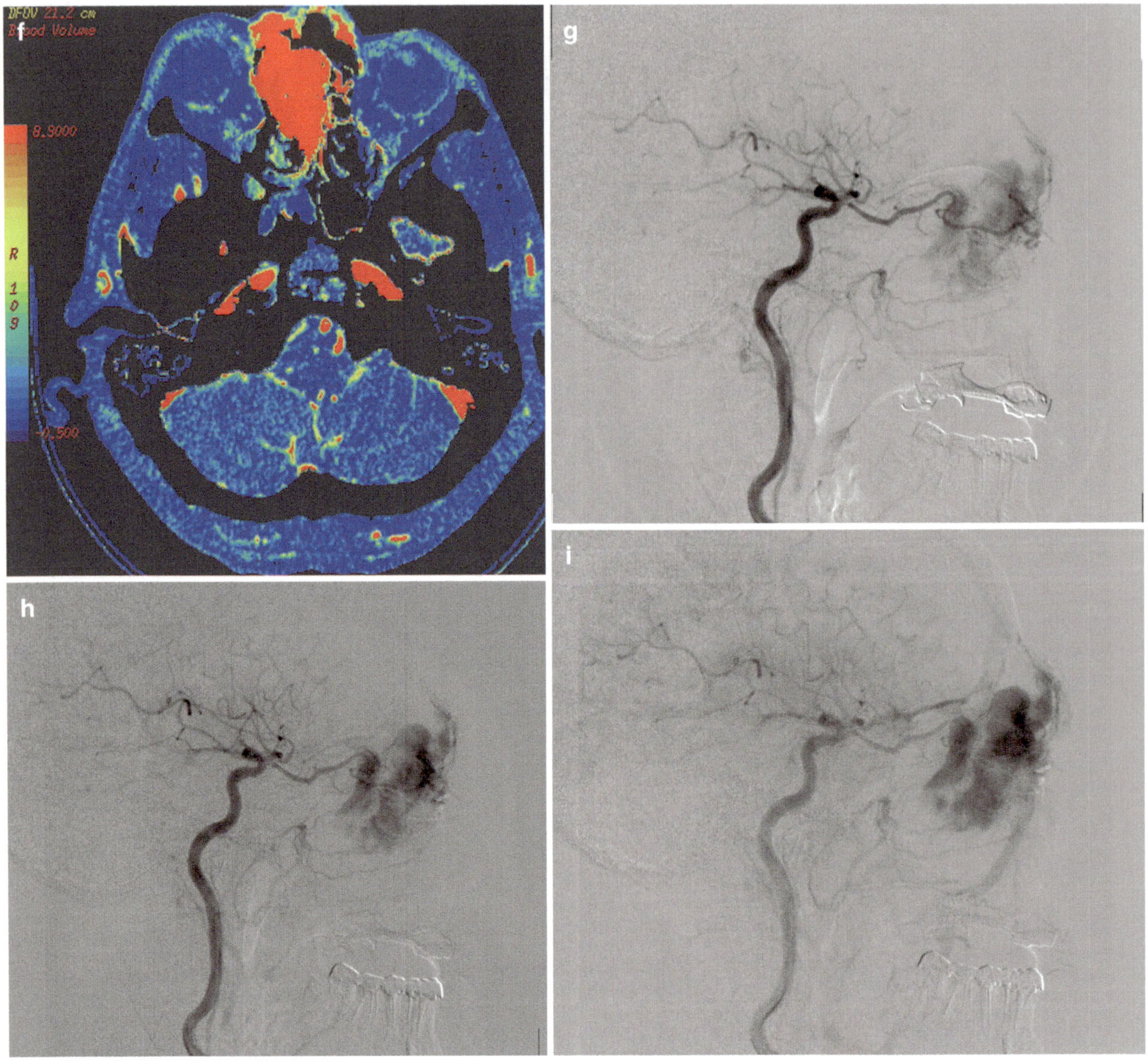

Fig. 11.33 (continued)

Inflammatory Diseases

12

Acute rhinosinusitis (AR) Acute rhinosinusitis is an acute inflammatory process in the sinonasal mucosa. In most cases, it is caused by a viral infection of the upper respiratory tract. The cause of sinusitis can also be a bacterial infection, vasomotor dysfunction, or their combination with a head trauma or barotrauma. Up to 90% of patients with common cold have viral or bacterial rhinosinusitis. Inflammation is most frequently observed in the ethmoid and maxillary sinuses. As a rule, it does not change the structure of the bony walls of paranasal sinuses.

Imaging On X-rays, there is opacification of the sinus, mucosal thickening. The "air-fluid" level can be detected only in the maxillary sinuses and is difficult to determine in other sinuses.

On CT, there is mucosal thickening detected in the sinuses on the axial and coronal planes. Inflamed tissues cause obstruction of the sinus drainage pathways, produce "air-fluid" levels. The mucosa is inflamed, thickened, and enhanced after intravenous contrast agents injection. The central part of the sinus cavity with secretion is not enhanced.

On T1-weighted MR images, thickened mucosa has an isointense MR-signal, the air-fluid level inside the sinus is clearly defined. Signal intensity from the secretion becomes higher with increasing protein content. The air in the sinus and the cortical bone layer appear as a low MR-signal area, outlining the margins of inflammatory changes in the mucosa. On T2-weighted MR images, fluid in the sinus cavity and mucosa thickening are hyperintense. The mucosa enhances and becomes bright on post-contrast images (especially with Fat-Sat sequences), the central part of inflamed sinus with secretion doesn't enhance (Figs. 12.1, 12.2 and 12.3). In the absence of secretion in the sinus, normal nasal mucous cycle is sometimes difficult to distinguish from mucosa thickening in acute rhinosinusitis on MRI (Brook 2003).

Chronic rhinosinusitis (ChR) is a group of diseases characterized by inflammation of the nasal cavities and sinuses lasting for more than 12 weeks, which appears as thickened mucosa, sometimes filling the cavity of the sinus with chronic secretion or without it. A combination of mucosal thickening with sclerosis of sinus bone walls can be seen. ChR is more frequently observed in the ethmoids and maxillary sinuses, they can have normal or reduced size. Its etiology can be a bacterial, fungal, vasomotor, or allergic (Benninger et al. 2003).

Imaging On CT images, mucosal thickening is detected in the sinus, with varying degrees of the sinus filling, without its dilation. Different density of secretion depends on the protein and water content, as well as on concomitant complications (fungal infection, etc.). Occasionally, there may be calcifications within the mucosa. Bone sinus walls get thickened with sclerotic changes. ChR can be combined with polyps (Fig. 12.4). The thickened and inflamed mucosa strongly enhances after intravenous contrast enhancement.

On T1-weighted MR images, isointense, thickened inflamed mucosa and a secretion in the sinus cavity have a varying MR-signal intensity depending on the stage of the disease (Som et al. 1989). Sinus bone walls thickening and sclerosis are often observed, but their visualization on MRI is more difficult than on CT. On T2-weighted images, mucosa is usually hyperintense (Figs. 12.5 and 12.6). MR-signal from the contents of the sinus cavity varies from hyper- to hypointense (with decreasing water content and increasing protein levels). Over time, the mucous contents become more viscous and MR-signal on T2-weighted sequence becomes high. With increasing protein content in the secretion, the MR-signal intensity on T1-weighted images also increases. At this stage, the MR-signal in the sinus cavity can be bright both on T1- and T2-weighted images. Further increase in the protein concentration determines a gradual decrease of the MR-signal is observed on T1- and T2-weighted images. When the protein concentration reaches 35%, a pronounced loss of MR-signal is detected, which can sometimes mimic the presence of air in the sinus cavities, even when the sinus is completely obstructed. Secretion has the consistency of fatty glue or may even be solid at this phase (Zinreich 2004).

Intracranial spreading of infection is clearly detected on MRI with contrast enhancement in the form of increasing of MR-signal from the adjacent dura mater, which is the most significant feature. An epidural abscess on T1-weighted images appears as an area with low MR-signal with contrast

I. Pronin, V. Kornienko, *CT and MRI of Skull Base Lesions*, https://doi.org/10.1007/978-3-319-65957-2_12

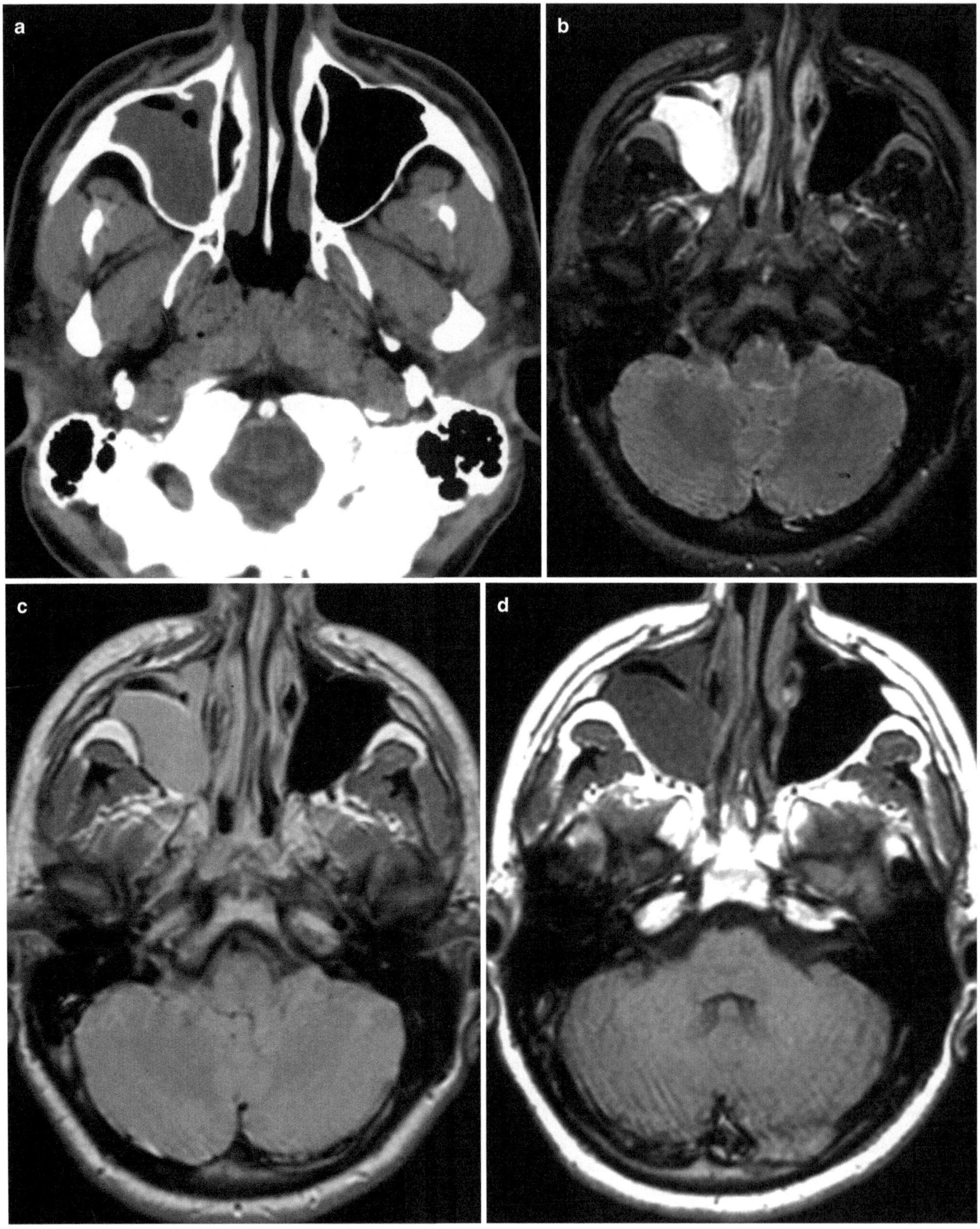

Fig. 12.1 Acute sinusitis. Axial CT scan (**a**) shows the right maxillary sinus filling with fluid content with the air-fluid level. T2-weighted (**b**) and T2-FLAIR (**c**) weighted MR images clearly demonstrate hyperintense content within the sinus. On T1-weighted image (**d**) the secretion is hypointense. Coronal T2-WI image shows the thickening of the mucosa into ethmoids as well (**e**)

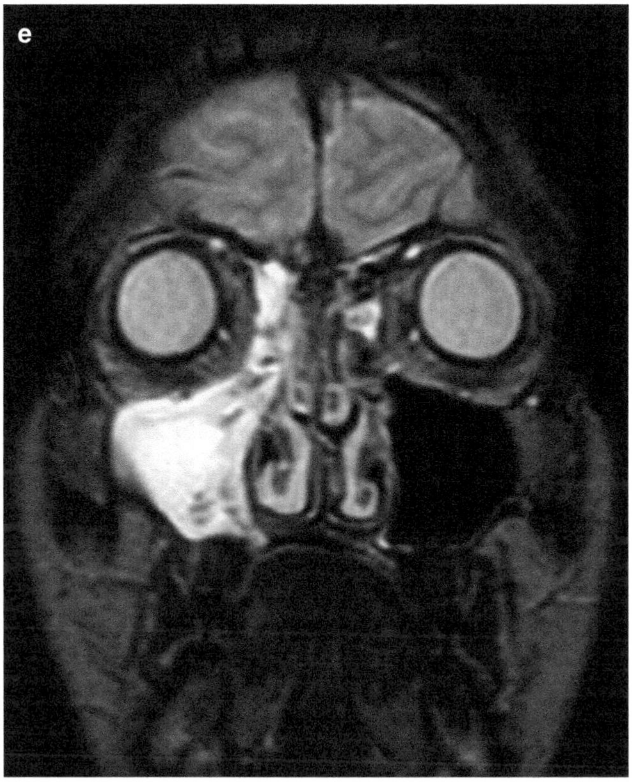

Fig. 12.1 (continued)

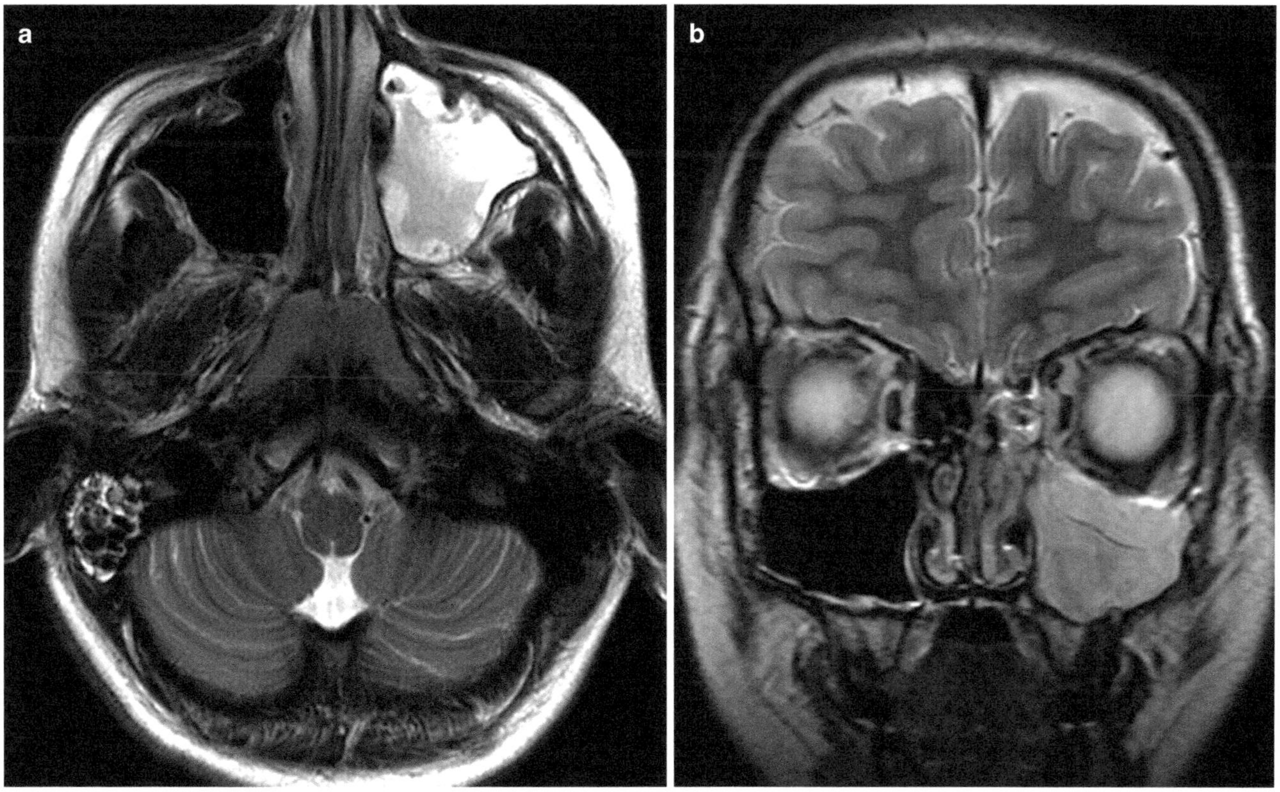

Fig. 12.2 Acute sinusitis. T2-weighted MRI (**a**, **b**) in axial and coronal projections show a hyperintense MR-signal from the fluid content and inflamed mucosa in the left maxillary sinus and from thickened mucosa in the ethmoids (on the *left*). There is similar hyperintense MR-signal from inflamed mucosa into mastoid air-cells of the right temporal bone. On T1-weighted MR image (**c**) secretion in the left maxillary sinus has reduced MR-signal comparing to the thickened mucosa

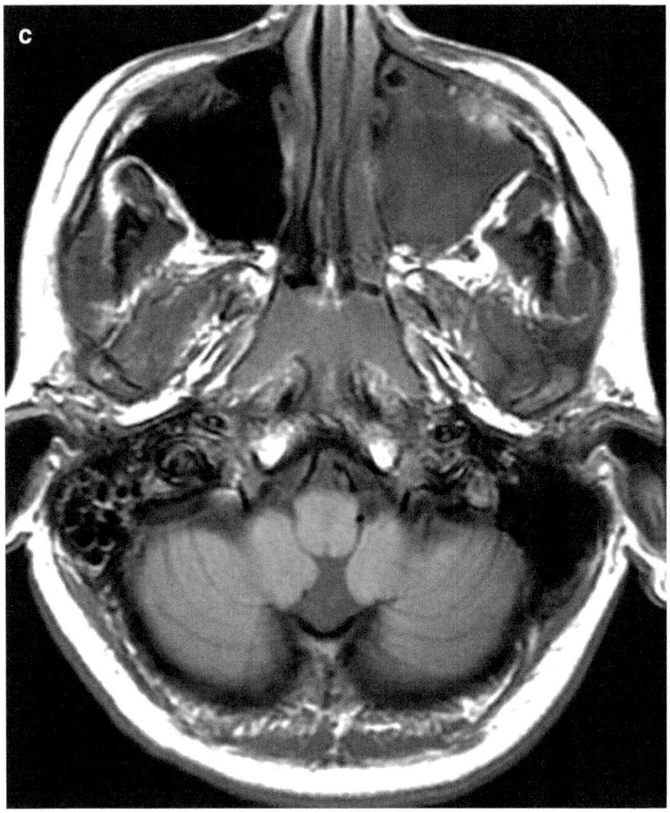

Fig. 12.2 (continued)

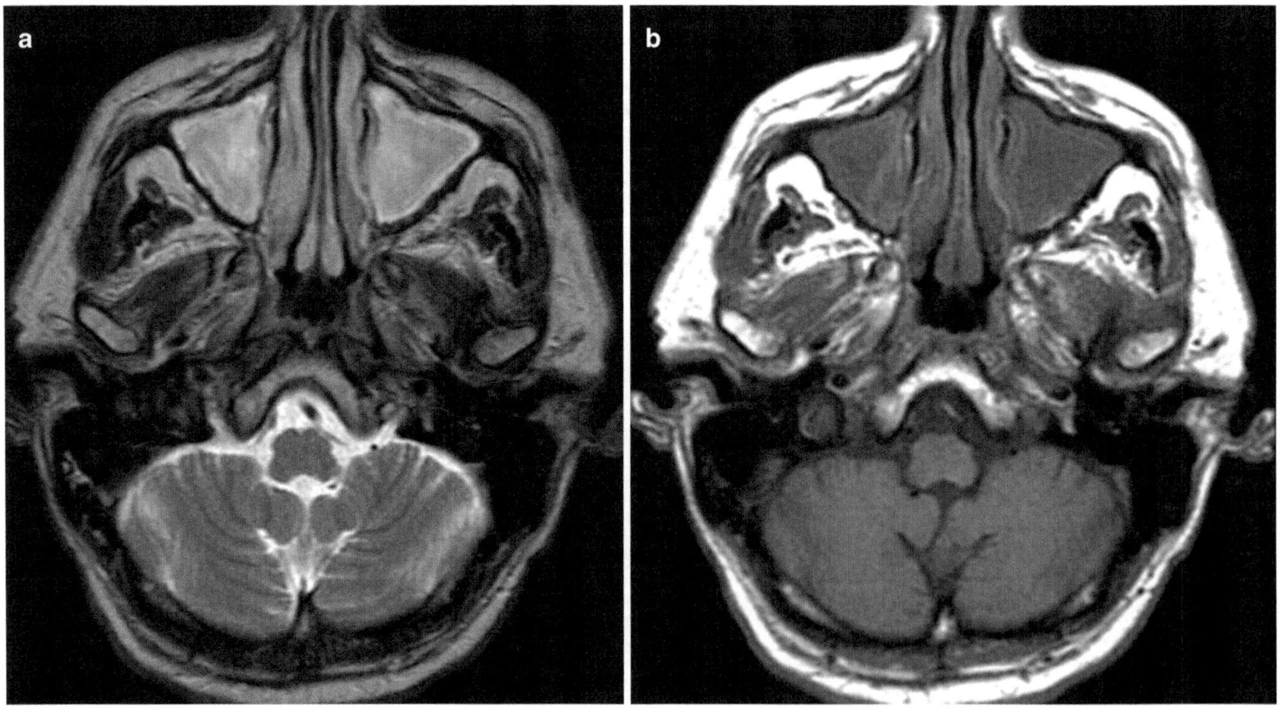

Fig. 12.3 Acute sinusitis. On T2-weighted (**a**), T1-WI (**b**), and T2-FLAIR (**c**) MR images both maxillary sinuses are filled with liquid contents. Post-enhanced T1-weighted scans in axial (**d**) and coronal (**e**) views show contrast enhancement in the thickened and inflamed mucosa. On diffusion-weighted image (**f**) there is bright signal in the sinuses cavities (**f**) due to purulent secretion

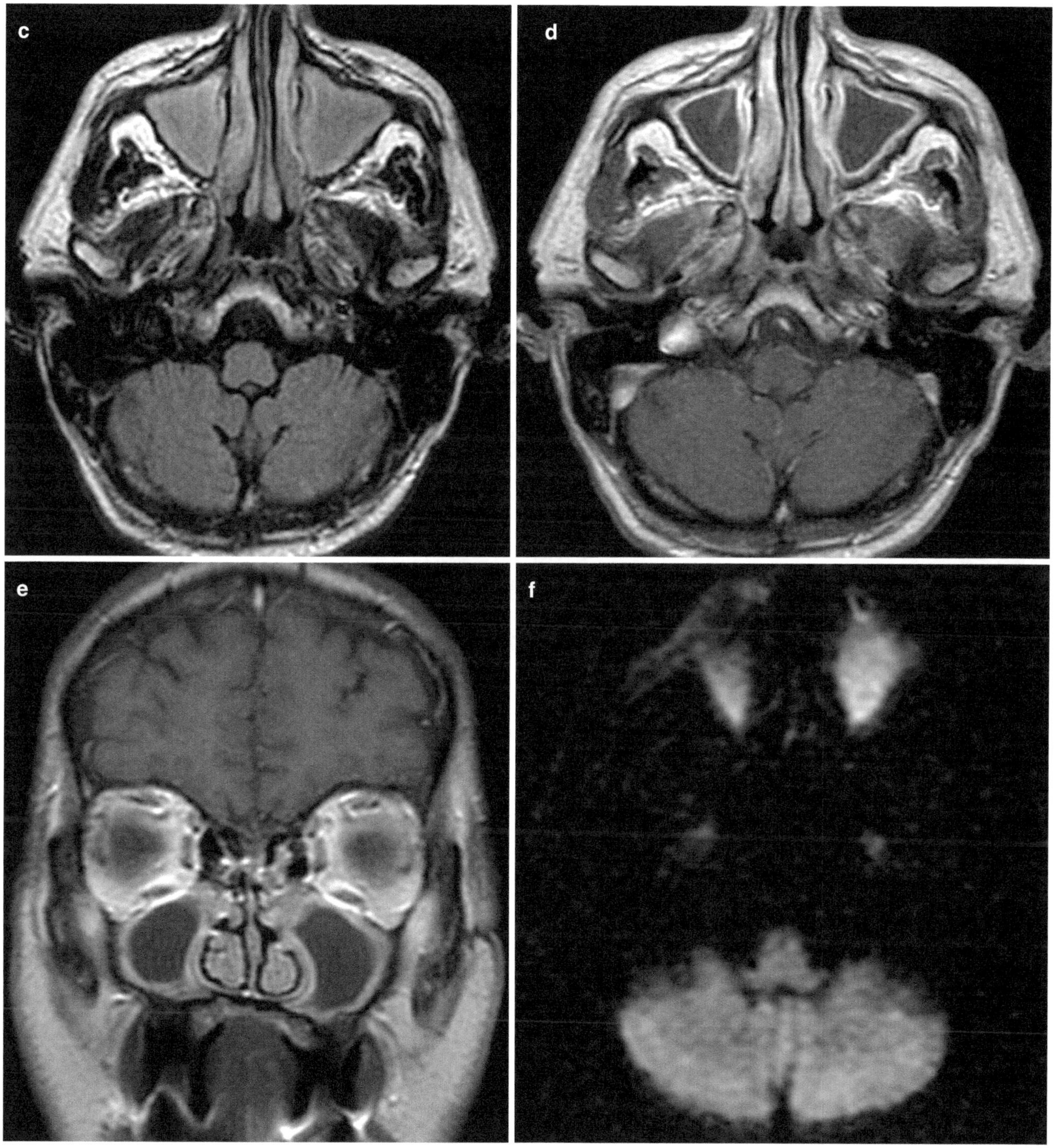

Fig. 12.3 (continued)

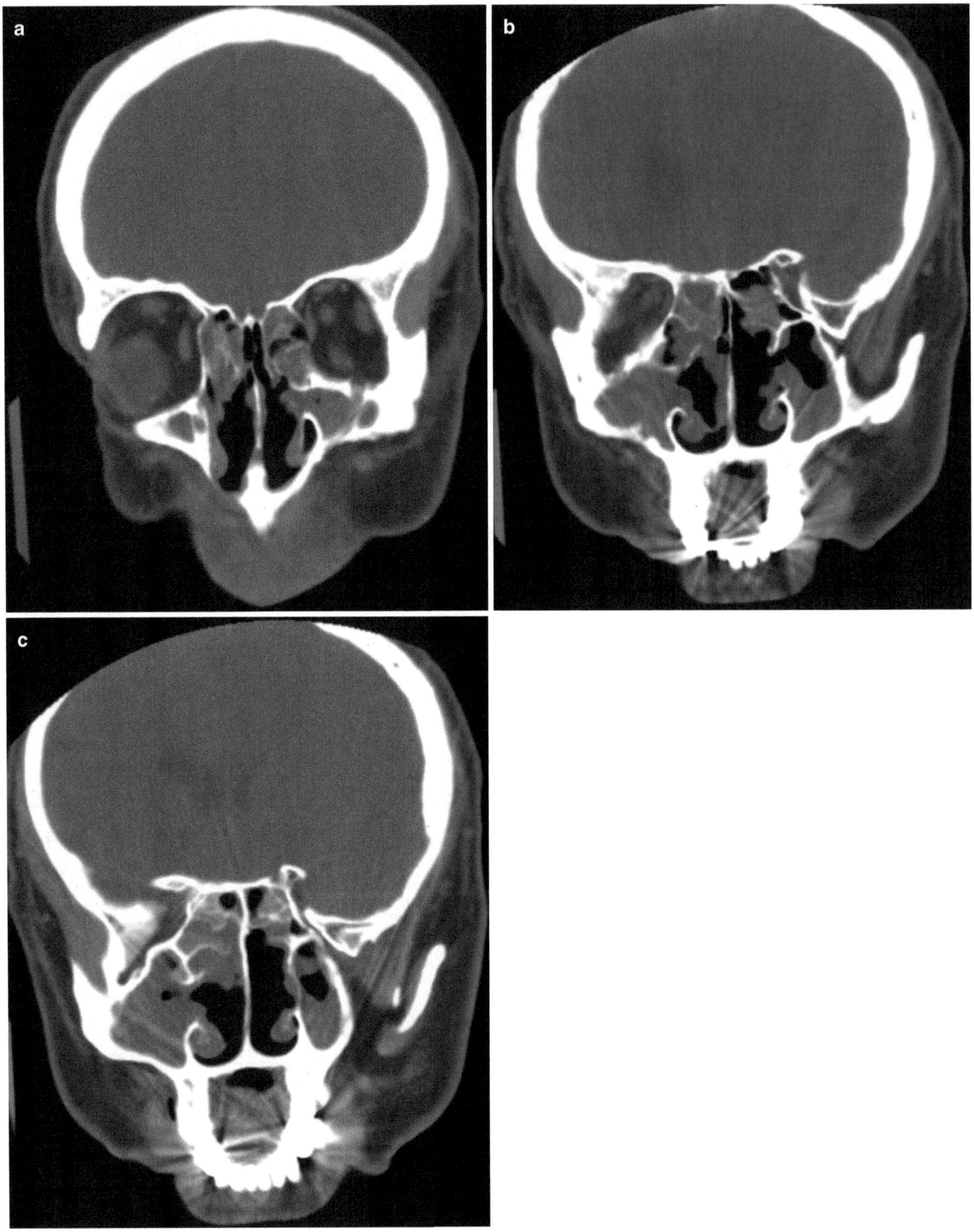

Fig. 12.4 Chronic sinusitis. On coronal CT scans (**a**–**c**) bone walls thickening of the maxillary sinuses in patient with chronic rhinosinusitis and polyposis is detected. There are changes of the mucosa into the left maxillary sinus cavity after endoscopic surgery

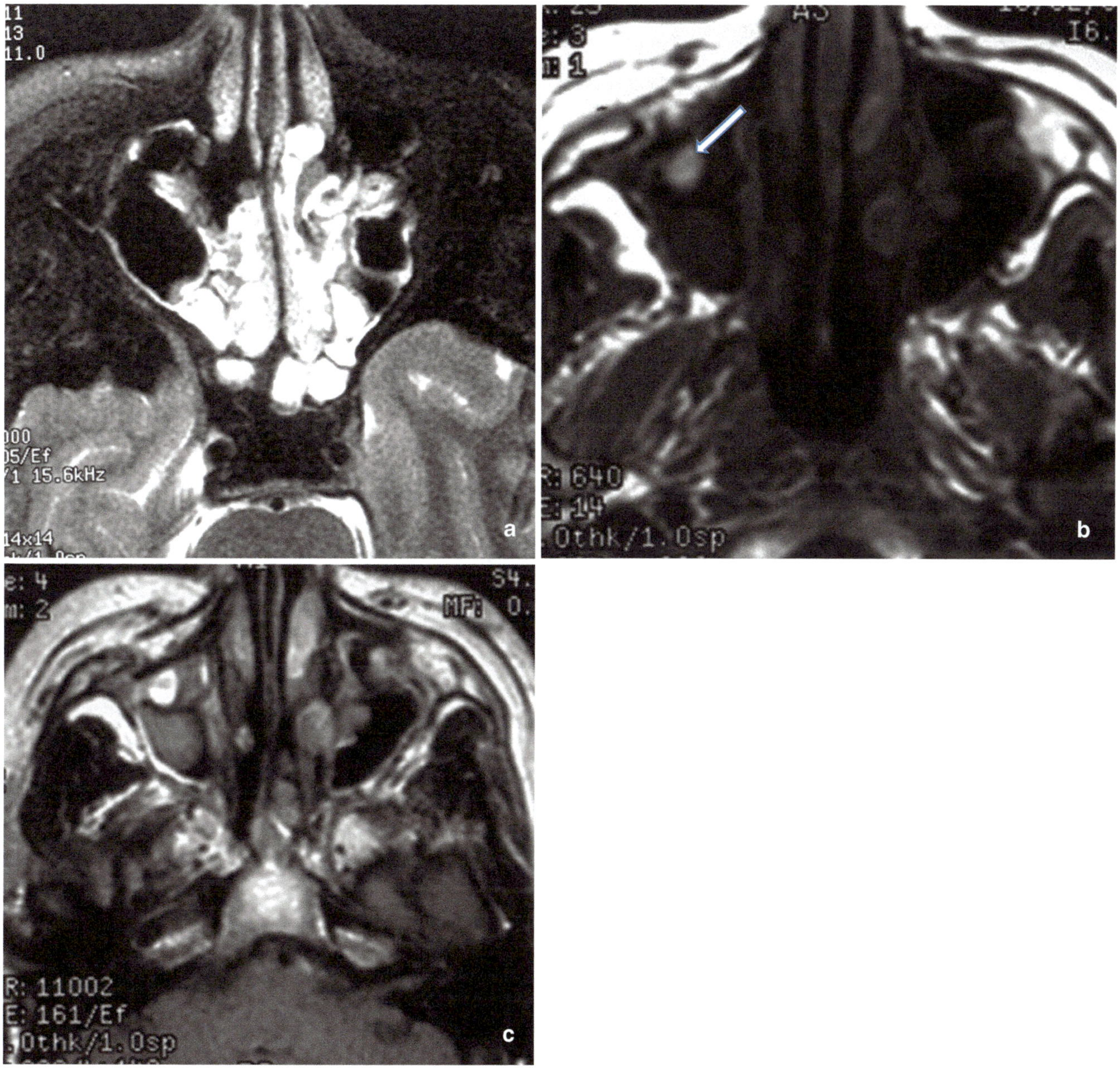

Fig. 12.5 Chronic sinusitis. On T2-weighted (**a**), T1-weighted (**b**), and T2-FLAIR (**c**) MR scans a thickening of mucosa in the both maxillary sinuses with polyps and small mucocele of the right maxillary sinus (*arrow*) are revealed

enhancement at the margins, representing the inflamed dura. Further development of the inflammation leads to formation of a brain abscess.

A low MR-signal intensity is often observed due to secondary infection with *Aspergillus fungus* caused by a chronically obstructed sinus cavity. These and other fungi accumulate various metal ions, producing a secondary paramagnetic effect and further reducing the MR-signal. In case of a relatively high signal on T1-weighted images, melanoma or tumor hemorrhage should be ruled out, but if a high signal is observed only in the sinus cavity, its inflammatory obstruction should be considered (Hamilos et al. 2004). Intravenous injection of contrast material helps better identify the lesions: in case of inflammatory changes, the mucosa of the sinuses accumulates contrast agents, while their central part filled with secretion doesn't. Tumors involving the sinus are usually diffusely enhanced (Som et al. 1988).

Mucocele is often a complication of sinusitis due to chronic sinus obstruction in its ostium, which results in filling the sinus cavity with mucus and causes the bulging of the sinus bone walls. It is often formed as a result of inflammation, trauma, endoscopic surgery, or presence of various space-occupying lesions. Constant mucus secretion in the obstructed sinus cavity leads to formation of a mucocele. There may be mild erosion of bone walls, an increased sinus volume towards the area of lower resistance. Symptoms of

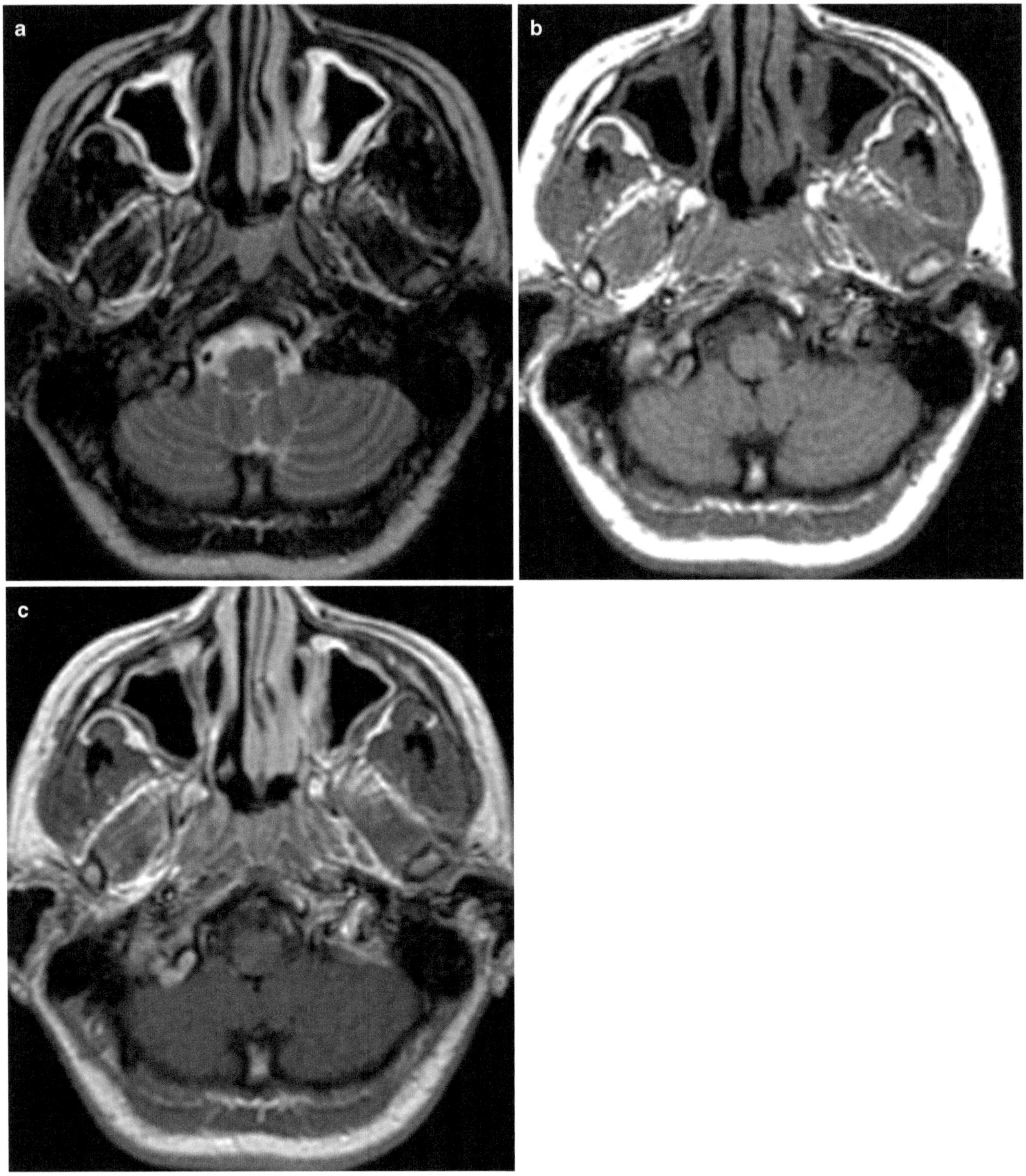

Fig. 12.6 Chronic sinusitis. T2- (**a**) and T1- (**b**) weighted MR images (**b**) show an irregular thickening of the mucosa within the maxillary sinuses. The mucosa accumulates the contrast agent and becomes bright on T1-weighted image (**c**)

mucocele depend on its localization. Mucocele is more frequently observed in the frontal sinus and ethmoid bone (90%), followed by the maxillary and sphenoid sinuses. It may develop in the sinuses separated by septas and in different anatomical variations. Sometimes mucocele of the frontal sinus extends under the skin of the forehead or into ACF. If mucocele is located in the ethmoid bone, thinning and changes in the lamina papyracea are observed with protrusion into the orbit. If mucocele is located in the maxillary sinus, it can extend into the nasal cavity, into the posterior portions of the ethmoid bone and the top of the orbit, and the sphenoid sinus (Iannetti et al. 1997; Har-El 2001).

Imaging CT detects a non-enhancing lesion in the affected sinus with low or soft tissue density; sometimes with areas of high density, if fungal invasion is present. Sinus bone walls are thinned, sometimes absent. Contrast enhancement is observed at the periphery in case of infection (mucopyocele). MR-signal characteristics of mucocele are variable: from low to high MR-signal on T1-weighted sequences (reflecting the protein concentration and the lesion "age"), high signal on T2-weighted sequences; however, hypointense areas can be detected as well (Lloyd et al. 2000a, b). Mucocele does not accumulate the contrast material, thickened surrounding mucosa is indicative of an infected mucocele. If there are contrast-enhanced foci, this is likely to be a tumor and secondary mucocele (Lanzieri et al. 1991). In our series of observations, mucocele in the frontal sinuses was characterized by a high MR-signal on T1-and T2-weighted sequences due to high protein concentrations in the fluid contents (Figs. 12.7 and 12.8). Aspergillus colonies in mucocele can also alter its MR-signal, reducing its intensity.

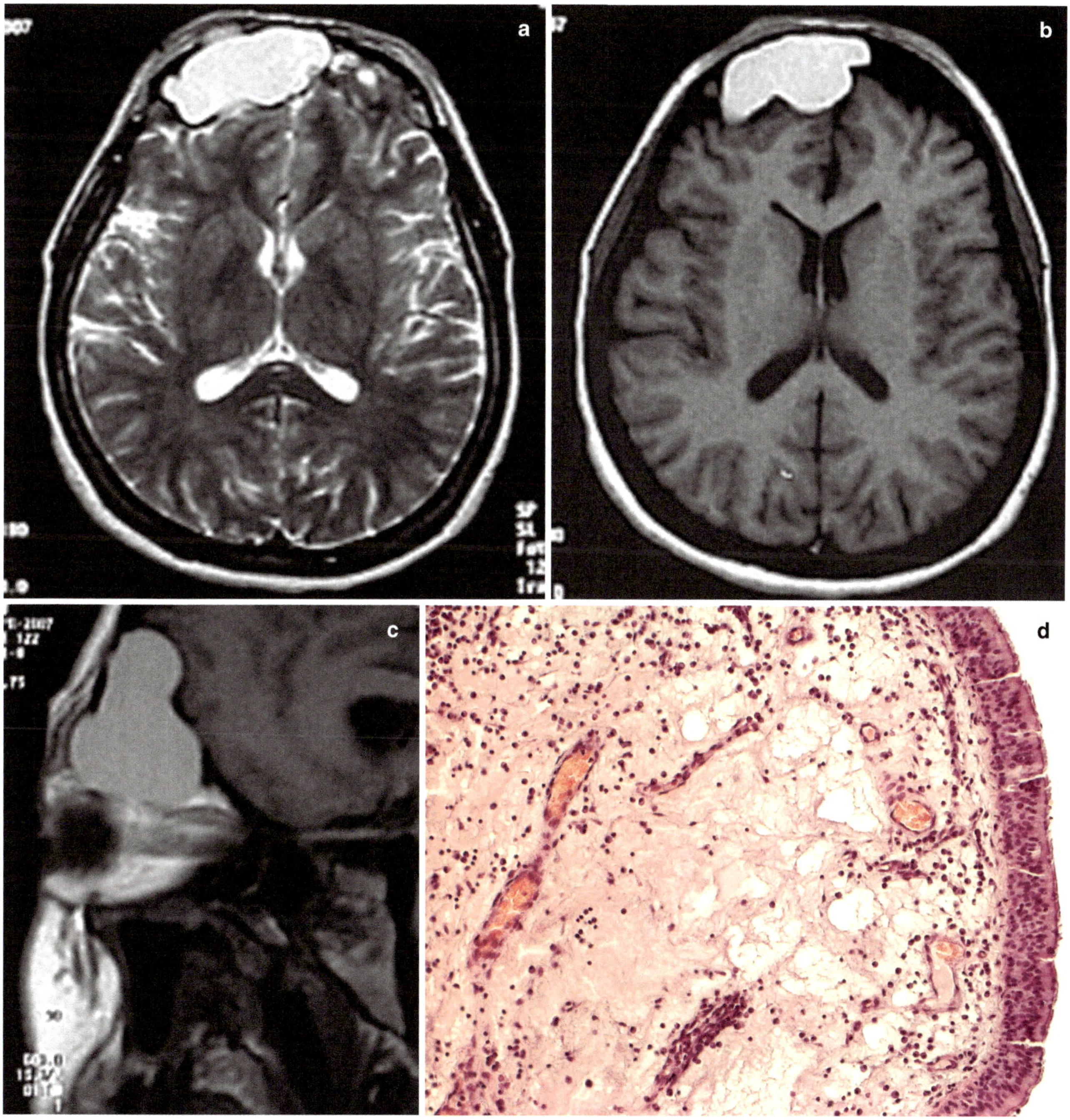

Fig. 12.7 Mucocele of the frontal sinus. T2-weighted (**a**) and T1-weighted (**b**, **c**) MR images demonstrate a large mucocele causing the extension of the frontal sinus with a high MR-signal in all sequences due to high content of proteins into secretion; (**d**) histological specimen

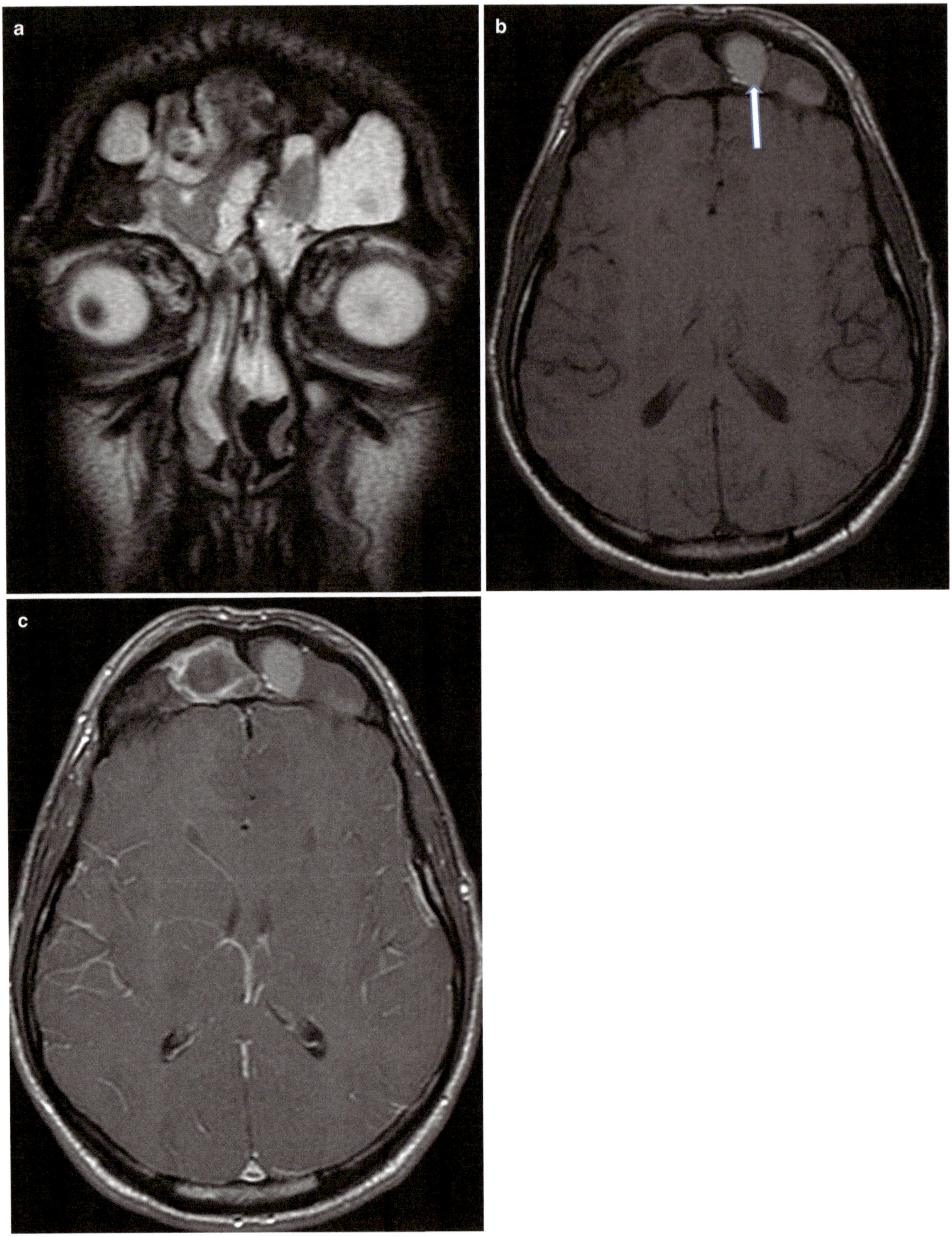

Fig. 12.8 Mucocele of the frontal sinus. T2-weighted (**a**) and T1 (**b**)-weighted MR images on the background of MR-signs of chronic inflammation, and polyps in the left parts of the frontal sinus demonstrate a small lesion with hyperintense MR-signal on T1-WI—focal mucocele (*arrow*). The contrast enhancement of inflamed mucosa within the right part of the frontal sinus on T1-weighted scan (**c**) can be seen

Differential diagnosis:

1. Fungal sinusitis involves several sinuses, high density on CT is a typical feature;
2. Sinonasal polyposis involves all sinuses;
3. Antrochoanal polyp is a dumbbell lesion that fills the maxillary sinus and prolapses through its ostium into the nasal cavity;
4. Any slow growing benign or malignant tumor can simulate mucocele on CT; tumors accumulate the contrast agent, while mucoceles don't.

Sinonasal polyps (SP) are one of the allergic sinusitis manifestations or the reflection of prior inflammatory disease in the sinus (Som et al. 2011). More often SPs arise from the maxillary sinus cavity and penetrate through the sinus ostium or accessory ostium into the nasal cavity. SPs can also be non-allergic nature and occur as a result of the inflamed mucosa hyperplasia. Large SPs are dumbbell-shaped lesions with a narrow stalk that arises from the maxillary infundibulum or an accessory ostium, connecting two globular polypous formations in the nasal cavity and the maxillary sinus. A solitary polypoid mass of large size can reach the nasopharynx. SPs are most frequently detected in the antrochoanal area and less frequently in nasochoanal, sphenochoanal, and ethmoidochoanal areas (Ozdek et al. 2002).

Imaging On CT, they appear as well-defined, dumbbell-shaped, soft tissue (close to that of mucosa) lesions with smooth borders, which extend from the maxillary sinus through the widened maxillary ostium into the nasal cavity and then into the nasopharynx. An increased density in the center may be present, depending on the protein content, or due to infection, stage of the process or the presence of fungal colonization (usually aspergillosis). There is a marked peripheral accumulation of contrast material by the surrounding mucosa without enhancement of the central part of the lesion. The widened sinus cavity or components of the nasal cavity get thinner as bone erosive changes develop in the anterior portions of the skull base (Chung et al. 2002).

On MRI, SPs have a low or increased intensity on T1-WI, depending on the stage of the process, on T2-WI MR-signal is high, always reflecting cystic content (Fig. 12.9). Differentiation between polyposis and cancer on MRI and CT is not always possible. Sometimes polyps accumulate contrast material, therefore, the use of CT-perfusion is appropriate in these cases allowing to differentiate these two entities in majority of the cases.

Retention cysts result from an obstruction of small submucosal mucinous glands, often in the maxillary sinus. In most cases, distinguishing polyps from retention cysts is impossible (Fig. 12.10).

Differential diagnosis:

1. Intranasal glioma is a soft tissue lesion that extends onto the skull base, rarely localized in the nasopharynx, the maxillary sinus being intact;
2. Naso-ethmoidal encephalocele—intracranial origin of the process; there is an obvious defect of the cribriform plate;
3. Juvenile angiofibroma—only boys are affected; the lesion accumulates contrast agent and locates in the posterior regions of the nasal cavity, prolapses into the pterygopalatine fossa, obstructs the maxillary sinus; high perfusion parameters are typical features;
4. Olfactory neuroblastoma—an aggressive, destructive lesion in the upper nasal cavity, diffusely enhancing, extending through the cribriform plate to ACF.

Abscess of CFR is a focal pyogenic infection and is usually a complication of an infection in the paranasal sinuses, mastoid cells, teeth infection, osteomyelitis, purulent meningitis. The abscess formation is induced by a direct invasion of infectious agent in cases with craniocerebral trauma or due to surgery. Posttraumatic abscesses may develop early or within years or even decades after an open head injury. Lesions are solitary in 70% of cases and multiple in 30% of cases (Berlit et al. 1996). Despite the fact that an inflammatory process goes through the four subsequent stages in its development: early cerebritis (1–3 days), late cerebritis (4–9 days), early formation of the capsule (10–13 days) and late formation of the capsule (day 14 and later) (Britt et al. 1984), radiologists usually observe in their practice an already formed capsule with necrotic core.

Imaging On CT and MRI, this is a round space-occupying lesion with a thin capsule that is also visible prior to intravenous contrast enhancement. There is a rim around the edge of the necrotic center, which is somewhat more hyperdense than the inner contents of the abscess on CT. On T1-weighted MR images, the capsule has a slightly hyperintense MR-signal compared to the central necrotic core and surrounding brain edema. On T2-weighted MR images, the abscess capsule is typically hypointense and clearly contoured due to a high signal from the pus inside and perifocal edema outside (Spreer 2009). The abscess capsule intensely enhances. The typical diagnostic features are a smooth inner contour of the capsule and a high MR-signal on diffusion-weighted images from the central core. In rare cases, it is possible to visualize a passage from the adjacent paranasal sinuses, where inflammatory changes are also observed (thickened mucosa, effusion, pus in the sinus cavity) (Figs. 12.11, 12.12, 12.13, 12.14 and 12.15).

All intracranial space-occupying lesions with central necrosis and enhancing rim (a "ring-like effect") can mimic

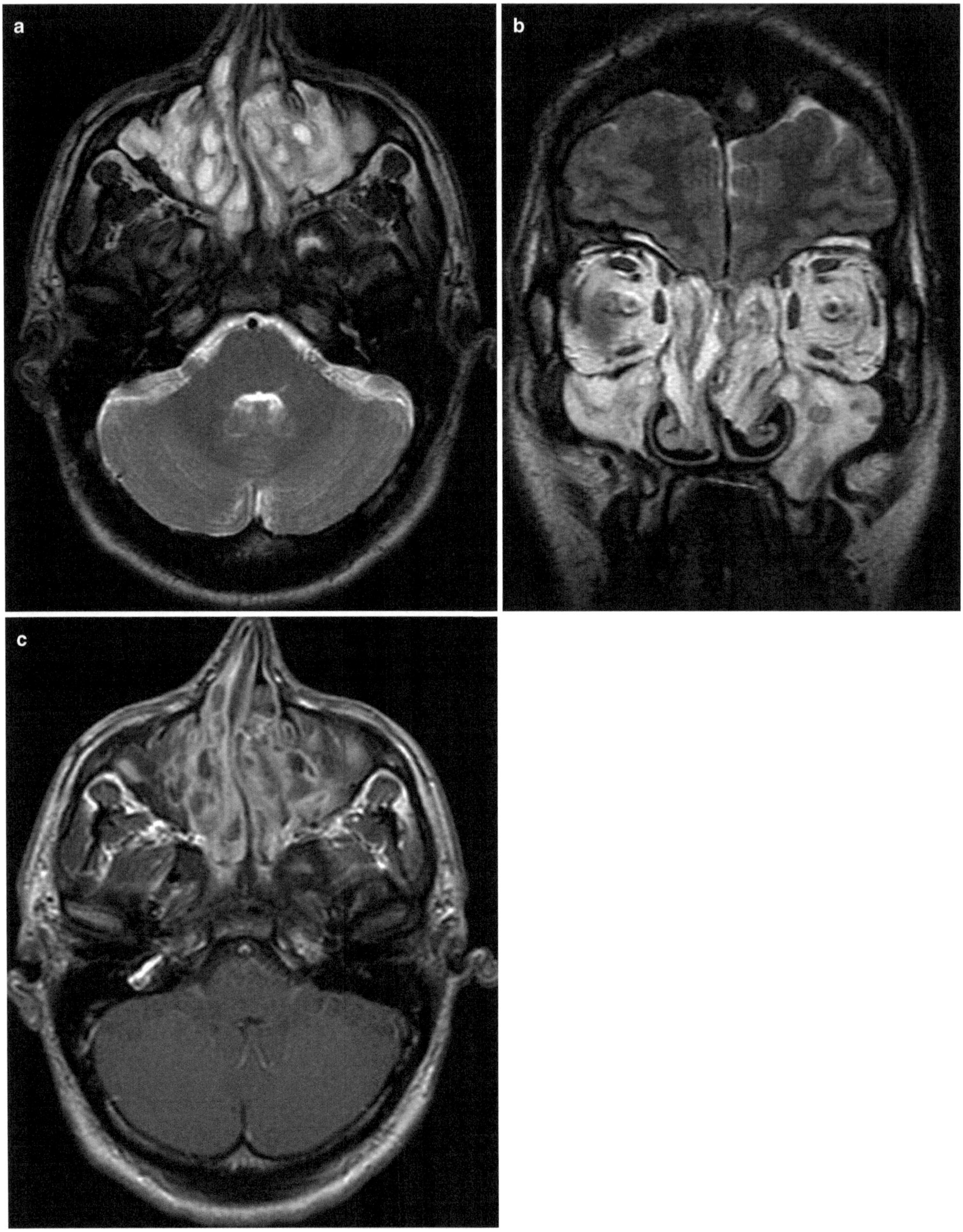

Fig. 12.9 Sinonasal antrochoanal polyps. T2-weighted MR images in axial (**a**) and coronal (**b**) projections show a hyperintense space-occupying masses (*polyps*) extending from the both maxillary sinuses into nasal cavities and the nasopharynx. After contrast enhancement the inflamed mucosa as well as polyps of the maxillary sinuses and nasal cavities demonstrates the prominent enhancement (**c**)

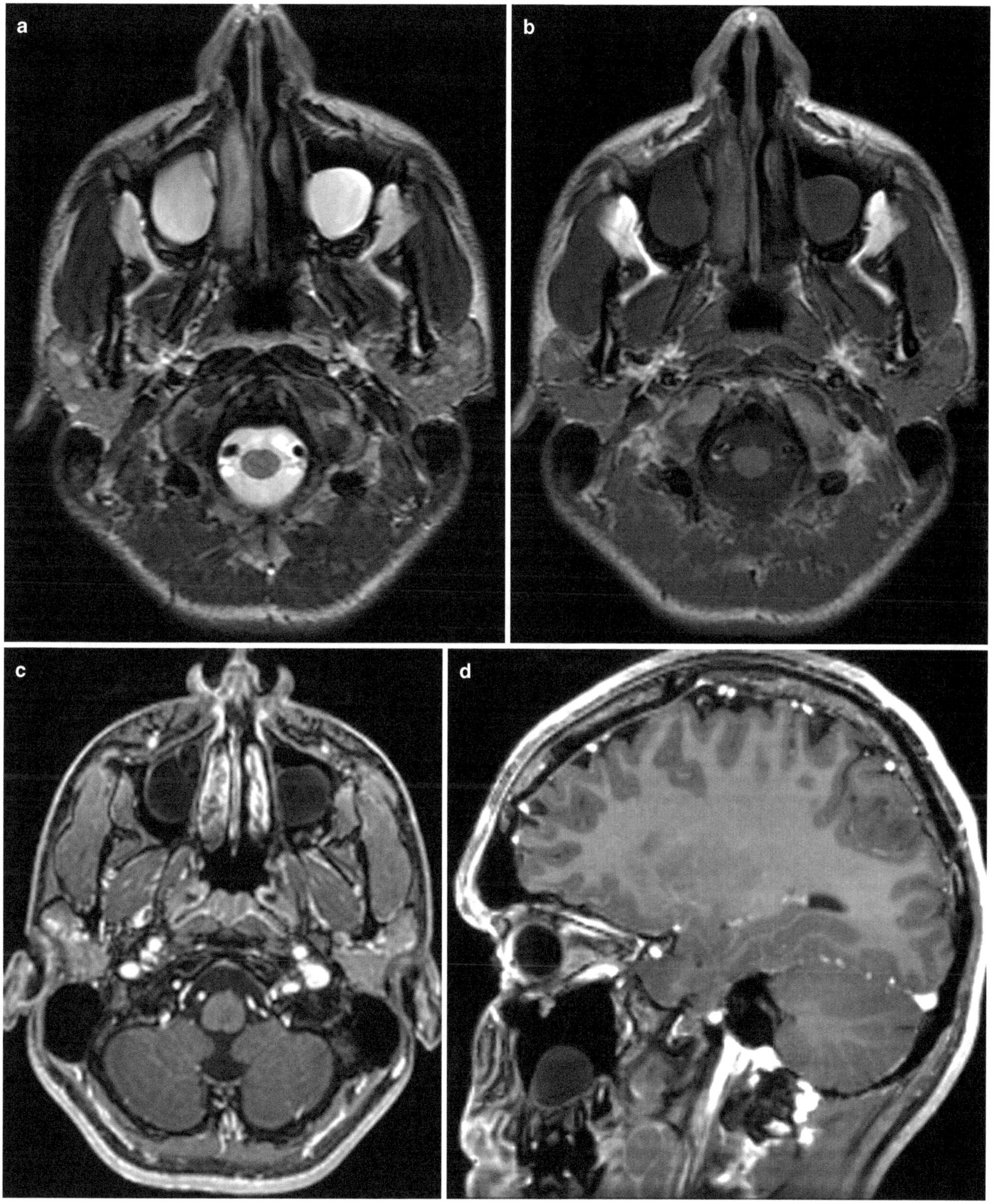

Fig. 12.10 Retention cysts of the maxillary sinuses. MR imaging with the use of T2- (**a**) and T1- (**b**) weighted scans demonstrates a uniform oval cystic lesions within both maxillary sinuses, with homogeneous MR-signal. There are difficulties in distinguishing these lesions from polyps. Contrast-enhanced MR-study clearly demonstrates the accumulation of contrast agent thickened mucosa of the maxillary sinuses (**c**, **d**) only, confirming the presence of retention cysts

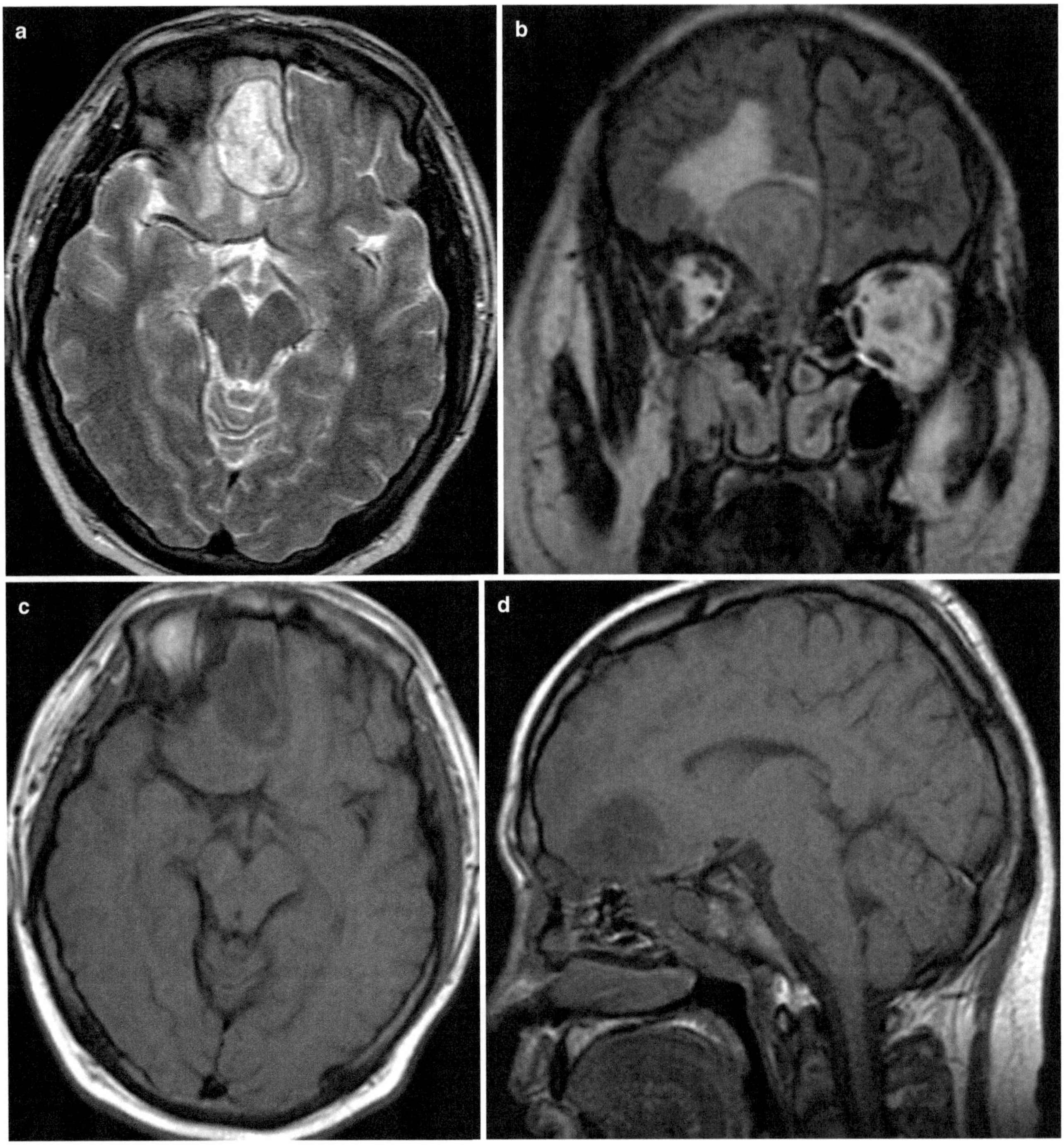

Fig. 12.11 Abscess of the right frontal lobe, a complication of the head trauma. T2-weighted (**a**), T2-FLAIR- (**b**) weighted MR images demonstrate a heterogeneous hyperintense on T2 oval mass extending from the ethmoid bone intracranially. On T1-weighted (**c**, **d**) images a lesion has hypointense MR-signal. Diffusion-weighted images (**e**, **f**) reveal a high MR-signal within the mass indicating the restriction of diffusion and the presence of purulent content

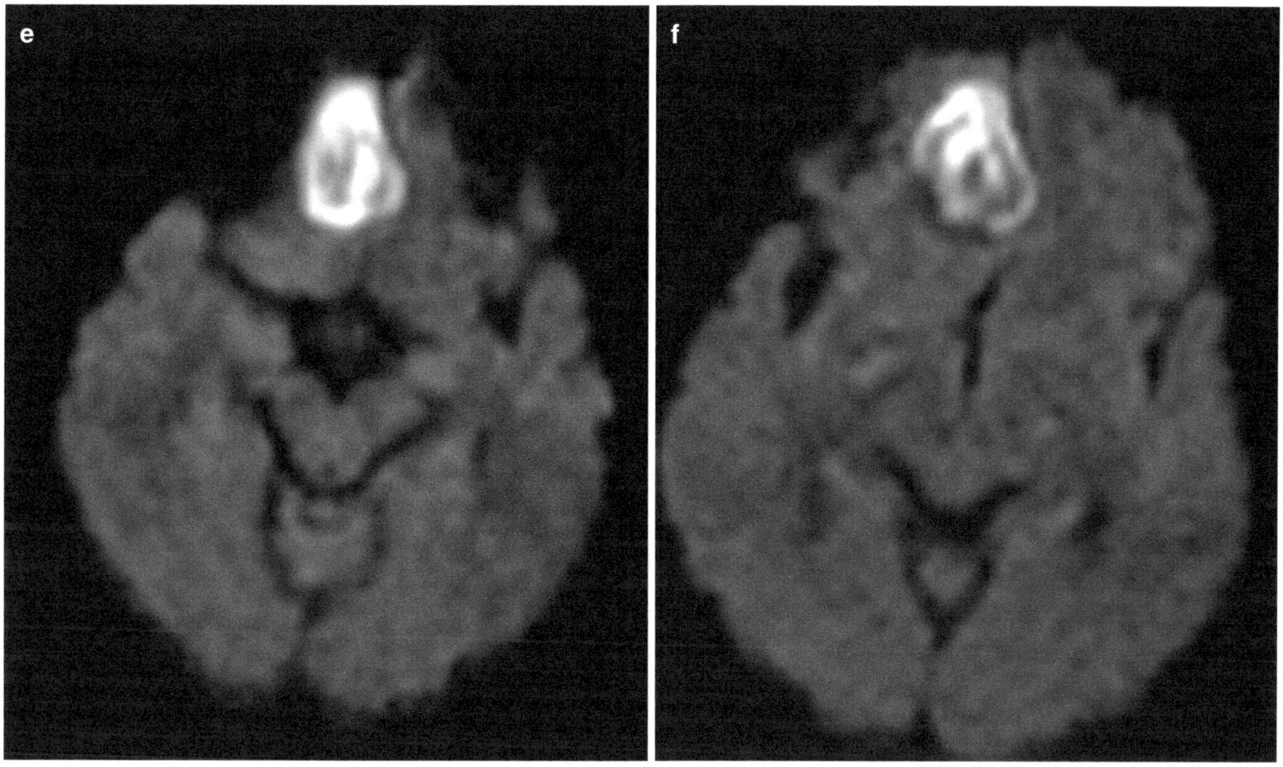

Fig. 12.11 (continued)

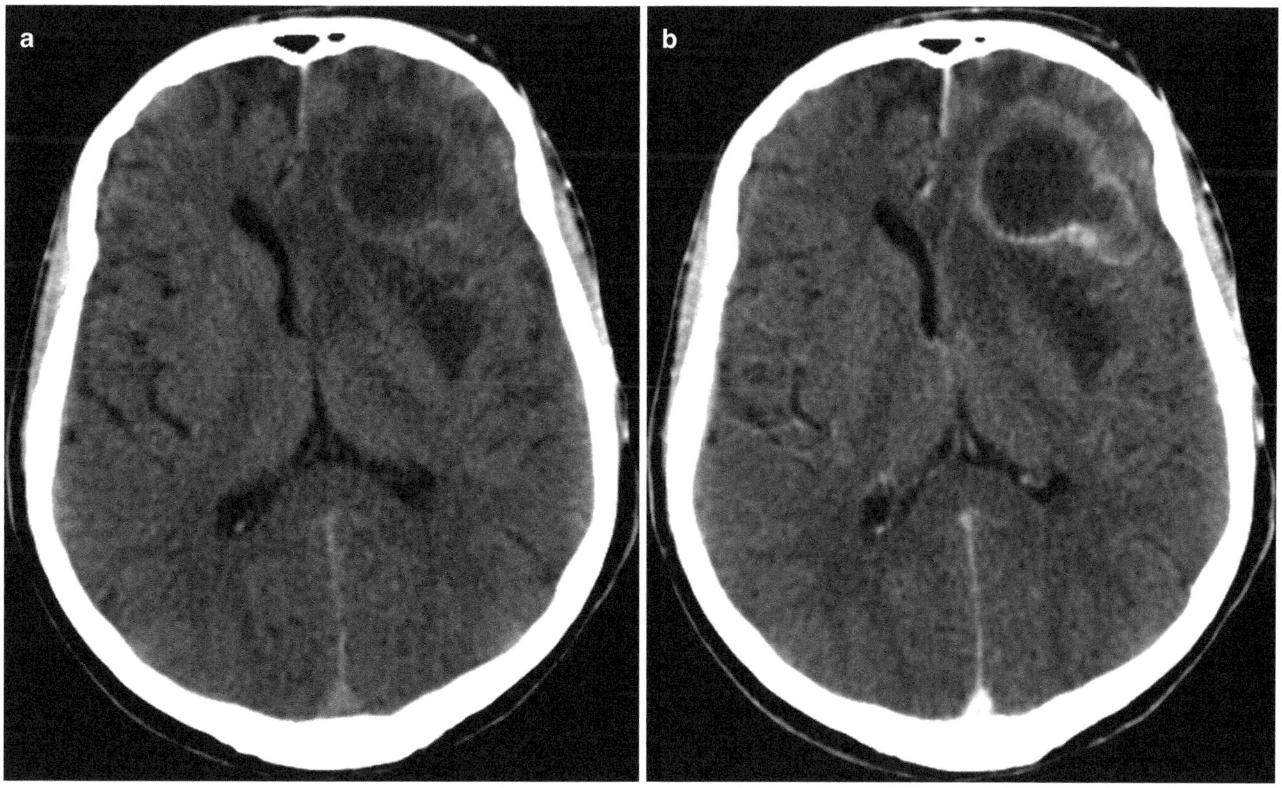

Fig. 12.12 Posttraumatic abscess of the left frontal lobe. Axial CT scans before (**a**) and after contrast enhancement demonstrate a ring-like enhancing lesion in the left frontal lobe with perifocal edema. CT-perfusion study (CBF-**c**) doesn't show elevation of blood flow as within the lesion as in capsule of the lesion. On T1-weighted (**d**) and T2-weighted (**e**) MR images a lesion has well-defined contours, with hyperintensity on T1 from the capsule of the abscess. Diffusion-weighted image (**e**) demonstrates a typical for pus within the lesion hyperintense MR-signal indicating a restriction of diffusion

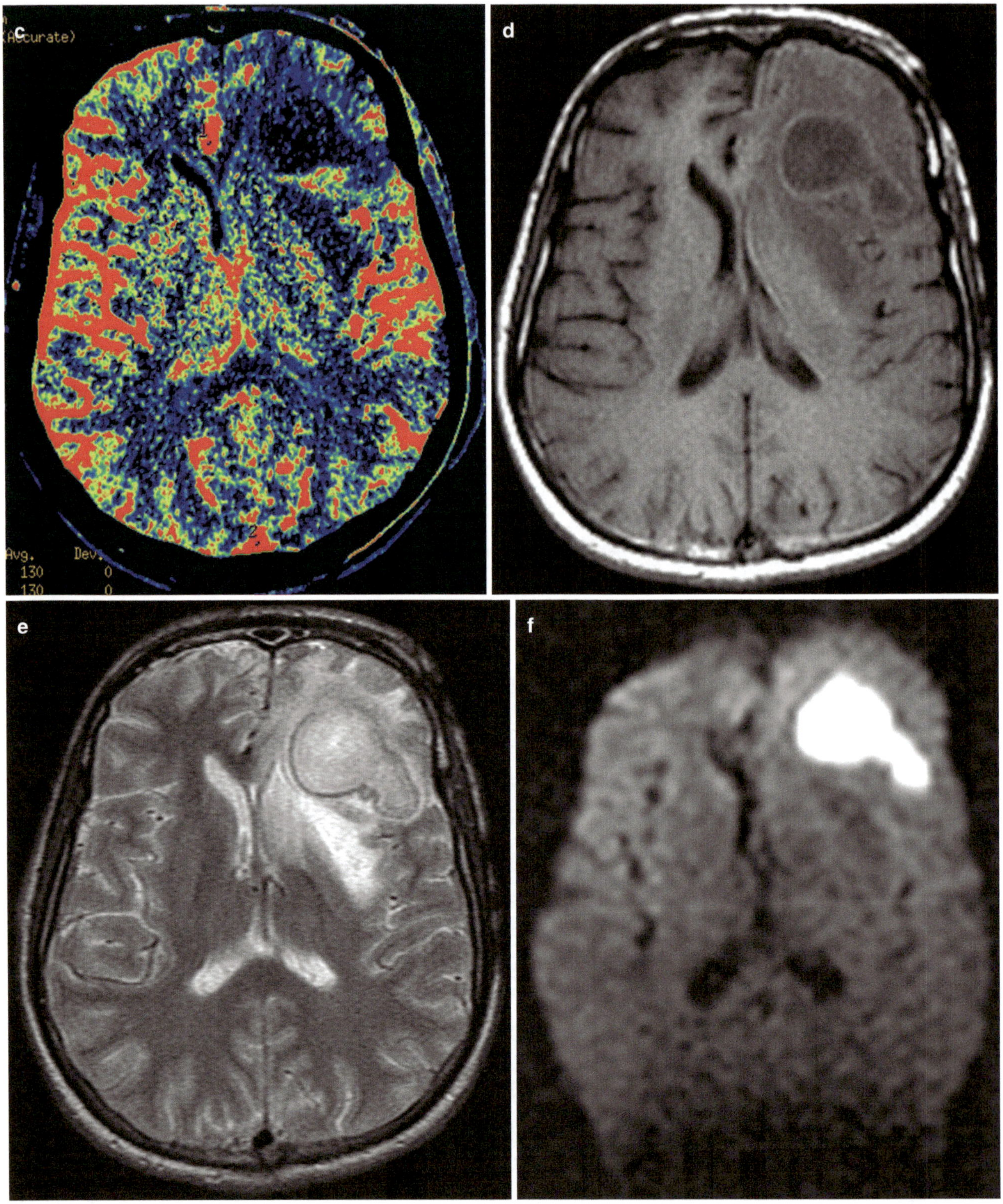

Fig. 12.12 (continued)

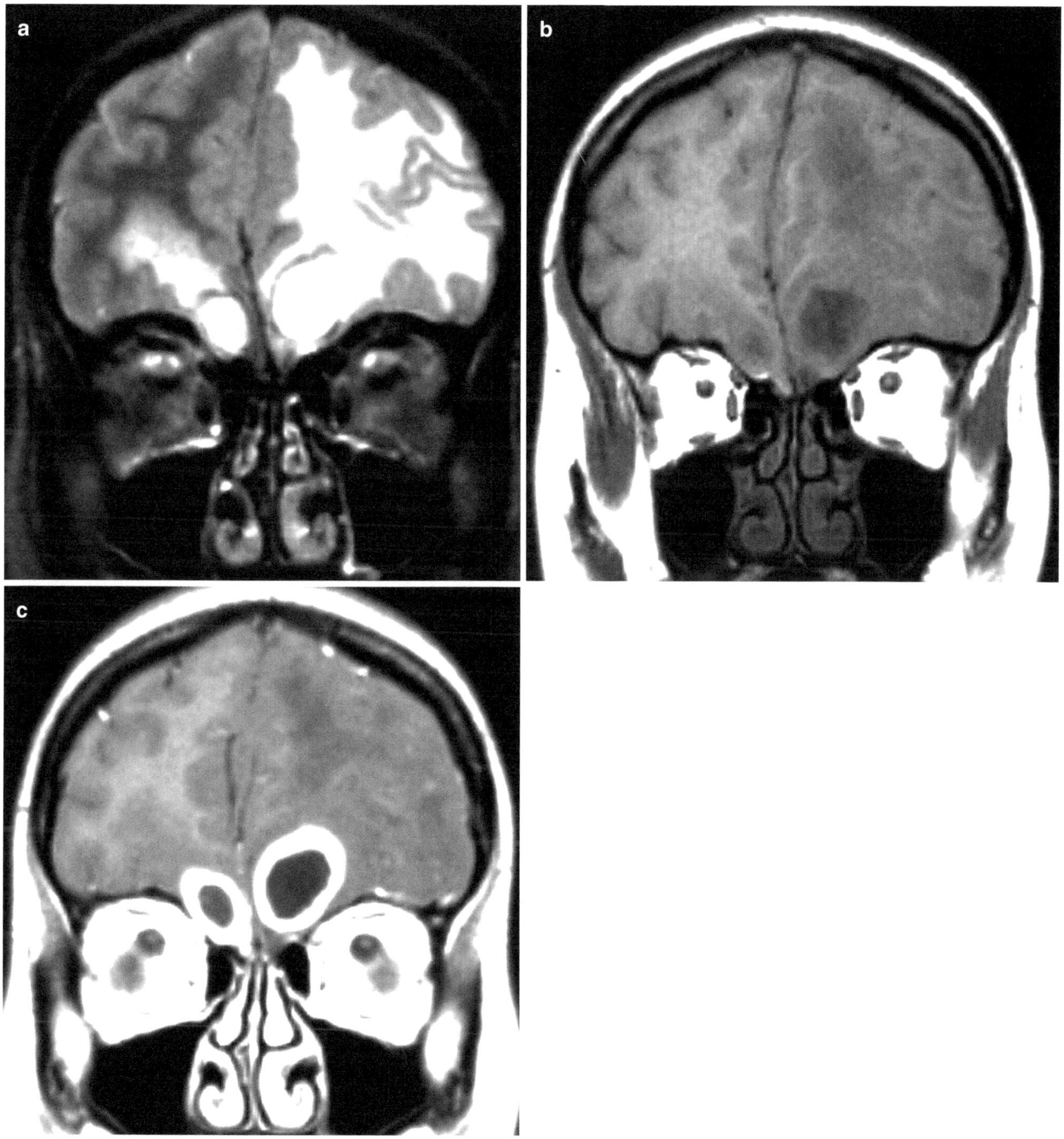

Fig. 12.13 Multiple abscesses of the frontal areas. T2-weighted (**a**) and T1-weighted MR images in coronal plane performed before (**b**) and after contrast enhancement (**c**) reveal both sides abscesses in fronto-basal areas with intense ring-like accumulation of contrast agent

abscesses. If the lesion is a solitary, then *differential diagnosis* with malignant gliomas and metastases should be made. However, contrast enhancement within the majority of the tumors is inhomogeneous, with wide brain infiltration and irregular internal contours as opposed to abscesses. An increased MR-signal on the diffusion-weighted sequences and a decrease in ADC of purulent contents of the abscess is a reliable sign of inflammatory origin, but is not absolutely specific sign. CT- or MR-perfusion studies are supplemental methods of differential diagnosis: the tumor tissue is rapidly hyperperfused, while the abscess capsule is weakly and low-perfused.

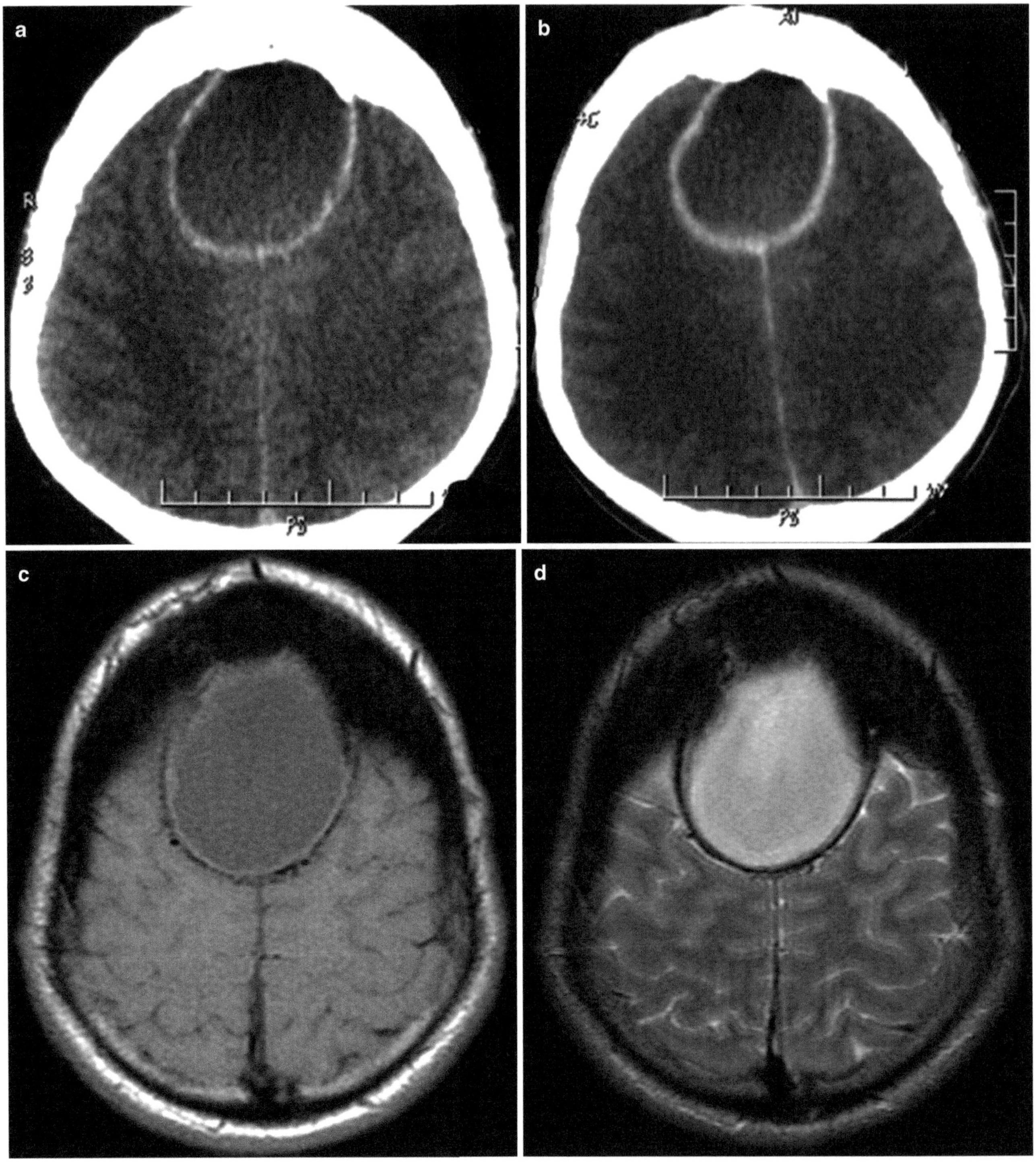

Fig. 12.14 Posttraumatic epidural abscess of interhemispheric fissure. A 45-year-old male was admitted at the hospital with headache and elevation of body temperature (up to 38). 4 years ago patient has got a head trauma (in supraorbital region) with formation of orbital phlegmon that was treated following polypectomy from sinus cavities. At the moment of admission axial CT scans before (**a**) and after (**b**) contrast enhancement show a large oval mass, which has calcified capsule. The capsule strongly accumulates contrast medium. MR imaging with using T1-weighted (**c**), T2-weighted (**d**), and T2-FLAIR (**e**) scans as well as post-contrast T1 study demonstrates a large lesion with prominent contrast enhancement (**f**, **g**) in projection of capsule with double-contour pattern; a lesion has hypointense on T1 and hyperintense on T2 and T2-FLAIR MR-signal. On diffusion-weighted image (**h**) there is a high MR-signal in the central part of the mass (diffusion restriction). An enhanced passage which is connected abscess cavity with frontal sinus cavity is clearly visible (*arrows*). T2-weighted coronal slice demonstrates chronic inflammation and polyps within maxillary sinuses and ethmoid complex

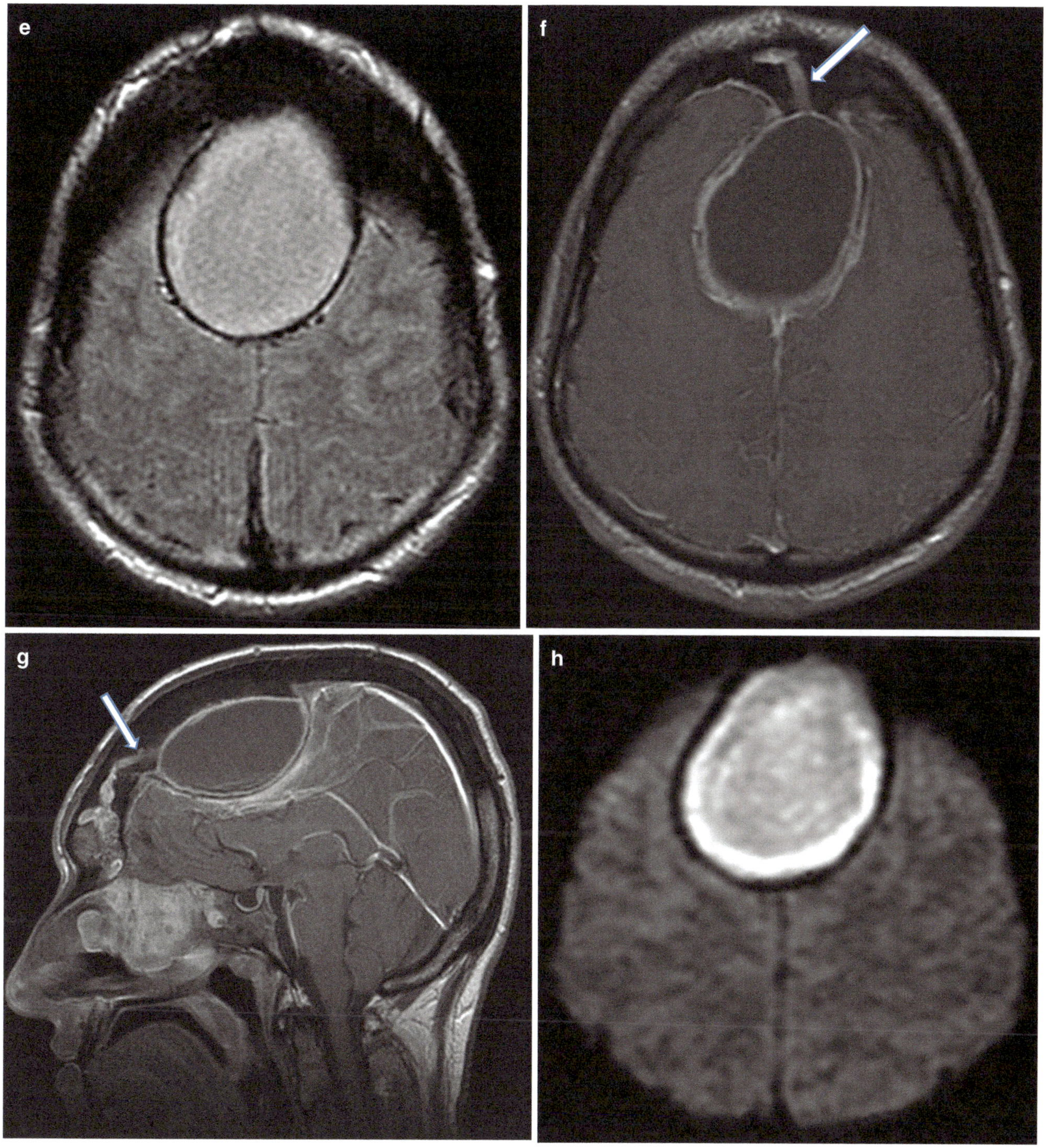

Fig. 12.14 (continued)

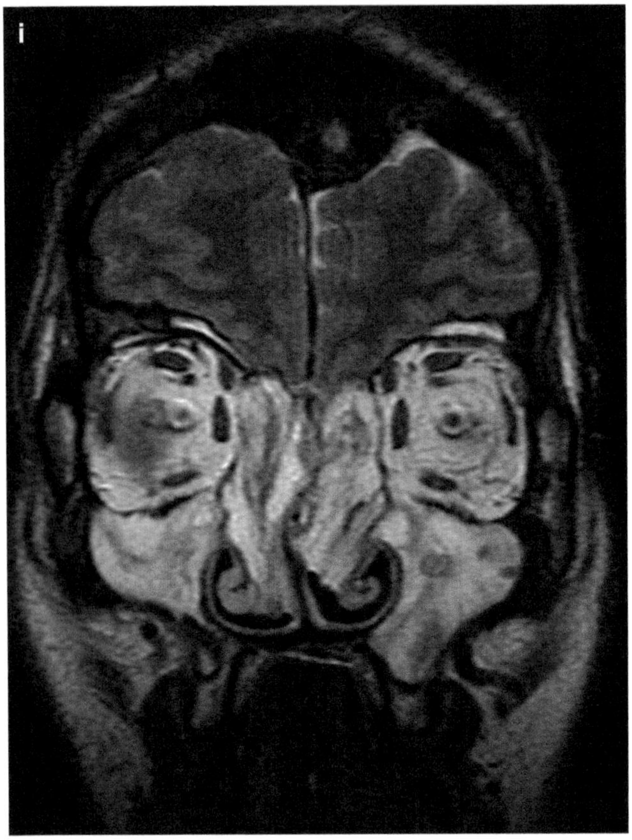

Fig. 12.14 (continued)

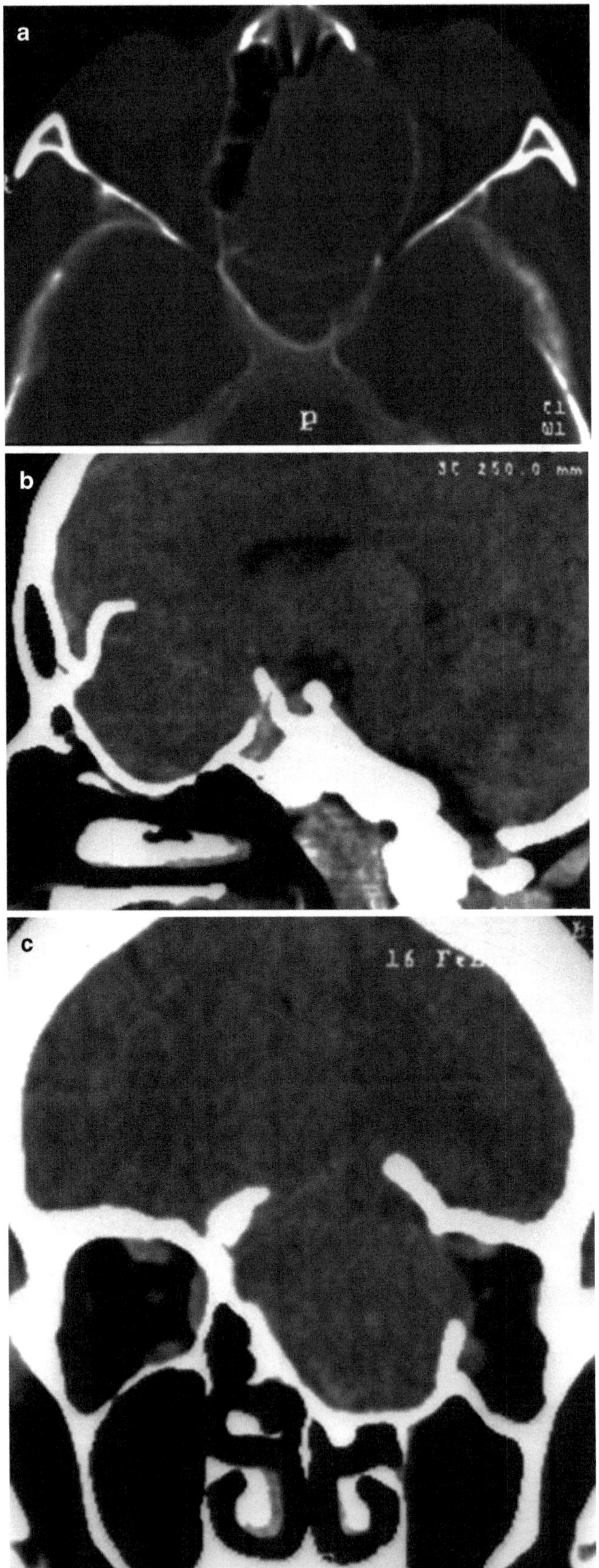

Fig. 12.15 Pyogenic granuloma. Axial CT scan (**a**) and sagittal (**b**), and coronal (**c**) reformats show a large expansile mass in projection of left ethmoid complex with bone remodel and deformation. A lesion protrudes into the left orbit. There is thickening of surrounding granuloma bones

13 Congenital Disorders

Meningoencephalocele (MEC) can be fronto-ethmoidal, fronto-nasal, naso-ethmoidal, and naso-orbital (Rojvachiranonda et al. 2003). MEC is a congenital protrusion of the meninges, brain tissue, cerebrospinal fluid through the calvarial or skull base defect in the ACF area and represents a lesion inside or outside the nasal cavity. Unlike occipital encephalocele, MEC has no association with neural tube defects. It develops common enough—1:4000 of births (Osborn et al. 2016). MCE can be combined with other developmental abnormalities, such as callosal dysgenesis, interhemispheric lipoma, neuronal migration anomalies, colloid cyst, median craniofacial dysraphism, etc. MEC is a soft tissue lesion "closely" adjacent to the brain parenchyma and extending extracranially through the skull base defect. It often occurs in the middle face, fronto-ethmoidal area near the dorsum of the nose or in naso-ethmoidal area, extending from the anterior cranial fossa. MEC is localized in the area of the midline defect (*foramen cecum*) in 90% and a double cleft in the cribriform plate divided along the midline by the bone bridge in 10% (Mahapatra et al. 2002).

Imaging On CT, MEC displaces the frontal bones upwards, whereas the nasal bones, frontal process of the maxilla, and nasal cartilage are pushed downwards. Nasal bones can be deformed, with the presence of a passage in the frontal part of the ethmoid bone (in cases with naso-ethmoidal MEC). The cribriform plate and portions of the frontal bones can be partially or completely absent. CT-cisternography in typical cases detects the subarachnoid spaces filled with contrast material around the soft tissue lesion prolapsing into the bone defect (Boonvisut et al. 1998). CT clearly demonstrates a prolapse of the brain tissue into the defect area (Fig. 13.1).

On T1-weighted MR images, this is a soft tissue lesion with heterogeneous MR-signal, isointense relative to the gray matter, extracranial content of protrusion is closely adjacent to the intracranial brain parenchyma, extending into the bone defect. T2-weighted MR images demonstrate hyperintense signal from CSF around the prolapsing soft tissue lesion. The brain substance may have an increased signal on T2-weighted images due to edema and gliosis. MEC content doesn't enhance (Fig. 13.2). Contrast enhancement can be observed in the surrounding membranes due to concomitant inflammatory (meningitis).

Differential diagnosis:

1. Nasal glioma is a soft tissue congenital non-neoplastic heterotopia, localized along the dorsum of the nose or under its bones, no association with intracranial contents;
2. Dermoid, epidermoid—focal masses on the dorsum of the nose or in the medial part of the orbit (fat density, if dermoid; fluid density and high signal on DWI, if epidermoid);
3. Nasal dermal sinus;
4. Dacryocystocele is a sharply marginated tense blue to blue-gray lesion situated just inferior to the medial canthi, not connected to the base of the skull, enlarged nasolacrimal duct.

Fibrous dysplasia (FD) is a congenital disorder with defect in osteoblastic differentiation, and maturation, and characterized by lesions with mixture of fibrous and bone tissue (Osborn et al. 2016).

It is often localized in the maxilla, less frequently in the mandible, frontal, ethmoid, and sphenoid bones. This is a slow-growing, expanding bone lesion, which is practically an immatured bone that can be accompanied by a variety of endocrine disorders, as well as painful swelling, obstruction of the sinuses and nasal cavity, and headache. If FD grows

I. Pronin, V. Kornienko, *CT and MRI of Skull Base Lesions*, https://doi.org/10.1007/978-3-319-65957-2_13

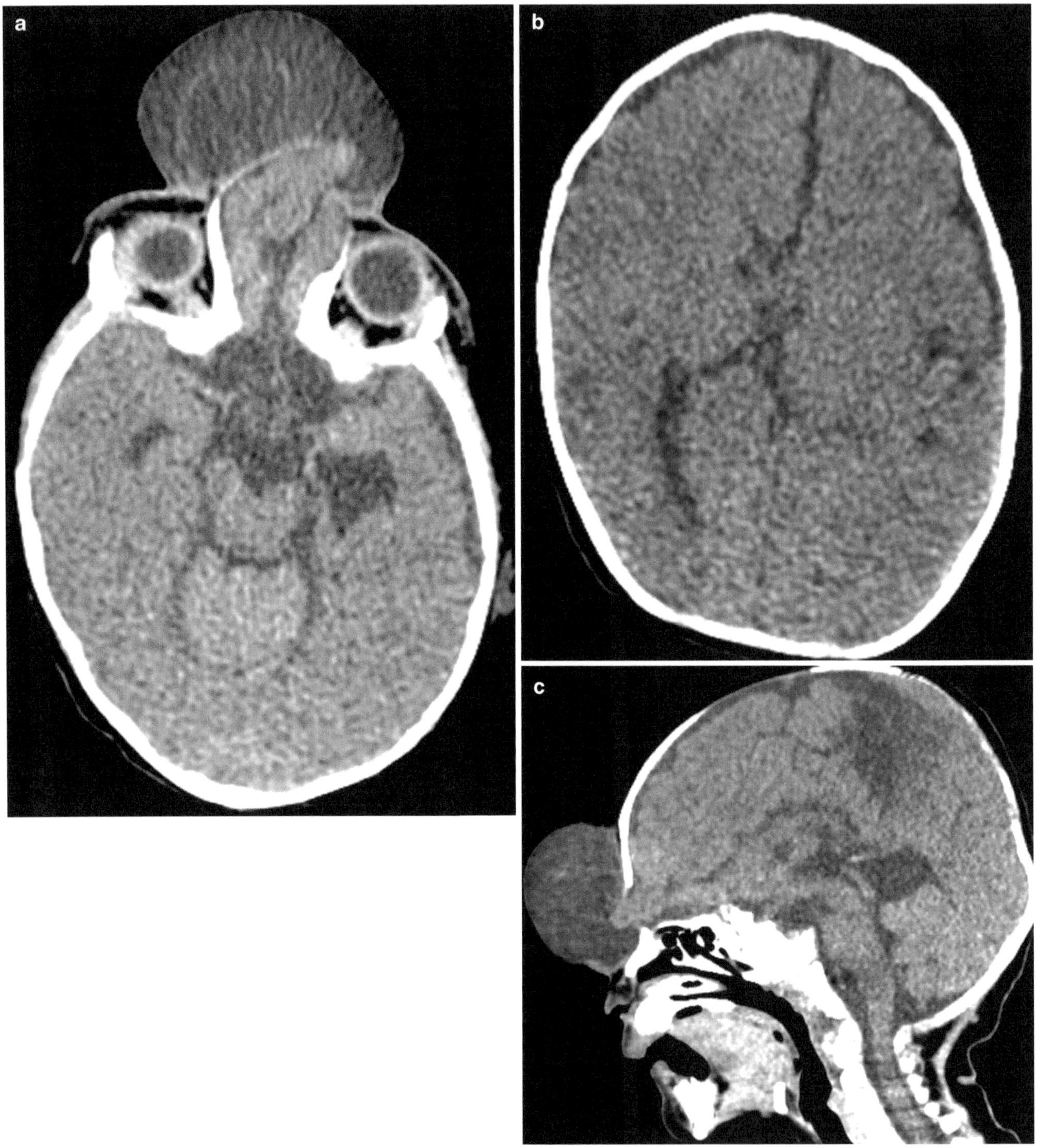

Fig. 13.1 Meningoencephalocele. Axial (**a**, **b**) CT scans and sagittal reformat (**c**) show an extracranial cystic mass in frontonasal area. There is a clearly visible protrusion of frontal lobe into the bone defect in frontonasal region. Axial CT scan (**c**) on the level of lateral ventricles reveals an agenesis of the corpus callosum also as a concomitant malformation

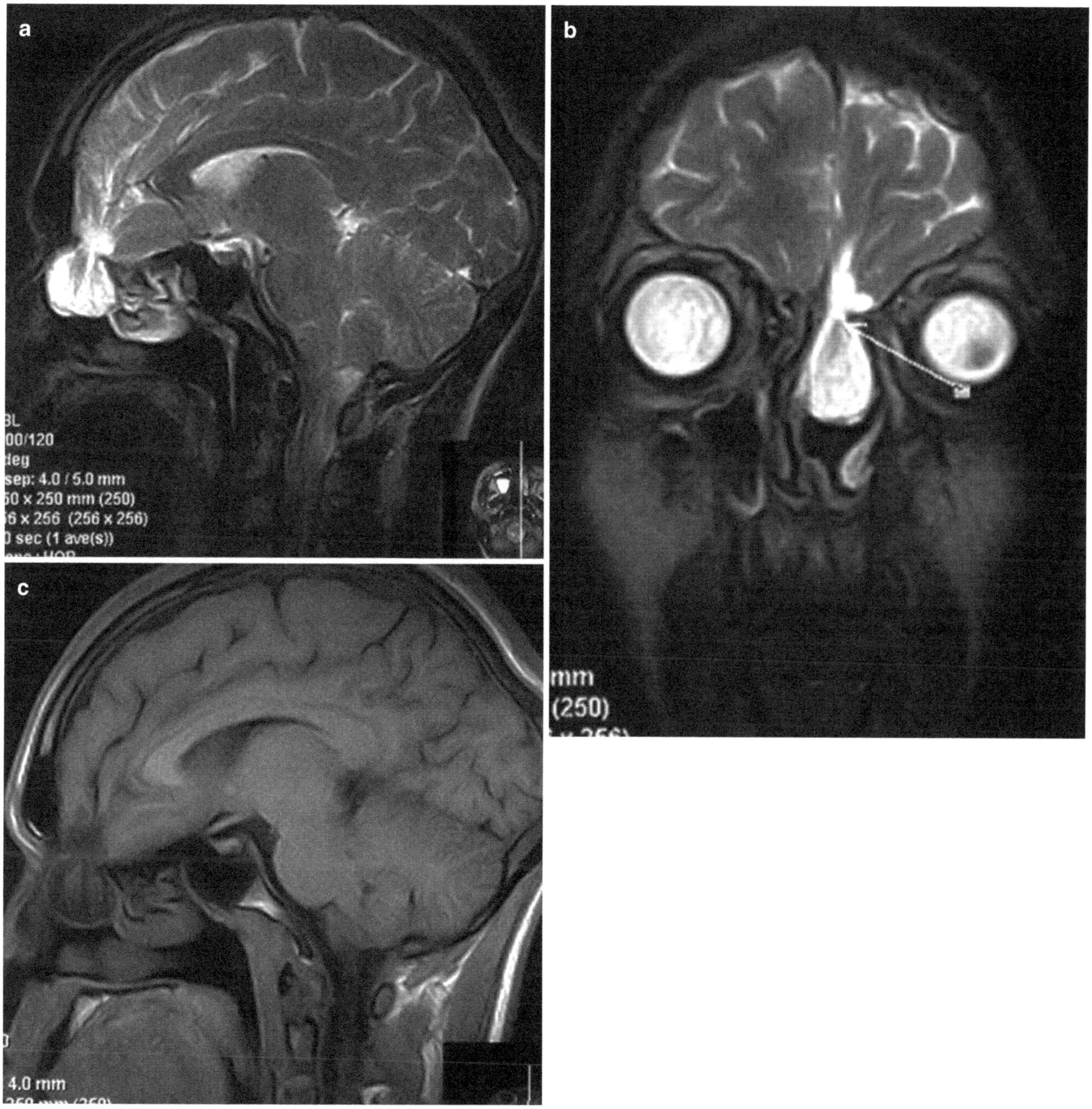

Fig. 13.2 Meningoencephalocele (naso-ethmoidal). Sagittal (**a**, **c**) and coronal (**b**) MRI with the use of T2- (**a**, **b**) and T1- (**c**) weighted slices demonstrates an expansile cystic mass with protrusion of meninges and brain tissue (partially) through the defect in the left part of anterior cranial fossa into the nasal cavity. High MR-signal on T2-WI can be seen due to the presence of CSF (predominantly) in the herniation sac

fast, the secondary osteogenic sarcoma, chondro- or fibrosarcoma should be differentiated. FD can be detected accidentally, when patients are treated for any other reason. It develops in people younger than 30 years old, often from 3 to 15 years old, in 75% of cases. There are monostotic and polyostotic forms of FD (Osborn et al. 2016).

Imaging CT picture is variable, consistent with the amount of fibrous tissue present in abnormal structures, but the main feature is repeating the bone contour, which makes the diagnosis more obvious. A classic CT-sign is the "ground-glass" effect and thickened bone. This is an expansile bone lesion with widened diploic space. FD may heterogeneously enhance, depending on the amount of fibrous tissue present. Bone changes can also be found around the foramina of the cranial nerves in the skull base, which are often displaced or narrowed, but are usually clearly identified (Figs. 13.3, 13.4, 13.5, 13.6 and 13.7).

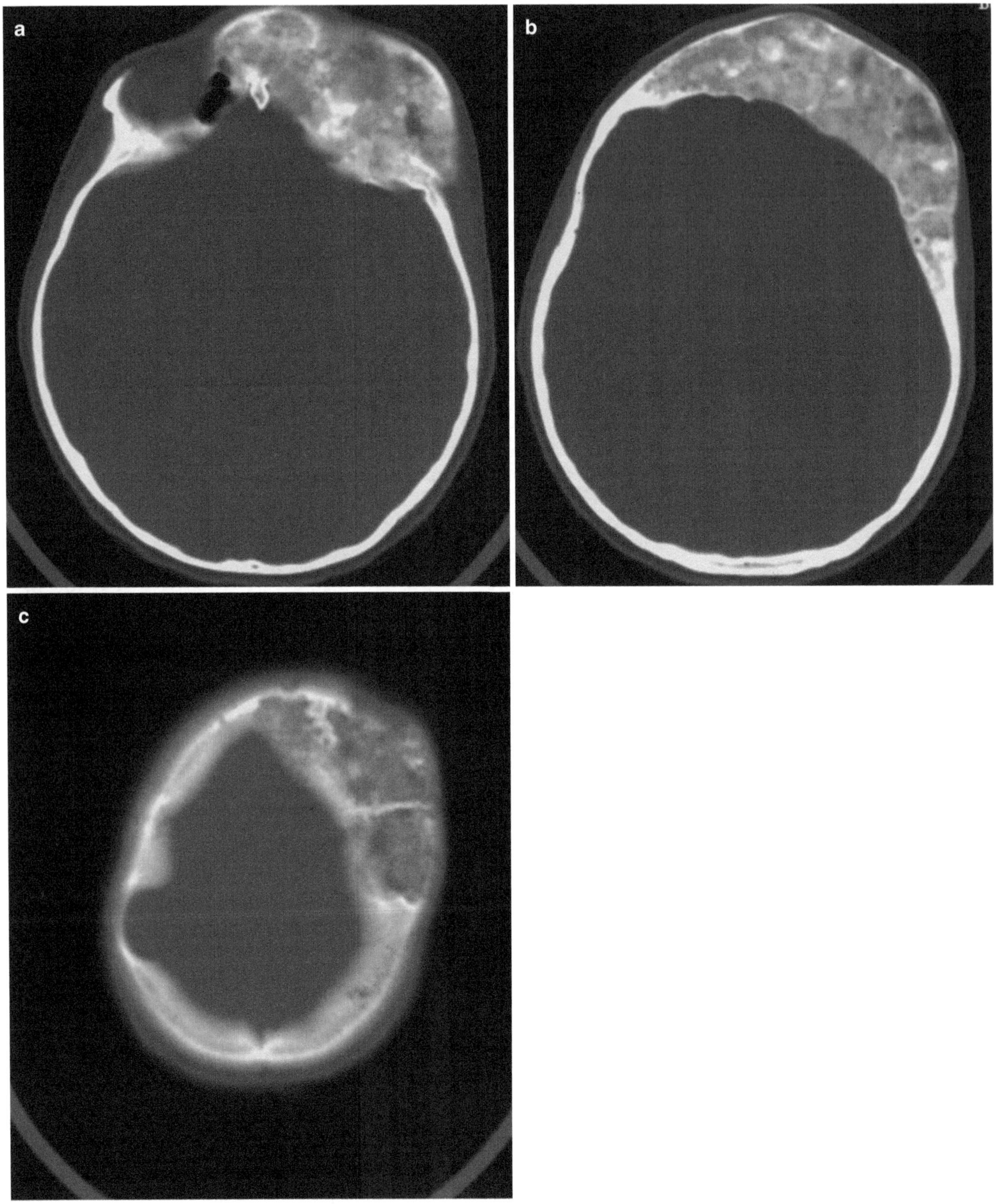

Fig. 13.3 Fibrous dysplasia. Axial CT scans (**a–c**) demonstrate a typical fibroosseous lesion with involvement of frontal, nasal, and ethmoid bones. The medullary cavity is expanded and there is good corticomedullary distinction

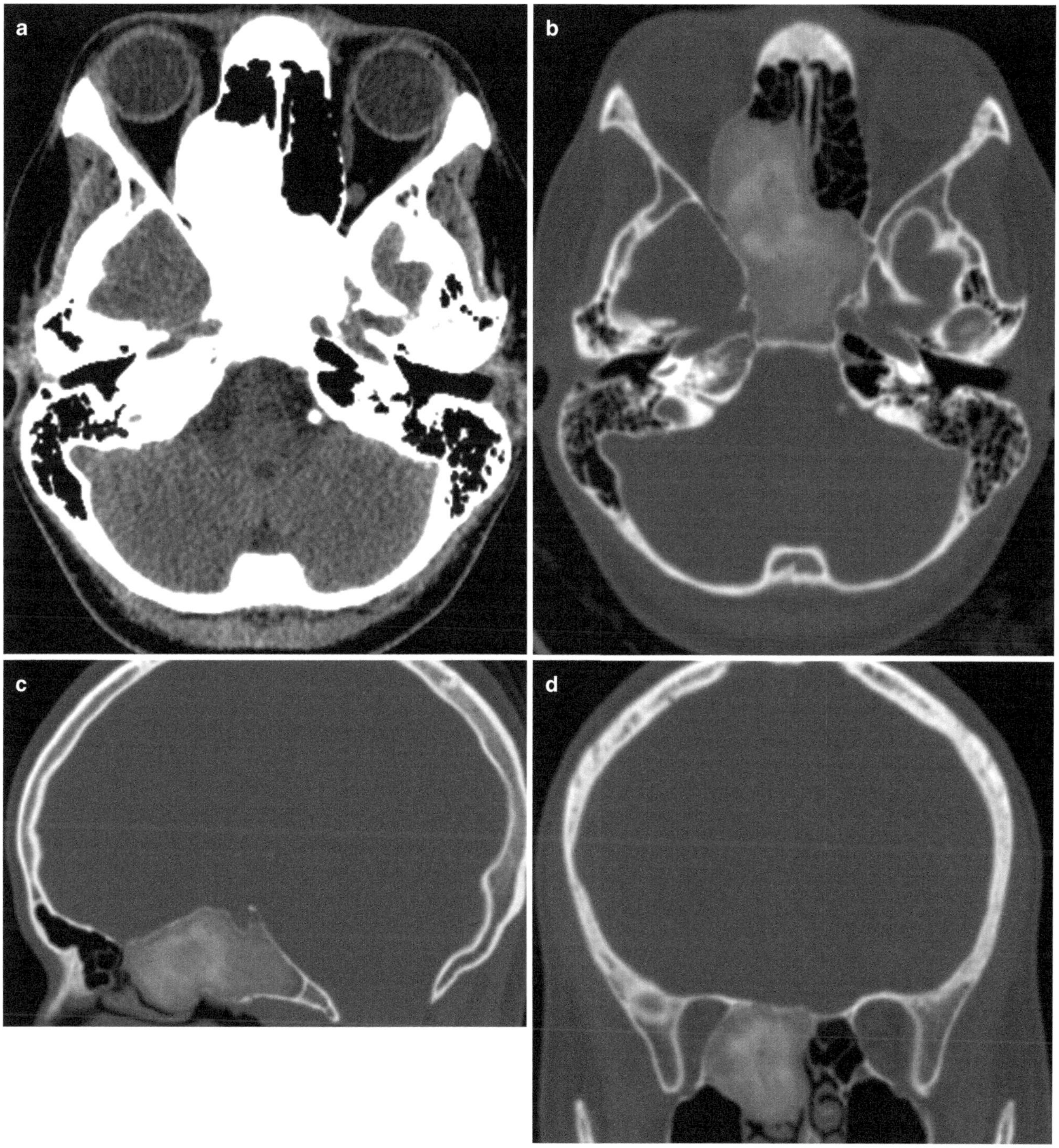

Fig. 13.4 Fibrous dysplasia. Axial CT scans (**a**, **b**) and sagittal (**c**), and coronal (**d**) reformats show a focal medullary mass with expanding ethmoid and sphenoid bones. There is a "ground glass" pattern. The medullary cavity is expanded and there is good corticomedullary distinction. (**e**) Histological specimen

Fig. 13.4 (continued)

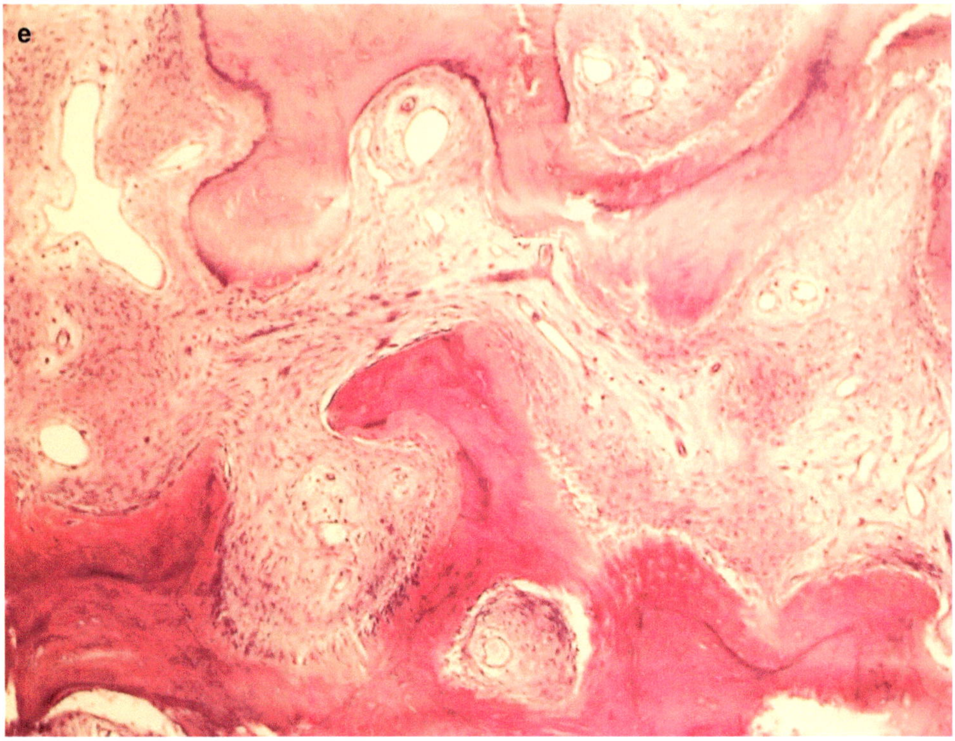

On T1-weighted MR images, this is an expansile, usually homogeneous bone lesion with an intermediate MR-signal intensity. On T2-weighted images, dense bony structures have low MR-signal, fibrous tissue or cysts produce hyperintensity and heterogeneity, small fragments of cartilage may also be present. Fibrotic component may intensely homogeneously or heterogeneously accumulate contrast material (Jee et al. 1996; Alawi 2002) (Fig. 13.8). But CT-perfusion demonstrates low perfusion parameters within osseous and fibrotic portions of the FD (Fig. 13.9).

Differential diagnosis:

1. Neo-osteogenesis—areas adjacent to the sites of surgery or chronic inflammation;
2. Ossifying fibroma is a solitary lesion with clear contours, bone density at the periphery and soft tissue density in the center;
3. Osteoma is a solitary, well-defined focal lesion with bone density.

Dermoid cyst (D) develops due to inclusion of cutaneous ectoderm at the time of neuronal tube closure or sequestration of surface ectoderm at the time of epithelial fusion along course of normal embryonic invagination. Dermoids contain squamous epithelium, keratinous material, and skin appendages (sweat glands, hair follicles, sebaceous glands). Dermoids are very rare and represent less than 0.5% of all intracranial tumors. They are often found in the 2nd and 3rd decades of life. Most frequently Ds are found in the lumbar spine, parasellar region, at the base of ACF and PCF (Barsi et al. 1992; Gupta et al. 1993; Roeder et al. 1995). Almost all Ds are localized at the midline, have the same CT and MR characteristics as fat due to the high cholesterol content (epidermoids contain solid cholesterol and, therefore, are hypointense on T1-WI) (Gupta et al. 1993; Castillo 2002). They may be complicated by "chemical" meningitis if rupture and spill their contents into the subarachnoid space (Barsi et al. 1992; Roeder et al. 1995). Midline lipomas are difficult to differentiate from Ds (Fig. 13.10). In cases with infectious complications Ds can enhance on the periphery and being difficult distinguished from malignant tumors (Fig. 13.11).

Epidermoid cyst (EC) (cholesteatoma) grows from the embryonic ectodermal elements, with their intracranial inclusion during neuronal tube closure. They occur ten folds more frequently than intracranial dermoid cysts. Epidermoids may contain epithelial remnants, but no dermal appendages. Most epidermoids are found in early adulthood. They grow very slowly. Most ECs are asymptomatic, but in case of a large size they may cause mass effect, compress the cranial nerves and rarely to be a cause of epileptic seizures. The most common EC sites are: cerebellopontine angle cisterns

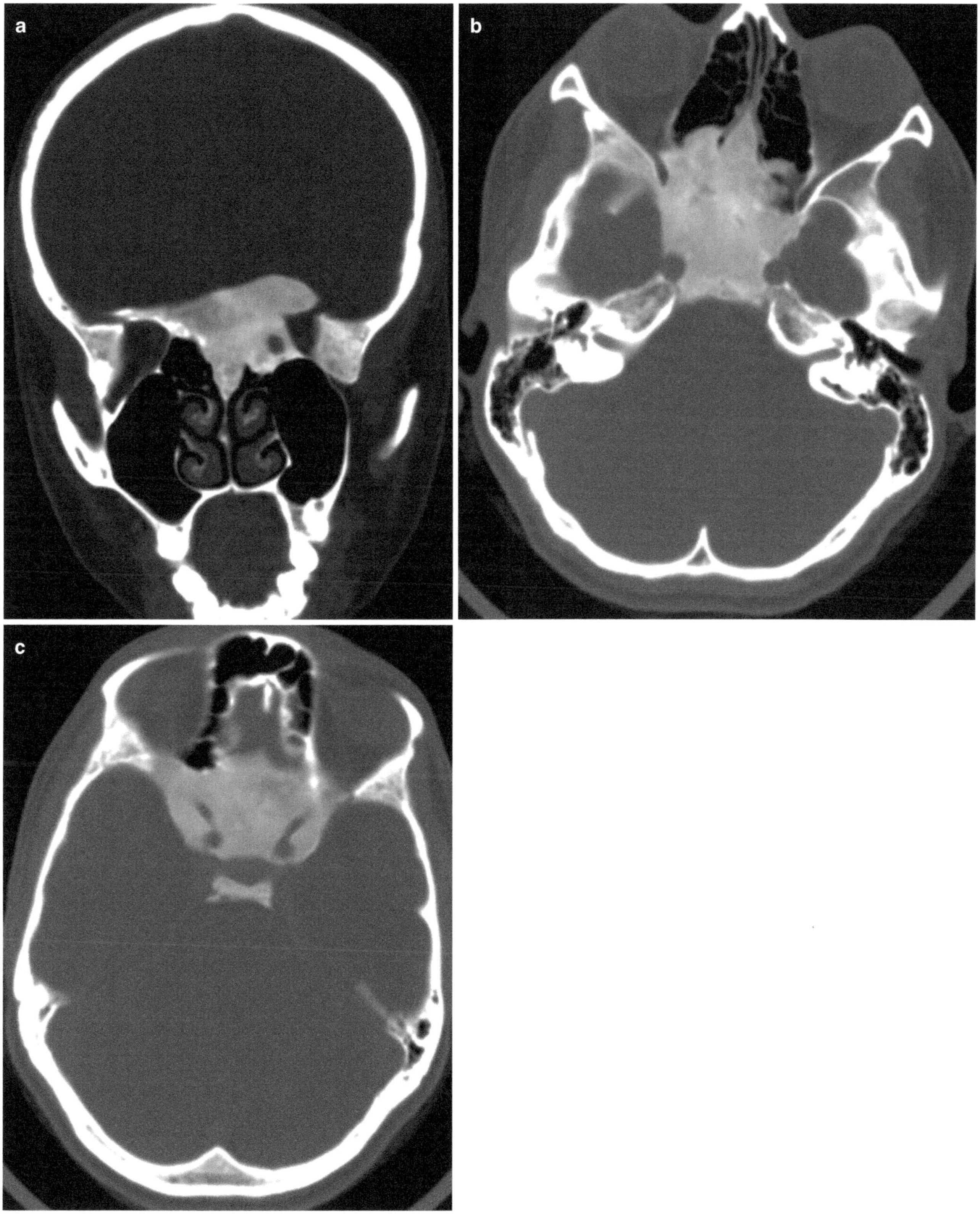

Fig. 13.5 Fibrous dysplasia of the sphenoid bone. Coronal (**a**) and axial (**b**, **c**) CT scans demonstrate a focally expanded sphenoid bone mass with typical "ground glass" appearance. Both optic canals are involved

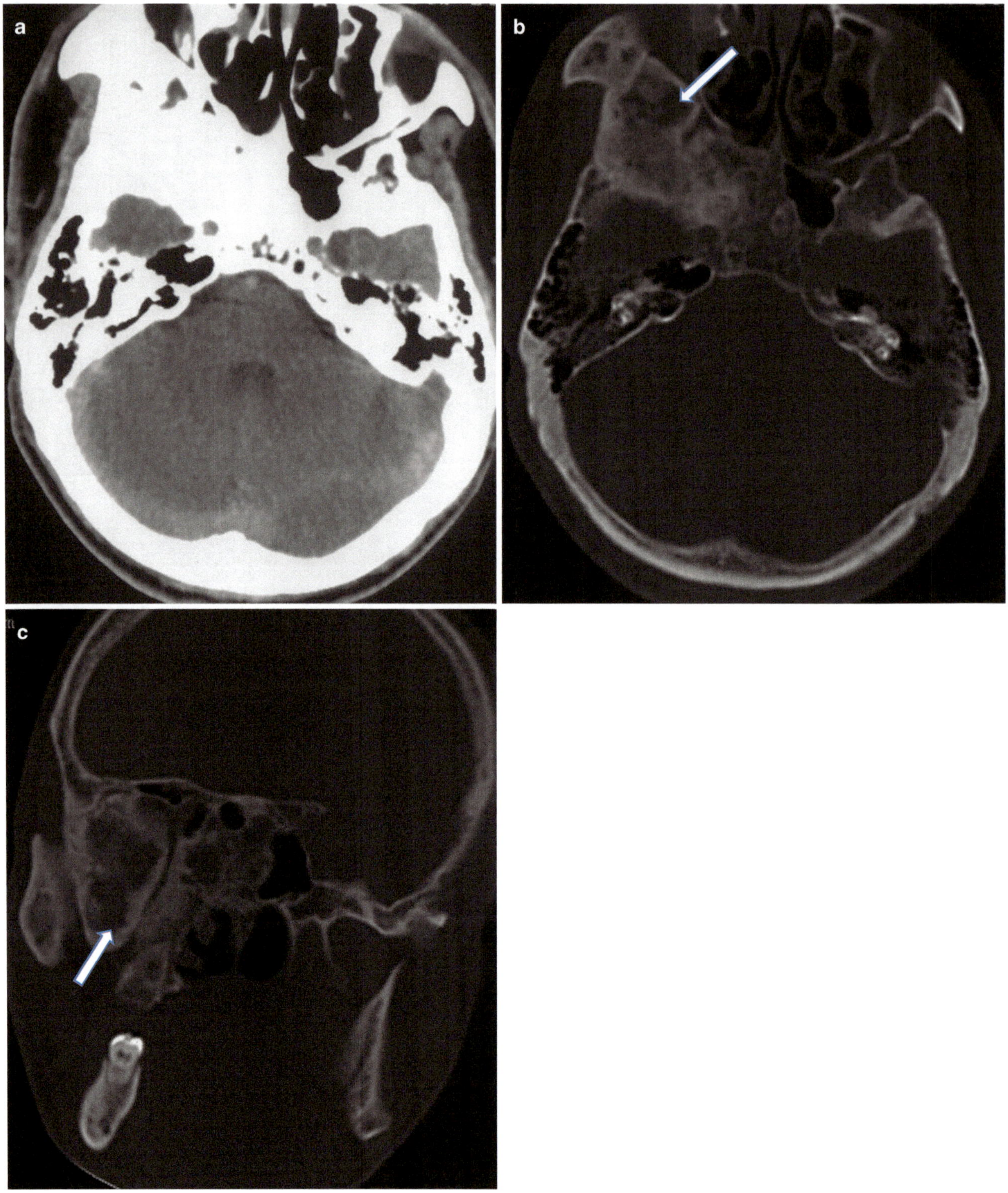

Fig. 13.6 Fibrous dysplasia of the craniofacial area. Axial (**a**, **b**) and coronal (**c**) CT images show a fibroosseous lesion with involvement of right medial cranial fosse base and sphenoid-ethmoid complex. An area of soft tissue CT-density from the central fibrous part of the dysplasia (*arrows*) can be seen

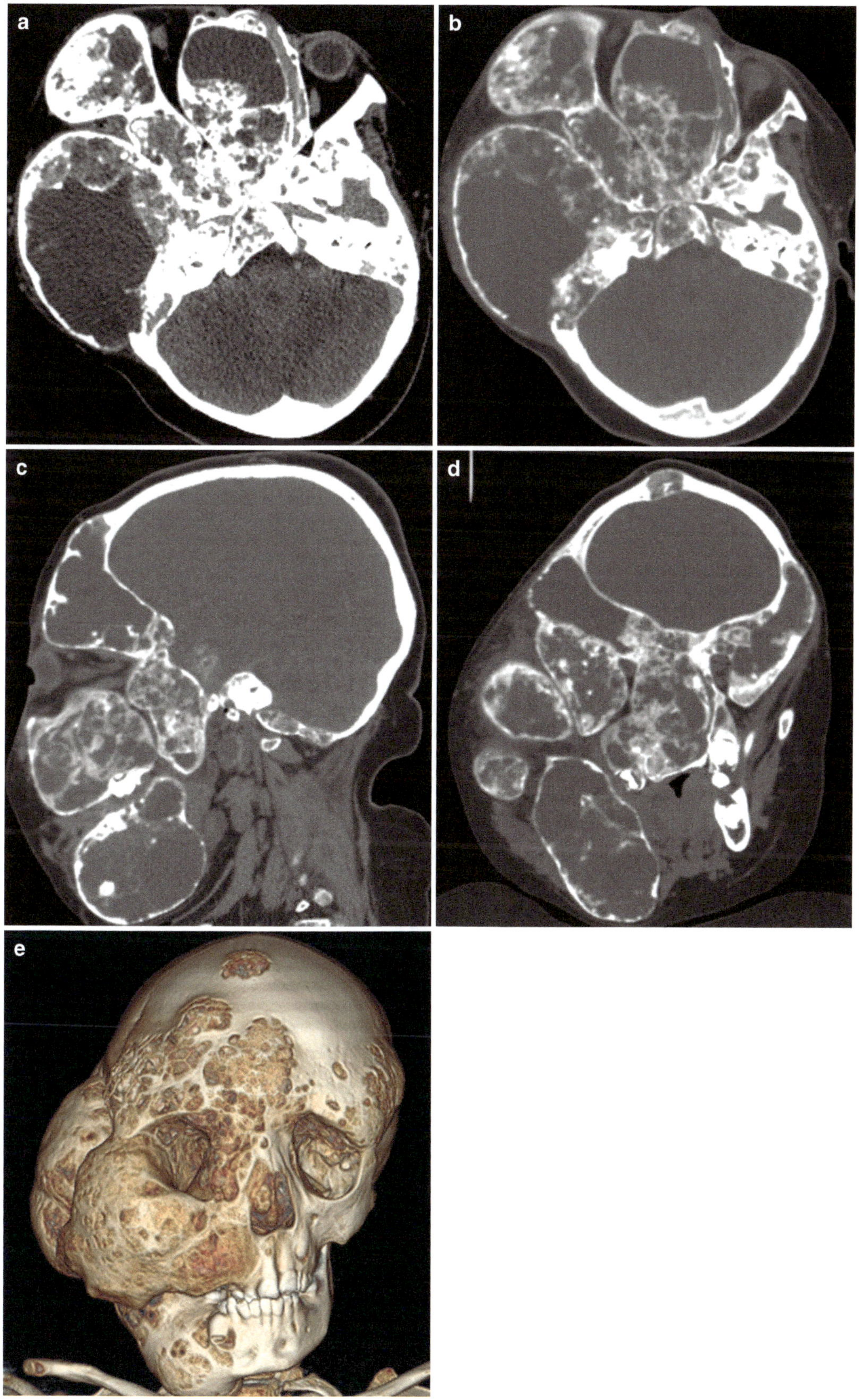

Fig. 13.7 Fibrous dysplasia. Axial CT scans (**a**, **b**) and sagittal (**c**), coronal (**d**) reformats as well as 3D reconstruction (**e**) show that all right-side facial and skull base bones are greatly expanded with intact cortices. The medullary spaces in these areas are filled with ossified and nonossified components. Some of bones demonstrate the cystic transformation

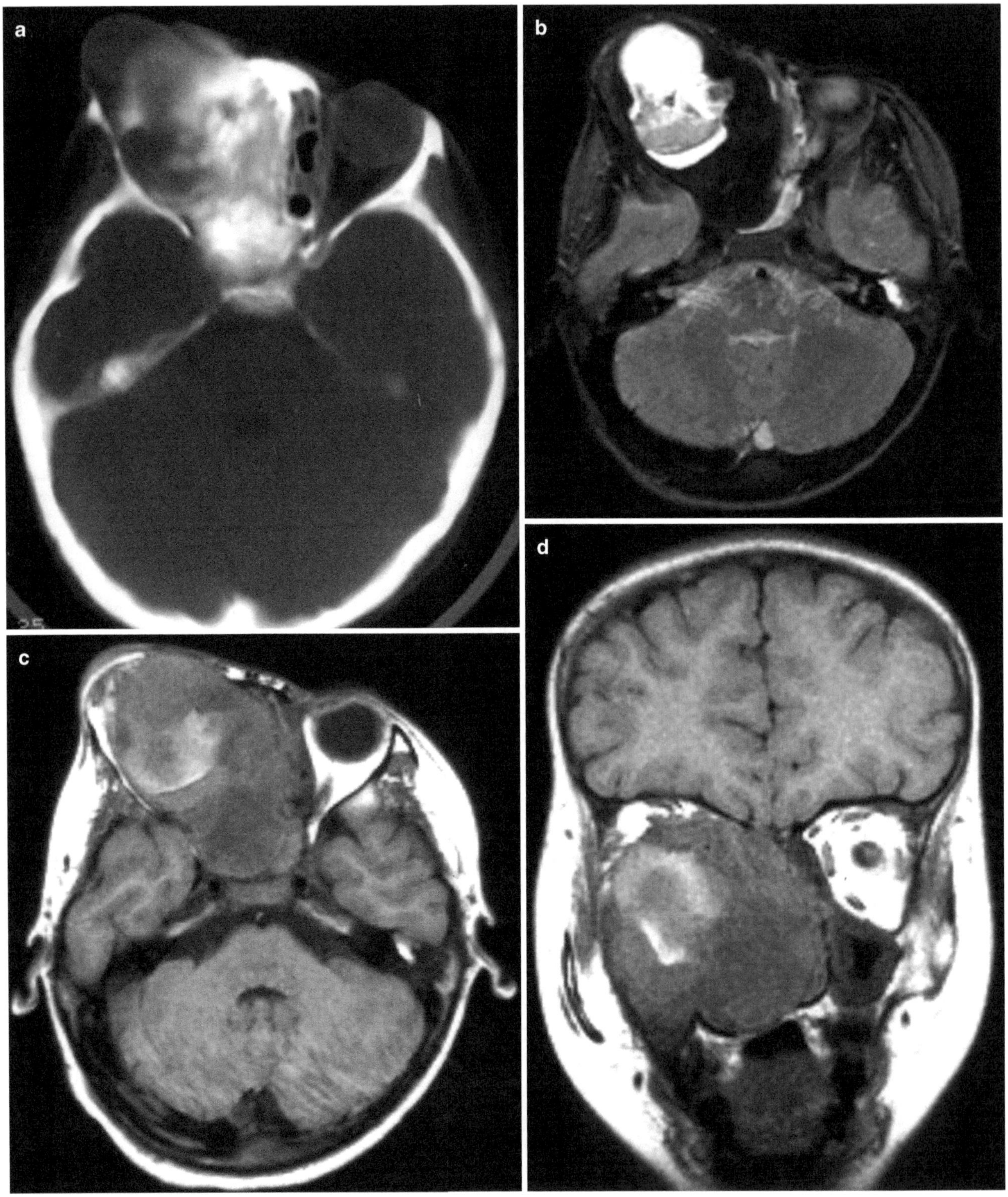

Fig. 13.8 Fibrous dysplasia of the right craniofacial region. Axial CT scan (**a**) shows a fibroosseous lesion with involvement of sphenoid-ethmoid complex, right orbit and maxilla. On T2-weighted (**b**) and T1-weighted MR images in axial (**c**) and coronal (**d**) planes the heterogeneous area of hypo- and hyperintensity is revealed (dark MR-signal from osseous and bright MR-signal from fibrous components). The intense inhomogeneous contrast enhancement of the fibrous component of dysplasia can be seen (**e**, **f**)

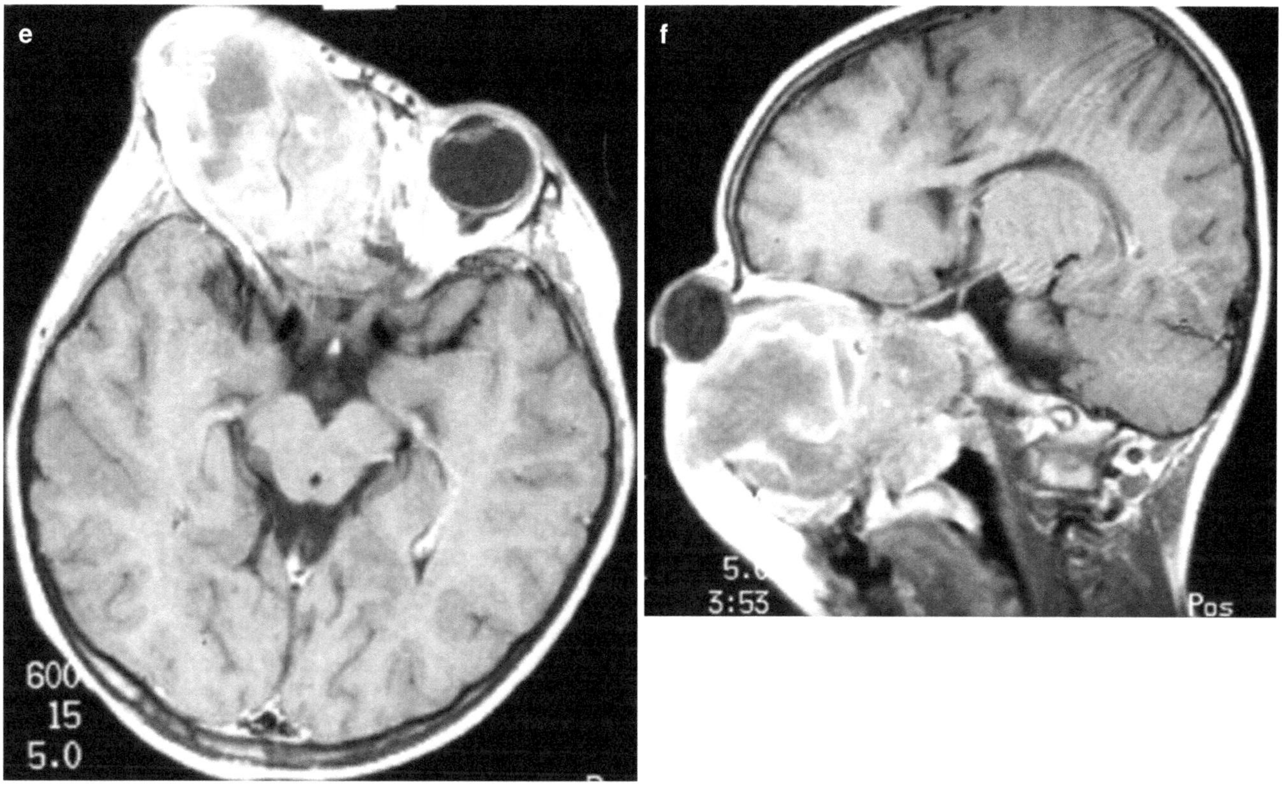

Fig. 13.8 (continued)

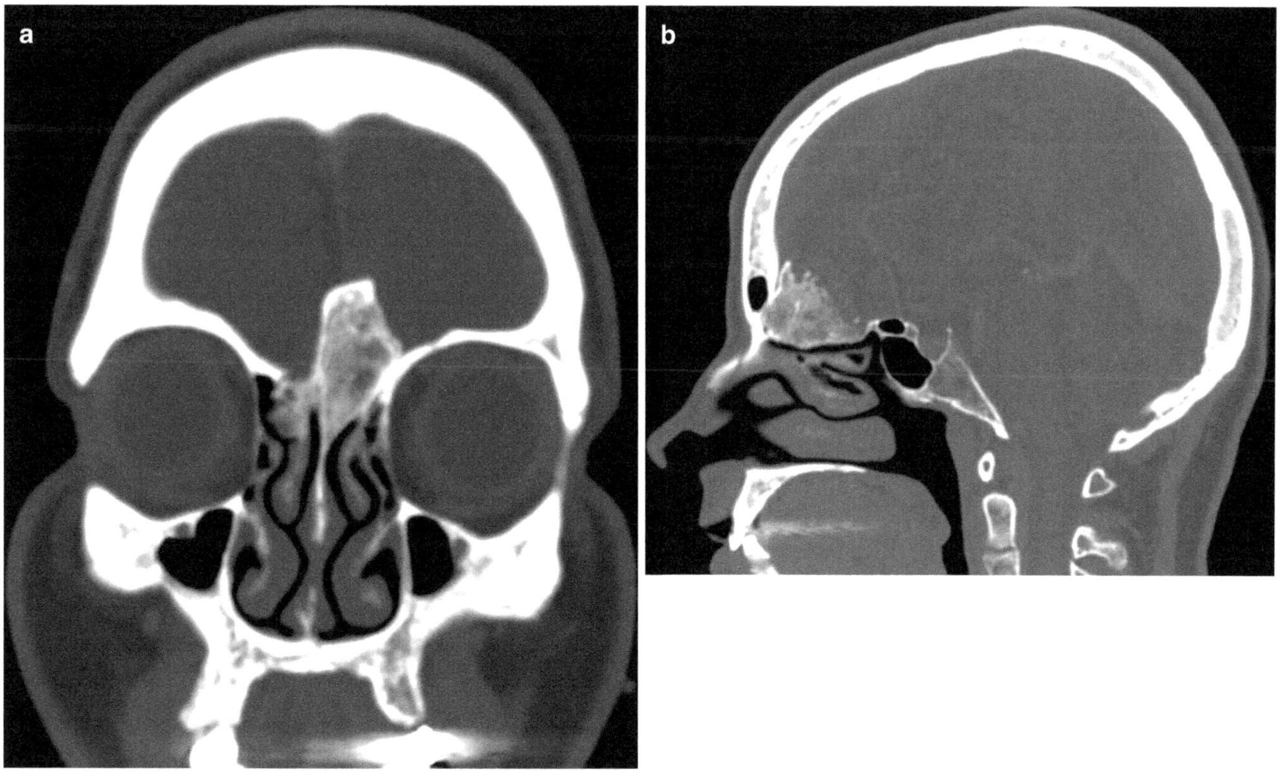

Fig. 13.9 Fibrous dysplasia. Coronal (**a**) and sagittal (**b**) CT reformats show a focal fibroosseous lesion with involvement of upper ethmoids, floor of the anterior cranial fossa and crista galli. There is a good corticomedullary distinction. CT-perfusion demonstrates low perfusion parameters (CBF map (**c**), PS map (**d**)) within osseous and fibrotic portions of the lesion. On T2 (**e**–**g**)-weighted images a lesion has a heterogeneous hypointense MR-signal with dark rim due to cortical bone. T1(**h**)- and T1 + fat-sat (**i**) weighted images demonstrate fat-contained mass without obvious contrast enhancement (**j**–**l**)

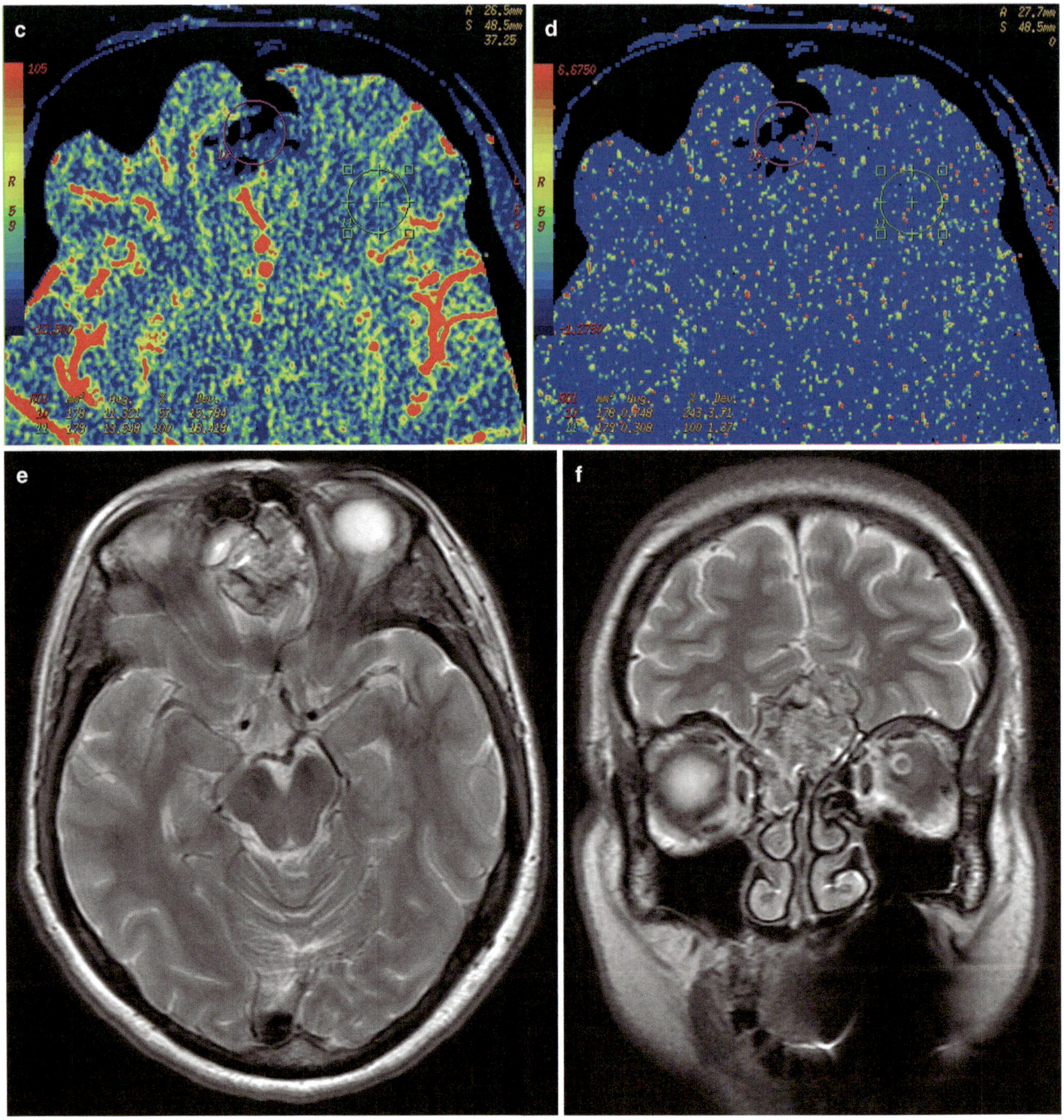

Fig. 13.9 (continued)

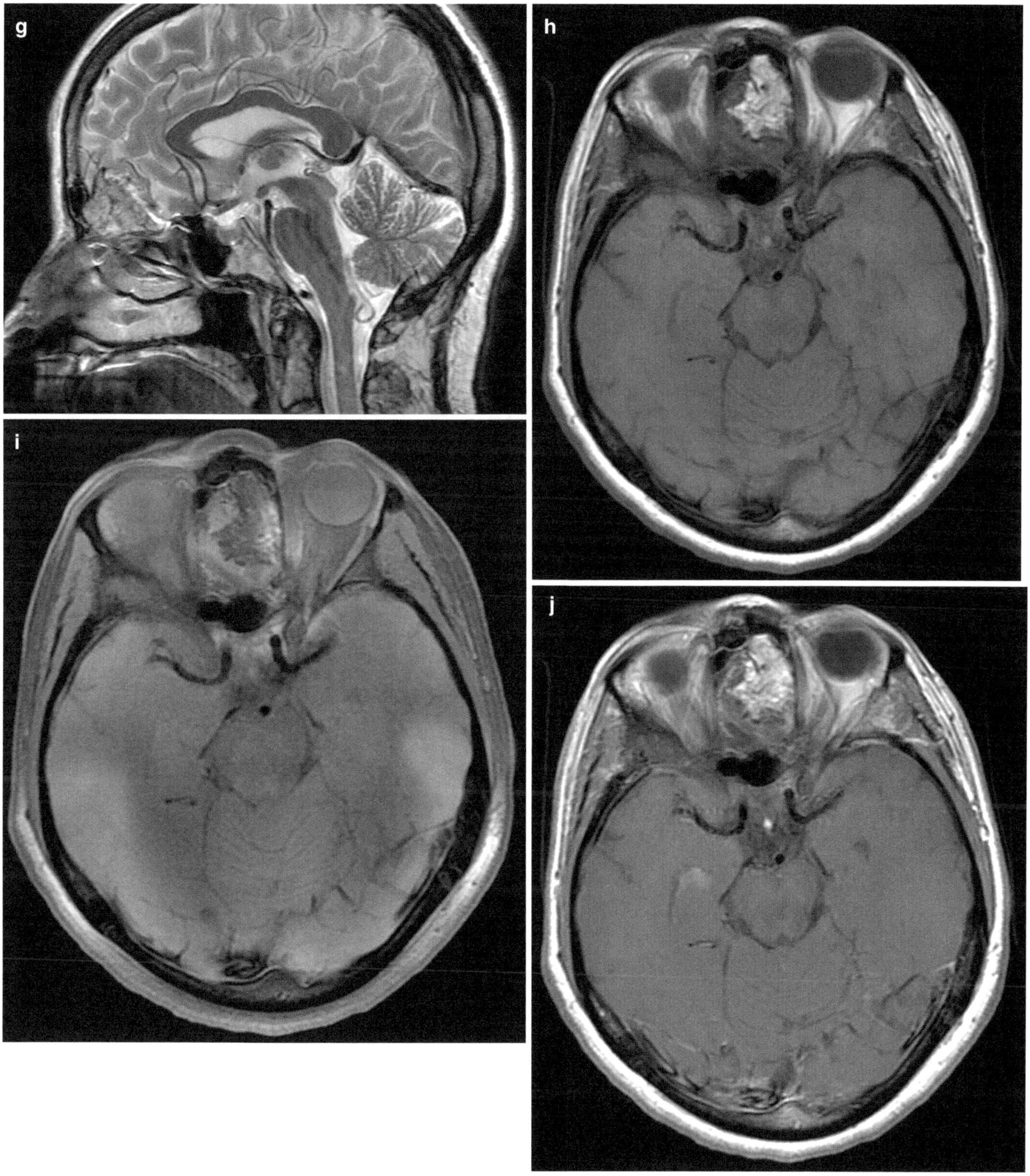

Fig. 13.9 (continued)

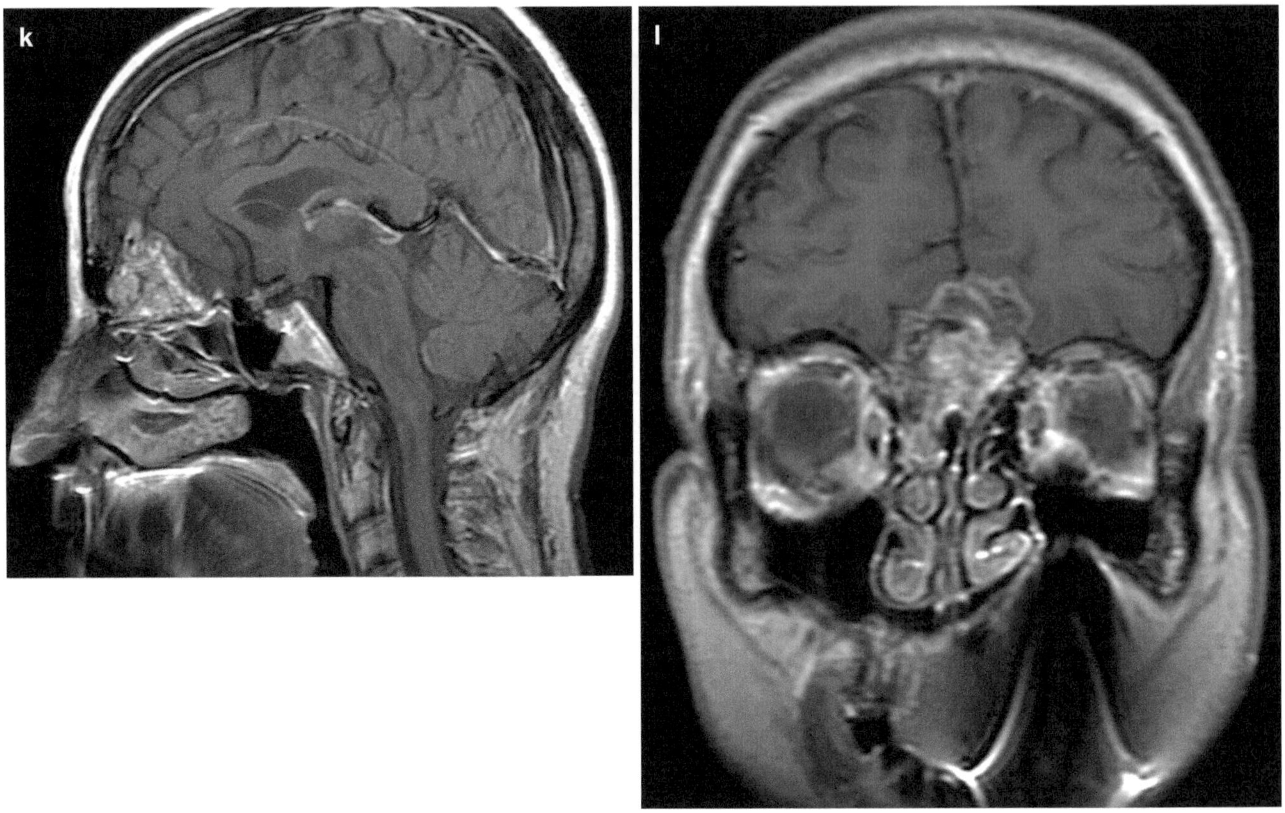

Fig. 13.9 (continued)

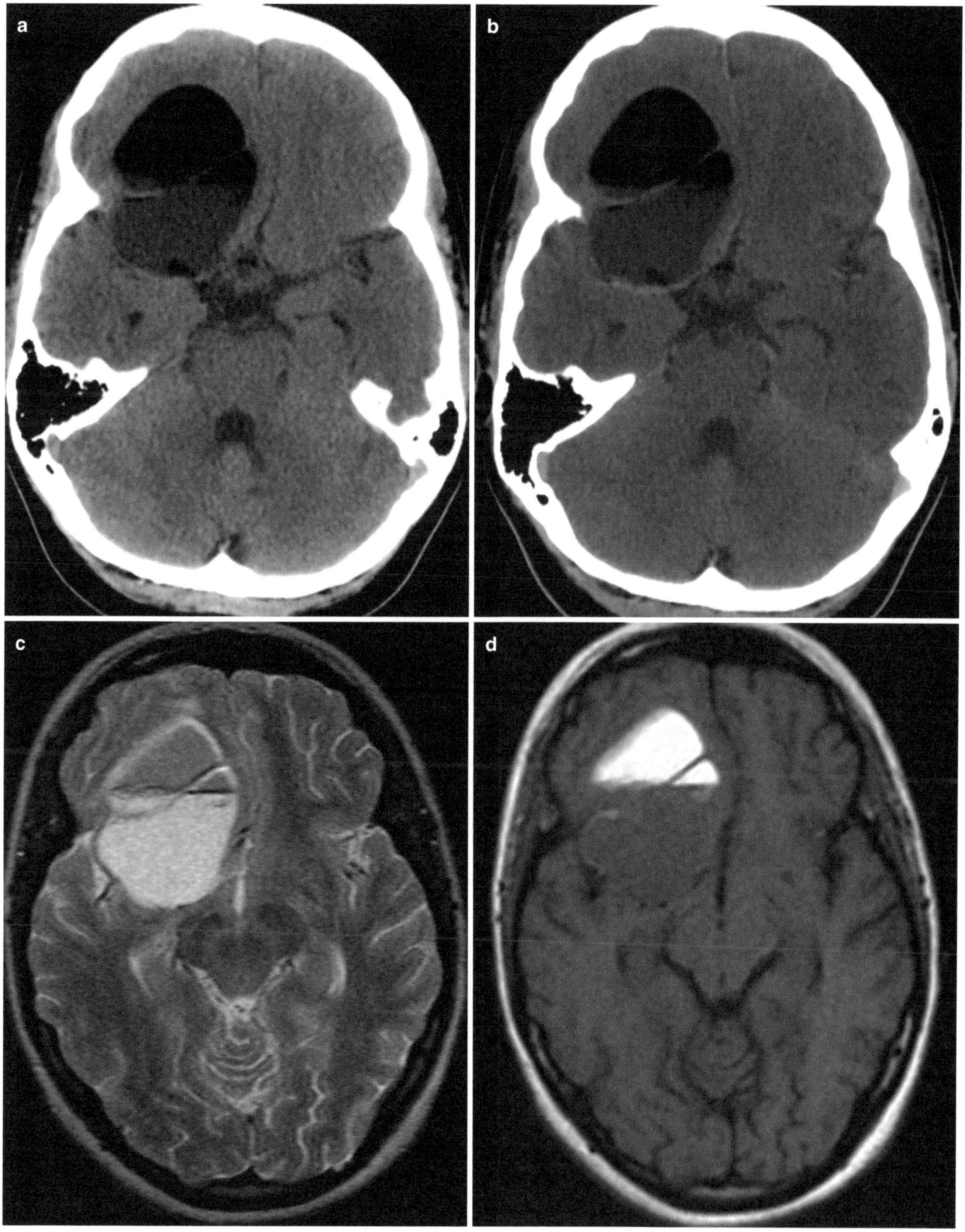

Fig. 13.10 Dermoid cyst of the right frontal region. Axial CT scans before (**a**) and after (**b**) contrast enhancement demonstrate a large heterogeneous hypodense (−60 HU) mass in the right frontal area without obvious contrast enhancement. Within the lesion the fat-fluid level in the middle can be seen. On T2- (**c**) and T1- (**d**, **e**)-weighted images a fat has a bright MR-signal on T1. After changing position of the patient from "back to face" (T1-WI (**f**)) a fat is moved to the "upper sections" of the cyst

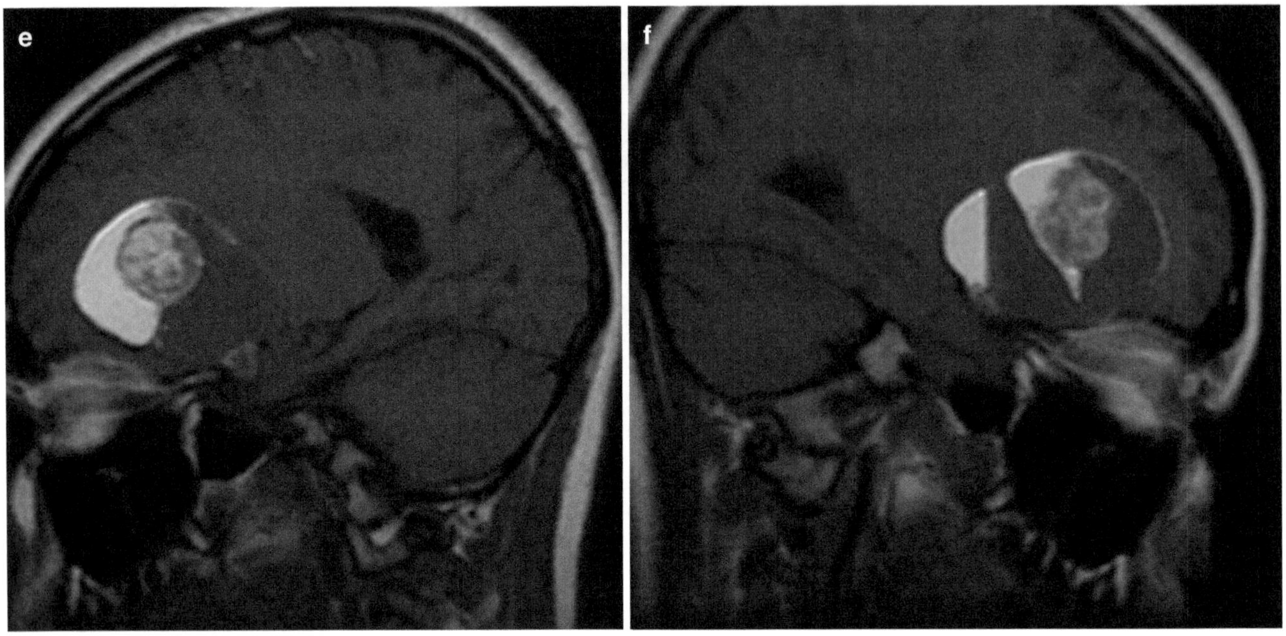

Fig. 13.10 (continued)

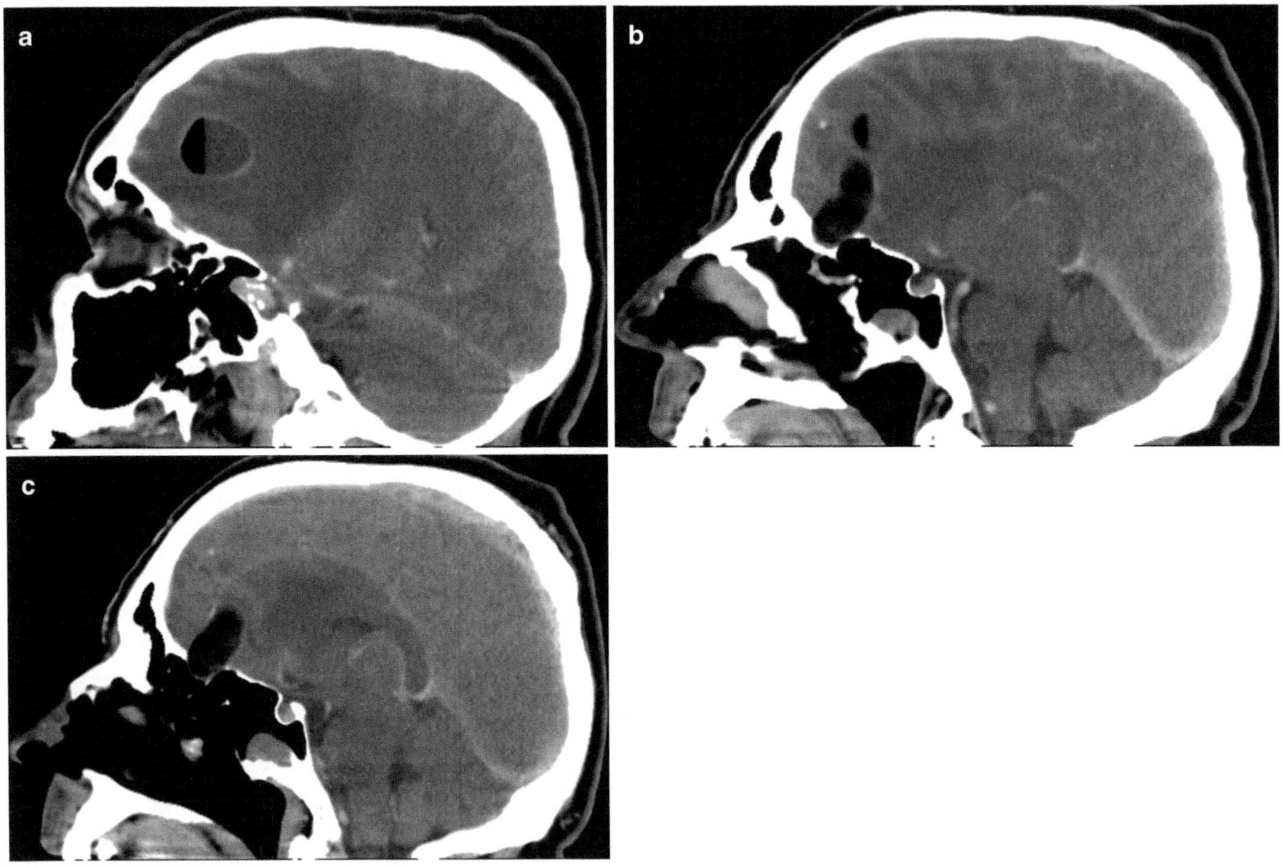

Fig. 13.11 Dermoid cyst of the right frontal region with inflammation. Contrast-enhanced series of sagittal CT reformats (**a**–**c**) demonstrate a large hypodense lesion in projection of right frontal lobe arising from the base of anterior cranial fossa. In the upper part of the lesion the fluid–fluid level sign can be seen. There is a thin rim of contrast enhancement around superior cystic lesion and ring-like elevation of blood volume parameters on the CT-perfusion mapping (**d**), simulating the malignant tumor. The dermoid cyst causes of extensive perifocal edema brain tissue. MR imaging with using T2- (**e**), T1- (**f**) and diffusion- (**g**) weighted sequences demonstrates fat-contained mass in right frontal lobe surrounding with perifocal edema. There is no restriction diffusion within the lesion. Contrast-enhanced MR-study in axial (**h**, **i**), sagittal (**k**, **i**), and coronal (**l**) planes shows hyperintense mass of unusual shape with peripheral contrast enhancement. Phenomena of sedimentation (fat-fluid level) within superior cystic lesion is clearly visible as well

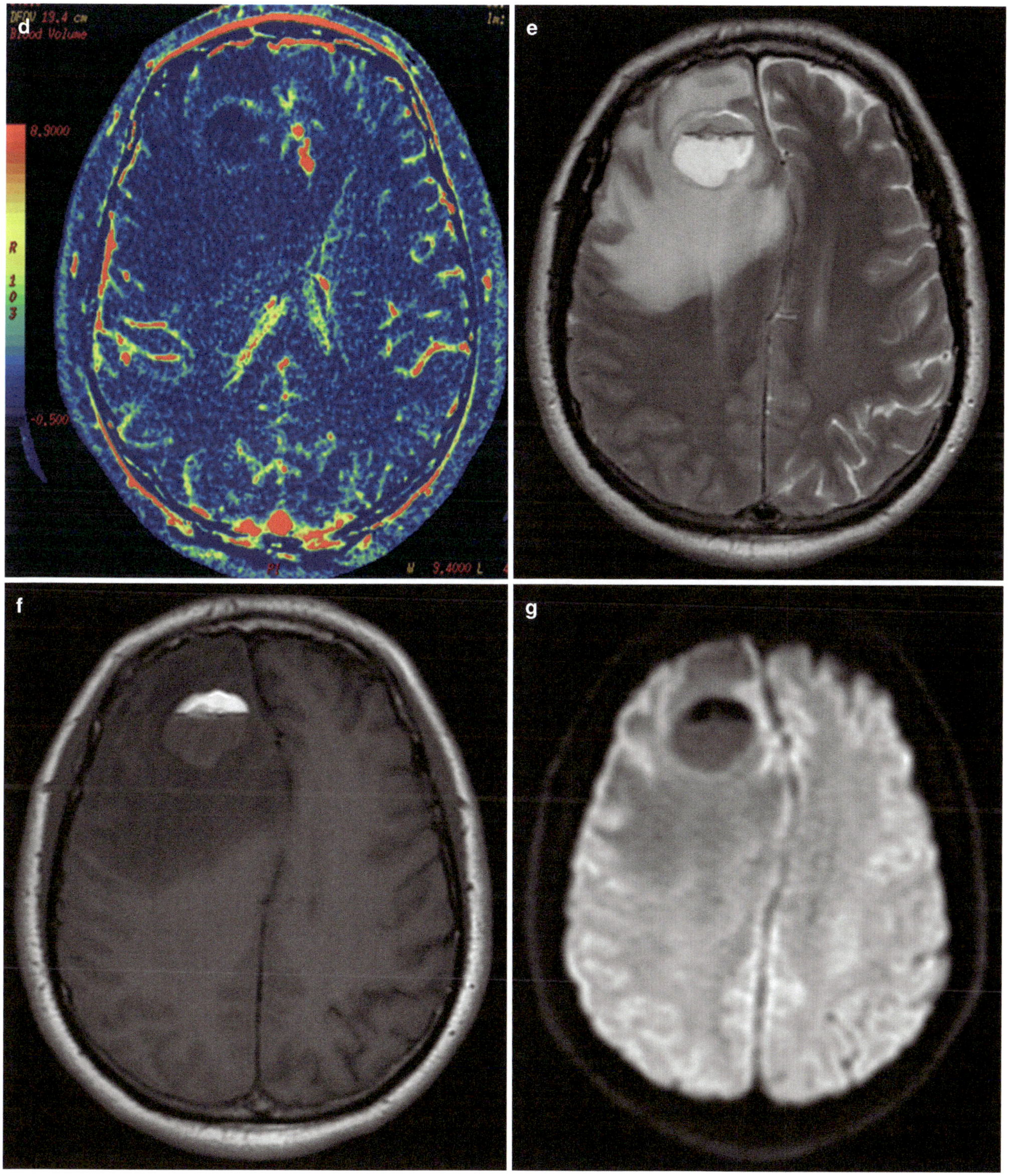

Fig. 13.11 (continued)

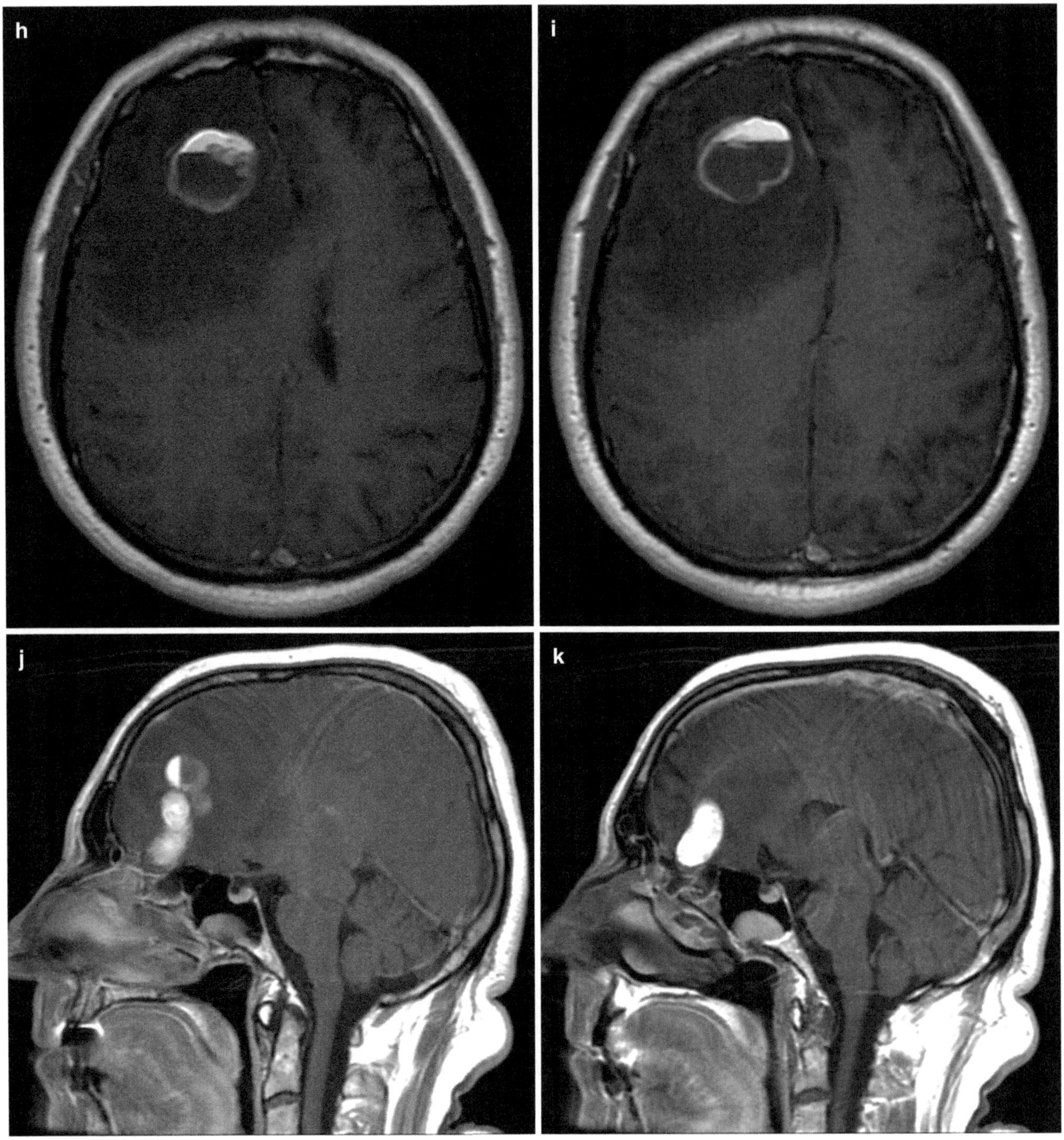

Fig. 13.11 (continued)

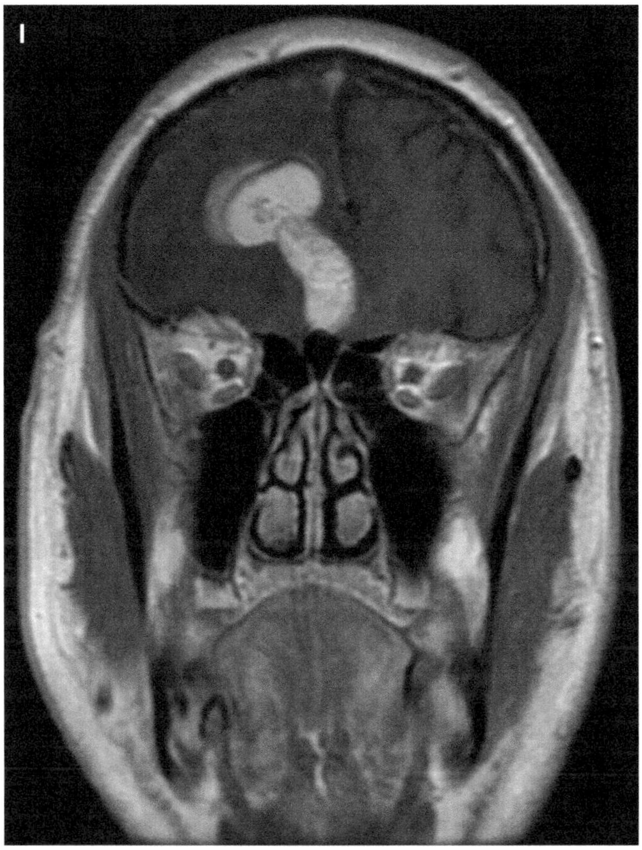

Fig. 13.11 (continued)

(50%), sellar and parasellar region (10–15%), fourth ventricle (17%), and prepontine cistern. All ECs are localized outside the midline (Tampieri et al. 1989; Castillo 2002). ECs can also be detected in the diploic layer of the skull (10%), extending the bone, with sharply cortical edges.

Imaging On MRI and CT, epidermoids may look similar to arachnoid cysts, and routine MRI sequences often fail to distinguish between these lesions. However, epidermoids are usually slightly hyperintense on T1- and T2-FLAIR-weighted sequences than arachnoid cysts. ECs may also contain areas of heterogeneous MR-signal intensity (although CSF pulsation in the arachnoid cyst can also produce heterogeneity of MR-signal). In some cases, MR-signal from ECs may be higher to the brain, due to the presence of a high protein, triglycerides and fatty acids content within the cystic lesion. The leading role in the diagnosis of epidermoids plays DWI: most epidermoids have a hyperintense MR-signal compared to CSF (Tsuruda et al. 1990; Kallmes et al. 1997) (Figs. 13.12 and 13.13). Epidermoids can show minimal peripheral contrast enhancement (in capsule) in some cases, complicating the differential diagnosis with other intracranial lesions. Also, the *differential diagnosis* is performed with arachnoid cysts, parasitic cysts, cystic tumors, dermoid cysts.

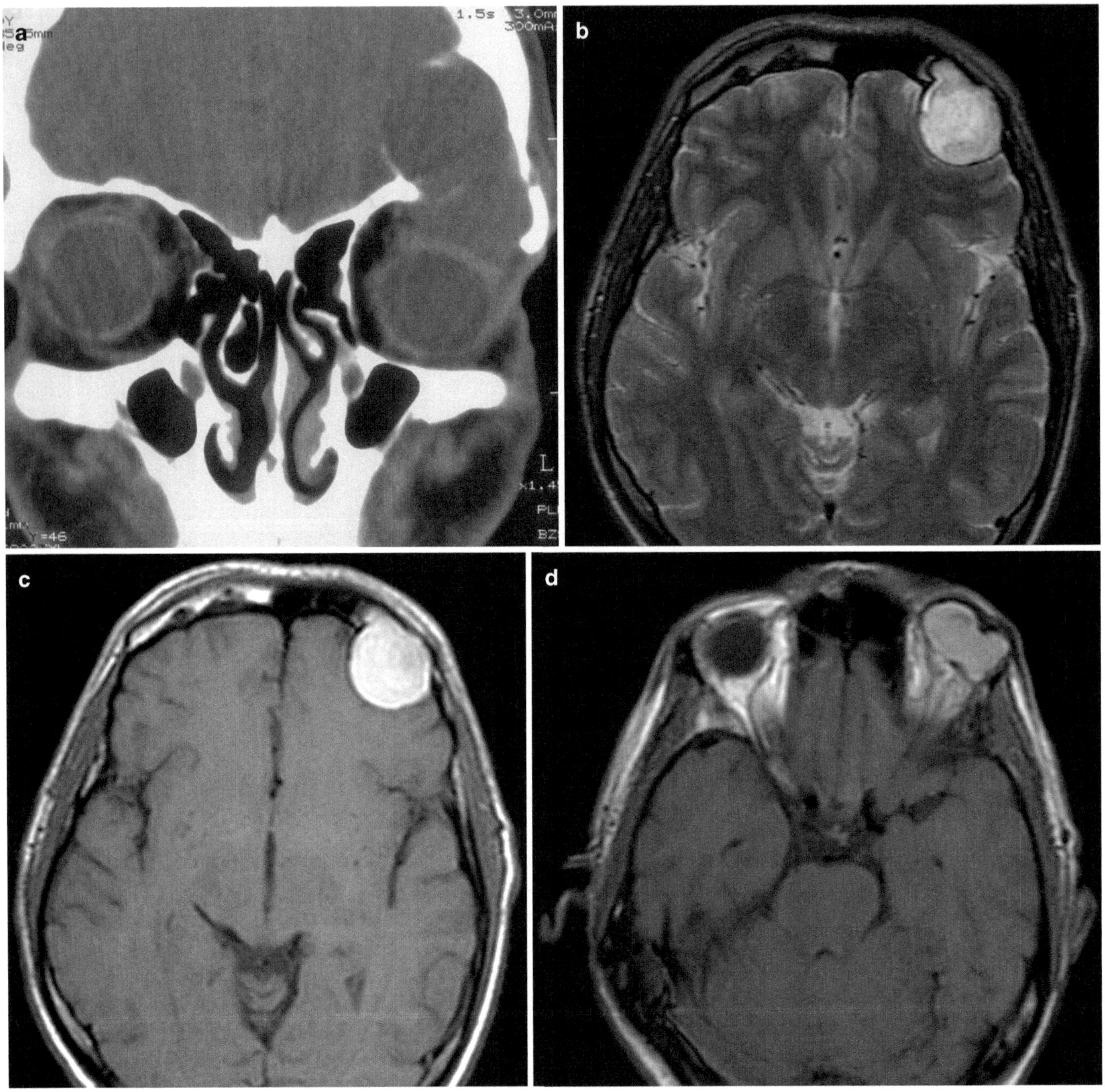

Fig. 13.12 Epidermoid cyst of the left fronto-orbital region. Coronal CT scan (**a**) shows an expansile hypodense mass in projection of orbital roof spreading intracranially. Series MR imaging with using T2- (**b**) and T1- (**c**– **e**) weighted scans demonstrates a hyperintense lesion with bone remodel. DWI defines a high MR-signal from the cyst (**f**)

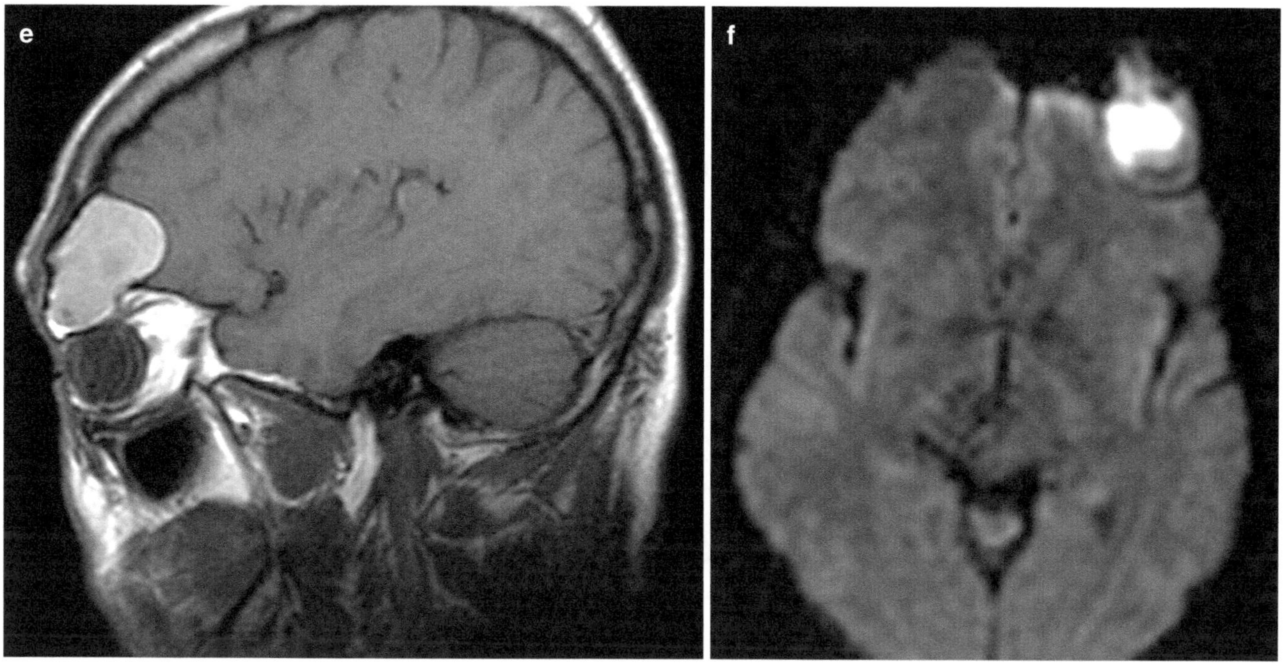

Fig. 13.12 (continued)

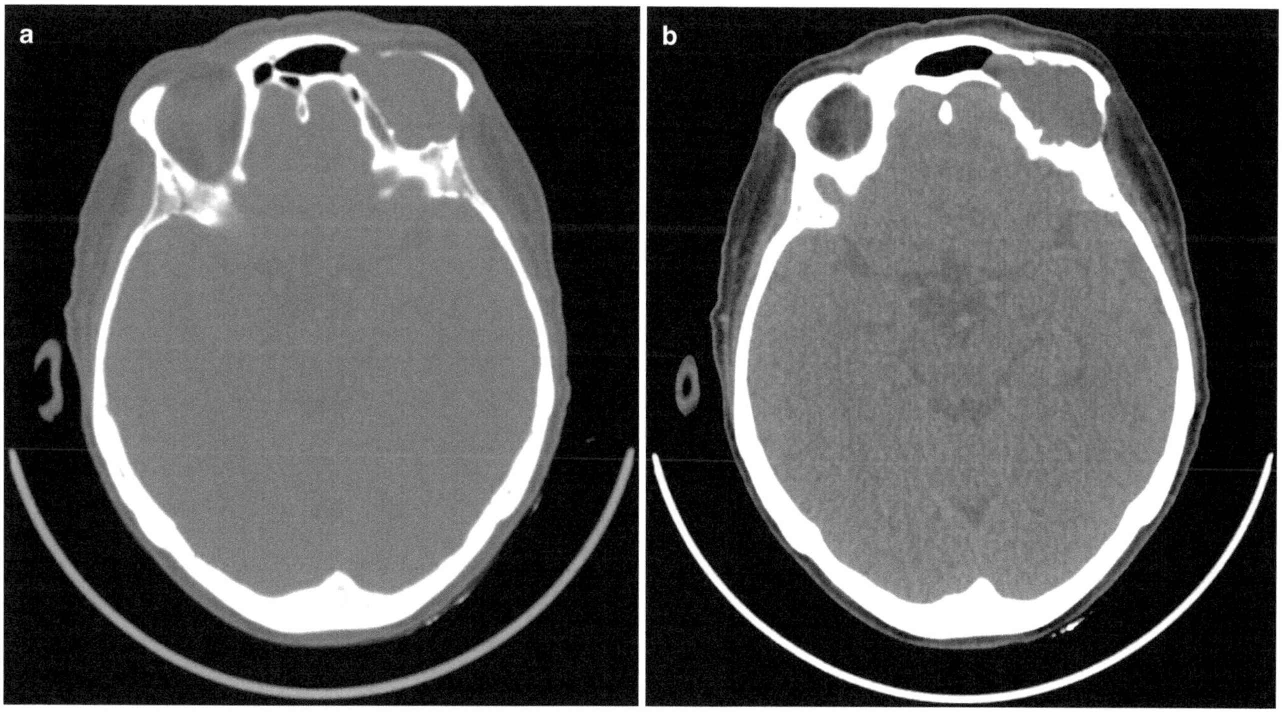

Fig. 13.13 Epidermoid cyst of the left fronto-orbital region. Axial CT scans before (**a**) and after (**b**–**e**) contrast enhancement show an expansile hypodense mass in projection of orbital roof and frontal bone spreading into frontal sinus. There is surrounding bone remodel and no enhancing within the lesion. Series MR scans with using T2 (**f**), T2-FLAIR (**g**), and T1-(**h**) weighted sequences demonstrate a hyperintense heterogeneous lesion with bone remodel. DWI defines a high MR-signal from the cyst (**i**) typical sign for epidermoid cyst

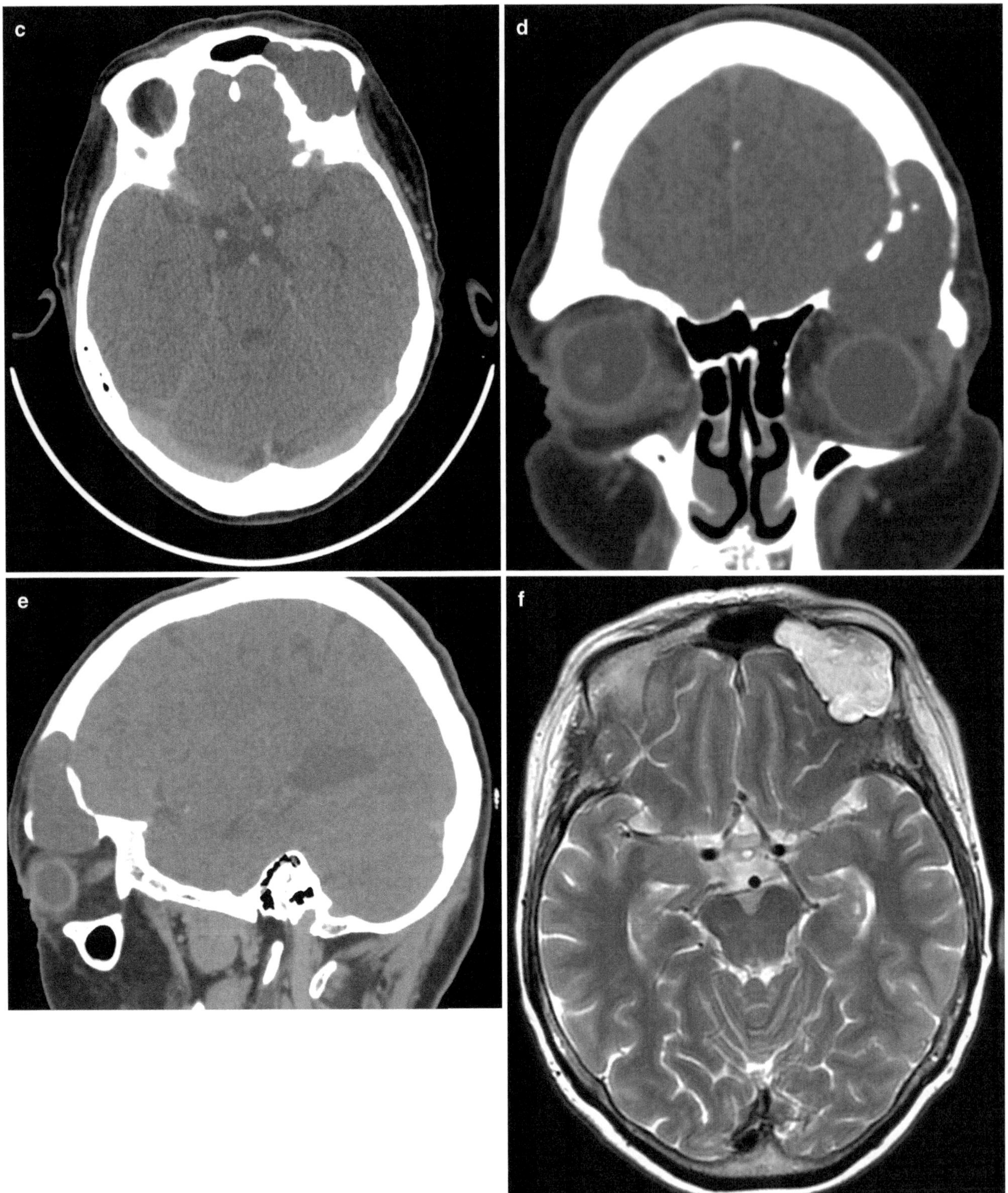

Fig. 13.13 (continued)

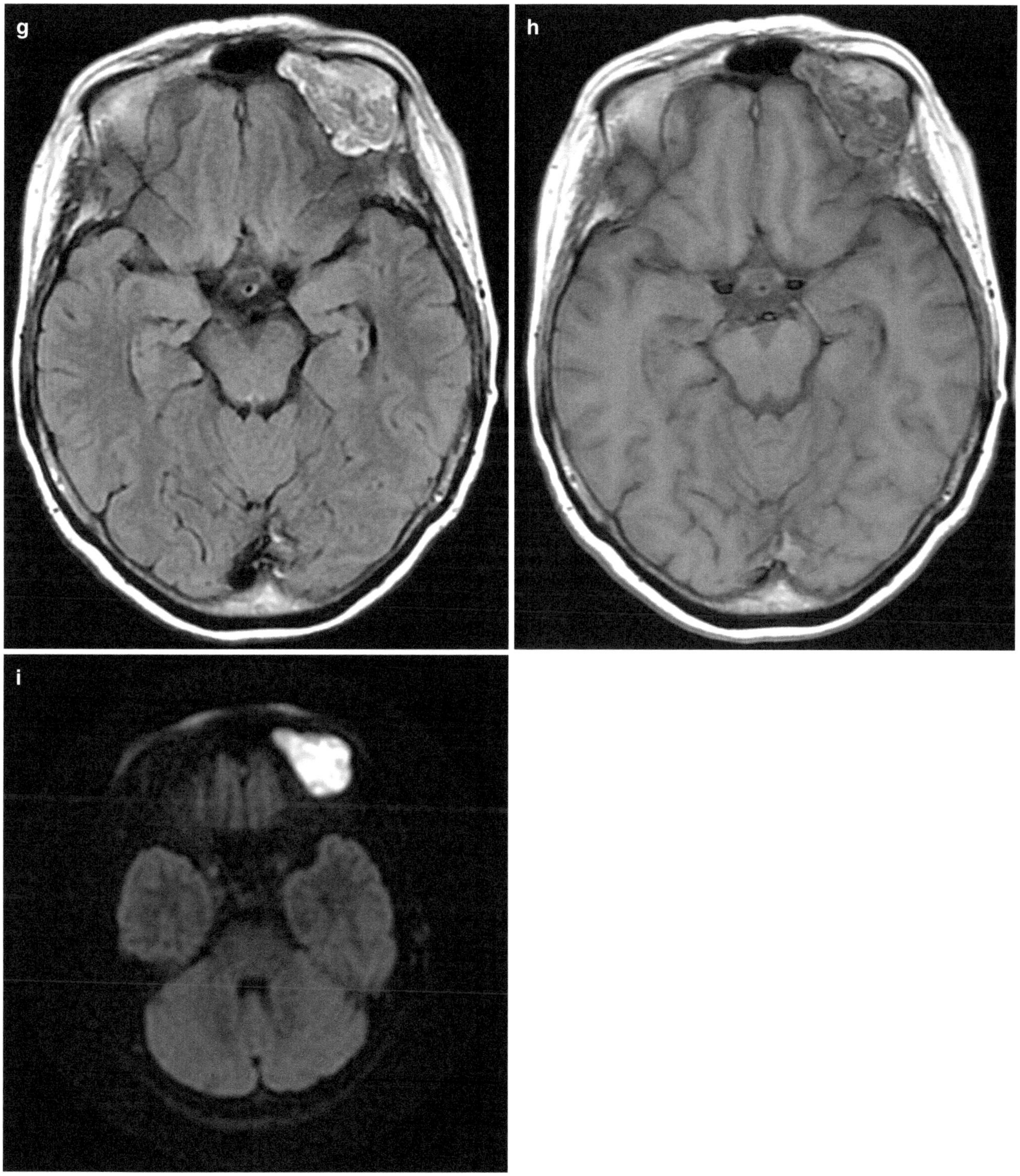

Fig. 13.13 (continued)

Presentation of Rare Cases of Anterior Cranial Fossa and Craniofacial Region Lesions

14

Contents

I. Pronin, V. Kornienko, *CT and MRI of Skull Base Lesions*, https://doi.org/10.1007/978-3-319-65957-2_14

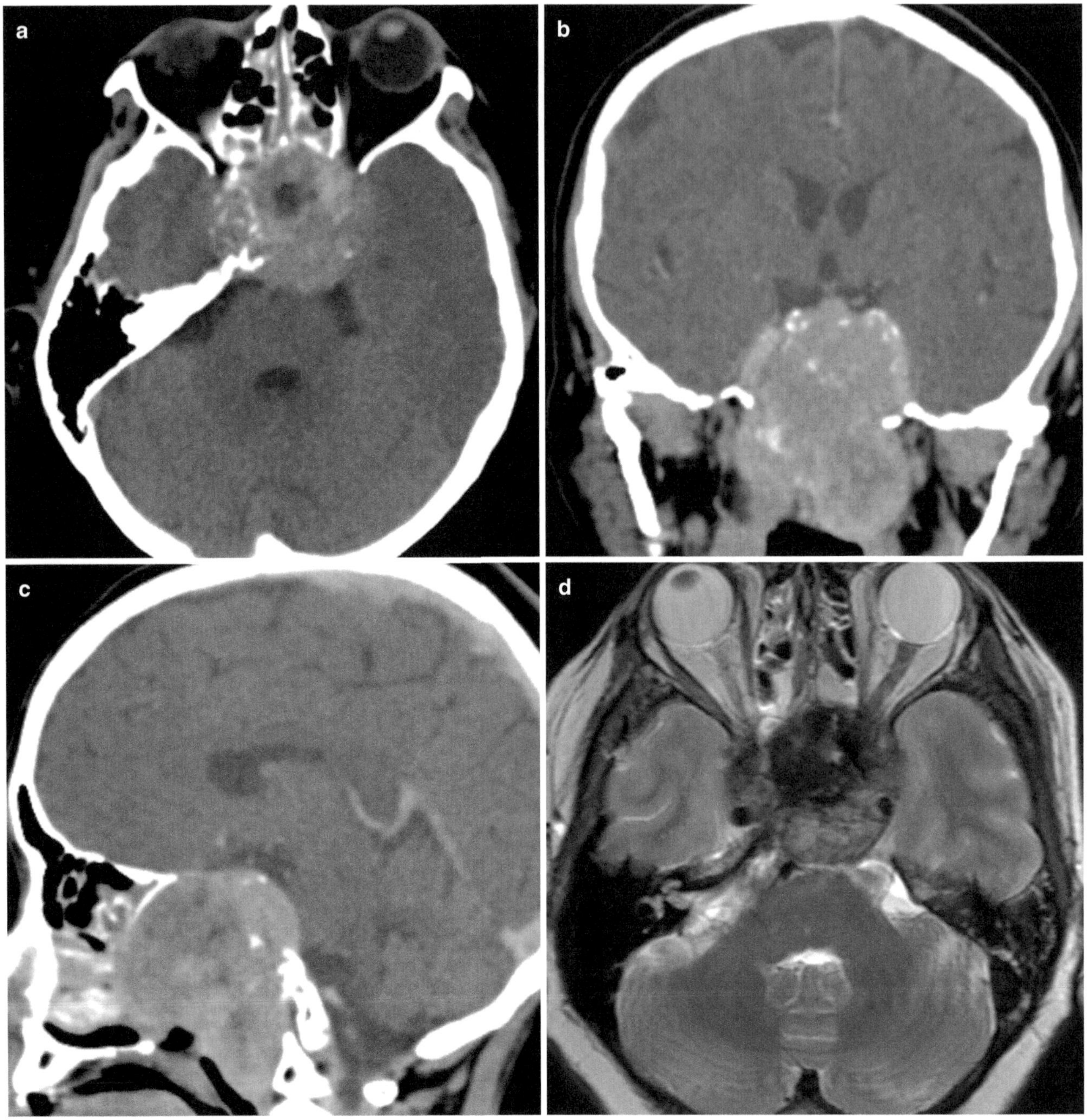

Fig. 14.1 Aspergillus granuloma. Contrast-enhanced CT scans in axial (**a**), coronal (**b**), and sagittal (**c**) projections demonstrate a large heterogeneous enhancing mass with wide bone destruction and remodel, it is predominantly located in sphenoid bone and sinus. A lesion has extension in ethmoid bone, nasal cavities, and nasopharynx. There are calcifications within the lesion. On T2- (**d**, **e**) weighted MR images a lesion has a hypointense MR-signal with area of dark signal in anterior part of the mass. T1-weighted images before (**f**) and after contrast enhancement (**g**, **h**) show a heterogeneously enhancing lesion. An area with dark T2 MR-signal doesn't enhance. (**i**) Histologic specimen

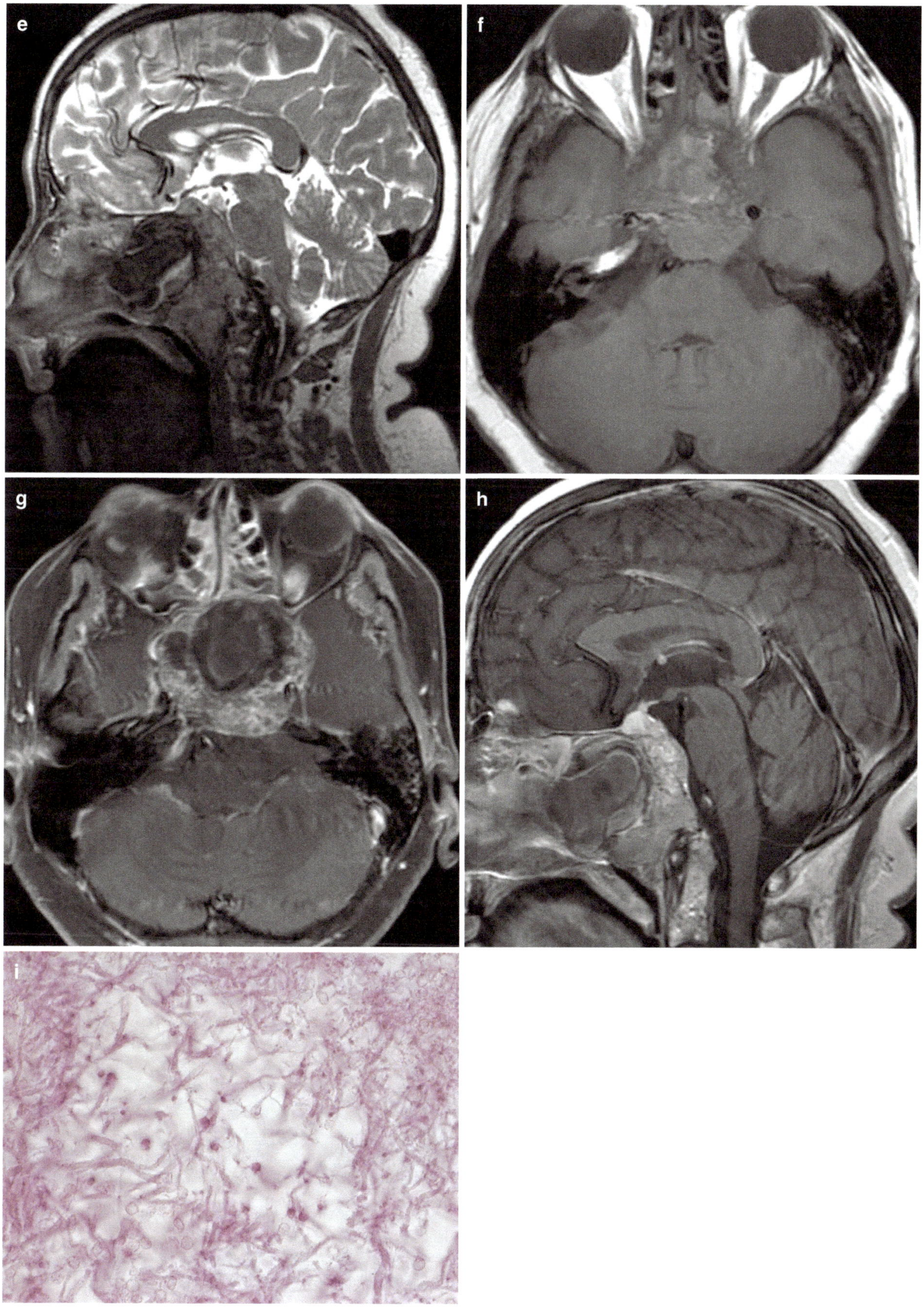

Fig. 14.1 (continued)

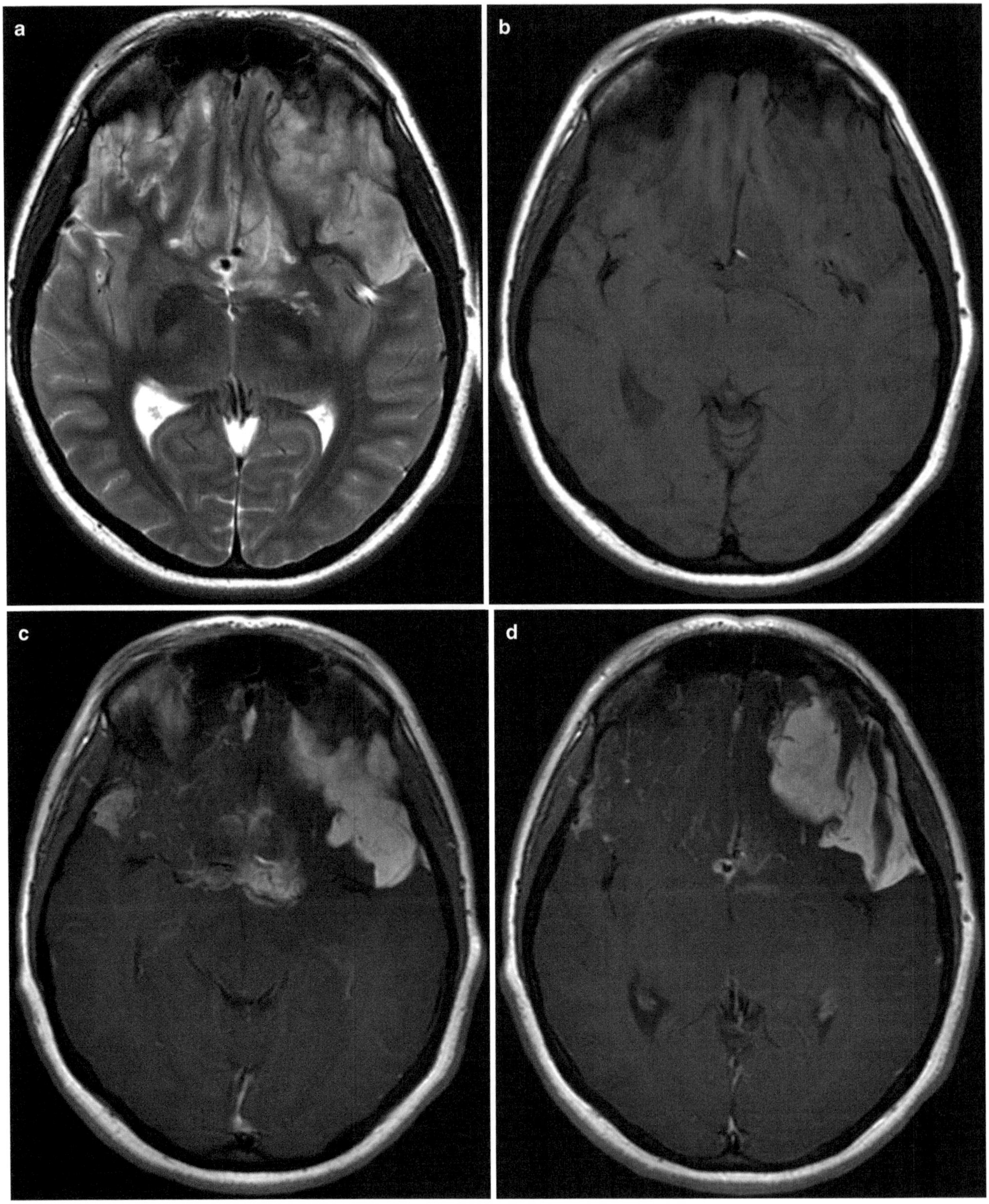

Fig. 14.2 Solitary fibrous tumor (hemangiopericytoma). MR imaging using T2 (**a**), T1 before (**b**) and after (**c**–**f**) contrast enhancement shows a strongly enhancing mass with wide extension along floor of anterior cranial fossa on the left. The contrast enhancement of leptomeninges of both frontal lobes can be seen as well. There is no perifocal edema of brain tissue. H1-MR-spectroscopy demonstrates the presence of lipid-lactate (*short arrow*) and alanine (*long arrow*) peaks (**g**). On axial CT scan (**h**) and CT-perfusion CBV map (**i**) a lesion has prominent enhancement and elevation of tumor blood volume

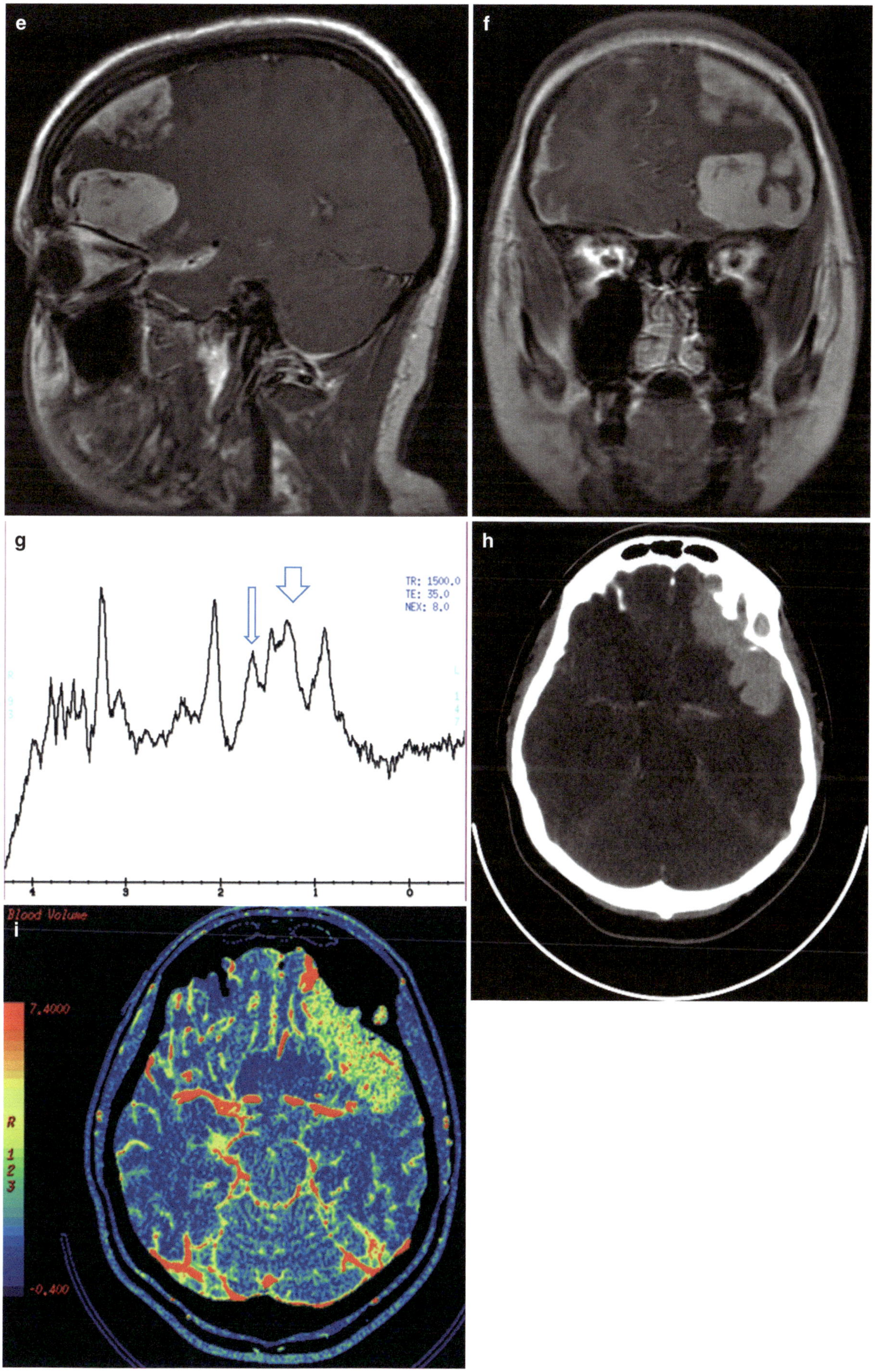

Fig. 14.2 (continued)

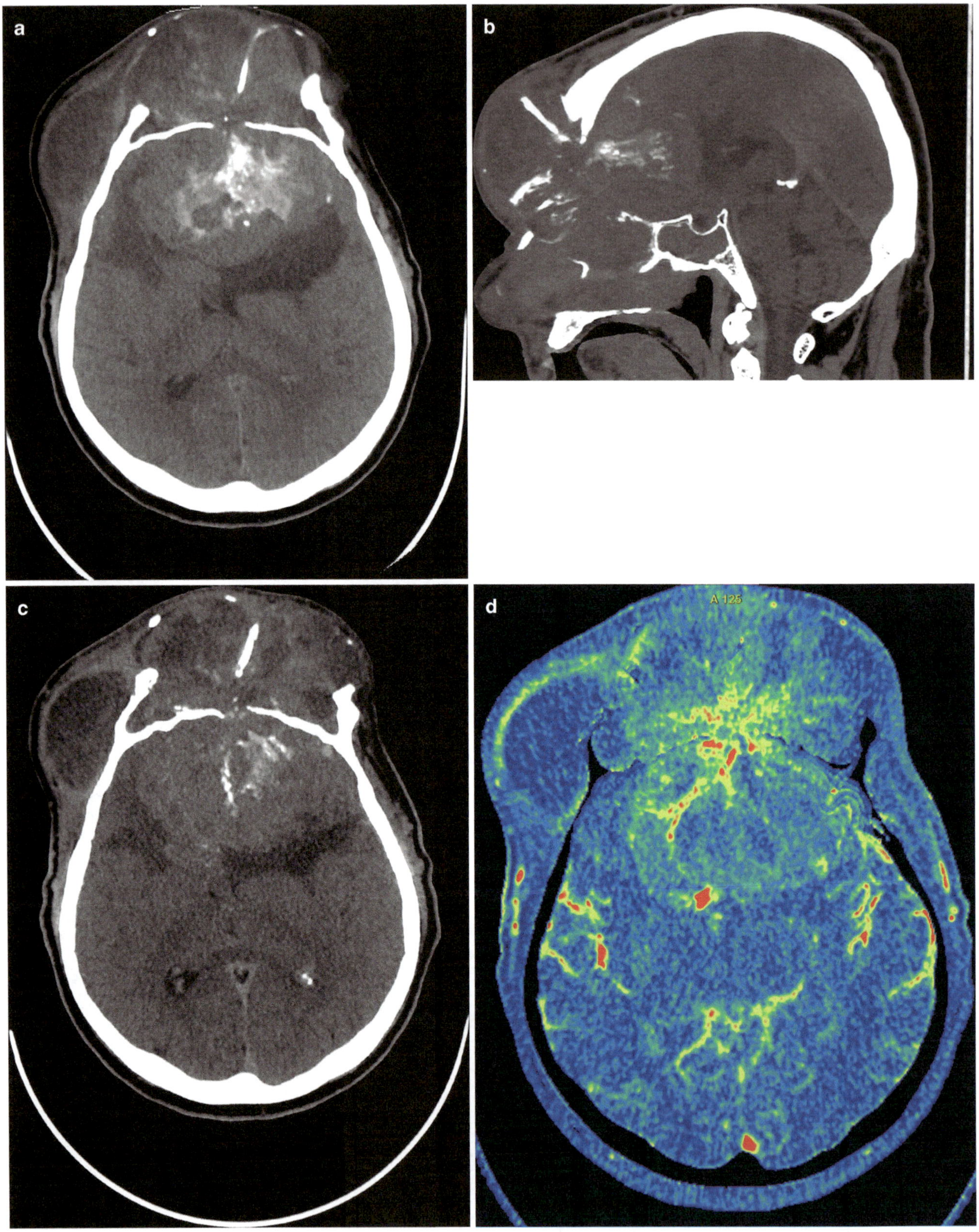

Fig. 14.3 Anaplastic meningioma of craniofacial region. Series CT scans in axial and sagittal projections before (**a**) and after (**b**, **c**) contrast enhancement demonstrate a huge heterogeneous enhancing mixed structure (soft-tissue and cystic) mass with massive calcifications. A lesion leads to extensive craniofacial bone destruction and remodel. "Whole brain" CT-perfusion study shows an increased perfusion parameters of tumor tissue, especially in area of matrix—central part of the tumor (**d**, **e**). On MR-imaging using T2- (**f**) and contrast-enhanced T1- (**g**) weighted scans a tumor has heterogeneous MR-signal and enhancement with well-defined matrix vessels. MR-angiography (3D TOF (**h**)) and DSA (**i**) revealed abundant vascular network with supplying from ophthalmic artery and fronto-polar arteries

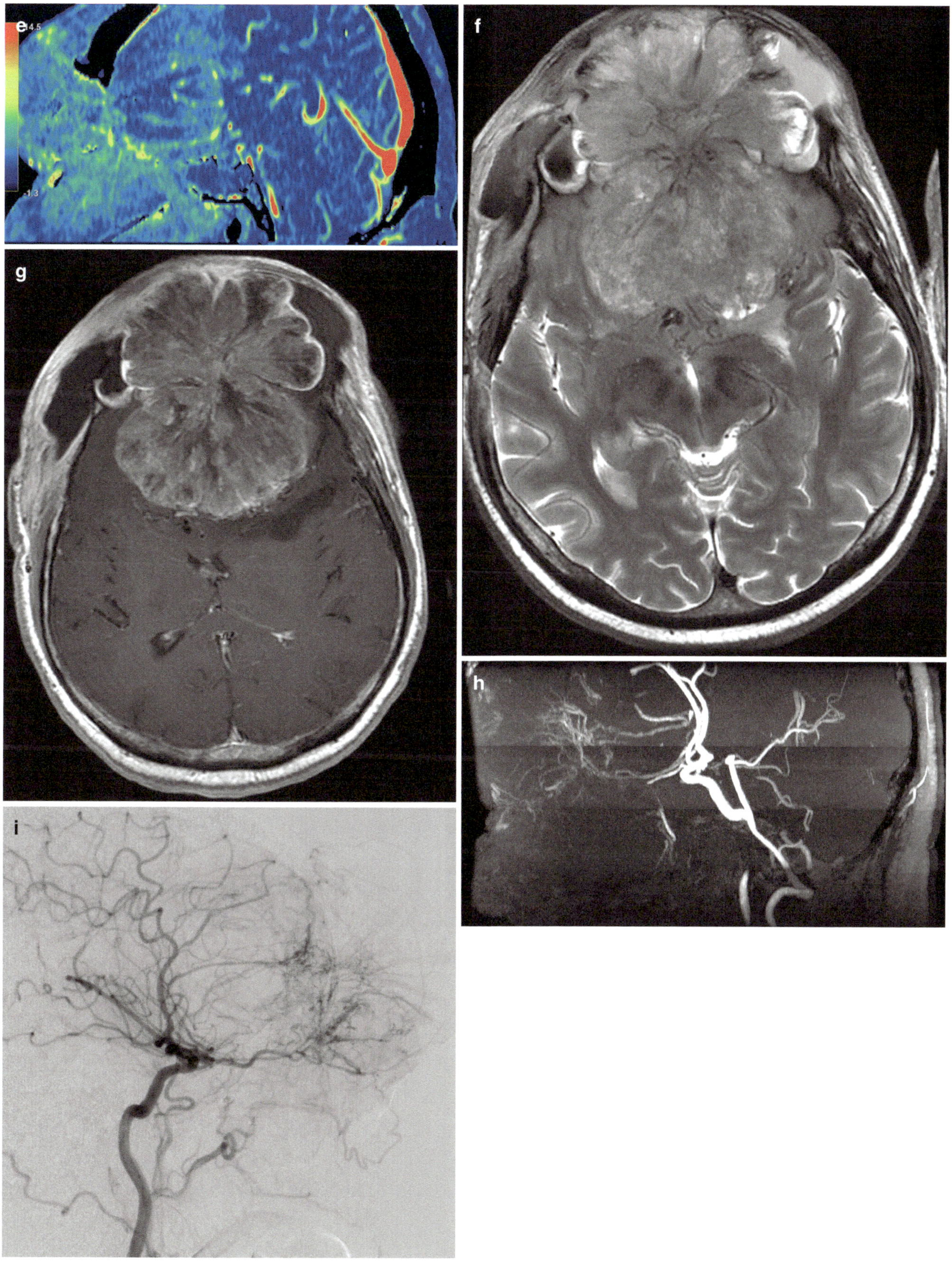

Fig. 14.3 (continued)

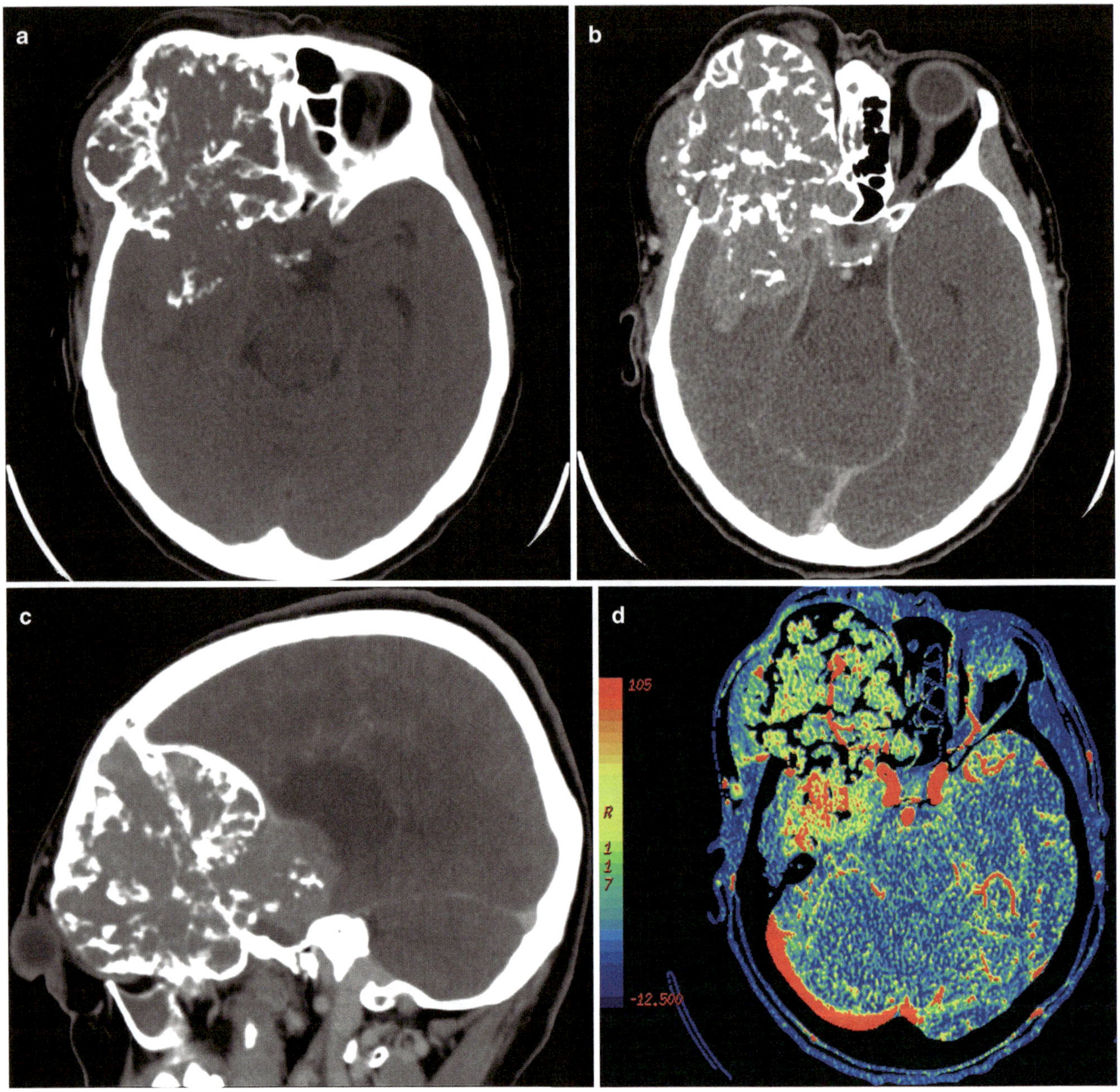

Fig. 14.4 Meningioma of craniofacial region with infiltrative growth. Axial and sagittal CT images before (**a**) and after (**b**, **c**) contrast enhancement demonstrate a large heterogeneous enhancing mass of right craniofacial region with calcifications and bone remodel. Soft tissue component strongly enhances. CT-perfusion study (CBF (**d**)) shows a hyperperfused lesion especially within intracranial portion. On MR imaging (T2- (**e**), T1 before (**f**) and after (**g**) enhancement) tumor has isointensity of MR-signal with brain and more homogeneous than on CT contrast enhancement. Calcification and bone remodel can be estimated better on CT compared to MRI. High resolution MR-angiography (**h**, **i**) 3D TOF demonstrates the different origins of tumor blood supply (predominantly from meningeal media artery, as well as short branches of a. maxillary and ICA)

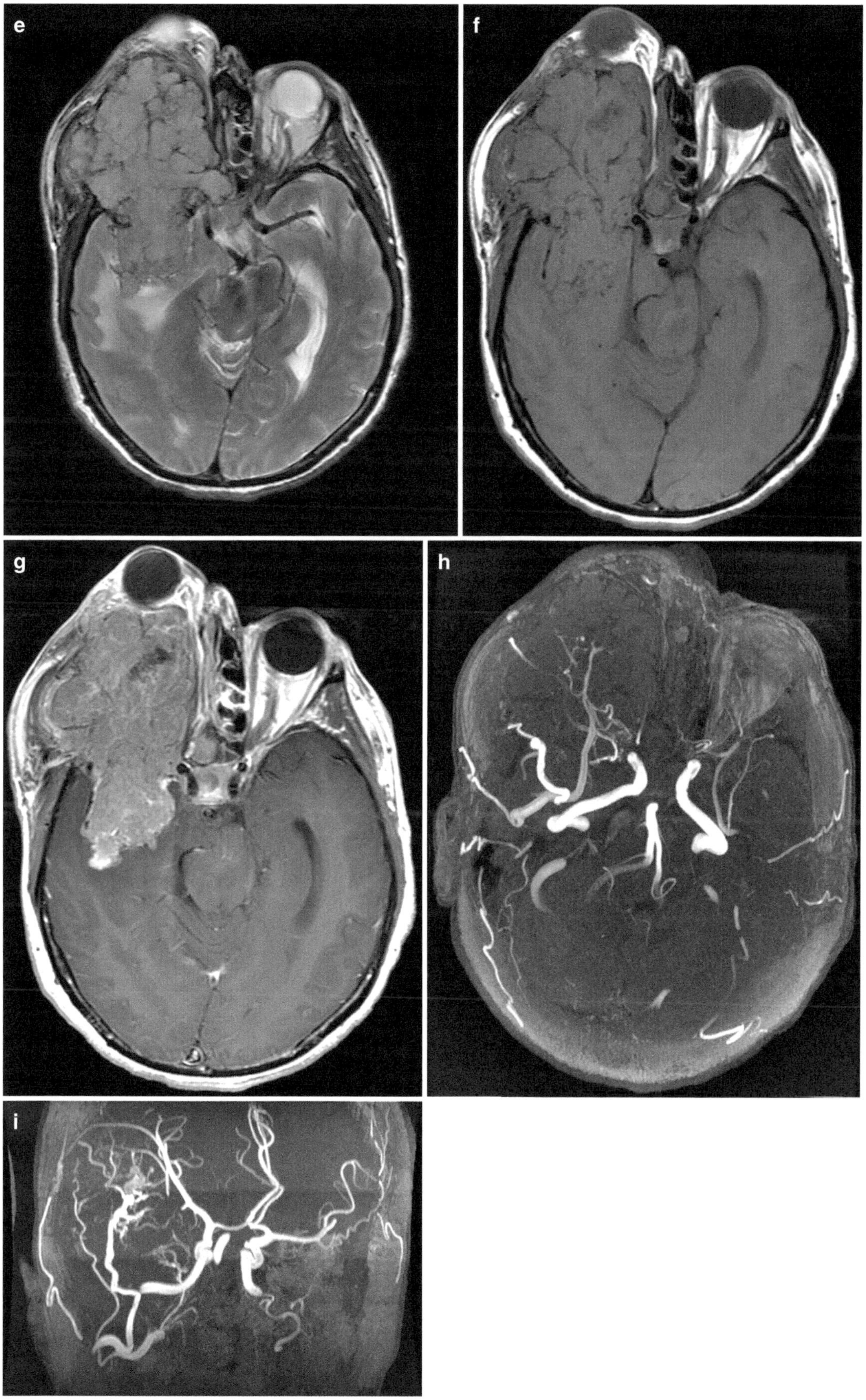

Fig. 14.4 (continued)

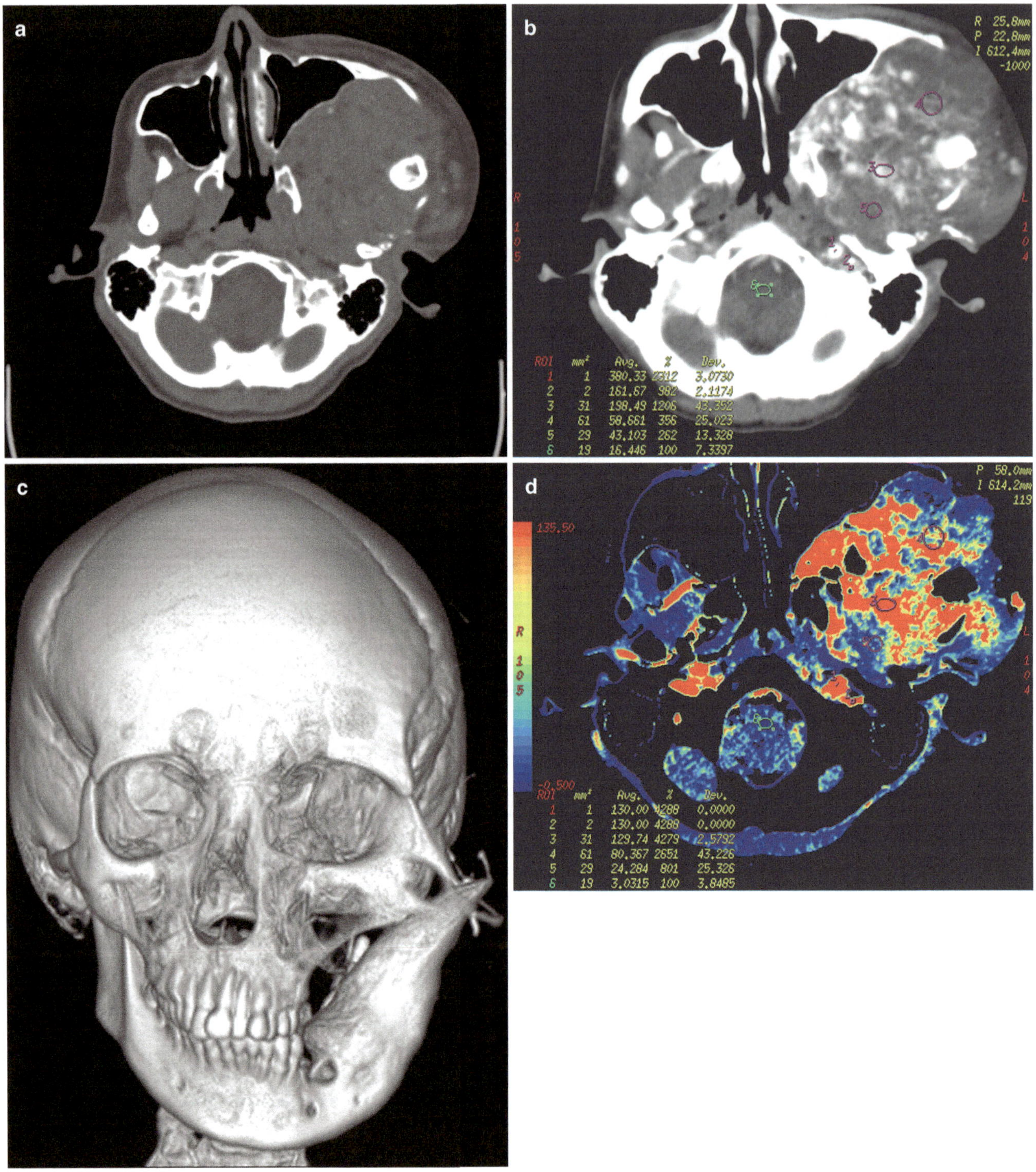

Fig. 14.5 Epithelioid hemangioma. Axial CT scans before (**a**) and after (**b**) contrast enhancement show a huge left side craniofacial soft tissue mass with heterogeneous enhancement in early stage of contrast-enhanced CT-perfusion study (**b**). A lesion causes of craniofacial bones remodel (3D (**c**)). CT-perfusion study demonstrates a prominent elevation of tumor blood flow (**d**) and blood volume (**e**) indicating an abundant blood supply. MR imaging (T2- (**f**) and contrast-enhanced T1- (**g**, **h**) weighted images) shows a large soft tissue mass with more homogeneous than on CT enhancement. Within the lesion areas of flow-void effect due to large vessels can be seen that was confirmed on dynamic time-resolved MR-angiography (TRICKS (**i**))

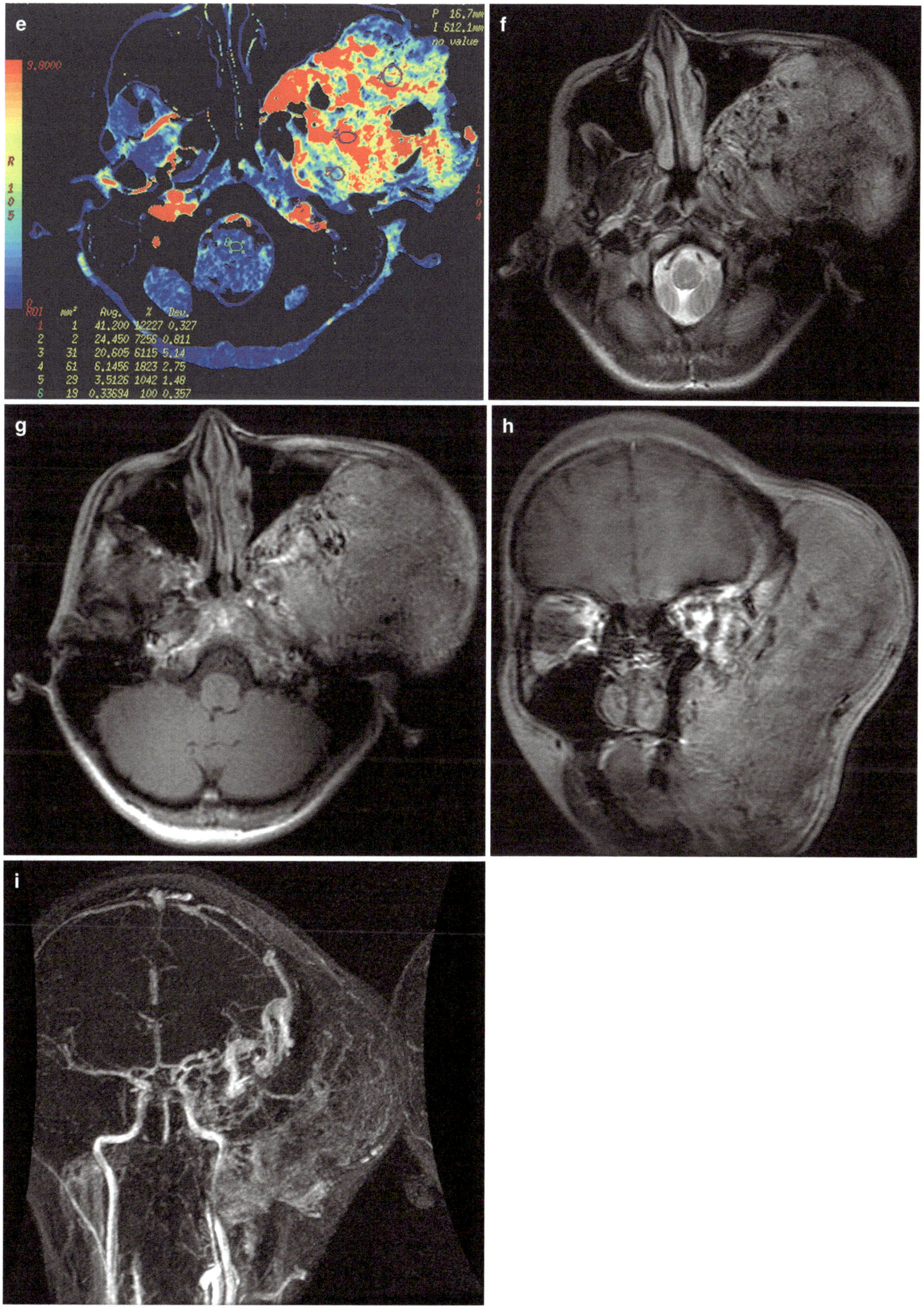

Fig. 14.5 (continued)

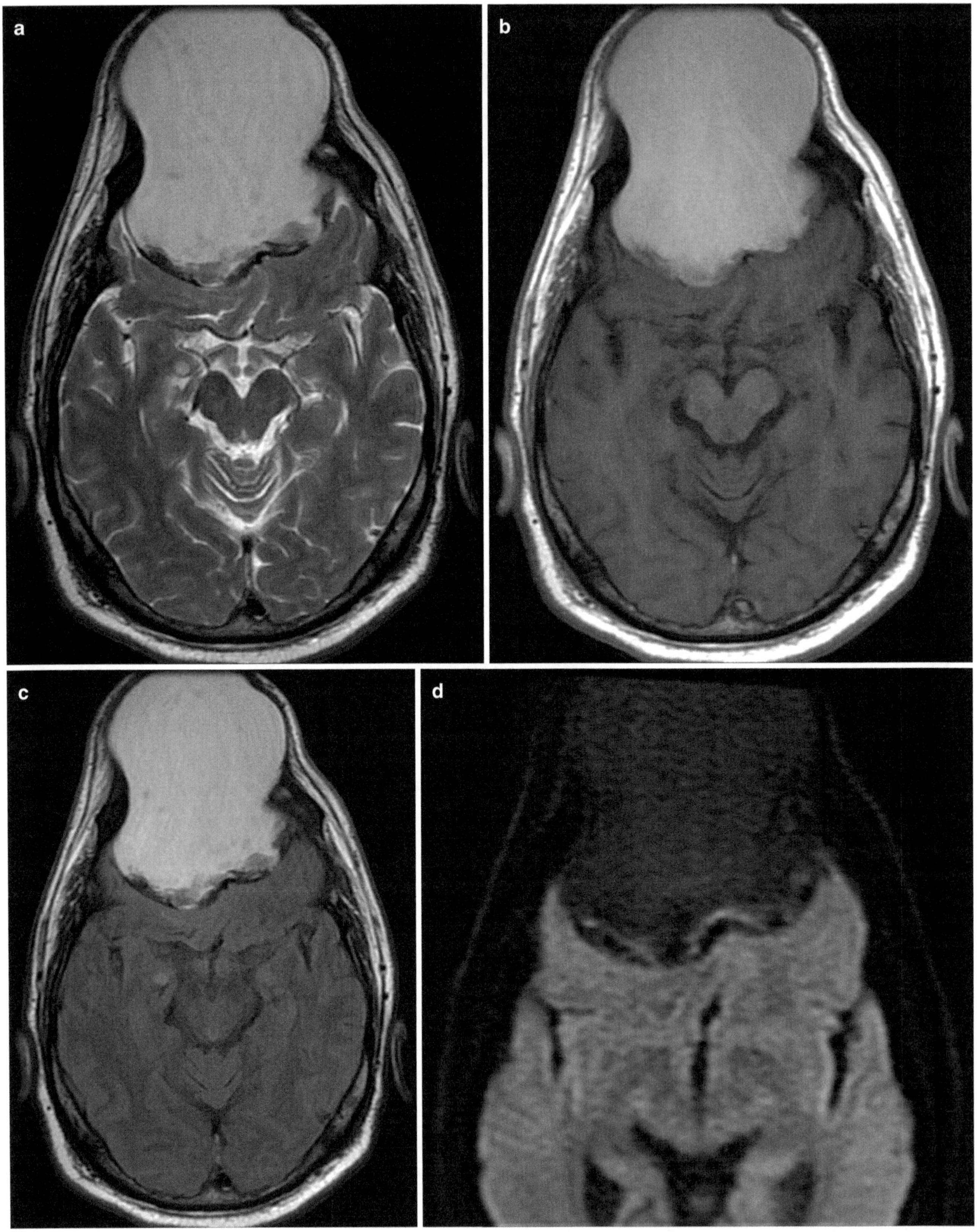

Fig. 14.6 Pyomucocele of frontal bone and sinus. MR imaging using T2- (**a**), T1- (**b**), and T2-FLAIR- (**c**) weighted scans demonstrates a huge homogeneous hyperintense expansile mass with destruction of frontal bones and with intra- and extracranial extension. DWI (**d**) shows low MR-signal within the lesion and excludes the pus presence inside. Post-contrast study (**e–h**) in axial and sagittal projections reveals a thin rim of contrast enhancement into the borderline area between lesion and brain tissue. There is no enhancement within the lesion and no blood flow in capsule of the lesion on ASL MR imaging (**i**)

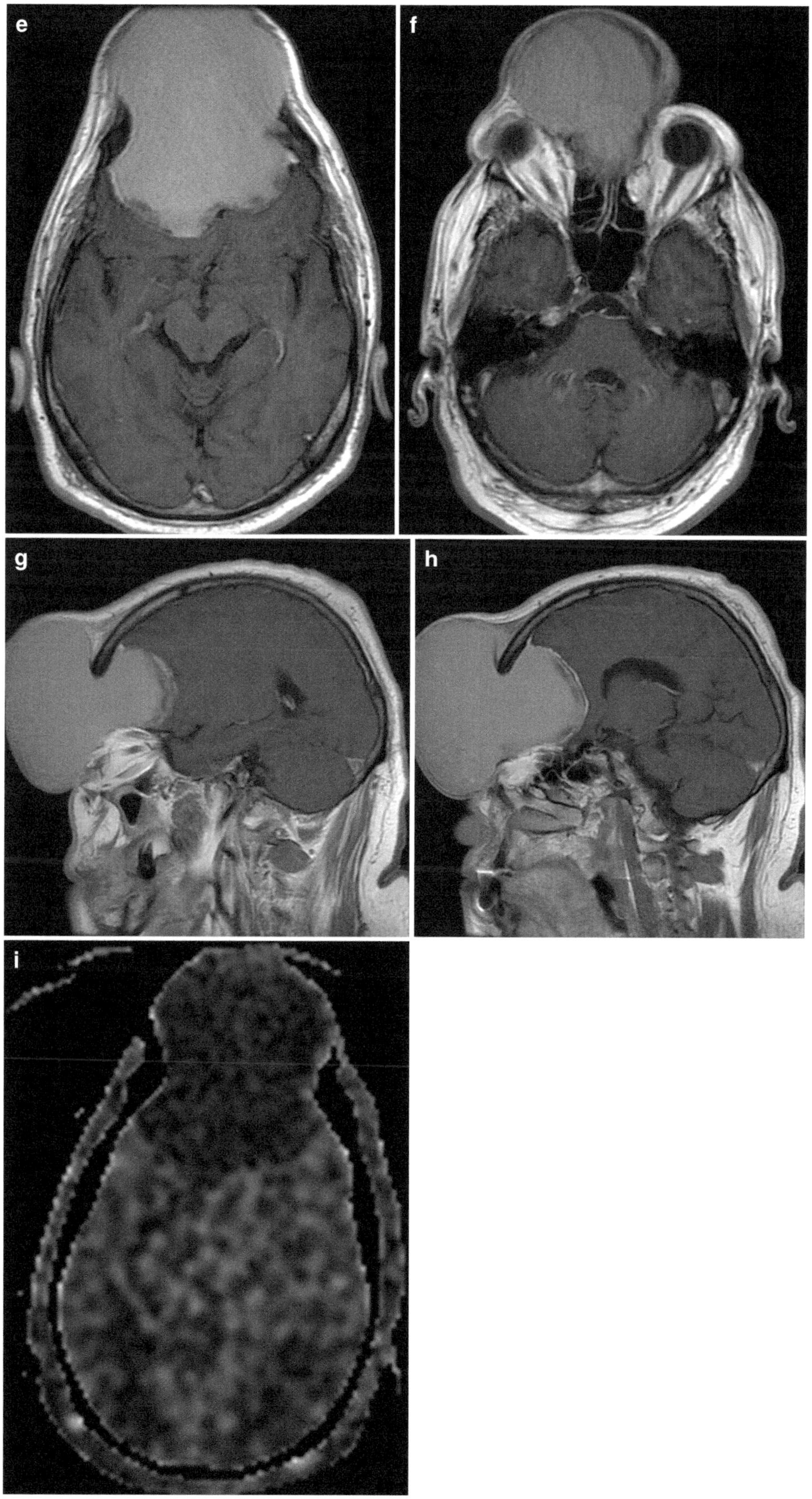

Fig. 14.6 (continued)

Part III

Middle Cranial Fossa and Sellar Region Lesions (in Collab. with N. Zakharova)

15 Sellar and Parasellar Tumors

Contents

15.1 Pituitary Adenomas

Pituitary adenoma is a benign, slow-growing epithelial tumor arising from the adenohypophysis. Pituitary adenomas consist of (according to most authors) 10–15% of all intracranial tumors. These are mainly adult cases; these tumors are rarely seen in children, less than 6% of intracranial tumor in adolescents, rare in children (Osborn et al. 2016). The peak incidence is between 20 and 40 years. In rare cases, pituitary carcinoma may grow from the anterior pituitary, but their histological criteria are still not clearly defined. Cellular polymorphism, atypical mitoses, hemorrhages and necrosis, signs of invasive growth may occur in benign adenomas. The presence of distant metastases is a sign of pituitary carcinoma. According to Kadashev (2007), among 1600 patients operated at the Burdenko Neurosurgery Institute within the period from 2000 to 2005, only in two cases was diagnosed a pituitary carcinoma with metastases.

Usually the pituitary adenomas are classified according to their size: less than 10 mm (microadenomas), greater than 10 mm (macroadenomas).

In our opinion, the most acceptable is the classification by incidence adopted at the Burdenko Neurosurgery Center (Kadashev 2007).

Intrasellar adenomas

1. Microadenoma (not causing an enlargement of the sella turcica)
2. Macroadenomas

Intraextrasellar adenomas

1. Intrasuprasellar adenomas (suprasellar deviation from the vertical axis of the sella turcica is not considered as an additional direction of growth)
2. Tumors invading the skull base structures
   (a) Infrasellar growth (into the sphenoid sinus, or nasopharynx)
   (b) Laterosellar growth (into the cavernous sinus, or under the dura of the middle cranial fossa, into the infratemporal fossa)

I. Pronin, V. Kornienko, *CT and MRI of Skull Base Lesions*, https://doi.org/10.1007/978-3-319-65957-2_15

(c) Antesellar growth (ethmoidal labyrinth, orbit)
(d) Retrosellar growth (behind the dorsum sella, onto the clivus with the formation of extra- or intradural nodes in the posterior cranial fossa).

Adenomas are considered small, intermediate, large, and giant, respectively, if they are smaller than 25 mm, of 26–35 mm, 36–59 mm, and larger than 60 mm. Giant adenomas are considered as a separate group, since they severely invade the hypothalamus, can cause development of obstructive hydrocephalus; surgical treatment becomes more complex; the rate of the incidence of severe postoperative complications and mortality rate increase.

An important component of the pituitary adenomas growth is their ability to infiltrate surrounding membranes and bones. Therefore, a concept of *infiltrative* adenomas is distinguished in literature (Chena et al. 2011). However, there are no obvious radiological differences between infiltrative and expansive tumor growth. There is also the term of ectopic pituitary adenoma; this lesion is clearly not associated with the contents of the sella turcica and locates completely outside the sella.

Clinicians subdivide adenomas according to presence, absence and, if present, the type of hormonal activity.

Clinical manifestations of adenomas depend on the size of a tumor, the type of a hormone produced and the extent of extrasellar expansion. In approximately 75% (Osborn et al. 2016) of patients with adenomas, there are clinical signs caused by secretion of various hormones, the remaining 25% of cases tumors are nonfunctioning. The most frequently seen tumor of the pituitary gland that is hormonally active is prolactinoma—a tumor that secretes prolactin, which constitutes approximately 30–40% of hormonally active adenomas and about 30% of all adenomas (Osborn et al. 2016). Prolactin hypersecretion may cause amenorrhea, galactorrhea, and infertility, reduction of libido or impotence. Among all patients with pituitary adenomas, children and adolescents account 2–6%. The most frequent tumors in children are prolactinomas, then corticotropinomas, somatotropinomas, thyroprolactinomas, and finally adenocarcinomas. Corticotropinomas and prolactinomas are more frequent in girls (2:1 and 3:1 respectively), and somatotropinomas are most frequent in boys (5:1).

Other frequently encountered and hormonally active tumors are somatotropinomas (20%) and adrenocorticotropinomas (10%), the latter produce ACTH. The tumors originating from cells producing the growth hormone (somatotrophs) cause acromegaly in adults and gigantism in children. The tumors originating from cells that produce ACTH (corticotrophs) cause Cushing's disease which is the most severe endocrine disorder. It is more frequently seen in females (75%) and is a severe multi-system disease of hypothalamic-pituitary origin (ACTH-dependent Cushing syndrome); its clinical manifestations are caused by hypersecretion of adrenal hormones. Nelson syndrome is also caused by ACTH hypersecretion and is the result of continued growth of ACTH-producing adenoma in patients after adrenalectomy. Continued secretion of ACTH causes stimulation of skin melanocytes with subsequent hyperpigmentation. Adenomas that cause Nelson syndrome often reach large size and expand beyond sella turcica. Nelson syndrome occurs in 10–80% of patients who underwent bilaterally adrenalectomy (Marova 1996; Rozhinskaya 2011). Thyrotropinoma is very rare (about 1%). There is also a group of poly-(or pluri-) hormonal pituitary adenomas that can be both hormonally active and "silent." They produce various combinations of seven hormonal products (STH, PRL, ACTH, LH, FSH, TSH, and α-subunit of glycoprotein hormones). Immunohistology reveals positive immunoreactivity to different hormones; however, this is not always accompanied by increase hormone concentrations in the serum and the corresponding clinical picture. Adenomas secreting prolactin and the growth hormone are the most frequent among the multihormonal adenomas.

Adenohypophysis cells producing different hormones are characterized by certain topography within the pituitary gland. Cells that secrete prolactin and the growth hormone are laterally positioned; ACTH-, TSH-, and FSH/LH-secreting cells are centrally positioned. These findings are of certain importance, as they indicate the sites of initial growth of various types of adenomas. In contrast to hormonally active tumors, which manifest by signs of a certain hormone hypersecretion, the cause of clinical manifestations of a nonfunctioning adenoma is compression or invasion of the adjacent structures. Hormonally inactive adenomas usually reach large size by the time of clinical signs appear. They expand upwards into the suprasellar cistern, laterally into cavernous sinuses, or downwards into the sphenoid sinus. Compression of optic nerves, chiasm, and optic tracts causes vision impairment. The continued upward growth causes compression of the third ventricle and occlusion of the foramina of Monro which contributes to obstructive hydrocephalus. Expansion into cavernous sinuses causes compression of cranial nerves that pass there, which may lead to diplopia and sensory disturbances on the face. Compression of the rest of pituitary gland mainly causes anterior lobe dysfunction. Involvement of neurohypophysis and the pituitary stalk may cause diabetes insipidus, which is a rare and late manifestation of adenomas of the posterior part of the pituitary gland. In rare cases the pituitary adenoma may be manifested by the pituitary apoplexy due to intratumoral hemorrhage.

Imaging MR imaging is the leading method for diagnosing pituitary microadenomas (Seidenwurm 2008). T1-weighted images are more informative due to better visualization of the anatomic structures of sellar-parasellar region. Preference is always given to a coronal thin-section scans.

Radiography almost lost its importance in the diagnosis of pituitary adenomas, as the increase in size of the sella turcica is usually observed at the "late" stages of tumor growth when the adenoma spreads beyond the bony walls of the sella turcica (Fig. 15.1).

Using CT, *microadenomas* in most cases can't be diagnosed. Intravenous contrast enhancement also doesn't give information in the majority of cases. Only in macroadenomas with an enlarge of the sella turcica and parasellar tumor growth, CT allows determining soft-tissue lesion that is iso- or slightly hyperdense as compared to the brain in the sella turcica, causing the partial destruction of the bony walls. Since differences in CT density of pituitary adenomas and the brain tissue are minor, the best imaging of the tumor is achieved after intravenous contrast agent injection. These are the following types of growth: laterosellar growth into the cavernous sinus and middle cranial fossa, antesellar growth anteriorly to the anterior cranial fossa, infrasellar growth into the sphenoid sinus cavity and ethmoid bone and retrosellar growth with compression of the brainstem. Most adenomas moderately enhance, which makes them hyperdense compared to the surrounding bone marrow (Figs. 15.2 and 15.3). Sometimes, e.g. in prolactinomas, there are cysts and calcifications detected in their structure or on the periphery. The sellar tumors with different components of growth are better seen when the study is performed in coronal plane or when using coronal and sagittal reformations.

Diagnosis of pituitary *microadenomas* (<10 mm in size) should be based on mainly clinical and endocrinological data, and neuroimaging techniques help additionally to confirm or to rule out the diagnosis. As the sizes of hormonally active microadenoma may comprise only a few millimeters, MRI should be done with high spatial resolution. If microadenoma is suspected, then slice thickness should be 2–3 mm for spin-echo pulse sequence, and 1–1.5 mm for spoiled gradient spin echo (SPGR) pulse sequence. The most informative are T1- and T2-weighted sequences. The use of T2-FLAIR is limited due to a presence of artifacts from the bones of the skull base and the cerebrospinal fluid pulsation in thc suprasellar cistern. FIESTA doesn't help in the visualization of prolactinomas excluding cases with cystic formation.

Neuroimaging of adenomas takes into account the direct feature of a tumor as well as indirect signs. The main direct and indirect signs of a pituitary microadenoma on MRI are an increasing size of the pituitary gland, presence of signal changes asymmetry of the upper adenohypophysis contour, displacement of infundibulum (not always in the opposite direction), asymmetrical descent of the floor sella, compression of adjacent portions of the cavernous sinus.

On MRI, the normal tissue of adenohypophysis is homogenous and isointense to brain tissue. Microadenomas are usually characterized by prolonged relaxation times and

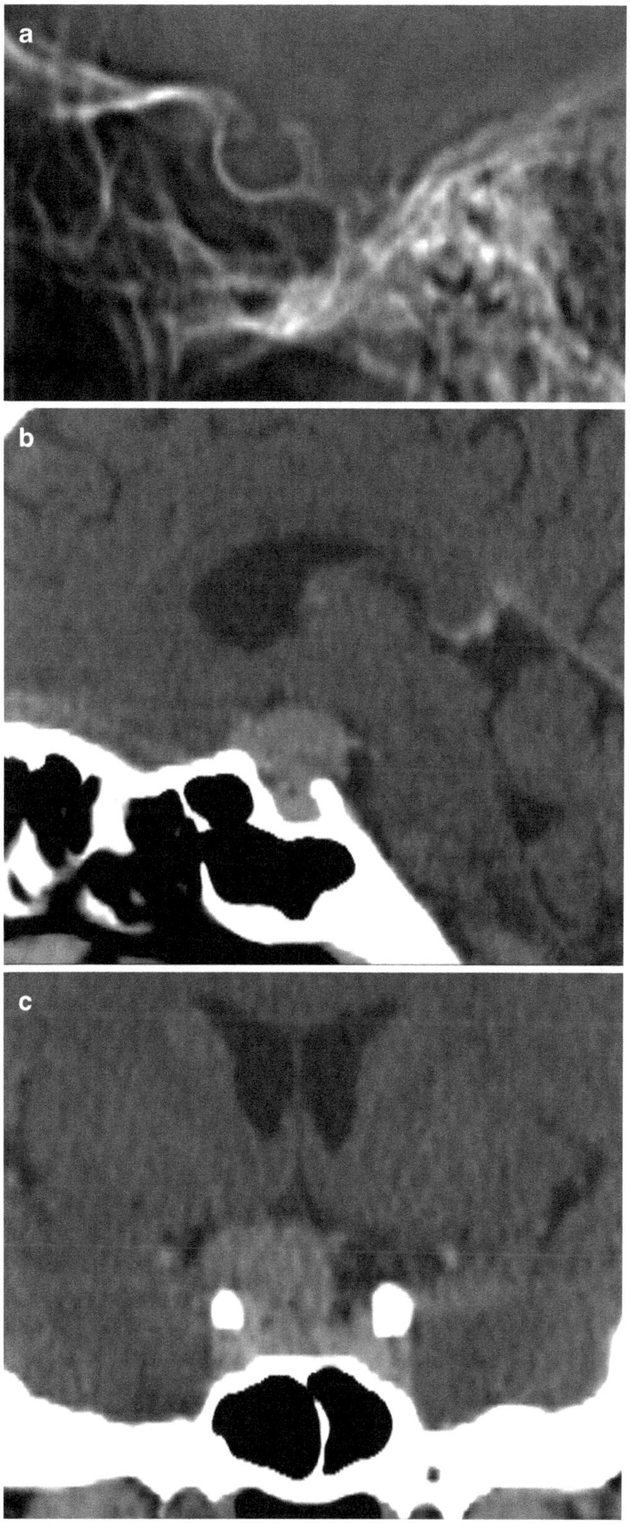

Fig. 15.1 Pituitary adenoma. X-ray examination (**a**) reveals moderate enlargement of the sella turcica. Sagittal (**b**) and coronal (**c**) CT reformats of axial with CE show a hyperdense sellar-suprasellar tumor with right-side laterosellar growth

appear on T1-weighted images as hypointense areas compared to the surrounding tissue of the adenohypophysis (Fig. 15.4). On T2-weighted images these areas are

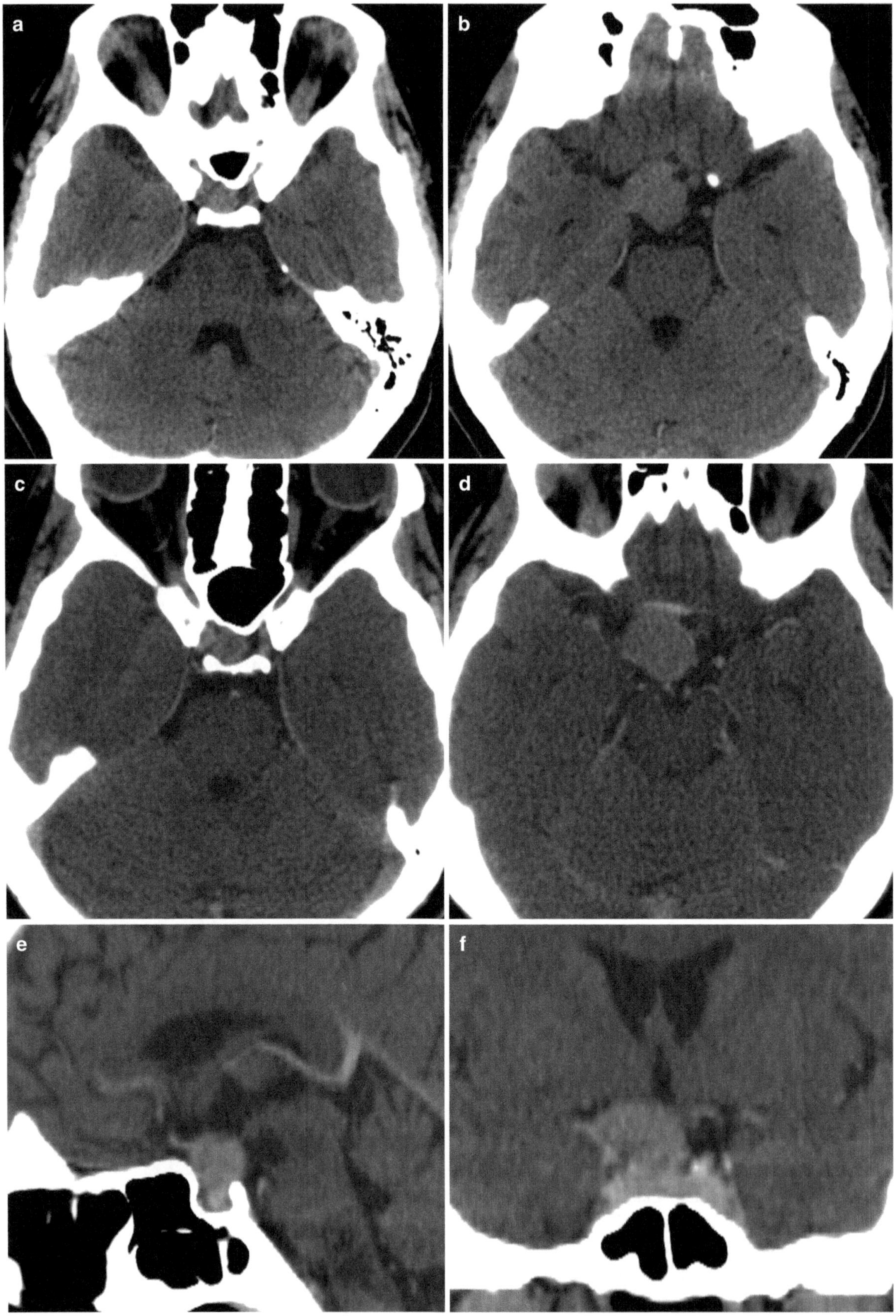

Fig. 15.2 Pituitary adenoma. Axial CT scans before (**a**, **b**) and after contrast enhancement (**c**, **d**) show a moderately enhanced tumor with suprasellar growth. Sella turcica is not enlarged. Sagittal (**e**) and coronal (**f**) CT reformations obtain additional information about the tumor growth

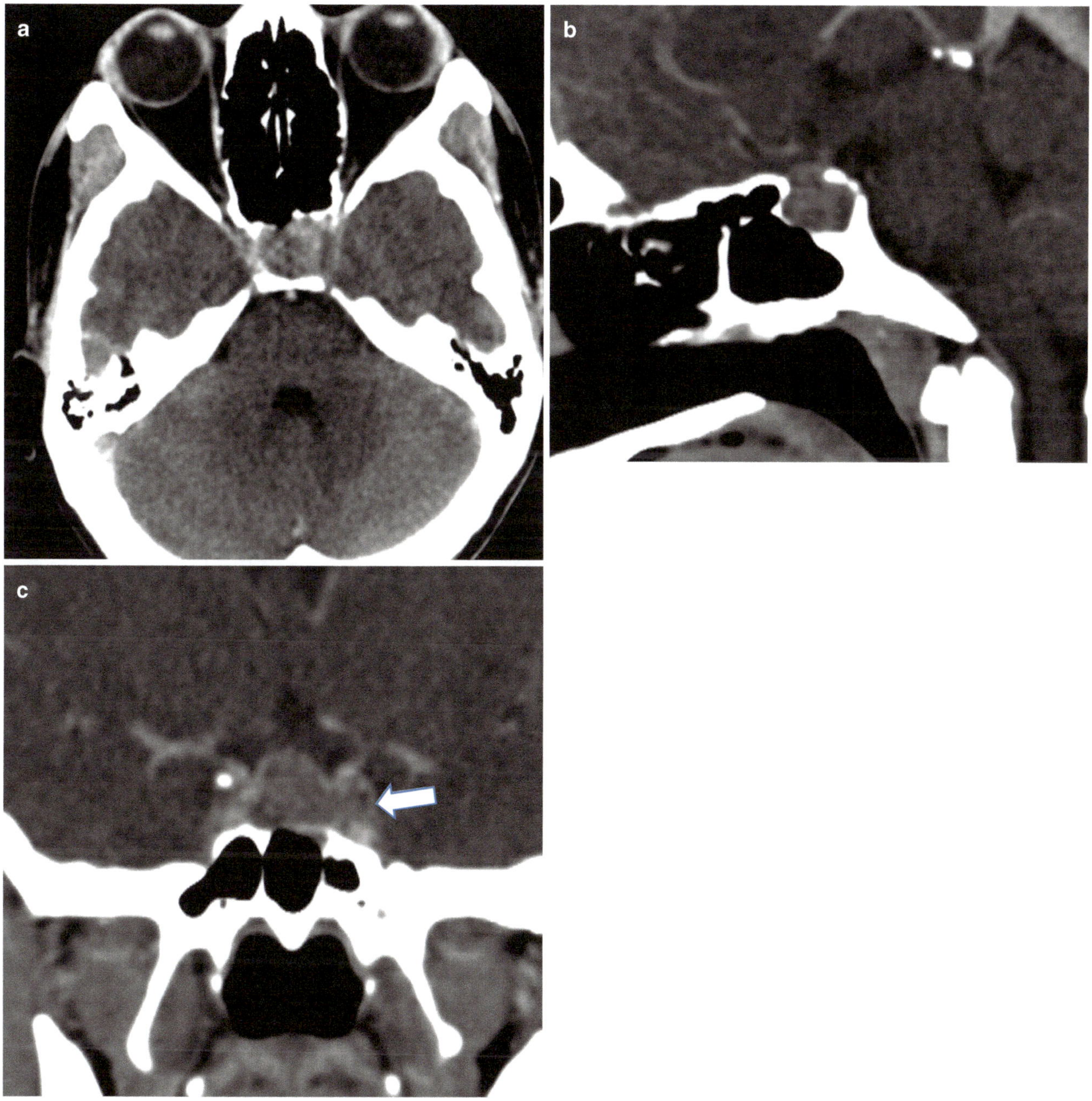

Fig. 15.3 Pituitary adenoma. Axial CT scan (**a**) after CE with sagittal (b) and coronal (c) reformations demonstrate a pituitary tumor with moderate enhancement. Coronal reformat is clearly visualized laterosellar growth of the tumor (*arrow*)

hyperintense. However, these changes may sometimes be mildly pronounced. According to our data, the sensitivity of T1-weigthed images in imaging of the tumor is higher than that of T2-weighted images. However, microcytic changes in the tumor are better identified on T2-weighted images. Prominent characteristic hyperintensity appears on T1-weighted images if a hemorrhage into the tumor tissue develops. However, the degree and characteristics of signal changes depend on the time after onset: in the hyperacute stage, blood looks dark in T1- and isointense in T2-weighted images (due to deoxyhemoglobin), which often mimics manifestations of a large parasellar saccular arterial aneurysm. In a subacute stage, predominant methemoglobin causes an increase in the MR signal on T1-weighted images, and then (in case of erythrocyte lysis) an increase in the signal on T2-weighted images (Fig. 15.5).

After contrast enhancement, the majority of microadenomas accumulates the contrast agent and expands into the adenohypophysis tissue. That is why borders between the tumor and the pituitary may smoothen on post-contrast

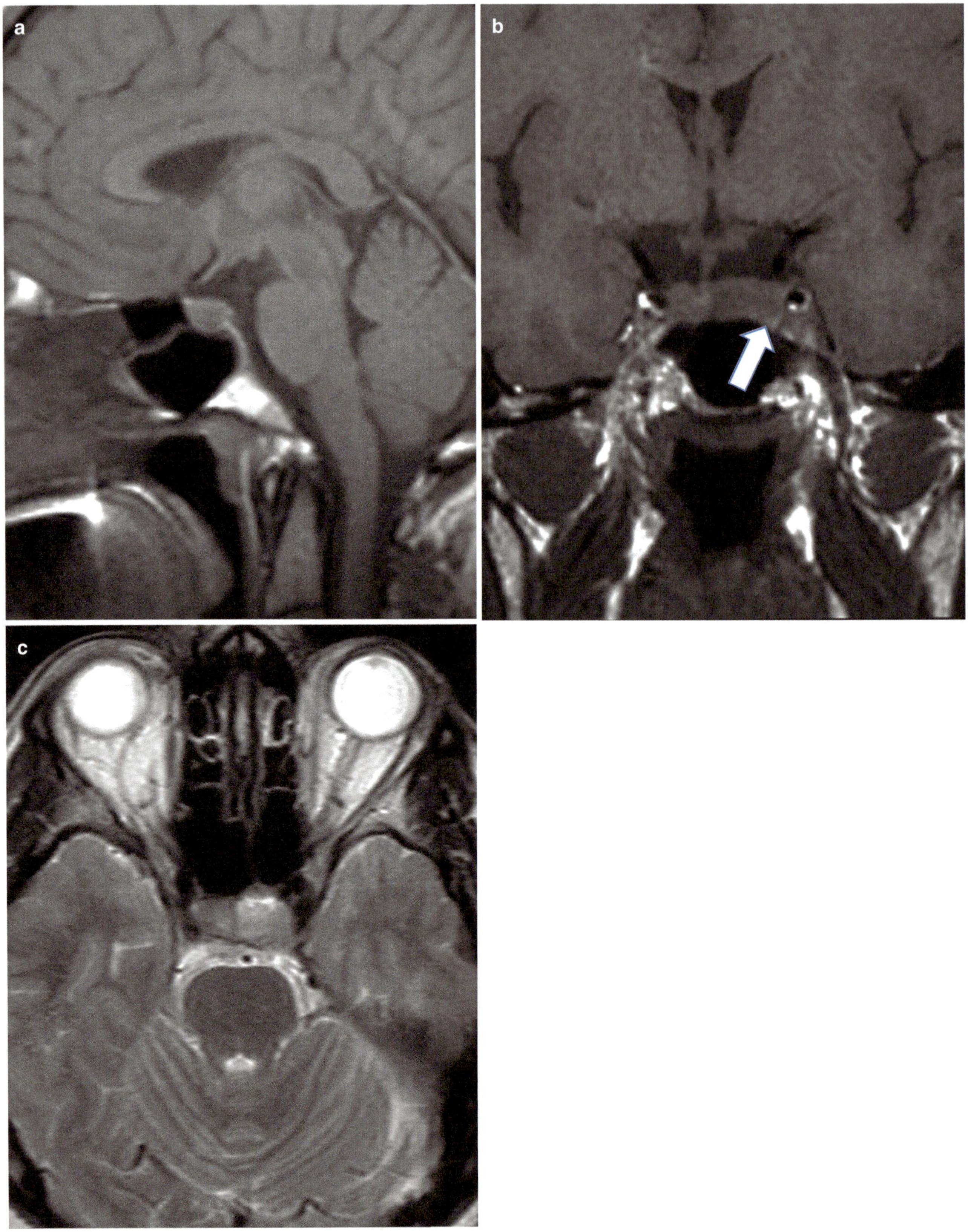

Fig. 15.4 Pituitary microadenoma. Sagittal (**a**) and coronal (**b**) T1-weighted images show a hypointense tumor in the left half of the adenohypophysis, which is inhomogeneous and moderately hyperintense on T2-weighted image (**c**). The tumor growths into the left cavernous sinus and particular envelops of the left internal carotid artery (*arrow*)

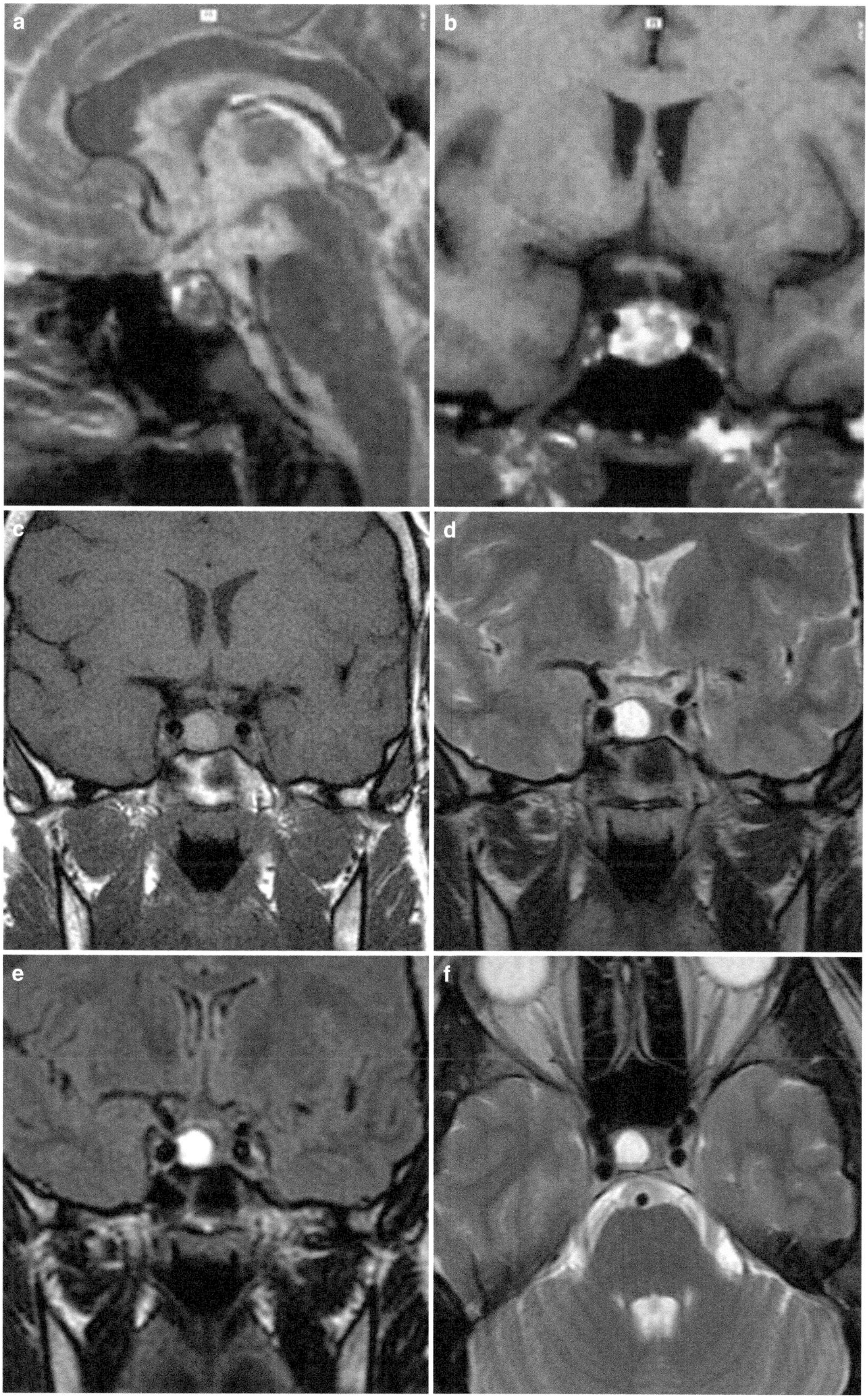

Fig. 15.5 Pituitary apoplexy. Case 1: T2- (**a**) and T1- (**b**) weighted images show sellar tumor with multiple microhemorrhagic areas. Case 2: Sellar pituitary adenoma with hemorrhagic cyst in the left part of adenohypophysis. On T1- (**c**), T2- (**d**), and T2-FLAIR (**e**) weighted images the hemorrhagic area has hyperintense signal. Axial T2-weighted image (**f**) reveals a blood-fluid level in the posterior part of the hemorrhagic cyst

images. In these cases bolus dynamic scanning becomes effective as it differentiates between microadenoma and the pituitary tissue more precisely—the former shows slow enhancement (Figs. 15.6 and 15.7). Especially informative is dynamic scanning in isointense tumors (Huk et al. 1990; Sakamoto et al. 1991; Rang et al. 2002; Kornienko and Pronin 2009).

It is noteworthy that if MR picture of microadenoma is present, then the clinical history should always be taken into account as well as clinical manifestations and endocrinological tests. Only this complex approach allows making a correct diagnosis, differentiating between Cushing's disease, Nelson syndrome, etc., and prescribing appropriate treatment. In literature, there are descriptions of cases with

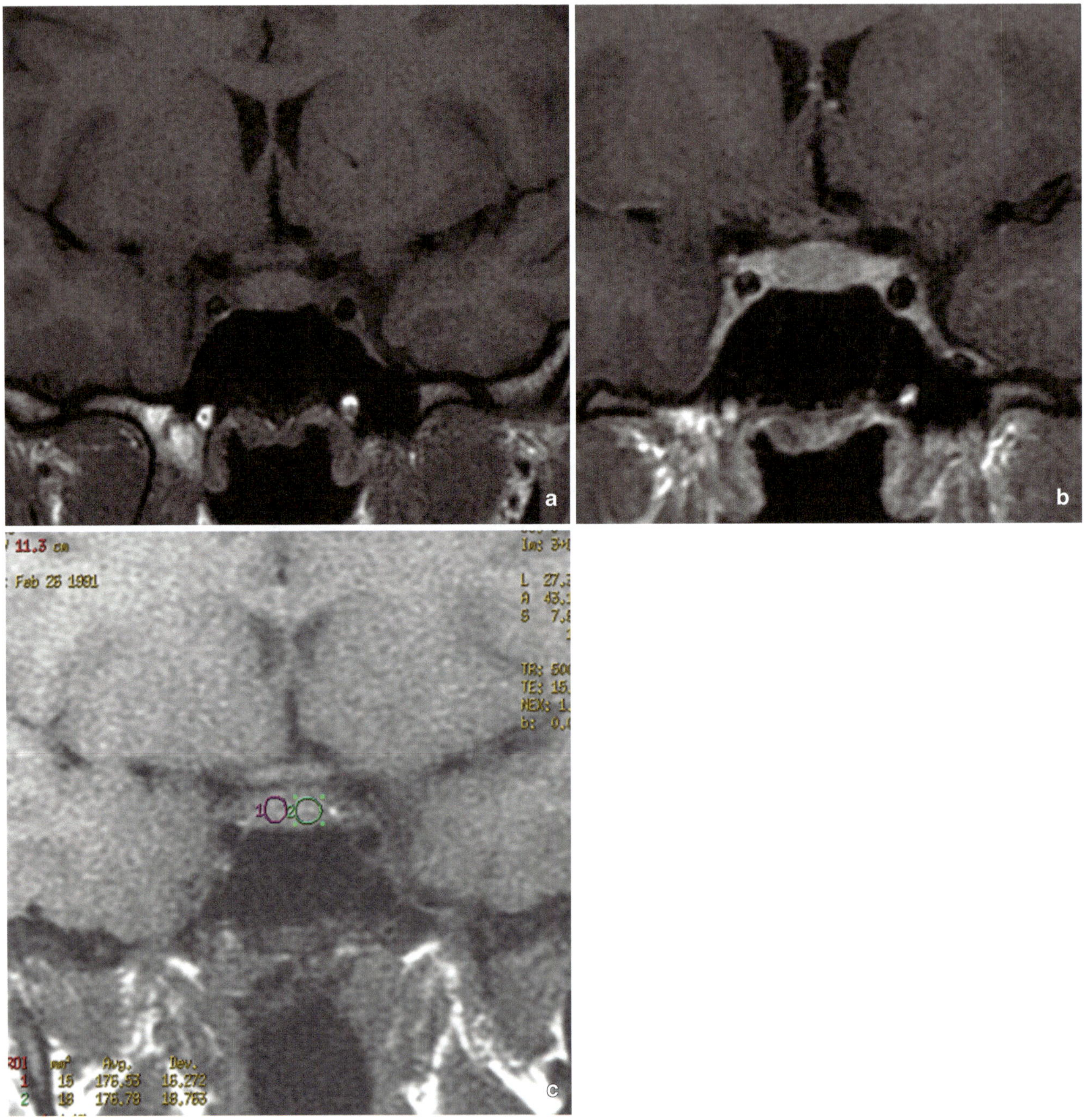

Fig. 15.6 MR imaging of adenohypophysis in healthy volunteer. Coronal T1-weighted images before (**a**) and after CE (**b**) demonstrate homogeneity of the adenohypophysis tissue. Dynamic coronal thin-section T1-weighted image (**c**) obtained following rapid bolus injection of contrast agent does not reveal any abnormalities of enhancement into adenohypophysis. Regions of interest (ROIs) are marked by the circles; the curves on diagram of contrast enhancement correspond to ROIs (**d**). Identical contrast enhancement patterns are detected in the left and right parts of adenohypophysis (**e**)

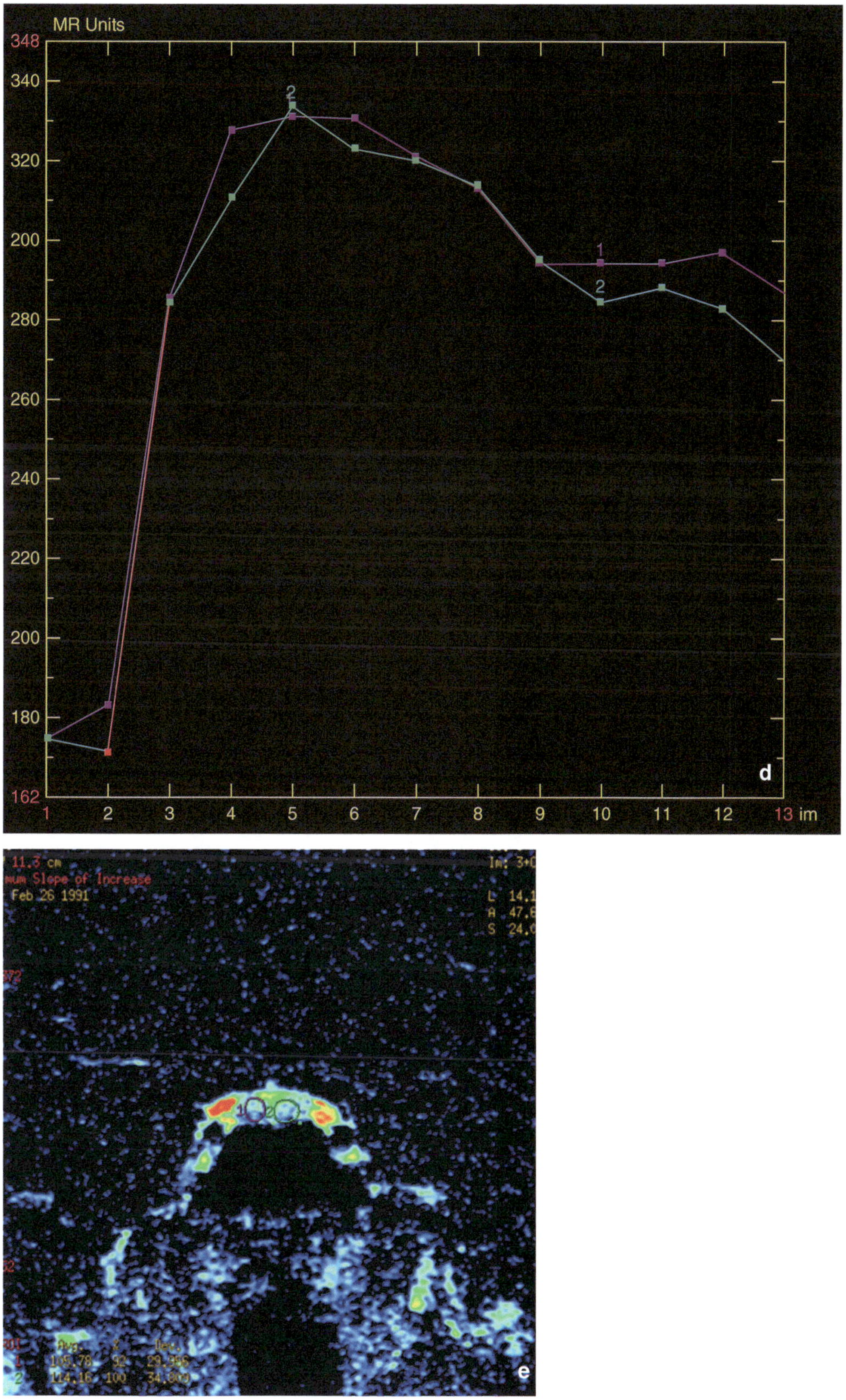

Fig. 15.6 (continued)

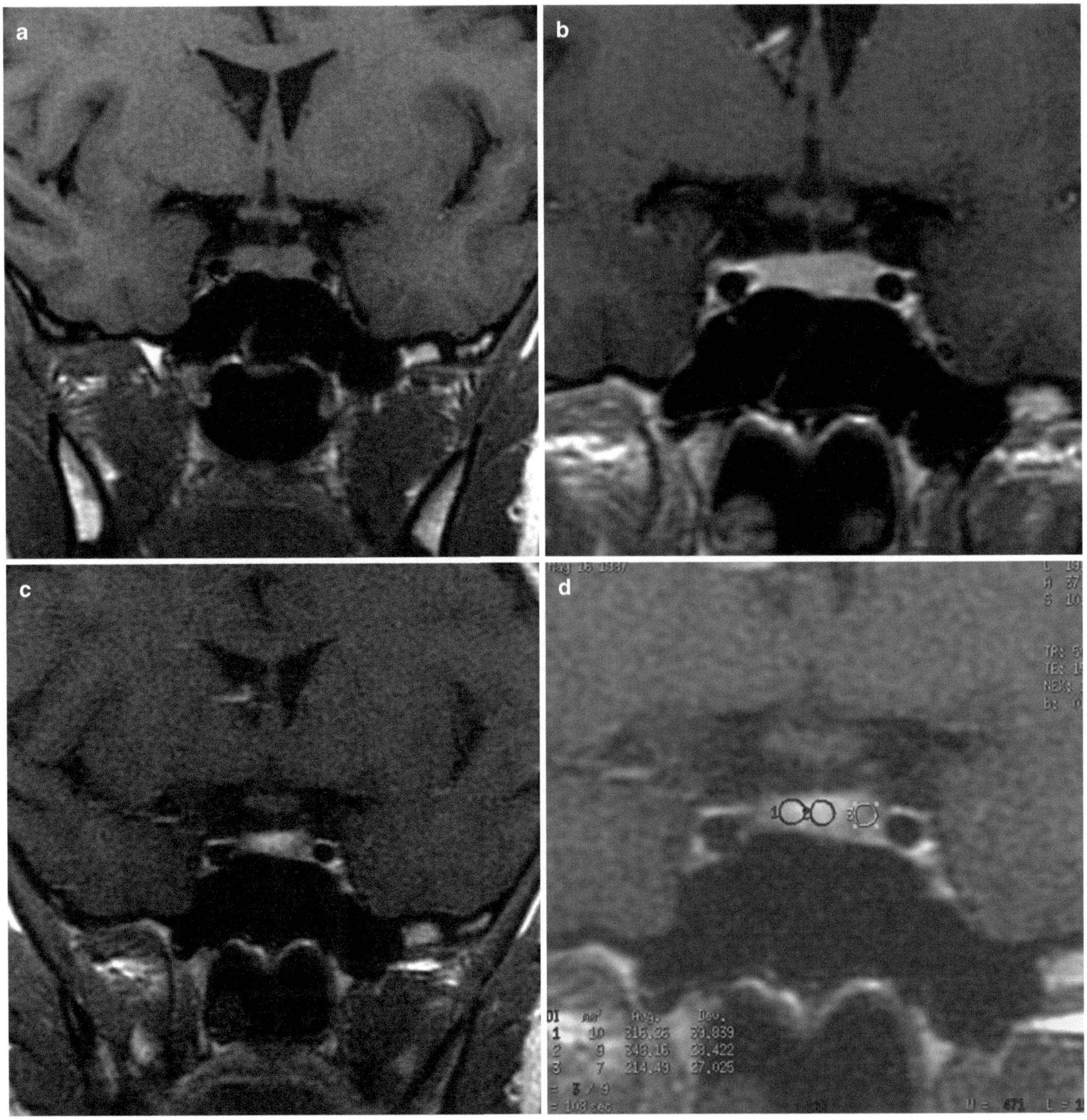

Fig. 15.7 Pituitary microadenoma. Coronal T1- (**a**) and post-contrast T1-weighted images (**b**) do not reveal any significant differences of the MR-signal between the two lobes of adenohypophysis. There is only slight enlargement of the left half of the adenohypophysis. The infundibulum of the pituitary gland is slightly displaced to the left. On dynamic T1-weighted image after contrast agent bolus injection a microadenoma is seen in the left half of the adenohypophysis presenting as a small hypointense area (**c**). Regions of interest on T1-weighted image from dynamic MRI series (**d**) correspond to the curves of enhancement on diagram (**e**). There is a delay of contrast agent accumulation in the microadenoma within the first minute after CE (curve 3); the distinction between normal adenohypophysis and lesion becomes less clear then. (**f**) MR-perfusion colored map

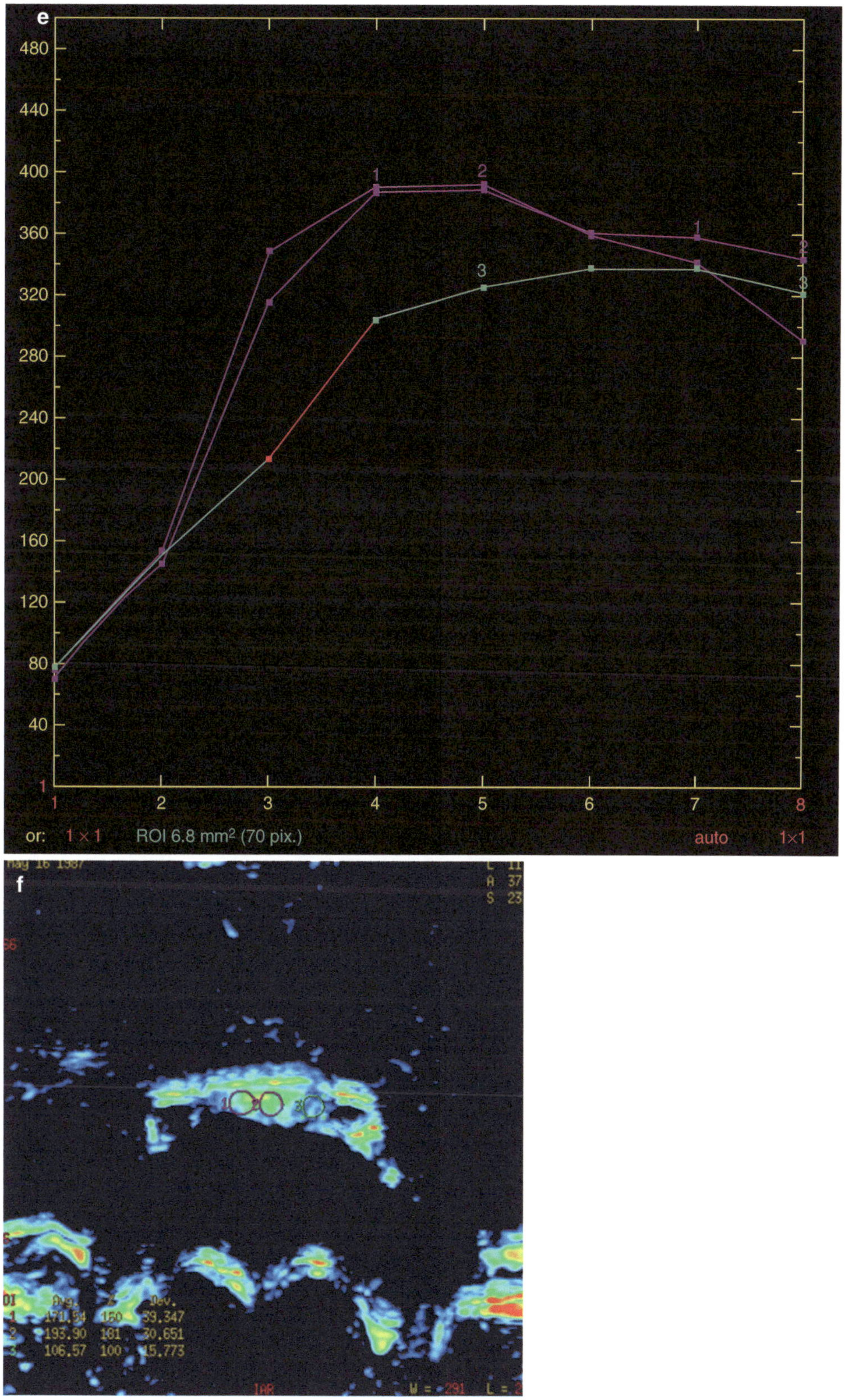

Fig. 15.7 (continued)

asymptomatic, non-progressive focal changes in the adenohypophysis, which are called *incidentalomas*. One reason for these changes is considered to be the presence of local artifacts with magnetic inhomogeneity observed in the inferior part of sella turcica at the site of the attachment of the sphenoid sinus septum. Such an artifact should not be interpreted as a microadenoma, especially if there are no clinical symptoms.

Tumors over 10 mm in size are considered as *macroadenomas*. It is easy to visualize them on modern CT and MR scanners (Kornienko and Ozerova 1993; Konovalov et al. 1997; Dedov 1997; Kornienko and Pronin 2009). More difficult is to make the differential diagnosis from other mass lesions of the chiasmal-sellar region (Asa 2008). If a tumor is relatively small, then it fills only sella turcica. However, in most of our observations, tumors had extrasellar growth. In such cases, the extension of the process should be estimated as well as its spatial relationship to parasellar structures, i.e. the chiasm, optic nerves, the internal carotid artery, the cavernous sinus and others. Optimal surgical access to the tumor is required: transcranial, transnasal or combined (Wolfsberger et al. 2004; Kadashev 2007).

Most pituitary macroadenomas are hormonally inactive and manifest clinical symptoms of an impact on the visual pathways, hypothalamus, cavernous sinuses, brainstem structures, depending on the size and predominant growth direction.

In typical cases MRI reveals a mass lesion originating from sella turcica, iso- or hypointense on T1 weighted images. The intact normal pituitary tissue can be traced along the contour of the adenoma and has more intense signal. On T2-weighted and T2-FLAIR images, macroadenomas are characterized by a high signal more often than microadenomas (Figs. 15.8 and 15.9). On diffusion-weighted images, the tumor has MR

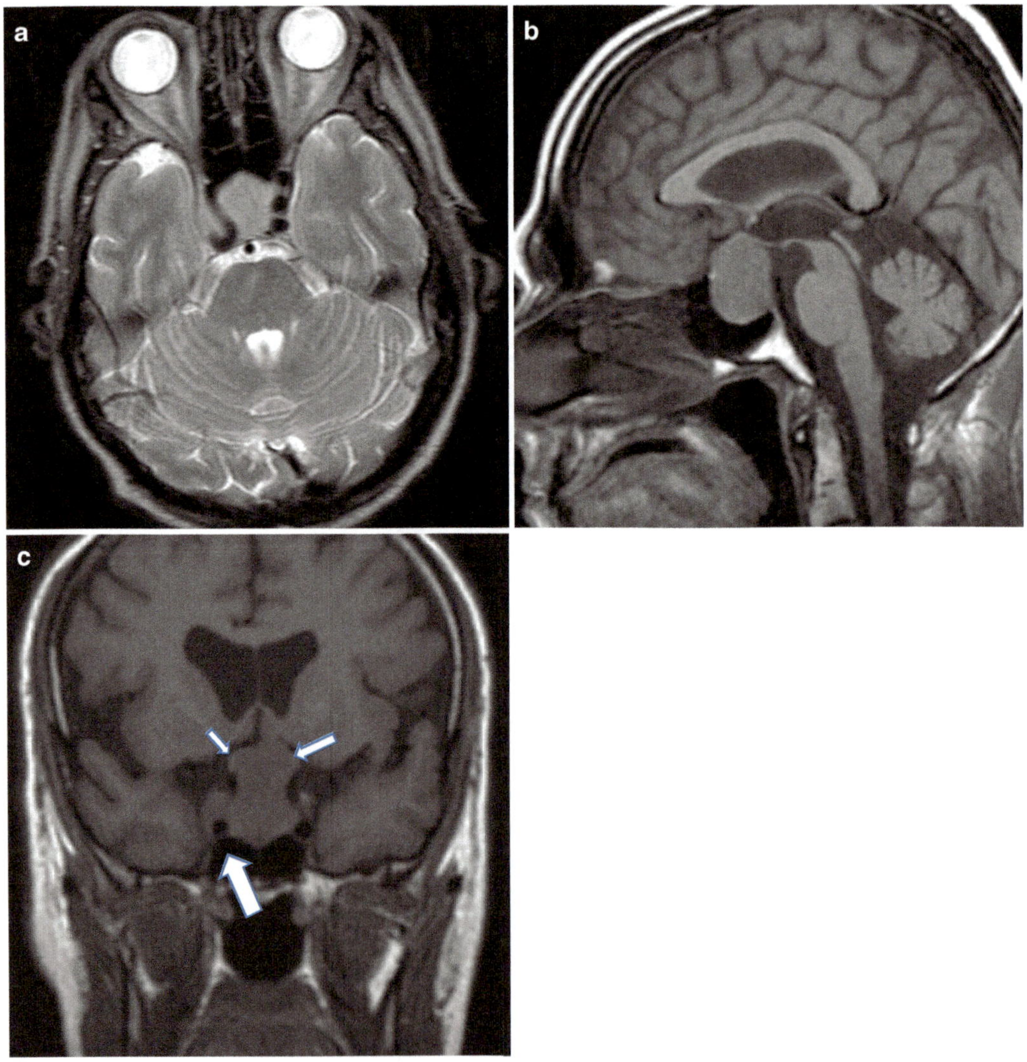

Fig. 15.8 Nonfunctioning pituitary adenoma with sellar, suprasellar, and laterosellar growth, which is characterized by isointense signal on T2-weighted image (**a**) and by slightly decreased signal intensity on T1-weighted images ((**b**)—sagittal, (**c**)—coronal). There is laterosellar tumor growth into the right cavernous sinus; the internal carotid artery is included into the tumor (*arrow*). The optic chiasm is compressed and displaced upward (*small arrows*)

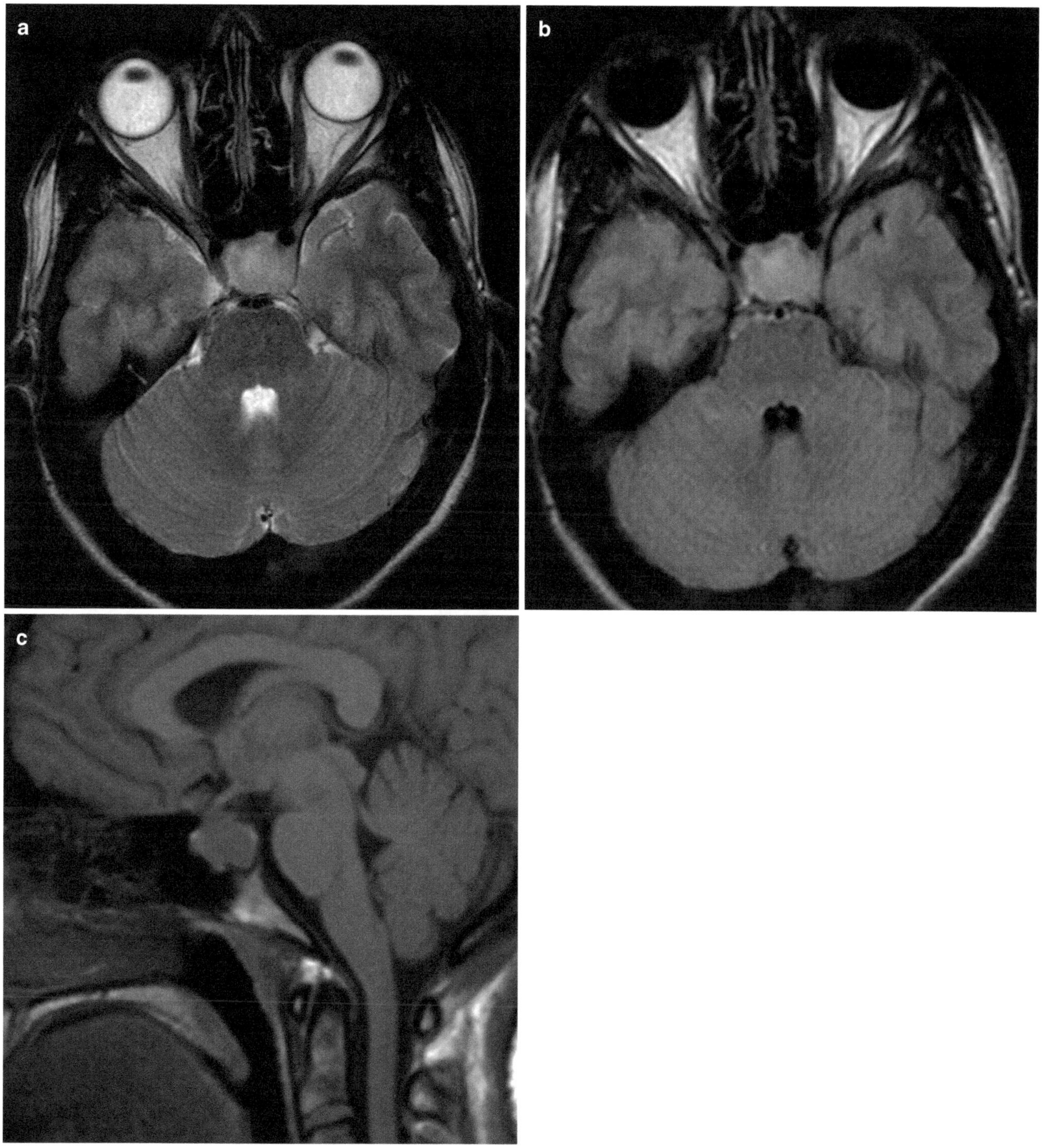

Fig. 15.9 Sellar pituitary adenoma with laterosellar left-sided growth. MR-signal of the tumor is slightly hyperintense on T2-weighted (**a**) and T2-FLAIR (**b**) images, and hypointense on T1-weighted image (**c**)

characteristics close to those of the brain with low ADC values (Fig. 15.10). On CE MRI adenoma intensively and rapidly accumulates contrast media, which makes it hyperintense relative to the brain, in most cases (Fig. 15.11). In rare cases, it is possible to visualize the margin between intact parenchyma of the anterior pituitary and the tumor due to a more pronounced contrast enhancement of the unaffected pituitary tissue (Figs. 15.12 and 15.13). A microcystic adenoma structure sometimes causes a speckled pattern in the tumor. In 20–30% of cases, macroadenomas can contain cystic and hemorrhagic areas, often without clinical manifestations (Fig. 15.14). A pituitary macroadenoma hemorrhage, as one of the possible complications of drug therapy, may occur in patients treated with cabergoline (from the group of dopamine antagonists). In

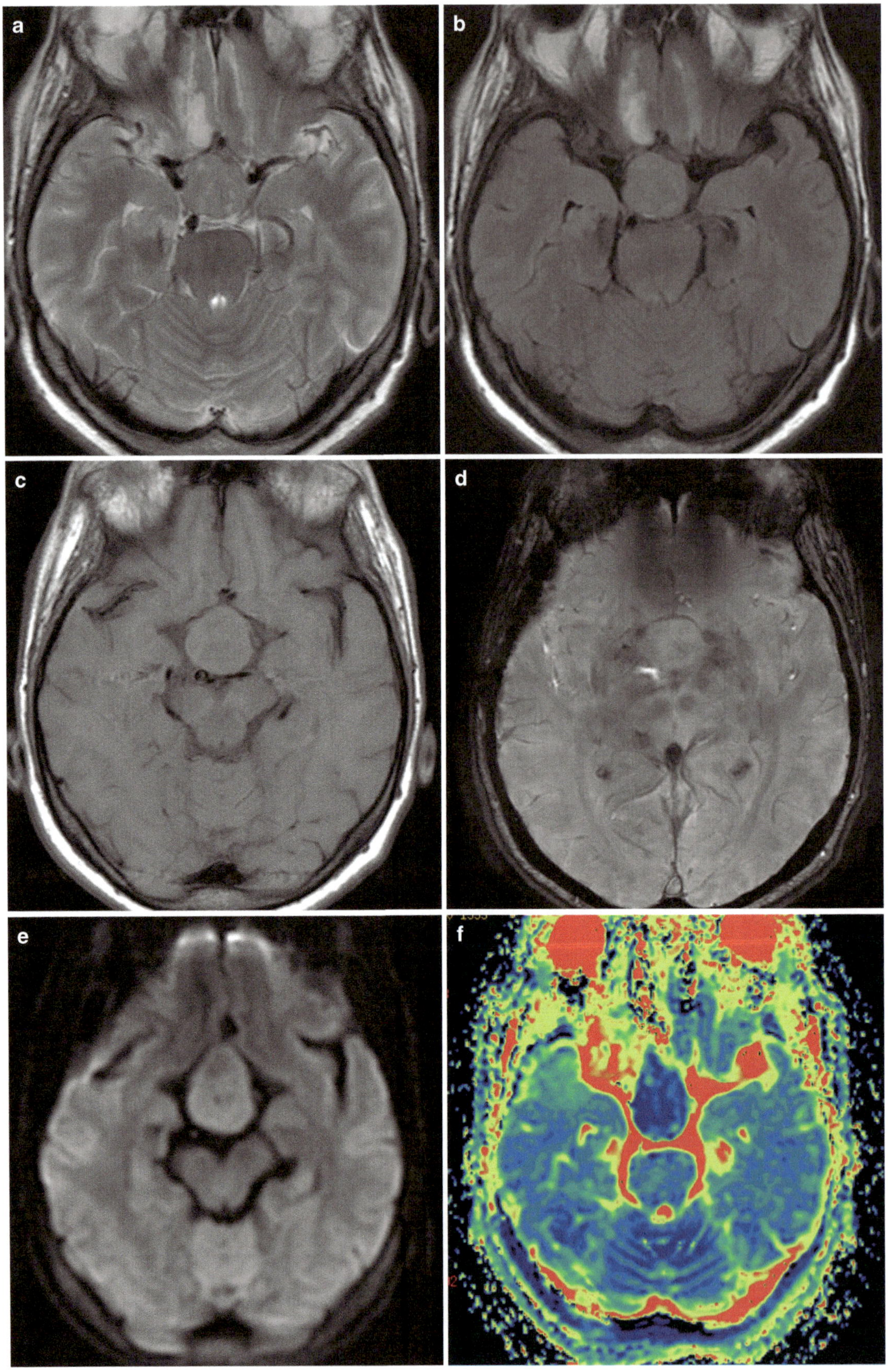

Fig. 15.10 Pituitary sellar-suprasellar adenoma. On T2-weighted image (**a**), T2-FLAIR (**b**), T1-weighted image (**c**), SWAN (**d**), DWI (**e**) an adenoma has homogeneously isointense MR-signal. A color map (**f**) demonstrates the low values of ADC

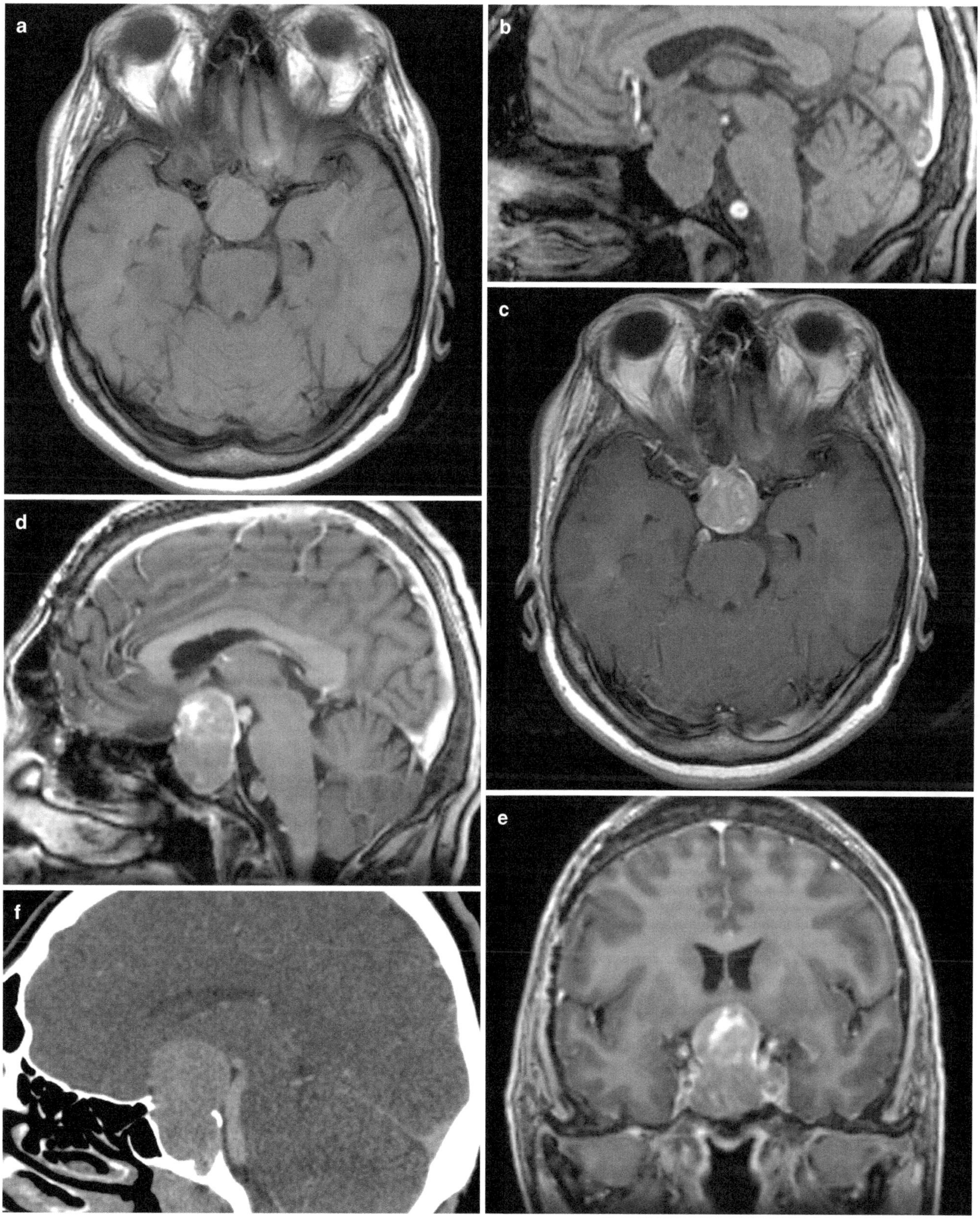

Fig. 15.11 Pituitary adenoma with sellar-supra-laterosellar growth. T1- (**a**, **b**) and post-contrast T1-weighted images (**c**–**e**) demonstrate an intensive contrast enhancement of the tumor mass. Left cavernous sinus is involved by the tumor. A hyperdense tumor within the expanded sella with the eroded floor and dorsum is revealed on CT sagittal reformation after CE (**f**)

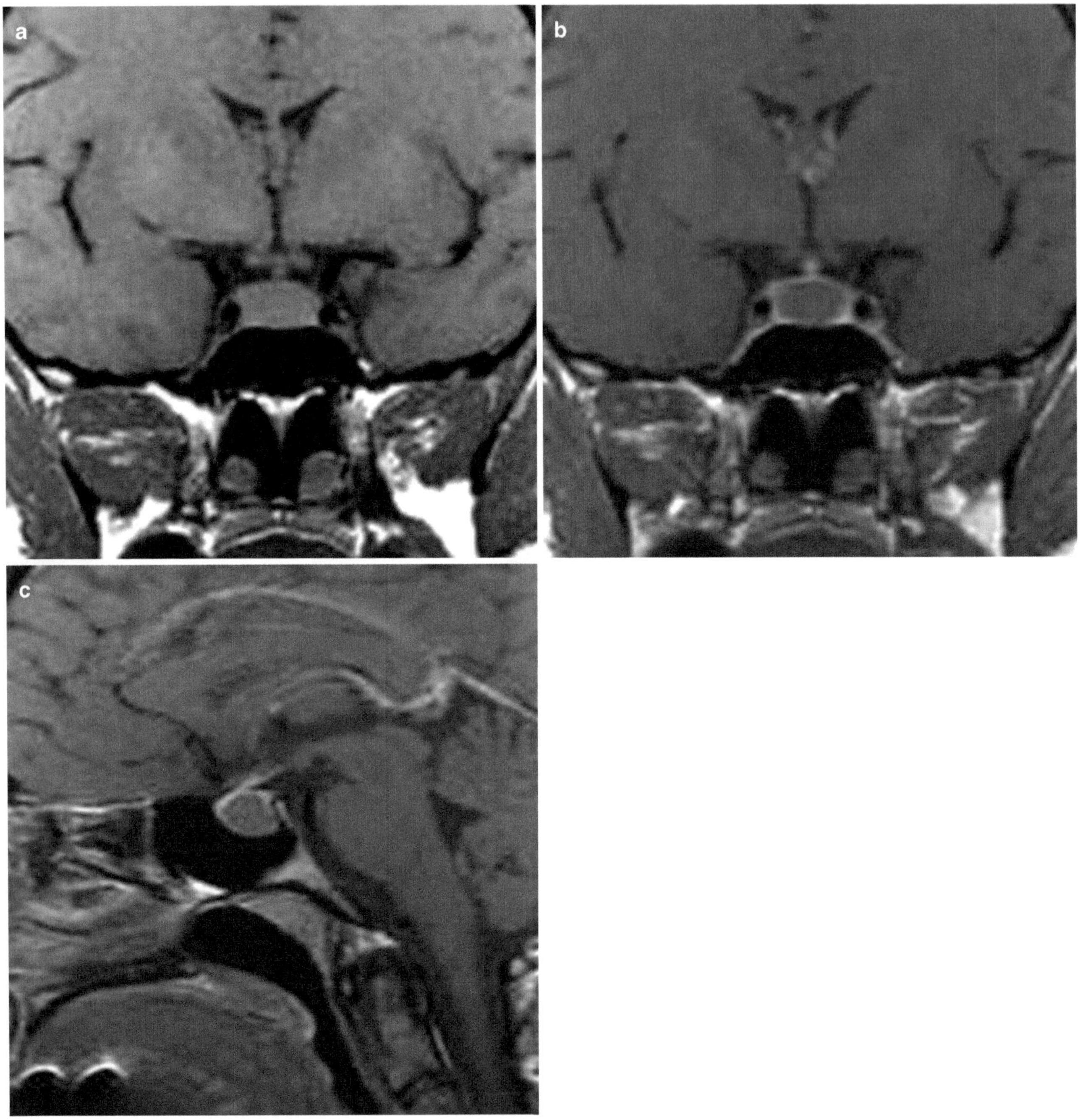

Fig. 15.12 Pituitary adenoma. On T1-weighted image (**a**) and post-contrast T1-weighted images (**b**, **c**) an intensive enhancement is detected in the remaining intact part of the adenohypophysis with better demarcation of the tumor compared with a non-contrast-enhanced MR image

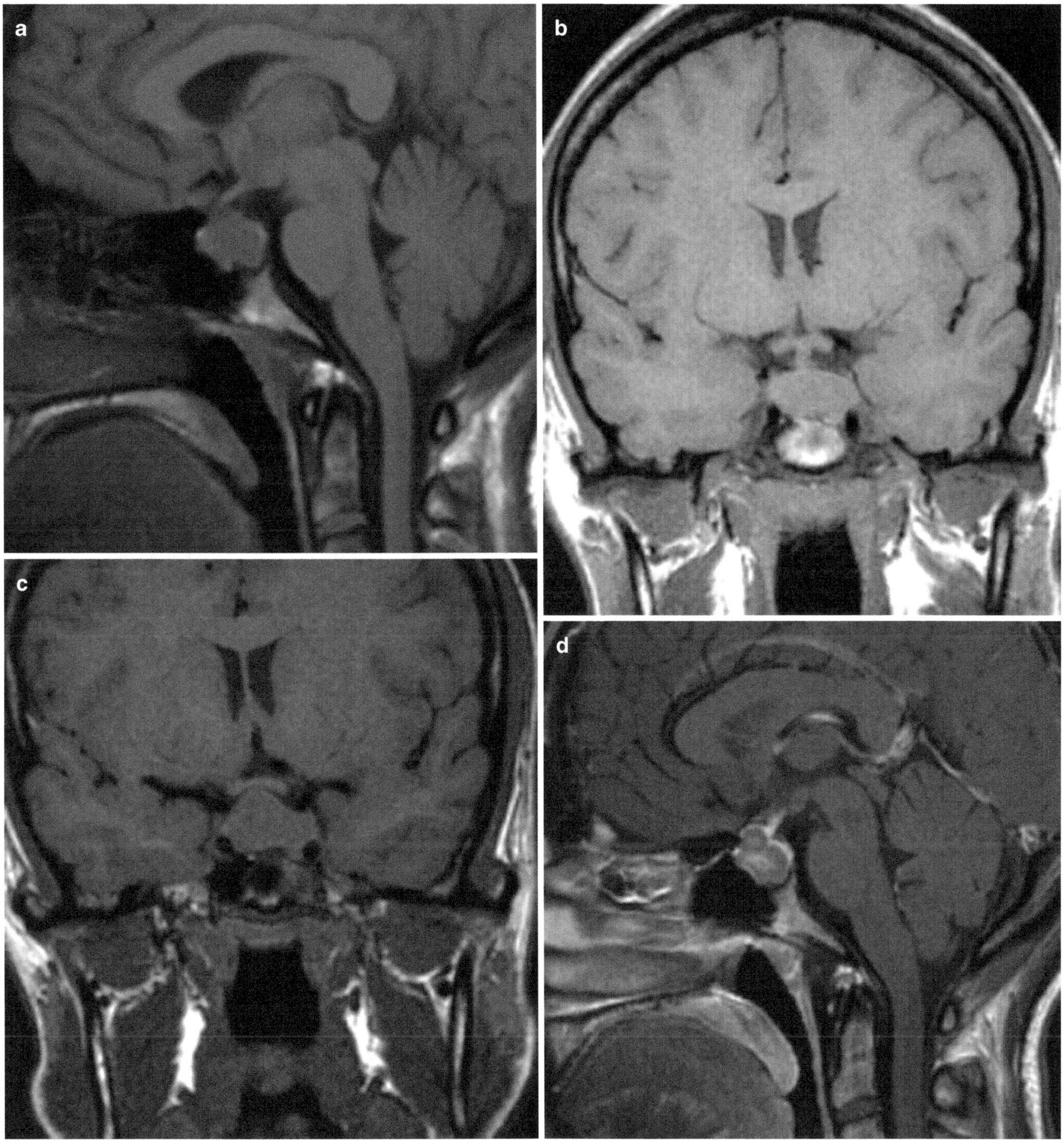

Fig. 15.13 Pituitary adenoma with sellar-suprasellar growth. T1-weighted images (**a–c**) and post-contrast T1-weighted images (**d–f**) demonstrate a heterogeneous enhancement in the tumor tissue and more intense enhancement into the pituitary stalk and remaining normal pituitary tissue at the right-upper margin of the adenoma

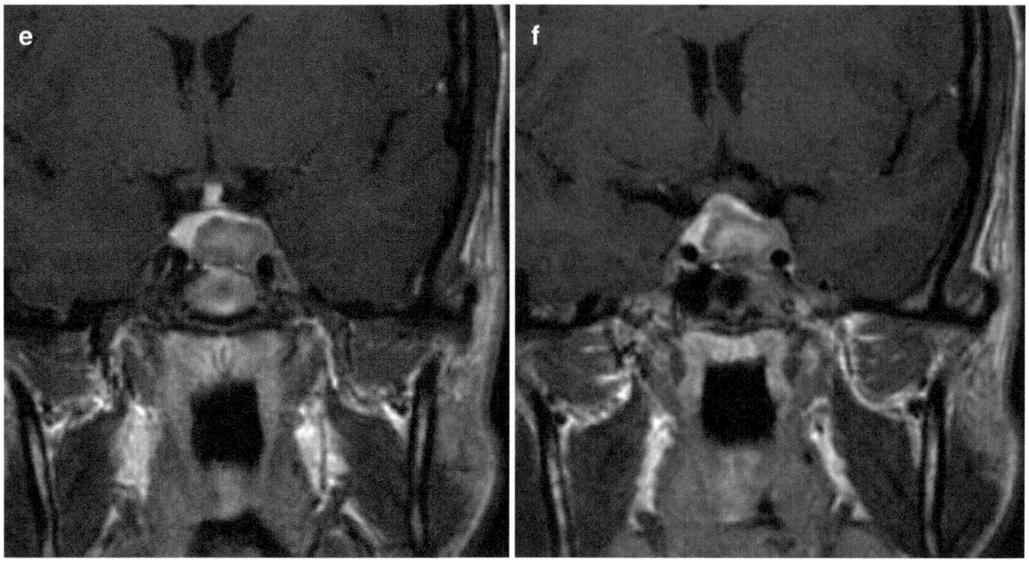

Fig. 15.13 (continued)

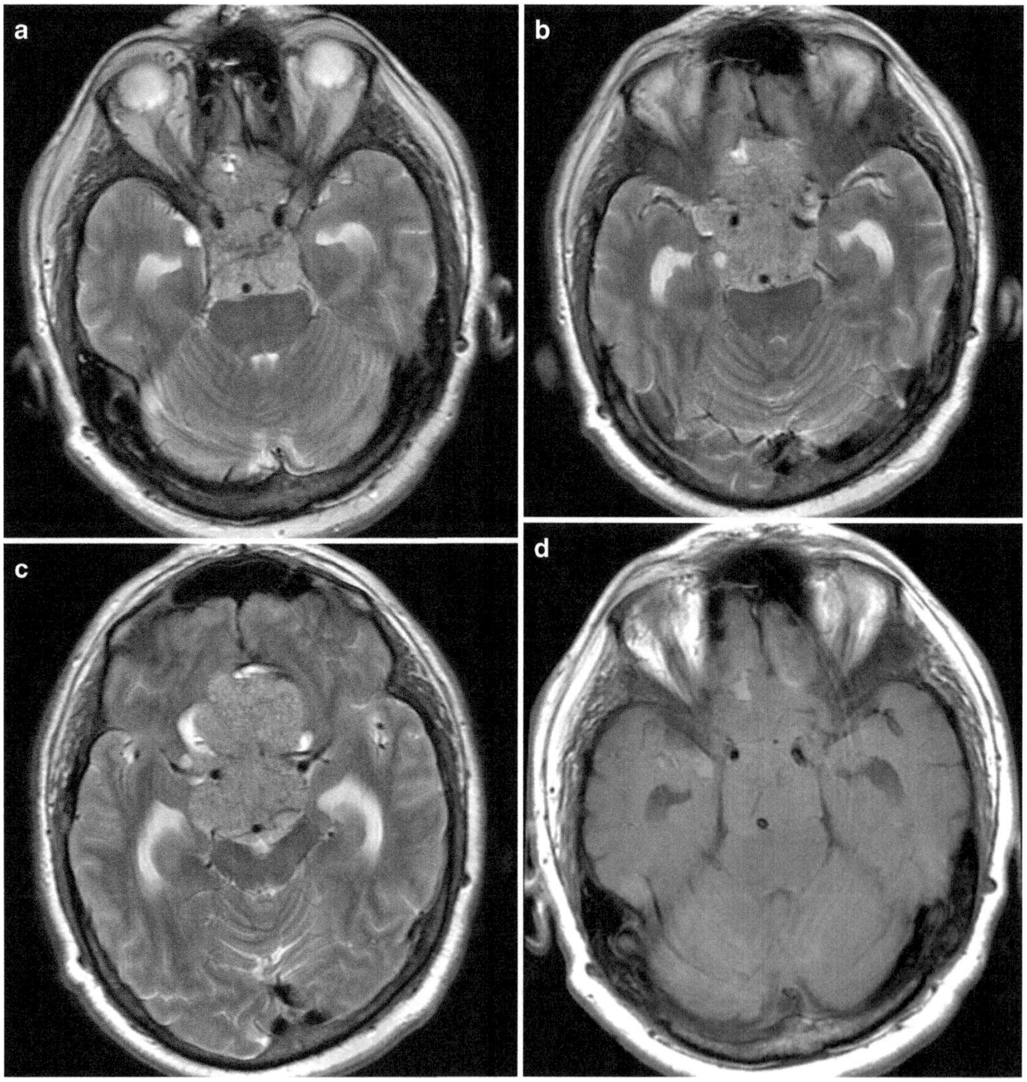

Fig. 15.14 Giant pituitary adenoma. A large sellar-supra-latero-infrasellar tumor with multiple hemorrhagic areas is seen on the series of T2-weighted (**a–c**) and T1-weighted images (**d–f**). Axial 3D T2* image (SWAN) shows the hypointense foci of hemosiderin deposition (**g**). The tumor intensively and heterogeneously enhances (**h, i**). Circle of Willis vessels enveloped by the tumor and have a typical "flow void" hypointense signal

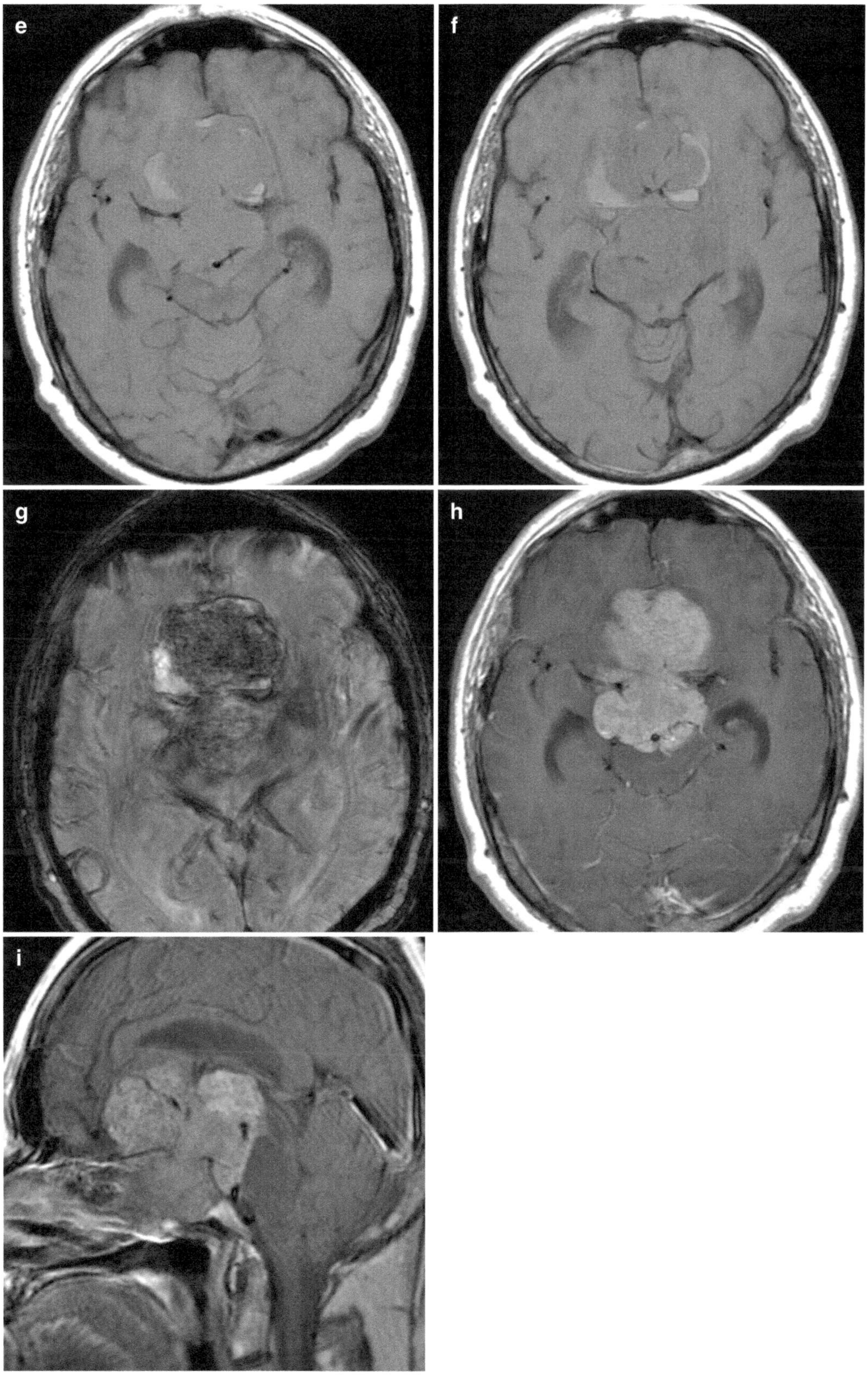

Fig. 15.14 (continued)

such cases, MRI is the method of choice in dynamic studies in patients receiving these drugs, allows monitoring the effectiveness of the treatment (Astafyeva et al. 2009, 2011). The drug administration for 3–24 months in patients with giant hormonally active pituitary adenomas (prolactinomas) turned out to achieve a tumor size reduction in 93% of cases. In 45% of cases, the tumor completely disappeared with formation of a secondary "empty" sella turcica (Fig. 15.15).

In 5–7% of cases the pituitary adenomas may be completely represented by cystic mass lesions. MR signal of the cystic part may vary from markedly hypointense to markedly hyperintense on T1-weighted imaging depending on protein content in the cystic fluid which is shortened T1 relaxation time. Sometimes the sedimentation phenomenon may be observed in the cavity of a cyst which is a specific sign of cystic degeneration (Fig. 15.16).

MR imaging allows accurately determining the relationship between adenoma and arteries, which is extremely important to know when choosing the treatment strategy: whether the tumor compresses or grows over the vessels that are clearly visible on routine scans due to a flow void signal from the artery. The arteries are better visualized using 3D TOF, 3D PC angiography. The arch-shaped displacement of the anterior cerebral artery, rectification and lateral displacement of the internal carotid artery siphon are the typical features of these tumors (Fig. 15.17). Tumor vasculature typically is not visualized. However, as clinical experience shows, pituitary adenoma is a poorly perfused lesion and conventional cerebral angiography is adopted if a giant pituitary adenomas and mass lesions with intratumoral hemorrhages are present. Hemorrhagic complications of pituitary adenomas (paratumoral hemorrhages, tears in the adenoma capsule with intracerebral or subarachnoid hemorrhages) are visualized using a modern gradient echo pulse sequences, such as SWI, SWAN, etc. (Figs. 15.18 and 15.19).

On CT, adenoma in the absence of intratumoral hemorrhage is usually iso- or moderate hyperdense relative to the brain matter. Hemorrhagic areas are hyperdense in the acute period. Cystic changes appear as hypodense areas. Contrast enhancement in all cases contributes to better visualization of the structure and margins of the macroadenomas (Abe et al. 2002). Imaging of the carotid arteries, their displacement or enveloping is best achieved using CT-angiography (Figs. 15.20 and 15.21).

The determining of the upward or *suprasellar* growth of macroadenoma on MRI and CT usually is very easy (Figs. 15.22 and 15.23). But, it is difficult to unequivocally

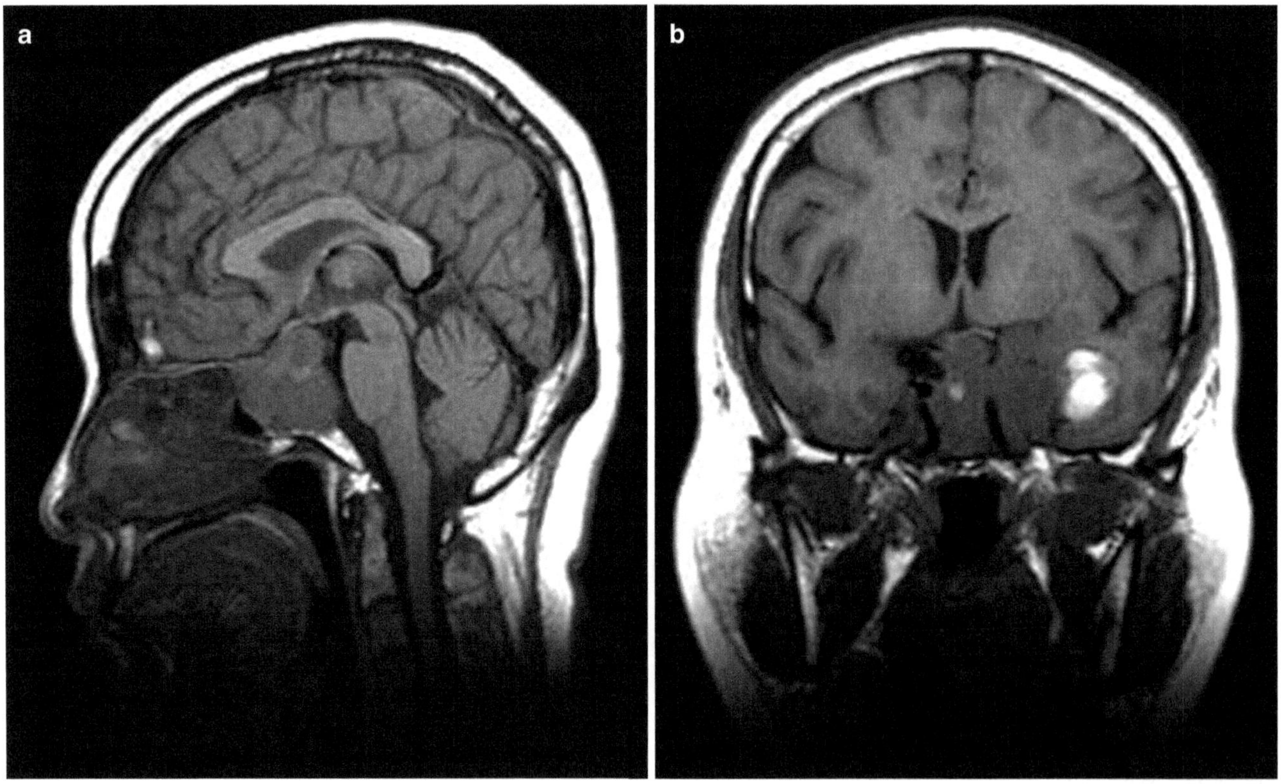

Fig. 15.15 Pituitary adenoma with hemorrhage. T1-weighted images before cabergoline therapy (**a**, **b**) demonstrate infra-supra-latero-sellar tumor with hemorrhagic areas in the left lateral and central part of the lesion. On MRI in 6 months after cabergoline therapy (**c**–**f**) the tumor volume is significantly decreased

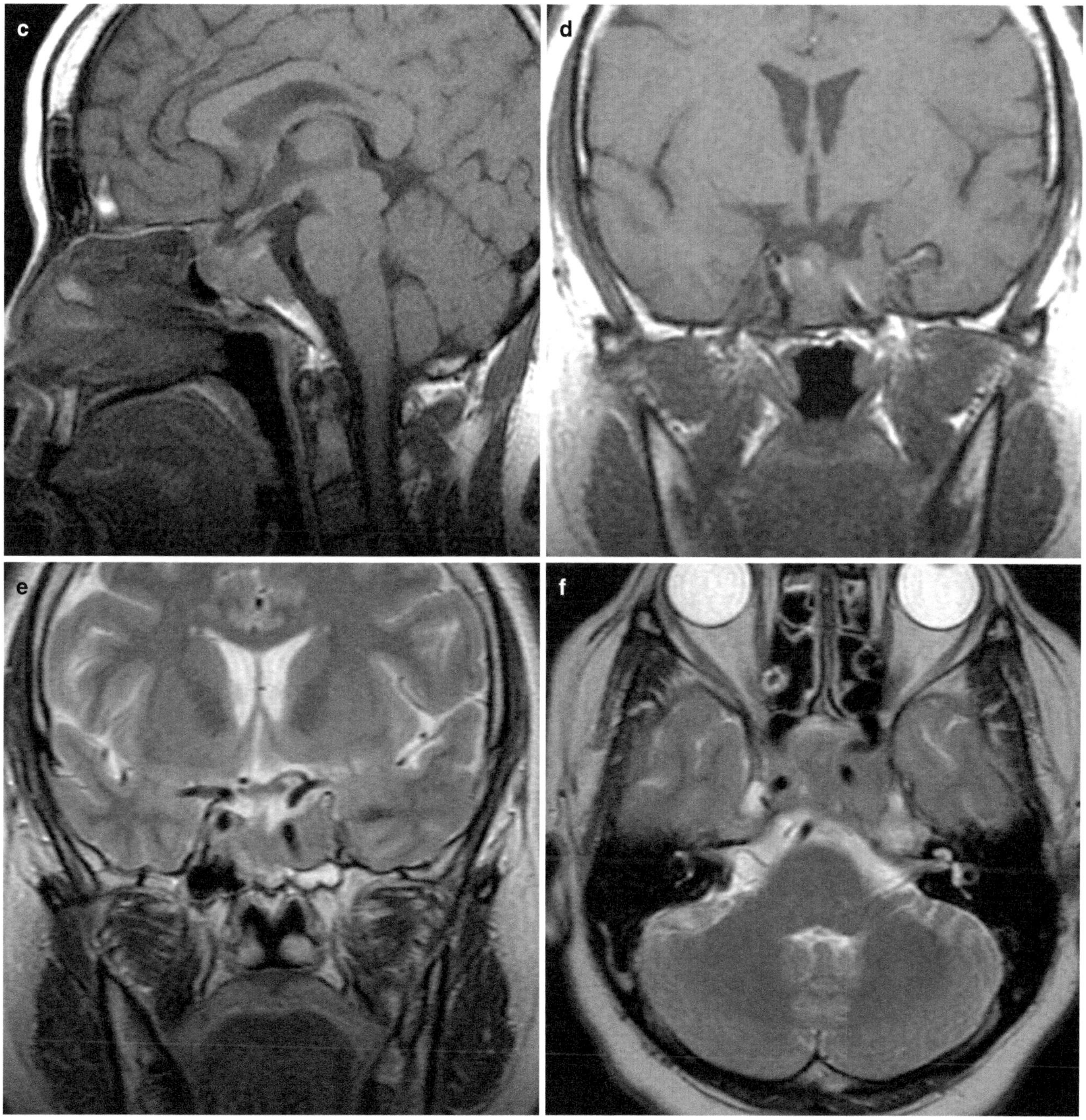

Fig. 15.15 (continued)

judge about the degree of adenoma infiltration of the surrounding capsule. Formation of secondary nodes and tumor growth into the ventricles can be considered as signs of adenoma growing beyond the capsule. It must be admitted that verification of adenoma growth pattern (infiltrative, non-infiltrative) is sometimes possible only after surgery or autopsy.

A *laterosellar* growth of adenomas into cavernous sinuses, in contrast to suprasellar growth, is less clearly identified by MRI (Ahmadi et al. 1985). The main reason for this is that the medial wall of the sinus is very thin and thus is not visualized in most cases. In many cases coronal MRI scans show how a tumor grows above and beneath the cavernous part of the internal carotid artery, but it is not possible to identify simultaneously whether an adenoma invades the cavernous sinus or it just compresses it. On the other hand, the lateral wall of the cavernous sinus is a reliable landmark—it is relatively thick and is clearly identified on MRI. The growth of a

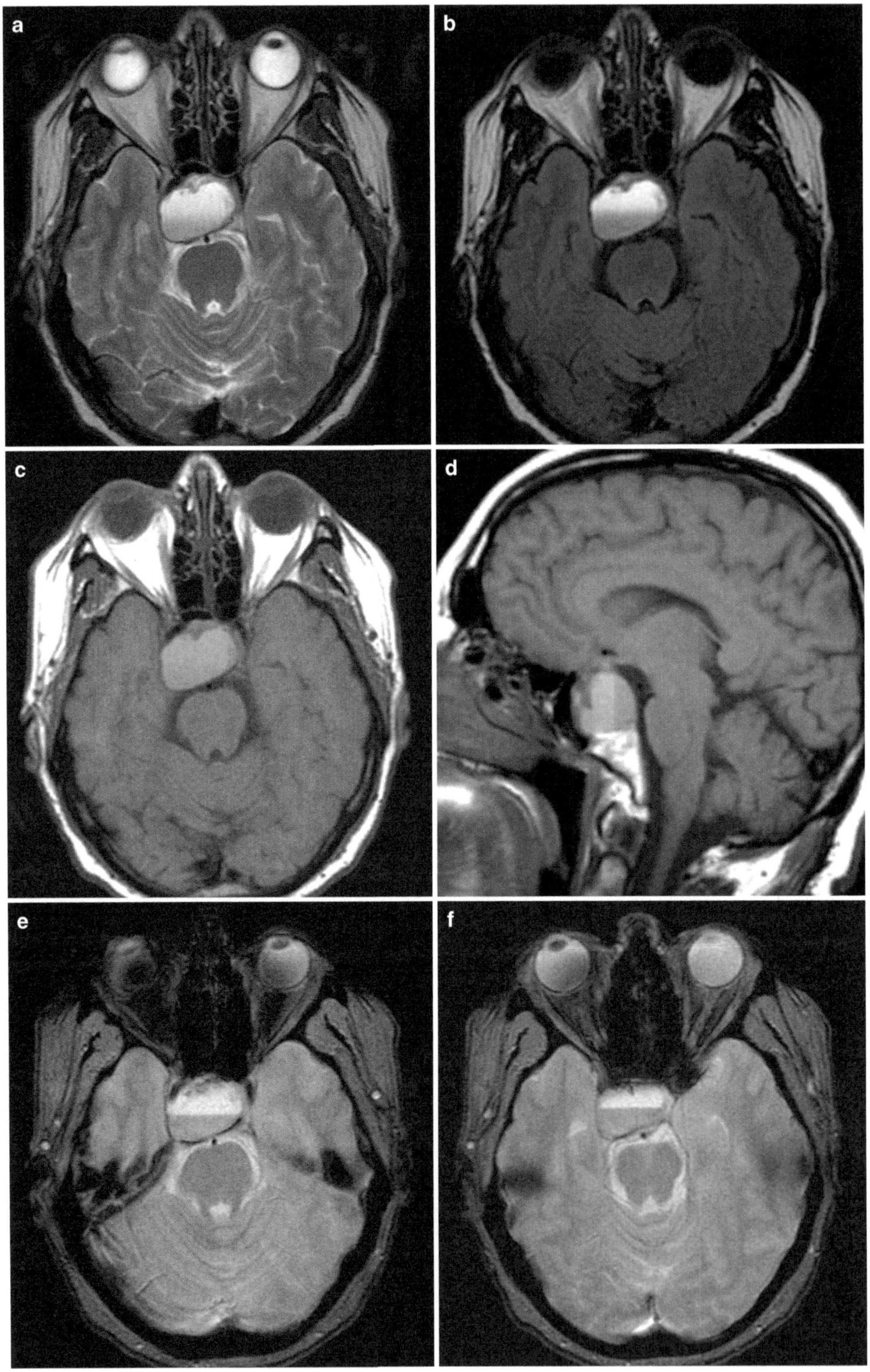

Fig. 15.16 Pituitary macroadenoma with hemorrhage. T2-weighted image (**a**), T2-FLAIR (**b**), T1-weighted images (**c**, **d**) and T2*GRE images (**e**, **f**) demonstrate a cystic structure within the tumor with a blood-fluid level

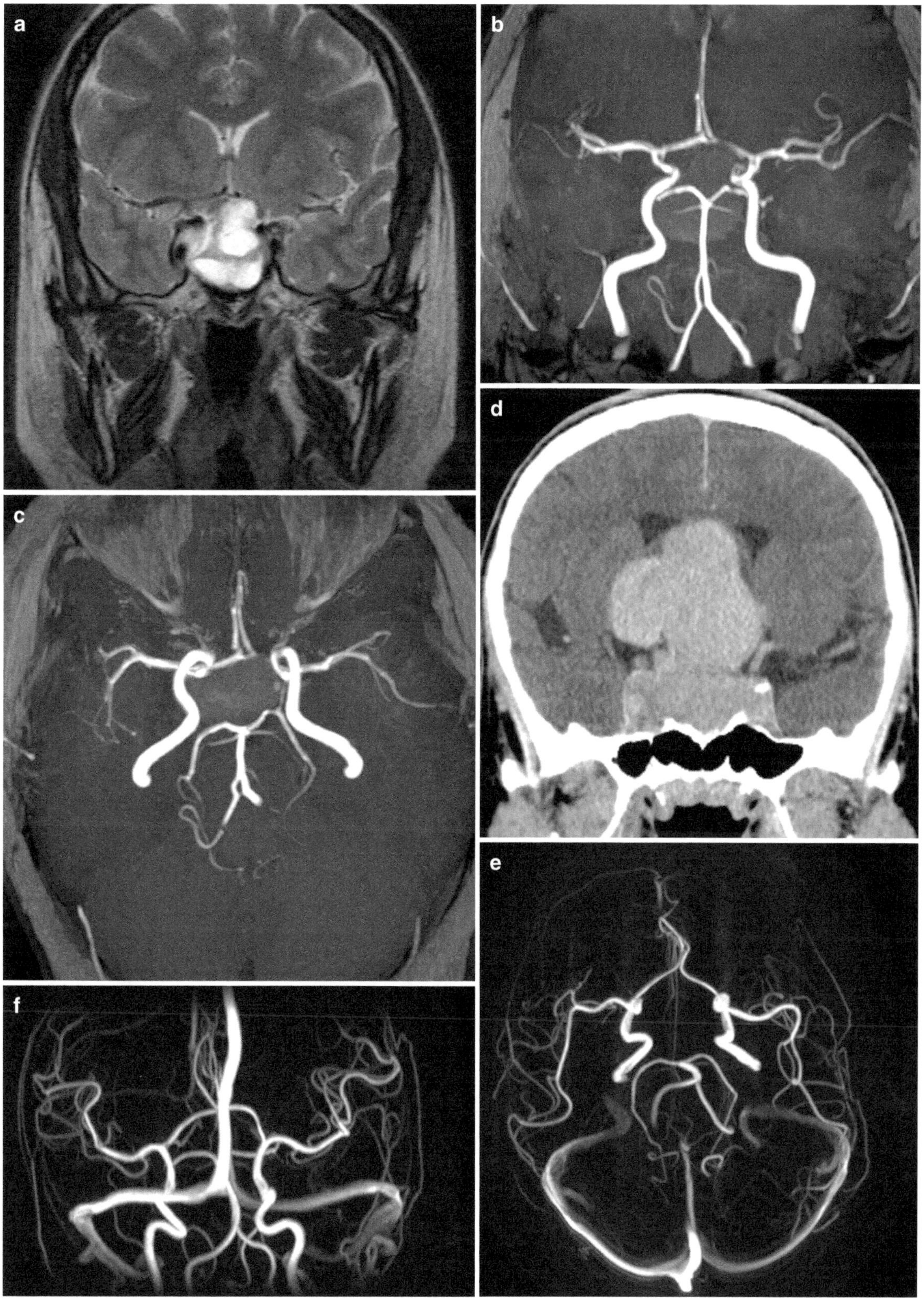

Fig. 15.17 Pituitary adenoma. Case 1. T2-weighted MR image (**a**) shows a supra-laterosellar tumor with heterogeneous structure. Cavernous sinuses are laterally displaced, mainly on the right side, where the tumor encases the carotid artery. 3D TOF angiography (**b**, **c**) reveals laterally displaced a right internal carotid artery. P1 segment of the posterior cerebral artery displays posteriorly and A1 segments of anterior cerebral arteries are displaced superiorly. The vasculature of the tumor is absent. Case 2. Giant pituitary adenoma. Coronal CT scan with CE detects a giant tumor with increased density (**d**). 3D PC MR angiography reveals arcuate superior displacement of the anterior cerebral arteries; a tumor displaces the internal carotid arteries as well. The tumor vasculature is not visible (**e–f**)

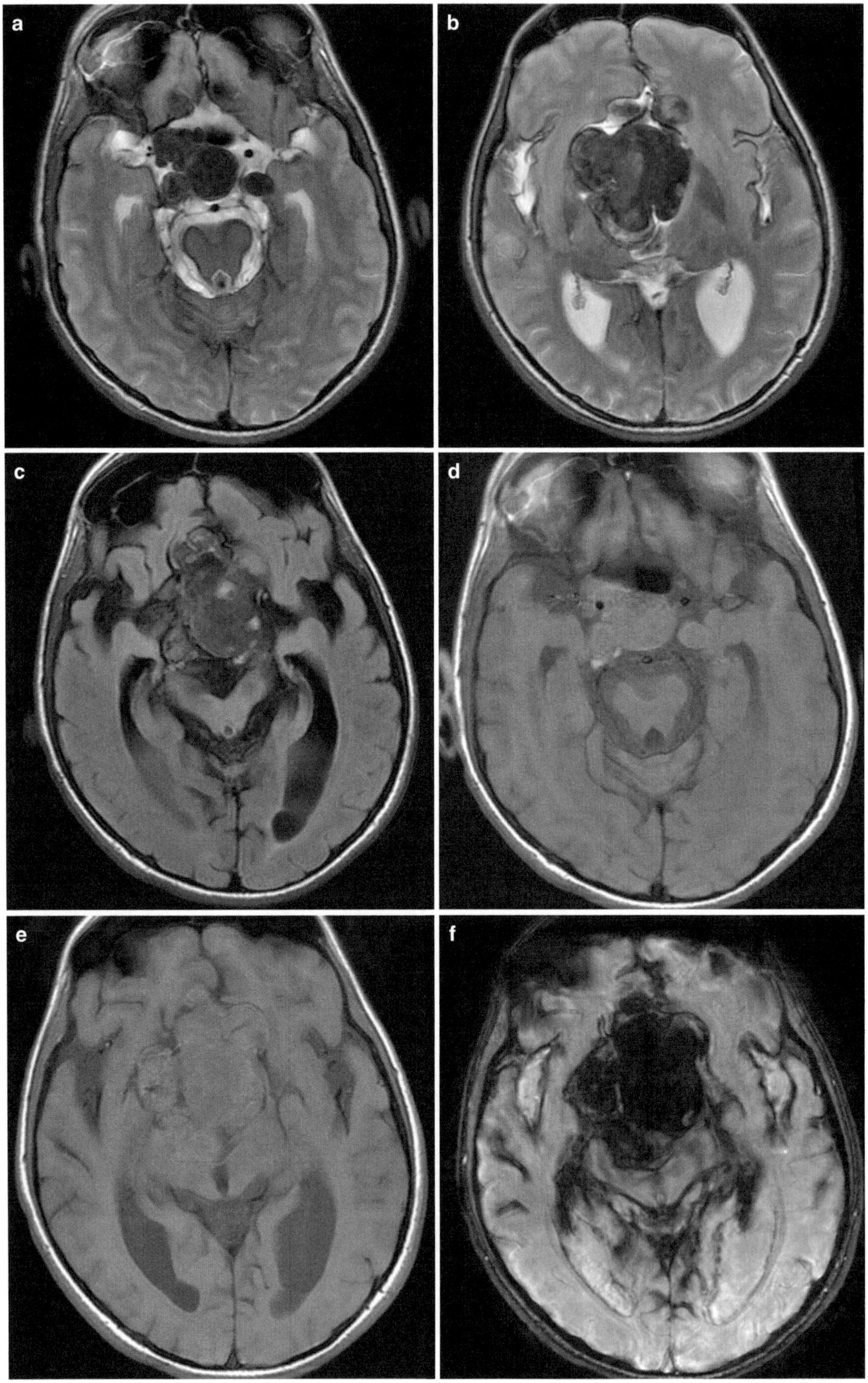

Fig. 15.18 Giant pituitary adenoma with hemorrhage. T2-weighted images (**a**, **b**), T2-FLAIR (**c**), T1-weighted images (**d**, **e**) demonstrate a diffuse hemorrhage within the pituitary adenoma mass. A low signal in adenoma tissue and in surrounding leptomeninges on 3D T2* (SWAN) (**f**) proves that there is not only the intratumoral but subarachnoid hemorrhage (probably due to adenoma capsule rupture) as well

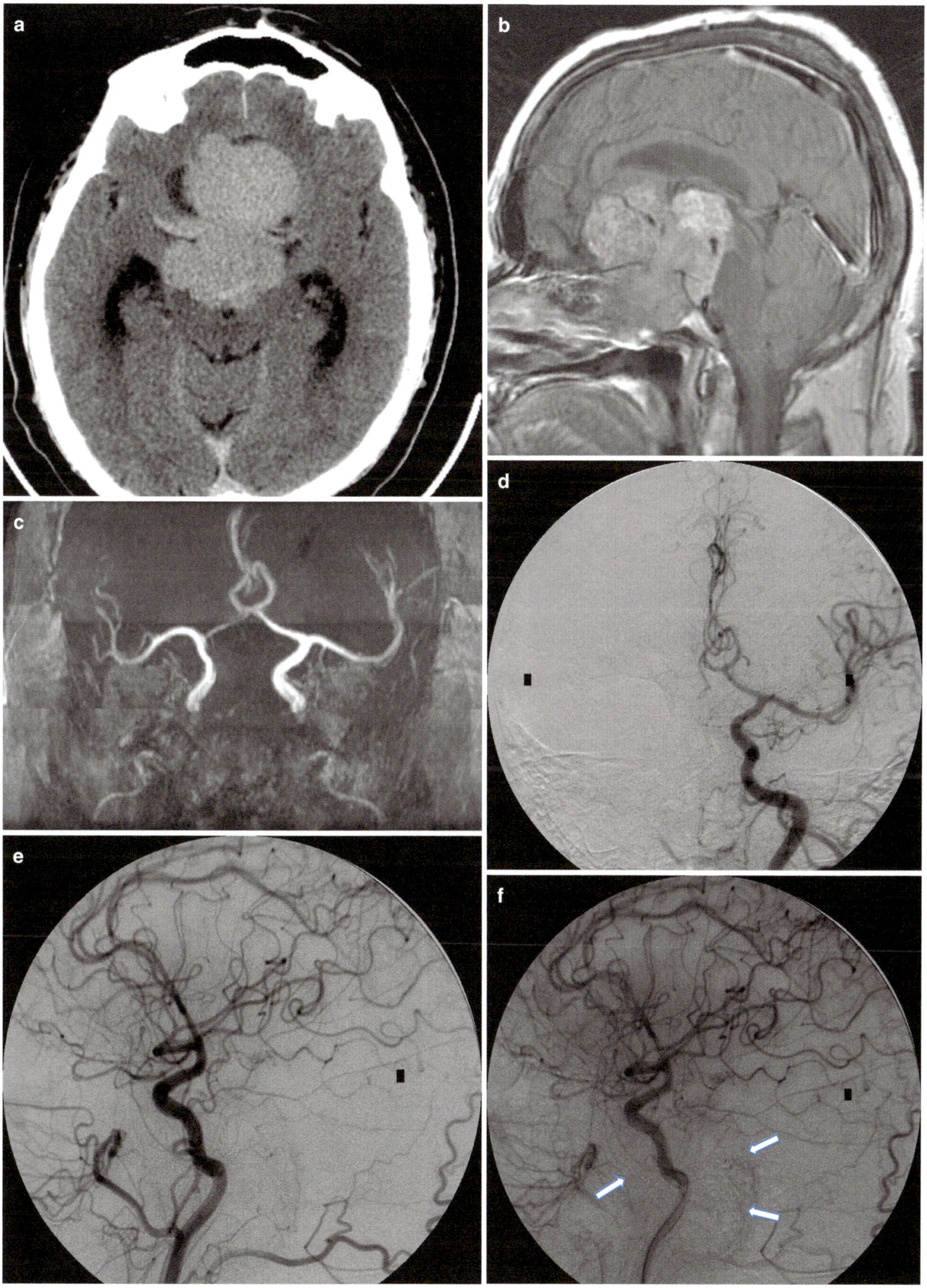

Fig. 15.19 Giant pituitary adenoma. Enhanced CT (**a**) and sagittal T1-weighted images (**b**) demonstrate a giant supra-infra-laterosellar tumor. 3D TOF angiography (**c**) detects arcuate superior displacement of the A1 segments of the anterior cerebral arteries; the tumor vasculature is not visualized. Conventional angiography in coronal (**d**) and sagittal (**e**, **f**) projections reveals a mild vasculature net of the tumor (*arrows*)

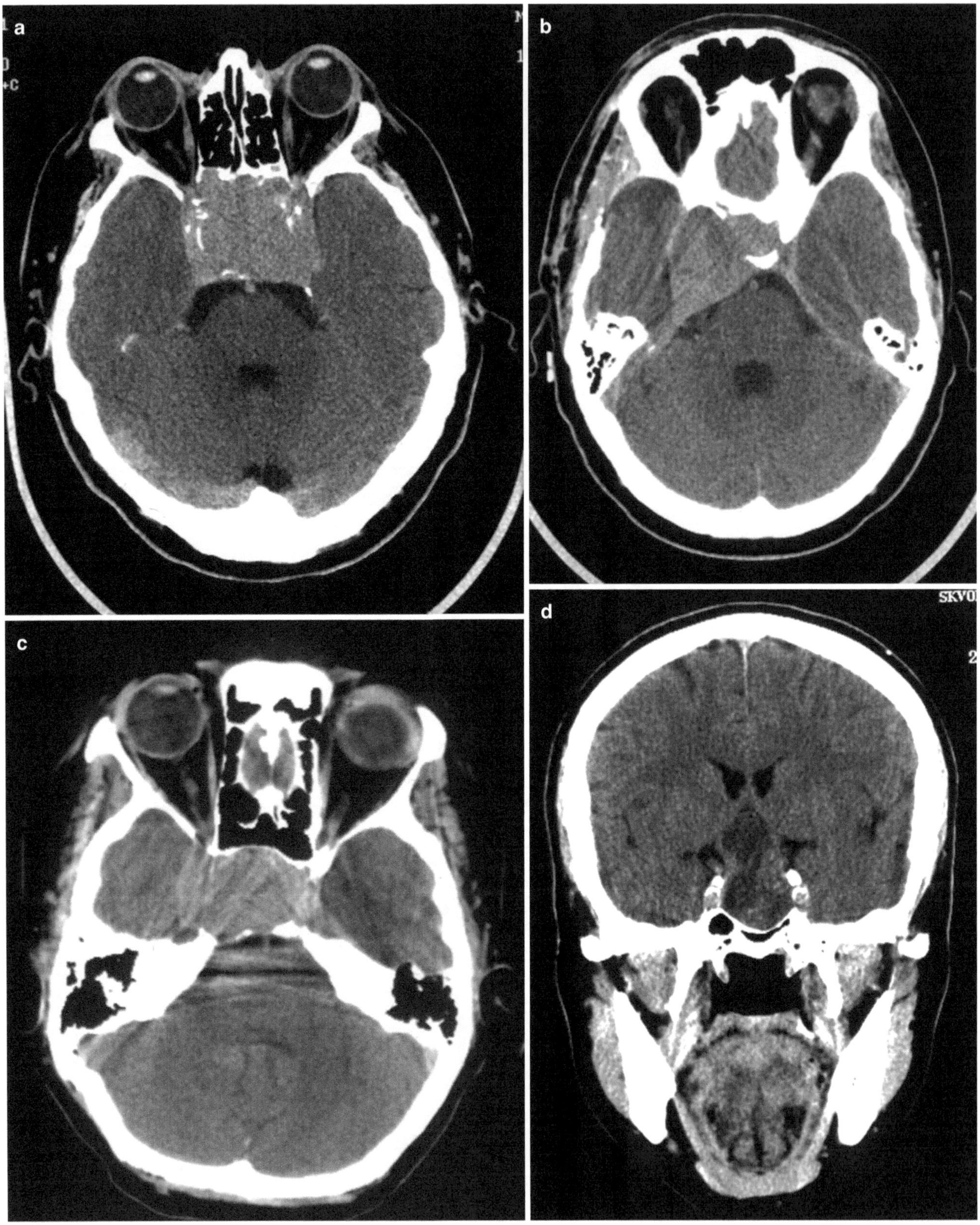

Fig. 15.20 Variants of pituitary adenoma growth in different patients on CE CT. Intravenous contrast agent injection improves a visualization of the tumor structure and delineates the borders between tumor and brain tissue. It gives additional information about the tumor (**a**–**f**)

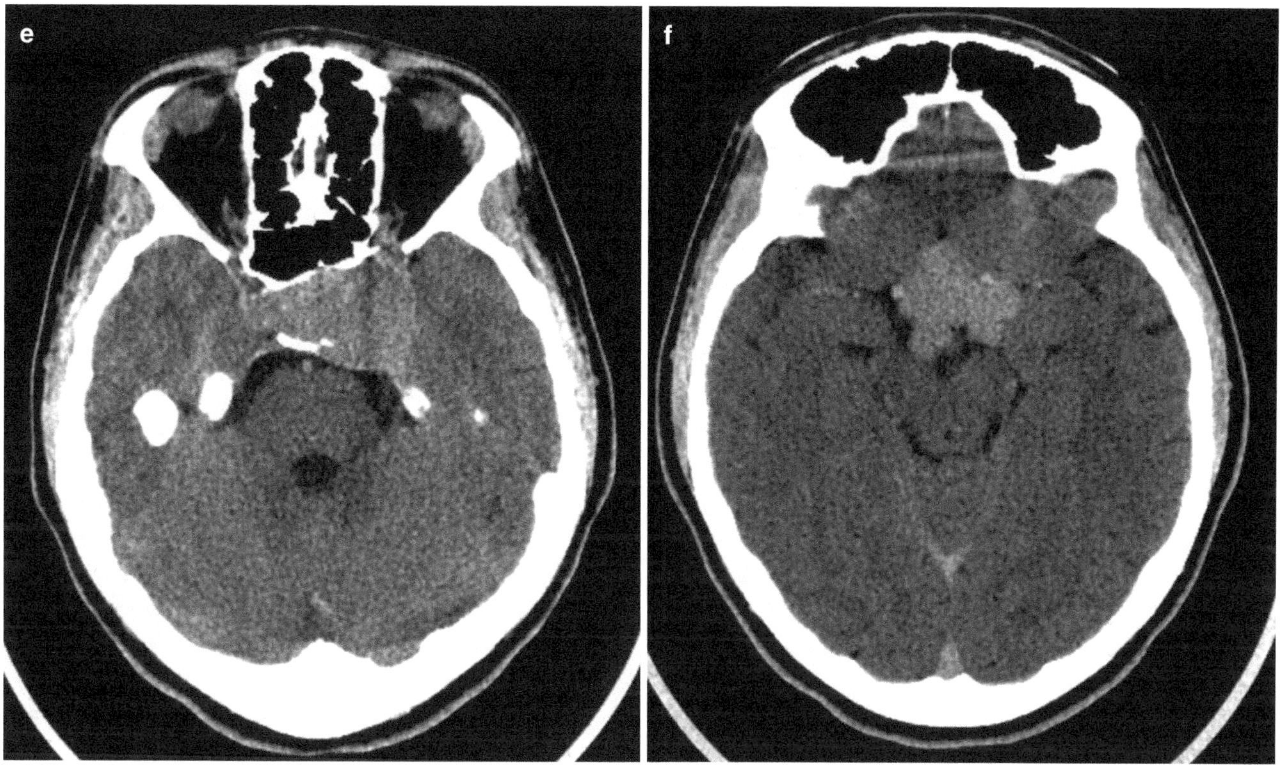

Fig. 15.20 (continued)

tumor between the lateral wall of the cavernous sinus and the internal carotid artery is the most reliable sign of the cavernous sinus invasion. Asymmetrical enlargement of one of the cavernous sinuses should lead to suspect sinus invasion. The tumor usually completely overgrows the infraclinoid portion of the internal carotid artery (Fig. 15.24). It is important to note that despite the fact that lateral invasion of cavernous sinuses is a frequent event, compression and occlusion of the cavernous segment of the internal carotid artery rarely occurs. This has diagnostic significance in the differential diagnosis between adenomas and meningiomas. By invading the sinus, adenoma can form secondary intradural nodes, extending from the primary tumor. This may occur at the entry point of the oculomotor nerve into the sinus wall. Separating the layers of the dura laterally to the sinus wall, the tumor can spread extradurally to the middle cranial fossa. Extracranial growth into the infratemporal fossa occurs due to destruction of the middle cranial fossa bones by the tumor growing from the cavernous sinus.

The *infrasellar* growth of a tumor is easily identified on sagittal and coronal T1-weighted images when the adenoma's tissue is revealed in the sphenoid sinus containing air, the tumor usually destroys the floor of the sella turcica, although sometimes it can remain almost intact (Fig. 15.25). The degree of bone destruction should be assessed using CT.

In case of *antesellar* growth, tumor infiltration into the ethmoid bone occurs through the lower anterior wall of the sella turcica and is usually associated with the presence of adenoma tissue in the sphenoid sinus. Antesellar adenoma growth into the orbit usually starts from the ethmoid bone and the cavernous sinus and leads to destruction of the medial or lateral orbital walls with extending along the optic canal into the superior orbital fissure along large veins.

Adenomas grow *retrosellarly* from the sella turcica or the cavernous sinus area. This may occur due to destruction of the dorsum sella and the upper parts of the clivus. In this case, the tumor extends extradurally along the clivus as a "tongue." Intradural penetration of tumor masses is also possible due to the growth along the cranial nerves, rarely due to invasion into the dura mater. In case of retrosellar growth from the cavernous sinus, extra- and intradural nodes are formed in the posterior cranial fossa (Fig. 15.26).

There is a well-accepted concept of *invasive or infiltrative pituitary adenoma* in literature. In the absence of obvious signs of anaplasia in the tumor tissue, adenoma affects the skull base bones (sphenoid bone, clivus, ethmoid bone, etc.) and occupies a large area by the time of diagnosis, which makes its total removal almost impossible (Figs. 15.27 and 15.28).

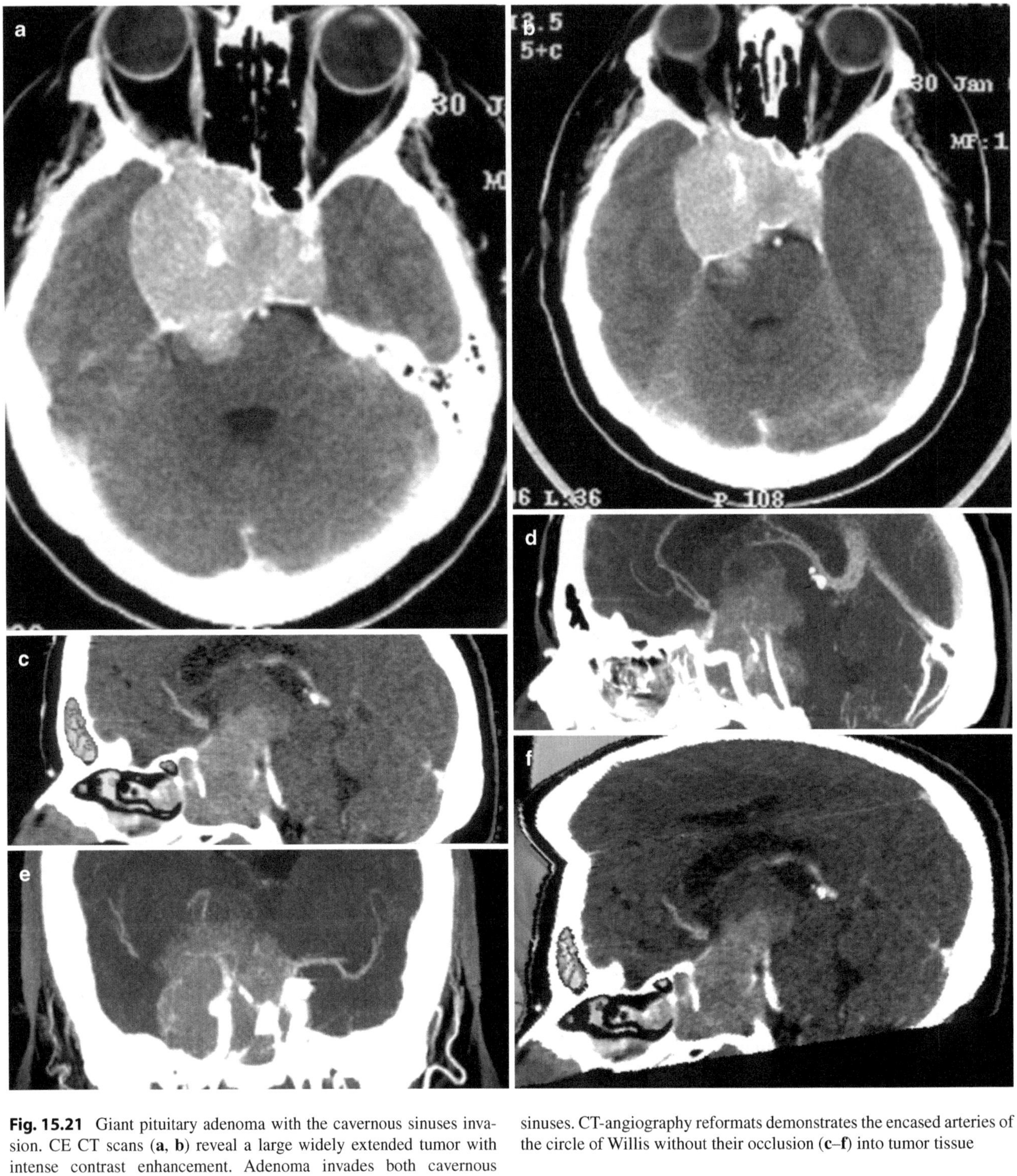

Fig. 15.21 Giant pituitary adenoma with the cavernous sinuses invasion. CE CT scans (**a**, **b**) reveal a large widely extended tumor with intense contrast enhancement. Adenoma invades both cavernous sinuses. CT-angiography reformats demonstrates the encased arteries of the circle of Willis without their occlusion (**c**–**f**) into tumor tissue

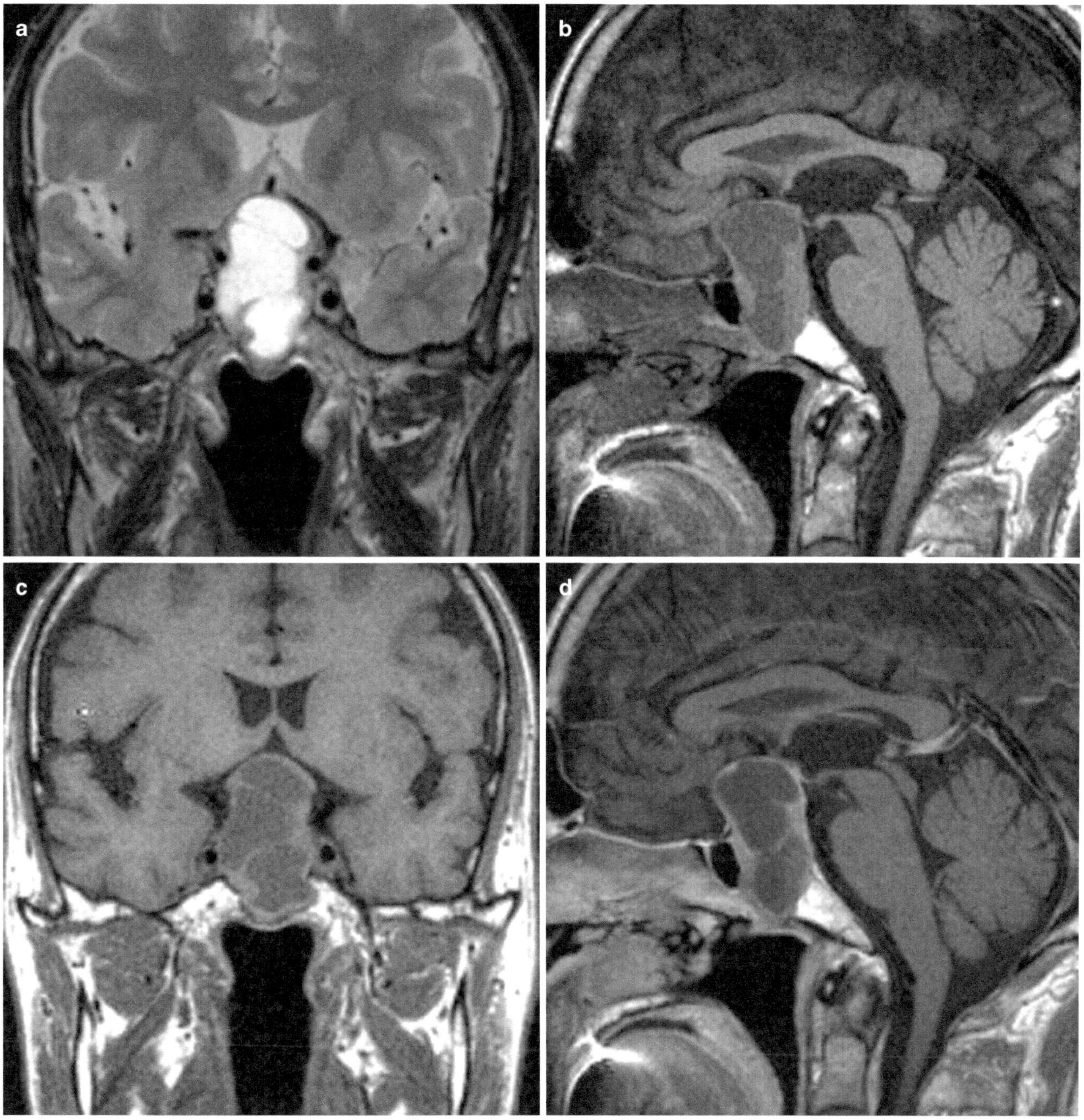

Fig. 15.22 Giant cystic sellar-suprasellar pituitary adenoma. T2-weighted image (**a**) and T1-weigted images (**b**, **c**) reveal a heterogeneous, mainly hyperintense tumor with sellar and suprasellar growth. There is no invasion into the cavernous sinuses. On post-contrast T1-weighted images a moderate enhancement predominantly in tumor capsule is seen (**d**–**f**) and multicystic structure of the adenoma is better visualized

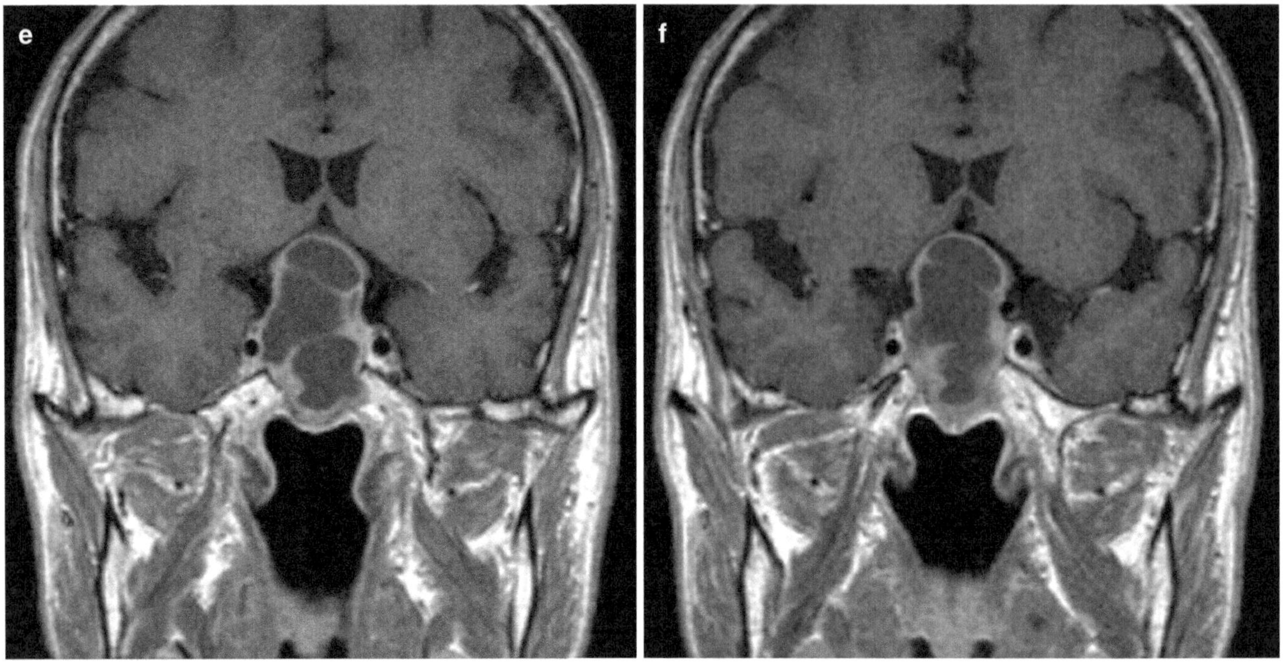

Fig. 15.22 (continued)

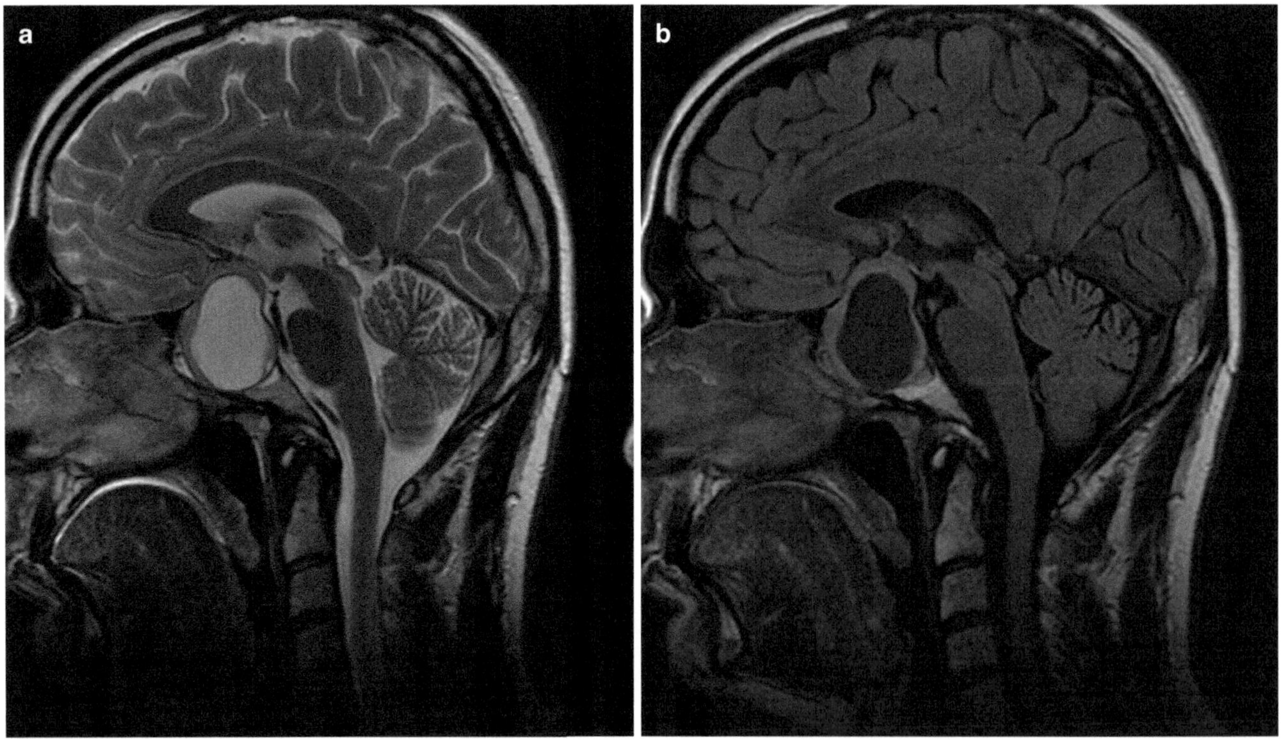

Fig. 15.23 Pituitary cystic sellar, infra- and suprasellar adenoma. Sagittal T2-weighted (**a**) and T1-weighted (**b**) images show a large tumor which compress and displaces the optic chiasm. CE CT scan (**c**) clearly demonstrates a soft-tissue enhanced component of the tumor. The central cystic component does not enhance

Fig. 15.23 (continued)

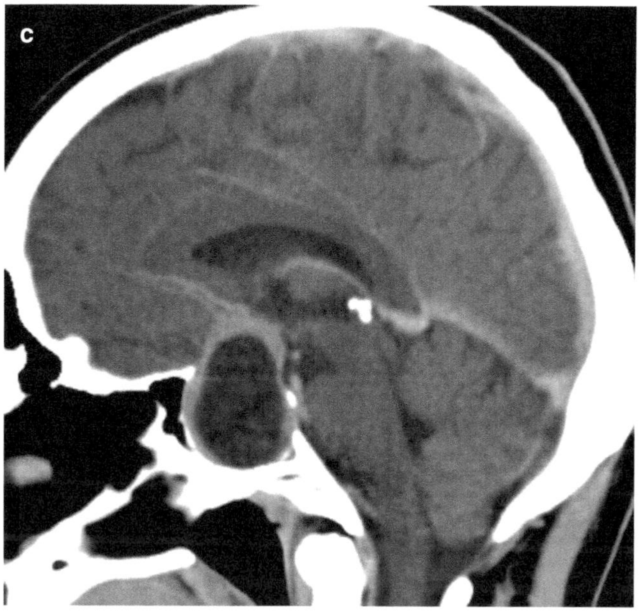

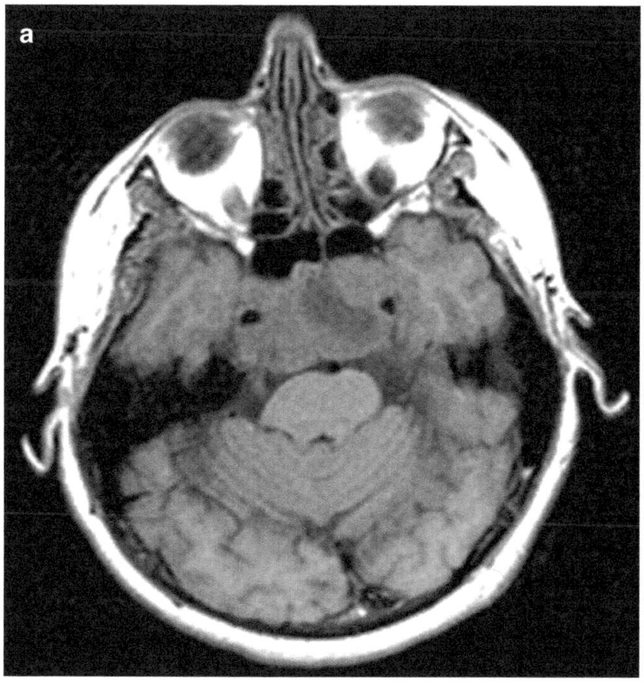

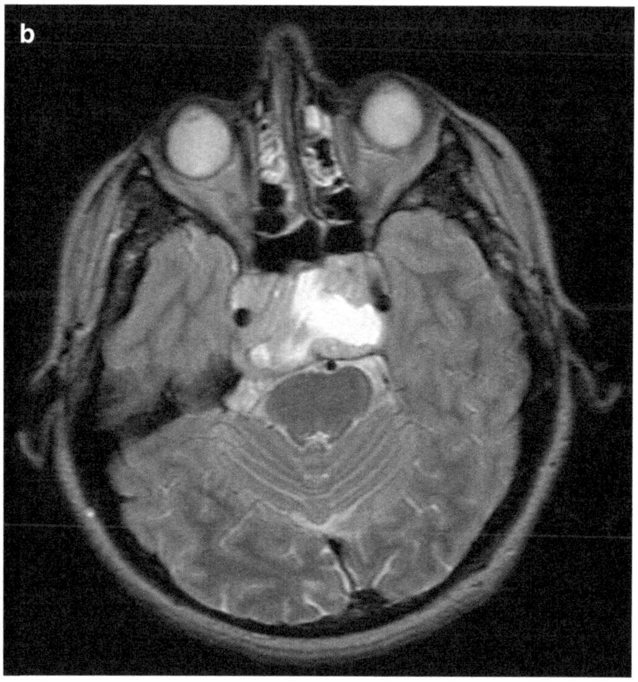

Fig. 15.24 Pituitary adenoma with supra-laterosellar growth. Axial T1-weighted (**a**) and T2-weighted (**b**) images reveal a heterogeneous signal throughout the large adenoma. The tumor invades both cavernous sinuses without the occlusion of involved internal carotid arteries. Post-contrast T1-weighted images (**c–f**) show an intensive heterogeneous enhancement and improve the visualization of the tumor structure and extension. Coronal T1-weighted images (**e**) show secondary node (*arrow*)

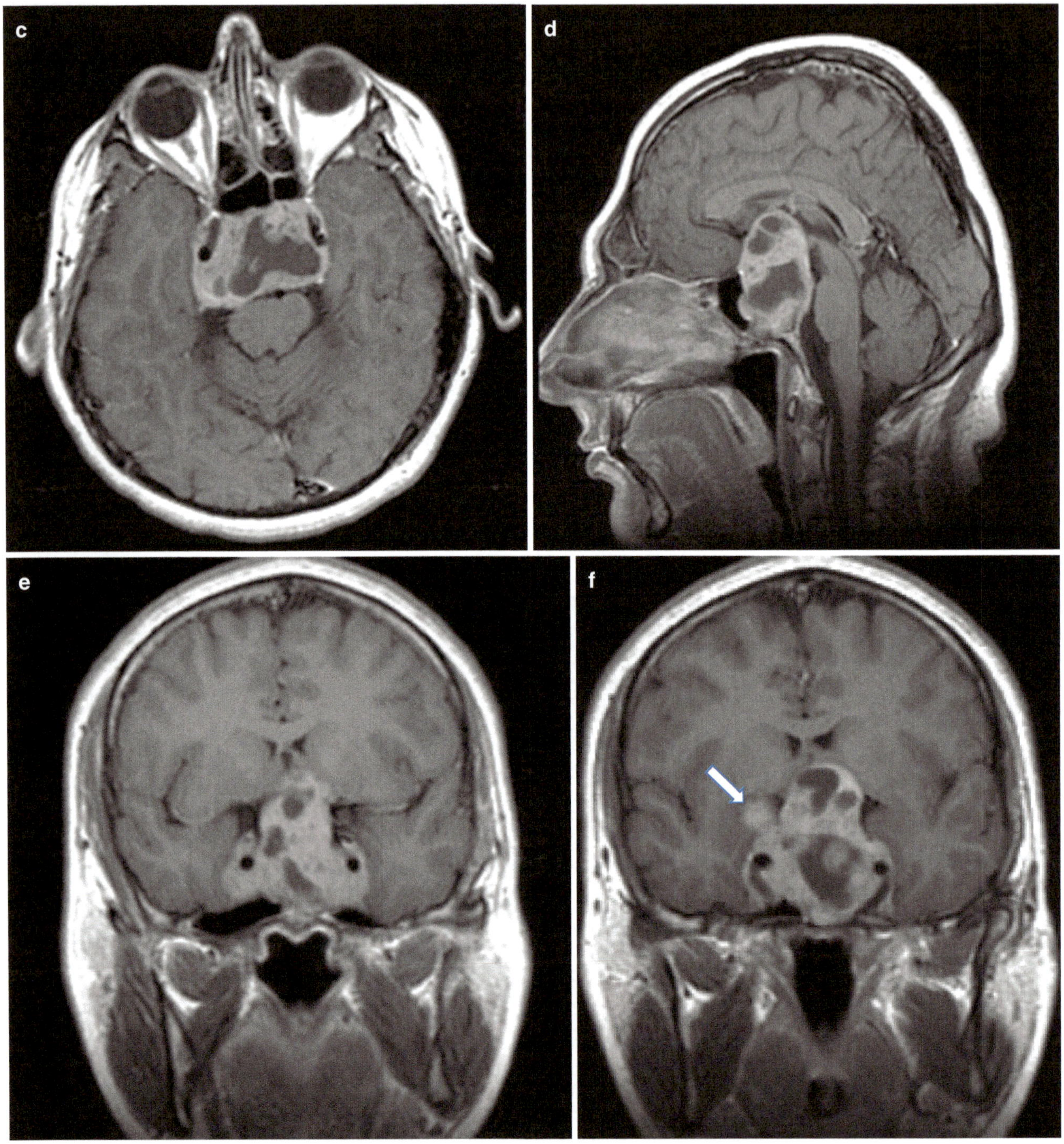

Fig. 15.24 (continued)

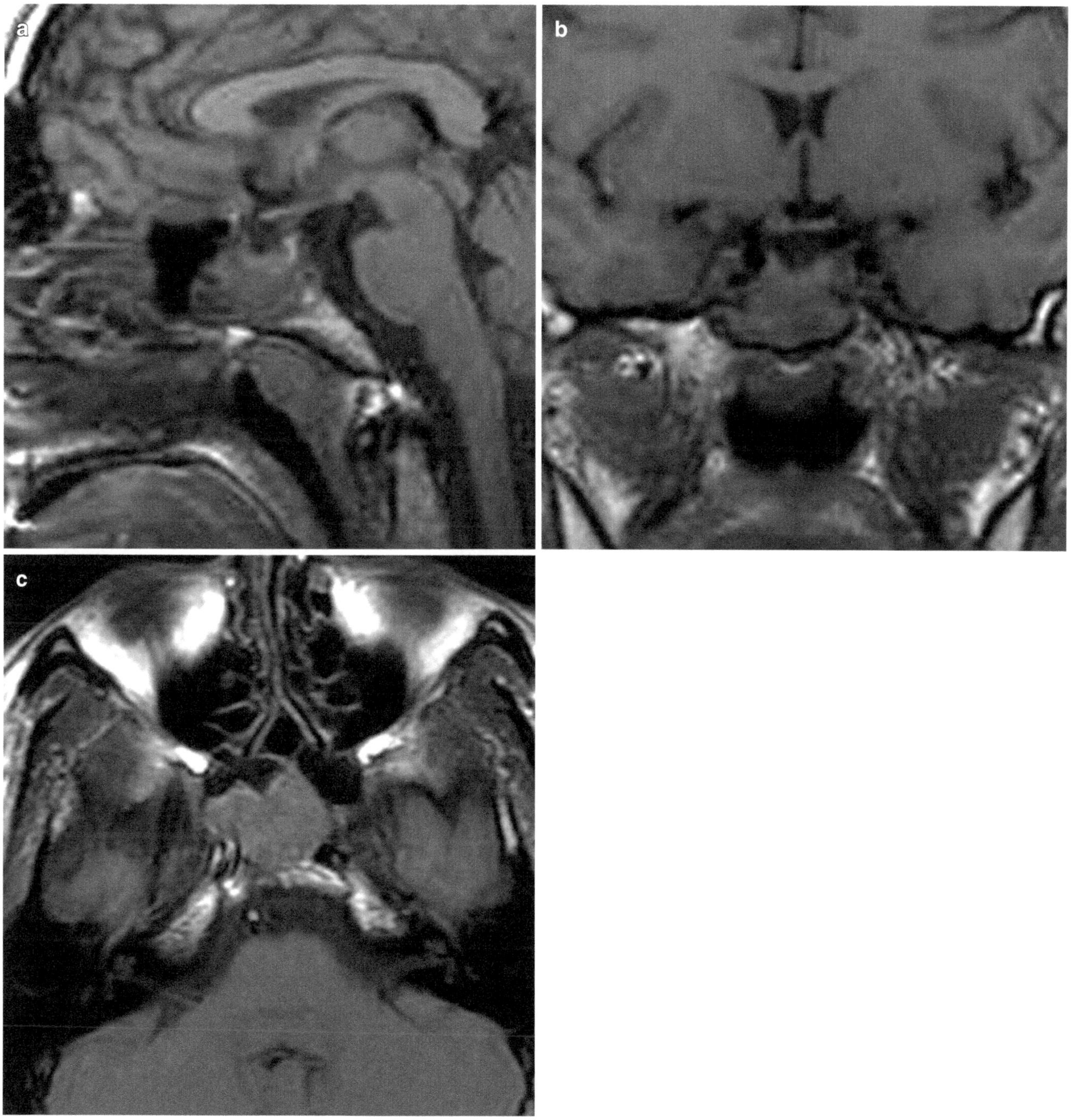

Fig. 15.25 Pituitary adenoma with infra-laterosellar growth. Sagittal (**a**), frontal (**b**), and axial (**c**) T1-weighted images demonstrate a tumor which is located predominantly at the sphenoid sinus

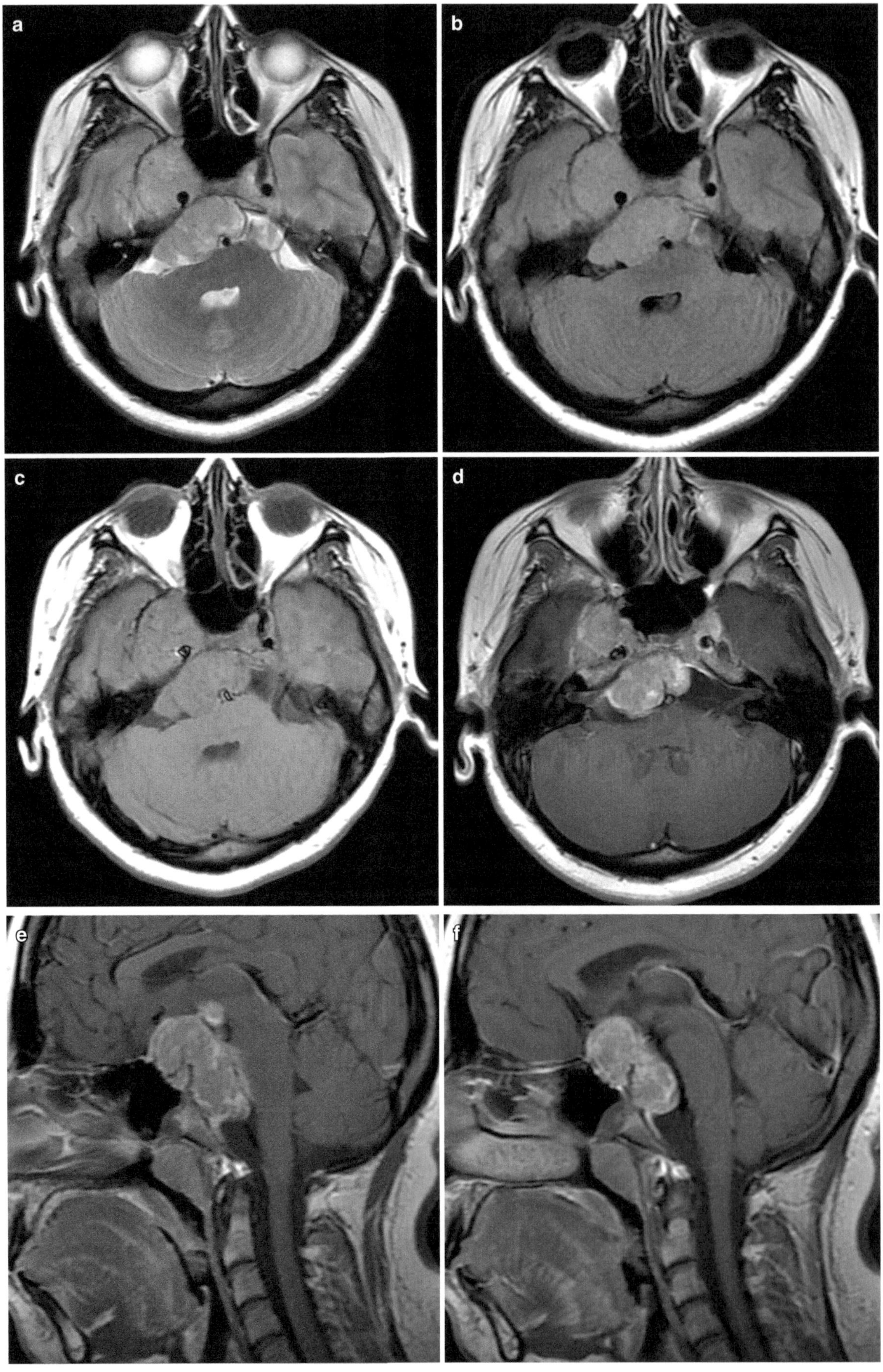
a
b
c
d
e
f

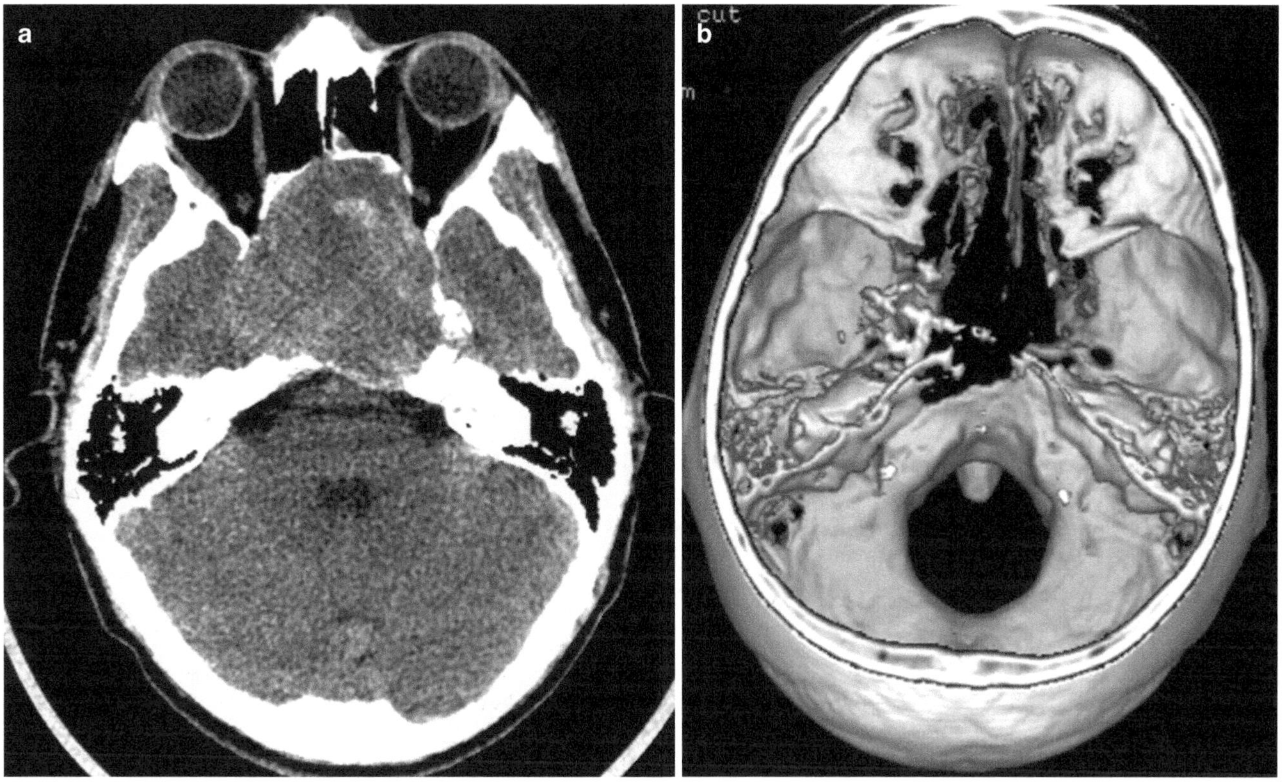

Fig. 15.27 Giant invasive pituitary adenoma with ante-laterosellar growth. A tumor causes the clivus destruction, fills the sphenoid sinus, and invades the cavernous sinuses and ethmoid bone. Axial CE CT scan (**a**) and 3D reconstruction (**b**) reveal a wide skull base bones destruction

Fig. 15.26 Giant pituitary adenoma with supra-retro-laterosellar growth. Axial T2-weighted (**a**), T2-FLAIR (**b**), and post-contrast T1-weighted images (**c**) show a moderately hyperintense on T2-weighted and T2-FLAIR images tumor. The laterosellar growth with cavernous sinuses invasion is clearly visualized. Internal carotid arteries are not occluded. The basilar artery is displaced by retrosellar part of the tumor. The tumor is extended into the clivus, compresses the brainstem. Post-contrast T1-weighted images show a strong heterogeneous enhancement. Secondary node is visualized at the upper margin of the adenoma (**d**–**f**)

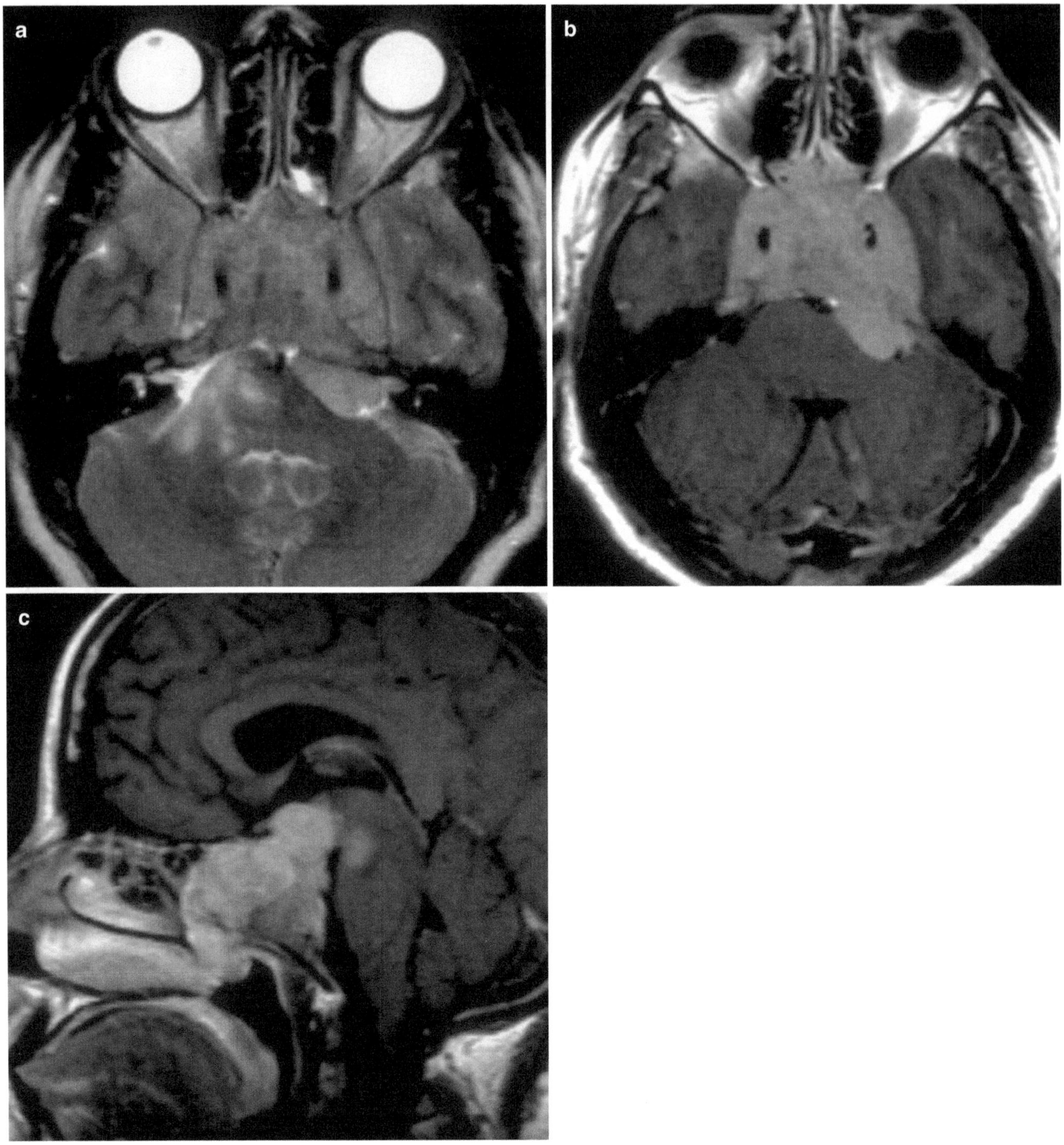

Fig. 15.28 Giant pituitary adenoma. T2-weighted (**a**) and post-contrast T1-weighted images (axial (**b**) and sagittal (**c**)) reveal a large invasive tumor that extends into the sphenoid sinus and basal cisterns of the brain, ethmoid bone and nasopharynx, invades the cavernous sinuses. T2-weighted image shows the local edema in the right part of the pons due to ischemia

Among modern techniques for the structural imaging of pituitary adenoma tissue, MR spectroscopy, 3D gradient echo sequence (SWI, SWAN) and CT-perfusion can be distinguished (Pinker et al. 2005; Kornienko and Pronin 2009). Although MR spectroscopy is widely used in evaluation of metabolites in various brain tumors, the best results have been mainly achieved in investigations of supratentorial lesions. Its use at the skull base is limited by technical issues, complexity of shimming and suppression of a negative influence of the bone structures on the MR signal quality. If the sellar tumor is less than 2–3 cm, the use of MR spectroscopy is unjustified. Large parasellar tumor nodules are evaluable. Using MR spectroscopy for pituitary adenomas, we identified the following findings: a marked increase in a choline peak, an increase in a lactate-lipid complex peak along with a decrease in an *N*-acetyl-aspartate peak (Fig. 15.29).

3D gradient echo (SWI, SWAN, etc.) sequence provides a different way of visualizing the pituitary adenomas structure. It was found that, while small tumors have an isointense MR signal relative to the brain on this sequence, the vast majority of large and giant tumors contain plenty of small hemorrhages. They are most likely to be the source of unexpected intra- and paratumoral hemorrhages. The latter are clearly seen on T1-weighted images as hyperintense areas (methemoglobin) and are characterized by a low (hemosiderin) or high (methemoglobin) MR signal on 3D gradient echo (SWI, SWAN) (Fig. 15.30).

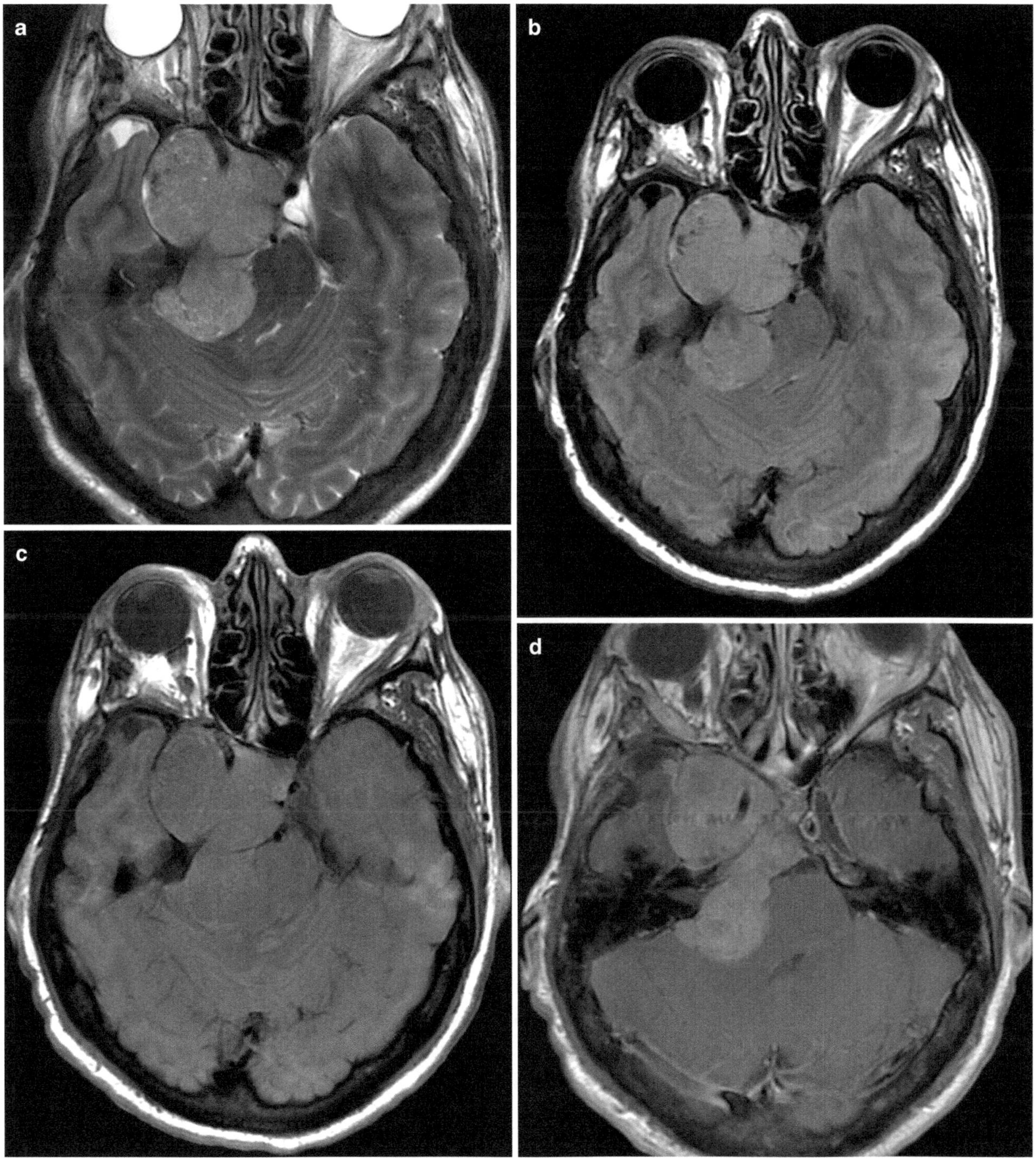

Fig. 15.29 Giant pituitary adenoma with supra-latero-retrosellar growth. T2-weighted image (**a**), T2-FLAIR (**b**), T1- (**c**) and post-contrast T1-weighted images (**d**, **e**) show an invasive adenoma with predominantly extending to the right-side of the skull base. Single-voxel (**f**) and multi-voxel (**g**, **h**) MR-spectroscopy reveals an elevation of choline peak, appearing lipids–lactate complex and decreasing the peak of N-acetyl aspartate. 2D colored map shows a high choline content into the infratentorial part of the tumor tissue (**i**)

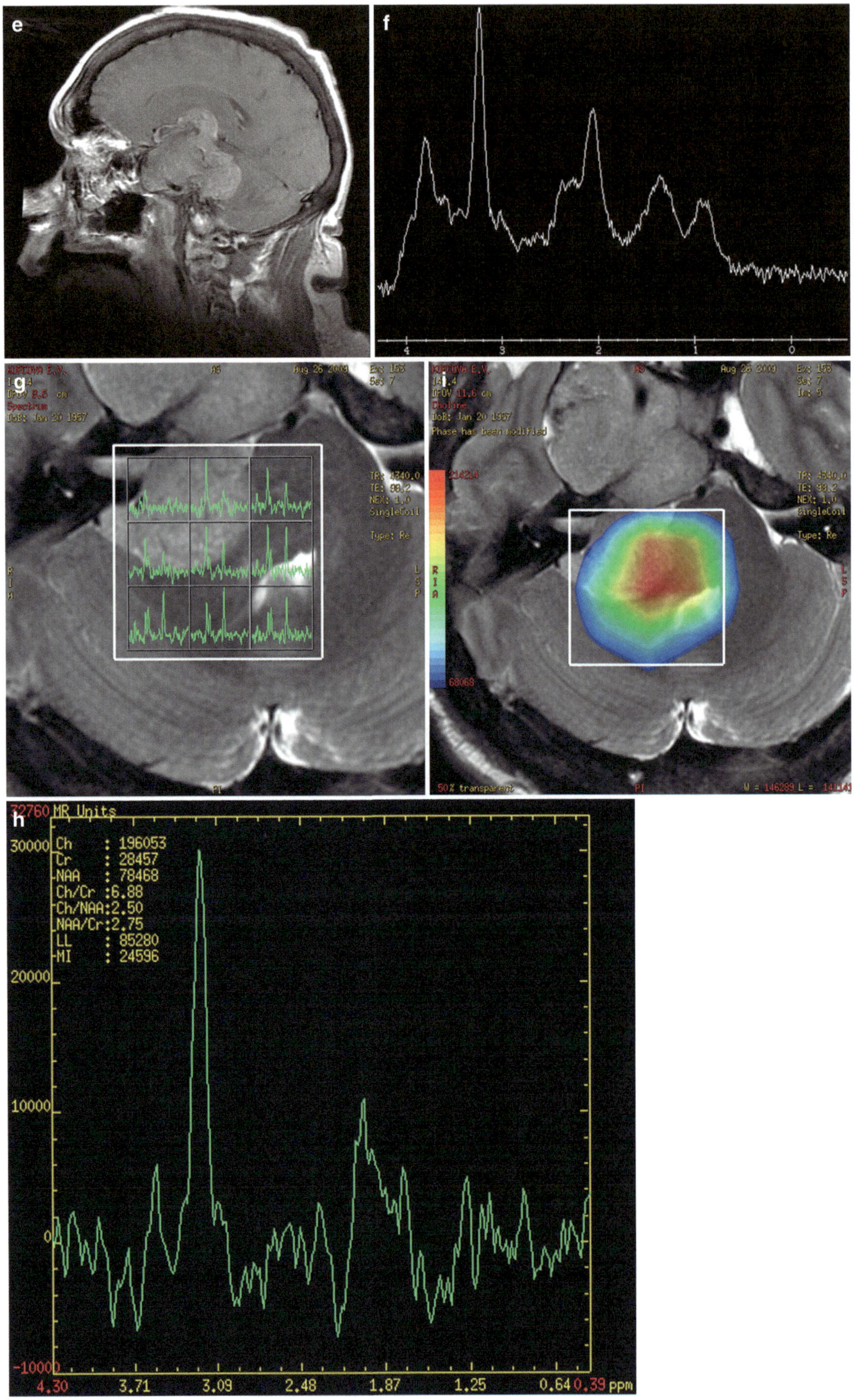

Fig. 15.29 (continued)

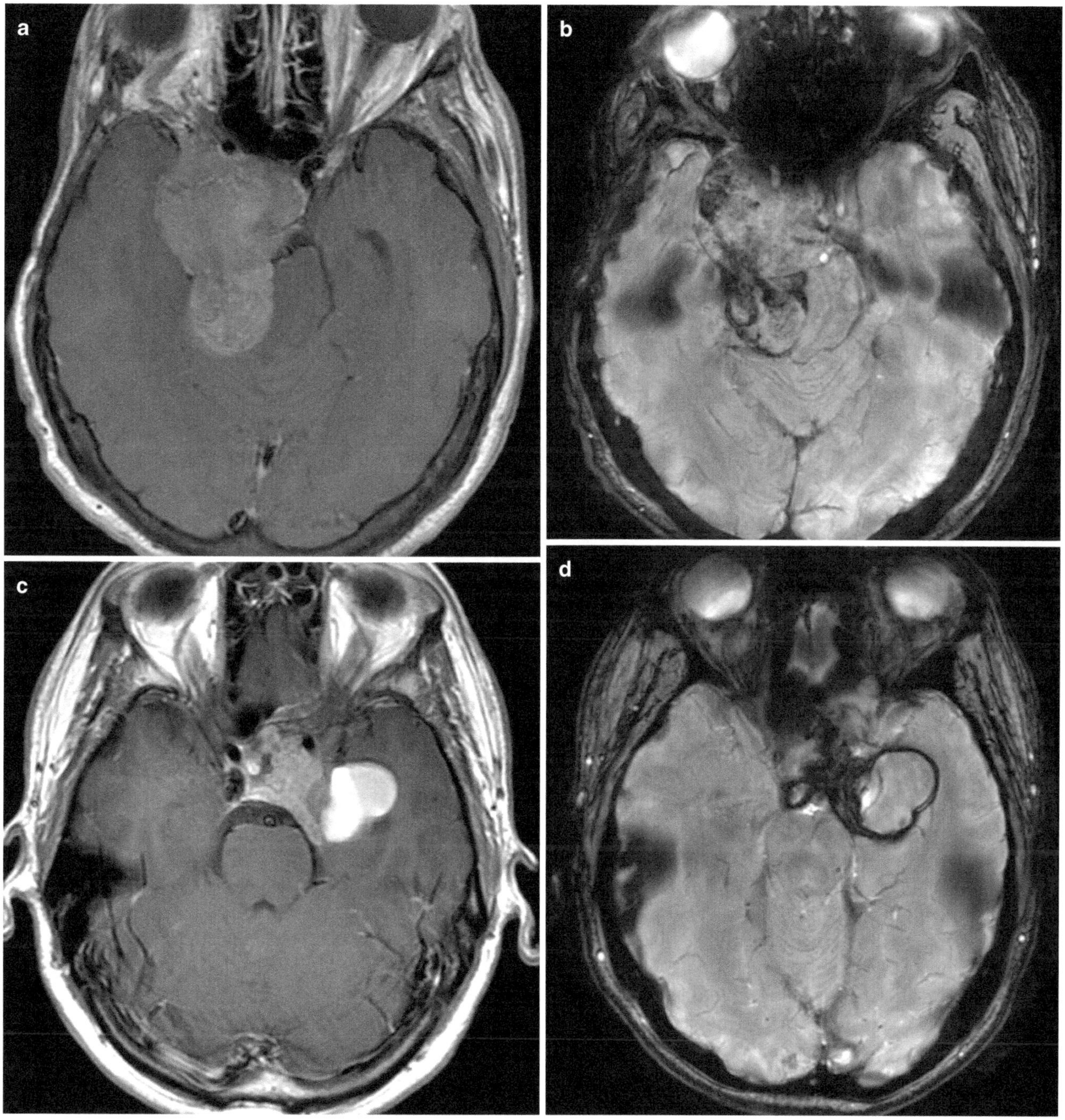

Fig. 15.30 Giant pituitary adenoma with hemorrhage. Case 1: post-contrast T1-weighted image (**a**), 3D T2* (SWAN) scan (**b**) show hemorrhagic macroadenoma which is characterized by hypointensity on T2*. Case 2: sellar-suprasellar-laterosellar macroadenoma with hemorrhage in the lateral aspect of the tumor. Post-contrast T1-weighted image (**c**) shows a heterogeneous hyperintense enhancement. SWAN (**d**) notes a total heterogeneous hypointensity in the tumor due to presence of blood product. Case 3: latero-retrosellar adenoma with heterogeneous enhancement on post-contrast T1-weighted image (**e**) and multiple microhemorrhages in the central aspect of the tumor on SWAN (**f**)

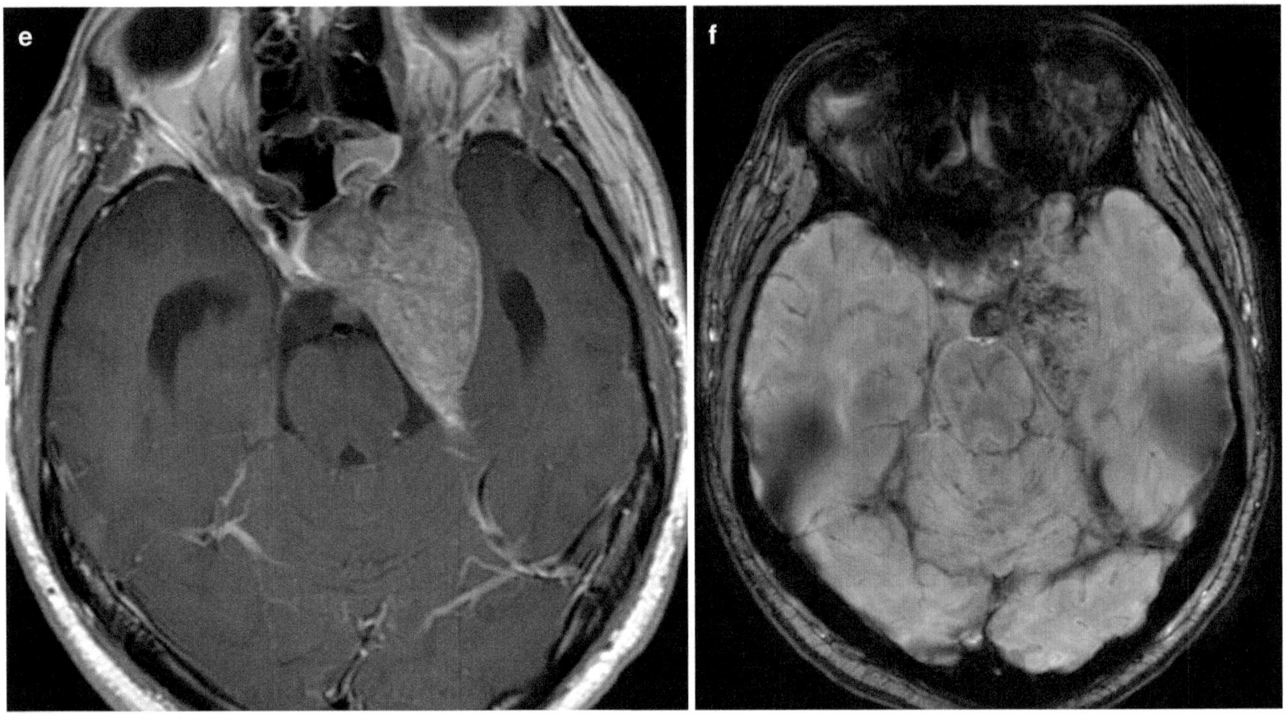

Fig. 15.30 (continued)

Tumor hemodynamics studies have become an important part of a comprehensive evaluation of pituitary adenomas, especially those that are accompanied by bleedings. In contrast to MR perfusion, bone structures of the skull base do not affect the quality of CT studies, and their images can be simply removed when constructing perfusion maps, without any spatial distortions. Now we widely use the CT-perfusion imaging for the diagnosis of skull base tumors and in particular in the differential diagnosis of pituitary adenomas, which showed high sensitivity and specificity in verification of the histological origin of neoplasms. Low values of tumor blood flow (sometimes comparable to those of the brain), a moderately increased CBV and very high values of mean transit time are typical for pituitary adenomas, no matter what size they reach. These properties help performing a differential diagnosis of pituitary adenomas and parasellar meningiomas in most cases (Figs. 15.31 and 15.32).

Multiple brain lesions, for example, multiple metastases, meningiomas, schwannomas, etc. are not an uncommon phenomenon in clinical practice. Underestimation of some of them may end up fatal during surgery. A combination of a pituitary adenoma and a parasellar saccular aneurysm of the carotid artery is a rare, but possible event (Fig. 15.33). In our clinical practice, we observed the combination of a giant pituitary adenoma and a large parasagittal meningioma. Differences in the MR characteristics between these two tumors allowed differentiating their histological identity (Fig. 15.34).

Ectopic pituitary adenomas are rather rare: the tumor is located entirely in the suprasellar region and is not connected with the contents of the sella turcica both radiologically and during surgery. We present the only one case of ectopic pituitary adenoma encountered in our long-standing practice, which was verified histologically, with the presence of signs of pronounced polymorphism and a high Ki-67 labeling index (7–8%). The absence of distant metastases did not allow classifying this tumor as pituitary carcinoma (Fig. 15.35).

Rare, but possible findings in clinical practice include complications of radiation therapy of sellar pituitary adenomas using rotational radiotherapy techniques or proton therapy. Clinical manifestations of the primary disease in such cases become insignificant, giving way to severe cerebral symptoms of involvement of the temporal lobes of the brain (Fig. 15.36).

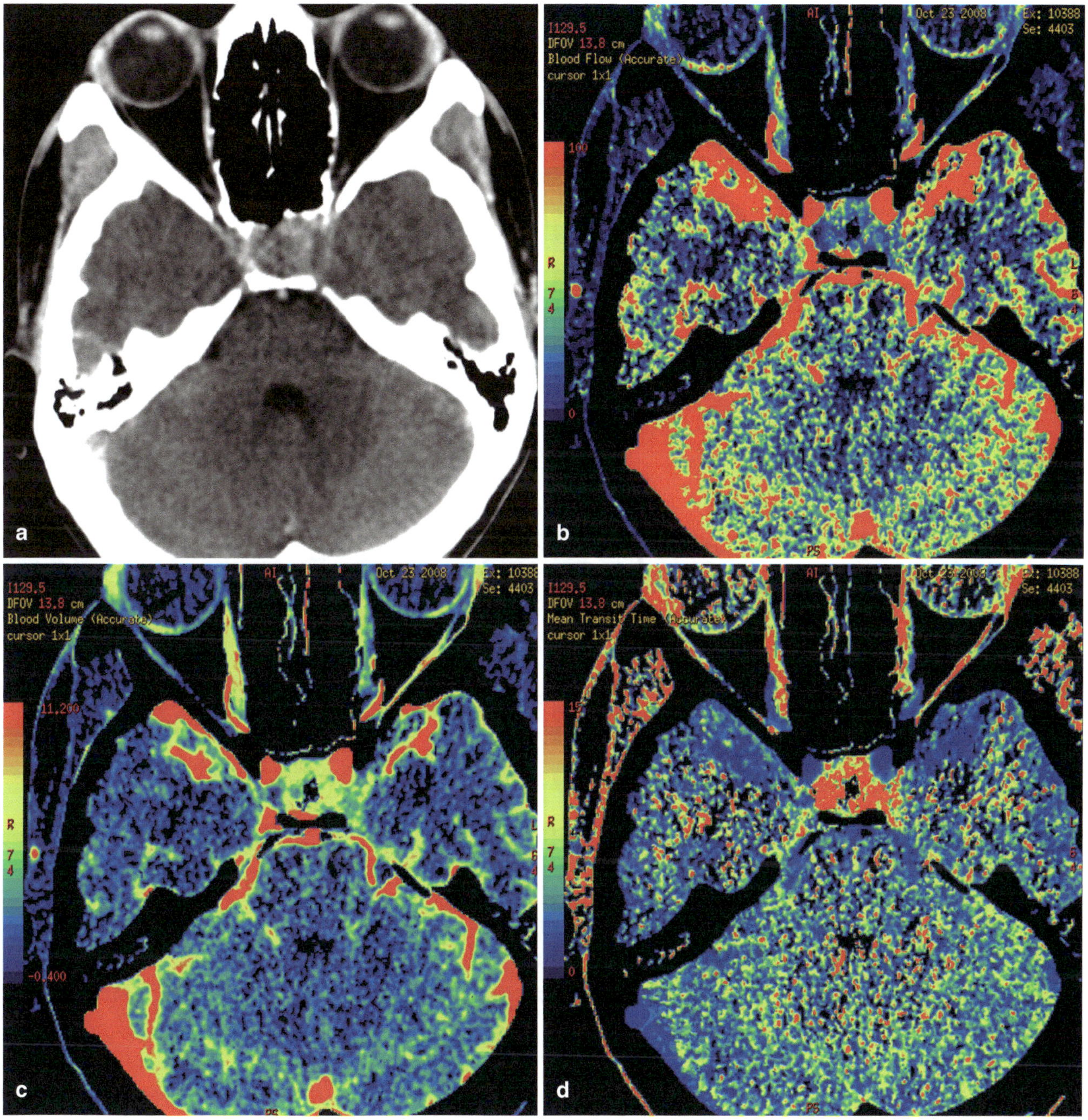

Fig. 15.31 Pituitary adenoma. Axial CT scan (**a**) reveals a tumor filling the sella with growth into the left cavernous sinus. Adenoma is characterized by low blood flow parameters (CBF map (**b**)), moderately increased CBV (**c**) and prolonged of MTT (**d**)

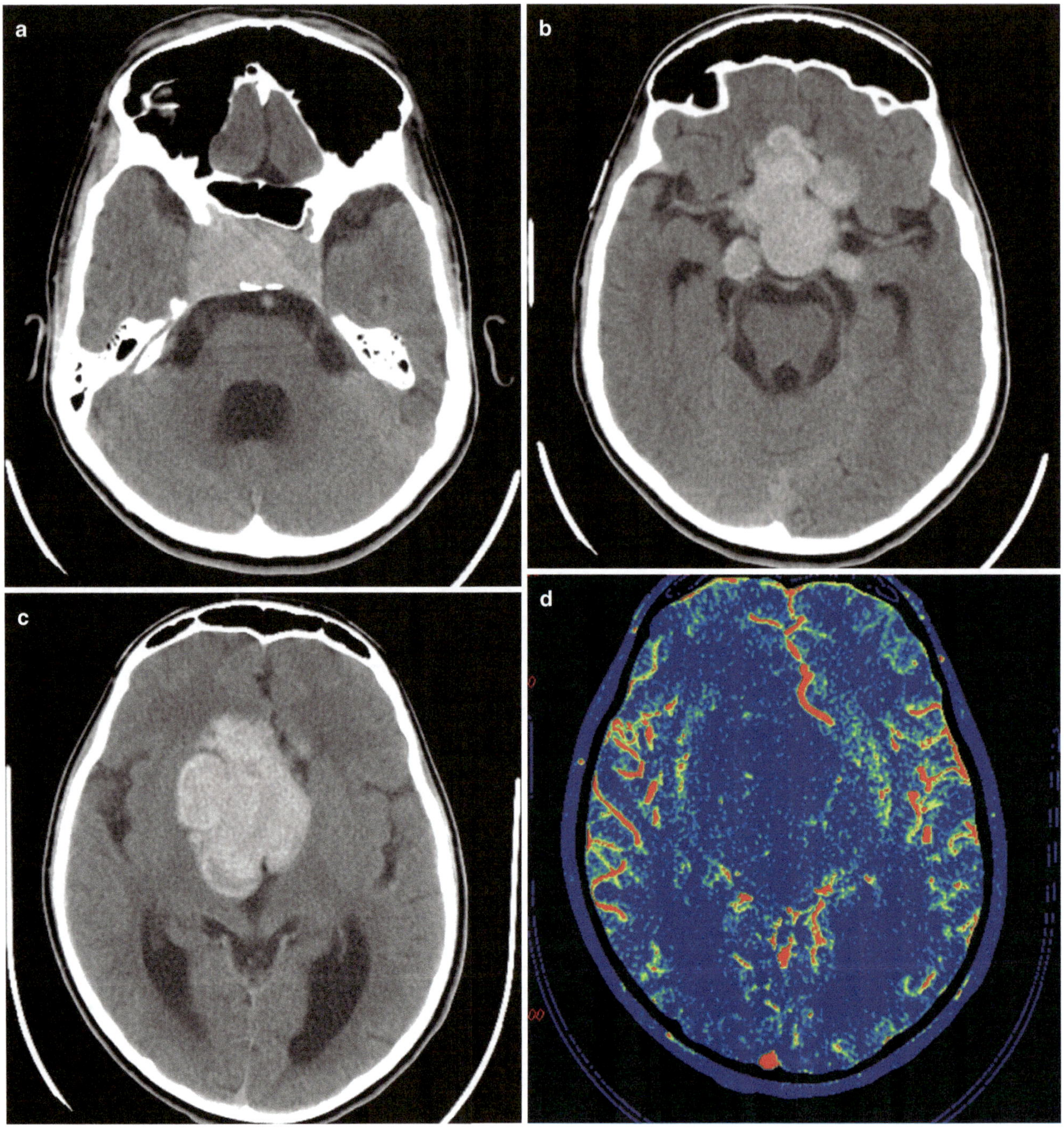

Fig. 15.32 Giant pituitary adenoma with the multiple secondary nodes. The tumor intensively enhances on CT series at different levels (**a**–**c**). Perfusion maps show low parameters of CBF (**d**), CBV (**e**) and a prolongation of transit time (**f**)

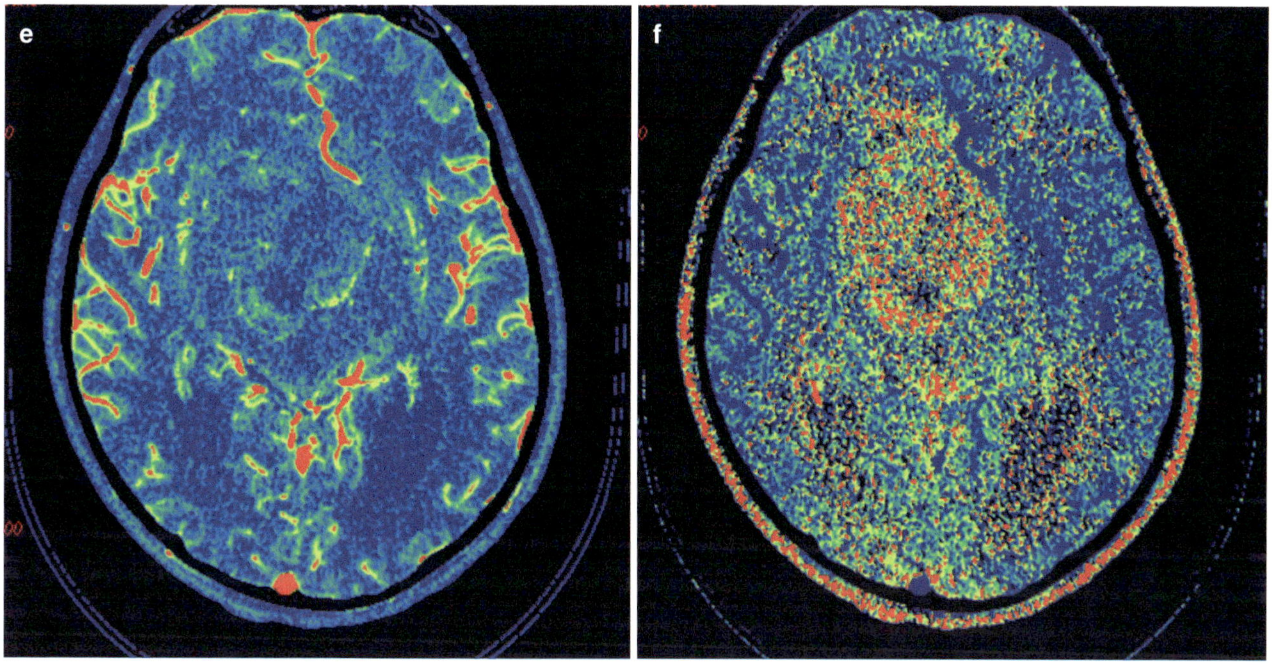

Fig. 15.32 (continued)

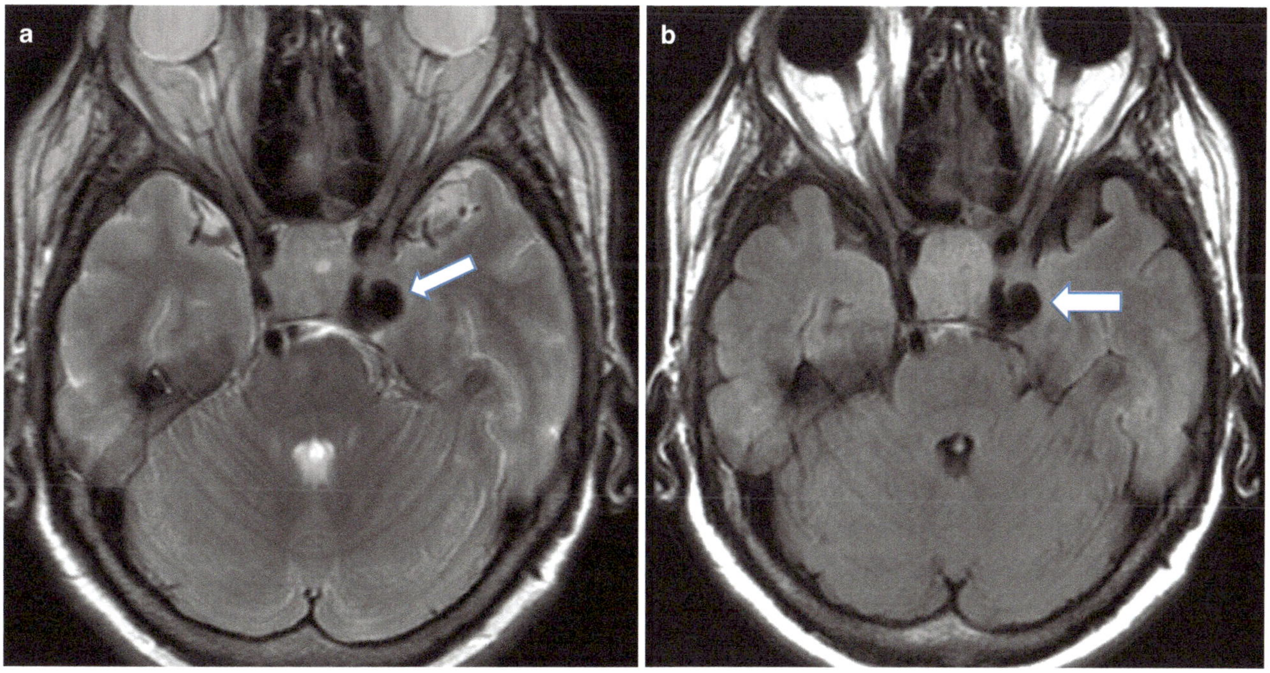

Fig. 15.33 Combination of sellar-suprasellar pituitary adenoma with functioning saccular arterial aneurysm in the infraclinoid part of left internal carotid artery. T2-weighted (**a**) and T2-FLAIR (**b**) images show a tumor occupying the sella turcica and laterosellar rounded hypointense “flow void” lesion: a saccular aneurysm (*arrow*). 3D TOF angiography (**c**) defines the location of the aneurysm more exactly (*arrow*)

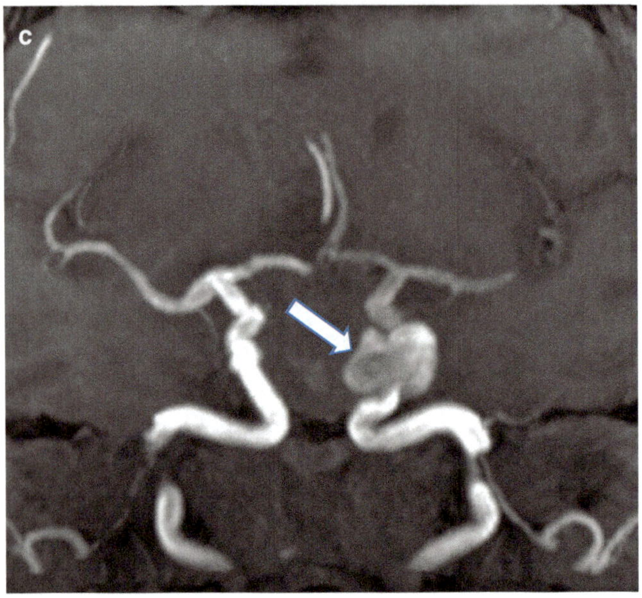

Fig. 15.33 (continued)

15.2 Hemorrhage in Pituitary Adenoma (Pituitary Apoplexy)

An acute hemorrhage or ischemic pituitary infarction in pituitary adenoma is responsible for the rapid development of the syndrome including severe headache, nausea, vomiting, and depression of consciousness, panhypopituitarism. Also ophthalmoplegia, visual impairment, and meningeal signs can be observed. Most of these symptoms are due to a direct hemorrhage into the tumor, and meningeal symptoms are caused by subarachnoid hemorrhage. The syndrome develops acutely and in rare cases may result in a sudden death.

Pituitary apoplexy occurs most often in patients with adenomas, and may be the first clinical manifestation of a pituitary tumor (Figs. 15.37, 15.38, and 15.39); hemorrhages rarely occur with normal pituitary gland. Anticoagulant therapy, radiation, bromocriptine, and cabergoline therapy for macroadenoma predispose to hemorrhage or infarction in adenomas. In rare cases, pituitary apoplexy causes "autohypophysectomy" with disappearance of clinical symptoms of acromegaly, Cushing's disease or hyperprolactinemia (a kind of "self-healing"). A more frequent consequence of hemorrhage is hypopituitarism. In rare cases diabetes insipidus develops. Pituitary apoplexy should be distinguished from a rupture of arterial aneurysm; such a situation often requires angiography (Sergides et al. 2007). Patients with acute pituitary apoplexy require monitoring by a neurosurgeon. Sometimes a surgical decompression of the pituitary gland may be required, which is usually performed via the transsphenoid approach.

Imaging Detection of changes with radiological methods depends on the time elapsed after the hemorrhage. In the acute phase, CT can show an area with an increased density in the pituitary adenoma without enhancement, the signs of subarachnoid hemorrhage may be identified. Over time, the density of a hemorrhagic area decreases. Stages of hemorrhage can be traced on MRI as well. In the early acute stage, hemorrhage in the pituitary gland appears as hypo- or isointense area on T1-weighted images. On T2-weighted images, hemorrhage is characterized by a pronounced hypointensity (Boellis et al. 2014). In case of optic chiasm and hypothalamus compression, diffuse signal changes along the optic tracts can be observed in the acute phase. There is a decrease of the diffusion coefficient in the affected area on diffusion maps. In late acute and early subacute stages, hyperintensity appears on T1-weighted images, while the signal on T2-weighted images can be variable depending on the degree of lysis of red blood cells. The changes remind the "empty" sella in the chronic stage. Following intravenous contrast agent injection, MRI detects heterogeneous enhancement in affected areas and adjacent dural enhancement in 50% of cases and also the thickened mucosa of the sphenoid sinus in up to 80% of cases (Osborn et al. 2016). Hypointense changes are observed in the chronic stage on T2* GRE images.

15.3 Pituicytoma

This tumor is also called infundibuloma. They are rare, arise from pituicytes (glial cells of the neurohypophysis and pituitary stalk) (Osborn et al. 2016).

Pituicytomas occur most frequently in adults, usually in the fifth decade of life; men are twice as likely to be affected as women (Osborn et al. 2016). They may be both asymptomatic and cause a number of clinical symptoms. Most often they are manifested by visual and endocrine dysfunctions, among which the signs of adenohypophysis compression (secondary hypocorticism, hypothyroidism, and hypogonadism) are prevalent.

Pituicytomas are localized in the posterior portions of the sella turcica and (or) pituitary stalk. They appear as well-circumscribed lesions, usually with homogeneous structure and rich blood supply. On MRI, they are visualized in the pituitary stalk area and posterior portions of the sella turcica. Pure sellar localization is rare. Their form is rounded or oval. Their sizes vary from a few millimeters to 4 cm. On T1-weighted images, pituicytomas look hypo- or isointense and usually uniformly enhance. Hyperintensity in the posterior pituitary is not observed. On T2-weighted images, they are heterogeneously hypointense or isointense (Fig. 15.40). They rarely infiltrate the optic chiasm and cavernous sinus (Osborn et al. 2016; Zygourakis et al. 2015).

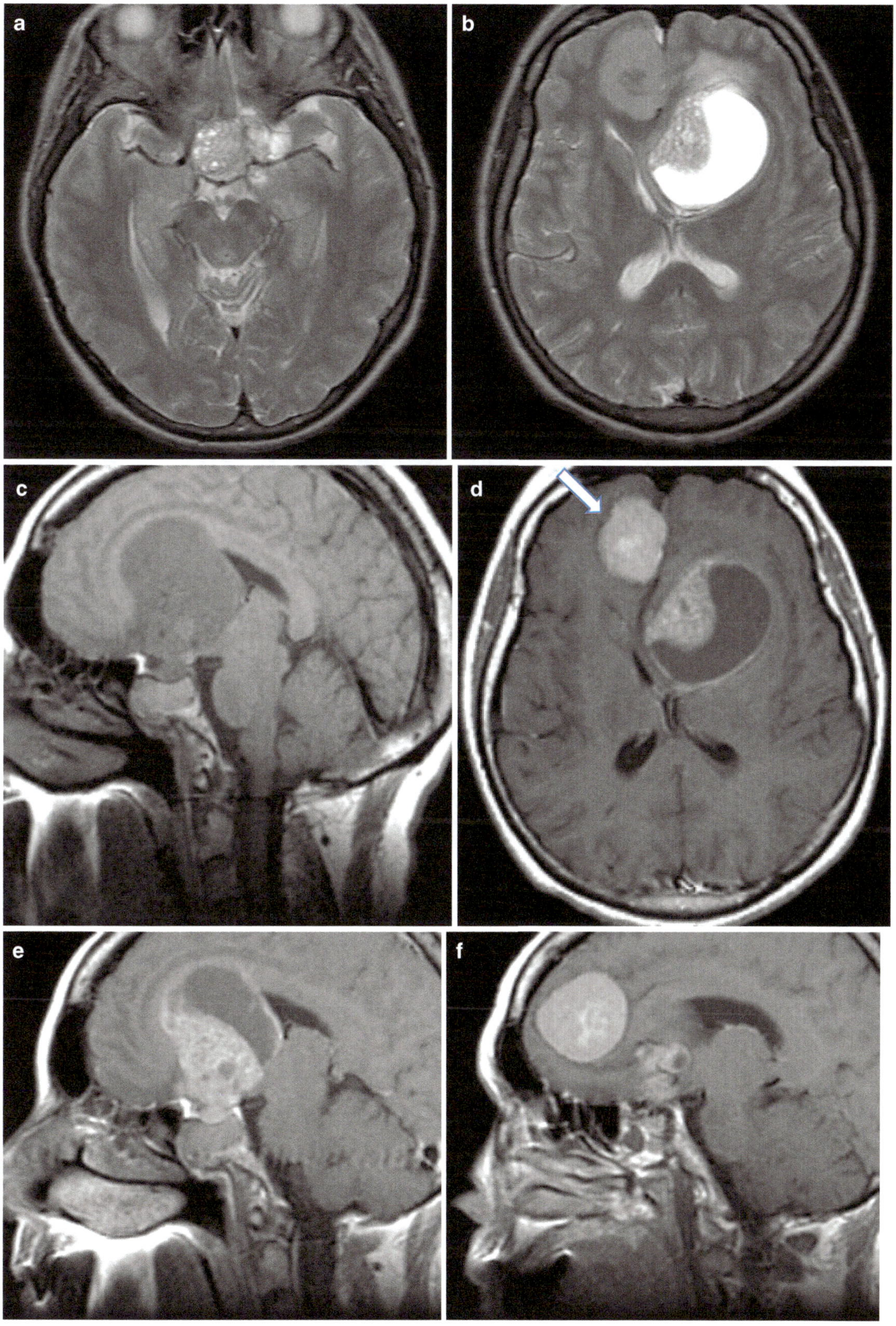

Fig. 15.34 Combination of the giant sellar-suprasellar pituitary adenoma extending into the third ventricle and anterior horn of the left lateral ventricle with meningioma of the falx cerebri (*arrow*). The differences between the tumors are better visualized on T2-weighted images (**a**, **b**) than on T1-weighted image (**c**). Both tumors intensively enhance (**d**–**f**). Adenoma has a more heterogeneous enhancement

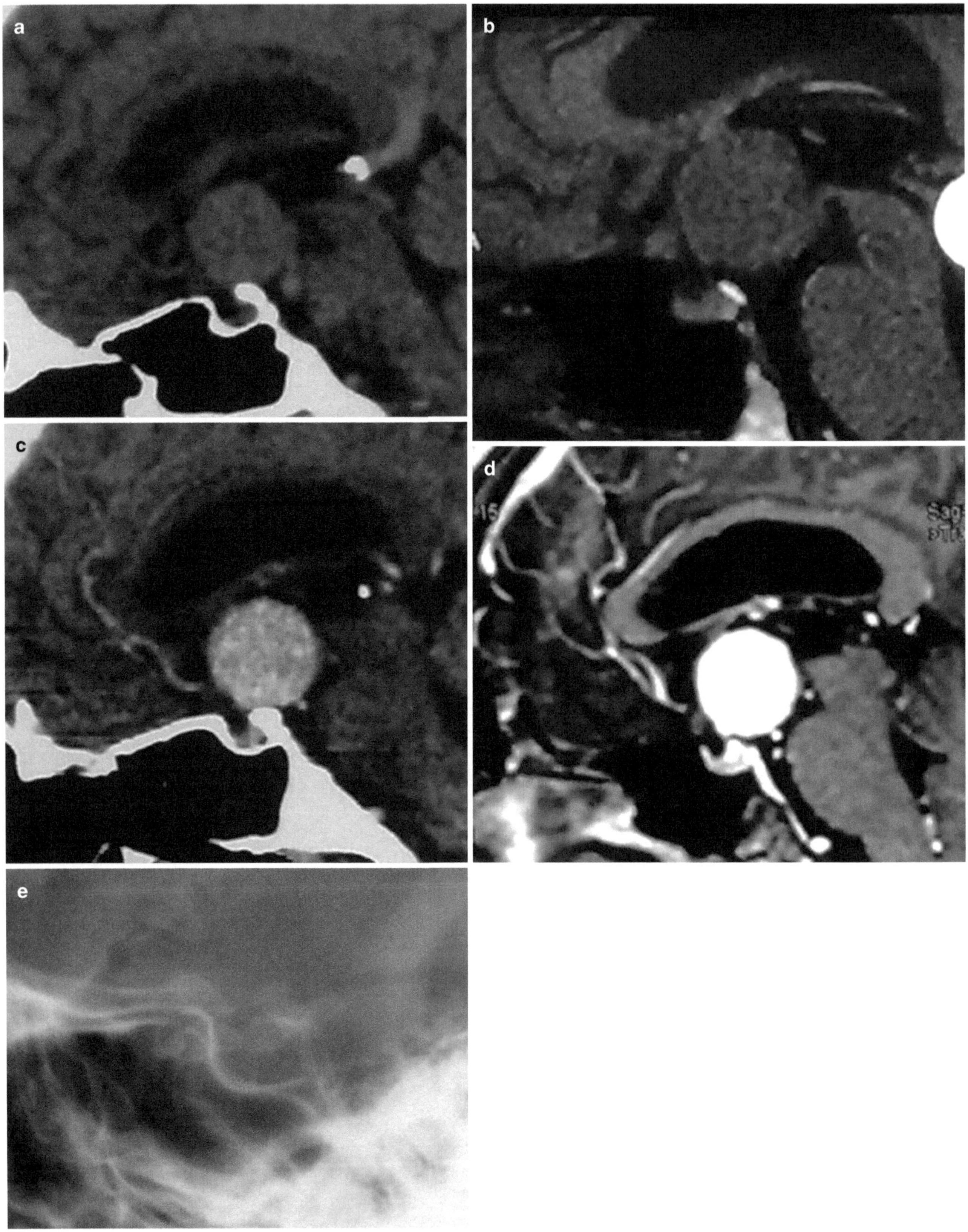

Fig. 15.35 Ectopic pituitary adenoma. Sagittal CT (**a**) and T1-weighted (**b**) and post-contrast T1-weighted images (**c**, **d**) identify a rounded tumor located above the dorsum of the sella. A tumor is intensively and homogeneously enhanced. There is no relationship between the tumor and pituitary gland in the non-enlarged sella turcica. Plan Rg doesn't show bone changes (**e**)

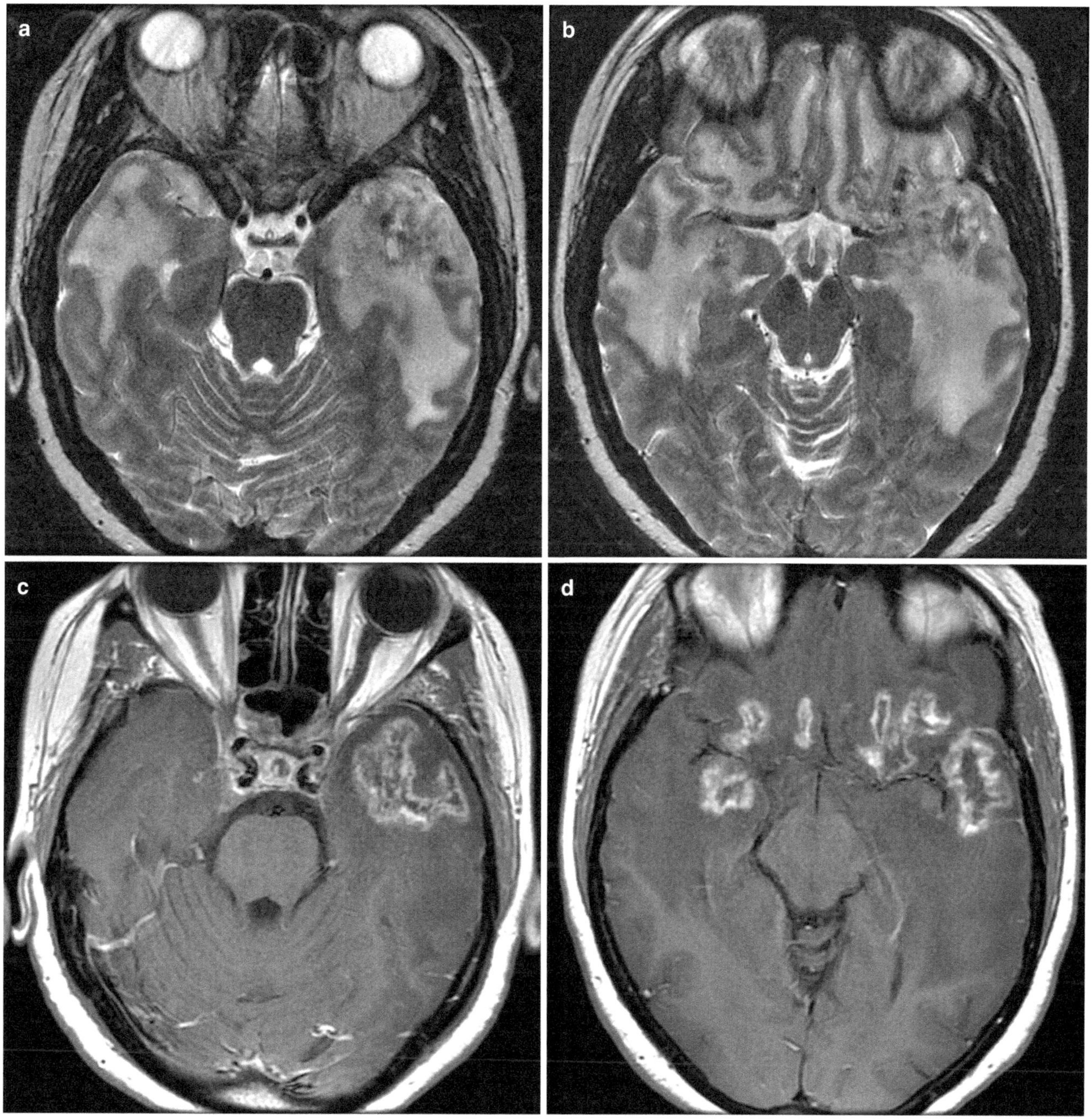

Fig. 15.36 Radiation necrosis in the temporal lobes after radiation therapy of the sellar pituitary adenoma. T2-weighted images (**a**, **b**) identify the extensive edema in the temporal lobes with hypointense areas within. T1-weighted images (**c**–**e**) reveal "Swiss cheese" or the heterogeneous prominent contrast enhancement in the frontotemporal area. CT-perfusion, CBF-map (**f**) shows a low blood flow parameters which are typical for the radiation necrosis

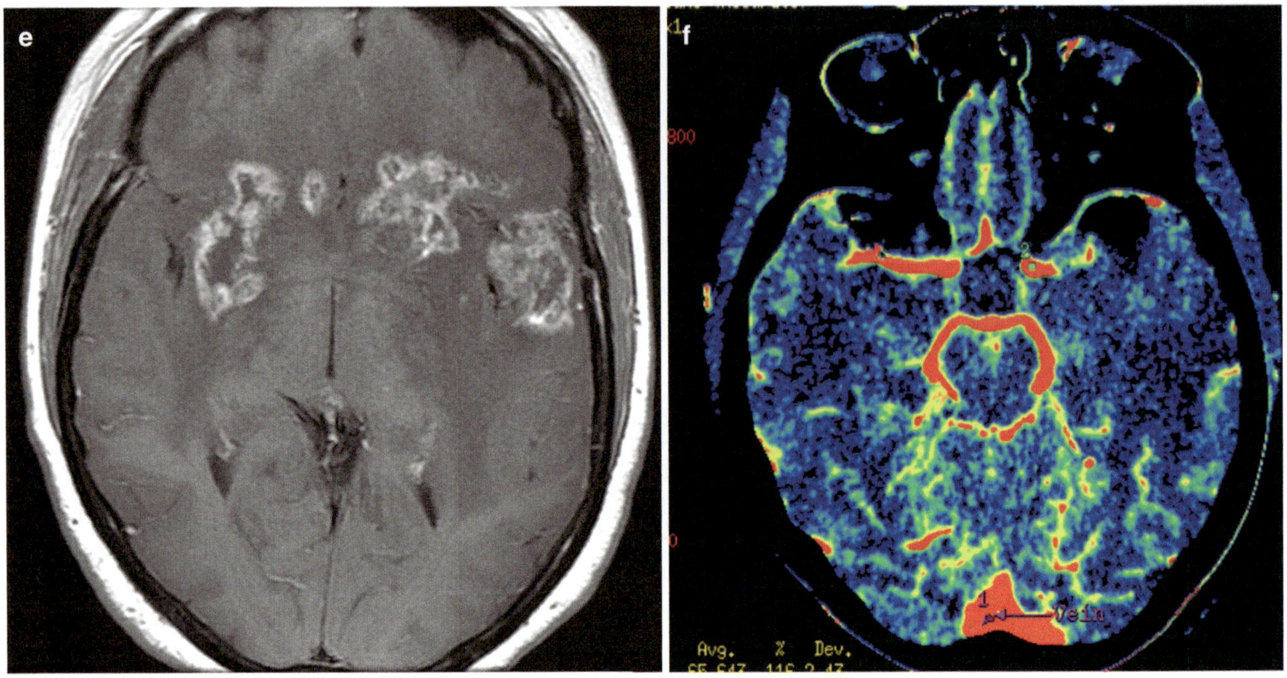

Fig. 15.36 (continued)

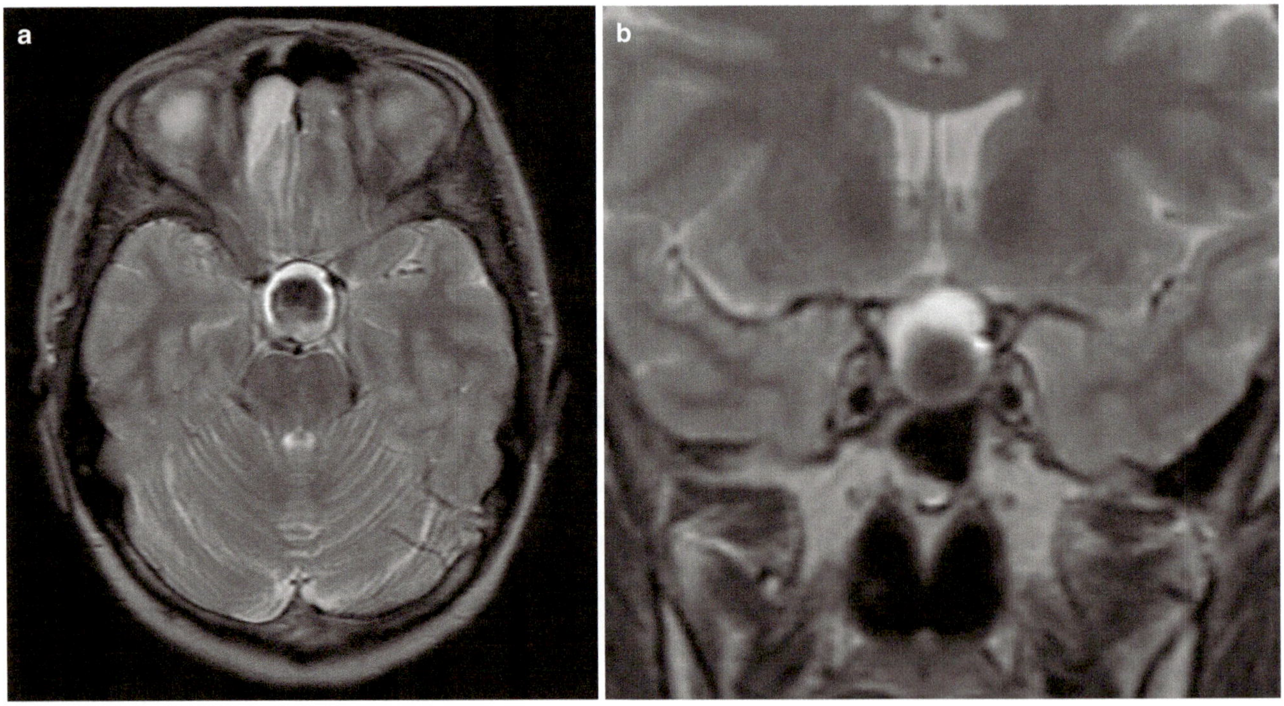

Fig. 15.37 Pituitary adenoma with hemorrhage in the early subacute stage. T2- (**a–c**) and T1-weighted images (**d–f**). Inferior aspect of the tumor is hypointense on T2- and hyperintense on T1-weighted images. These signal characteristics are related to the intracellular methemoglobin indicating the subacute stage of hemorrhage

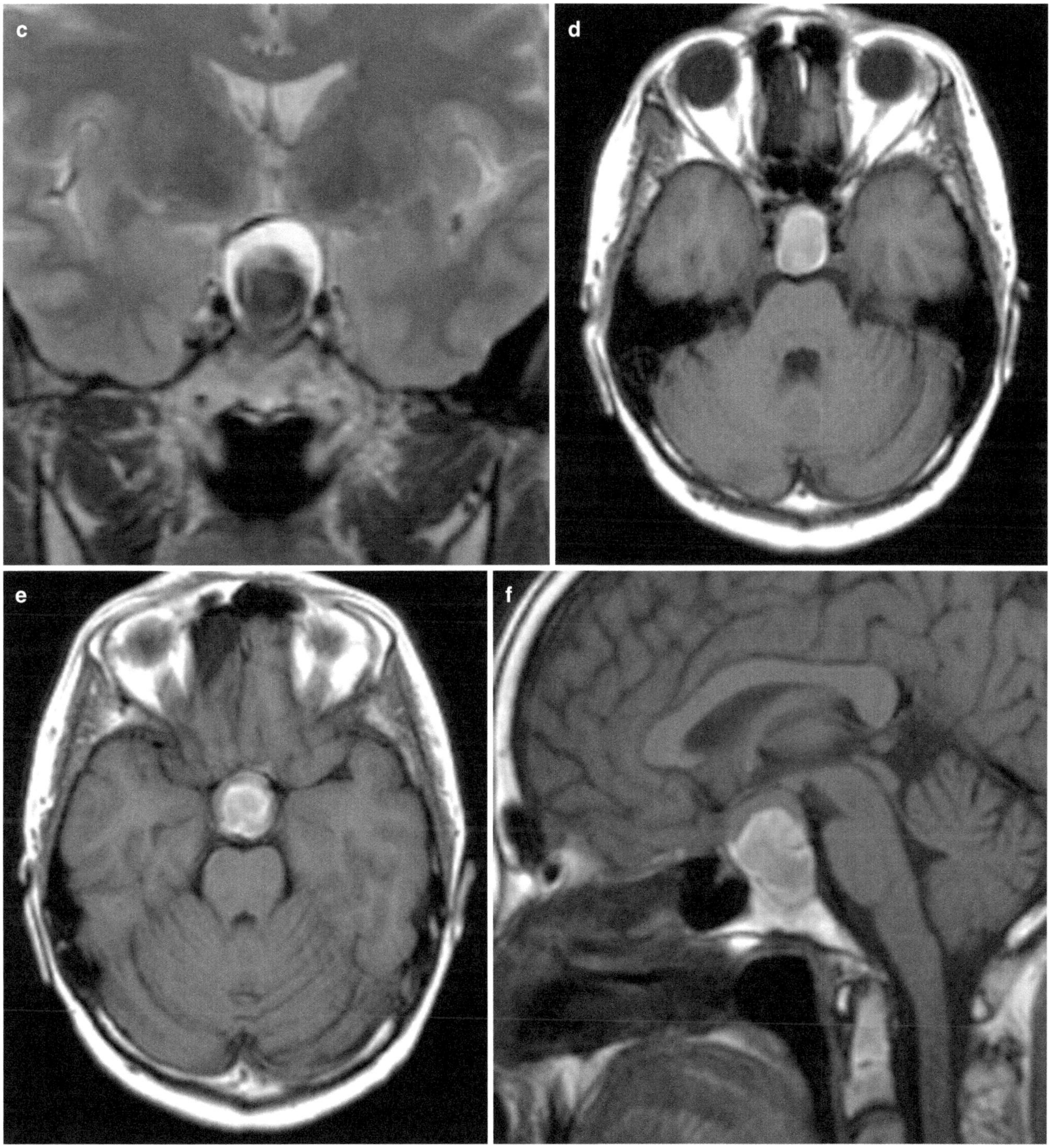

Fig. 15.37 (continued)

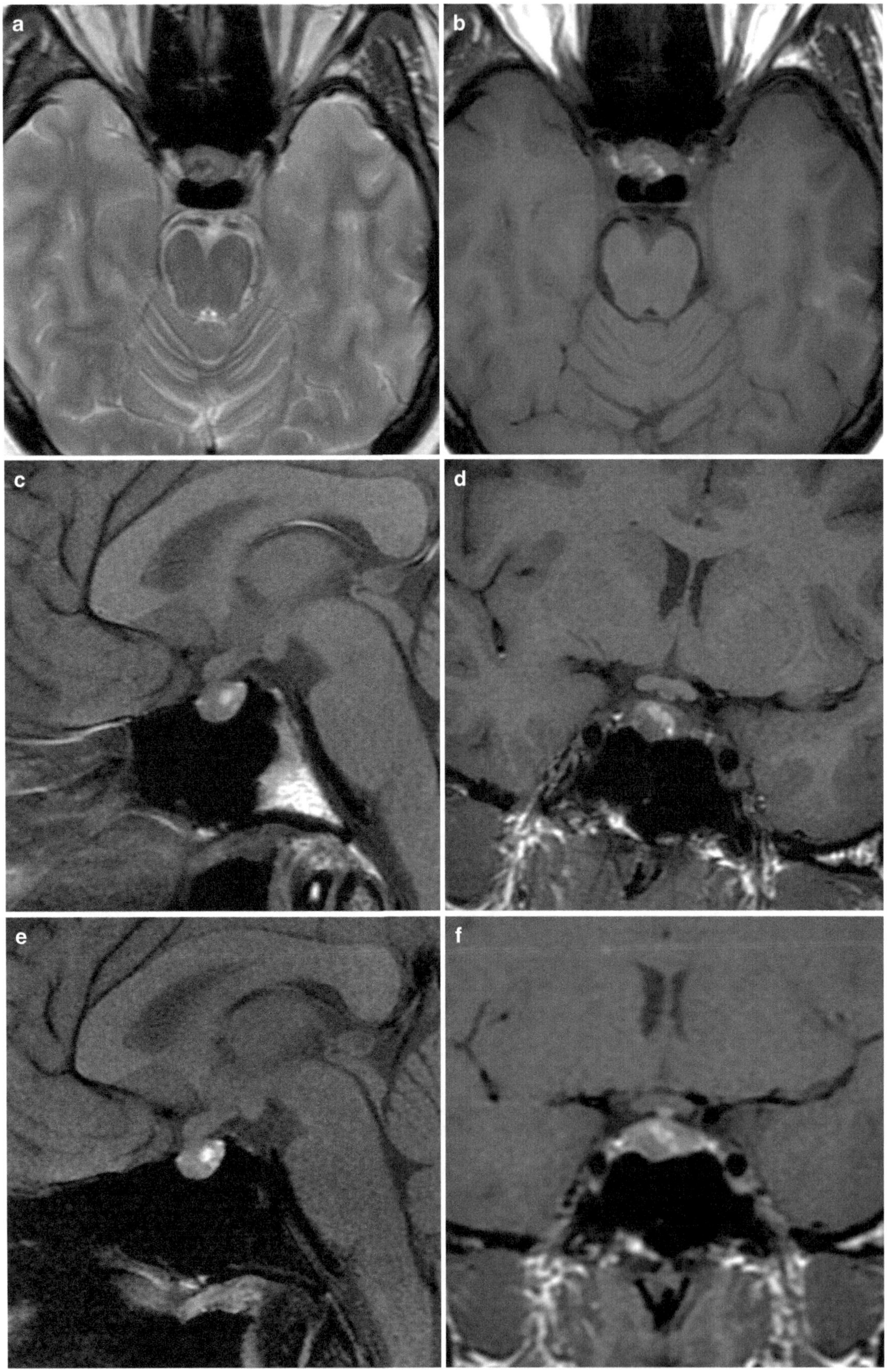

Fig. 15.38 Hemorrhage into the pituitary adenoma. T2- (**a**) and T1-weighted images (**b–e**): an area of hemorrhage in the sellar tumor is hypointense on T2-weighted image and hyperintense on T1-weighted image. The intensity of the signal from hemorrhage is not change on T1 fat-sat image (**e**) and on post-contrast MRI (**f**)

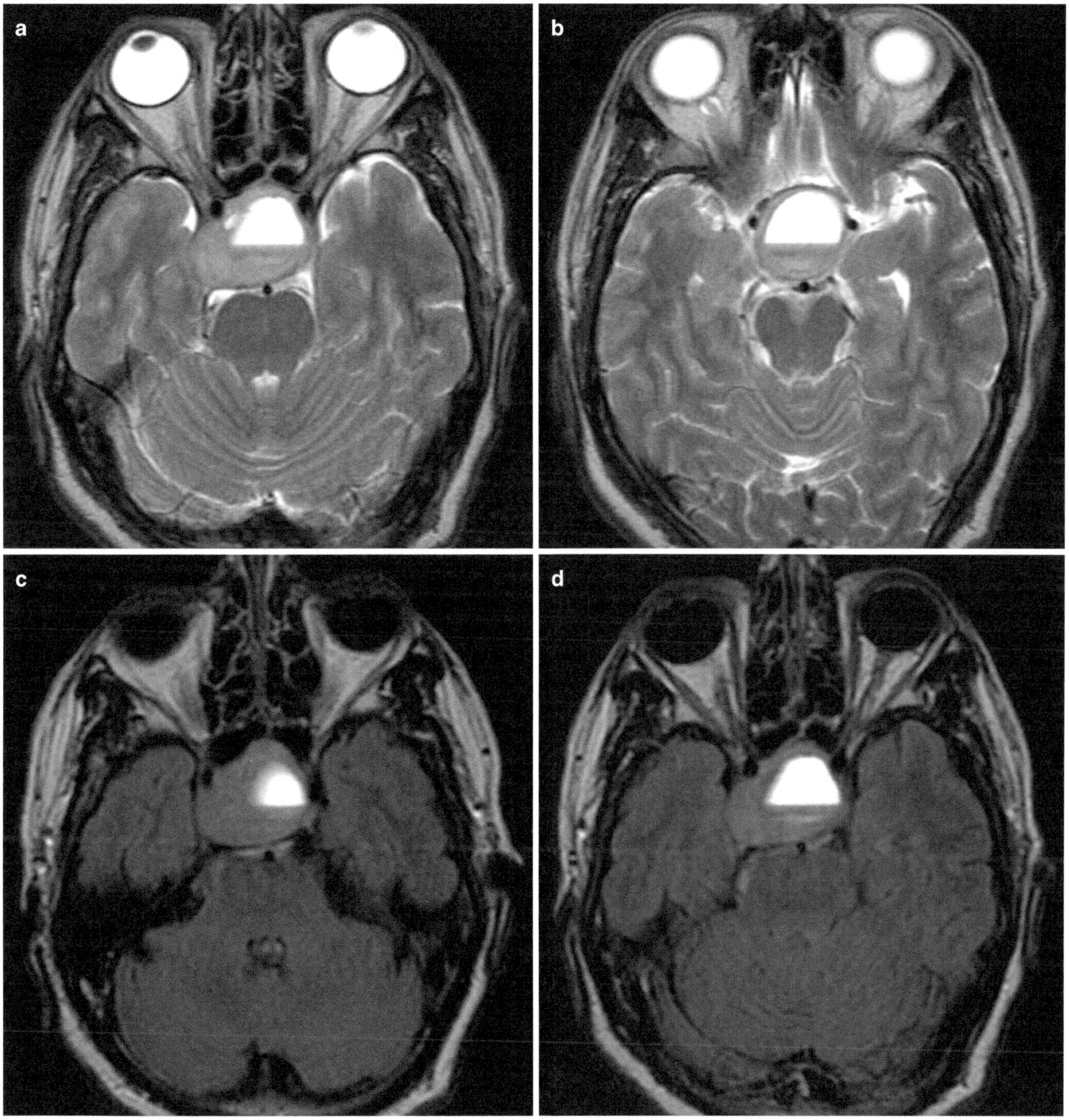

Fig. 15.39 Pituitary apoplexy. Axial T2- (**a**, **b**), T2-FLAIR (**c**, **d**), T1-weighted images (**e**, **f**) and sagittal T1-weighted images (**g**, **h**). Sellar, infrasellar, suprasellar large pituitary adenoma is clearly visible. The cystic cavity with hemorrhagic content and blood-fluid level can be seen in the superior aspect of the tumor. After the head position changing the blood-fluid level displaces (**i**). There is a rim enhancement in the remaining adenoma tissue (**h**, **i**)

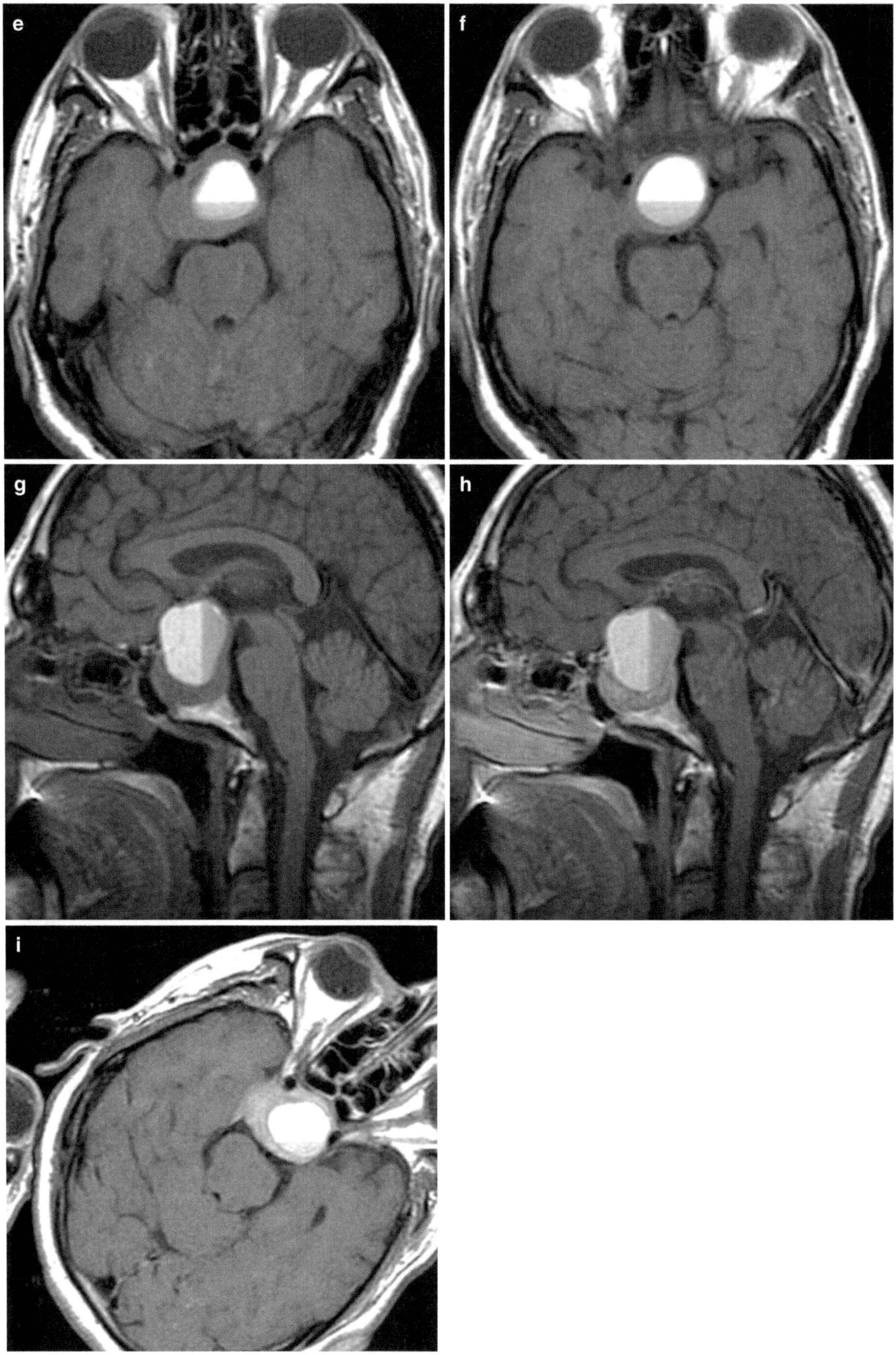

Fig. 15.39 (continued)

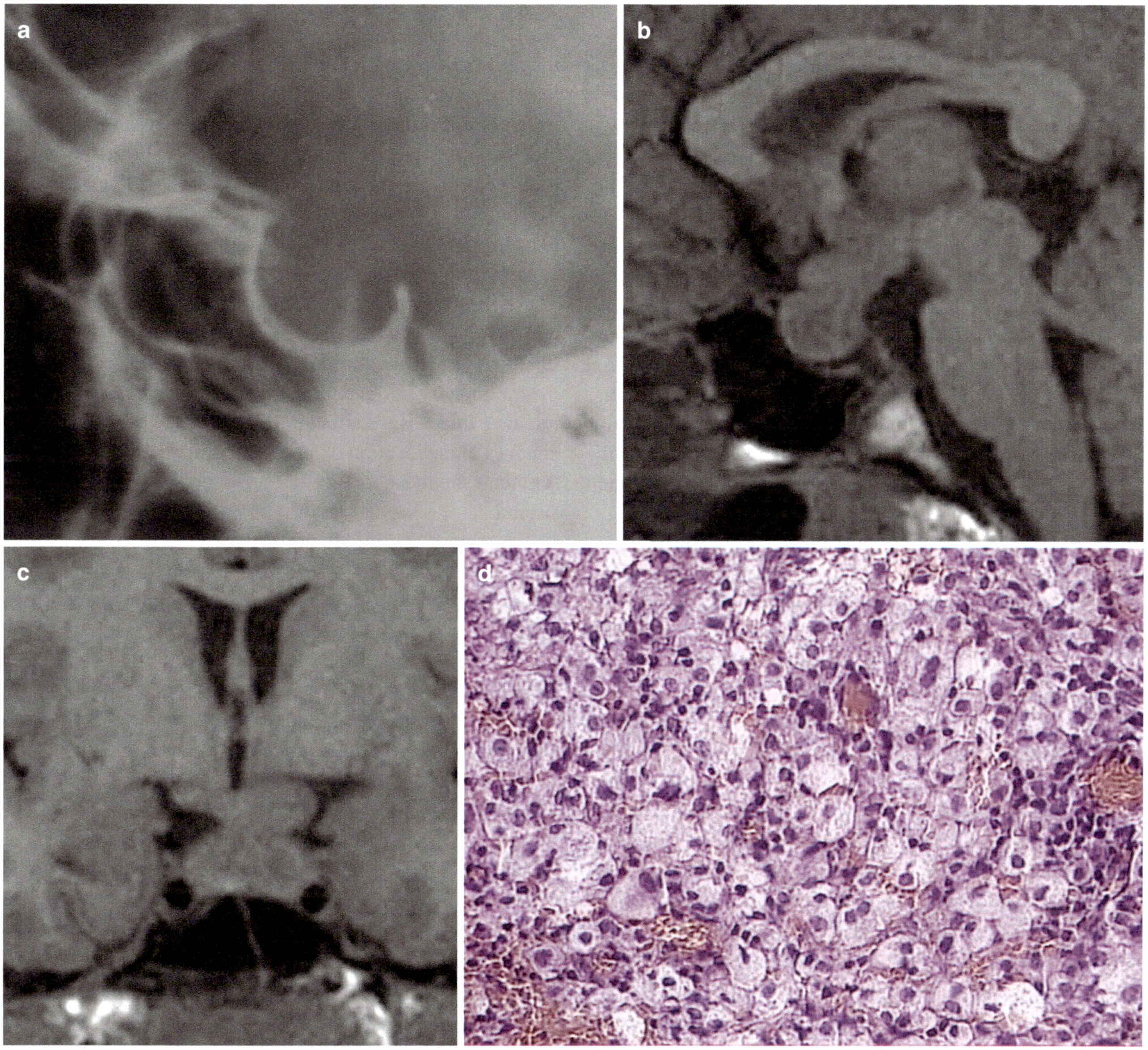

Fig. 15.40 Pituicytoma of the sellar-suprasellar area. X-ray craniogram shows an enlarged sellar turcica, eroded anterior clinoid processes and dorsum sella (**a**). Sagittal (**b**) and coronal (**c**) T1-weighted images show a sellar-suprasellar isointense mass with the small hypointense zone within the sella. Superior margin of the isointense tumor is poorly differentiated. Histopathologic specimen (**d**)

15.4 Craniopharyngiomas

Craniopharyngioma (CPH) is a benign neuroepithelial dysembriogenic neoplasm. There are two proposed theories of the sources of craniopharyngioma growth: from the remnants of the embryonic epithelium of the craniopharyngeal duct (Rathke pouch epithelium) and from squamous epithelial cells in pars tuberalis of adenohypophysis (Osborn et al. 2016). Craniopharyngiomas (CPH) account for 2.1–4.6% of all brain tumors, and they are more frequently found in children (5–10% of all cases of brain tumors in children), accounting for 17–21.4% of all supratentorial tumors and up to 56% of all tumors of the chiasmal-sellar region in children (Miller 1994; Muller 2013). The distribution of craniopharyngiomas (CPH) according to age is characterized by two peaks: between 5 and 10 years, and, the smaller group, on the fifth or sixth decade of life (Carmel et al. 1982; Hoffman et al. 1992; Van Effenterre et al. 2002).

Craniopharyngiomas are represented by two main histological variants, adamantinomatous and papillomatous types, which are not only pathologically, but also clinically different.

The most frequent is the adamantinomatous variant of CPH (up to 90% of cases). Typical features of this variant are polymorphism of pathological structure, invasive growth, glial capsule, and marked degenerative processes. Calcifications in the solid part of adamantinomatous CPH (from small to coral-shaped) are seen over than in 90% of cases. The macrostructure of craniopharyngiomas varies from completely calcified to completely cystic. The cystic components of the tumor have different content: opalescent or xanthochromic fluid in the thin-walled cysts, or brownish-green fritter-like masses (depending on the presence of protein, cholesterol, epithelium, keratin and fat) with thick walls with calcifications in its depth.

Papillary CPH (about 10%) is more common in adults; have mainly a compact structure; rarely they are represented by small uni-chambered cysts with thick walls. Their viscous consistency includes a good deal of cholesterol, detritus, and fat. The usual location of these CPH is intra-extraventricular; the type of growth is expansive with well-defined borders with adjacent brain structures. They rarely recur after a total removal. Calcifications are seen much less frequently than with adamantinomatous CPH.

These are the following types of craniopharyngiomas depending on their localization: intrasuprasellar, infundibular (suprasellar), intraventricular, and giant (Fig. 15.41).

Intrasuprasellar CPHs initially compress the pituitary tissue and the sella turcica as they originate from epithelial cells located within the adenohypophysis. Along with the tumor growth, the optic nerves, the internal carotid arteries and their branches are displaced upwards and laterally, the third ventricle becomes fissure-like due to its upward lifting. Miscommunication between the pituitary tissue and its stalk occurs, the latter, after detachment from the infundibular part of the floor of the third ventricle, becomes inseparable from the upper layers of the tumor capsule.

The infundibular CPHs originate from the epithelial cells located along the pituitary stalk in the space between the sella turcica diaphragm and the floor of the third ventricle. These tumors are usually located along the brain base—in the ante-, para-, and retrosellar region, they lift up the floor of the third ventricle as well as the previously discussed group of craniopharyngiomas does; however, the pituitary tissue remains intact. Infundibular CPHs cause the most severe changes in the location of arteries of brain base; infrequently, segments of the optic nerves are included into the tumor stroma.

Intraventricular CPHs originate from the epithelial cells of the floor of the third ventricle separate it in ventral and the dorsal layers. The bulk of the tumor lies within the cavity of the third ventricle; the pituitary stalk and the pituitary tissue remain intact under these circumstances. Intraventricular CPH has been observed spreading into the lateral ventricles or along the brain base—intra- and extraventricular tumors. Intra-infrasellar craniopharyngiomas are very rare.

Giant CPHs consist of a special group. CPHs of all topographic types are related to this group. The typical features of CPHs are their wider expansion, penetration into the ventricular system, and development of hydrocephalus, often obstructive. The blood supply of CPH proceeds via the posterior cerebral arteries and the internal carotid arteries. In some cases arteries follow along the tumor capsule and supply it with blood, in other cases, arteries that are located within the tumor stroma take part in the tumor and the adjacent structures blood supply, and in some instances arteries are situated on the surface of the CPH capsule but do not supply it with blood.

Clinical manifestations of CPH depend mainly on the anatomic variant of the location of a tumor and involve the following: ophthalmological signs, hydrocephalus with raised intracranial pressure, the hypothalamus–pituitary–suprarenal system disturbances, the cranial nerves impairment, and if a tumor invades the posterior cranial fossa, the brainstem symptoms. The extent of these symptoms and their sequence of their development depend on the anatomic variant of the tumor. The latter are not hormonally active tumors, but as they compress the pituitary gland or the hypothalamus they cause symptoms such as growth retardation, hypothyroidism, and diabetes insipidus.

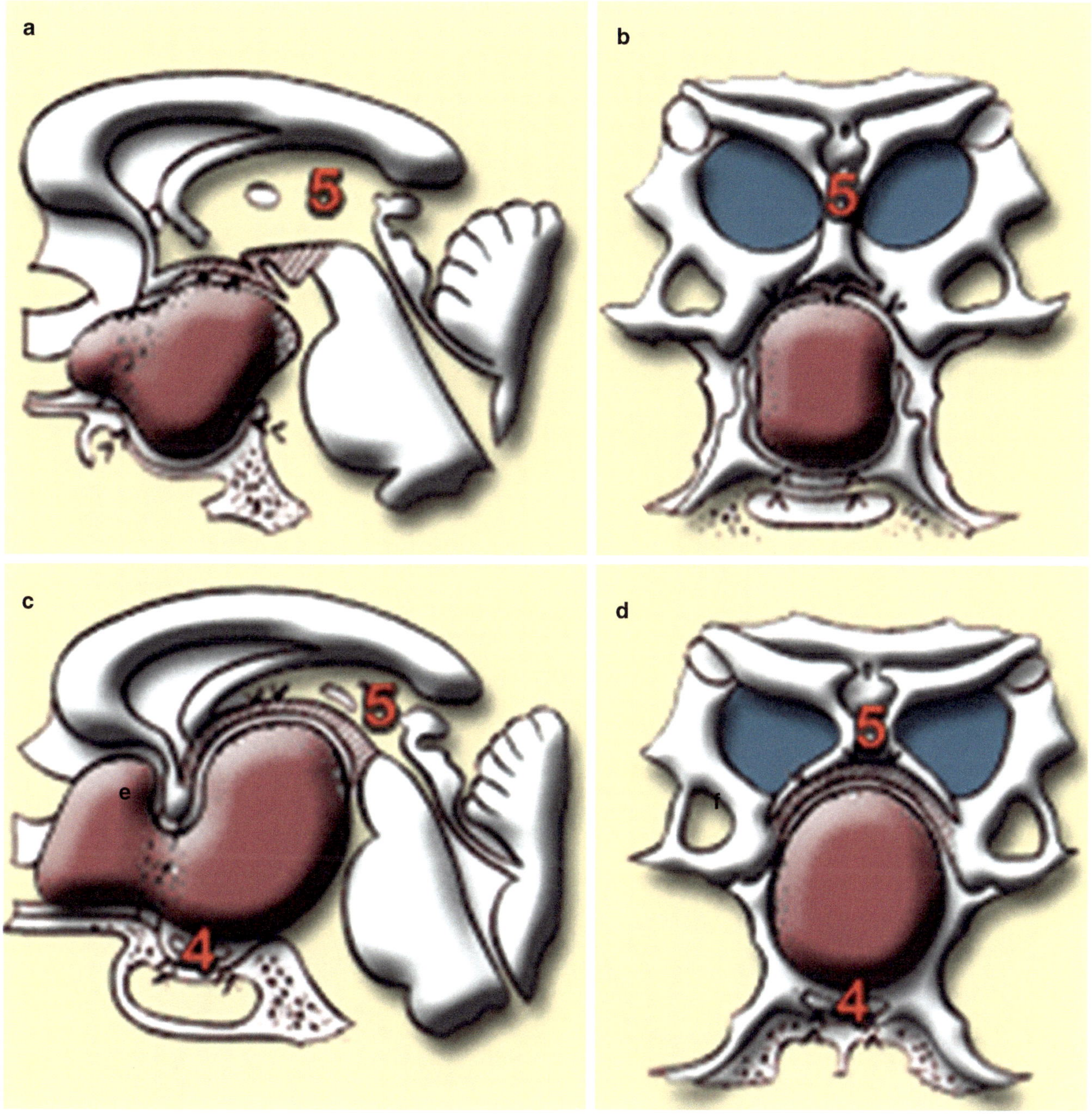

Fig. 15.41 Graphics of craniopharyngiomas variants location (coronal and sagittal projections): (**a**, **b**)—intra-suprasellar; (**c**, **d**)—infundibular; (**e**, **f**)—intraventricular; (**g**, **h**)—intra-extraventricular

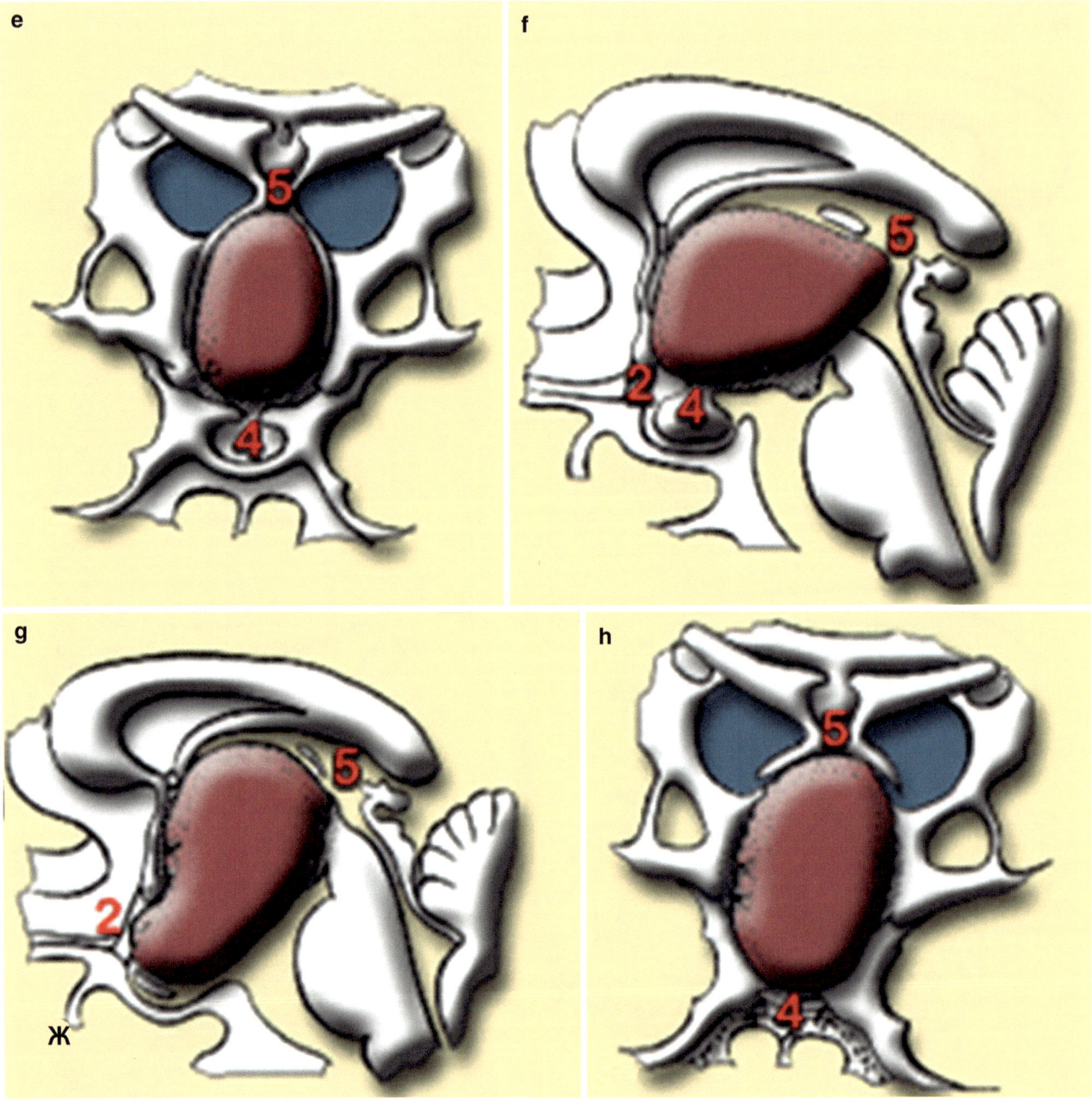

Fig. 15.41 (continued)

Imaging Neuroimaging findings depend on the type and anatomic variant of a tumor. X-ray exam reveals typical signs of CPH such as changes in shape, sizes of the sella turcica, and calcifications in the chiasmal-sellar region (Kopylov 1968). The shape and the size of calcifications vary, from small, crumb-like and poorly distinguishable to large, lump-like, and vivid coral-like ones. Laminar calcifications are frequent, which are usually situated in a tumor capsule.

Intrasuprasellar CPHs cause changes in the sella turcica: increase in size, deepening of the floor, widening of the entry and deformity (thinning, lifting, shortening) of the anterior clinoid processes. Calcifications are usually found within the cavity of sella and above it.

Intraventricular CPHs do not usually cause severe changes of the sella turcica; its size remains almost intact. However, in the majority of cases the dorsum sella turcica shortens. Being situated close to the CSF circulation pathways CPH causes of changes in the ventricular system and increase of intracranial pressure, which is observed on X-ray exams as a "fingerprints" pattern in the cranial vault bones, widening of cranial sutures, and changes in the sella turcica elements. Calcifications of CPH may be found in the third and in the lateral ventricles projection.

The navicular shape of sella turcica, which is sometimes combined with shortening of its dorsum, is typical for infundibular CPH. Calcifications are usually located in the chiasmal and adjacent regions. Lifting the floor of the third ventricle, these CPHs cause hydrocephalus and rise of intracranial pressure, which can be seen on X-ray exams. However, today the significance of X-ray examination in the primary diagnosis of CPHs is substantially limited. CT and MRI methods allow completely excluding plain radiography from the primary diagnostic algorithm.

On cerebral angiography, the vascular net of a tumor is not usually detected; only displacement of vessels may be seen—the arteries of the circle of Willis, and the anterior and middle cerebral arteries, which depends on a tumor location. At present, direct angiography is almost never performed as a method of identification for the location of vessels in cases of CPHs. The information presented by CT and MR -angiography is sufficient for presurgical planning.

CT and MRI identify the precise size of a tumor, the ratio between the cystic and the solid part of a tumor, and their sizes and location, and the state of the ventricular system (the extent of concomitant hydrocephalus and in most cases, the level of occlusion of the CSF pathways), and spatial relation of the tumor to the third ventricle cavity; the extent of expansion beyond the ventricular system is seen. On coronal CT scans with or without reformation, the upward displacement of the third ventricle is detected clearly; calcifications in the tumor being observed in up to 93% (Konovalov et al. 1983). In intrasuprasellar CPH, the sizes of sella turcica are usually enlarged (Fig. 15.42). The intrasellar part of a tumor is usually nodular with presence of calcifications. Growing upwards, the tumor fills the region of chiasmal cisterns (partially or completely), with elevation of the third ventricle floor. The suprasellar part of a tumor is usually cystic, but may be solid. Cysts may be located on the base of the anterior cranial fossa, in the paraventricular region (giant CPHs), and be identified in the depth of the nodular part.

Papillary tumors are usually well-delineated from the adjacent brain on CT and appear as a solid nodule in the suprasellar region. The nodular part of the tumor has almost the same density as the brain, intravenous injection of contrast material in most cases increases the CPH density by 20–25 HU, which makes it sufficiently separated from the surrounding brain tissue. In papillary CPH, calcifications are rarely found (Figs. 15.43 and 15.44).

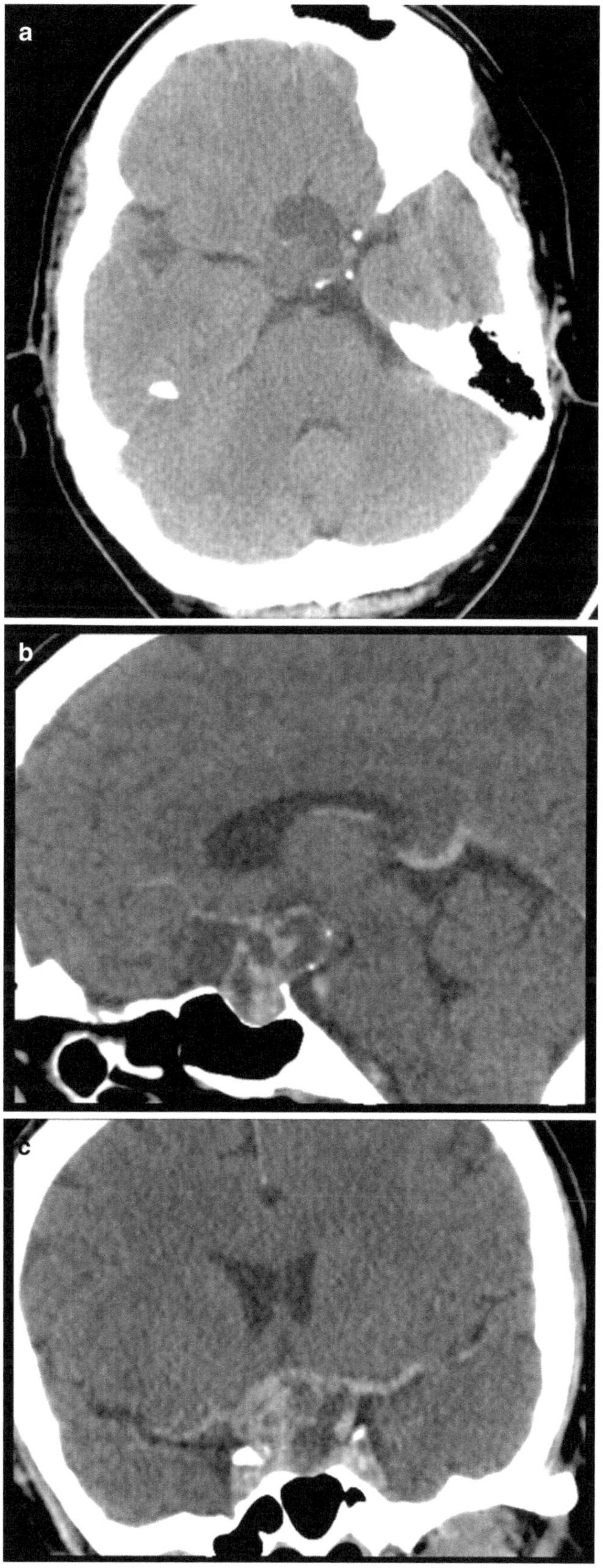

Fig. 15.42 Sellar-suprasellar craniopharyngioma. CT scans before (**a**) and after CE (**b**, **c**) show a suprasellar multicystic tumor with intrasellar component. There are small calcifications in the tumor capsule. The solid component of the tumor heterogeneously enhances

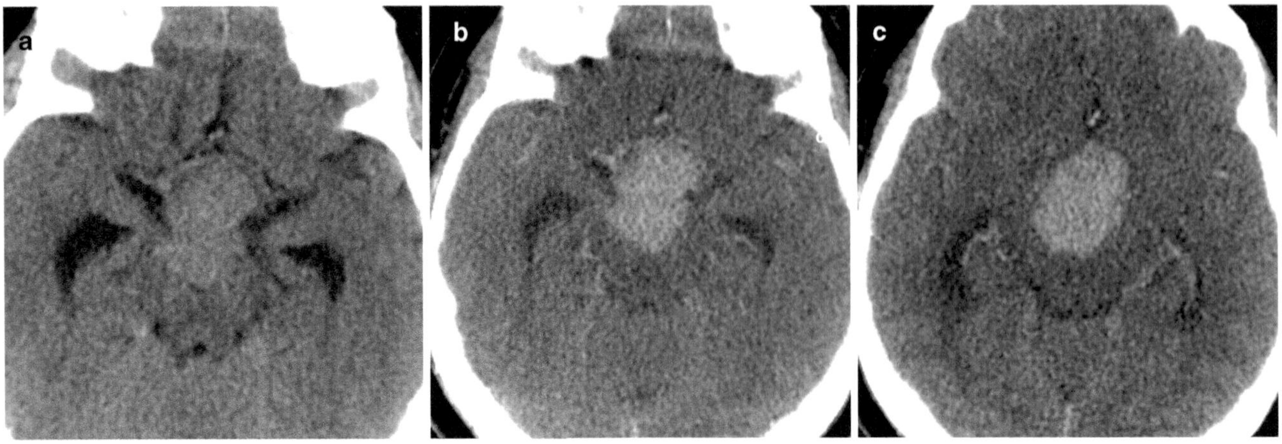

Fig. 15.43 Papillary craniopharyngioma. Axial CT scan (**a**) shows a solid isodense suprasellar tumor. CT scans after CE (**b**, **c**) demonstrate a homogeneous contrast enhancement of the tumor

Intraventricular CPHs are predominantly cystic and are located in the third ventricle cavity; they penetrate into the lateral ventricles, and often reach giant sizes. The density of cystic areas of CPH is usually higher than that of brain tissue, but isodense or mildly hyperdense cysts may be found. After CE, the walls of cysts moderately accumulate contrast medium. Intraventricular CPHs in most cases cause hydrocephalus.

Infundibular CPH has typical asymmetry, marked sizes, and expansion along the brain base with frequent invasion into the lateral ventricles cavity. If cysts are situated in the cavity of the third ventricle, then they usually completely fill its anterior portion. Sometimes cystic tumors are represented by a system of cysts, which are hardly differentiated and may be distinguished only on axial images (Fig. 15.45 and 15.46).

CPH with many calcifications in the nodular part located in the sella turcica and in the suprasellar space (predominantly adamantinomatous) are well differentiated on 3D CT. The spatial relationship between the tumor and the adjacent bone structures can be seen as well.

CT-perfusion study demonstrates differences in hemodynamic properties of different histological CPH types. Adamantinomatous CPHs show low CBV and CBF parameters, while papillary CPHs are characterized by a moderately increase in CBF with high CBV values. Mean transit time parameter (MTT) in the structure of these CPH types appeared to be prolonged and close to the absolute values (Figs. 15.47 and 15.48).

On T1-weighted imaging, the nodular part of the tumor is isointense; the signal of cysts may be hypo- or hyperintense (this depends on the protein content, cholesterol, and blood products within) (Kornienko and Ozerova 1993). On T2-weighted imaging the signal of the nodular part is isointense, and the signal of cysts may be hypointense or markedly hyperintense (Figs. 15.49 and 15.50). The extent of hydrocephalus depends on the spatial relation between the tumor and the ventricular system. Intravenous CE causes heterogeneous hyperintensity in the compact part of the tumor. Papillary CPHs are strongly enhanced, as most of the tumors consist of soft tissue elements; however, adamantinomatous CPHs are also enhanced by the capsule and separate compact tumor nodes (Figs. 15.51 and 15.52).

The cystic CPHs located only in the sella turcica cavity (hypointense on T1- weighted images and hyperintense on T2-weighted images) should be differentiated from the mucocele of the sphenoid sinus, the signal of which may be similar to the CPH (Fig. 15.53). Apart from differences in clinical manifestations and course, there are differences in their location. Mucocele lies under the floor of sella turcica inside the sphenoid sinus cavity, which appears enlarged and as if inflated, whereas the intact pituitary gland is located above the cystic mass lesion.

In rare cases, CPHs with atypical growth have to be differentiated from chordoma, chondrosarcoma, invasive pituitary adenoma, malignant mesenchymal tumor, germ cells tumors (Lee et al. 2015), etc. (Fig. 15.54).

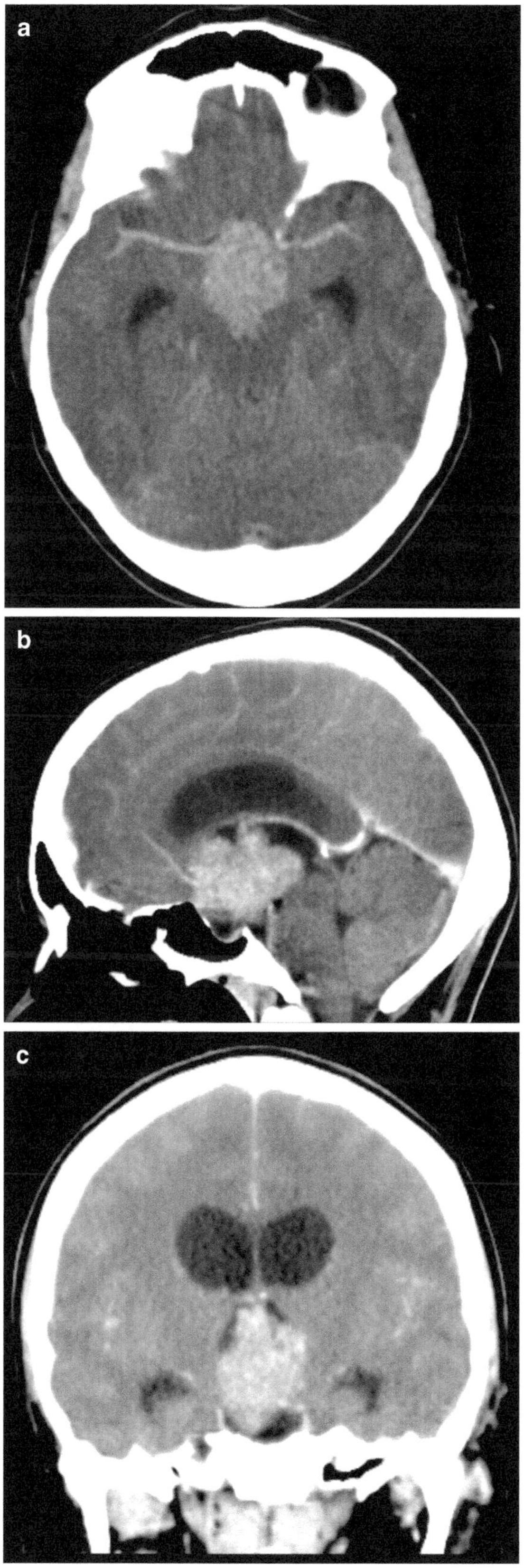

Fig. 15.44 Papillary infundibular craniopharyngioma. CT scans after CE (**a**–**c**) show the suprasellar tumor with an intensive heterogeneous contrast enhancement and irregular borders

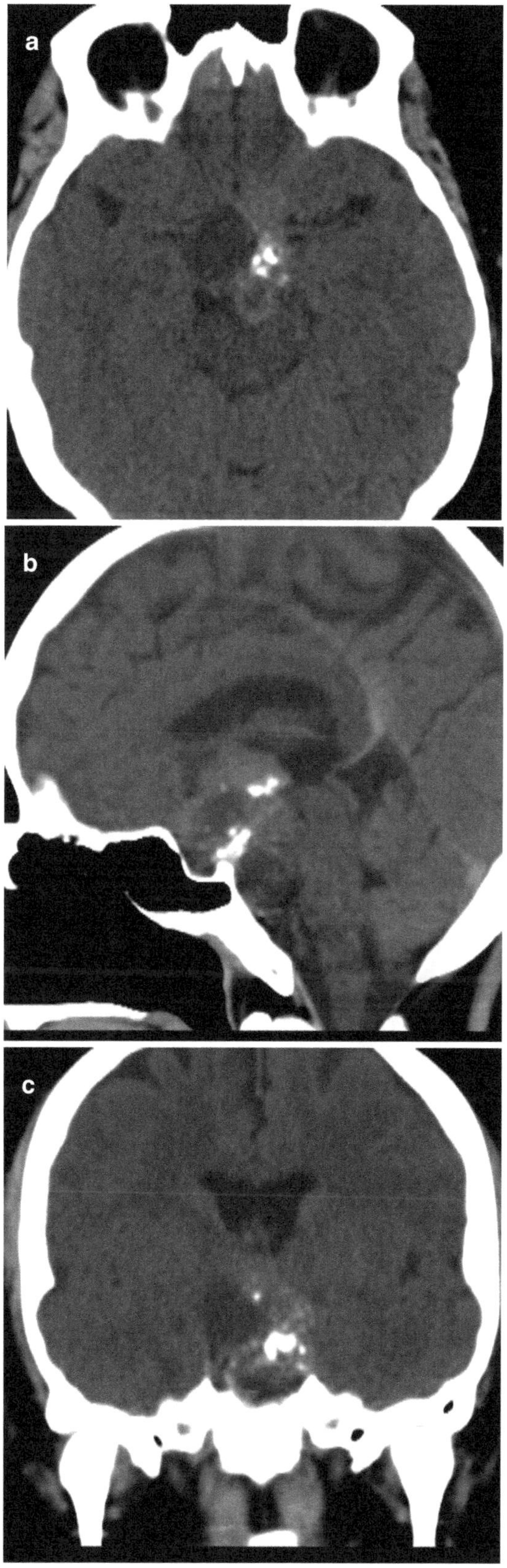

Fig. 15.45 Infundibular craniopharyngioma. Axial (**a**), coronal (**c**), and sagittal (**b**) CT images after CE demonstrate a tumor in the suprasellar cistern and anterior part of the third ventricle. Craniopharyngioma consists of the cystic and solid parts with calcifications

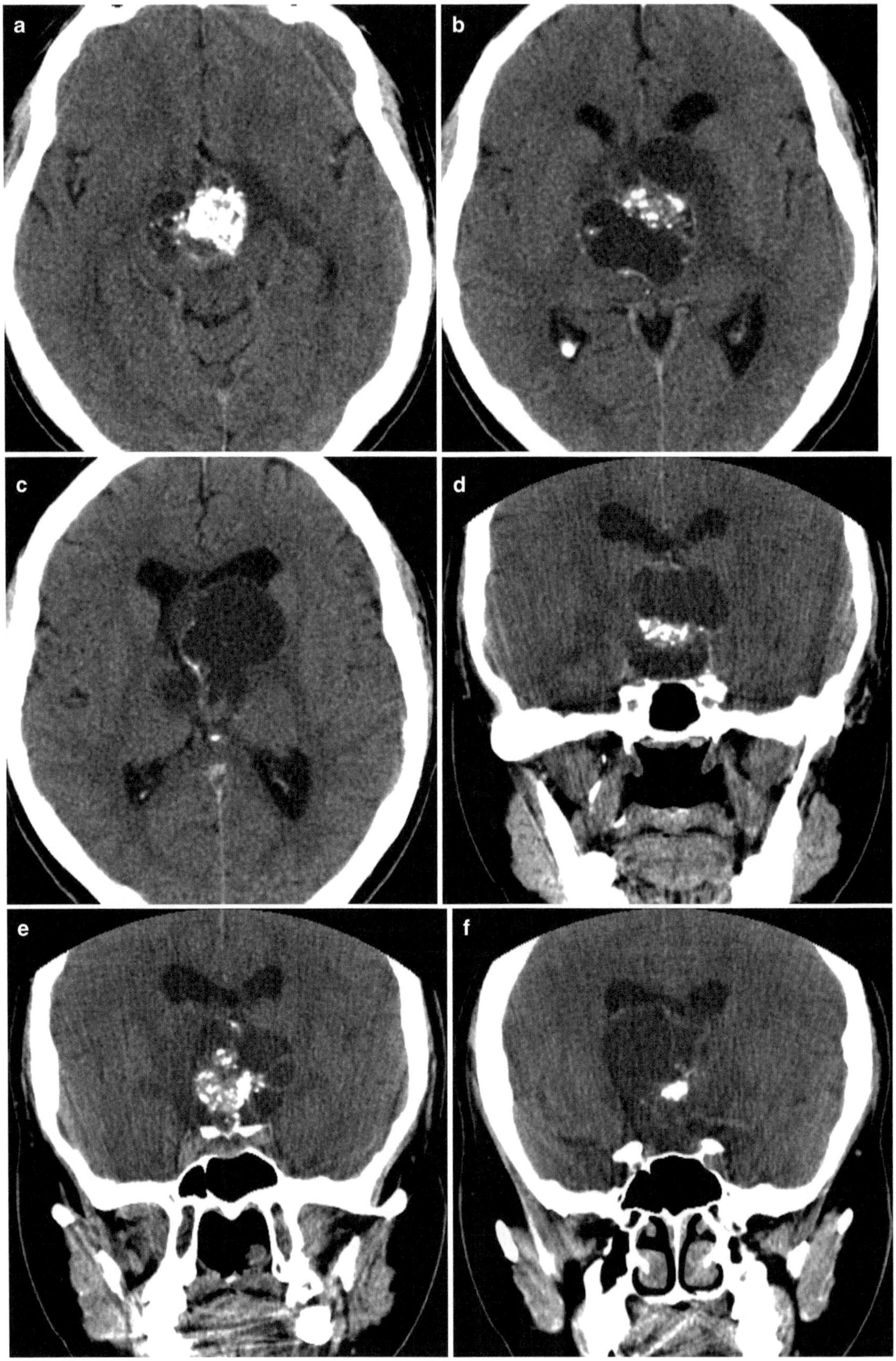

Fig. 15.46 Adamantinomatous craniopharyngioma. Axial CT-scans (**a**–**c**) with coronal reformations (**d**–**f**) visualize a large multicystic tumor, which extends into suprasellar cistern and the third ventricle. The tumor has a typical heterogeneous cystic structure with the focal rim calcifications and calcified central part. The cystic part of the tumor extends into the frontal horn of the left lateral ventricle

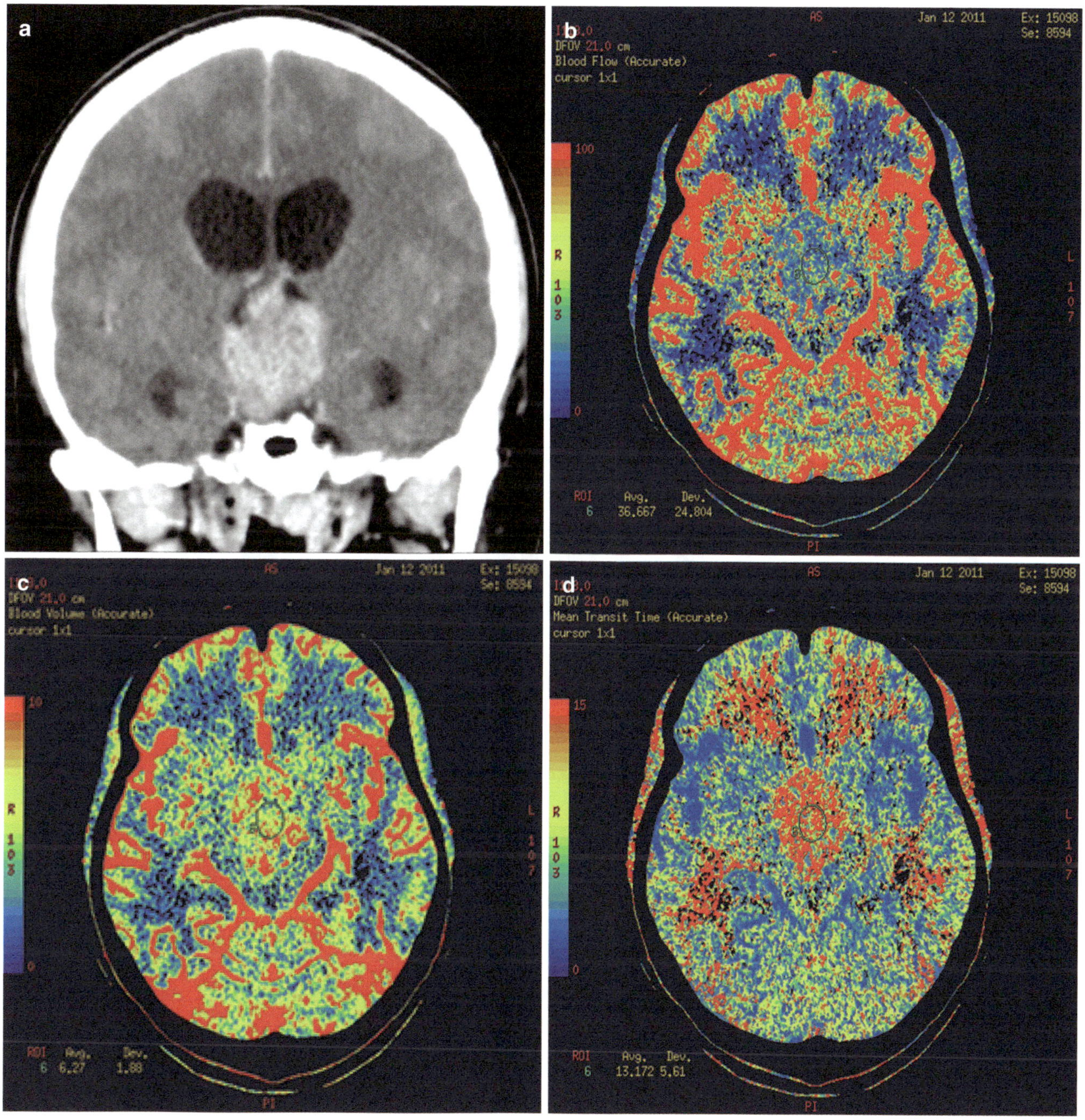

Fig. 15.47 Papillary craniopharyngioma. CT scan (**a**) demonstrates strongly enhanced suprasellar tumor. Perfusion CT mapping detects the low values of blood flow (CBF—**b**), moderately increased CBV (**c**), and prolonged MTT (**d**)

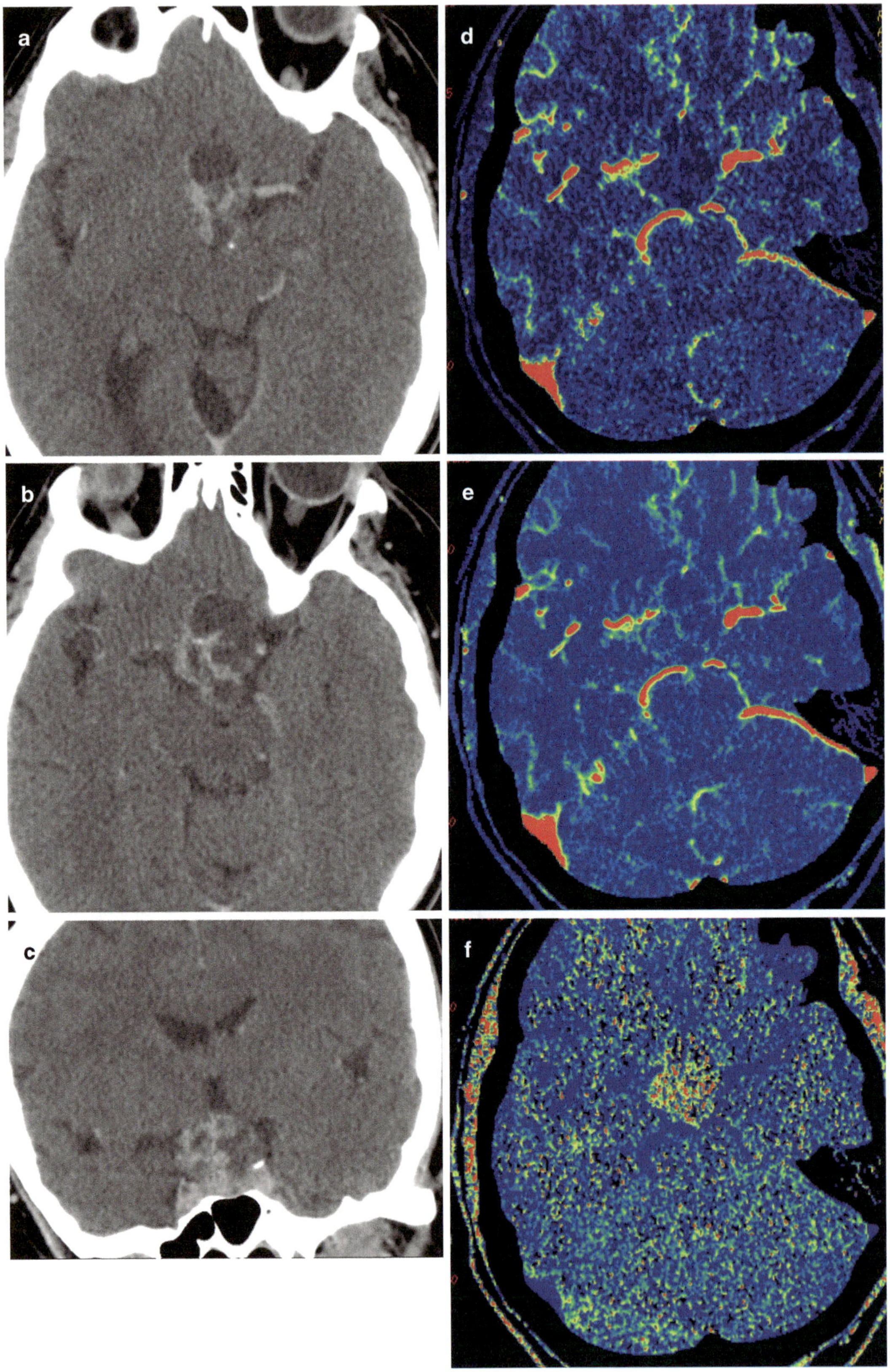

Fig. 15.48 Adamantinomatous craniopharyngioma. Axial CT scans (**a**, **b**) with coronal reformation (**c**) after CE demonstrate an intra-suprasellar heterogeneous tumor. Perfusion maps (CBF, CBV, MTT) reveal the low values of blood flow (**d**) and blood volume (**e**), and increased mean transit time, MTT (**f**), in the solid part of the tumor

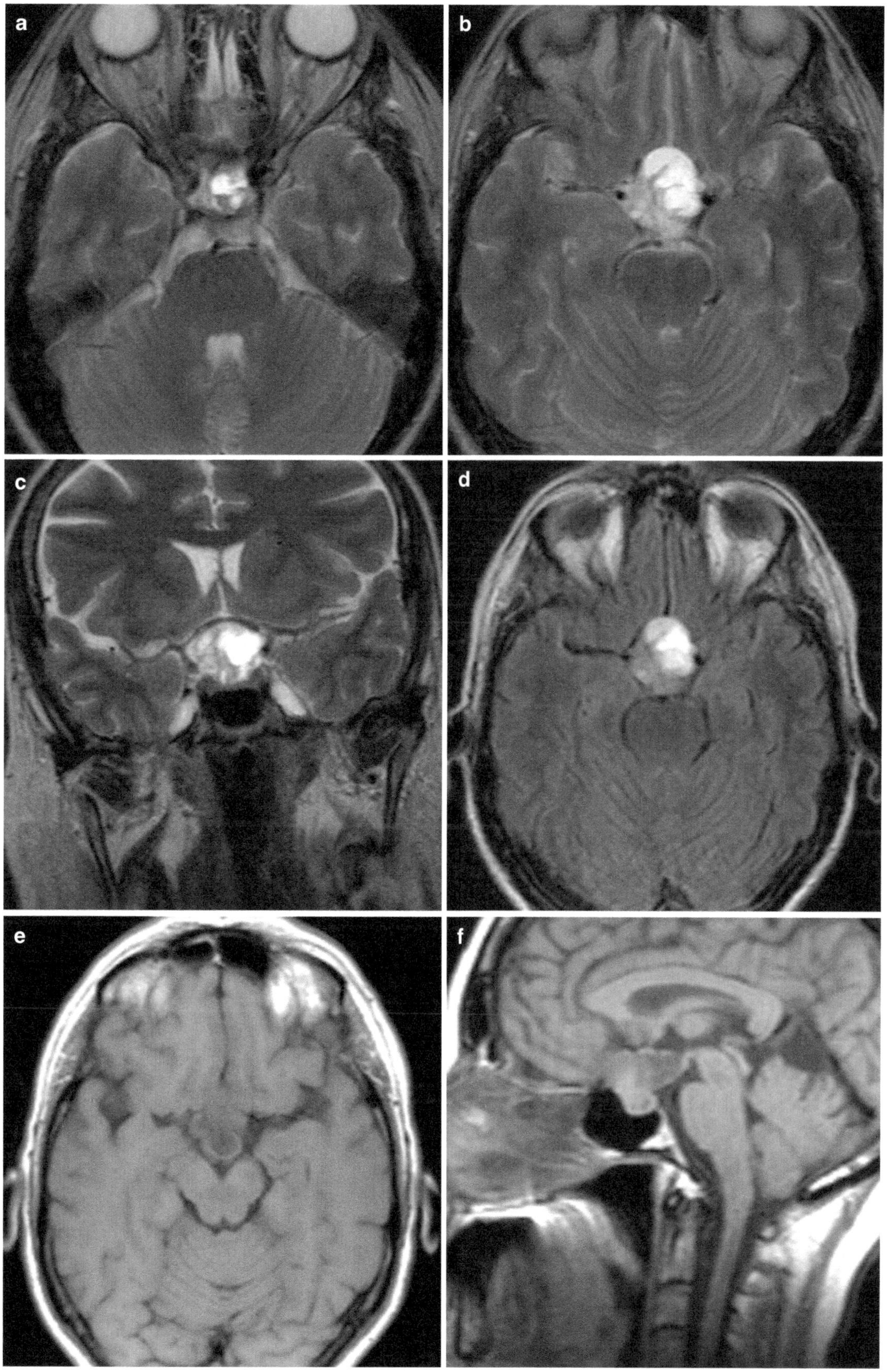

Fig. 15.49 Intra-suprasellar craniopharyngioma with the solid and cystic components. A cystic part is hyperintense on T2-weighted images (**a–c**). The cysts contain fluid of different signal intensities, T2-FLAIR (**d**). On T1-weighted images cysts have hypointense signal (**e**, **f**)

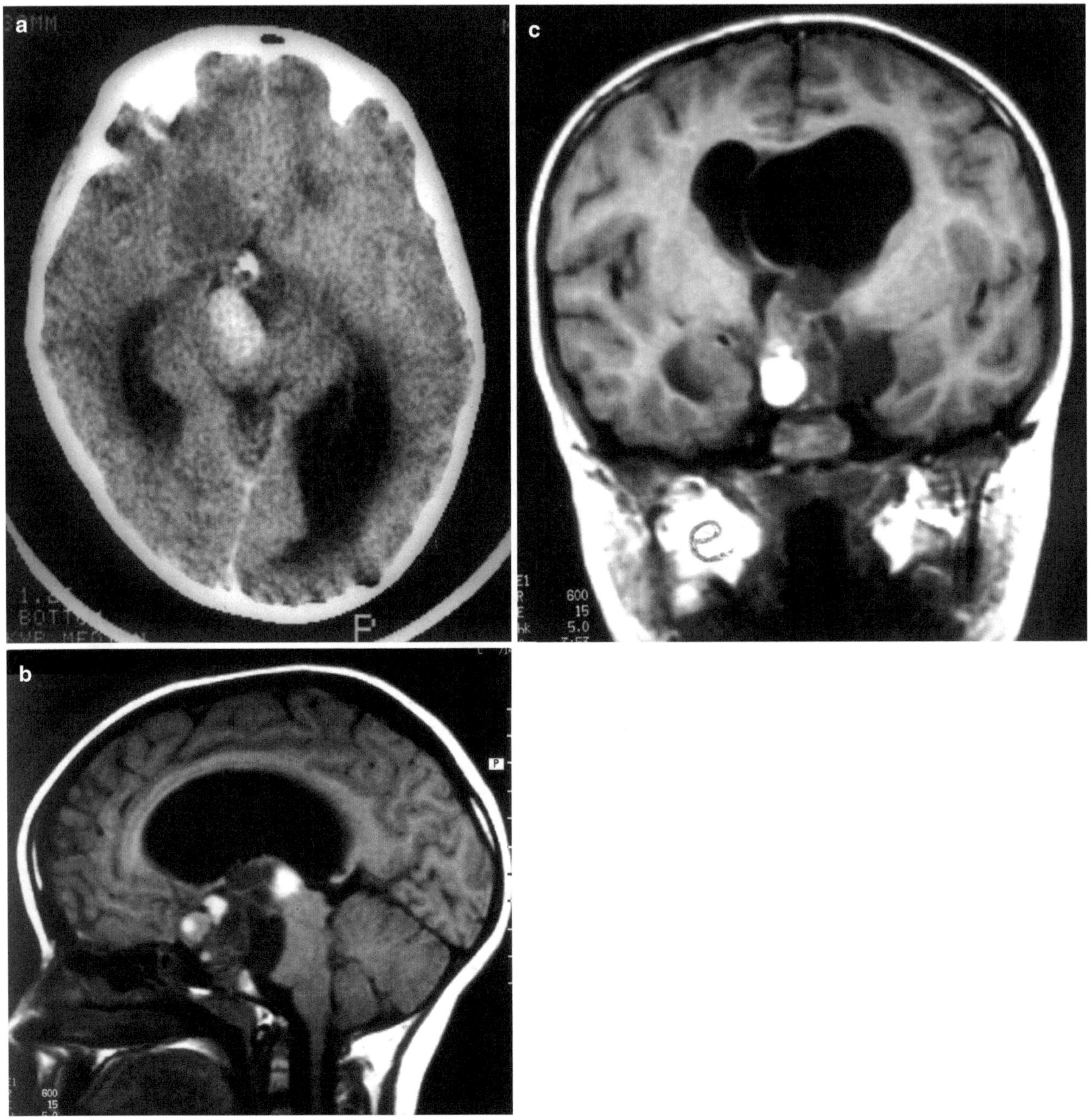

Fig. 15.50 Intra-suprasellar craniopharyngioma. CT (**a**) and T1-weighted MRI (**b**, **c**) visualize a large multicystic tumor. The cysts contain a fluid of different density and intensity from hypodense/hypointense to hyperdense/hyperintense

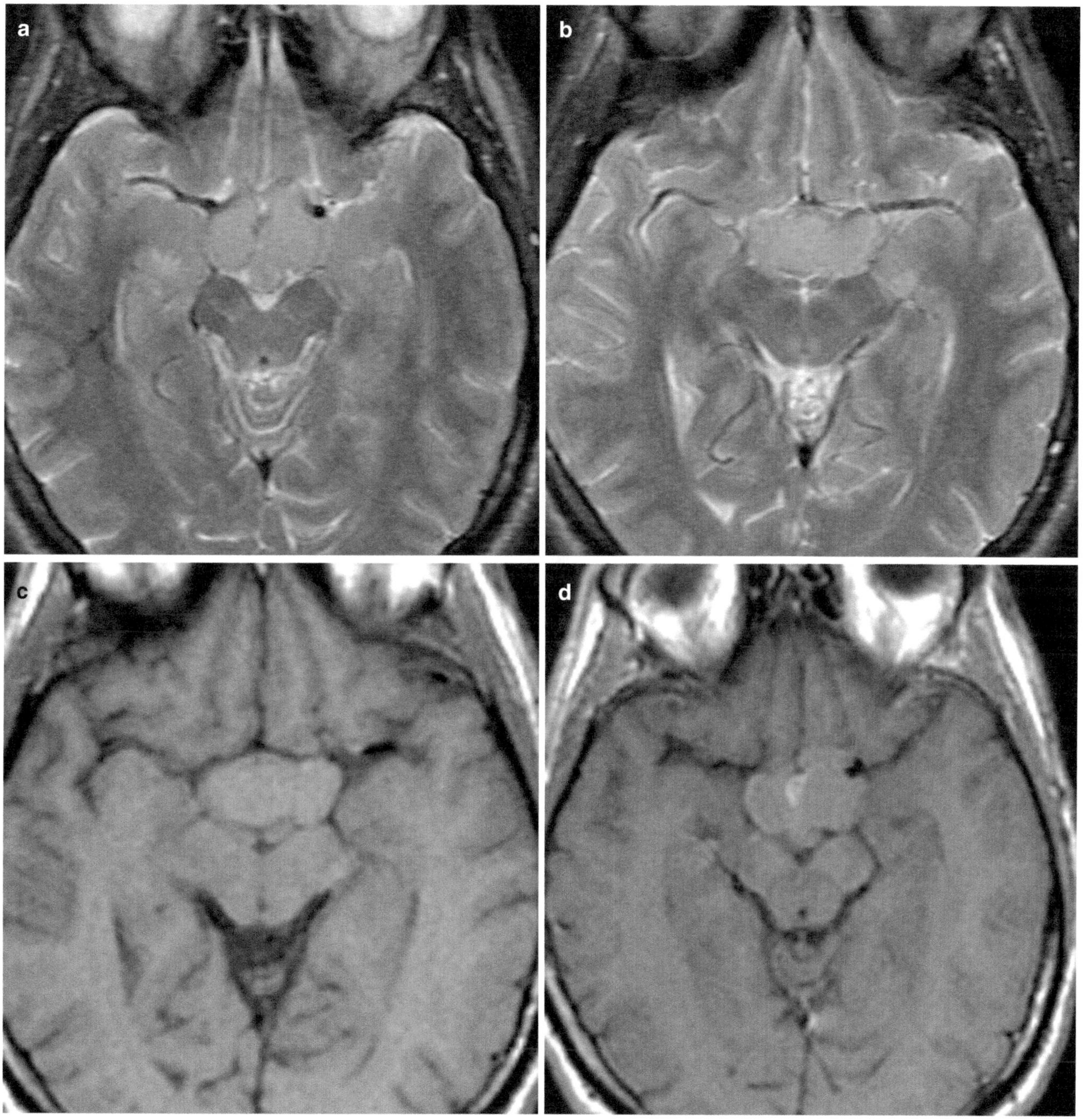

Fig. 15.51 Adamantinomatous suprasellar craniopharyngioma. T2-weighted (**a**, **b**), axial (**c**, **d**), sagittal (**e**), and coronal (**f**) T1-weighted images show an almost homogeneous suprasellar tumor. Axial, coronal, and sagittal CT images (**g–i**) after CE reveal a relatively homogeneous contrast enhancement. There are focal rim calcifications and the calcifications in the central part of the tumor. Calcifications are better visualized on CT, than on MRI

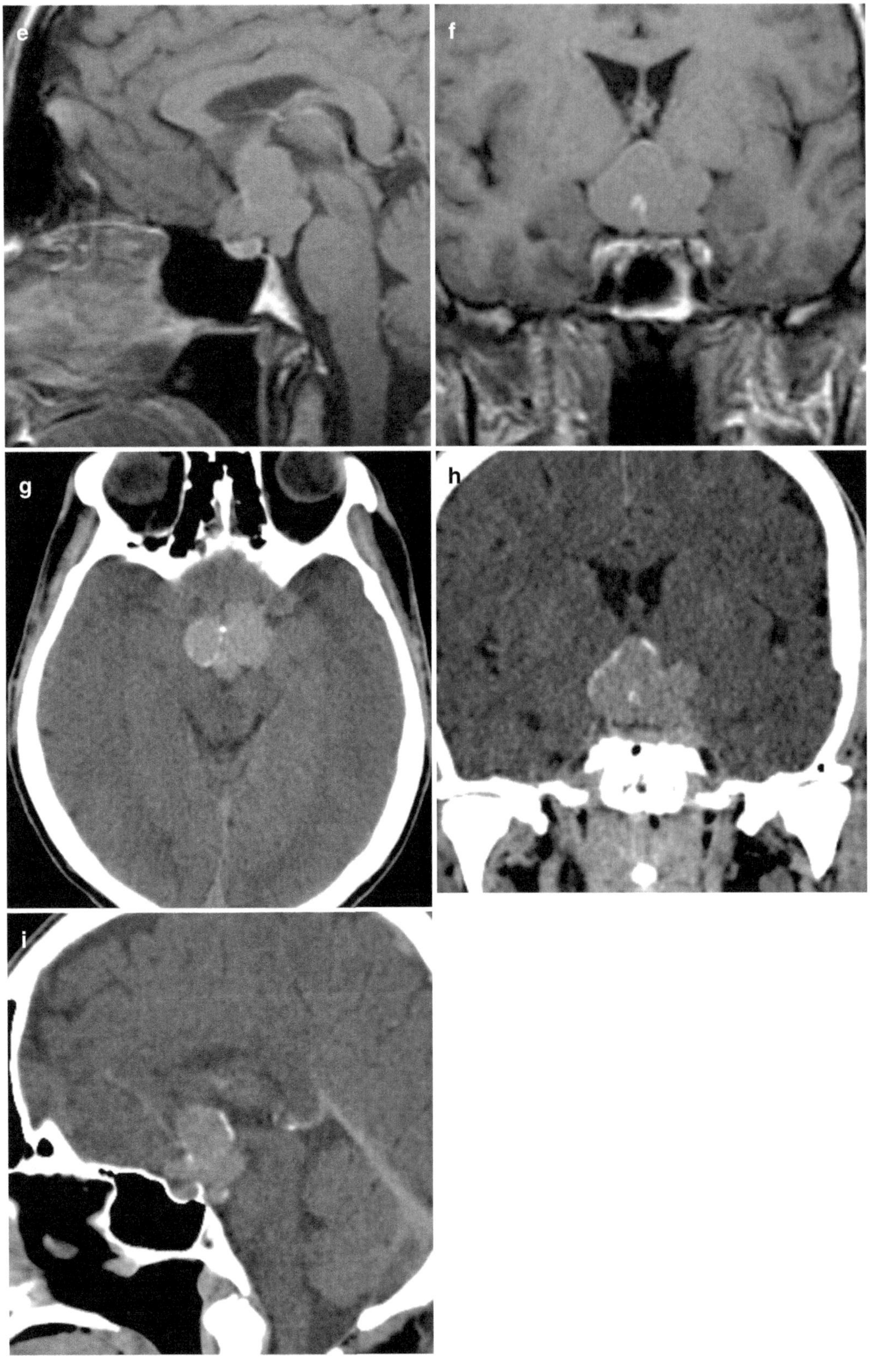

Fig. 15.51 (continued)

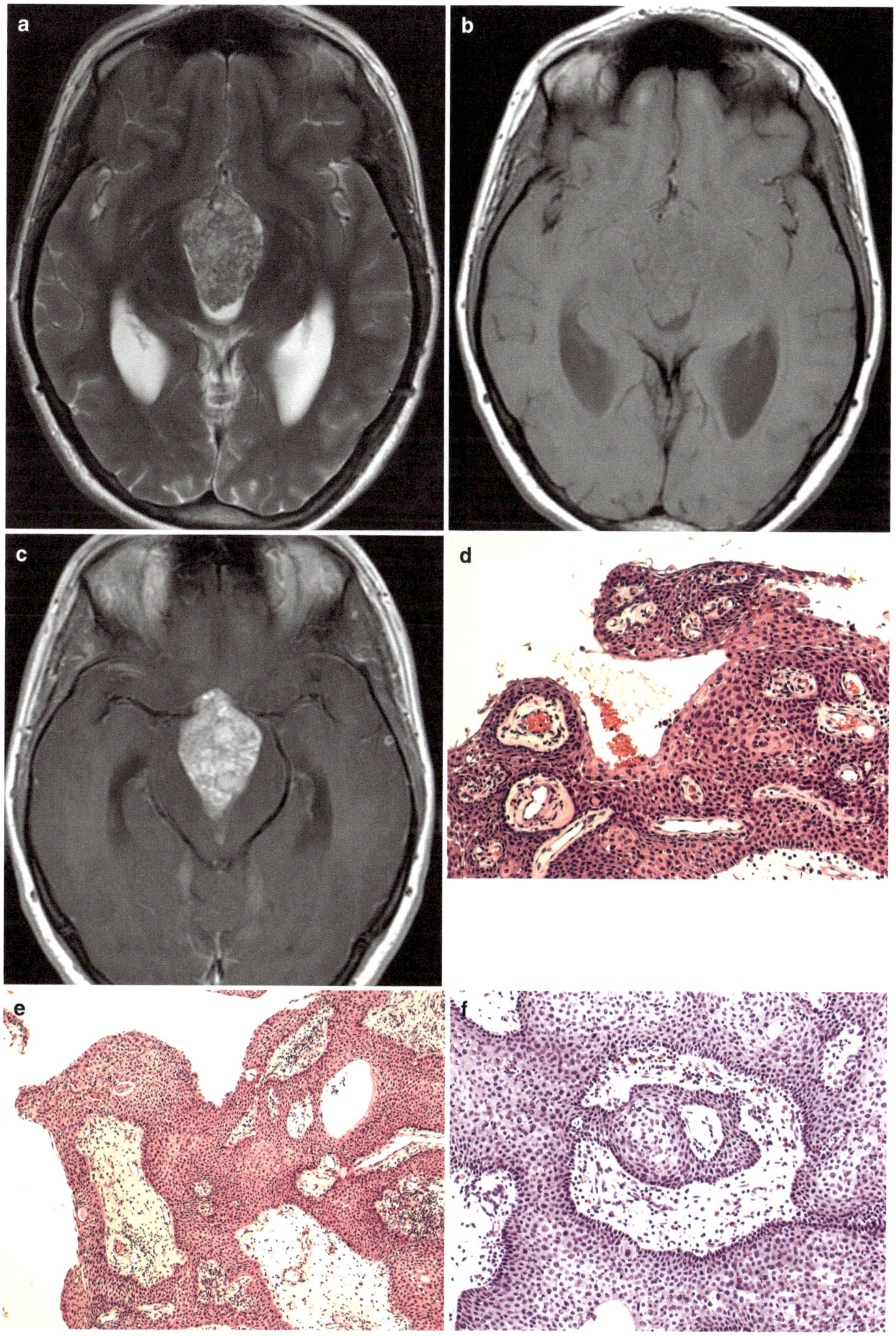

Fig. 15.52 Papillary craniopharyngioma. Axial T2-weighted (**a**), T1-weighted images (**b**) and post-contrast T1-weighted image (**c**) visualize a suprasellar tumor with multiple microcysts and hemorrhages. A craniopharyngioma intensively enhances. (**d**–**f**)—histopathologic tumor samples

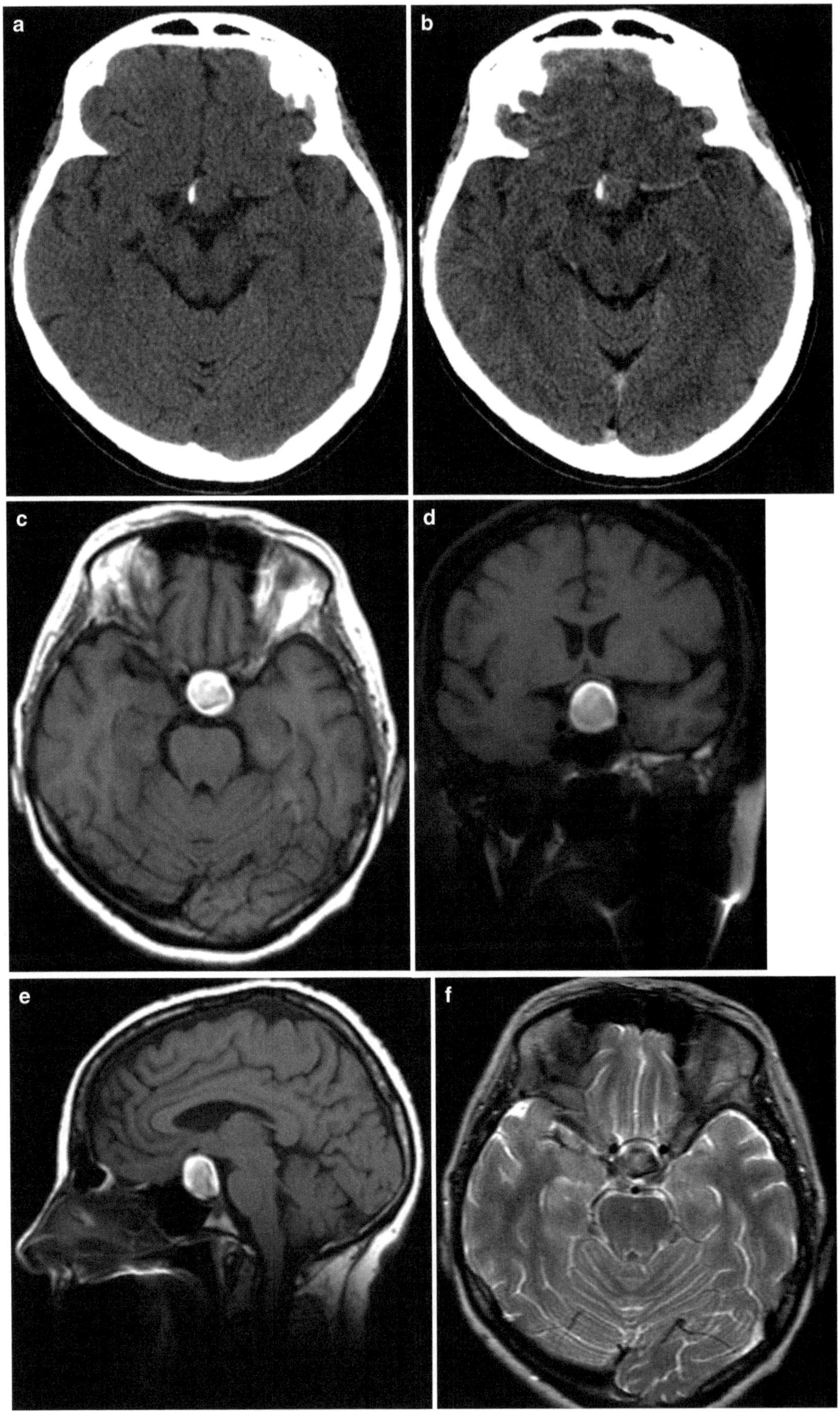

Fig. 15.53 Cystic suprasellar craniopharyngioma. Axial CT images before (**a**) and after (**b**) CE detects an isodense tumor with calcifications in the capsule. There are no signs of enhancement in the central part of the tumor. On T1- (**c**, **e**) and T1-weighted images with fat-sat (**d**) a cyst within the craniopharyngioma has a hyperintense signal. On T2-weighted image (**f**) a cystic part is heterogeneously hypo- and hyperintense

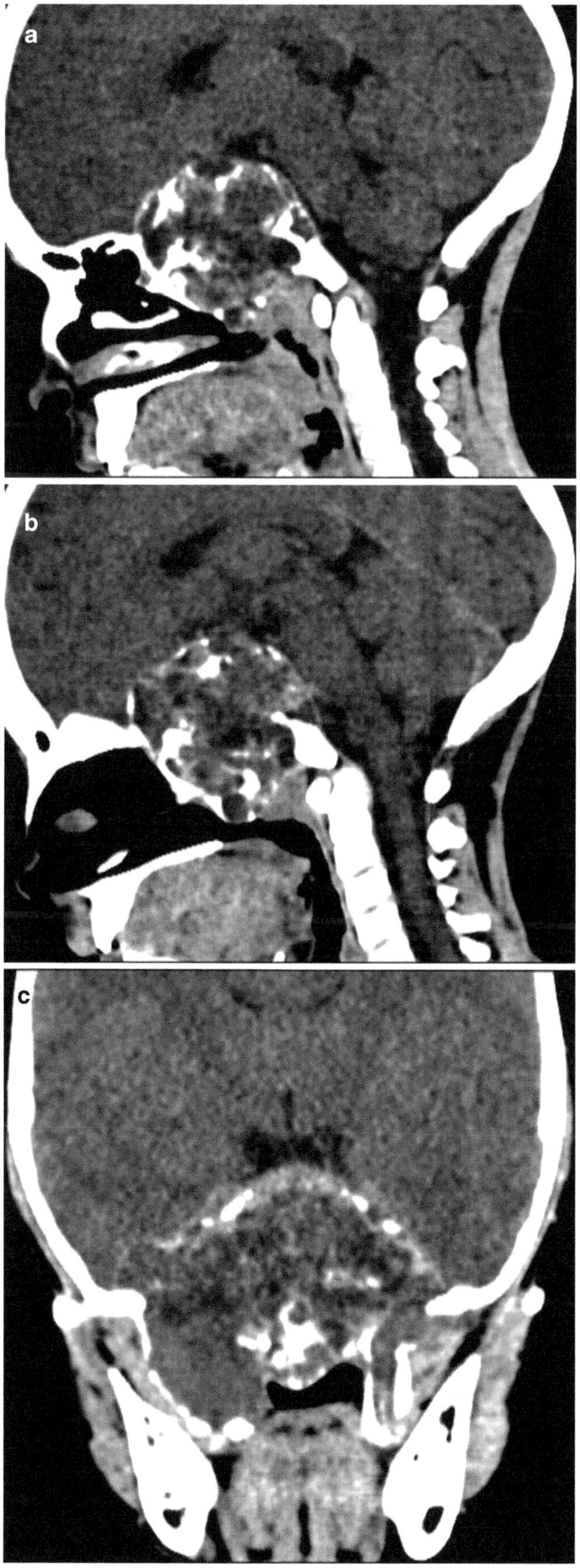

Fig. 15.54 Atypical craniopharyngioma. Sagittal (**a**, **b**) and coronal (**c**) CT-images show a large tumor in the sphenoid bone with the extending to the nasopharyngeal space. This craniopharyngioma simulates a malignant tumor of the skull base

15.5 Meningiomas

Meningioma (parasellar, sphenoid wing meningioma, pterional). Meningiomas are the most common intracranial tumors of non-glial origin (Buetow et al. 1991; Osborn 2004a, b). According to different authors, meningiomas account from 13% to 20% of all primary brain tumors (Russell and Rubinstein 1989; Orrison and Hart 2000). In addition, they rank first place in the group of tumors originating from meninges. Meningiomas are usually diagnosed in adults, with a peak incidence between 40 and 60 years, more often in women, with a male to female ratio of 1:2 to 1:4 (Buetow et al. 1991; Kozlov 2001). Only 1–2% of meningiomas occur in children under the age of 16 years old, often at atypical sites, such as the posterior cranial fossa or lateral ventricles (Tufan et al. 2005). In contrast to adults, malignant and giant forms prevail in children (Deen et al. 1982). Pediatric meningiomas are often combined with neurofibromatosis. Multiple meningiomas in older age groups are found in 1–9% of cases, which is confirmed by CT and autopsy findings.

In a number of cases, meningiomas of the lateral MCF area are clinically asymptomatic for a long time and may be an accidental radiological finding. Most often early neurological symptoms occur in tumors of the medial MCF area. Symptoms of the disease are very diverse and depend on tumor localization. Meningiomas of the sphenoid bone wings are most commonly characterized by the visual fields deficit, whereas tumors of the cavernous sinus usually cause cranial nerves III–VI neuropathy. Tumors of the II nerve sheath in the orbit or in the optic canal cause visual disturbances to the visual loss on the affected side. Neoplasms of the greater wing of the sphenoid bone can grow into the orbit and compress its contents with development of visual disturbances and exophthalmos. Large tumors cause pronounced mass effect on the surrounding brain structures and the ventricular system. By their morphology, meningiomas are subdivided into two main groups. The first group includes rounded, globular, and well-demarcated with wide dural attachment tumors (Osborn et al. 2016); these are mostly meningiomas of the cavernous sinus. The second group tumors have a typical flat-like extension (meningiomas of the sphenoid bone wings) with infiltration to the adjacent dura and often the bone. MCF meningiomas are usually well demarcated from the adjacent brain tissue. The surface of most tumors is smooth or lobular. They are often pronounced CSF clefts with compressed vessels and arachnoid elements between the brain and tumor. If the tumor is located in the cavernous sinus area, its margins are more difficult to differentiate. Tumors of the sphenoid bone wings, even small ones, can cause the development of an extensive peritumoral edema of the temporal lobe of the brain.

Parasellar meningiomas, according to the scientific research of the Burdenko Neurosurgery Institute, comprise about 12% of all intracranial meningiomas. They typically arise from the tuberculum sella, anterior clinoid process, medial portions of the greater wings, cavernous sinus, rarely dorsum sella and diaphragm areas. Meningiomas initially growing from the optic nerve sheath may also grow into the cavernous sinus. Olfactory fossa meningiomas often grow into the tuberculum sella region and directly into the sella.

Clinical symptoms caused by parasellar meningiomas depends on tumor site and by possible compression of the optic nerve, optic chiasm, optic tracts, cranial nerves involvement in the cavernous sinus or venous congestion in the orbit.

Imaging Direct angiography continues to play an important role in identifying the vessels which supply lesion in the parasellar region and MCF (Figs. 15.55, 15.56, and 15.57). Undoubted benefits of angiography include the possibility of separate visualizing of vessels supplying blood to the tumor, for example, branches of the internal and external carotid arteries. Unfortunately, with DSA data, the degree of anaplasia in meningioma tissue cannot be differentiated. Based on direct angiography, there are two main sources of blood supply to the tumor. Most frequent source includes groups of dural vessels, for example, such as the middle meningeal artery and ophthalmic artery. Below we present a table of the most frequent supplying meningeal arteries, depending on the site of MCF meningioma (Table 15.1).

It should be noted that large, long-term meningiomas with invasive growth or anaplastic meningiomas may be additionally supplied from the pial vessels. This is the second source of blood supply for tumors. This finding often combines with the presence of a pronounced peritumoral edema around even small meningiomas.

CE CT is one of the main methods of primary imaging for meningiomas, allowing diagnosing at least 95% of intracranial meningiomas (Konovalov and Kornienko 1985). Meningiomas are most often identified as sharply circumscribed lesions due to intense (40–45 HU) contrast enhancement (Figs. 15.58 and 15.59). Therefore, the use of contrast enhancement is one of the principal elements of meningioma CT diagnosis. In 10–15% of cases (Osborn et al. 2016), meningiomas weakly accumulate contrast material. In general, meningiomas have initially more or less hyperdense characteristics in up to 75% of all cases. Up to 25% of meningiomas contain calcifications in their structures, which can be single or multiple, punctate, and very large. In rare cases, there are completely calcified tumors that are clearly revealed even on X-ray exams and especially on CT (Figs. 15.60 and 15.61). In one third of cases, meningiomas of the sphenoid

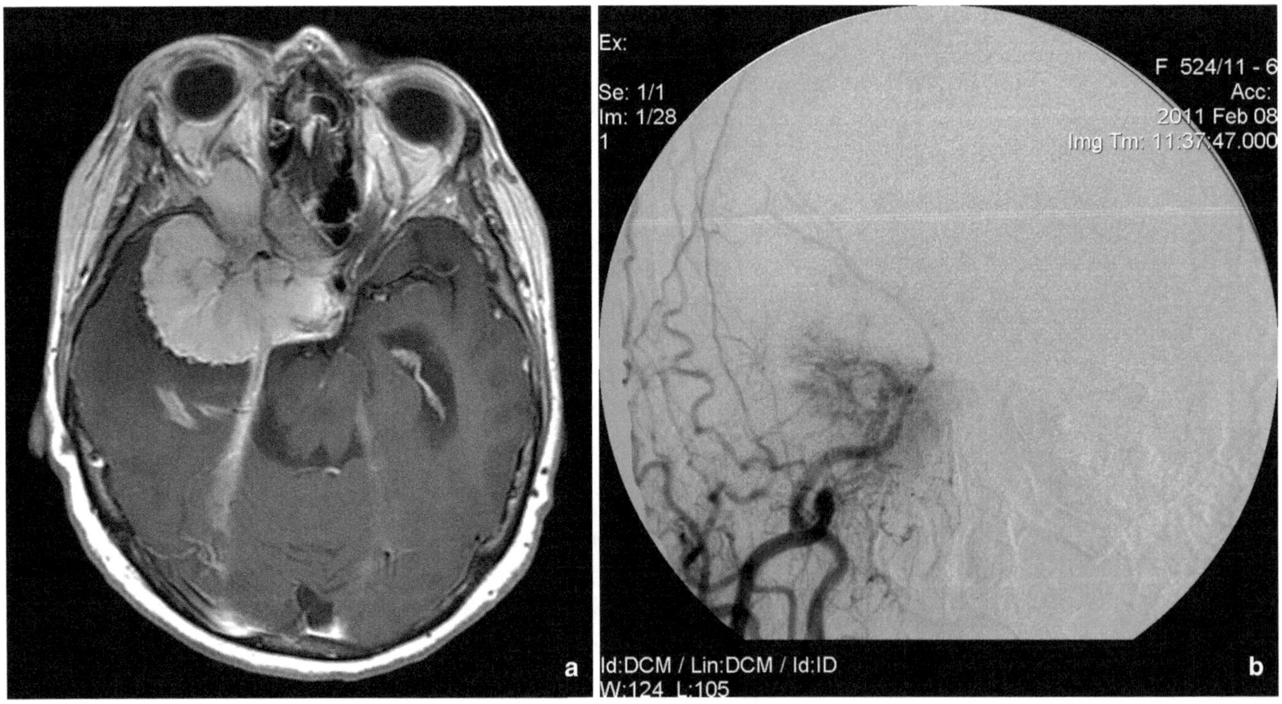

Fig. 15.55 Meningioma of the right greater sphenoid wing. Post-contrast T1-weighted image (**a**) demonstrates a widely extended tumor involving the orbit, cavernous sinus, middle cranial fossa, and sellar region. Anterior-posterior (**b**, **c**) and lateral (**d**–**g**) DSA show an abounded tumor vascular net with the supplying superior maxillary artery. The internal carotid artery is narrowed due to tumor compression

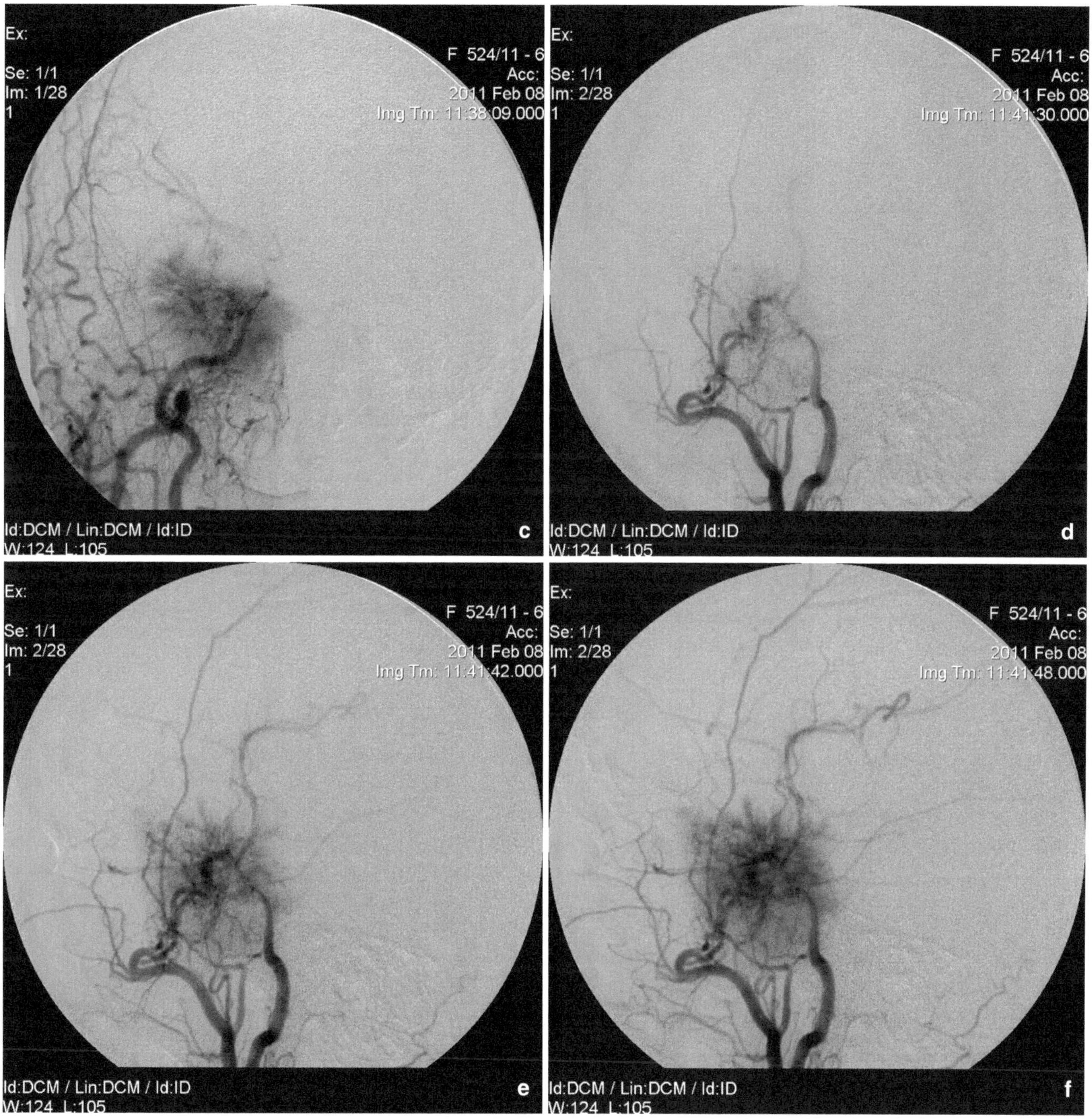

Fig. 15.55 (continued)

bone wings have a peritumoral area of low density, which is caused by a brain edema. The latter is not always associated with anaplastic changes in the tumor structure, but is probably due to pial blood supply. CT fairly easily identifies bone changes encountered in meningiomas, in particular, irregular cortex, bone destruction, intraosseous component, and hyperostosis. The latter changes are frequently diagnosed in meningiomas of the sphenoid bone wings and tuberculum sella (Fig. 15.62). It is believed that meningiomas arise from arachnoid meningothelial cells in the diploic layer of the bones of the cranial vault and the base of the skull, while the whole tumor is located in the extradural area, infiltrating and destroying the bone. These are so-called hyperostotic meningiomas characterized by a combination of widespread cranial bone infiltration, their thickening with the presence of a flat soft-tissue extension. Invasive growth of meningiomas in the bone tissue is accompanied by bone destruction or spicule-shaped changes. Severity of these changes is not dependent on the degree of tumor anaplasia. The method of choice for such tumors is CT.

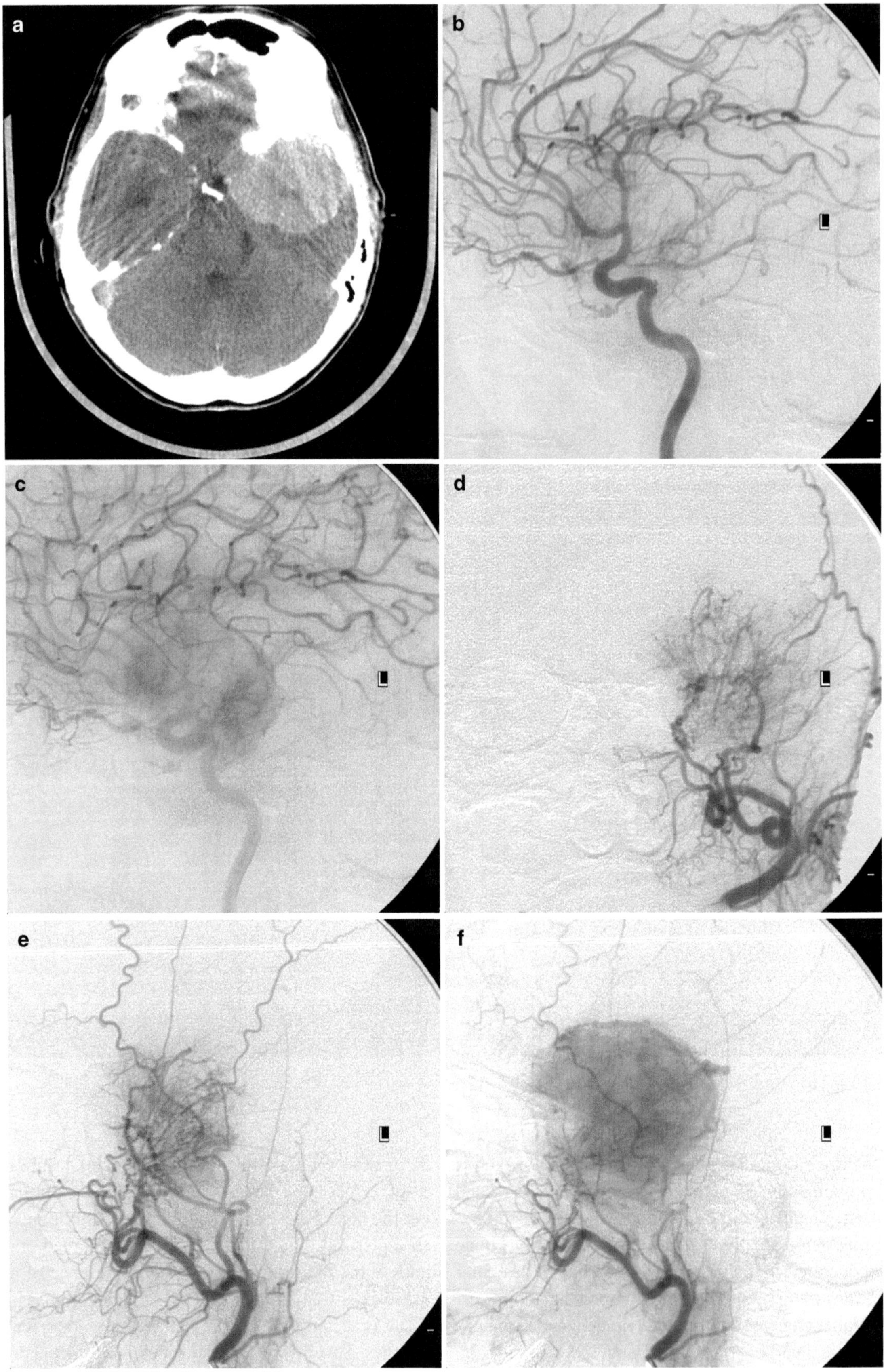

Fig. 15.56 Meningioma of the left greater sphenoid wing. (**a**) CE CT scan. Lateral angiograms of the internal carotid artery (**b**, **c**) and external carotid artery (**d**–**f**) demonstrate the multiple sources of tumor supplying from the short meningeal branches of internal carotid artery as well as from superior maxillary artery

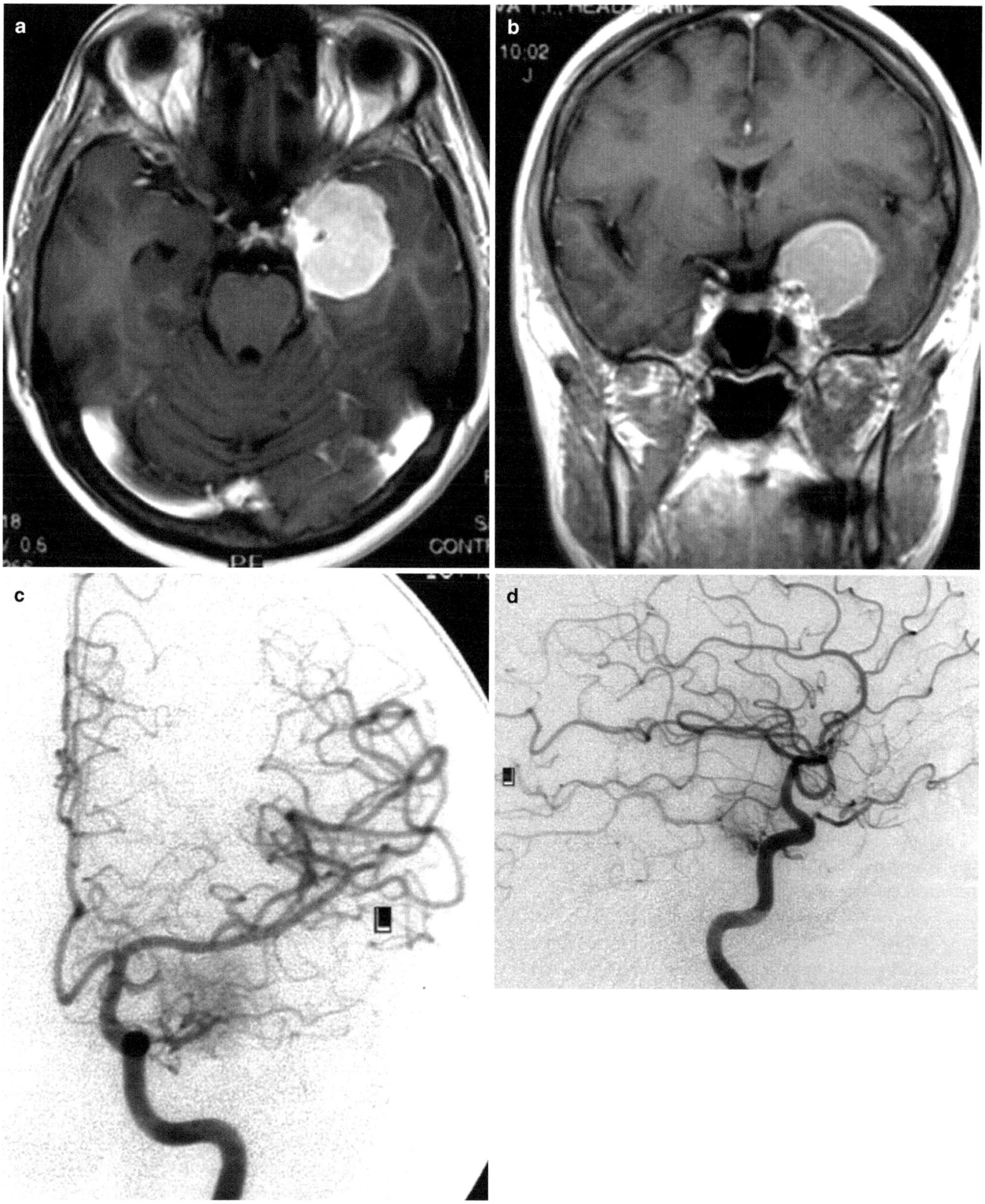

Fig. 15.57 Meningioma of the left anterior clinoid process and cavernous sinus. Post-contrast axial (**a**) and coronal (**b**) T1 weighted images reveal a homogeneously and intensively enhancing tumor. Anterior–posterior (**c**) and lateral (**d**–**f**) DSA of the internal carotid artery in arterial, capillary and venous phases demonstrate a meningioma blood supplying from the short meningeal branches of internal carotid artery

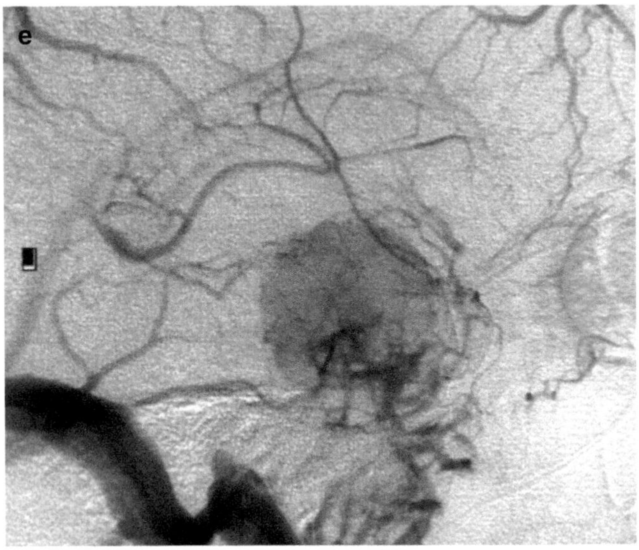

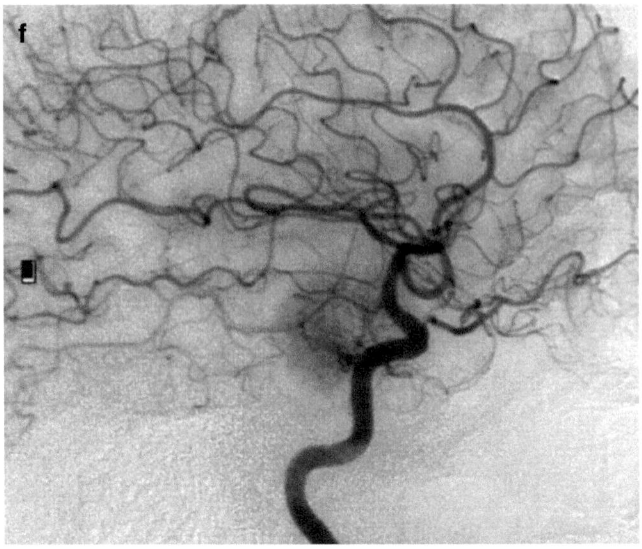

Fig. 15.57 (continued)

Table 15.1 The most frequent sources of blood supply to MCF meningiomas

Location	Supply artery
Sphenoid bone wing	Superior maxillary artery
	Middle meningeal artery
Tuberculum sella and jugum sphenoidale	Ophthalmic artery
Clinoid process, cavernous sinus	Meningeal branches of carotid siphon

The typical feature of meningiomas at the tuberculum sella and anterior clinoid processes is hyperpneumatization of the sphenoid sinus. Both hyperostosis in the meningioma matrix and hyperpneumatization of the adjacent sinus may be simultaneously observed (Fig. 15.63).

The use of CT-angiography in the diagnosis as the imaging method for tumor blood supply has a number of limitations related to the location of supplying arteries. In most cases of sphenoid wing meningiomas, supplying arteries are located either in the bones of the skull base, or on the dura surface, which significantly complicates further post-processing, since both arteries and bones have high density. This is why evaluation of meningioma blood supply sources when using this technique is difficult task (Fig. 15.64).

Currently, most researchers consider MRI as the "gold standard" in the evaluation of sphenoid wing meningiomas. Majority of studies have demonstrated a high accuracy and efficacy of MRI in determining the degree of vascularization, status of adjacent arteries, invasion into the venous sinuses, visualizing the margins of the tumor and its expansion, especially in assessing the degree of intracranial and extracranial extension.

MR signal changes in different histological forms of meningiomas are heterogeneous and variable. It is noted that in many cases changes in MR signal on T2-weighted images can correlate with histological subtypes of meningiomas. Up to 90% of fibrous and transitional (mixed) subtypes, as well as psammomatous meningiomas have lower signal intensity on T1- and T2-weighted images as compared to the white matter of the brain, while two thirds of meningothelial tumors are hyperintense on T2-weighted images (Elster et al. 1989; Daemerel et al. 1991; Kaplan et al. 1992; Konovalov et al. 1997). Regardless of their histological type, most meningiomas appear as iso- or hypointense lesions compared to the cerebral cortex on T1-weighted images. In general, MR features of meningiomas are distinguished by a relative homogeneity of the MR-signal, even despite their large sizes. Heterogeneity of the meningioma structure can be determined by several factors, such as tumor blood supply, presence of calcifications, and inhomogeneity of the tumors structure due to cystic lesions.

In case of large meningiomas, MR imaging can detect radially running small branches of the supplying dural vessels in the tumor ("sunburst" pattern), representing the tumor matrix. On T1- and T2-weighted images, they represent as areas with a vascular flow voids, appearing as radial rays from the site of the tumor attachment to the dura mater. Calcifications are determined as areas with low signal intensity on T1- and T2-weighted images. Completely calcified meningiomas occur in 5% of cases, they have a hypointense MR signal in all sequences, being more evident on T2-weighted and T2*-weighted images. This feature is typical for psammomatous meningiomas. Hyperpneumatized sinuses and hyperostosis at the site of meningioma attachment is better visualized on CT (Fig. 15.65). However, MRI better

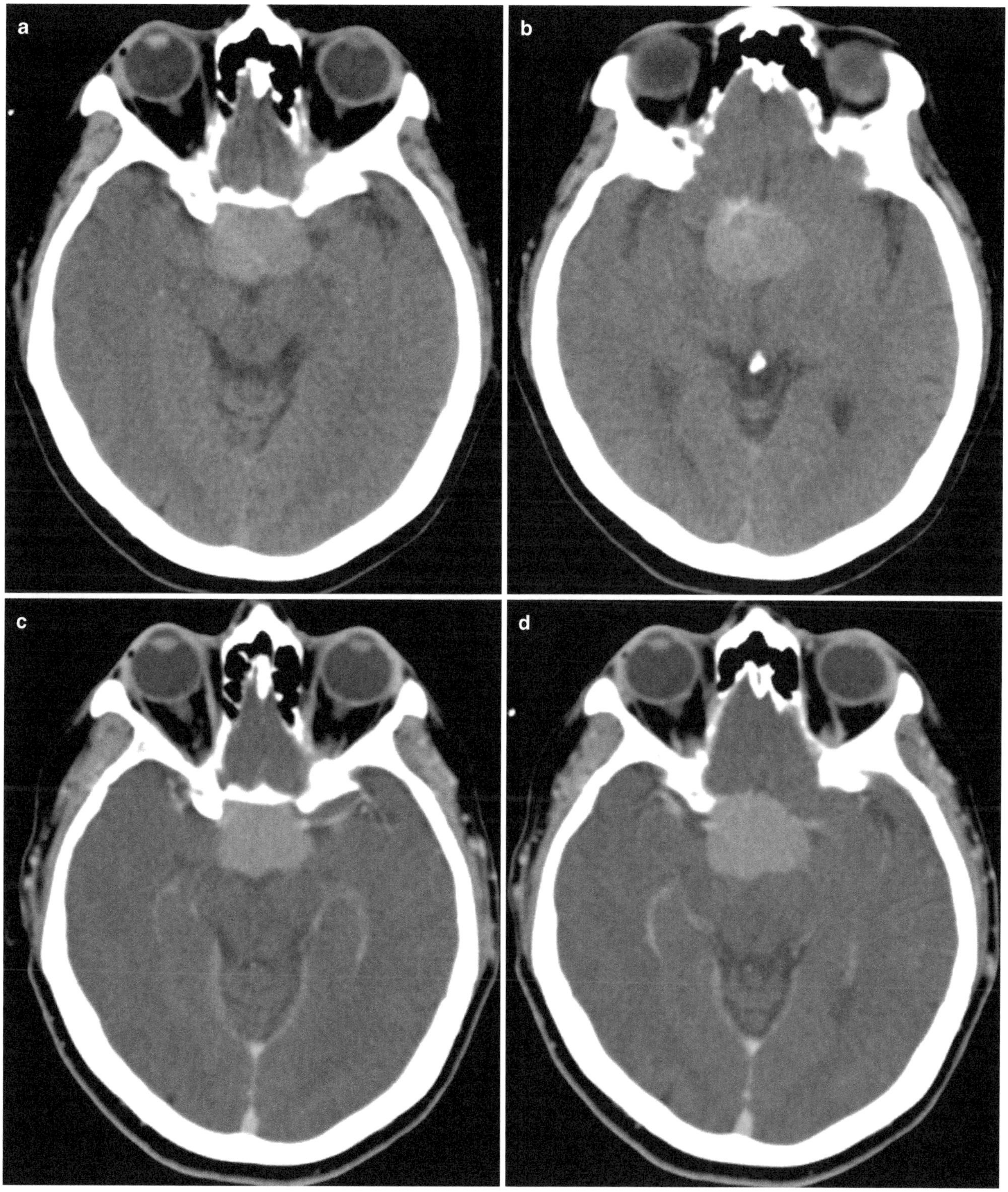

Fig. 15.58 Meningioma of the diaphragm and tuberculum sella with extending to the sellar and suprasellar area. Axial CT scans before (**a**, **b**) and after CE (**c**, **d**), sagittal (**e**) and coronal (**f**) reformats show a suprasellar homogeneously and intensively enhancing tumor. A local hyperostosis of the tuberculum sella is visualized on a sagittal reformat

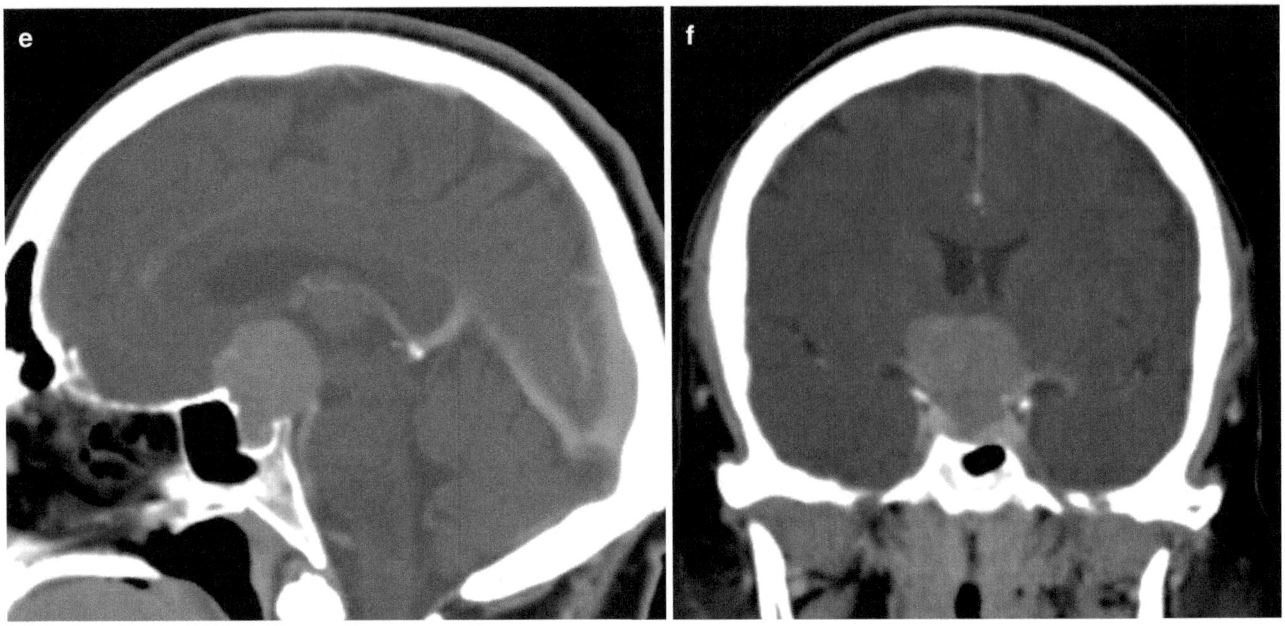

Fig. 15.58 (continued)

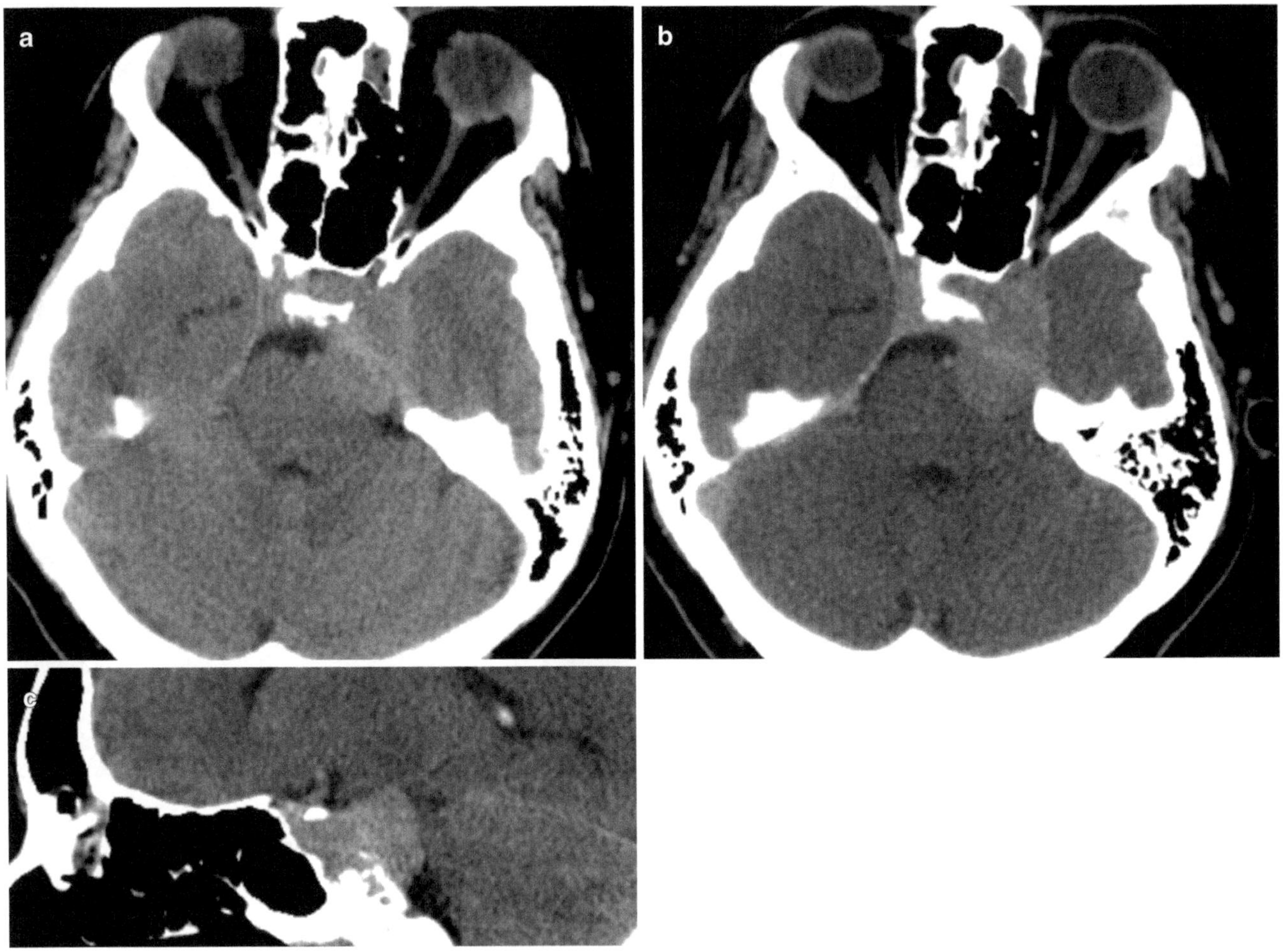

Fig. 15.59 Meningioma of the left cavernous sinus with extending to the clivus and the apex of the temporal bone. Axial CT scans before CE (**a**) shows a hyperdense tumor in the medial part of the left middle cranial fossa and petroclival area. After CE the tumor becomes more hyperdense (**b**, **c**)

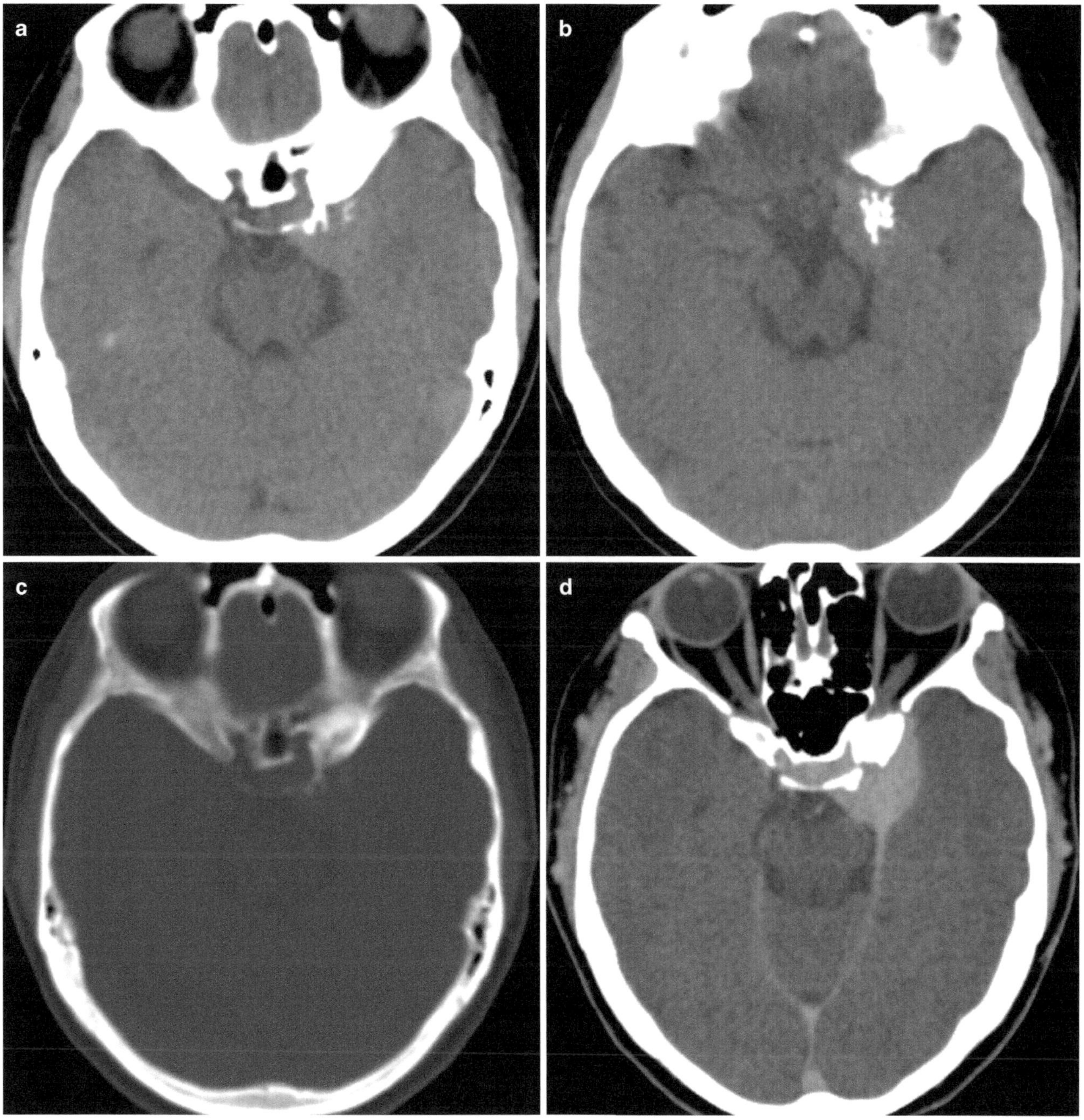

Fig. 15.60 Meningioma of the left cavernous sinus and anterior clinoid process with the hyperostosis and calcifications. Axial CT scans (**a**–**c**) reveal a mildly hyperdense tumor in the left cavernous sinus area with calcifications and the hyperostosis of anterior clinoid process. CT-imaging after CE (**d**–**f**) shows a well-delineated, strongly enhancing mass

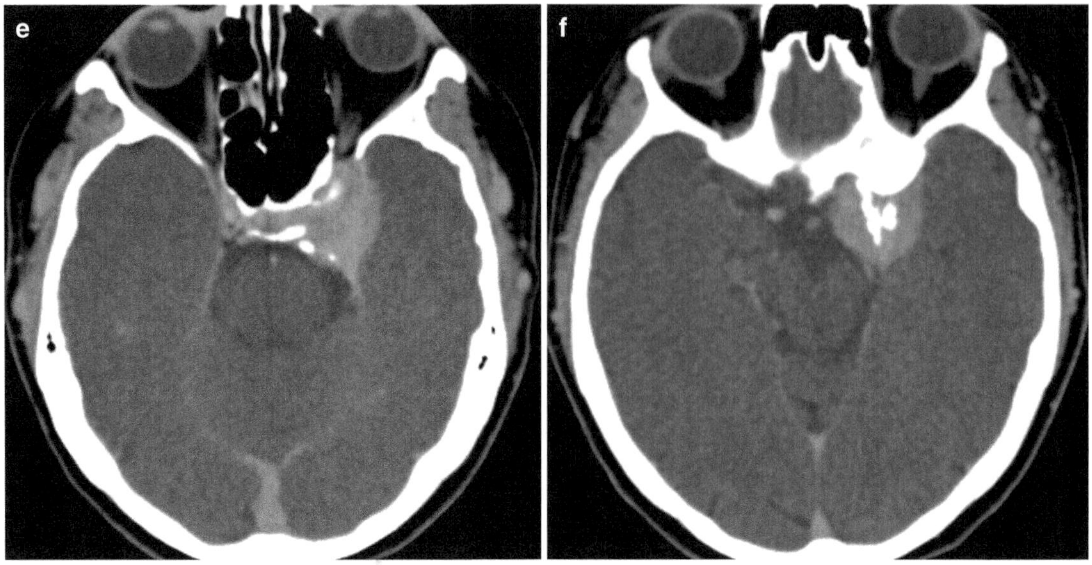

Fig. 15.60 (continued)

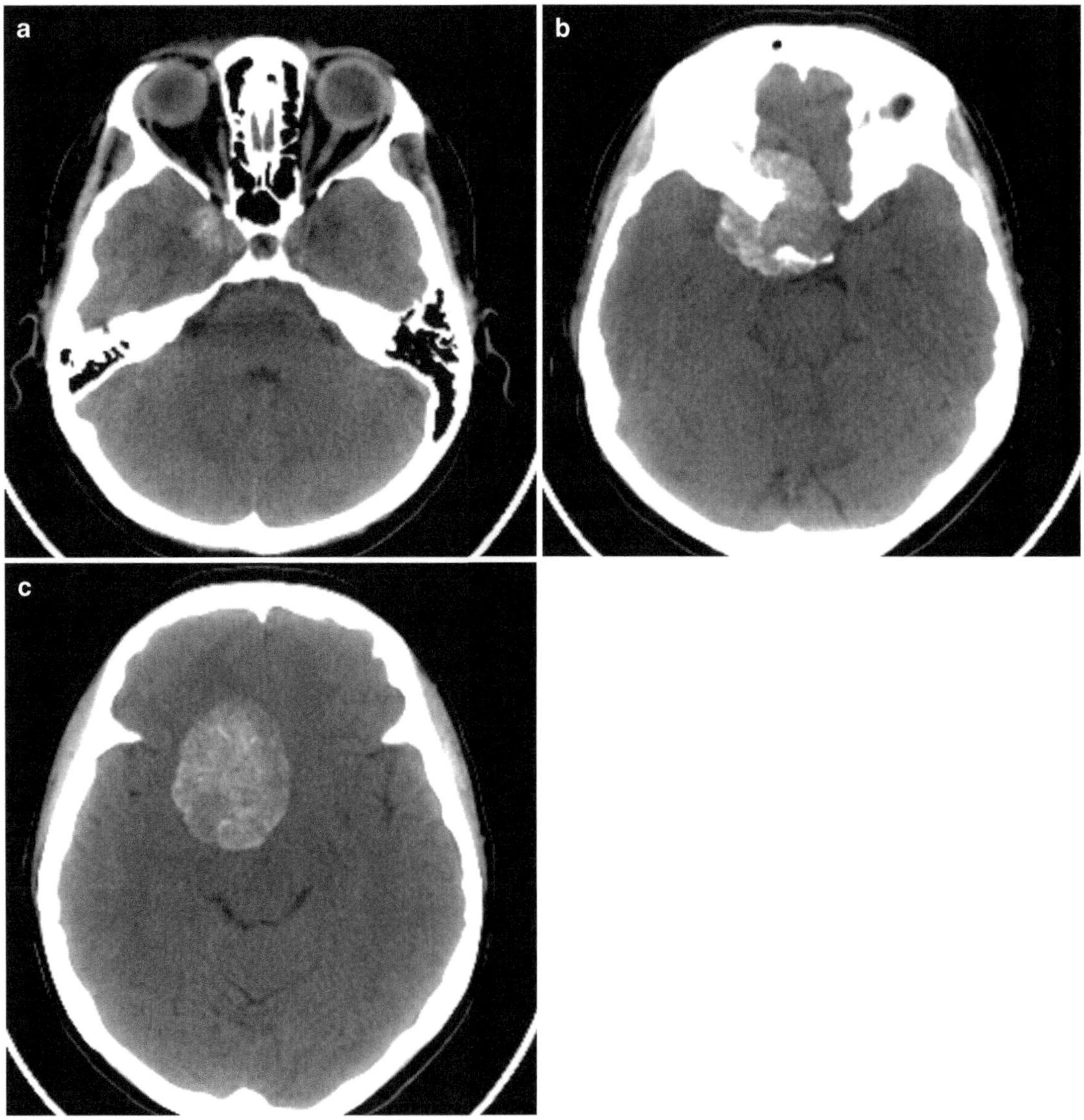

Fig. 15.61 Meningioma of the greater sphenoid wind and anterior clinoid process. Axial CT scans (**a**–**c**) show the meningioma with hyperdense structure and calcifications

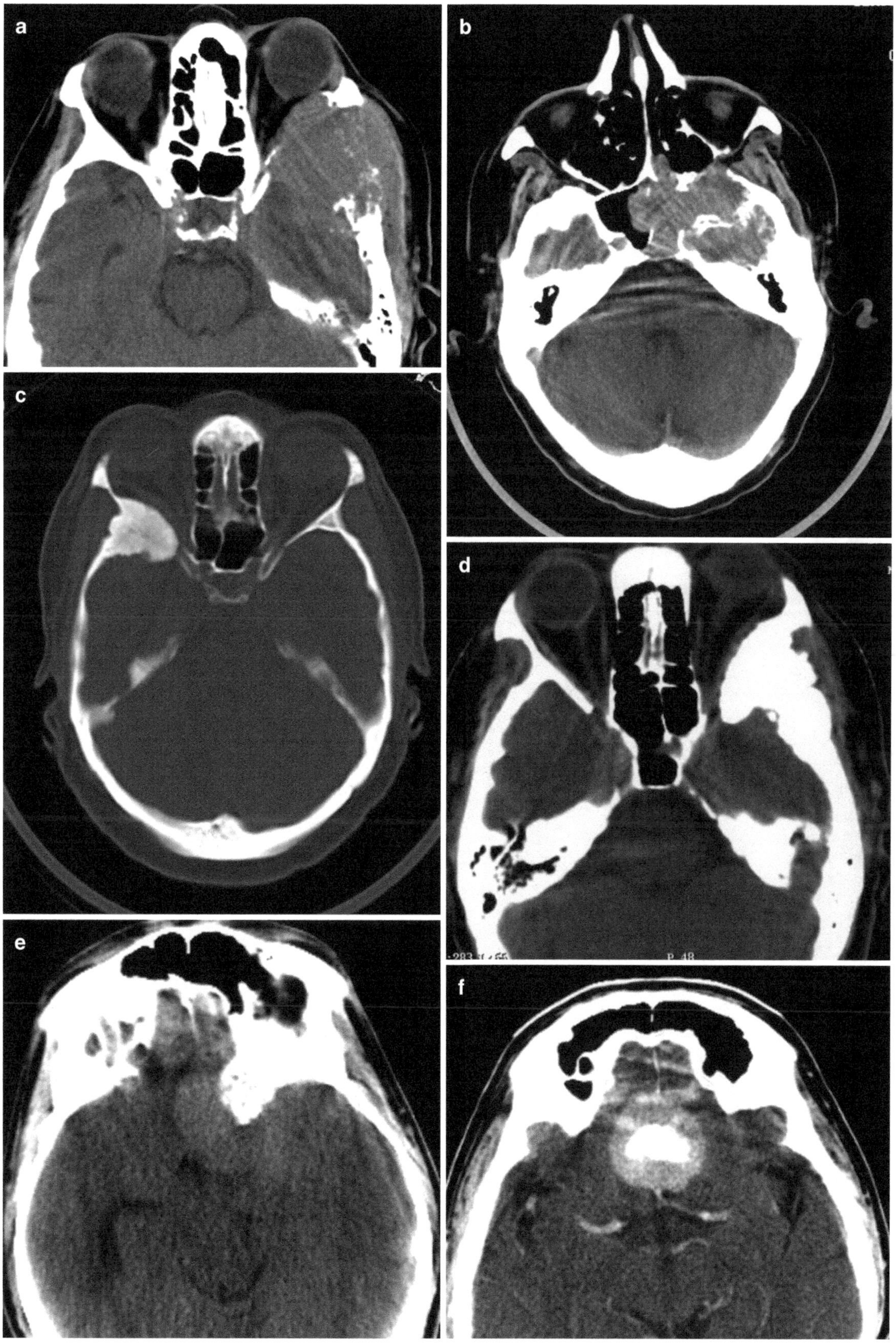

Fig. 15.62 Meningiomas of the skull base (different patients). Meningiomas of the pterional location (**a**) and the floor of the middle cranial fossa (**b**) cause the bone-destructive changes. Meningiomas of the greater sphenoid wing and temporal bone on the right (**c**), and on the left (**d**) are presented mainly by the hyperostosis. Meningioma of the anterior clinoid process and the roof of the orbit (**e**) and meningioma of the tuberculum sella (**f**) consist of the hyperostosis and a soft tissue component

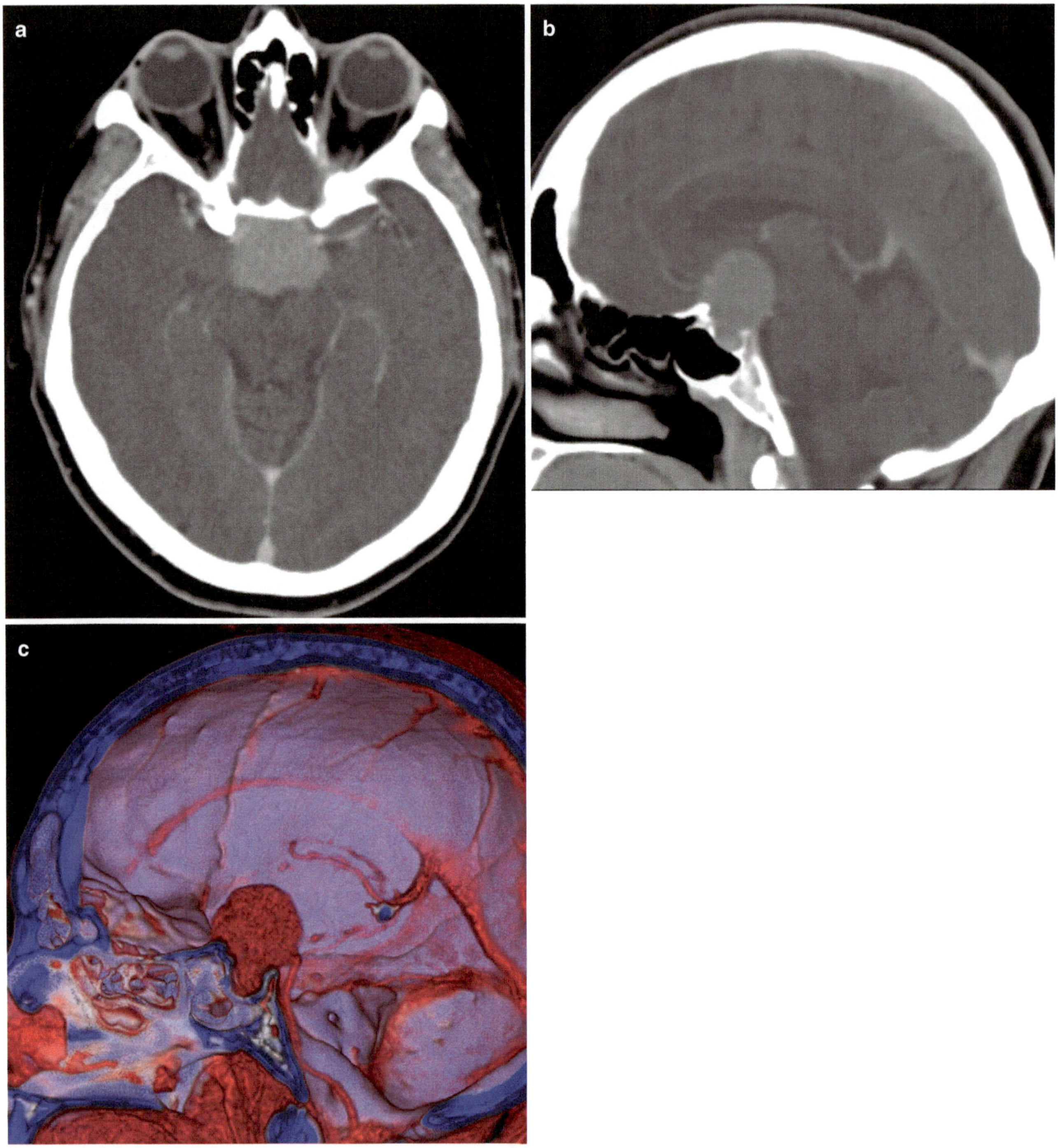

Fig. 15.63 Meningioma of the tuberculum sella with the extending into the chiasmal cistern and sella turcica. CE CT scans (**a**, **b**) and 3D reconstruction (**c**) visualize the hyperpneumatized sphenoid sinus, ethmoid bone and focal hyperostosis of the tuberculum sella in the meningioma matrix

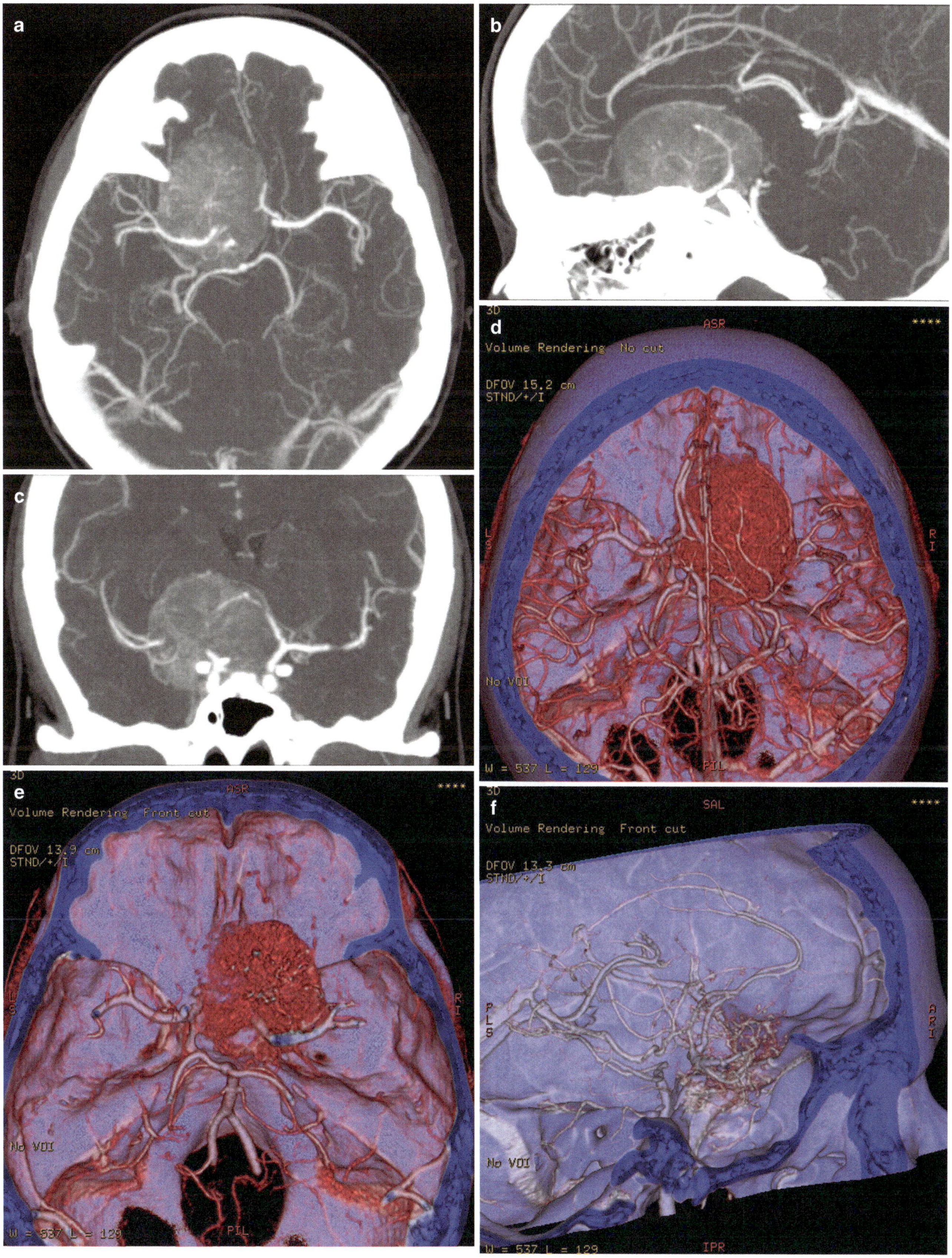

Fig. 15.64 Meningioma of the anterior clinoid process and greater sphenoid wing on the right. CT-angiograms demonstrate a large tumor, which invades into the right cavernous sinus and encase the anterior cerebral artery (**a**–**c**). 3D reconstructions of the CT angiography with various thresholds values show a different visualization of the tumor and vessels relationship (**d**–**f**)

evaluates other features, for example, the relationship of the tumor margin, optic chiasm, and vessels of the circle of Willis, dural infiltration at the jugum sphenoidale, etc. When meningioma is localized in the cavernous sinus and medial portions of the middle cranial fossa, the information about characteristics of its growth, the degree of cavernous sinus invasion and its expansion on the skull base is very important. Post-contrast MRI should be recognized as the best method: it clearly visualizes the typical feature of cavernous sinus meningiomas, i.e. compression of the carotid artery encased by the tumor.

Dura enhancement at the MCF and along the clivus of the sphenoid bone can be identified only by MRI (Figs. 15.66, 15.67, and 15.68). Sometimes after contrast enhancement,

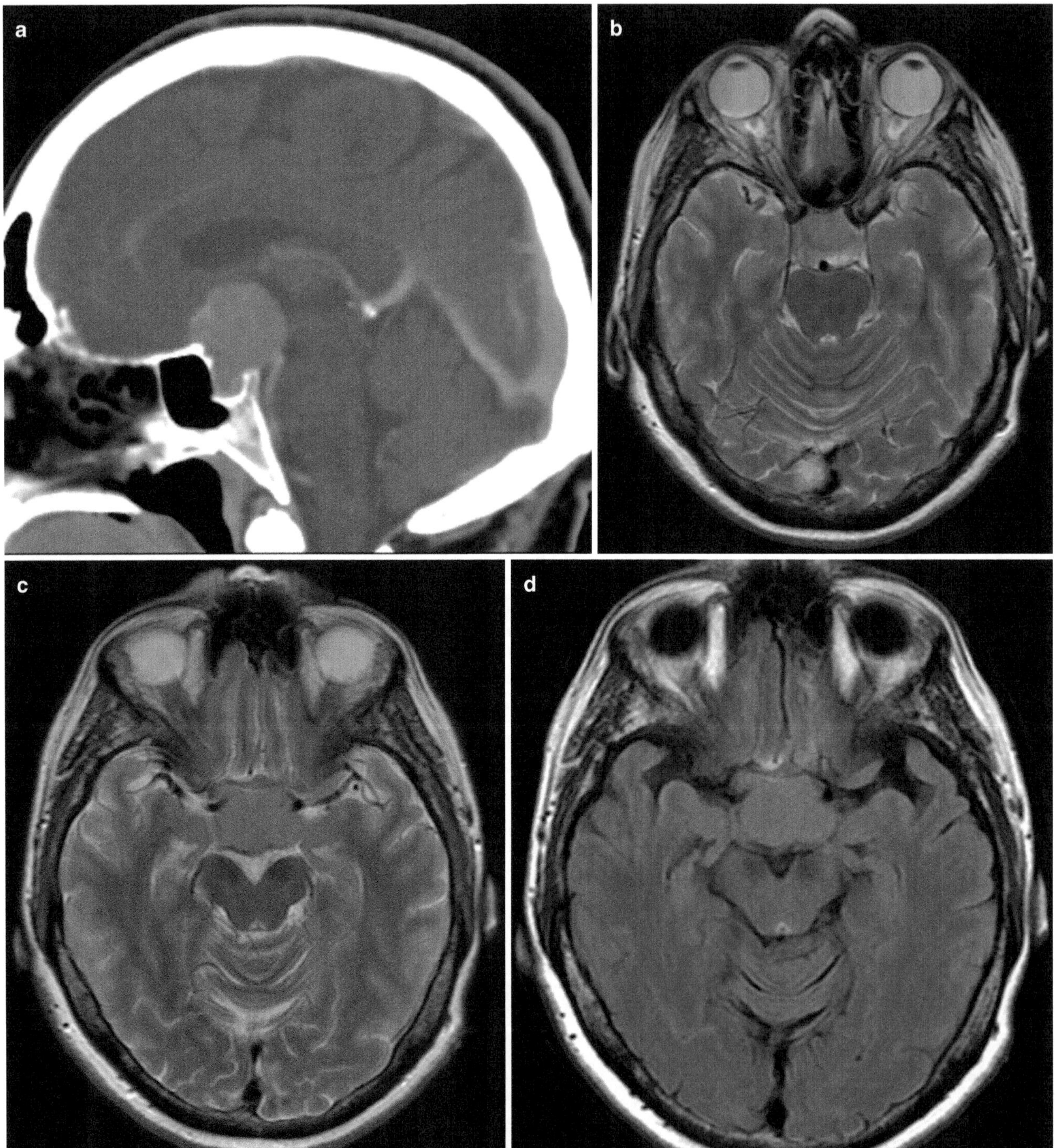

Fig. 15.65 Meningioma of the tuberculum sella. Sagittal CT scan (**a**) shows a large suprasellar tumor with the homogeneous enhancement. A hyperostosis of the tuberculum sella is clearly defined (more CT scans are presented on Fig. 15.58). On T2- (**b**, **c**), T2-FLAIR (**d**), T1-weighted images (**e**), and diffusion-weighted image (**f**) a meningioma has isointense MR-signal relative to grey matter. Post-contrast T1-weighted images (**g**–**i**) show a prominent contrast enhancement

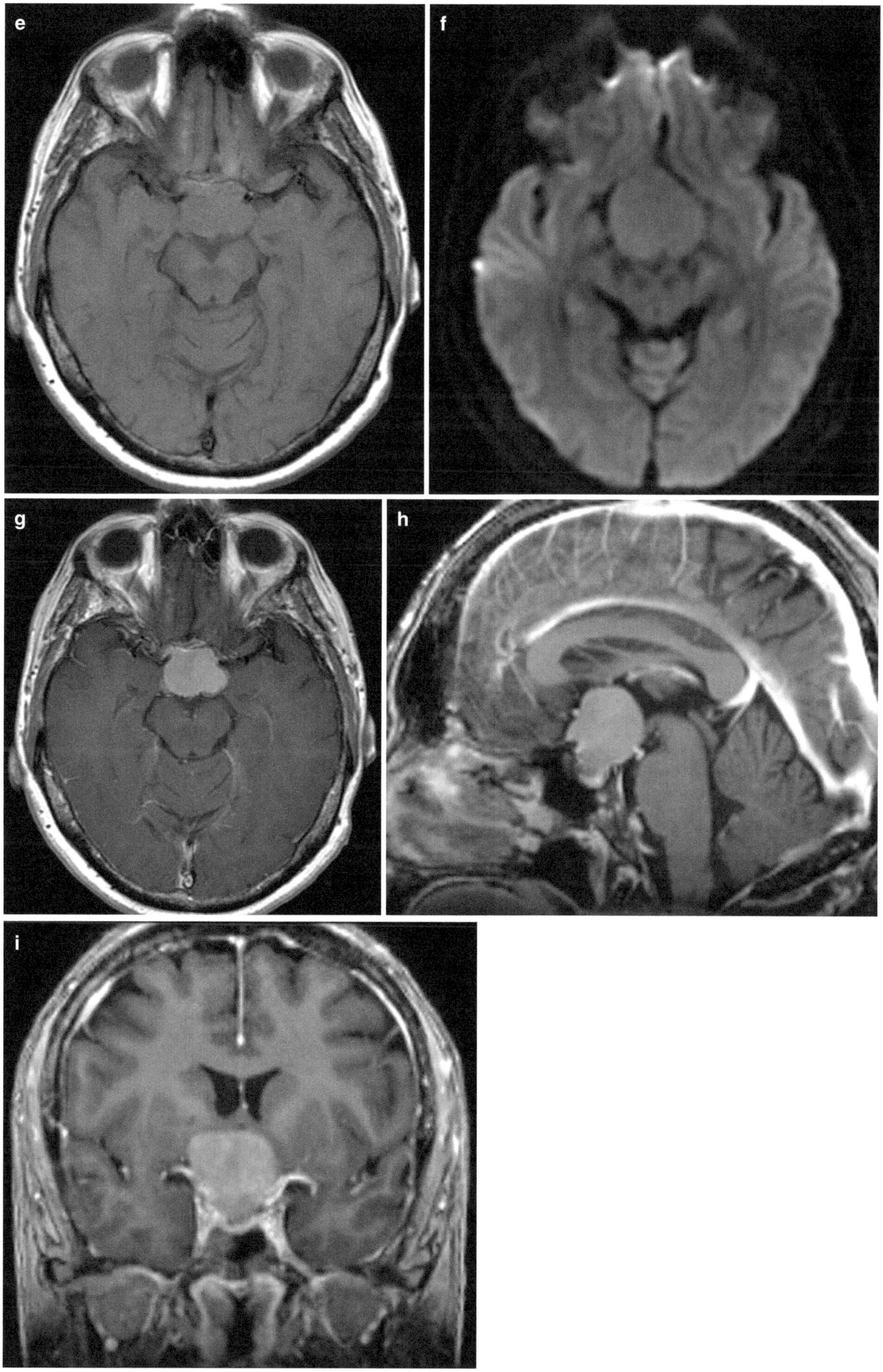

Fig. 15.65 (continued)

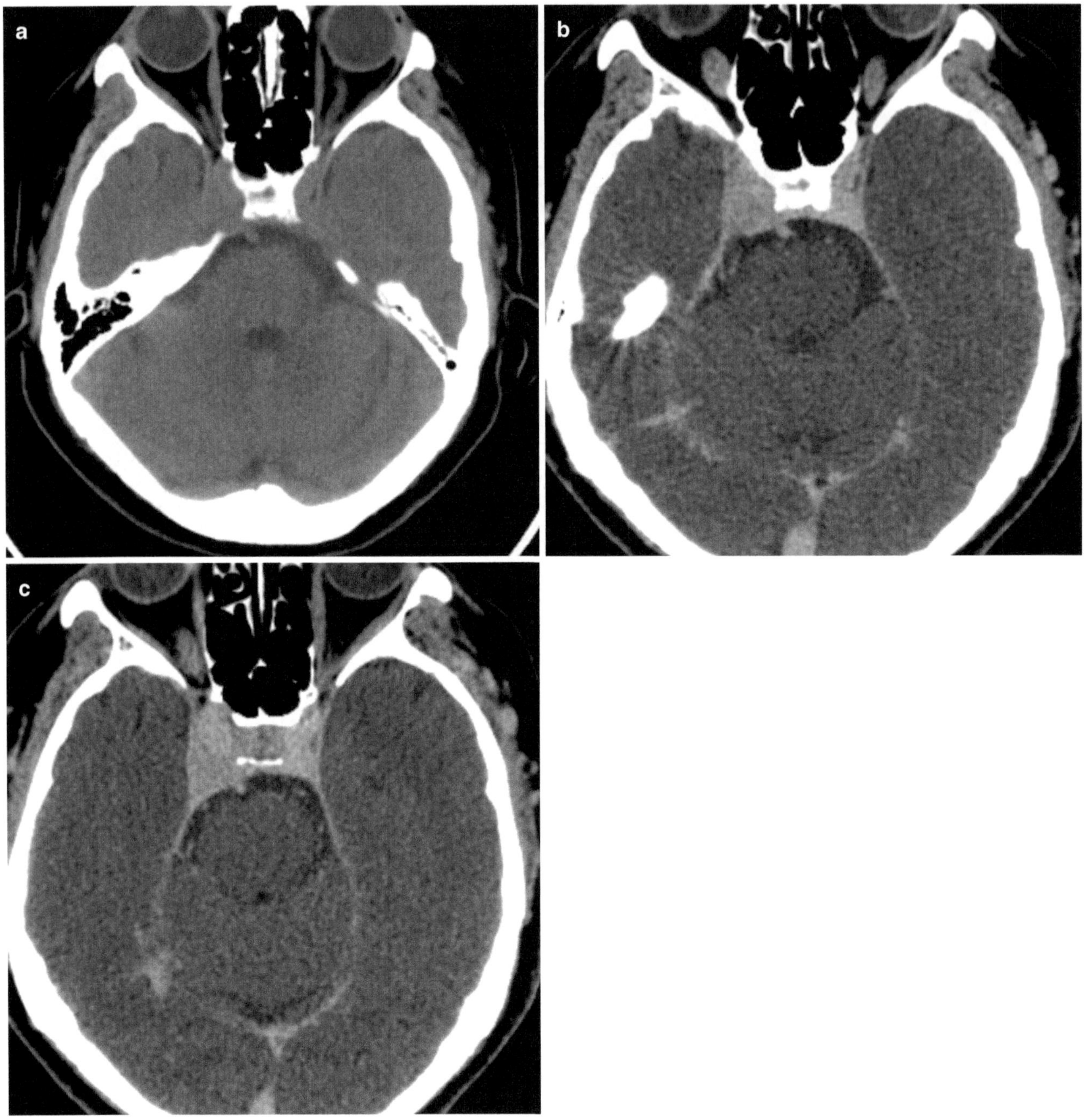

Fig. 15.66 Meningioma of the right cavernous sinus. CT scans before (**a**) and after CE in axial (**b**, **c**), coronal (**d**), and oblique projections (**e**) reveal a small meningioma with the strong and homogeneous contrast enhancement. 3D CT reconstructions (**f**, **g**) supplement with the information about a tumor and skull base bones relationship. Post-contrast coronal (**h**) and axial (**i**) T1-weighted images show a homogeneously and strongly enhancing meningioma. MRI is better for visualizing of the tumor extending along the tentorium

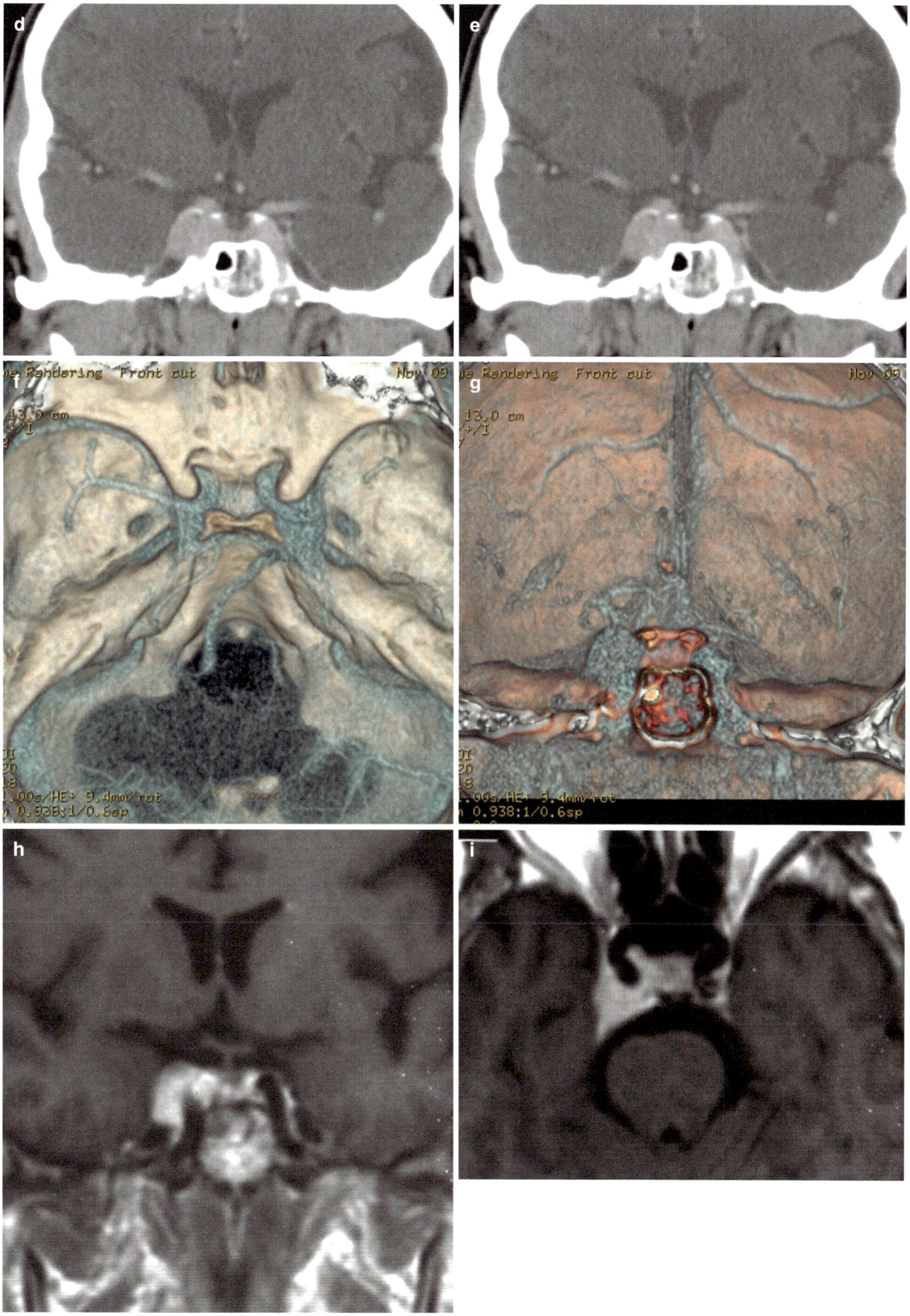

Fig. 15.66 (continued)

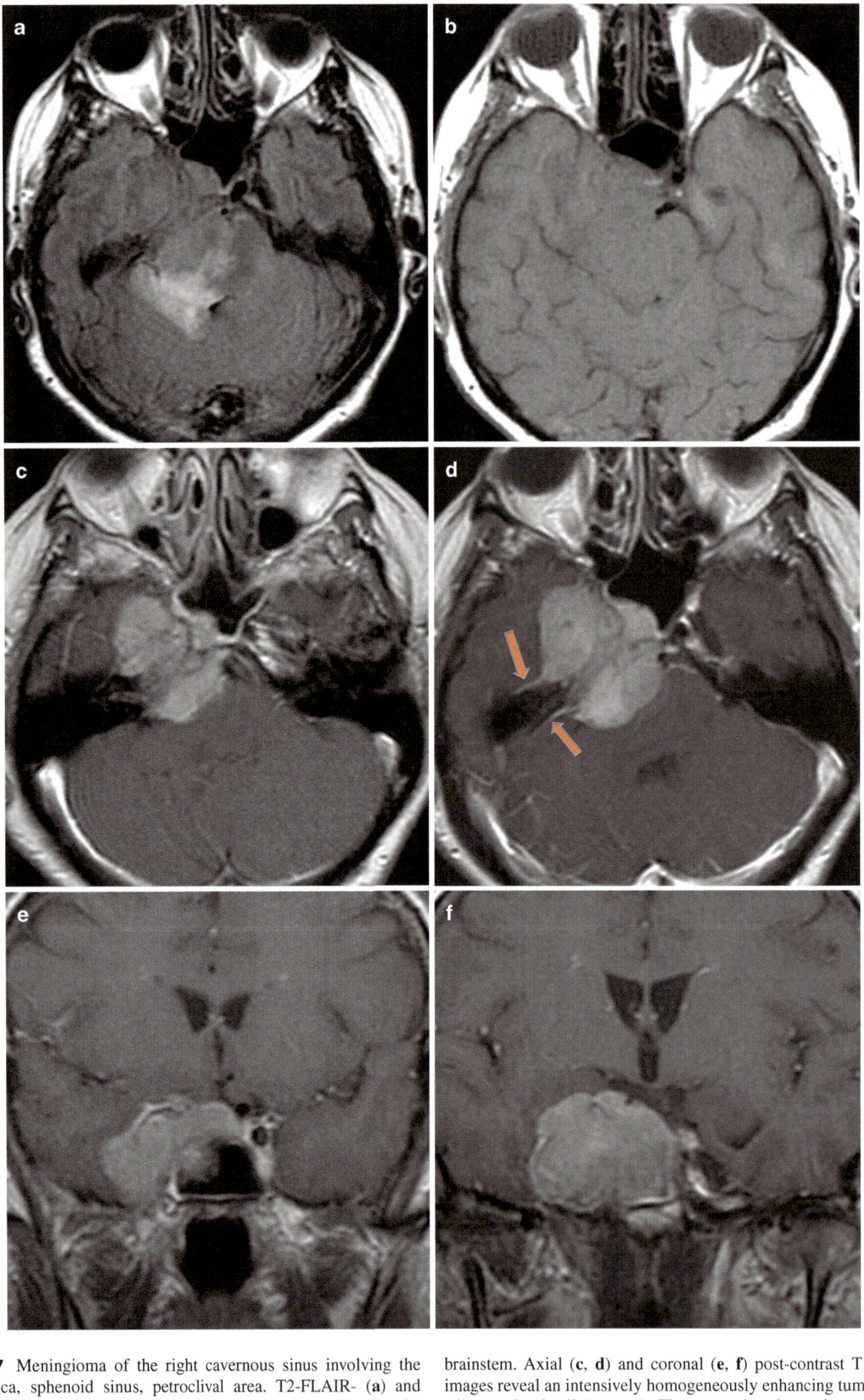

Fig. 15.67 Meningioma of the right cavernous sinus involving the sella turcica, sphenoid sinus, petroclival area. T2-FLAIR- (**a**) and T1-weighted images (**b**) demonstrate an extensive tumor infiltrating the apex of the temporal bone pyramid on the right and compressing the brainstem. Axial (**c**, **d**) and coronal (**e**, **f**) post-contrast T1-weighted images reveal an intensively homogeneously enhancing tumor with the adjacent dural tail (*arrows*). The tumor invades and compresses an internal carotid artery

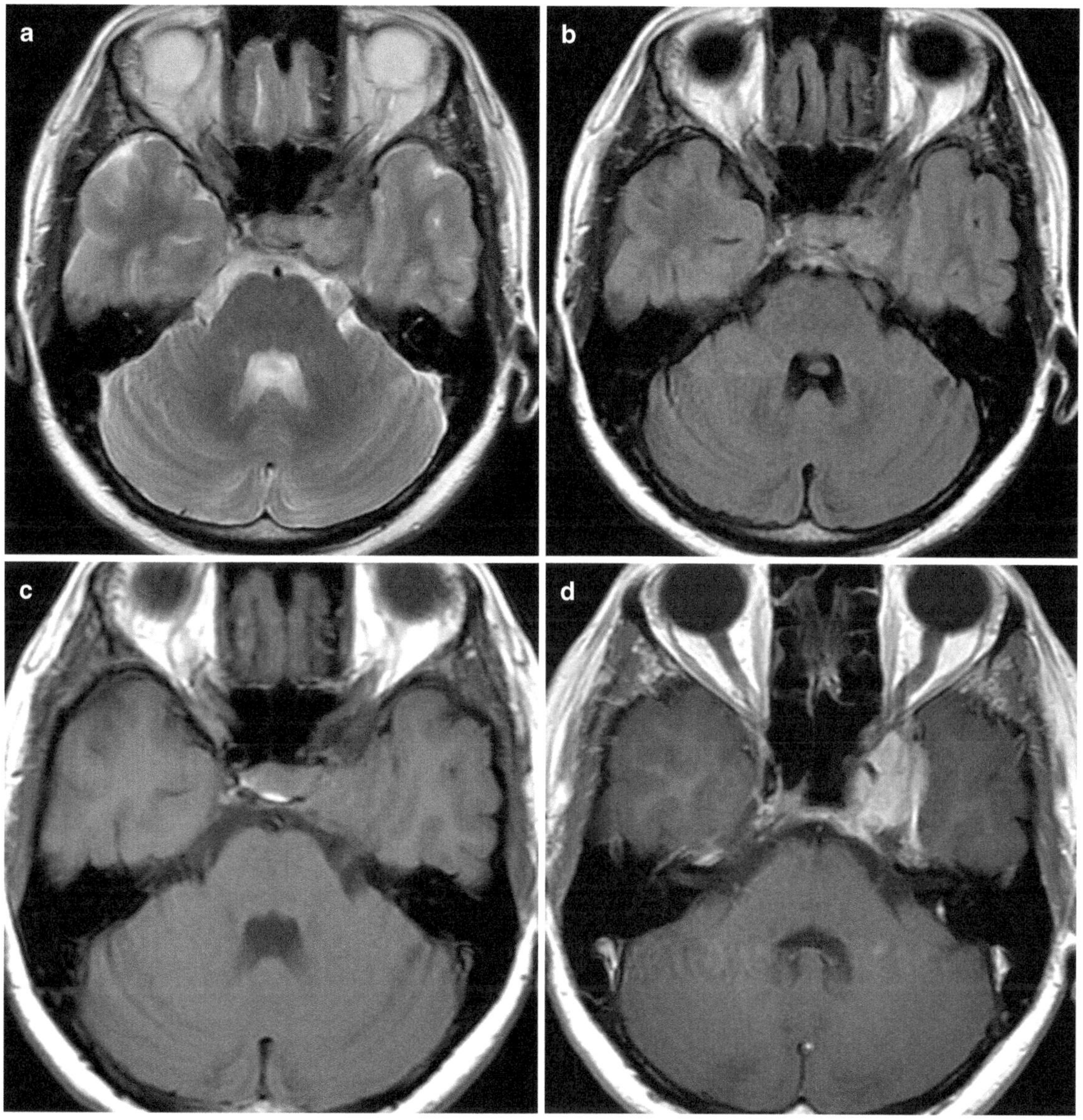

Fig. 15.68 Meningioma of the left cavernous sinus extending into the sella turcica. T2-weighted (**a**), T2-FLAIR- (**b**), T1-weighted images (**c**), FIESTA (**i**) visualize a tumor located in the medial part of the middle cranial fossa with the growth into the sella turcica. Post-contrast T1-weighted images (**d–h**) show a homogeneously enhancing tumor locally invading dura at the temporal bone pyramid, along the greater wing of sphenoid bone, along the tentorium and anterior cranial fossa area. Post-contrast T1-weighted image (**d**) clearly shows a hypointense lateral wall of the cavernous sinus which invades by the tumor

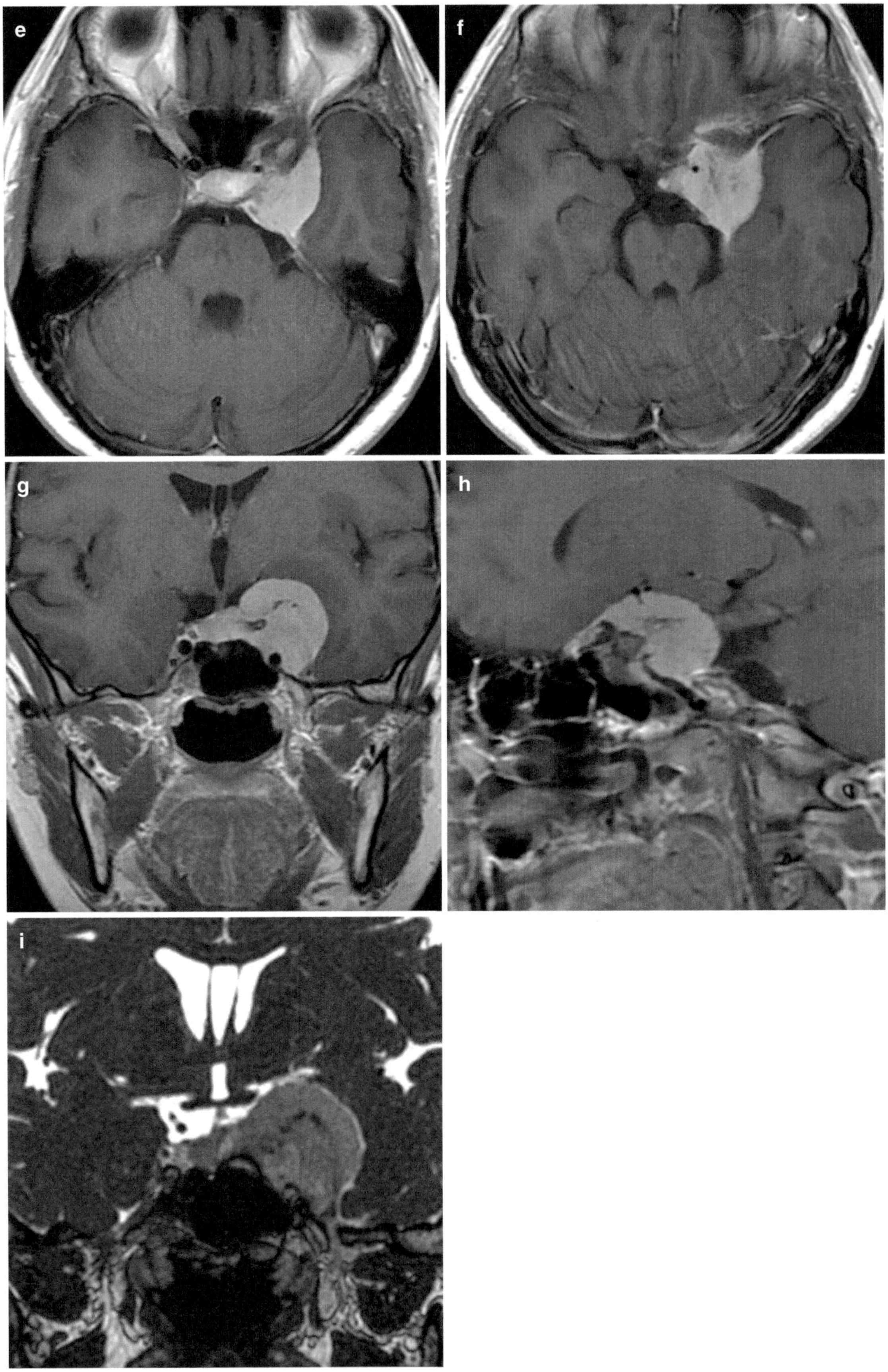

Fig. 15.68 (continued)

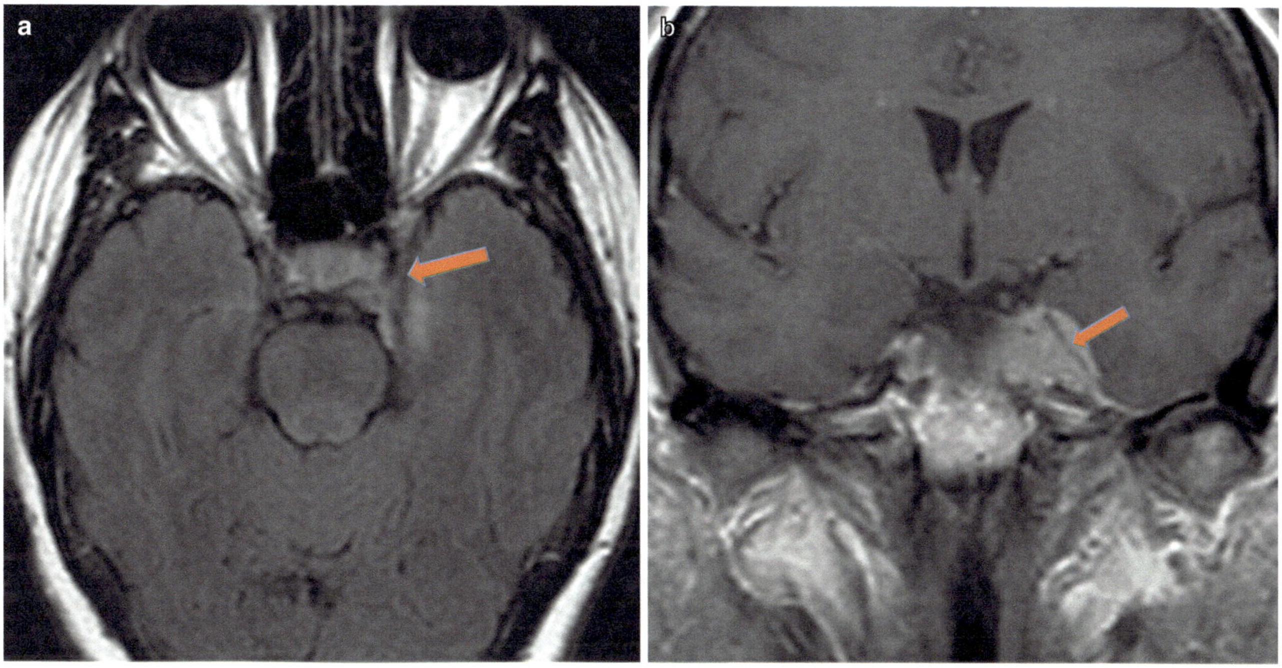

Fig. 15.69 Meningioma of the left cavernous sinus. Axial T2-FLAIR (**a**) and coronal post-contrast T1-weighted images (**b**) show an infiltrating of the lateral wall of the left cavernous sinus (*arrows*)

the outer wall of the cavernous sinus can be visualized, if the tumor mass pushes it outwards, lateral margin of the tumor is usually smooth and oval (meningioma grows within the sinus from the inner layer of the dura mater). If decreased MR signal band from the sinus wall is included in the tumor and the outer contour appears uneven on MRI, these are typical features of the cavernous sinus invasion with involvement of both dura mater layers (Fig. 15.69).

When using SWAN sequence, despite the artifacts from the skull base bones, meningiomas (at least benign) showed no hemorrhages. These findings sometimes allow performing a differential diagnosis with trigeminal nerve schwannomas. According to our data, the latter, by the contrast, are characterized by the presence of multiple intratumoral microhemorrhages. Unlike adenomas, meningiomas encase the large arteries cause their stenosis, which may also serve as a criterion for differential diagnosis. Rarely, meningiomas of the anterior cranial fossa and tuberculum sella can grow towards the sphenoid sinus and ethmoid bone cells.

CT-perfusion imaging may be useful for a differential diagnosis of parasellar pituitary adenomas and cavernous sinus meningiomas, as CBF and CBV values are significantly higher in meningiomas, while pituitary adenomas are mostly characterized by increased of MTT values (Figs. 15.70 and 15.71).

New opportunities in the assessment of tumor blood supply emerged with the implementation of 3.0T MRI. High spatial resolution and a new design of the pulse sequence in angiography protocol (3D TOF with 0.2 × 0.2 × 1.0 mm voxel) allow obtaining high quality images of supplying tumor vessels in the diagnosis of sphenoid meningiomas. Our series of comparisons with the results from direct cerebral angiography demonstrated identity in imaging the tumor vasculature and meningioma blood supply sources (Fig. 15.72).

In our clinical practice, we encountered giant forms of meningiomas of the middle cranial fossa base. They were benign and did not show infiltrative growth. These tumors had no clinical manifestations for a long time (usually patients were followed up for several years). This resulted in patients' refusal of surgical treatment (Figs. 15.73 and 15.74). In one of the rare cases, a patient was diagnosed with two histologically different groups of tumors (without evidence of neurofibromatosis) or a combination of oncologic and vascular disorders (Fig. 15.75).

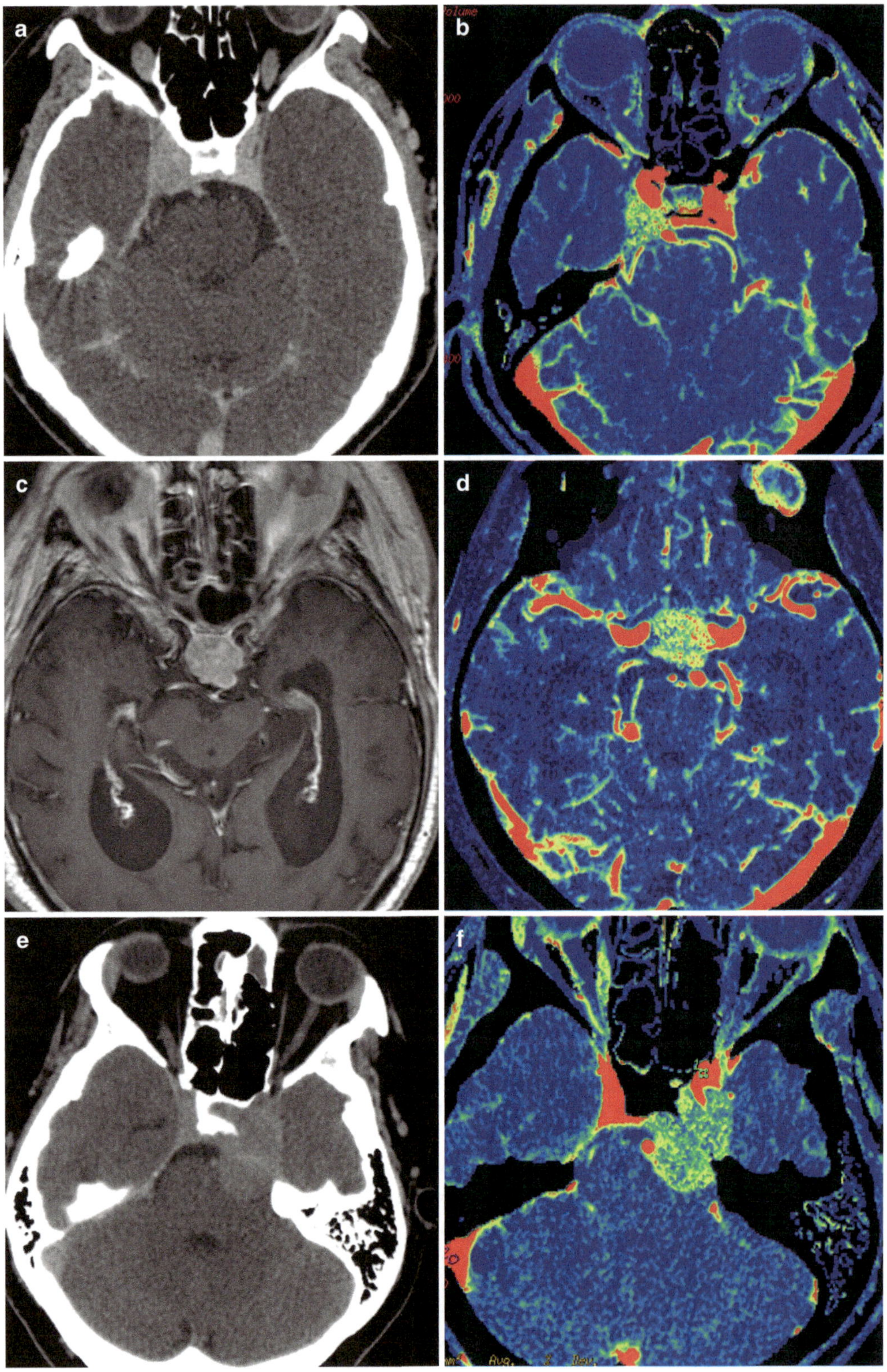

Fig. 15.70 Perfusion CT studies in meningiomas of the sellar-suprasellar area. Case 1. Meningioma of the left cavernous sinus. CE CT scan (**a**) and CBV map (**b**) demonstrate a small tumor with a high blood volume level. Case 2. Meningioma of the tuberculum sella. Axial T1-weighted image (**c**) and CBV map (**d**) reveal intensively enhancing suprasellar tumor with the high value of CBV. Case 3. Meningioma of the left cavernous sinus extending into the posterior cranial fossa. Post-contrast CT scan (**e**) and CBV map (**f**) show the high values of the blood volume in the tumor

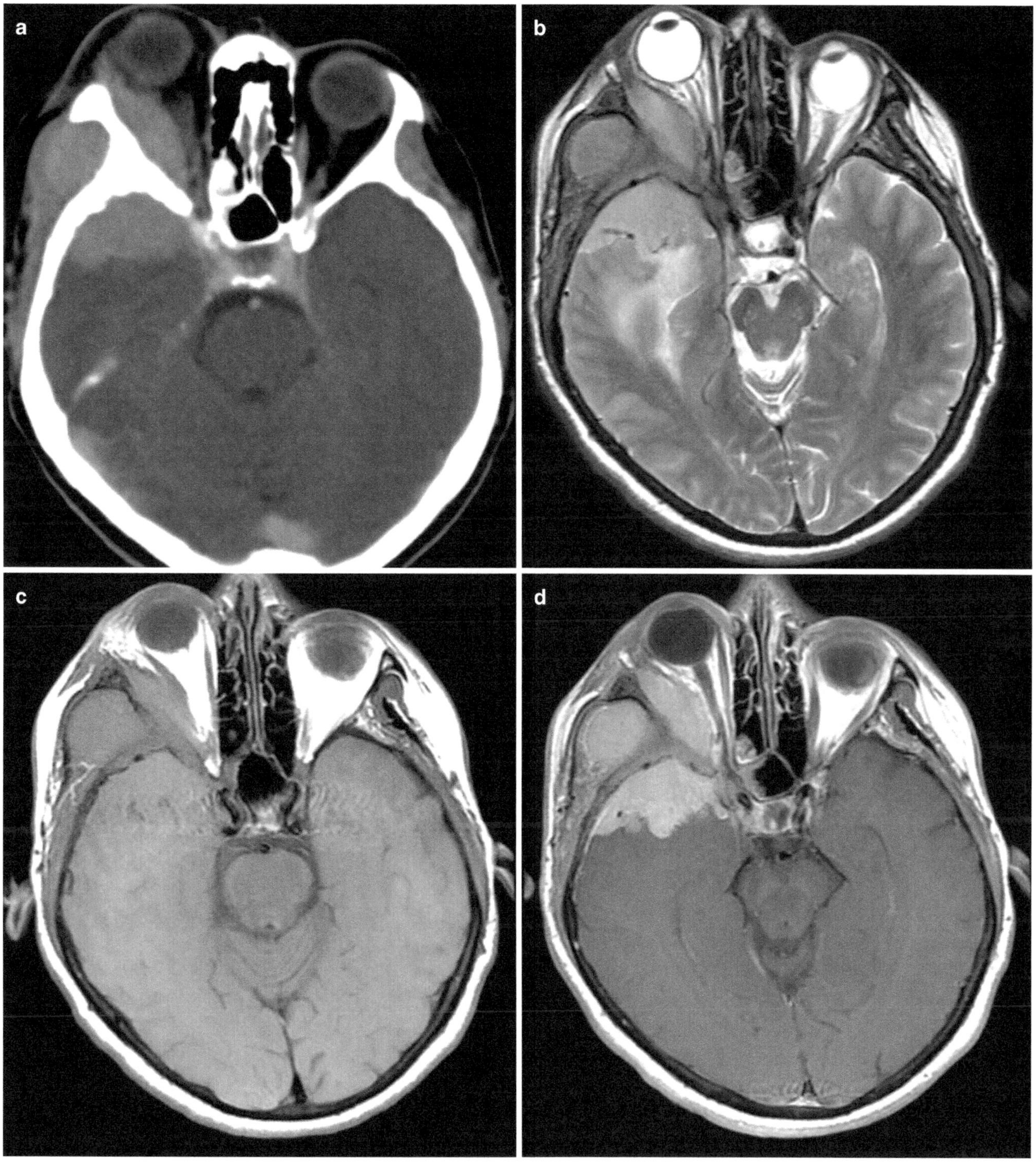

Fig. 15.71 Meningioma of the right pterional area. Axial CE CT scan (**a**), T2-weighted (**b**), T1-weighted (**c**), and post-contrast T1-weighted (**d**) images show a large meningioma with intracranial and extracranial components involving the infratemporal fossa and orbit. Perfusion CT mapping (**e**—CBF, **f**—CBV, **g**—MTT), ASL-perfusion (**h**) and DSE-map (**i**) reveal the high values of the blood volume and blood flow in the meningioma, whereas a mean transit time is decreased (typical hemodynamic features of meningiomas)

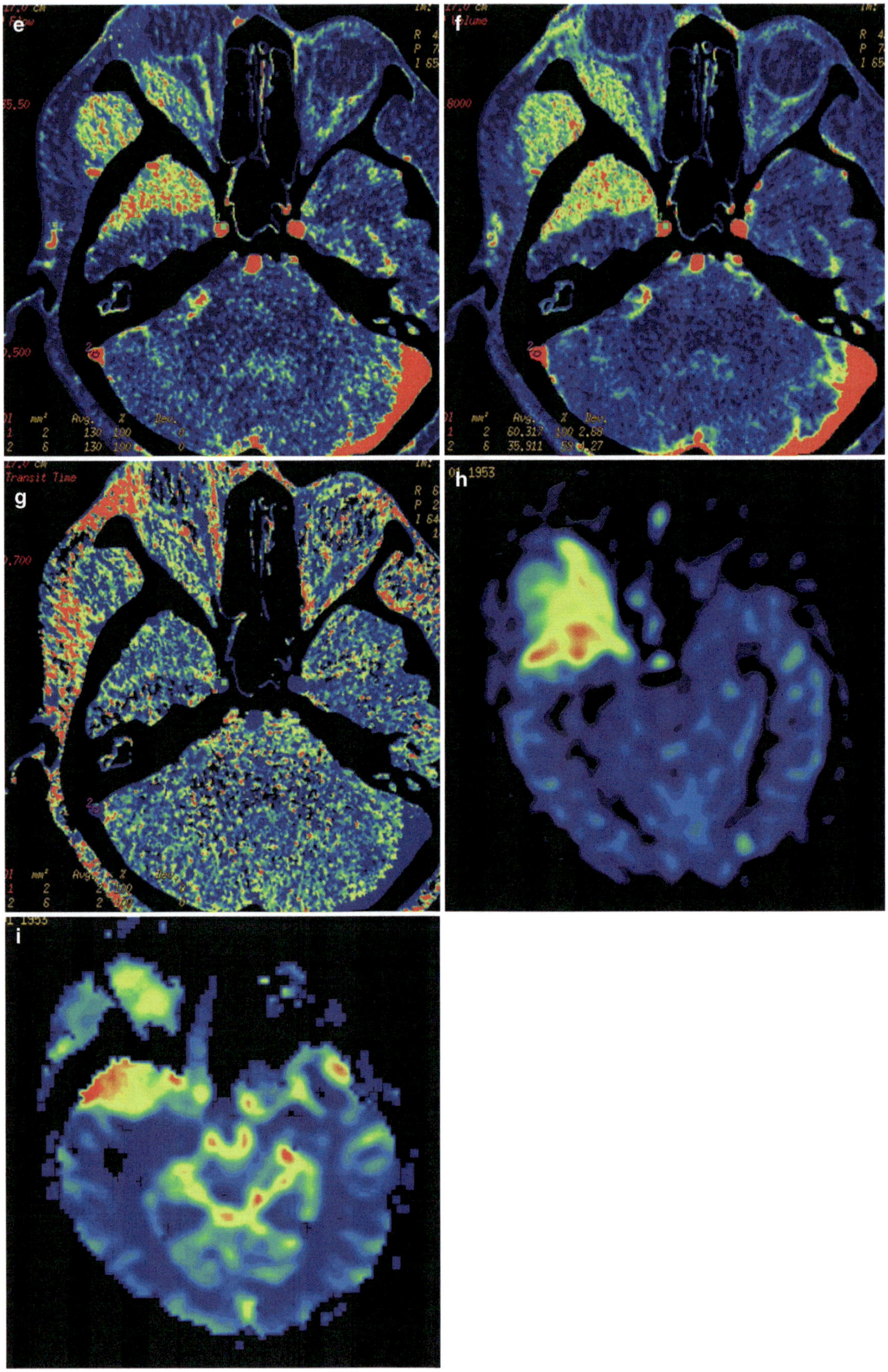

Fig. 15.71 (continued)

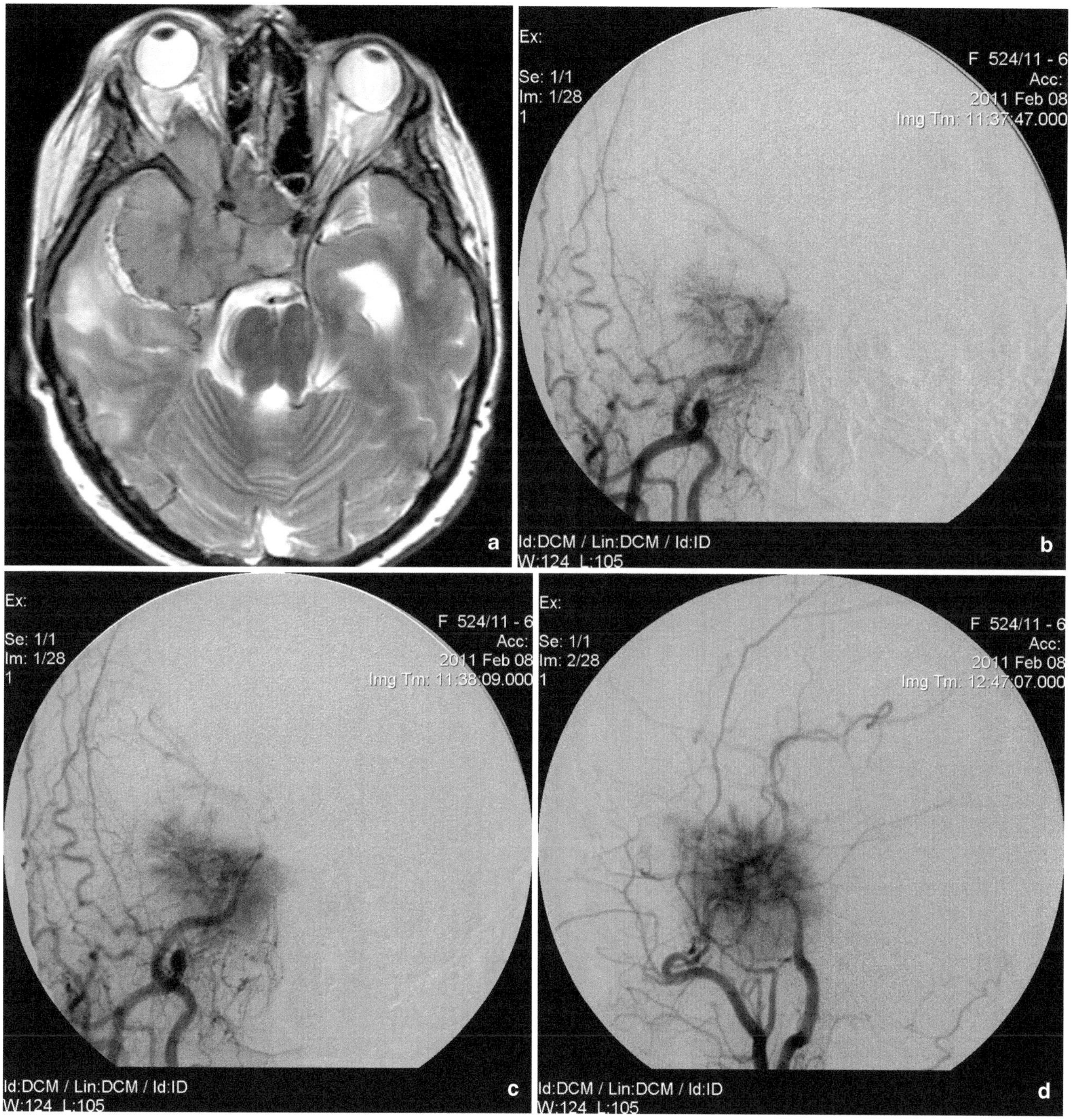

Fig. 15.72 Giant meningioma of the middle cranial fossa on the right involving the orbit and sphenoid sinus. Axial T2-weighted image (**a**) demonstrates a large meningioma. DSA (**b**–**d**) shows an abundant tumor vasculature, which is supplied by the branches of the upper maxillary artery, middle meningeal artery and short branches of internal carotid artery. 3D TOF MRA (**e**–**i**) visualizes the tumor vasculature with the equal accuracy

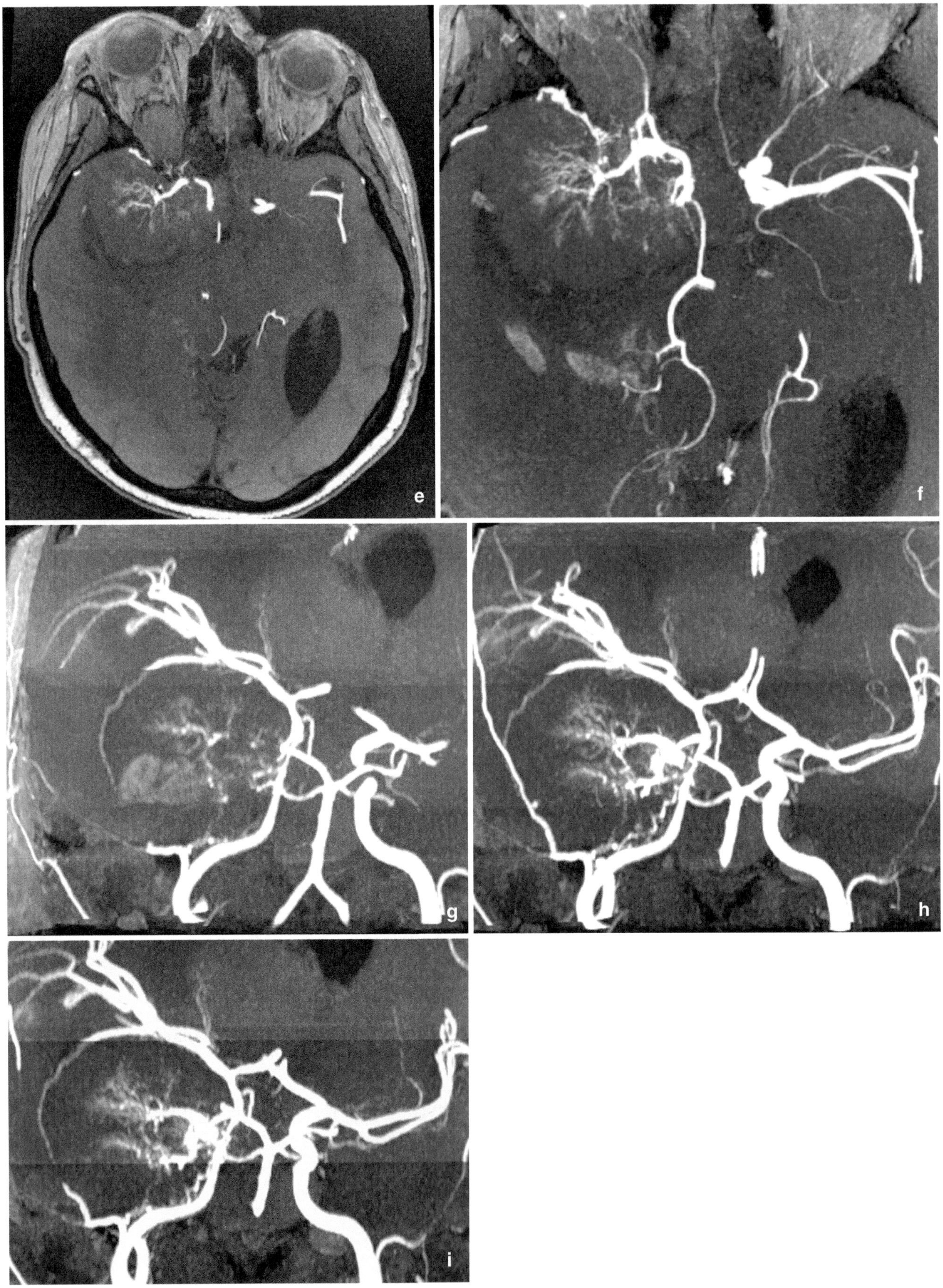

Fig. 15.72 (continued)

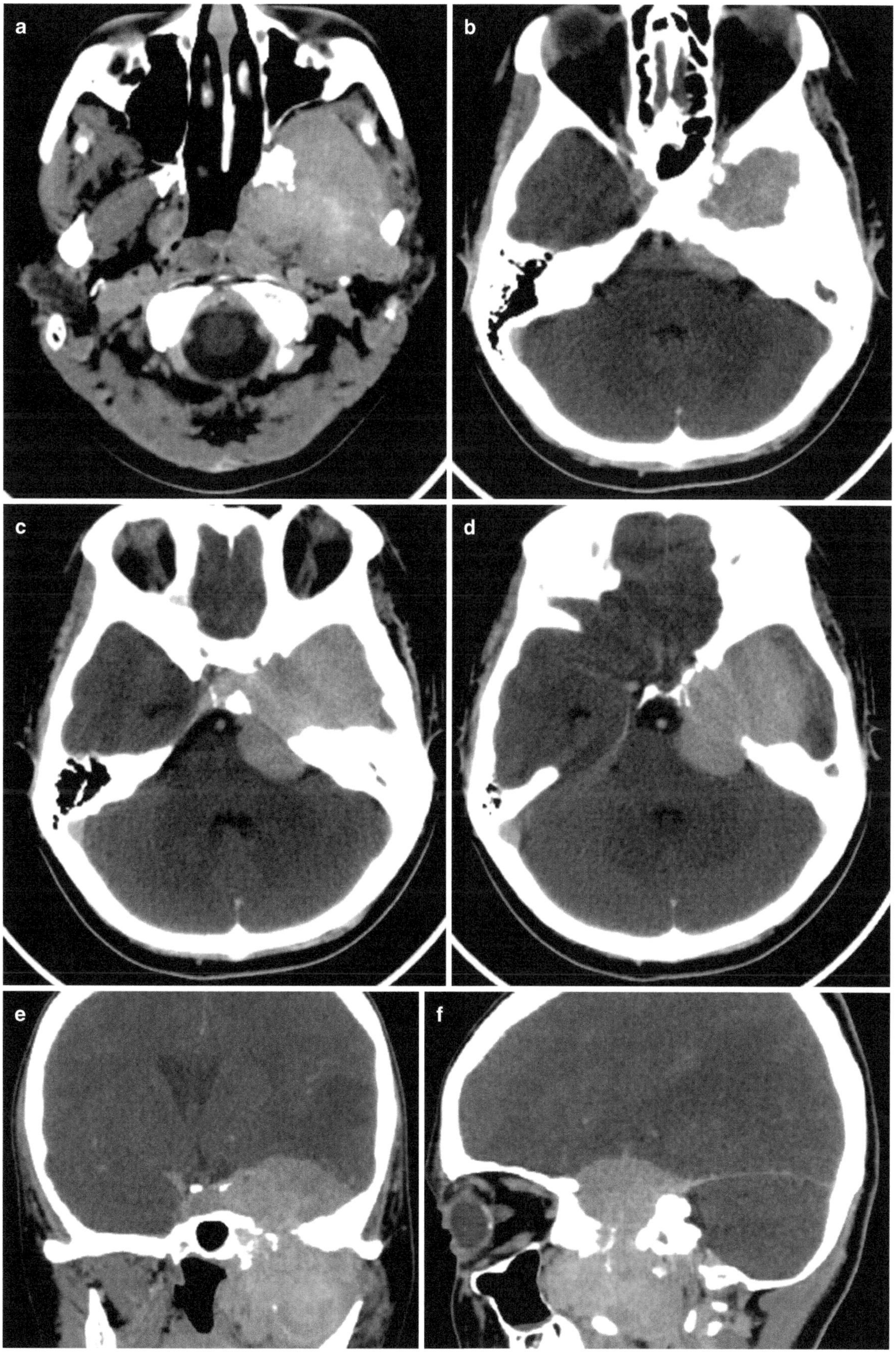

Fig. 15.73 Giant meningioma of the middle cranial fossa on the left with the destructive changes of the surrounding bones and spreading into the pterygopalatine and infratemporal fossae, petroclival region and sella turcica. Axial CE CT scans (**a**–**d**), coronal (**e**) and sagittal (**f**) reformations clearly visualize all tumor growth extension

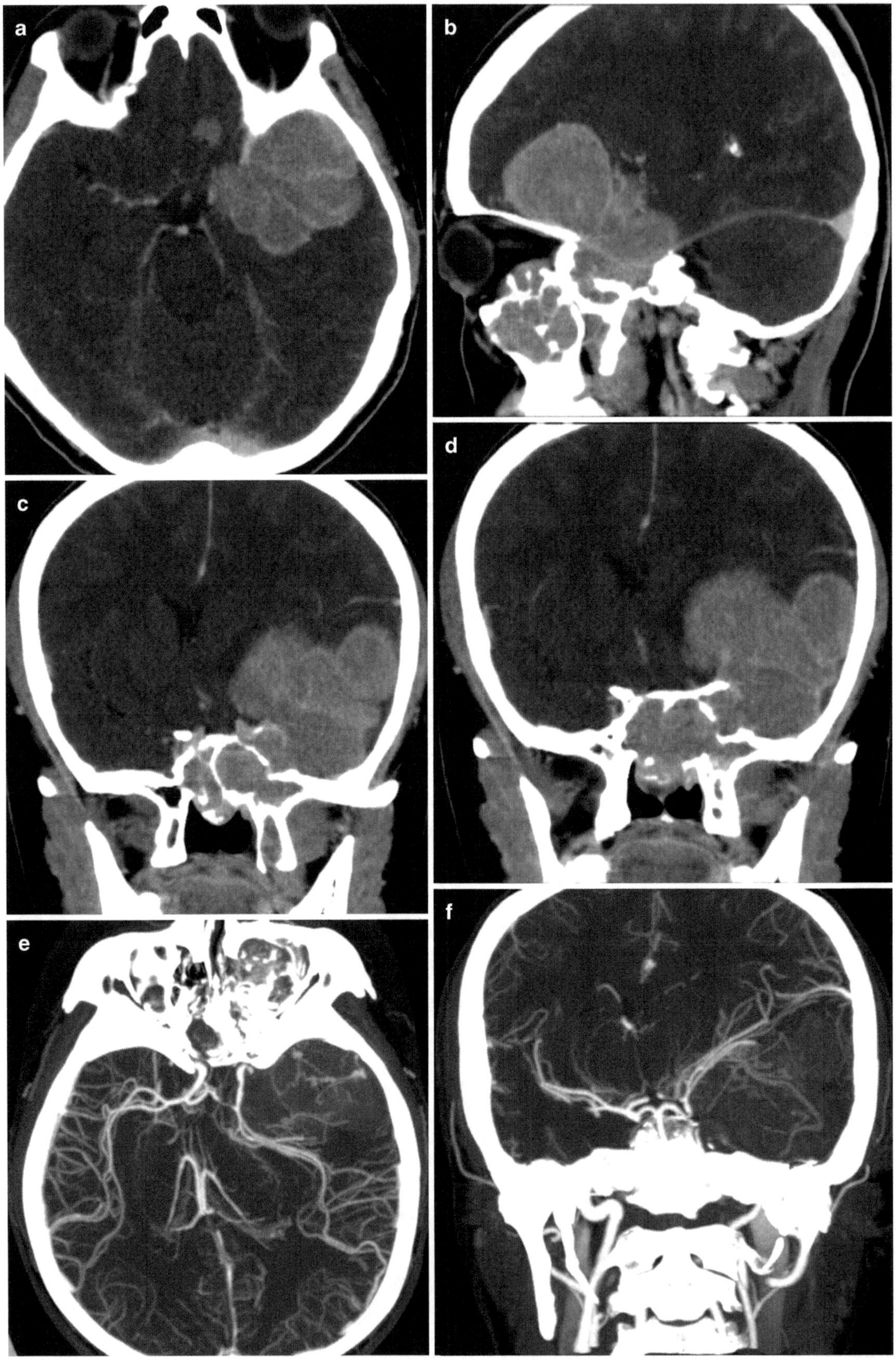

Fig. 15.74 Giant meningioma of the middle cranial fossa spreading into the anterior cranial fossa, sphenoid and maxillary sinuses. The tumor is intensively enhanced, which allows visualizing all tumor growth directions using CT (**a**–**d**). On CTA (**e**–**g**), a meningioma causes the displacement of the left middle and anterior cerebral arteries. 3D CT reformation (**h**) provides with the information about intracranial tumor extension. Perfusion CT (CBV—**i**) detects the moderately increased blood flow values in the tumor

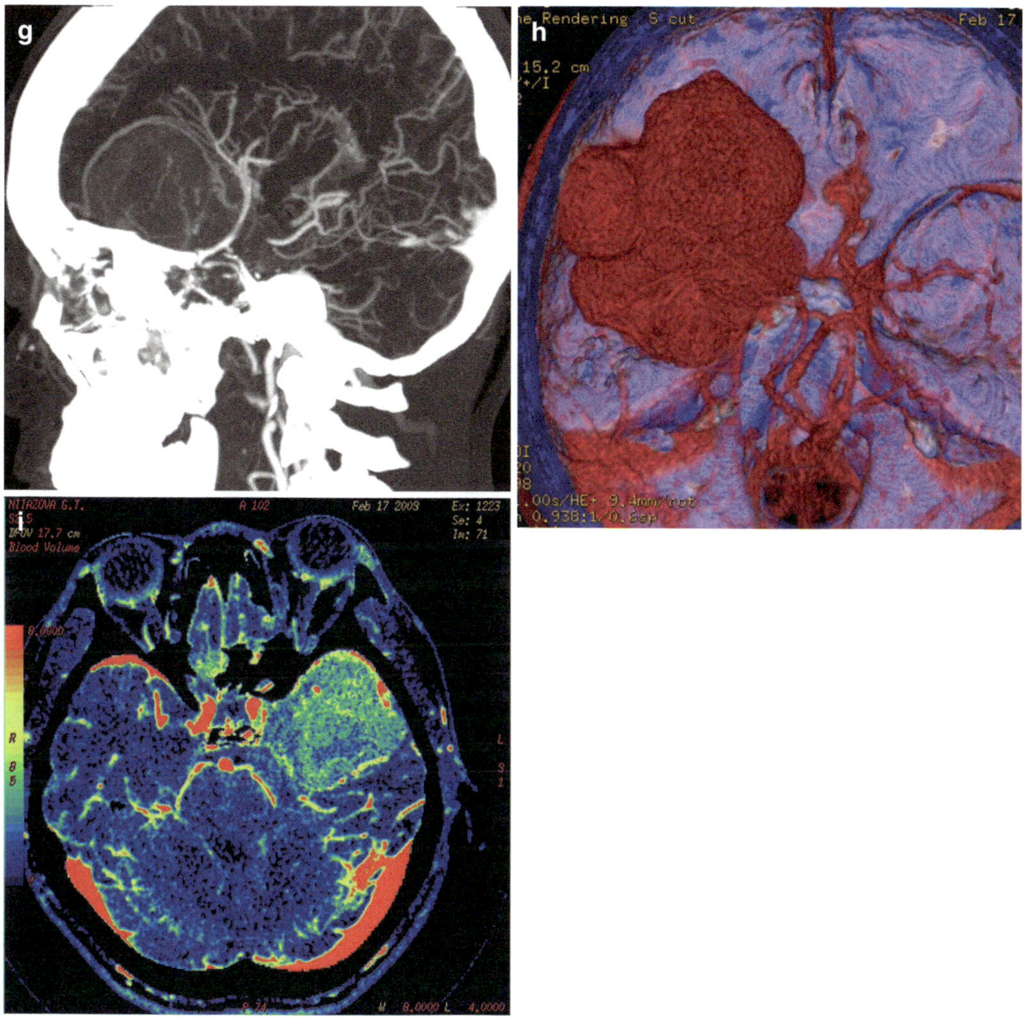

Fig. 15.74 (continued)

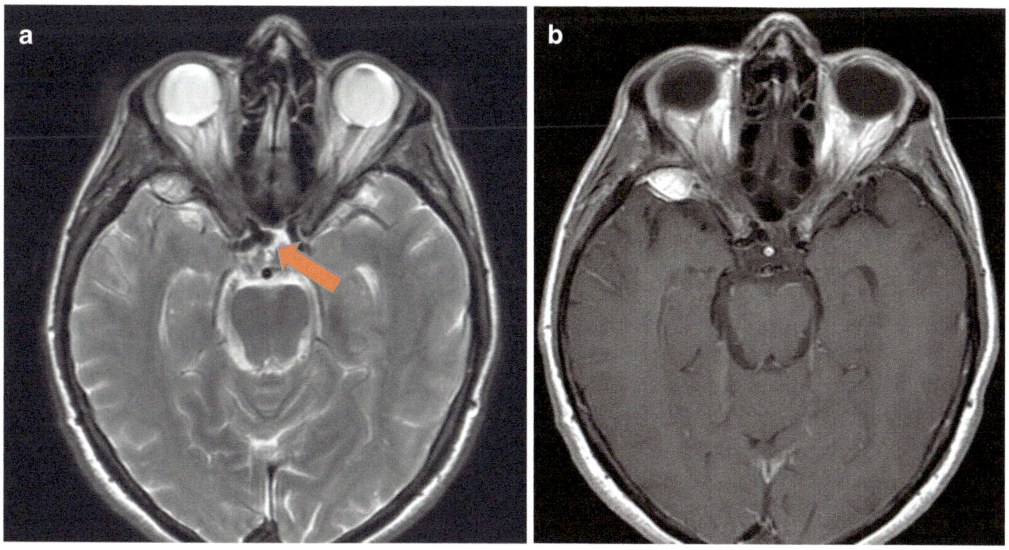

Fig. 15.75 A combination of the small meningioma of the sphenoid wing on the right with the right-sided vestibular schwannoma and the saccular aneurysm of the right internal carotid artery. T2-weighted (**a**), T1-weighted images (**b**) and CE CT scans (**c**, **d**) show multiple tumors with the different perfusion patterns. Perfusion parameters in the meningioma are higher, than in the vestibular schwannoma (**e**). Saccular aneurysm is visible on the routine MRI (*arrow*) and on 3D TOF MR-angiography (**f**)

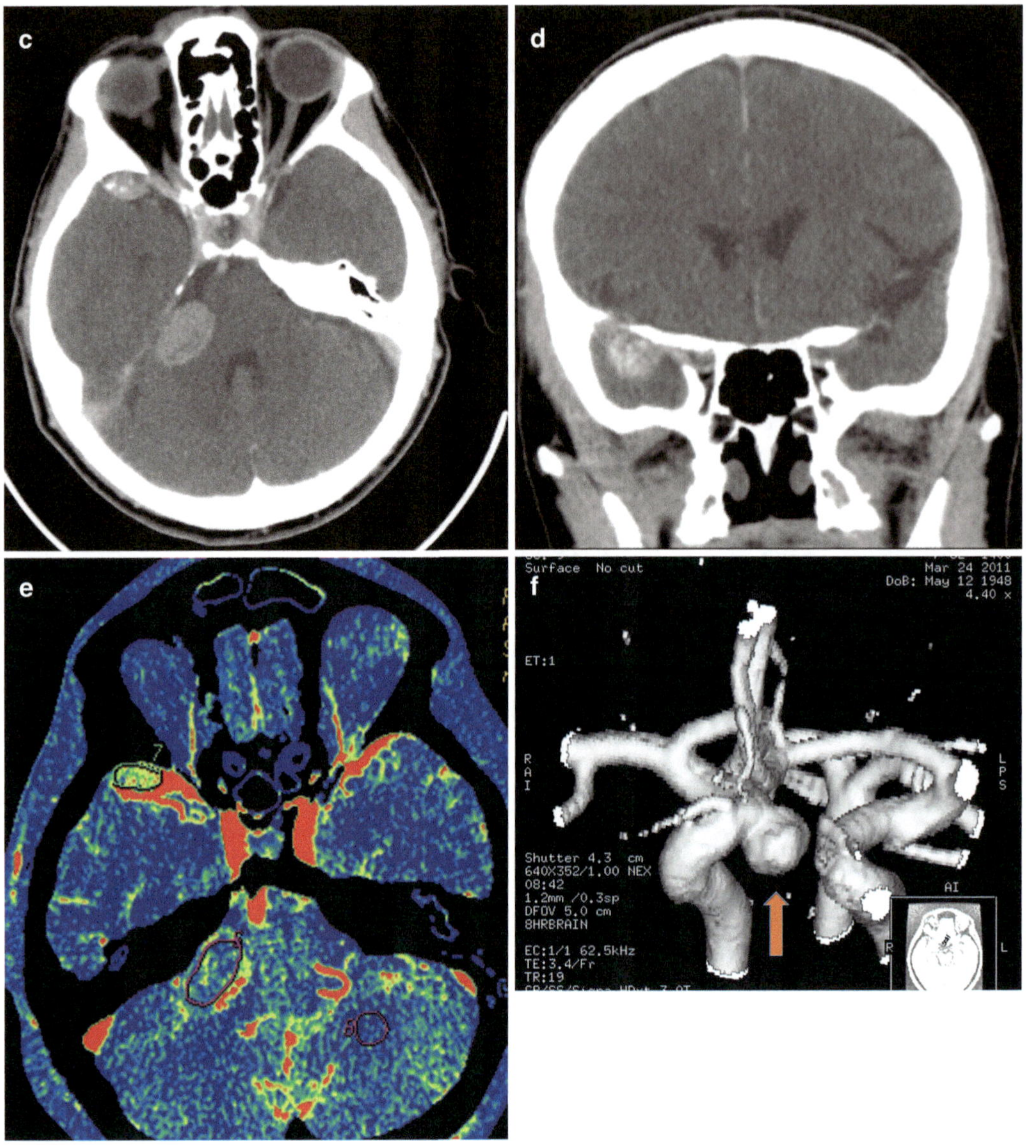

Fig. 15.75 (continued)

15.6 Gliomas of Optic Chiasm and Hypothalamus

These gliomas account for 3–5% of all intracranial tumors and 25–30% of the chiasmal-sellar region tumors in children. In 20–50% of cases these tumors are found in neurofibromatosis type I von Recklinghausen disease (Menor et al. 1991). Tumors of the optic chiasm frequently involve the hypothalamus and the third ventricle. Histologically, they are pilocytic astrocytomas in 75% of cases, but despite their benign nature, they are often unfavorable in terms of location and expansion (Collins et al. 2015). Tumors originating from the hypothalamus grow towards the chiasm, affect it, and expand into the third ventricle. On the other hand, tumors originating from the chiasm may expand not only along optic tracts, but also into the third ventricle. As it is difficult to identify the origin of these tumors growth according to neurological examination or neuroimaging, we discuss them together.

Clinical findings are as follows: progressive visual loss, hypothalamic-pituitary dysfunction, and increase of intracranial pressure.

According to clinical, neuroimaging, and surgical data five groups of tumors are distinguished:

(1) Tumors of the anterior angle of the chiasm and one of the optic nerves with predominant anterior growth; (2) antechiasmal gliomas invading into the cavity of the third ventricle; the origin of their growth is the lateral part of the chiasm; (3) tumors of the posterior parts of the chiasm, growing predominantly into the third ventricle; (4) tumors of the optic tract; (5) tumors of the third ventricle, growing into its lumen and causing occlusion of the CSF pathways (Fig. 15.76).

Imaging Cases of the optic nerve tumor with dilatation of the optic canal on the ipsilateral side occur. If both optic nerves are affected, then the dilatation occurs bilaterally (symmetrical or asymmetrical). If the chiasm is affected—changes of sella turcica may be found in giant tumors–changes of sella turcica and rise of intracranial pressure are the typical signs.

Angiography is helpful in those cases in which there are giant and rapidly growing tumors with signs of malignant transformation. Displacement of cerebral vessels and enhancement of the abnormal vascular tumor net are seen on angiography in these cases.

The involvement of the orbital portion (on CT) leads to thickening of the optic nerve of variable shape and size. The

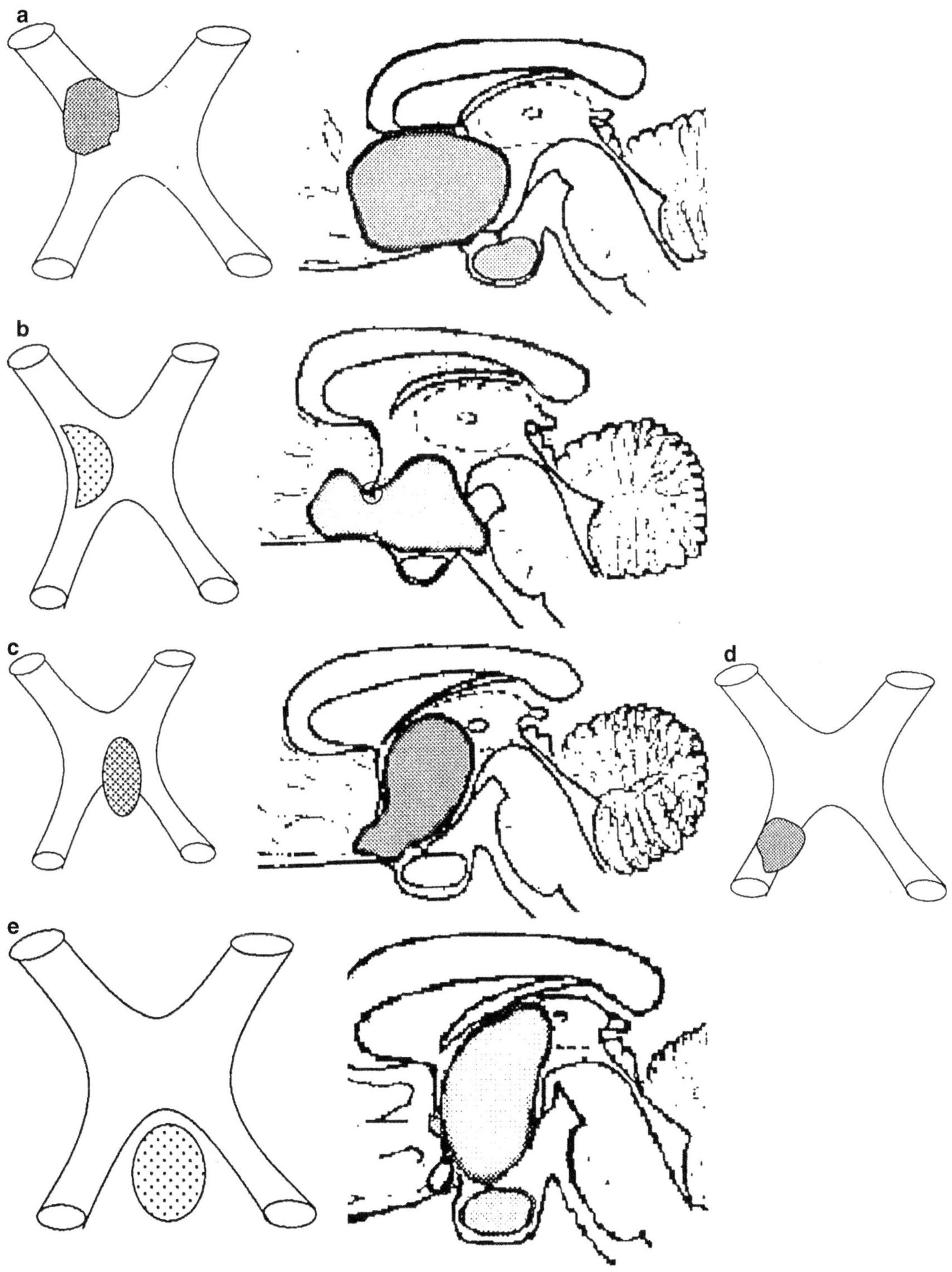

Fig. 15.76 Axial and sagittal graphics of the different types of the optical tract and hypothalamus tumors relationship. A growth site point and location of the tumor: (**a**) type 1, (**b**) type 2, (**c**) type 3, (**d**) type 4, (**e**) type 5

most frequent variants are fusiform, cylindrical or oval enlargement of the optic nerve. A tumor of the optic nerve expanding into its canal part causes dilatation of the optic canal and is clearly identified on CT. The density of the optic nerve gliomas on CT is within the range of 25–60 HU. After contrast enhancement, it can remain unchanged in the group of diffuse astrocytomas, while their density increases at varying degrees (10–15 HU) in other tumors. CE is necessary in cases in which the tumor expansion into the intracranial part of the optic nerve is suspected. In these cases, the solid part of the tumor originating from the orbit is seen, with involvement of the chiasmal cistern.

If the chiasm, optic nerves, and the hypothalamus are affected, then an iso- or hypodense mass lesion that mildly accumulates contrast medium is seen. In cases with widely expanded tumors, CE is observed along the optic tracts up to the lateral geniculate bodies and often within the third ventricle (Figs. 15.77 and 15.78). Several observations were made in our institution when the tumor reached the optic cortex. Obstruction of the CSF pathways causes

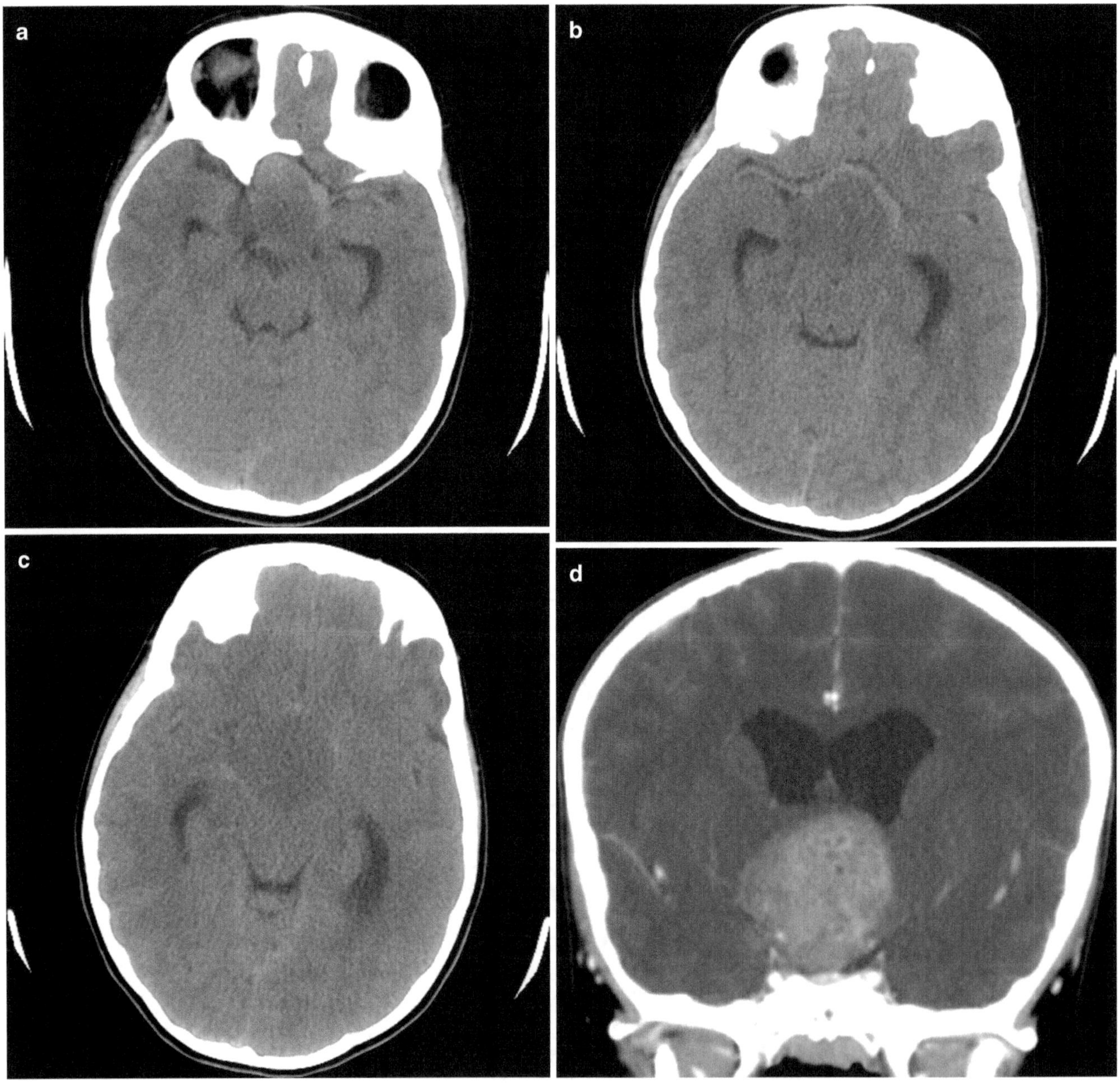

Fig. 15.77 Glioma of the chiasm and the bottom of the third ventricle area. Axial CT scans (**a**–**c**) show a hypodense tumor in the suprasellar area. Coronal (**d**, **e**) and sagittal (**f**) reformations after CE demonstrate an intensively enhancing tumor

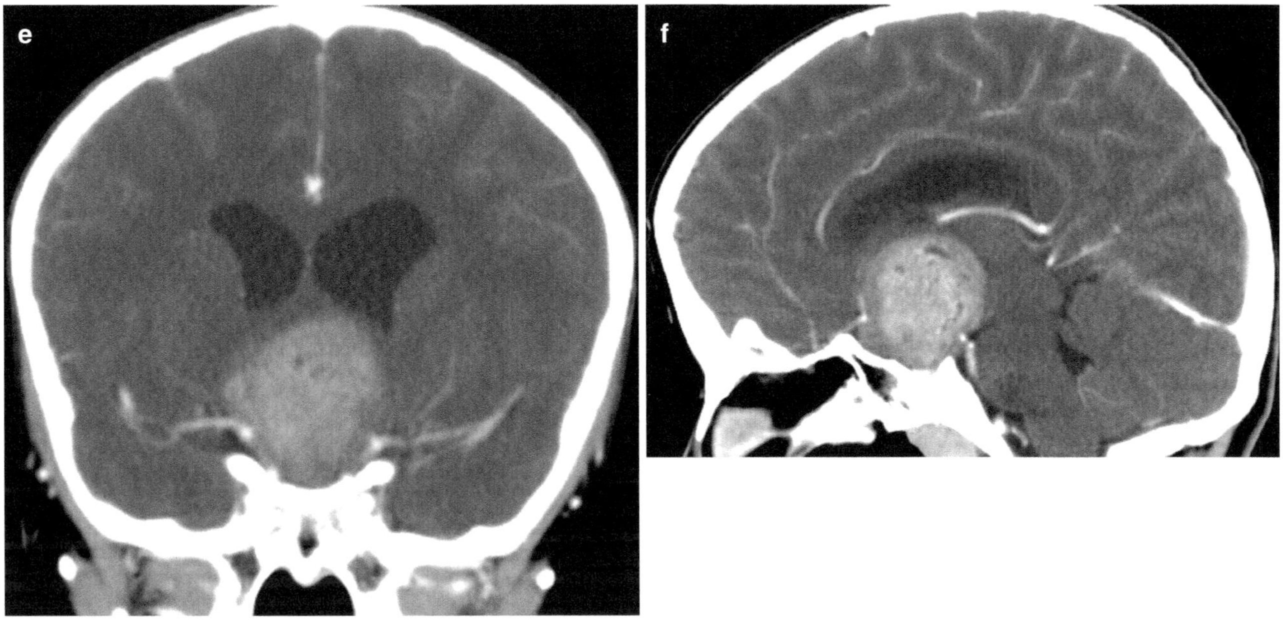

Fig. 15.77 (continued)

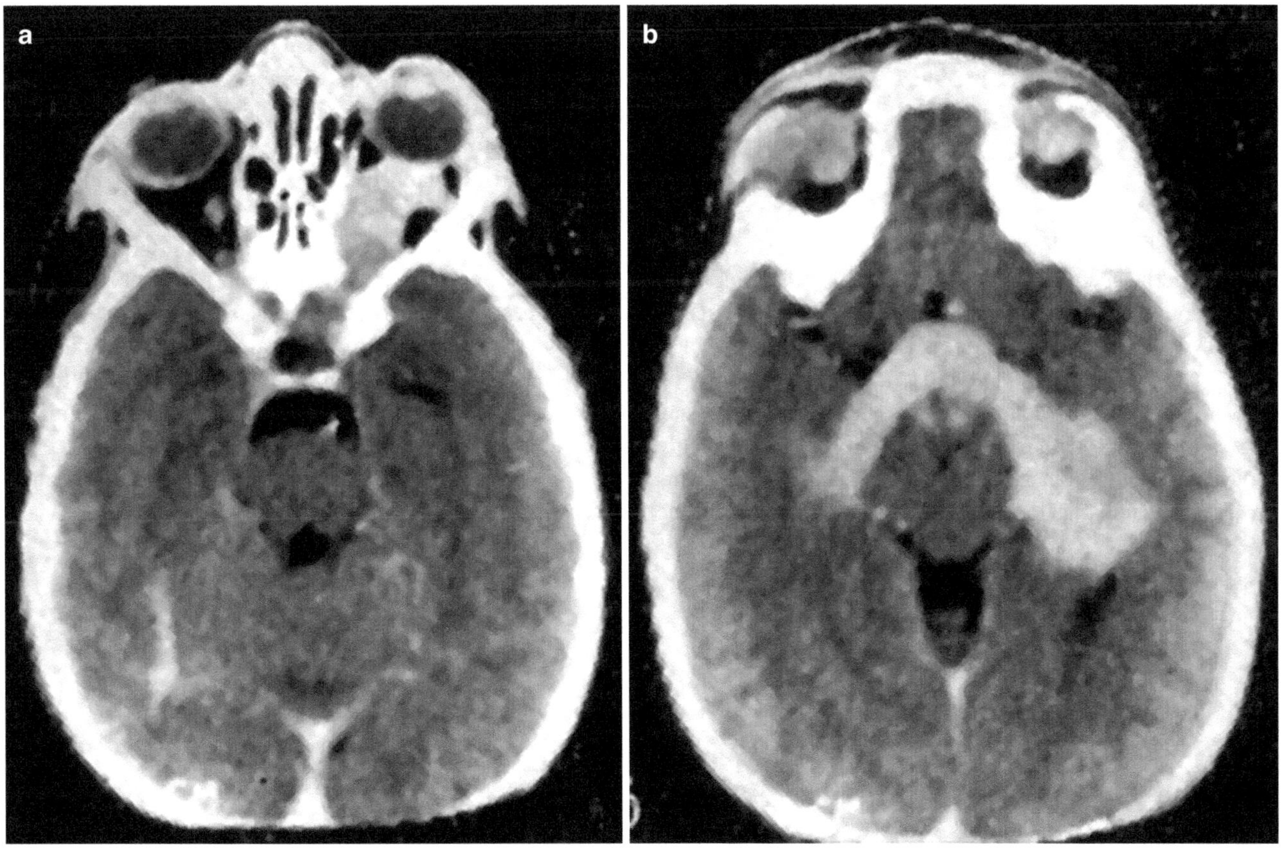

Fig. 15.78 Glioma of the left optic nerve, chiasm and optic tracts on both sides, which shows intense enhancement on CT (**a–c**)

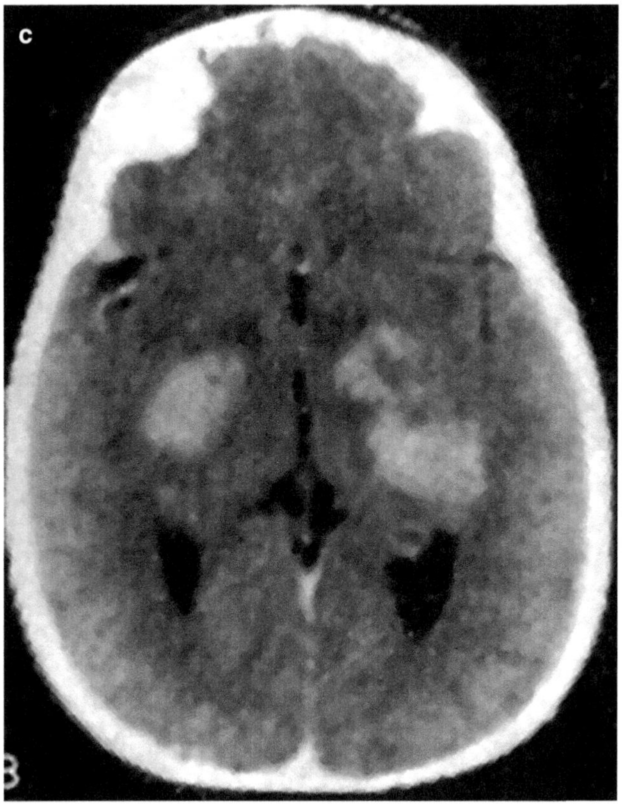

Fig. 15.78 (continued)

hydrocephalus of various extents. In several cases, calcifications could be seen within the stroma of hypothalamic gliomas, which makes them resembling craniopharyngiomas.

On MRI the signal of a tumor is isointense or hypointense on T1-weighted images and moderately hyperintense on T2-weighted images compared with that of brain tissue. Cysts often form within tumors or nearby, which is more typical for giant gliomas. The density of cystic components on CT and their signal intensity on MRI is equal to that of the CSF. Expansion of tumors along the optic tracts is well seen with T2-weighted images, whereas CT sometimes fails clearly to identify these changes. Identification of glioma invading into the optic nerve or along the optic tract is an important component of a correct interpretation of the tumor localization, even in large and giant size tumors. Intravenous CE reveals the accumulation of contrast medium in the tumor stroma which may be mild or homogenously intensive (Figs. 15.79, 15.80, and 15.81). Pilocytic astrocytomas most often are intensely enhanced. High level of contrast enhancement also distinguishes anaplastic gliomas located at this site. However, unlike benign forms, the latter are characterized by the presence of necrotic changes in the tumor structure and extensive perifocal brain edema. It should be remembered that malignant neoplasms are characterized by rapid, often invasive growth, presence of hemorrhages in the stroma, early metastases to the ependyma of the ventricles and subarachnoid space of the brain and spinal cord (Figs. 15.82, 15.83, 15.84, and 15.85).

Sometimes glial neoplasms from adjacent regions of cerebral hemispheres can invade into the optic chiasm and sellar region. These are usually astrocytomas of the uncus and medial temporal lobe and, less frequently, frontobasal astrocytomas. In the presence of contrast enhancement in the tumor, necrotic areas, perifocal edema and rapid progression of clinical symptoms of diencephalic area involvement, anaplastic forms of gliomas should be suspected, and the treatment should be planned based on the obtained diagnostic findings (Fig. 15.86).

Giant tumors of the optic chiasm in children (Fig. 15.87) should be differentiated with craniopharyngioma, arachnoid cyst, epidermoid and dermoid cysts, teratoma, chordoma, carcinoma, giant aneurysm, vascular malformations, inflammatory disorders (abscess, granuloma), and pituitary tumor. CT and MRI with CE are the most informative in the differential diagnosis of all tumors of this location (Alkonyi et al. 2015). If vascular lesions are suspected, then cerebral angiography is obligatory method.

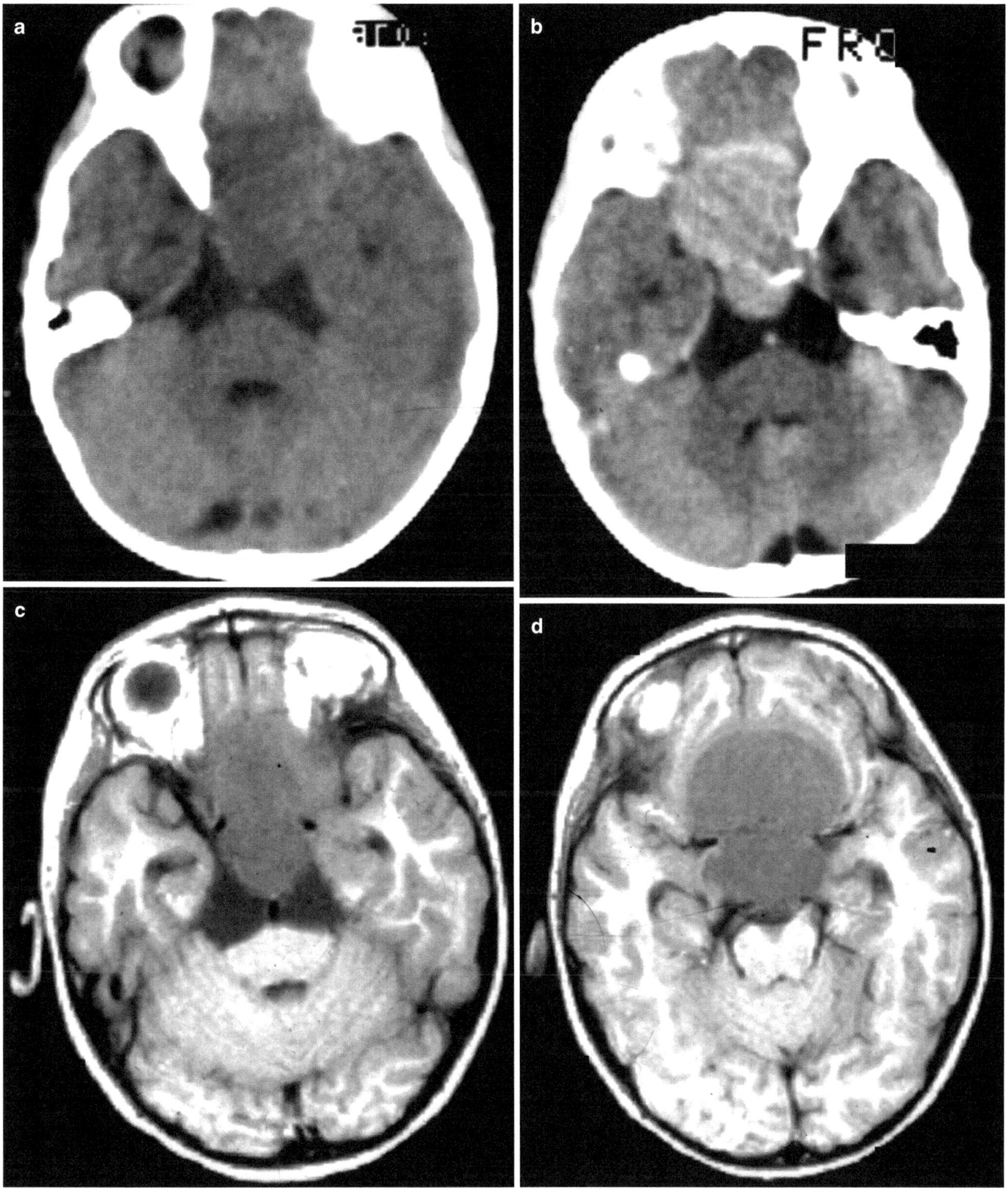

Fig. 15.79 Giant glioma of the chiasm and the third ventricle area. NE CT scan (**a**) shows a hypodense tumor. CE CT scan (**b**) demonstrates a homogeneous contrast enhancement in the tumor. Axial and sagittal T1-weighted (**c–e**) and T2-weighted images (**f**) show a well-delineated mass, which consists of the larger solid and the smaller cystic parts (prepontine)

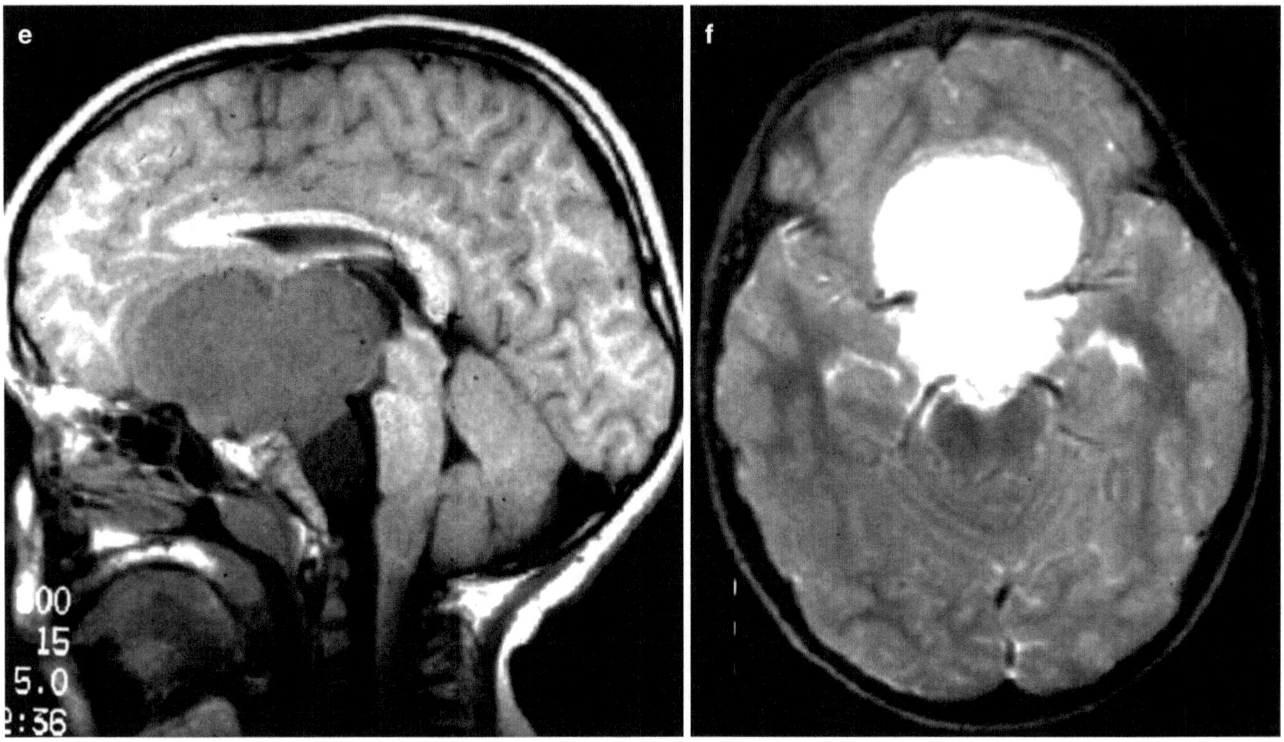

Fig. 15.79 (continued)

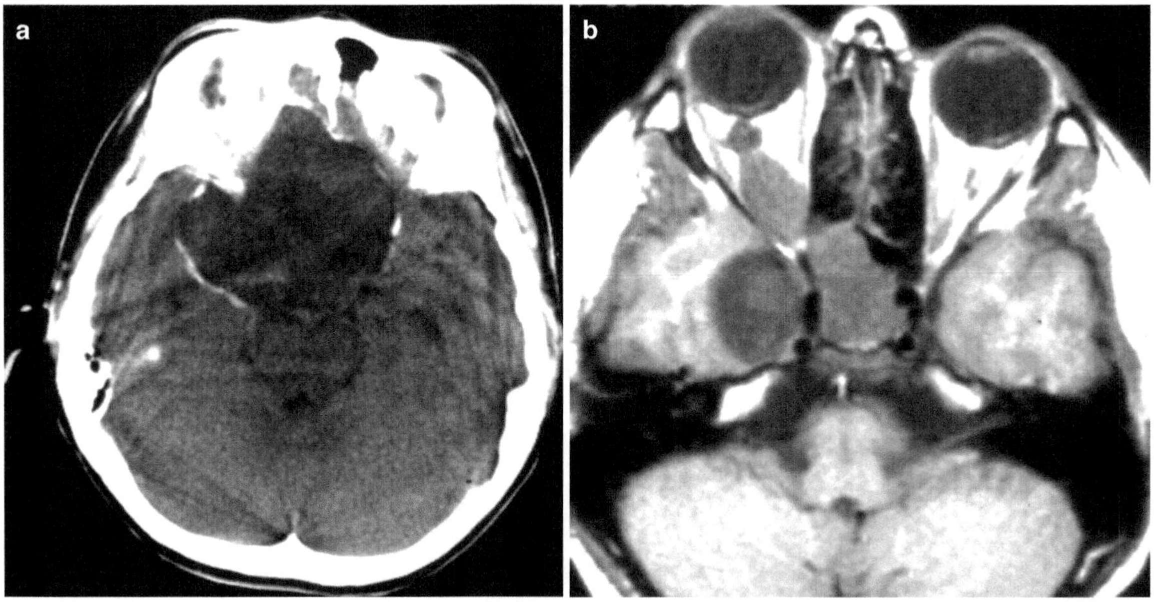

Fig. 15.80 Giant glioma of the chiasm and the right optic nerve. CT scan shows a homogeneous hypointense tumor with the calcifications in the capsule (**a**). On T1-weighted images (**b**, **c**) the tumor has hypointense MR-signal

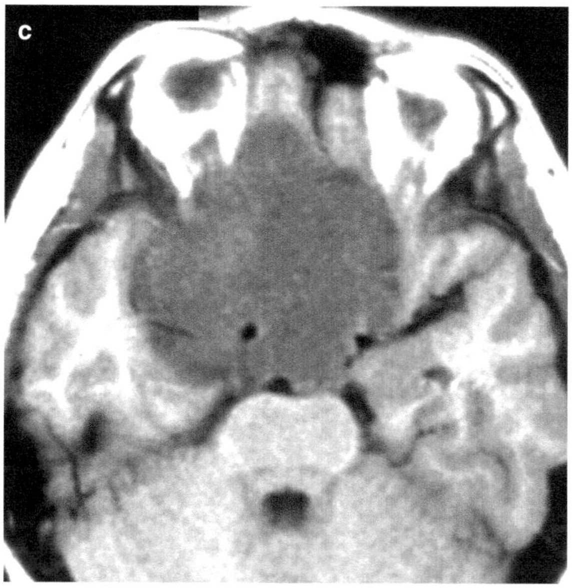

Fig. 15.80 (continued)

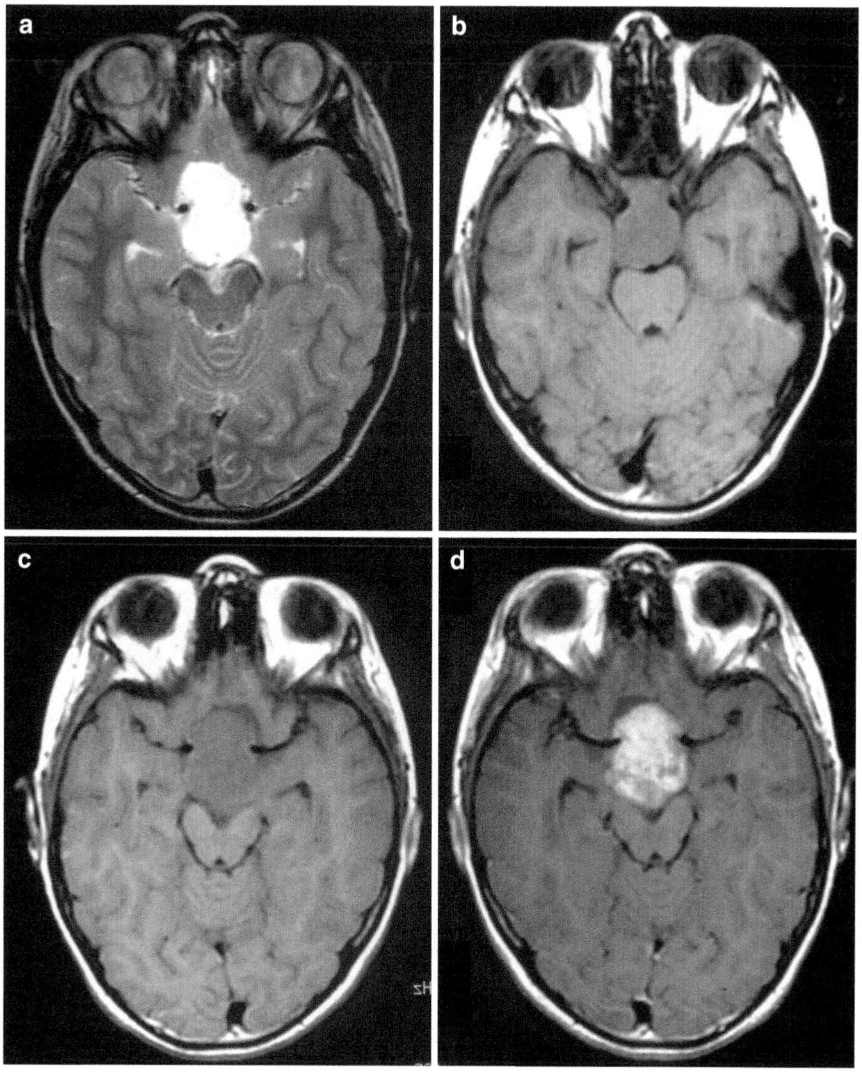

Fig. 15.81 Glioma of chiasm and the third ventricle area (pilocytic astrocytoma). MRI: the glioma has increased signal on T2-weighted image (**a**) and slightly decreased signal on T1-weighted images (**b**, **c**). Post-contrast axial (**d**), coronal (**e**) and sagittal (**f**) T1-weighted images show a heterogeneous, intense enhancement in the tumor

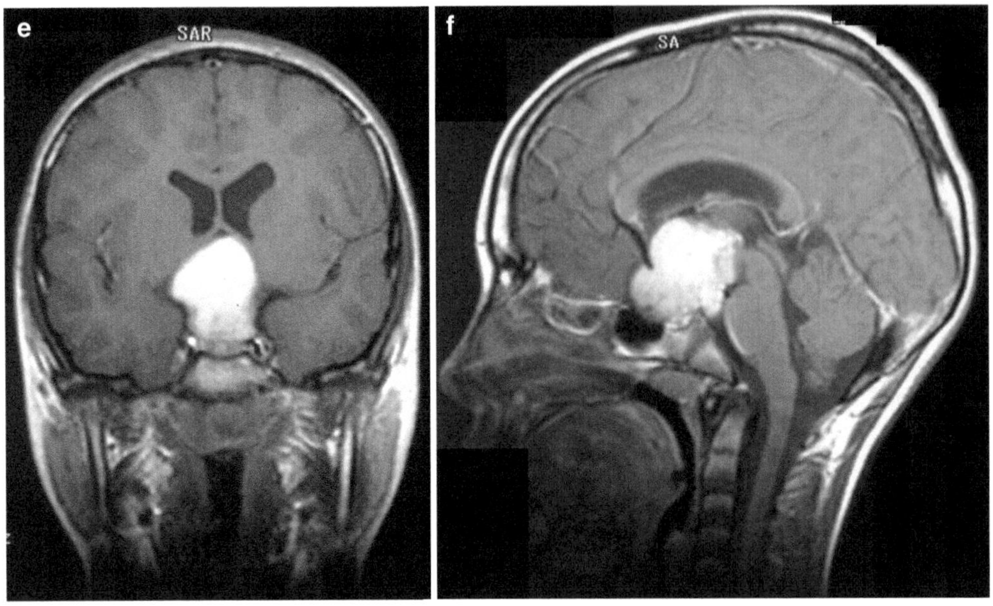

Fig. 15.81 (continued)

Fig. 15.82 Anaplastic astrocytoma of the third ventricle area. T2-weighted image (**a**) shows a hypointense mass in the third ventricle area with the surrounding vasogenic edema. Post-contrast T1-weighted images (**b**, **c**) show a well-delineated intensively enhancing tumor

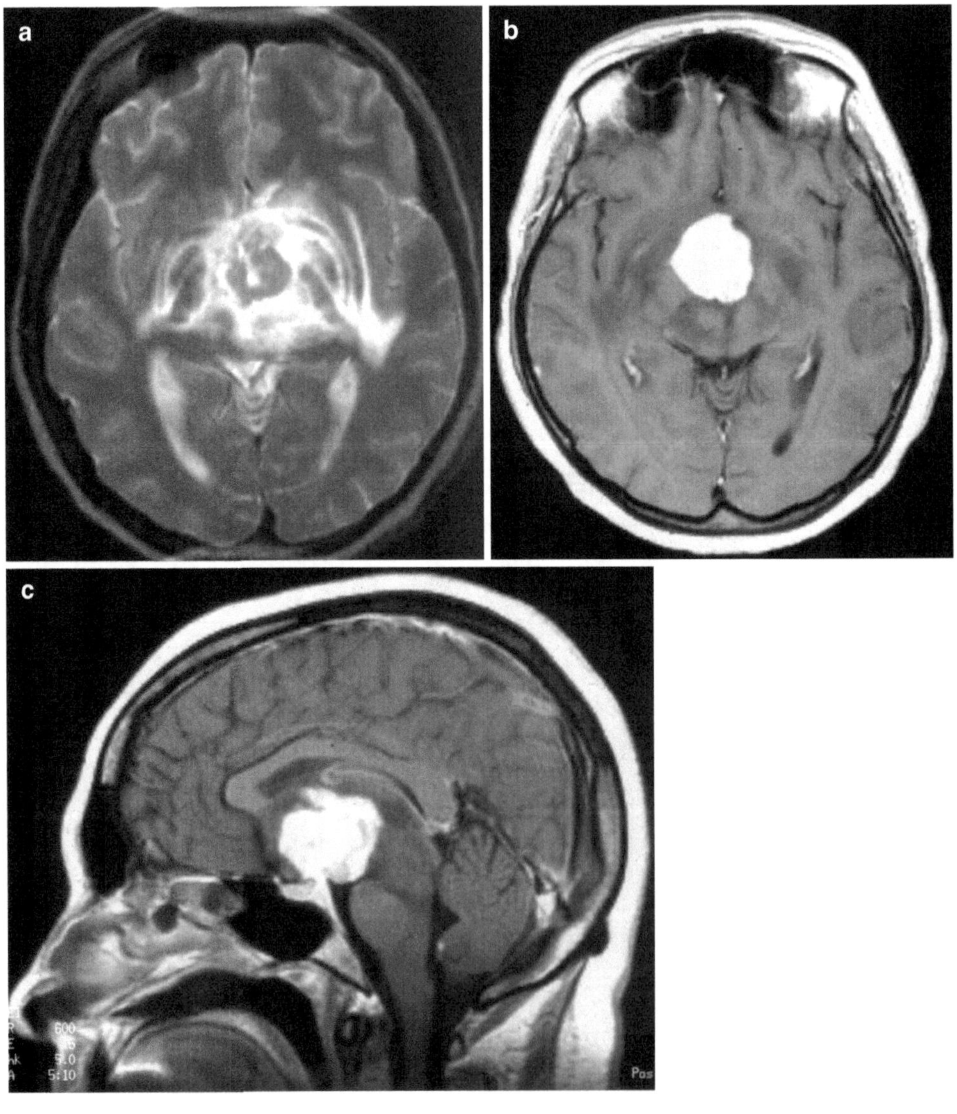

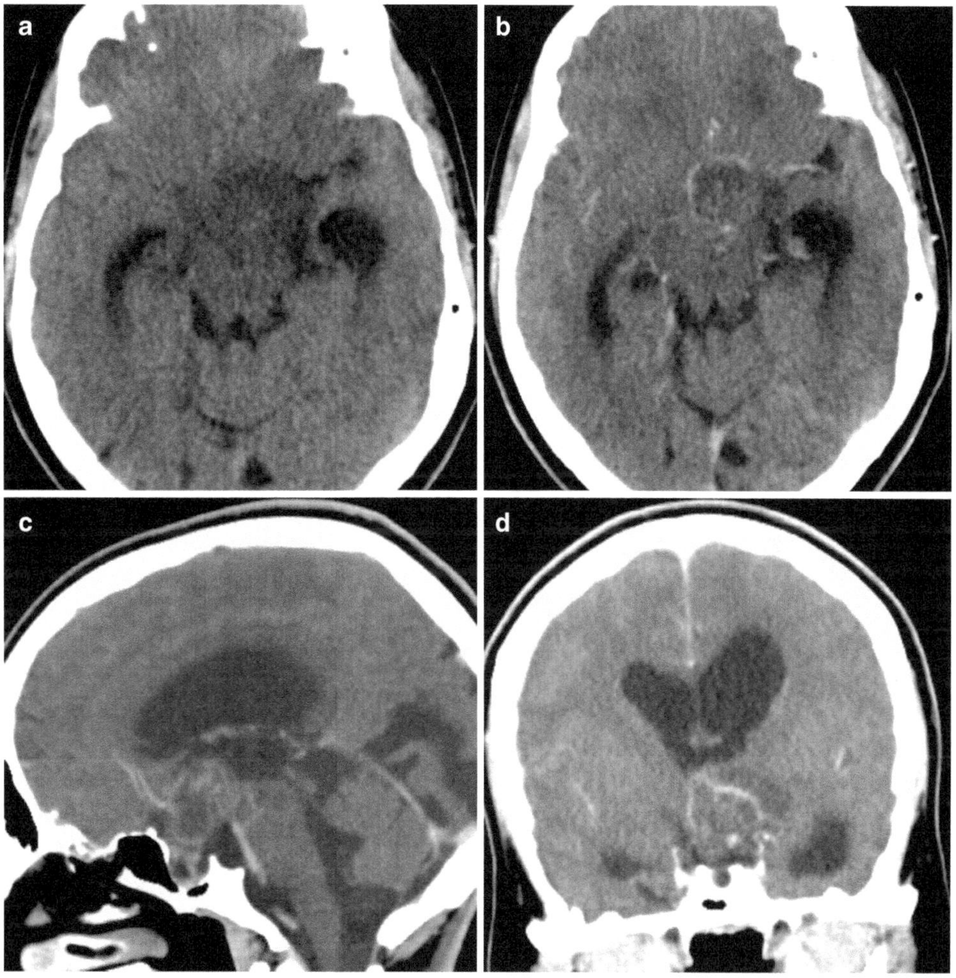

Fig. 15.83 Anaplastic astrocytoma of the optic chiasm, third ventricle and interpeduncular cistern areas. CT scans before (**a**) and after (**b–d**) CE reveal the hypodense mass in the suprasellar region with the heterogeneous enhancement. The communicating hydrocephalus is seen on the CT

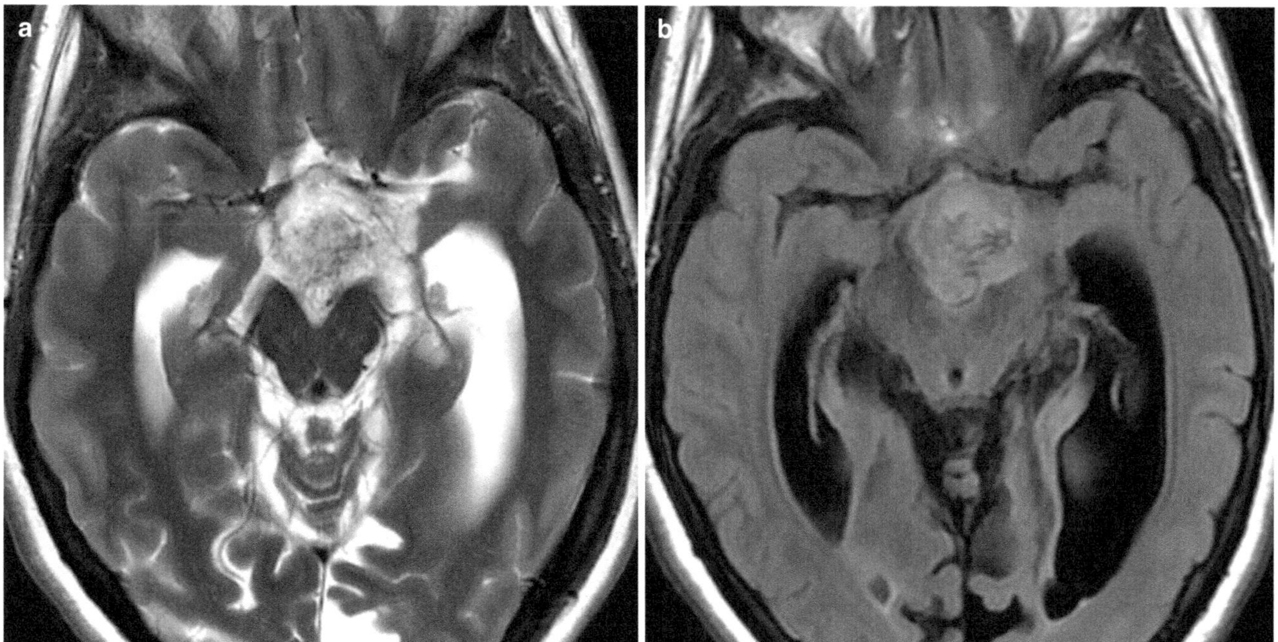

Fig. 15.84 Anaplastic astrocytoma of the optic chiasm, third ventricle area and interpeduncular cistern (see Fig. 15.83 for CT data). T2-weighted- (**a**), T2-FLAIR- (**b**), T1-weighted images (**c**) and SWAN (**d**) demonstrate a relatively homogeneous tumor with hemorrhagic areas (*arrow*) in its structure. Post-contrast T1-weighted images (**e**, **f**) show a heterogeneous enhancement with necrotic central part of the tumor. Glioma invades into the interpeduncular cistern and infiltrates the uncus of the left temporal lobe

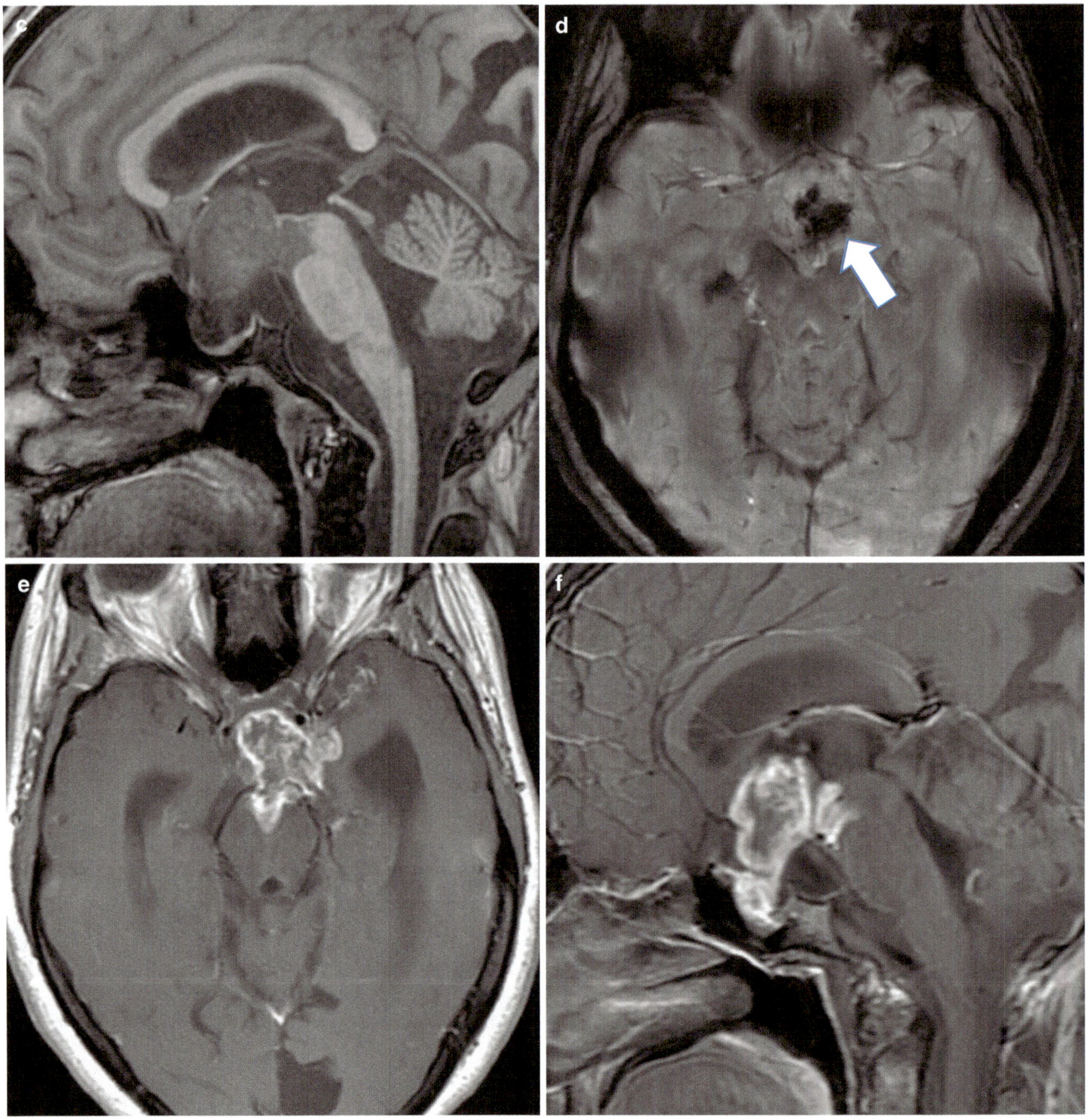

Fig. 15.84 (continued)

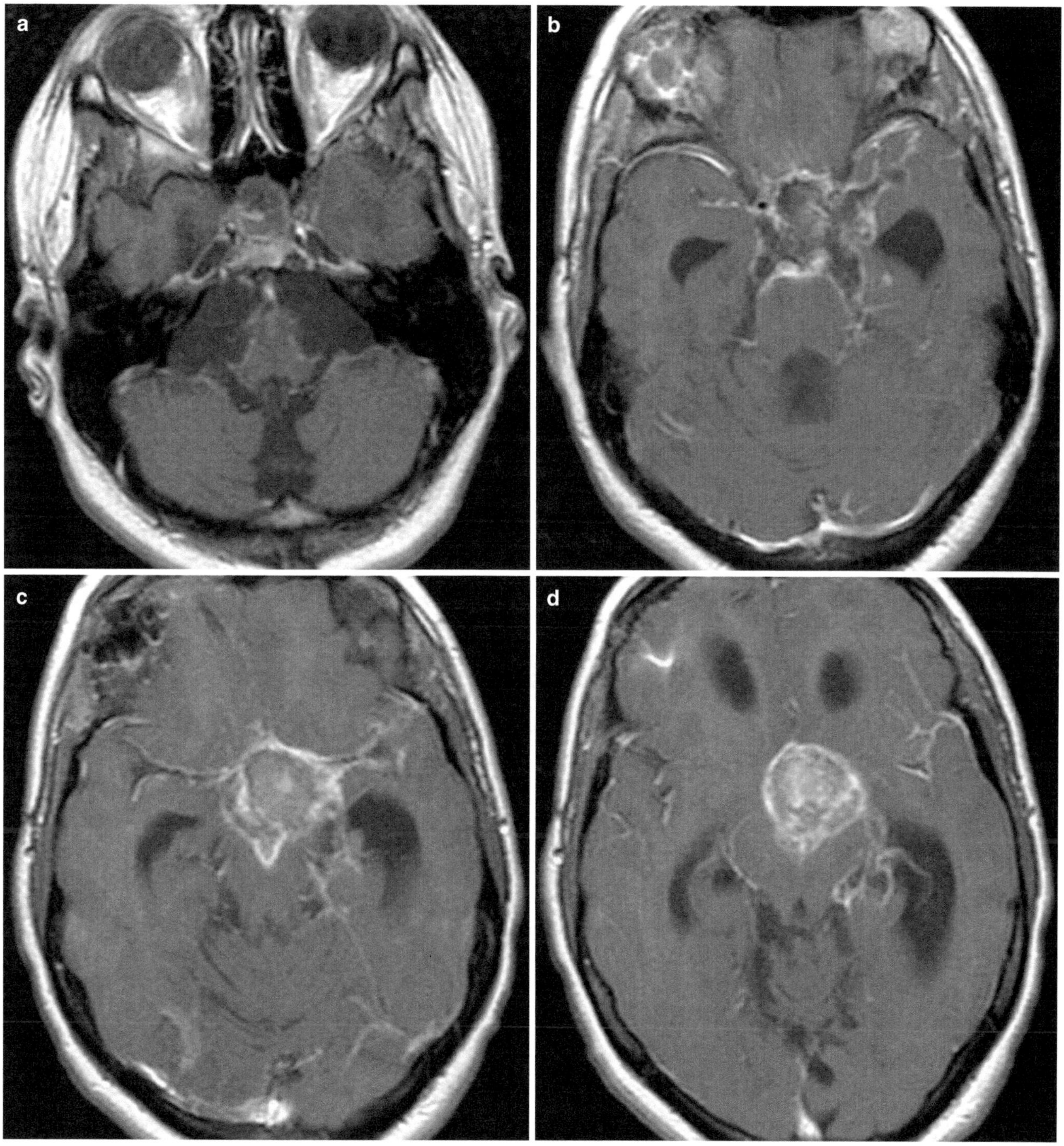

Fig. 15.85 MRI in the same patient (Fig. 15.84). Post-contrast T1-weighted images in 6 months after chemotherapy (**a**–**f**) demonstrate leptomeningeal metastases filling the subarachnoid spaces in the lateral fissures area, around the brainstem and the spinal cord

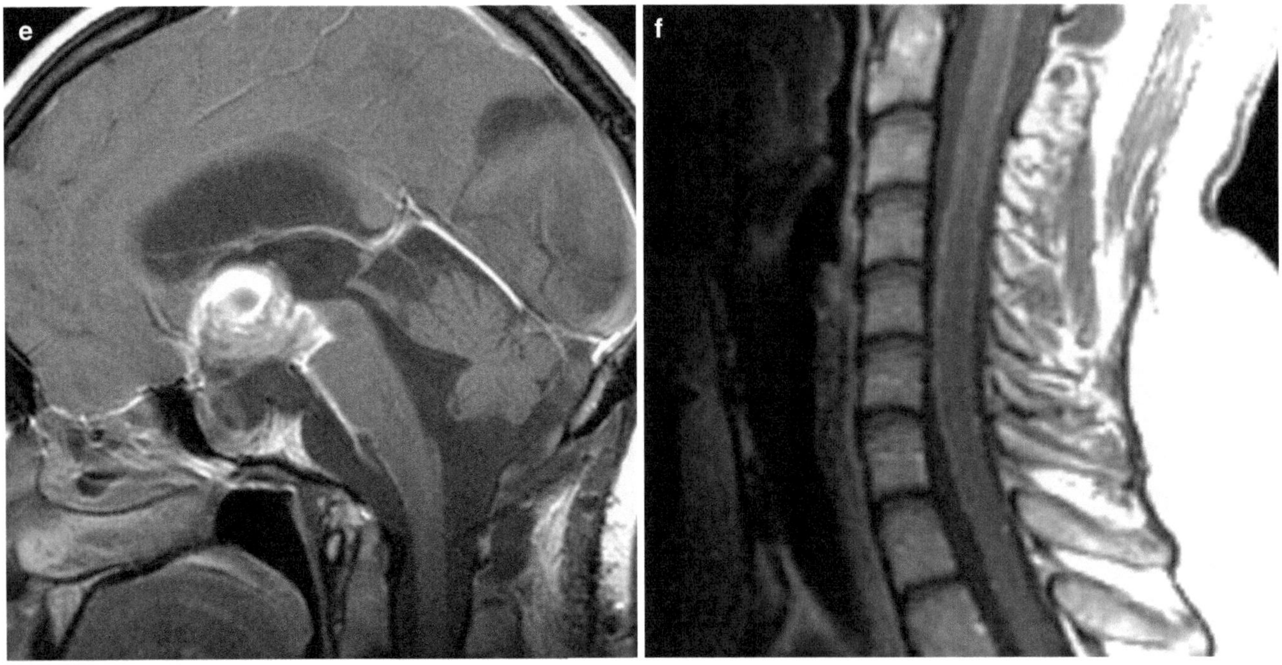

Fig. 15.85 (continued)

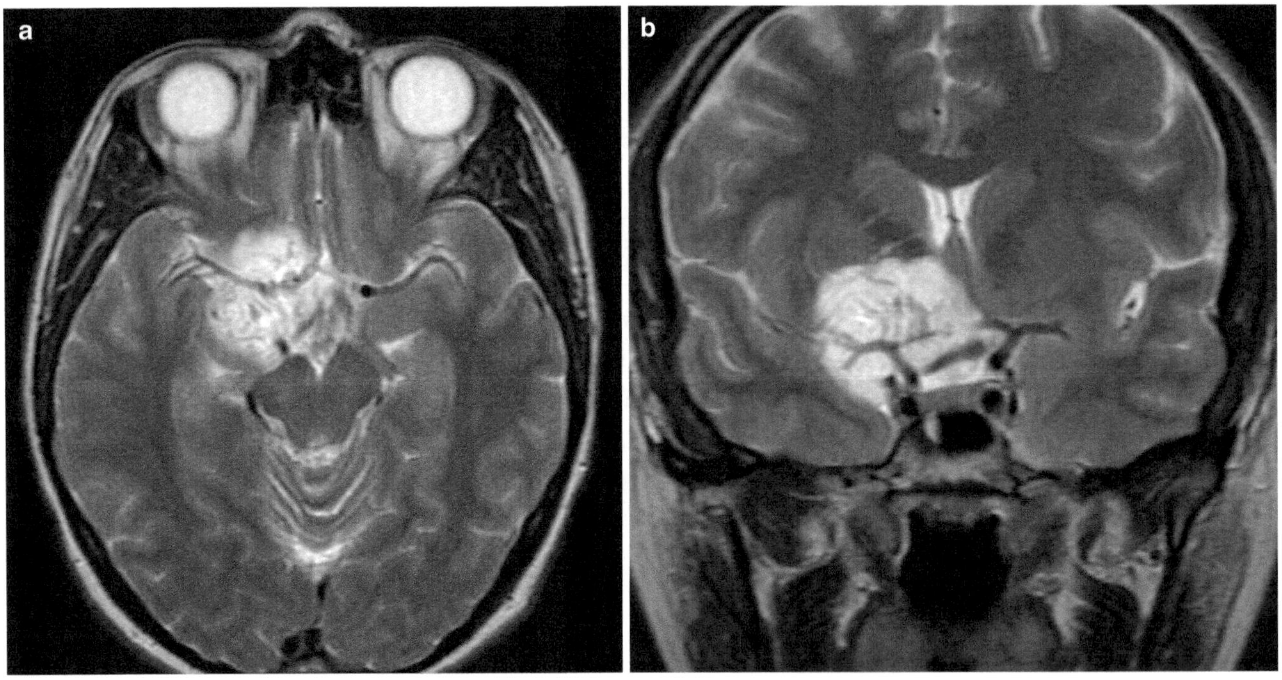

Fig. 15.86 Anaplastic astrocytoma of the medial part of the right temporal lobe invading the optic chiasm and suprasellar cistern. T2-weighted images (**a–c**) show a hyperintense tumor encasing the internal carotid, anterior and middle cerebral arteries (A1 and M1 segments, respectively). Post-contrast axial (**d**) and coronal (**e**, **f**) T1-weighted images demonstrate the intense contrast enhancement and a necrotic area in the lateral part of the tumor. The medial part of the tumor is moderately enhanced

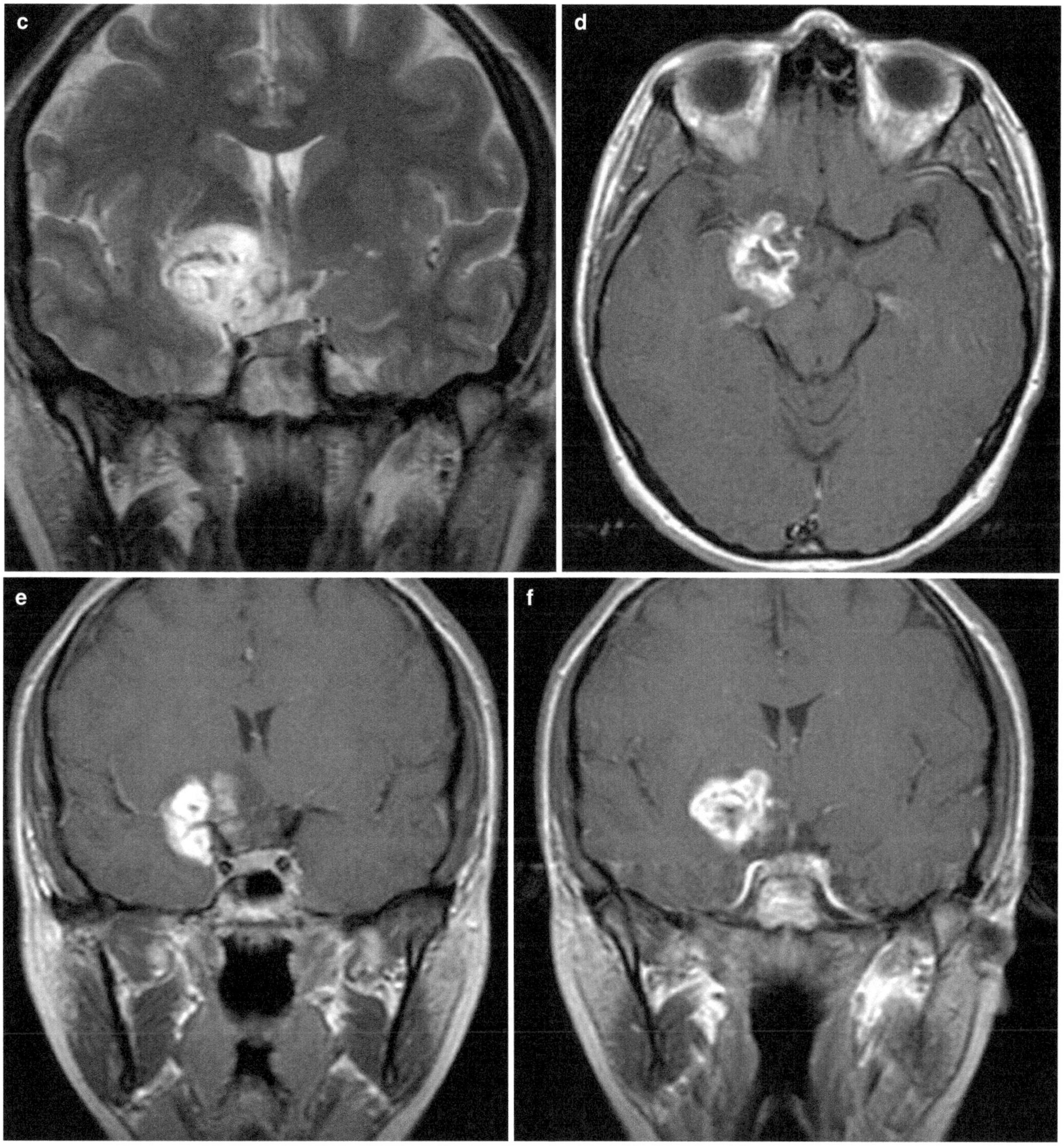

Fig. 15.86 (continued)

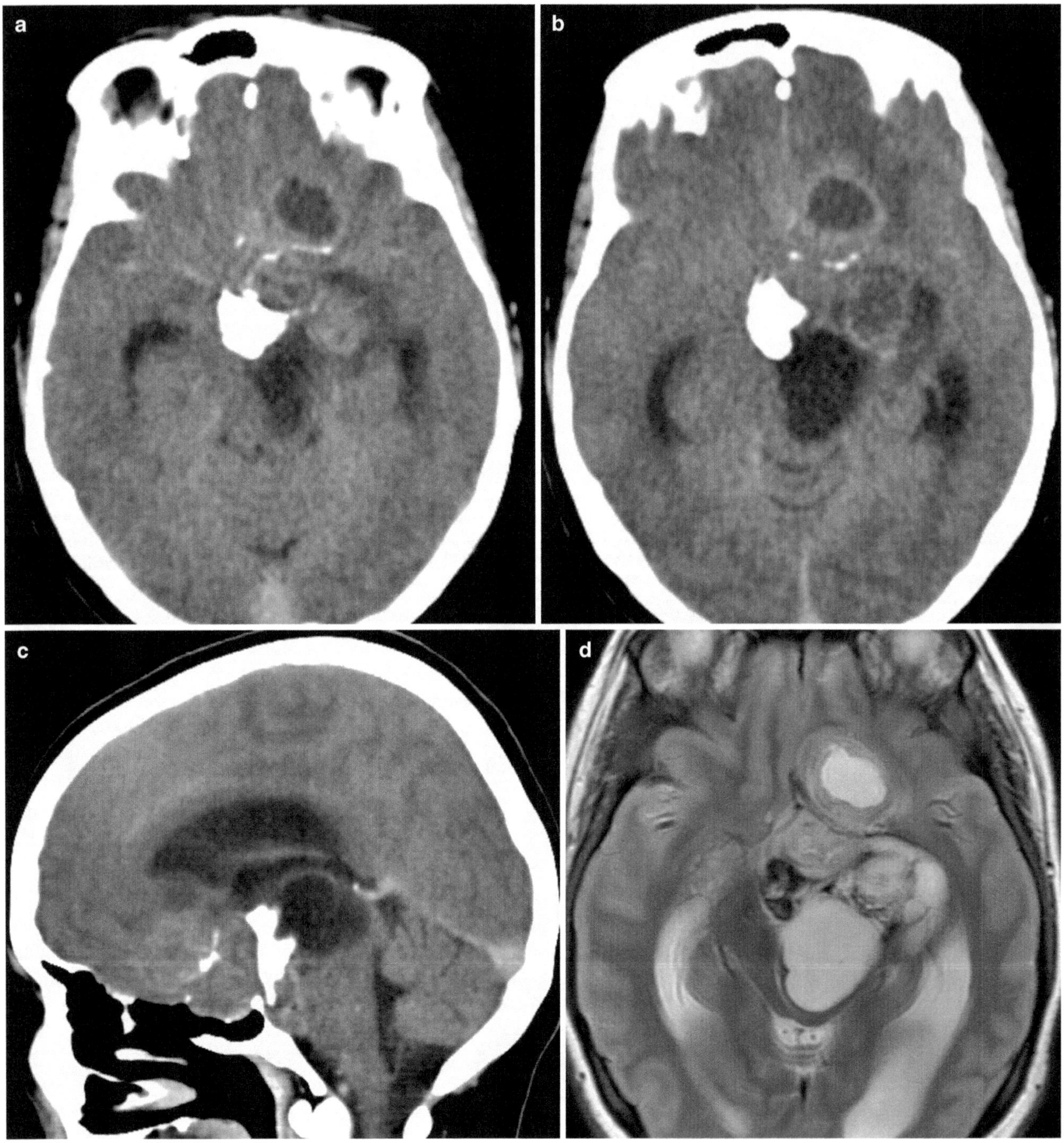

Fig. 15.87 Giant glioma of the optic chiasm and the third ventricle area (pilocytic astrocytoma). Axial CE CT scans (**a**, **b**) with sagittal reformation (**c**) demonstrate a heterogeneous tumor with multiple cysts and large calcification, a contrast enhancement is minimal. T2-weighted- (**d**), T2-FLAIR- (**e**), and T1-weighted images (**f**) show a huge heterogeneous mass with the solid and cystic components. A contrast enhancement is intensive and heterogeneous (**g–i**)

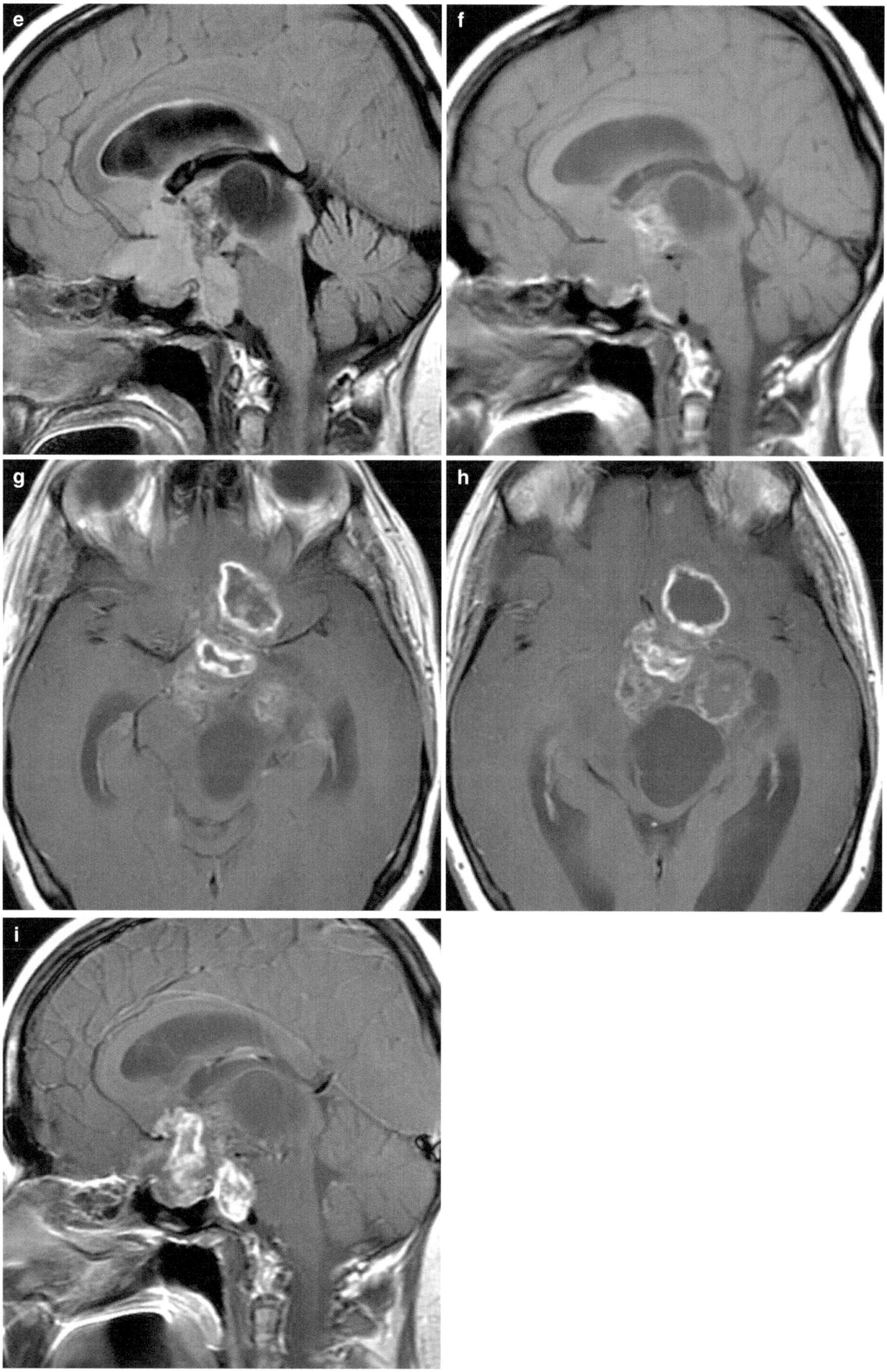

Fig. 15.87 (continued)

15.7 Germinomas

Germinoma is one of the most frequent tumors of the pineal region, and only in 20% of cases they are found in the suprasellar cistern and much less frequently in the pituitary fossa. Suprasellar germinomas may be primary and originate from the suprasellar cistern, or they may be metastases from the pineal region germinomas. Germinomas consist of large polygonal embryonic cells, accumulations of lymphocytes and thick connective tissue stroma. The suprasellar germinomas are nonencapsulated tumors with infiltrative growth; they may embed metastases into the walls of the lateral ventricles and the basal cisterns.

Germinomas are tumors of children and young adults (5–30 years). They are manifested by endocrinological dysfunction such as diabetes insipidus or panhypopituitarism. Such manifestation confirms that the tumor involves the walls of the third ventricle. Defects of visual fields and optic nerve atrophy are usual. If the CSF pathways are blocked hydrocephalus occurs. Oculomotor signs may develop if a tumor grows into the parasellar space. There is a notion of occult neurohypophyseal germinomas in literature (Kato et al. 1998). In such cases, diabetes insipidus is not accompanied by any lesion in the optic chiasm and sellar area, and thickening of the stalk without a normal MR signal from the posterior pituitary is detected. A decrease in blood growth hormone levels or an elevated in blood human chorionic gonadotropin levels can be found.

Imaging On CT without CE, germinomas are hyperdense and homogenously enhanced (Fig. 15.88). Calcifications are not usual for these tumors. Primary germinoma of the pineal region may be identified. The described characteristics are similar to those of lymphoma, differences can include age, clinical history and presence of a tumor in the pineal region.

Most of suprasellar germinomas are clearly detected on MRI, as their sizes are usually large by the time clinical manifestations occur. They are typically located along the median axis in the floor of the third ventricle. In contrast to craniopharyngiomas, the structure of germinomas is homogenous, and only in rare cases are small cysts revealed in a tumor stroma, usually located on the periphery. The signal of germinomas moderately differs from that of brain tissue. Germinomas are iso- or mildly hypointense on T1-weighted images and are iso- or hyperintense on T2-weighted images (Figs. 15.89 and 15.90). Usually, germinomas strongly enhance (Fig. 15.91) and metastases may be revealed along the lateral ventricles ependyma and in the subarachnoid space. In case of a tumor hemorrhage, preferable is the use of 3D gradient echo sequence (SWAN, SWI). In such cases, the tumors become markedly hypointense (Fig. 15.92).

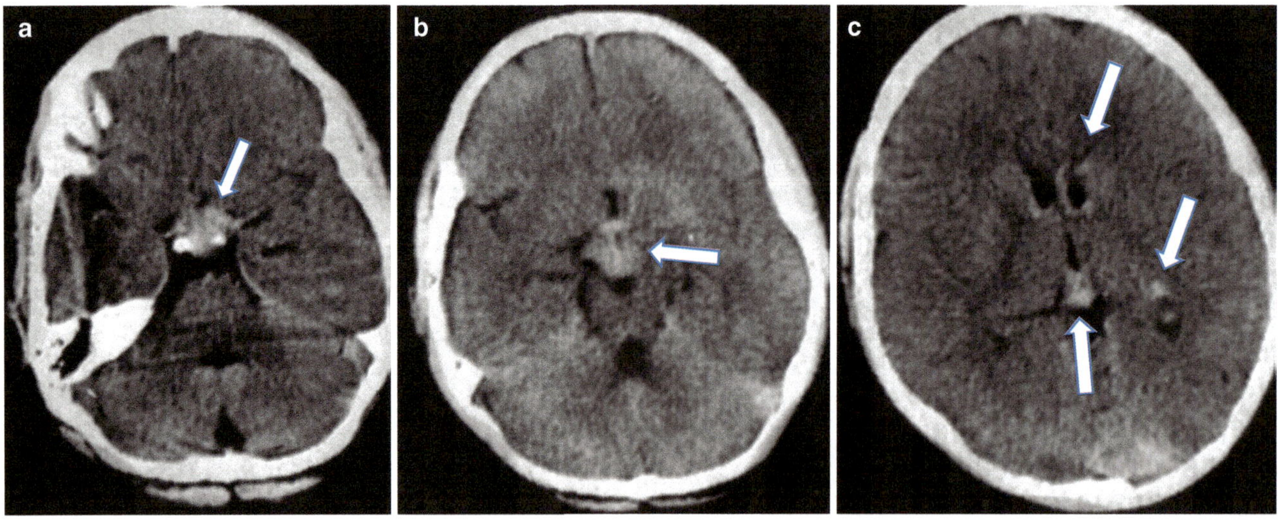

Fig. 15.88 Germinoma of the pineal region with dissemination into the suprasellar region and lateral ventricles. CE CT scans (**a**–**c**) show multiple foci of the contrast enhancement (*arrows*)—tumor in pineal region and metastases

Fig. 15.89 Germinoma in the suprasellar region. Sagittal (**a**) and coronal (**b**) T1-weighted images detect intra-suprasellar tumor, which mimics a pituitary adenoma

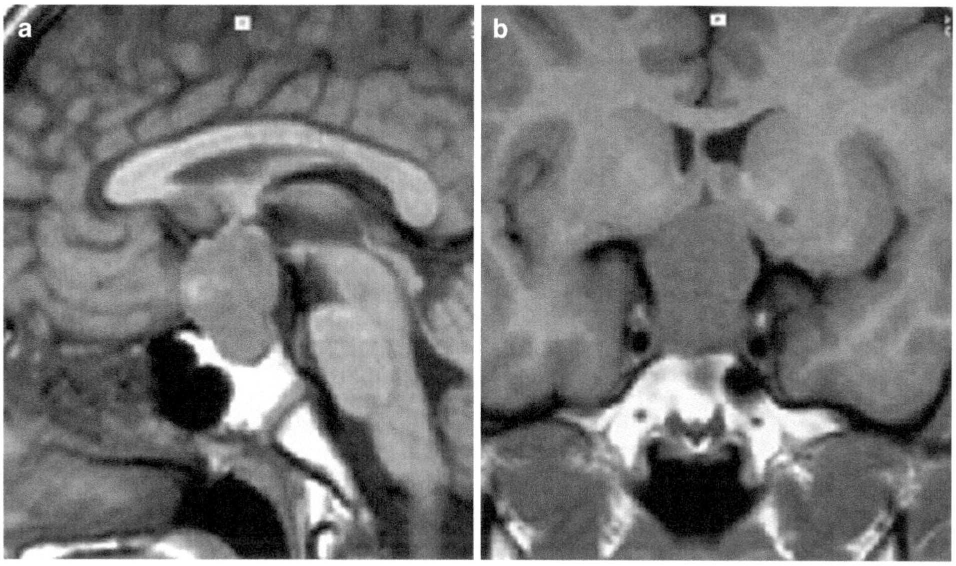

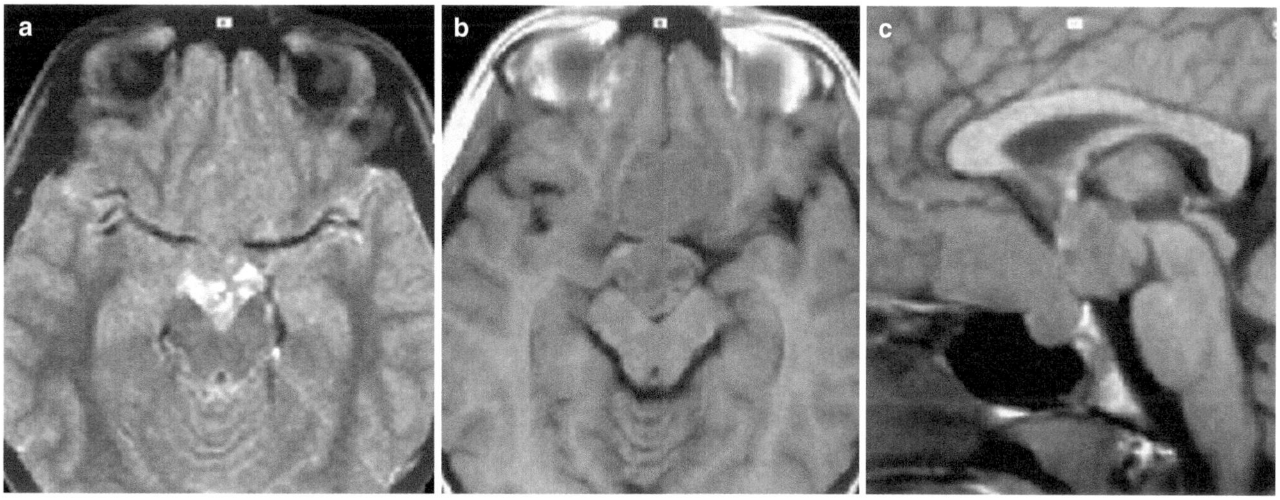

Fig. 15.90 Germinoma of the sellar, supra-ante-retrosellar region. A tumor has isointense MR-signal on T2-weighted image (**a**) and poorly visualized. T1-weighted images (**b**, **c**) show a hypointense signal from the tumor relative to white matter

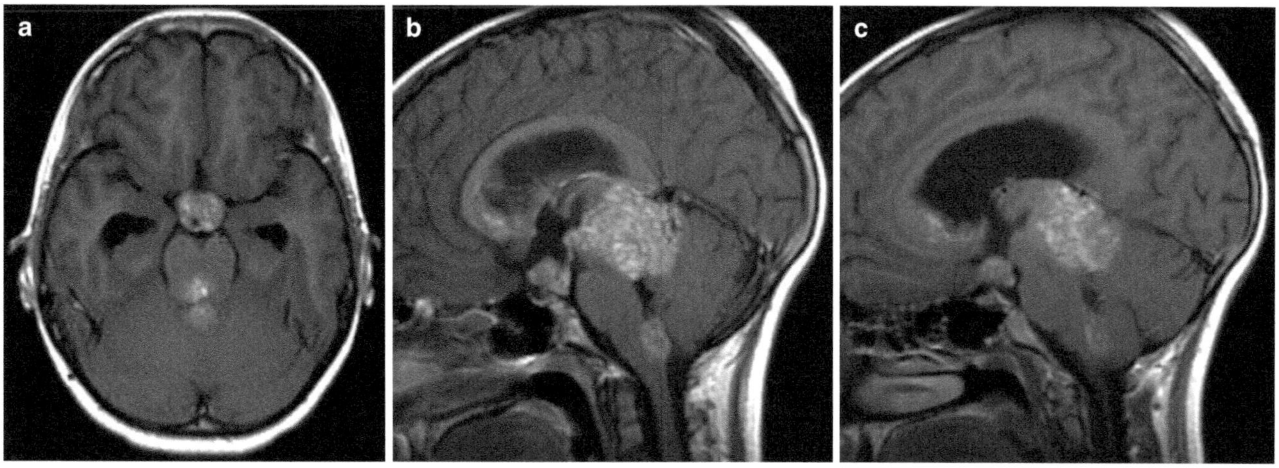

Fig. 15.91 Giant germinoma of the pineal and suprasellar region with metastases into the lateral, third, and fourth ventricles. Post-contrast axial (**a**) and sagittal T1-weighted images (**b**, **c**) reveal multiple mass with uniform enhancement

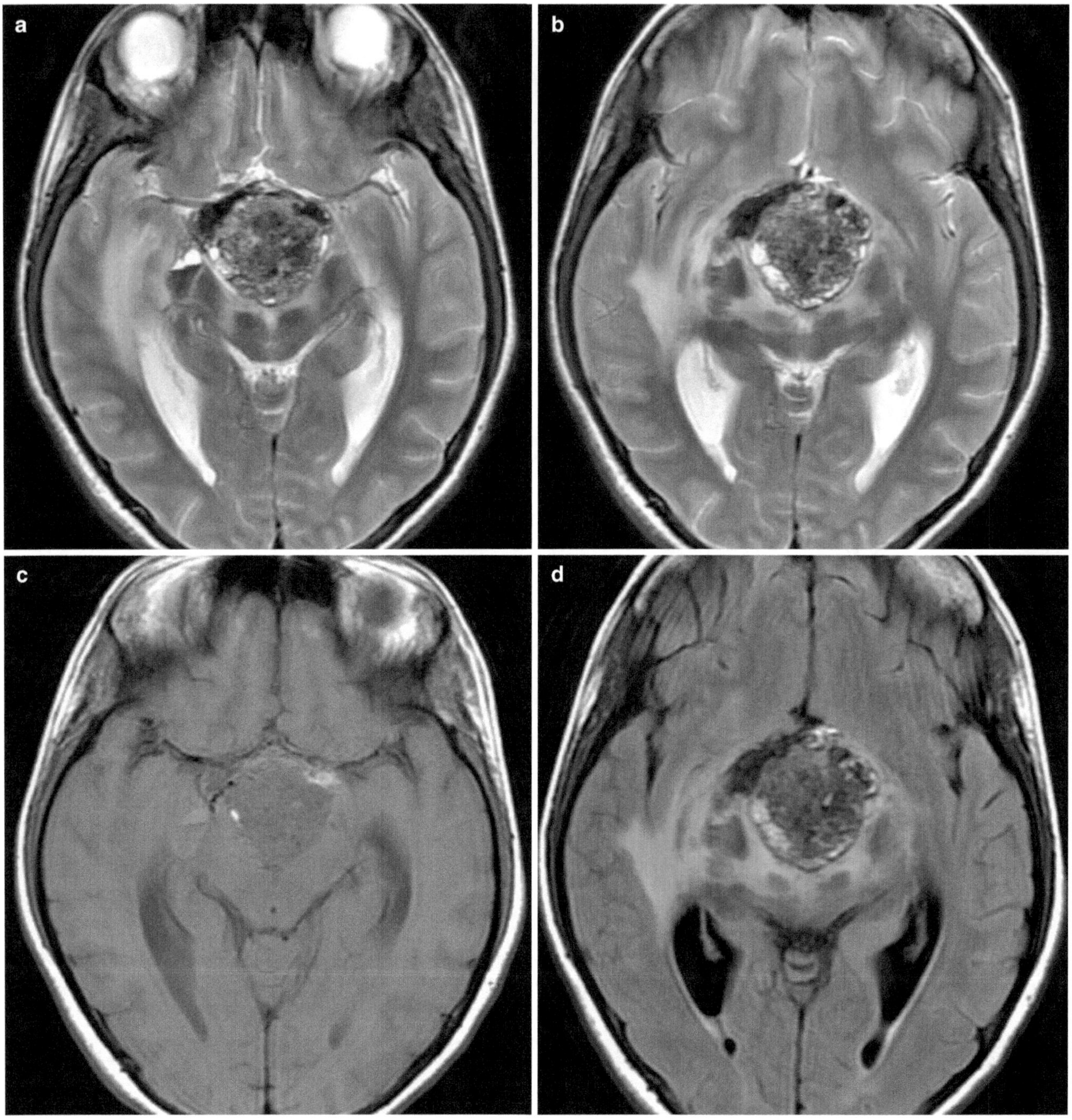

Fig. 15.92 Germinoma of the suprasellar area with hemorrhages. T2-weighted (**a**, **b**), T1-weighted images (**c**), T2-FLAIR (**d**) reveal a heterogeneous tumor with subacute hemorrhages visible on T1-weighted image (a hyperintense signal) and peritumoral edema (hypointense signal) on T2-weighted and T2-FLAIR images. On T2* (SWAN) image (**e**) a germinoma is strongly hypointense due to chronic hemorrhages. Contrast enhancement is moderate and heterogeneous (**f**)

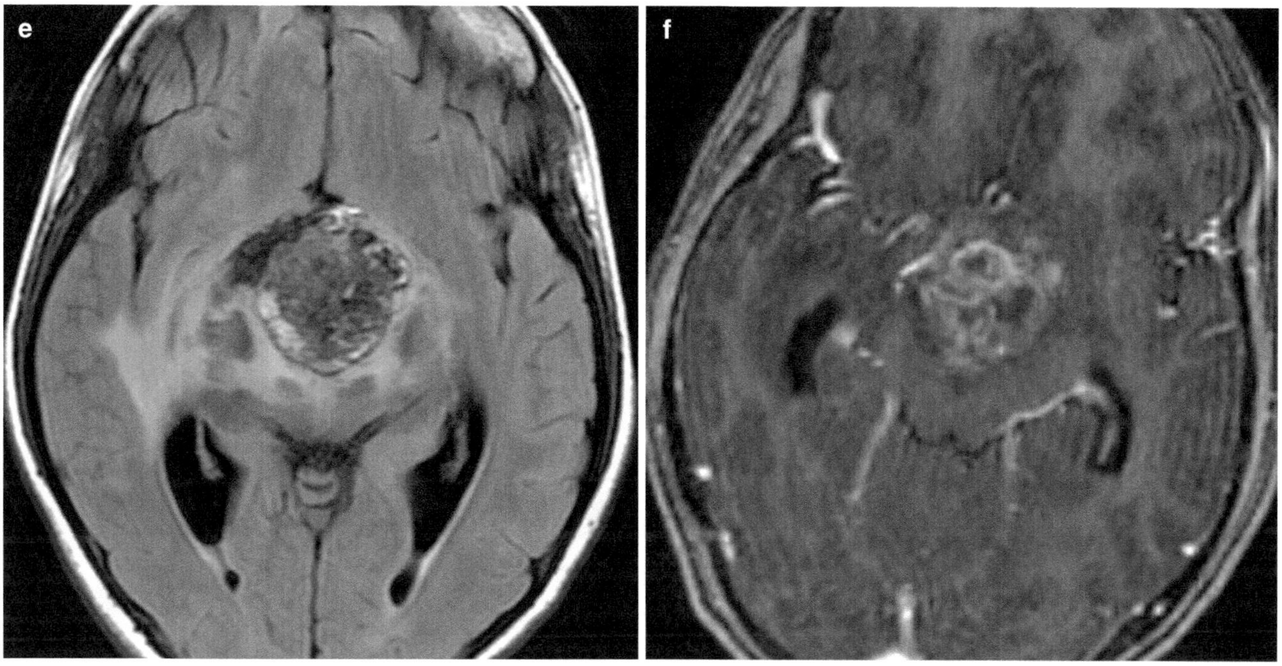

Fig. 15.92 (continued)

15.8 Schwannomas (Neurinomas)

Schwannomas (neurinomas and neurilemmomas) account for approximately one third of primary tumors of the trigeminal nerve and tumors of Meckel cavity (Yuh et al. 1988). Specifically, they make up less than 0.4% of all primary brain tumors. Schwannomas of the third, fourth, and sixth cranial nerves are less frequently observed. More frequently, schwannomas affecting the central part of the skull base and the cavernous sinus are tumors of the trigeminal nerve. As these tumors may originate from any part of the nerve between the root and the terminal extracranial branches, their clinical manifestations and neuroimaging findings differ depending on the direction and the growth of a tumor.

The most frequent clinical manifestation is sensory loss within the innervation area of the affected cranial nerve. Weakness of mastication muscles and facial pain are less frequently found. Due to compression of the adjacent cranial nerves, diplopia may ensue. The most typical growth of schwannomas is a growth along an affected nerve.

Imaging Schwannomas are isodense on routine CT scans, and hyperdense after CE, CT, especially with bone window mode, is more helpful in the assessment of erosion of the pyramid apical part at the typical site of the trigeminal ganglion. This fact supports the long-term growth of benign tumors. Contrast enhancement helps determine the shape and typical expansion along the nerve. All solid schwannomas intensively, but not homogeneously enhance. Contrast enhancement of cystic forms of schwannomas is peripheral. The Meckel cave on the affected side is usually not visualized. On CT-perfusion studies, schwannomas with this localization have typical features for the group of nerve root tumors with relatively low CBV and CBF values and increased MTT. Hemodynamic characteristics of schwannomas are important in differential diagnosis with the cavernous sinus meningiomas (Figs. 15.93, 15.94, and 15.95).

On MRI schwannomas are hypo- or isointense to brain tissue on T1-weighted imaging and hyperintense on T2-weighted imaging. Neurofibromas on T2-weighted sequences are characterized by hypointense MR signal, while schwannomas are usually hyperintense. Small tumors are homogenous, and larger ones usually have heterogeneous signal intensity (due to large or small cysts). Multiplanar MRI is helpful to identify a tumor extension. With meningiomas, neurinomas intensively accumulate contrast medium. Clinical symptoms, the structure of schwannoma and CT-perfusion parameters are useful in the differential diagnosis with meningiomas. A possibility of using MR-perfusion is limited due to artifacts from the bones of the skull base (Figs. 15.96, 15.97, 15.98, 15.99, 15.100, and 15.101).

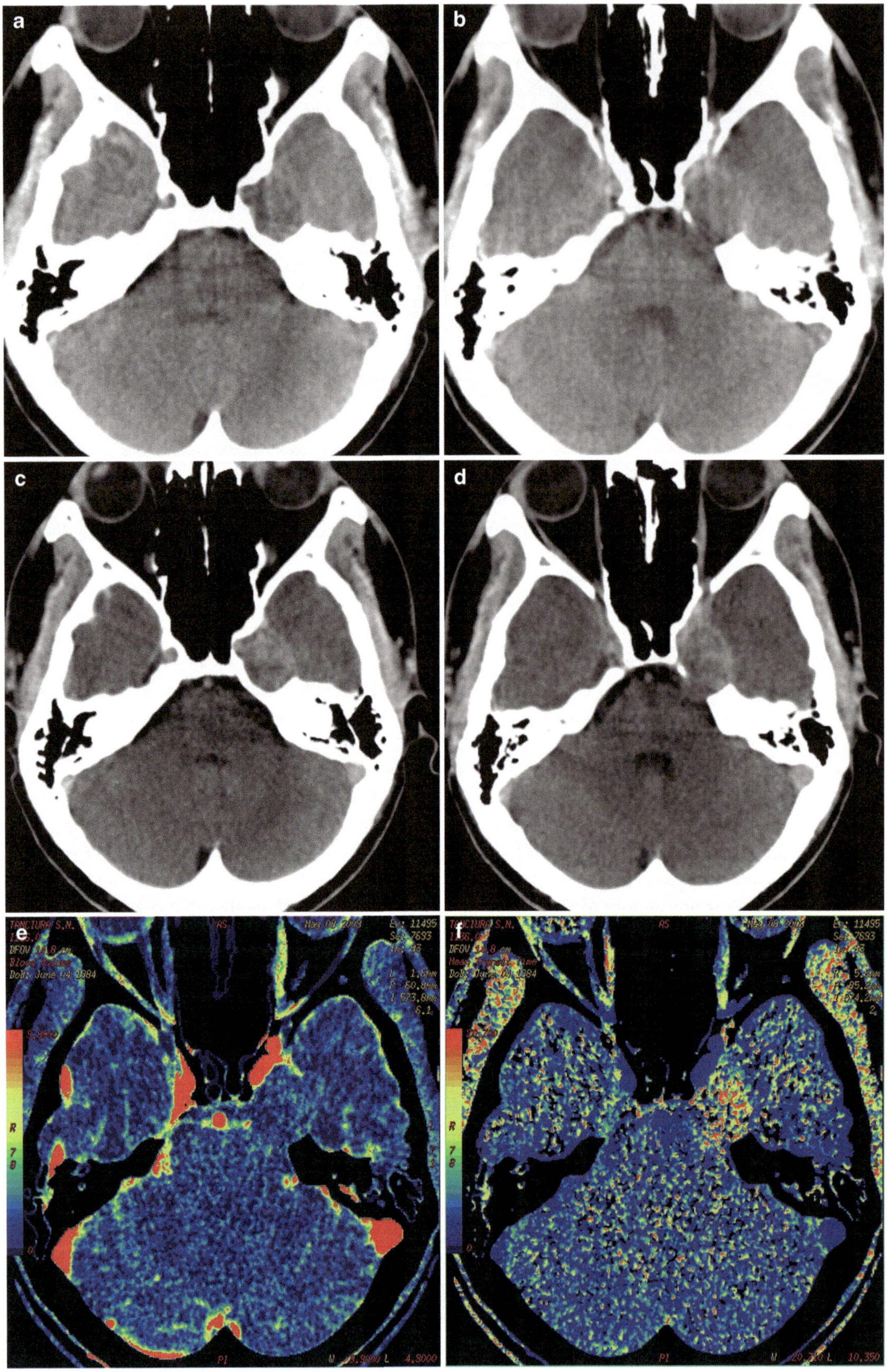

Fig. 15.93 Left trigeminal nerve schwannoma. CT scans before (**a**, **b**) and after CE (**c**, **d**) show a moderately and heterogeneously enhancing tumor originates from trigeminal cave. A tumor erodes the apex of pyramid and medial part of the sphenoid bone. Perfusion CT study reveals a similar to the brain CBV (**e**) and prolonged MTT (**f**)

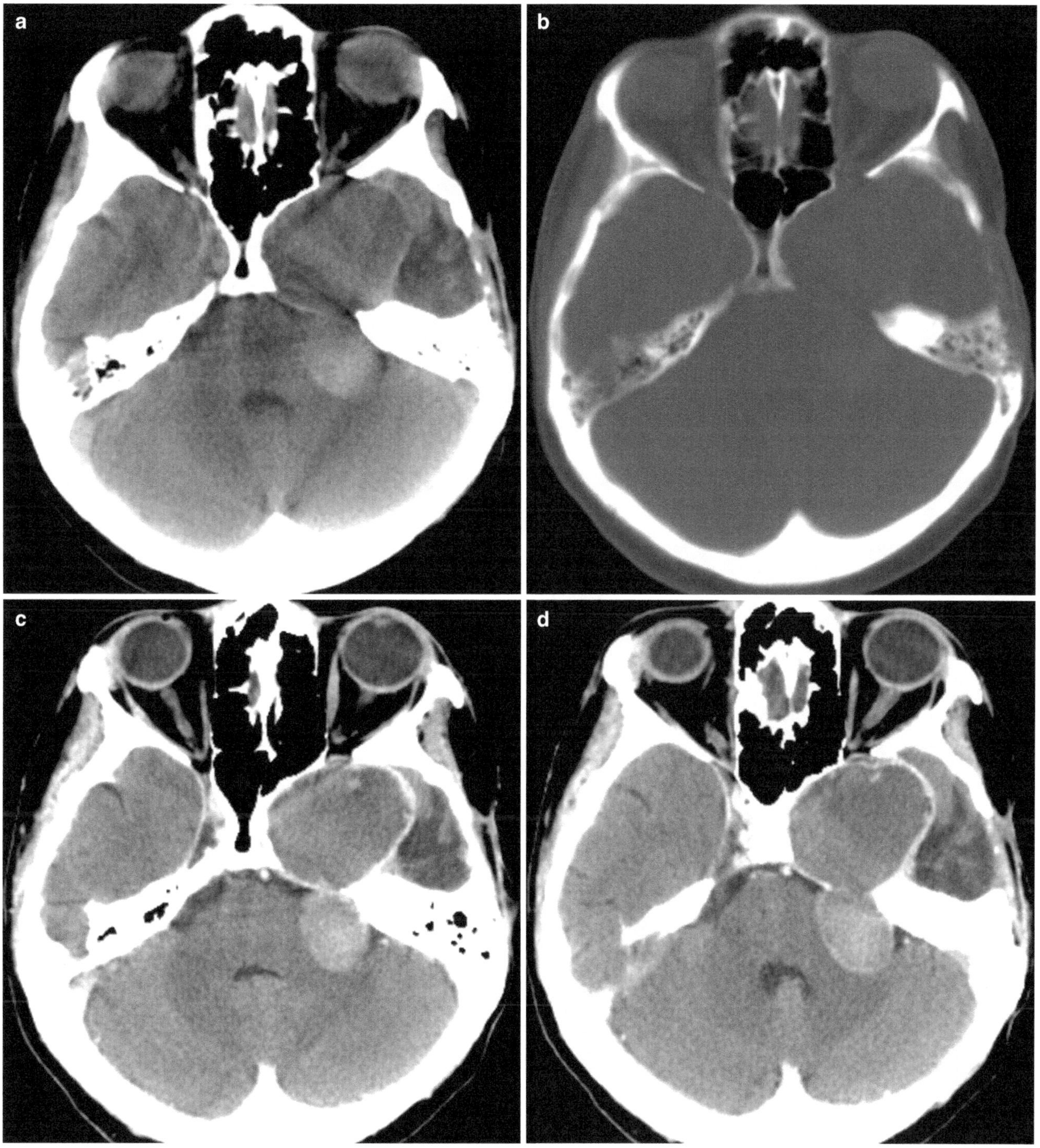

Fig. 15.94 Giant schwannoma of the left trigeminal nerve with spreading into the middle and posterior cranial fossae. Axial CT scan (**a**) and image in bone window (**b**) shows a large hyper- and hypodense tumor, which eroded the sphenoid bone and apex of the pyramid on the left. A subtentorial part of the tumor is hyperdense due to hemorrhage. CE CT scans (**c–d**) detect a prominent enhancement by tumor capsule. A cystic structure in the center doesn't enhance

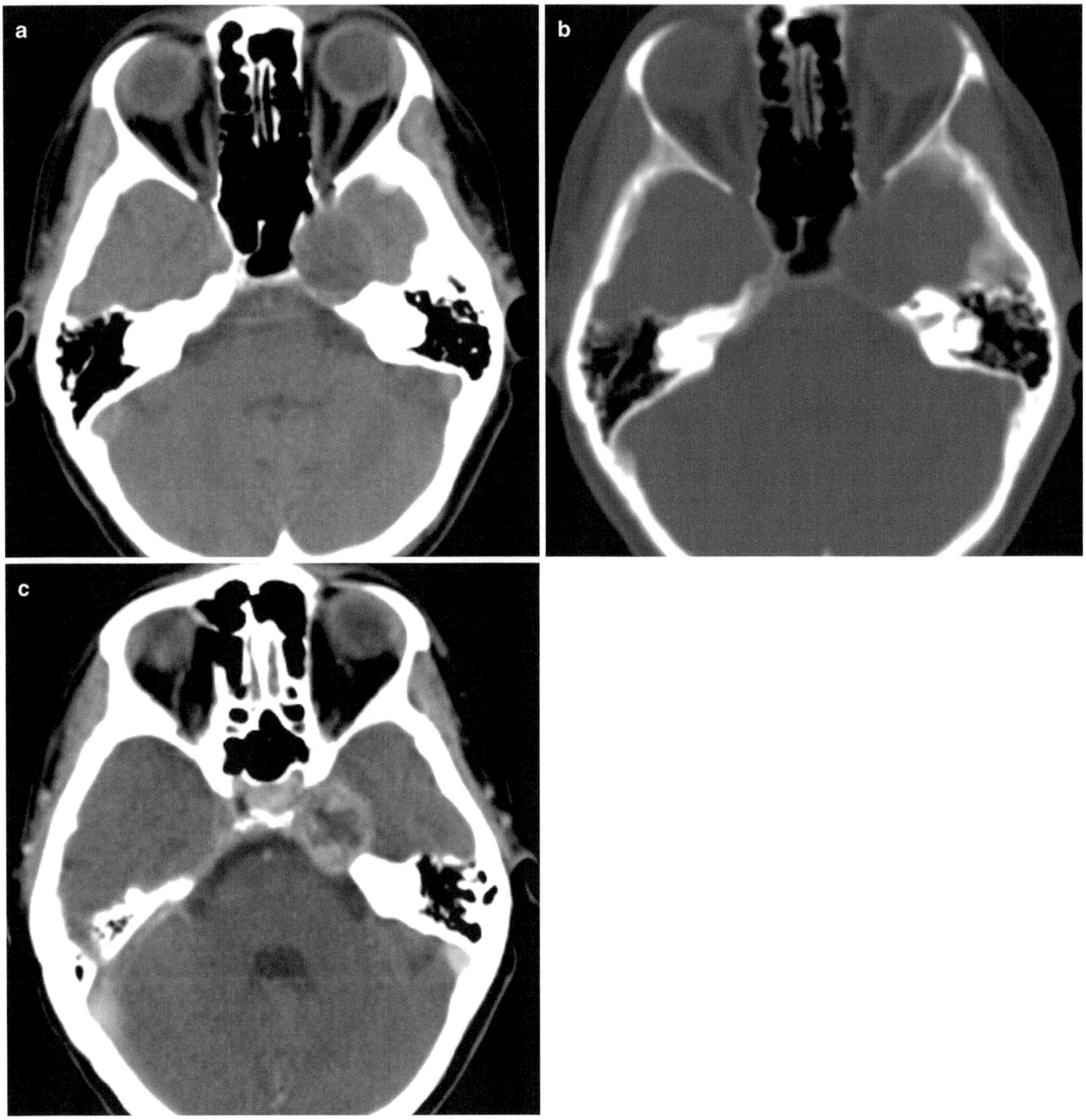

Fig. 15.95 Schwannoma of the left trigeminal nerve. CT scan (**a**) shows a hypodense tumor relative to brain in the trigeminal cave area. On CT scan in bone window mode (**b**) the expansive bone changes of the temporal bone pyramid are visualized. CE CT scan (**c**) demonstrates a heterogeneous (peripheral) contrast enhancement

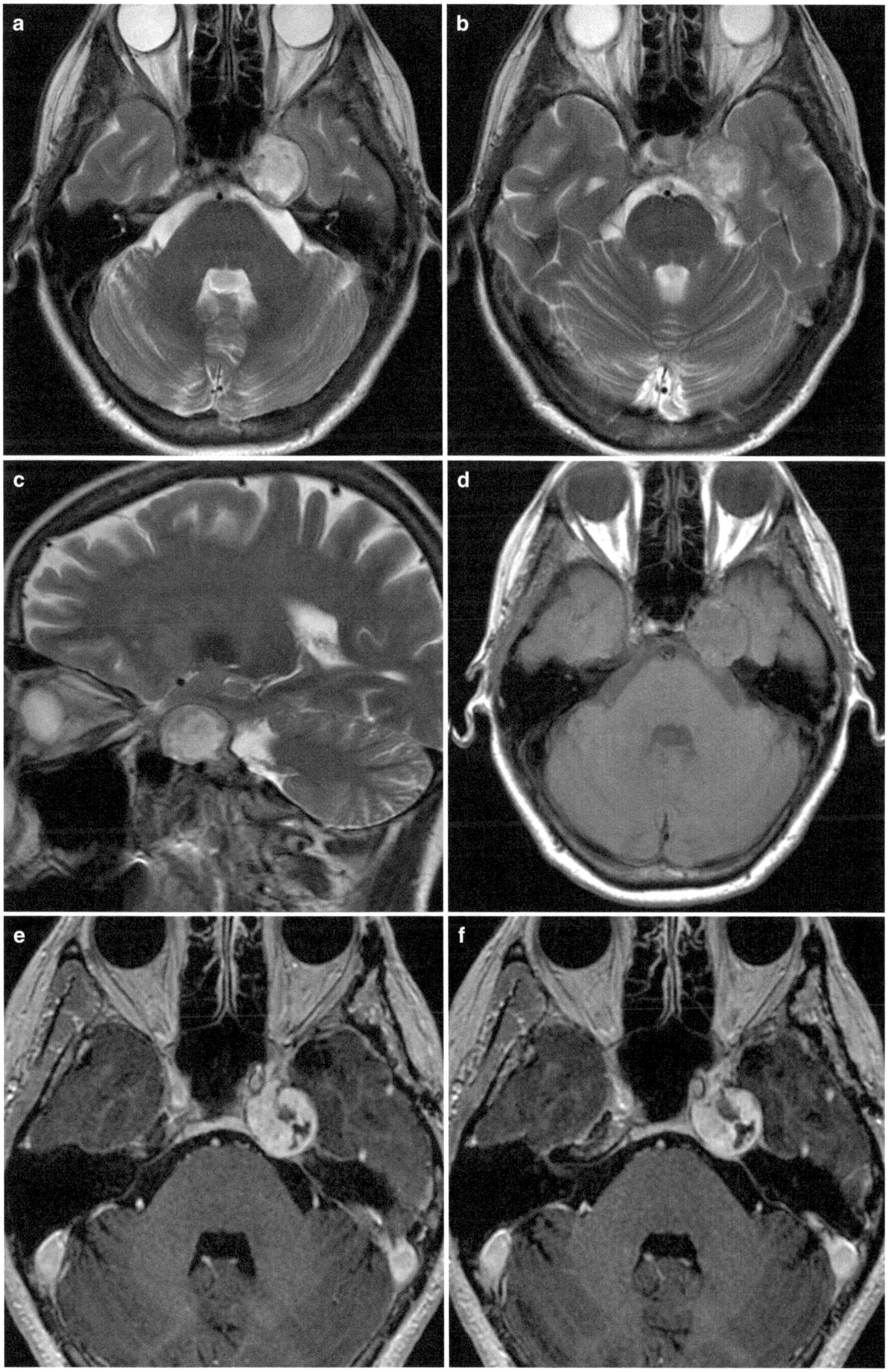

Fig. 15.96 Schwannoma in the left trigeminal cave area. T2-weighted images (**a–c**), T1-weighted images before (**d**) and after contrast enhancement (**e**, **f**). In the left trigeminal cave area a small heterogeneous tumor with intensive and heterogeneous enhancement is detected

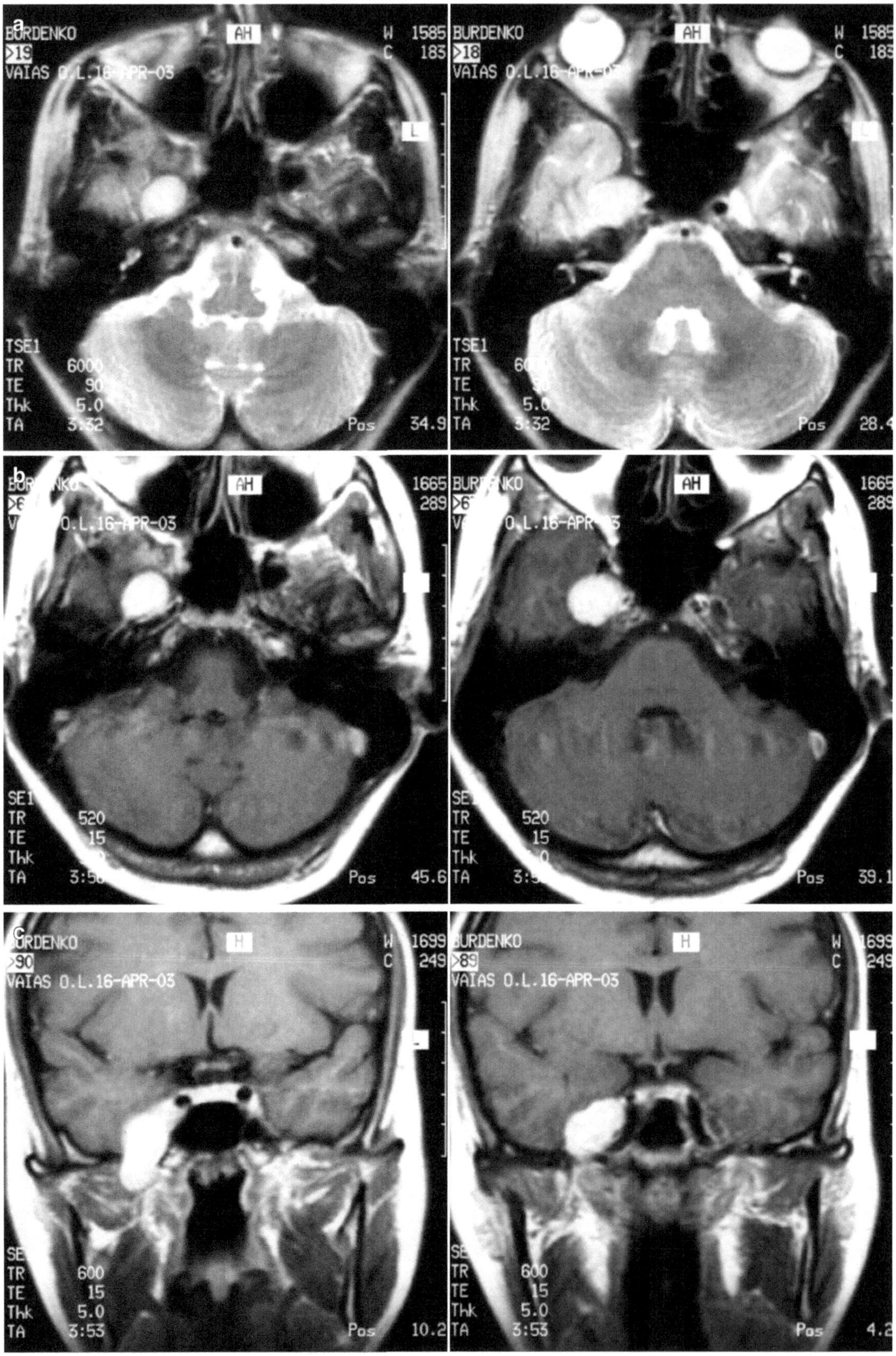

Fig. 15.97 Schwannoma of the right trigeminal nerve extending into the foramen ovale. A tumor has an increased MR-signal on T2-weighted image (**a**) and an intense homogeneous enhancement (**b**, **c**). Coronal T1-weighted image (**c**) clearly demonstrates an extracranial spreading of the schwannoma

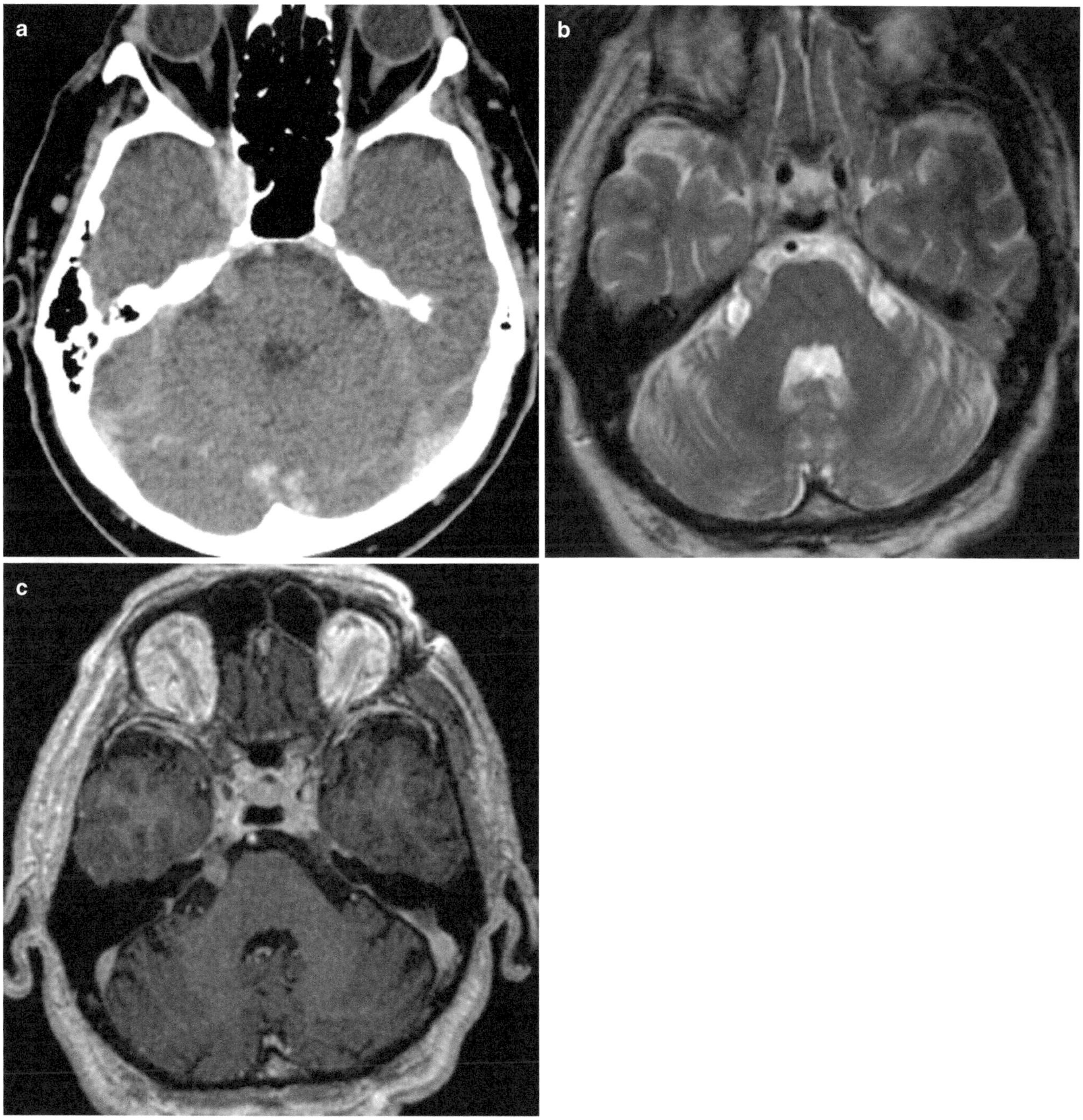

Fig. 15.98 Schwannoma of the right trigeminal nerve. CE CT scan (**a**) demonstrates a small enhancing schwannoma of the CN5 root in the lateral cistern of the pons. Axial T2 (**b**) and post-contrast T1-weighted images (**c**) add information regarding tumor location

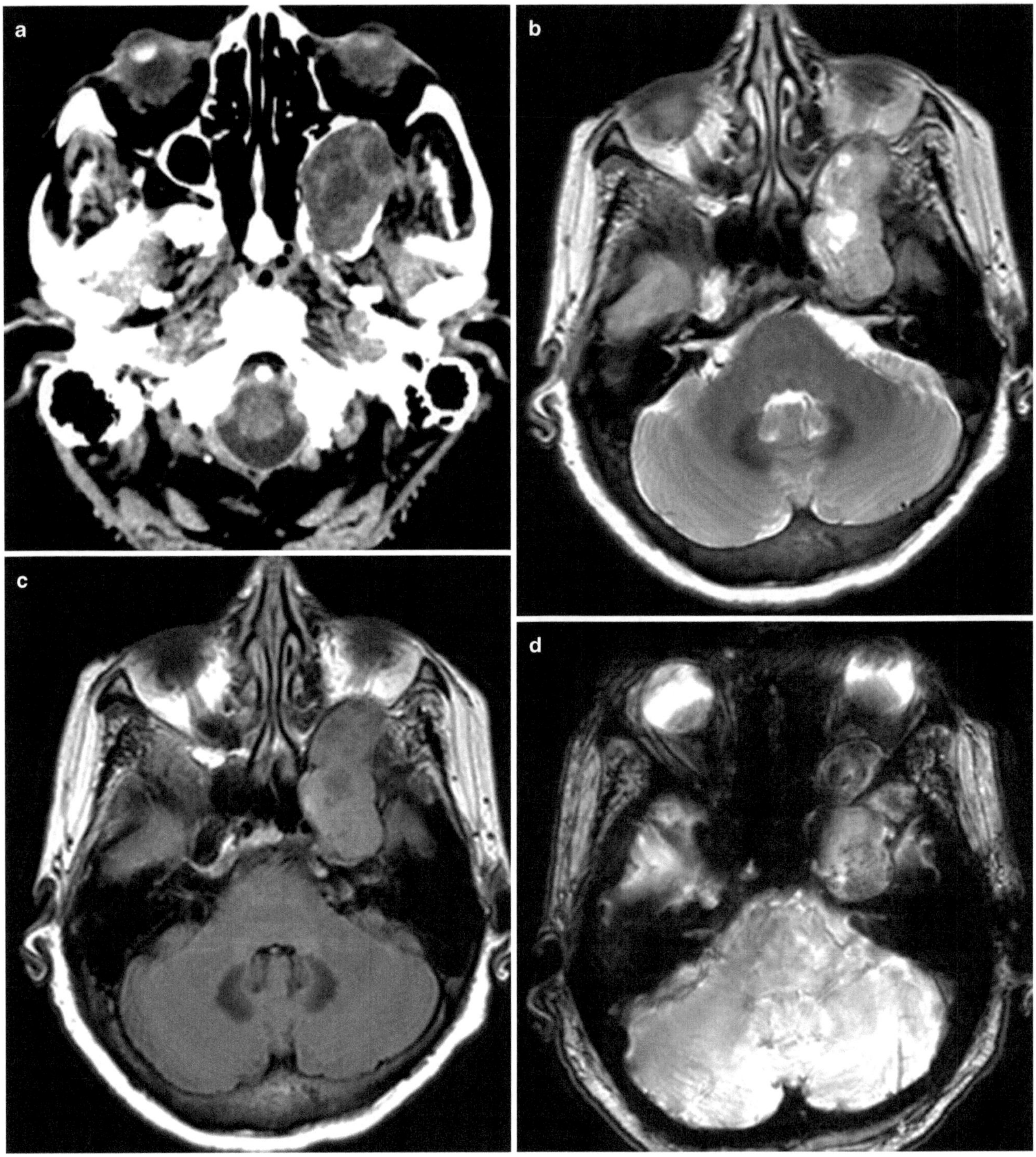

Fig. 15.99 Large schwannoma of the left trigeminal nerve extending into the middle cranial, infratemporal, pterygopalatine fossae and to the orbit. Axial CT scan (**a**), T2-weighted image (**b**), T2-FLAIR (**c**) and T2* (SWAN) (**d**) reveal a large tumor isointense to brain. A tumor has many hypointense petechial hemorrhages (**d**). A tumor is characterized by an intense and heterogeneous enhancement that clarifies of the structure and extending of the lesion (**e**, **f**)

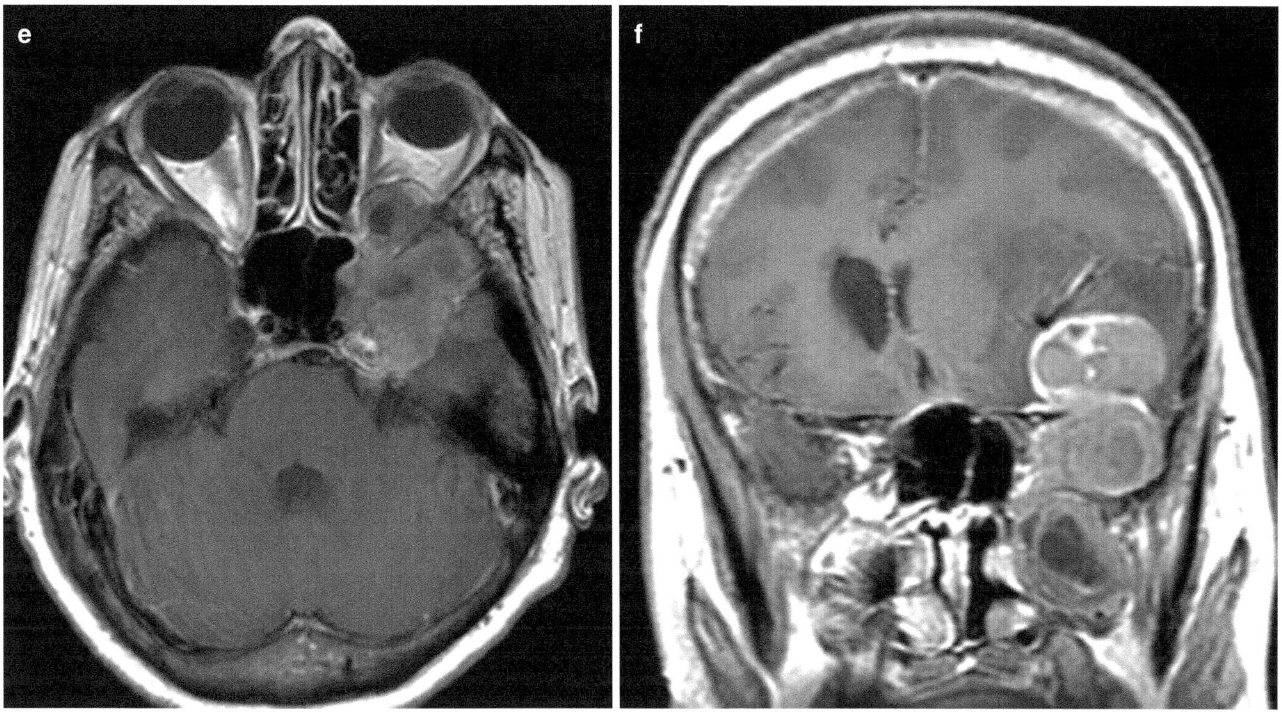

Fig. 15.99 (continued)

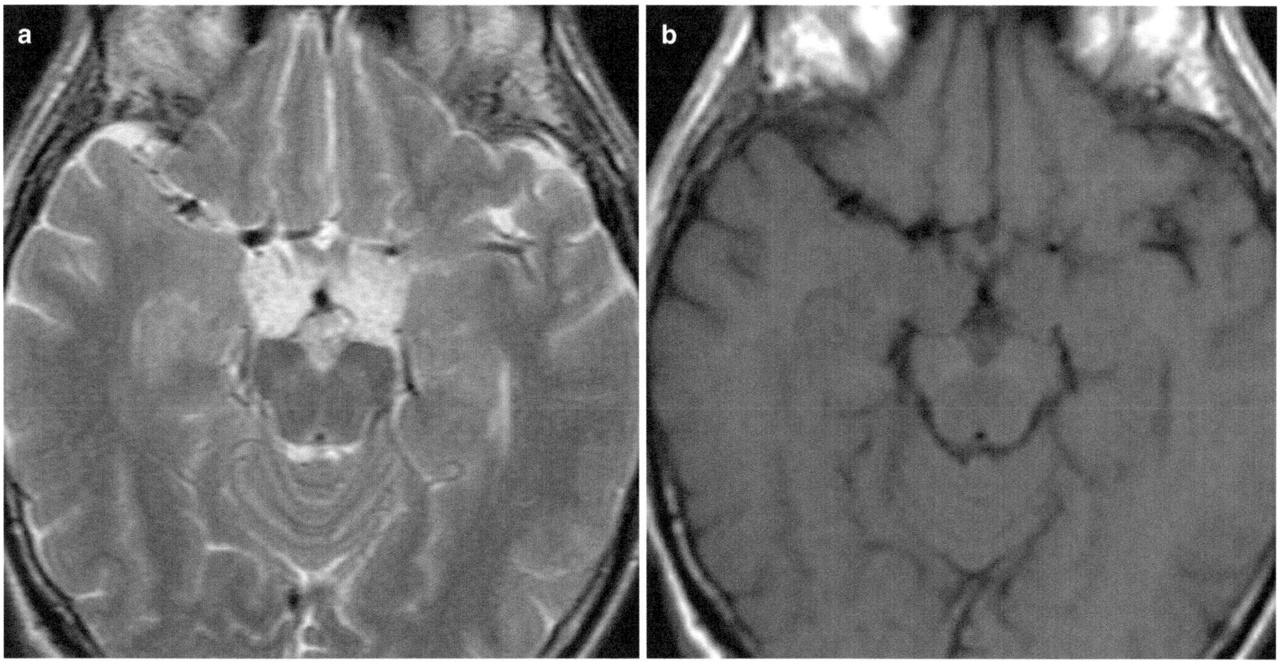

Fig. 15.100 Bilateral schwannomas of the oculomotor nerves. The disease was manifested in the childhood by divergent strabismus, which is slowly progressed. Axial T2-weighted (**a**), T1-weighted images before (**b**) and after CE (**c**) reveal the two suprasellar tumors with irregular shape, which are located along oculomotor nerve. The tumors are intensively and homogeneously enhanced

Fig. 15.100 (continued)

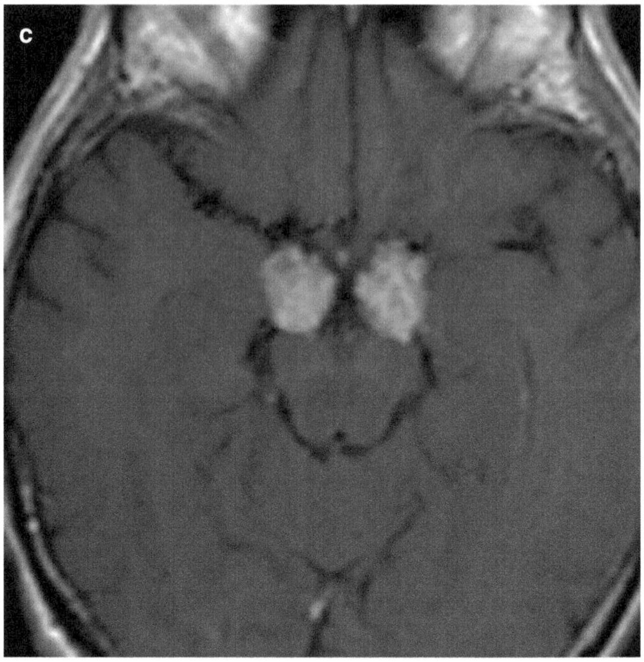

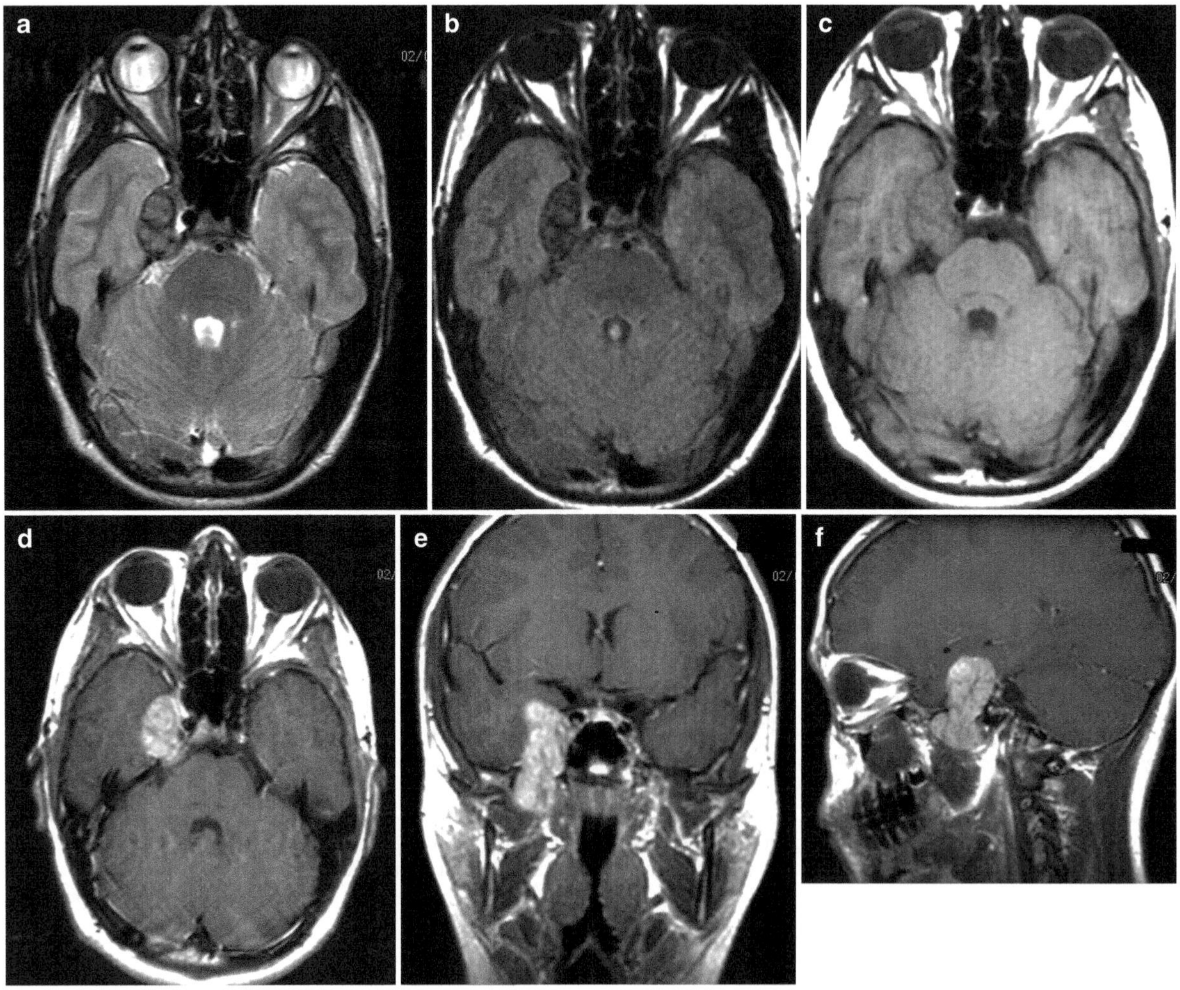

Fig. 15.101 Neurofibroma in the right trigeminal cave extending into the middle cranial fossa. A tumor is hypointense on T2-weighted (**a**) and T2-FLAIR (**b**) images and isointense on T1-weighted image (**c**). Neurofibroma is characterized by intense and homogeneous enhancement (**d**–**f**). Coronal MRI is clearly visualized the extracranial extending of the tumor along the third branch of the trigeminal nerve

15.9 Metastases

In 1–5% of cancer patients with symptomatic metastases latter in the pituitary gland are found (Kucharczyk and Montanera 1991). Prostate, lung, and breast cancers spread metastases to the skull base more frequently. Metastases from prostate cancer are osteoplastic and may mimic meningiomas, whereas metastases of lung cancer and breast cancer are usually osteolytic. Metastases in the pituitary affect the posterior lobe and infundibulum more frequently than the anterior lobe, which may be due to the direct blood supply of neurohypophysis. Pathological studies reveal high incidence of pituitary involvement—up to 28.1% of all brain metastases; however, these lesions are small and often asymptomatic.

Imaging A number of both clinical and diagnostic criteria should be taken into account in assessing the radiological picture of secondary focal lesions in the chiasmal-sellar region. Age and presence of extra- and intracranial malignancies must be taken into account, especially if there is an evidence of a primary tumor. It is advisable to perform blood tests for tumor markers (e.g., α-fetoprotein, etc.) to rule out germ cell neoplasms. Although radiological manifestations of metastatic lesions in the chiasmal-sellar region have no specific features, in most cases, metastases on CT and MRI appear as solid tumors. They are iso- or hyperdense on CT images, usually isointense on T1-weighted images and iso-hypointense on T2-weighted images. When the tumor is located in the floor of the third ventricle area and in the hypothalamus, a perifocal edema due to local invasion of the surrounding brain can be visualized on T2-weighted and T2-FLAIR images (Fig. 15.102). In case of primary sellar invasion, the tumor typically grows into the suprasellar region, acquiring a dumbbell shape with the presence of both sellar and suprasellar components. The sella turcica may partially enlarge, but not as much as with pituitary adenomas. In case of a suprasellar location, the tumor compresses the contents of the sella turcica. This is best determined on coronal MR images.

The metastasis stroma contains no calcifications, which distinguishes these tumors from craniopharyngioma. Approximately 1/3 of cases on T2- and T1-weighted images, microhemorrhagic inclusions can be visualized in the tumor (Fig. 15.103). Metastatic lesions in almost 100% of cases are

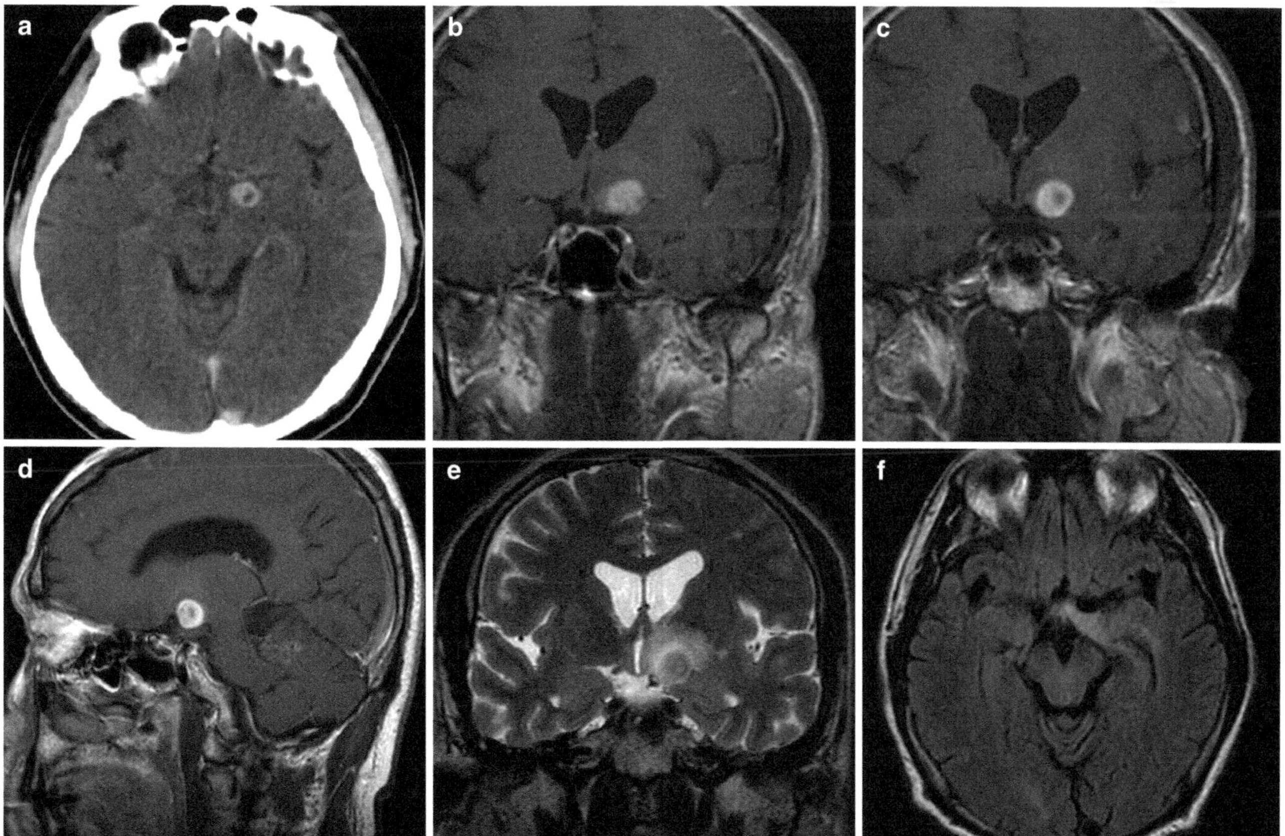

Fig. 15.102 Solitary metastasis from lung carcinoma in the hypothalamic region on the left. The lesion is characterized by intense enhancement on CT scan (**a**) and on MR T1-weighted images (**b–d**). Surrounding edema is better visualized on T2-weighted (**e**) and T2-FLAIR (**f**) images

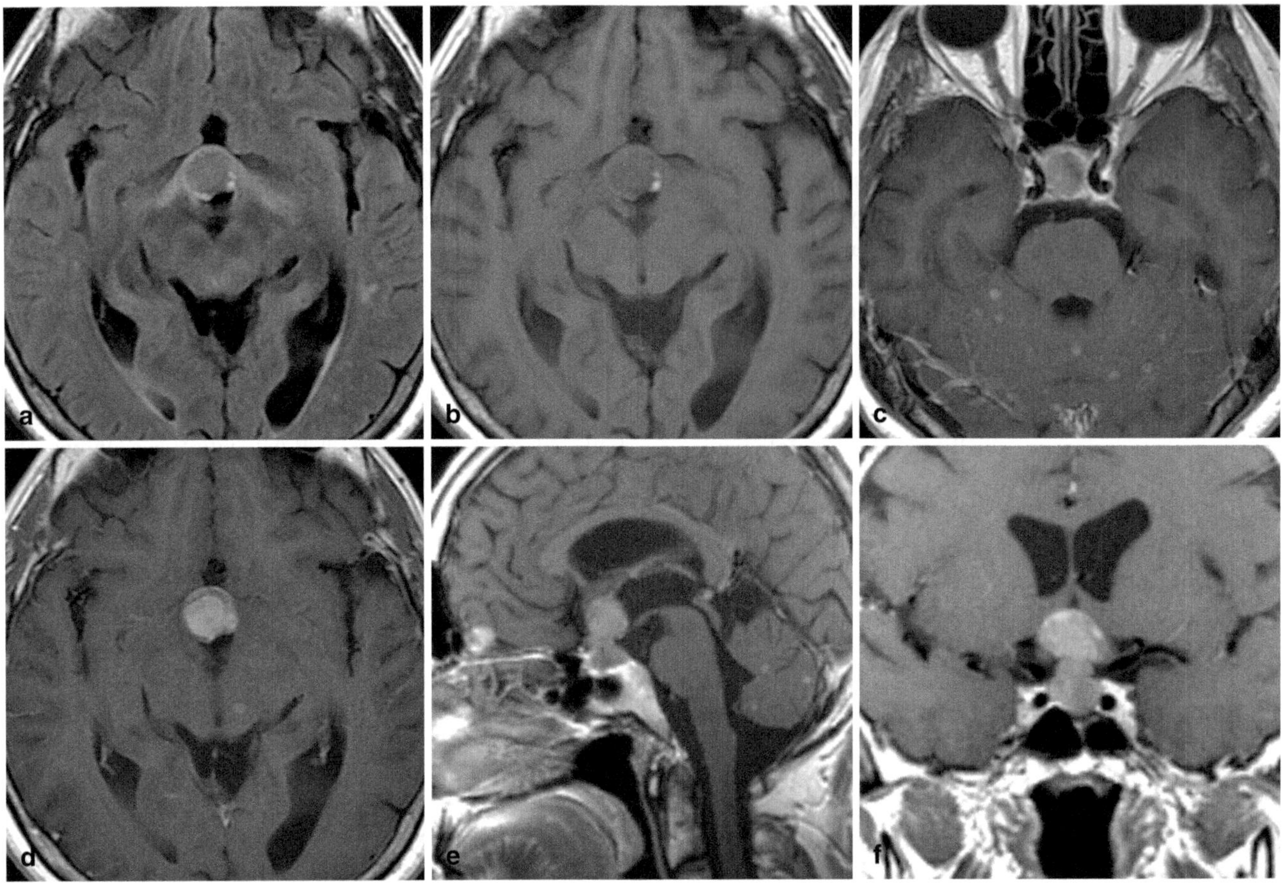

Fig. 15.103 Multiple metastases from breast carcinoma. Axial T2-FLAIR (**a**) and T1-weighted images (**b**) show a heterogeneous tumor in the infundibulum stalk area with small hemorrhages (hyperintense signal). Chiasma is compressed by the tumor; surrounding edema along the optic tracts is visualized. Contrast enhancement in the tumor is strong and homogeneous (**c**–**f**). The tumor has an intrasellar component as well. Multiple small metastases into the hemispheres of the cerebellum and midbrain are clearly visible on images with contrast enhancement (**c**–**f**)

characterized by marked contrast enhancement. On CT, density of metastatic tumors increases by 30–40%. CE MRI allows obtaining more precise information about the location of the lesion, its relationship with the surrounding structures and to better identifying the multiple metastatic brain lesions. An isolated lesion of the roots of the third and fifth nerves can be observed only on MRI using thin slices and intravenous contrast enhancement (Figs. 15.104 and 15.105).

In case of involvement of the middle cranial fossa bone structures, the majority of metastases on CT are characterized by a combination of osseous destruction foci with a soft tissue component, which is intensely enhanced. In such cases, MRI should be used with fat suppression sequences before and after contrast injection. When a metastatic lesion grows into the dura, capabilities of CE CT and MRI are, in general, identical, except for visualization of a "dural tail" symptom observed on MRI in case of the local dura mater invasion on the periphery of the main lesion (Figs. 15.106 and 15.107). Substantial help in differential diagnosis of metastases of the chiasmal-sellar region offers CT- perfusion. With relatively high CBV and CBF values, most metastases are characterized by an increased MTT. In contrast, meningiomas have higher values of CBV and CBF with shortening of the MTT, while pituitary adenomas show low CBF values along with increased MTT (Fig. 15.108). Rarely glial tumors may metastasize to the chiasmal recess of the third ventricle; these are mainly anaplastic astrocytomas and ependymomas (Fig. 15.109).

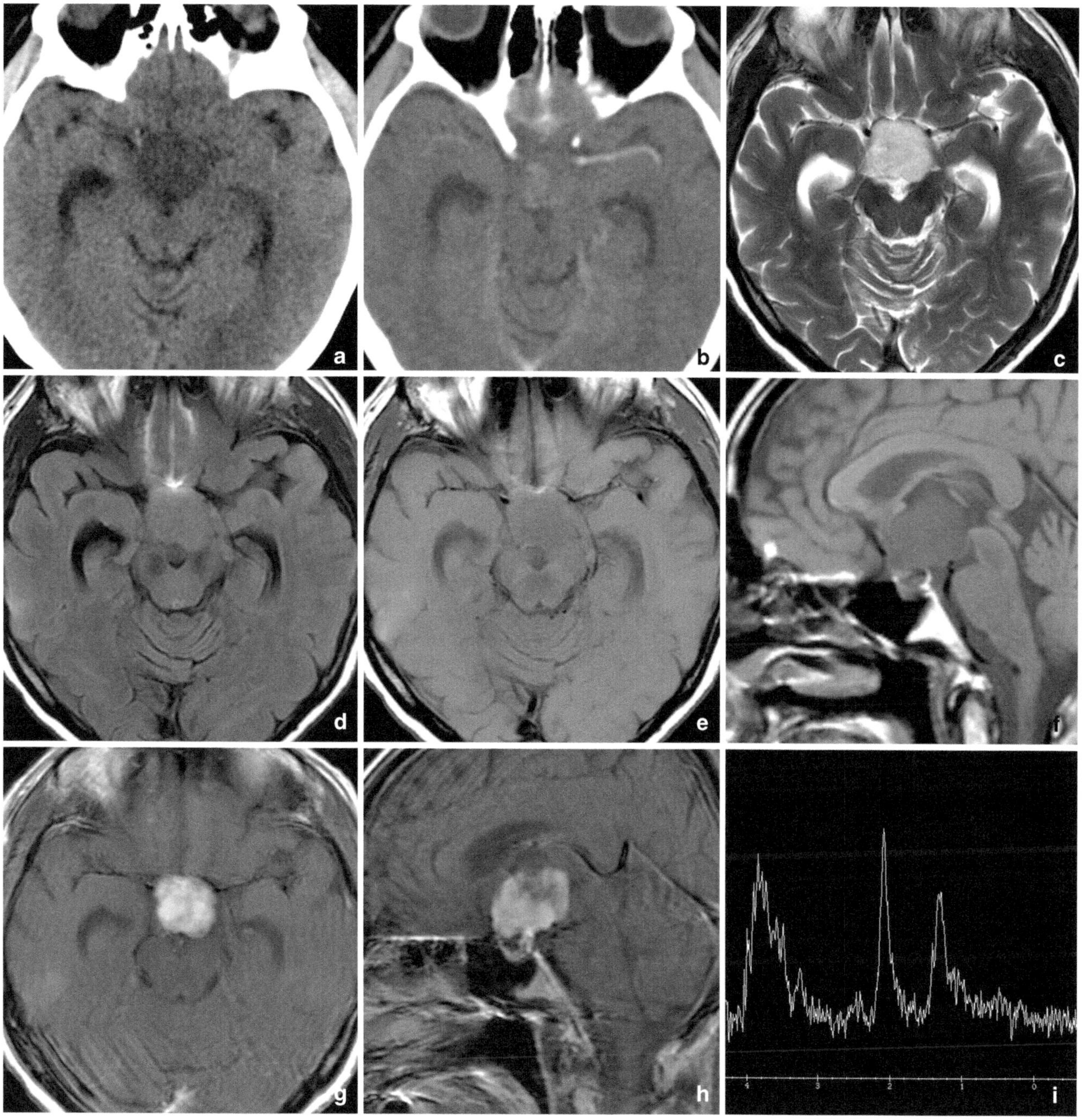

Fig. 15.104 Metastasis from breast carcinoma in the suprasellar region. Axial CT scans before (**a**) and after CE (**b**) show the hypodense mass in the suprasellar area with moderate enhancement makes the tumor less visible. T2-weighted (**c**), T2-FLAIR (**d**), T1-weighted images (**e**, **f**), and post-contrast T1-weighted images (**g**, **h**) show a hyperintense on T2 mass with heterogeneous prominent enhancement. Single-voxel MR-spectroscopy (**i**) shows a high lipids and lactate peak and decreased NAA peak

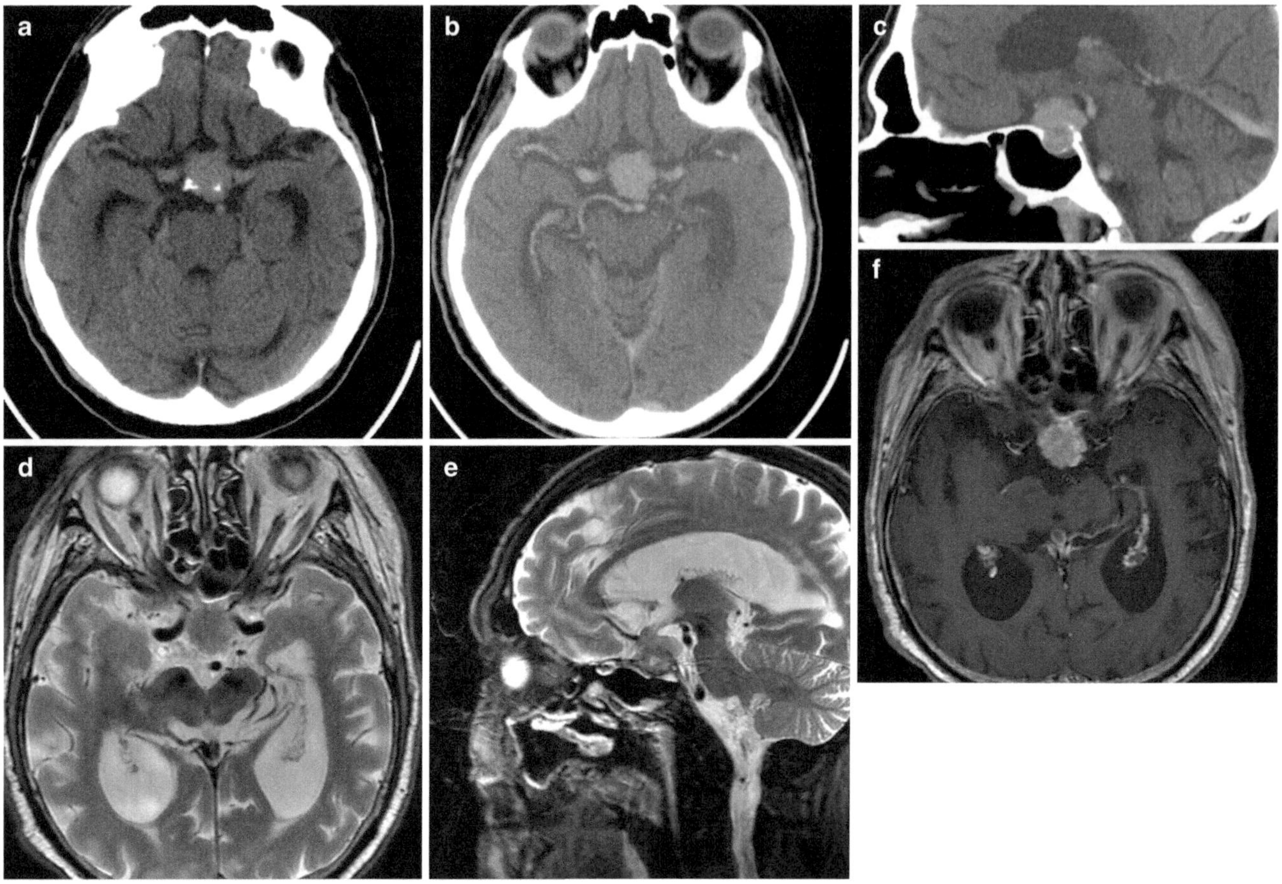

Fig. 15.105 Metastasis in the sellar-suprasellar region. CT scans before (**a**) and after CE (**b**—axial, **c**—sagittal) demonstrates an intensively enhancing mass in the suprasellar area spreading into the sella turcica. On T2-weighted images (**d, e**) the metastasis is isointense relative to the brain. Post-contrast T1-weighted image (**f**) shows a scalloped contour of the tumor, which is not typical for meningiomas of this location

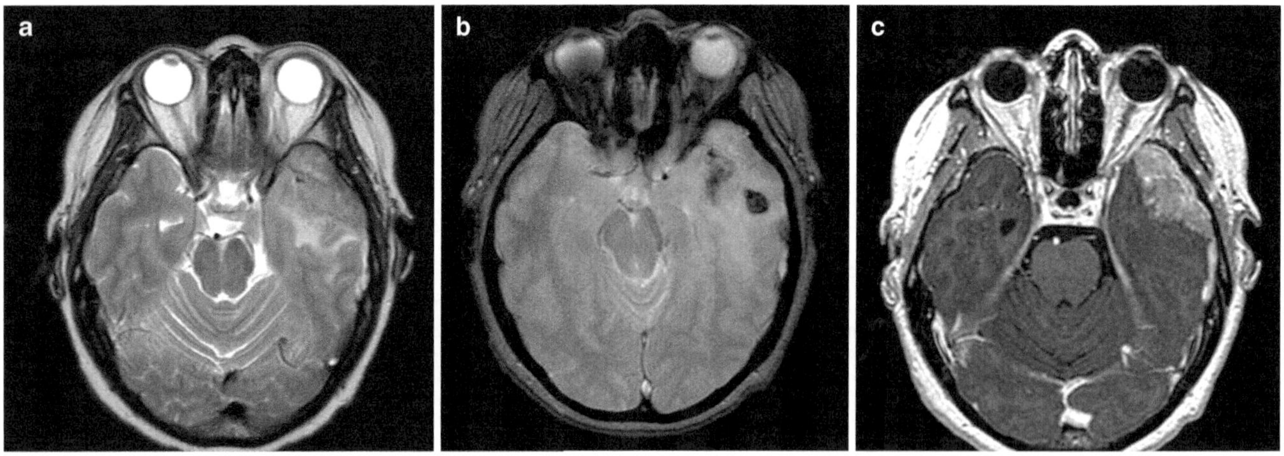

Fig. 15.106 Metastases in the left middle cranial fossa. T2-weighted (**a**) and T2* images (**b**) show an isointense relative to brain mass with surrounding edema and small hemorrhages on the periphery. Post-contrast T1-weighted image (**c**) allows visualizing the tumor localization and invasion the underlying dura

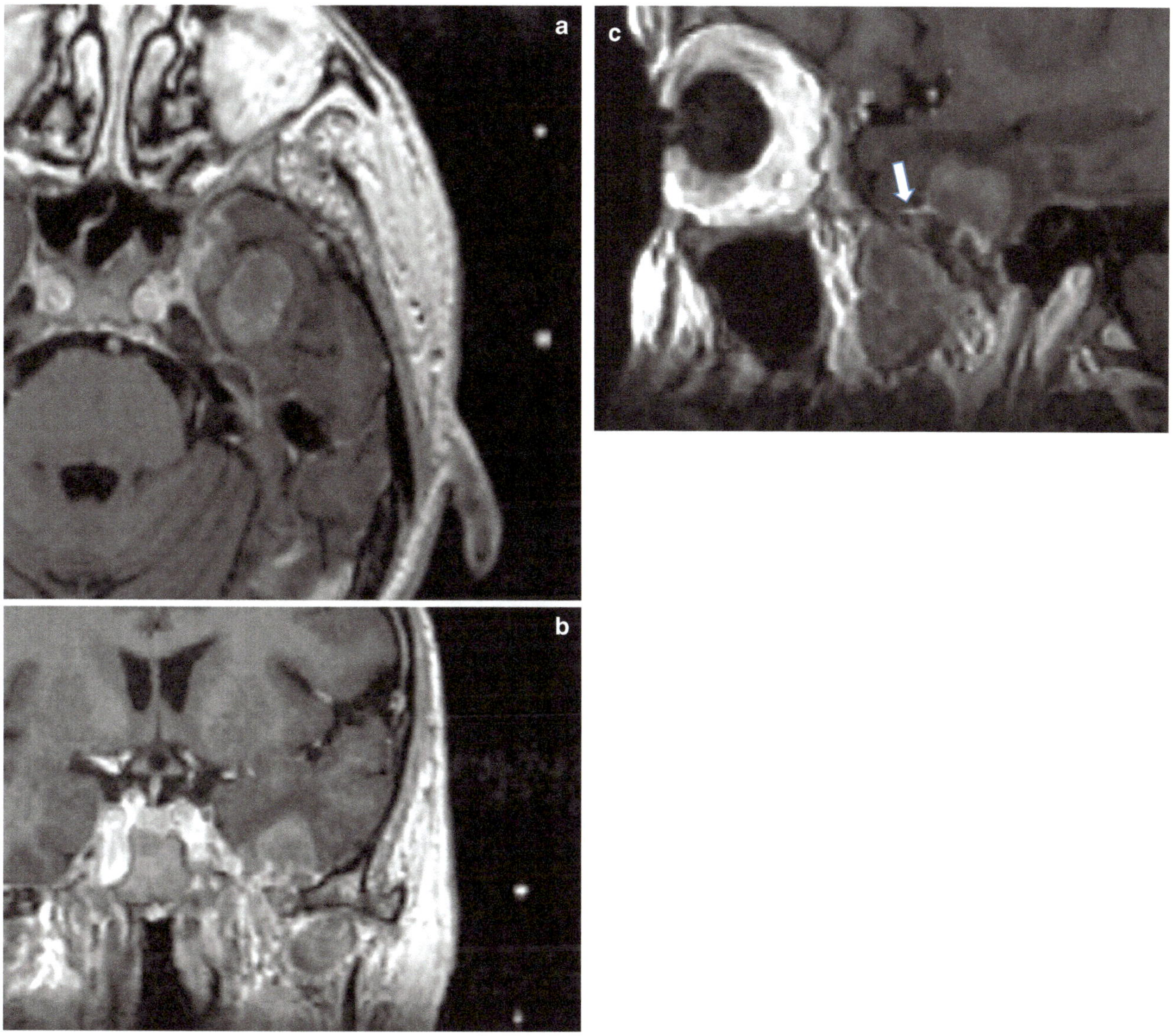

Fig. 15.107 Metastasis from testicular carcinoma into the left middle cranial fossa. Post-contrast T1-weighted images reveal a tumor, which is widely invades the dura of the middle cranial fossa (**a**–**c**). There are adjacent intensively enhancing "dural tails" (*arrow*)

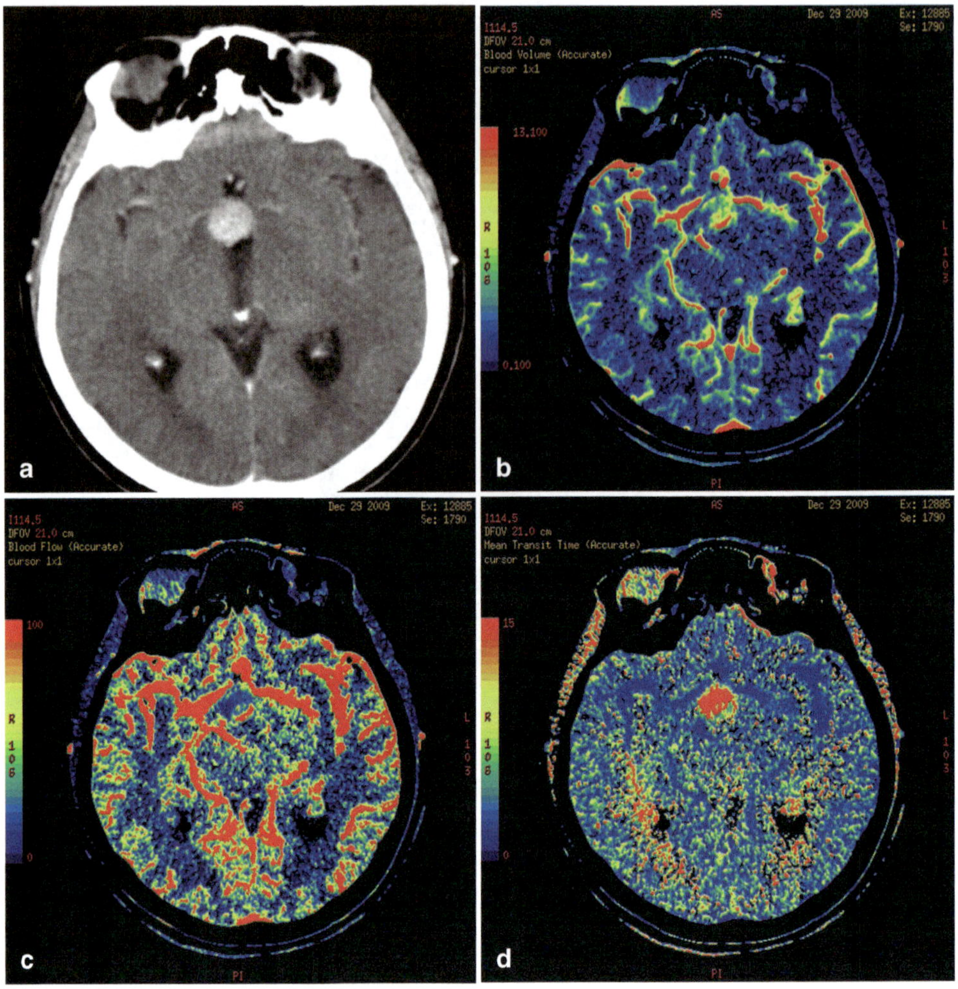

Fig. 15.108 Metastasis into the floor of the third ventricle. (**a**) CE CT scan. Perfusion CT study reveals increased values of CBV (**b**), decreased CBF (**c**) and prolonged MTT values (**d**) in the tumor

15.10 Paragangliomas

Paragangliomas are rarely found in the chiasmal-sellar region but if present they demonstrate sellar and parasellar growth. Differential diagnosis by CT or MRI is difficult. On MRI these tumors are clearly delineated from the adjacent tissues, they are round, and moderately homogenously hypointense on T1-weighted imaging and hyperintense on T2-weighted imaging. In case of sellar growth, MRI allows differentiating hypointense paragangliomas from compressed tissue of the anterior pituitary in the cavity of the sella turcica on T1-weighted images (Fig. 15.110). The pivotal distinguishing features are homogenous and marked CE and abundant vascular net on direct angiograms. Nowadays, CT-perfusion may be helpful in identification of paragangliomas of this region. Large arteries can also be visualized in the stroma of tumors on MRI as areas with flow void signal. Similar to invasive pituitary adenomas, paragangliomas can invade carotid siphons, without their compression, and can widely invade the skull base. Expansive growth and destructive bone changes can be observed (Figs. 15.111 and 15.112).

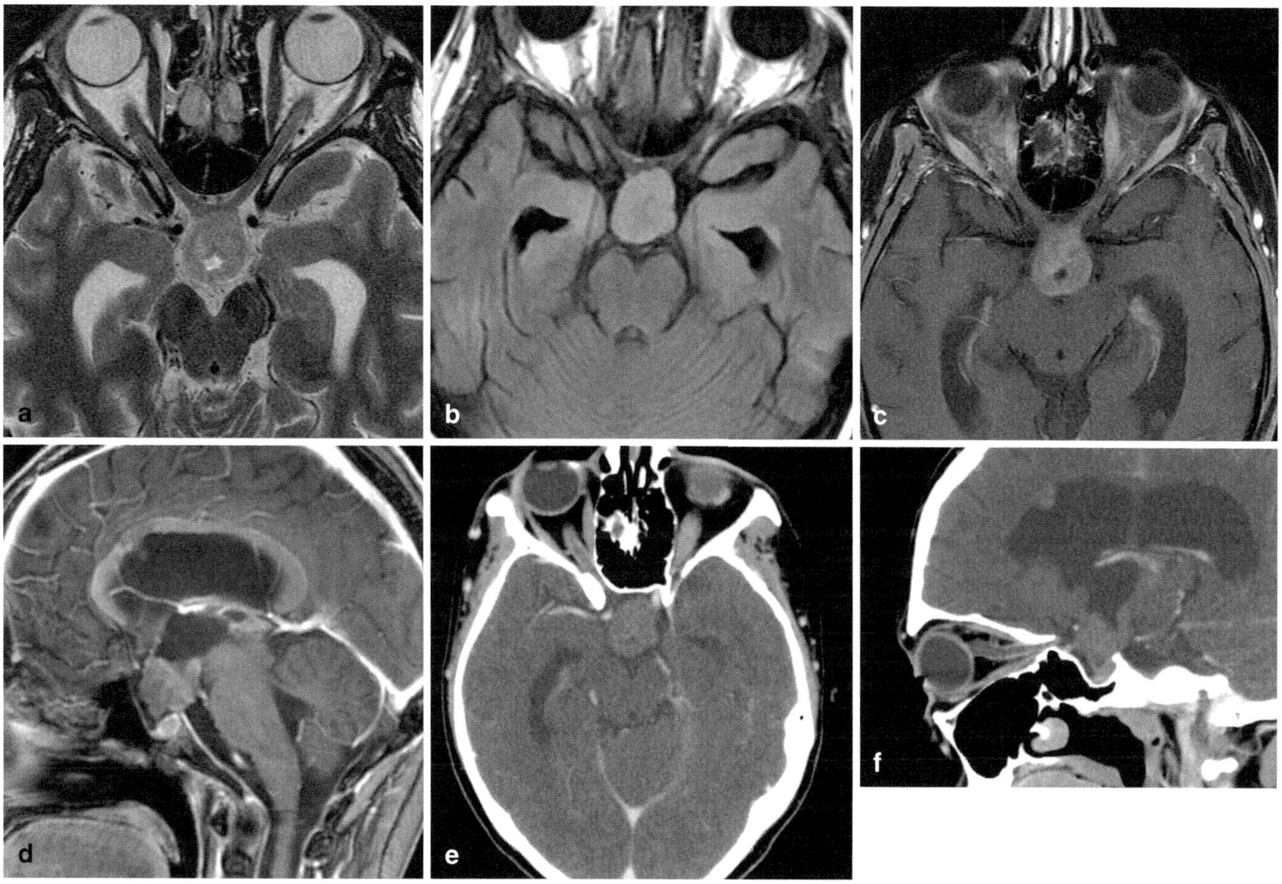

Fig. 15.109 Metastasis from anaplastic astrocytoma into the floor of the third ventricle. T2-weighted image (**a**), T2-FLAIR (**b**), post-contrast T1-weighted images (**c**, **d**) and CE CT (**e**, **f**) show a moderately enhancing solid mass in the suprasellar region. MR images reveal the ependymal enhancement along the wall of the lateral ventricles and along the both optic nerves

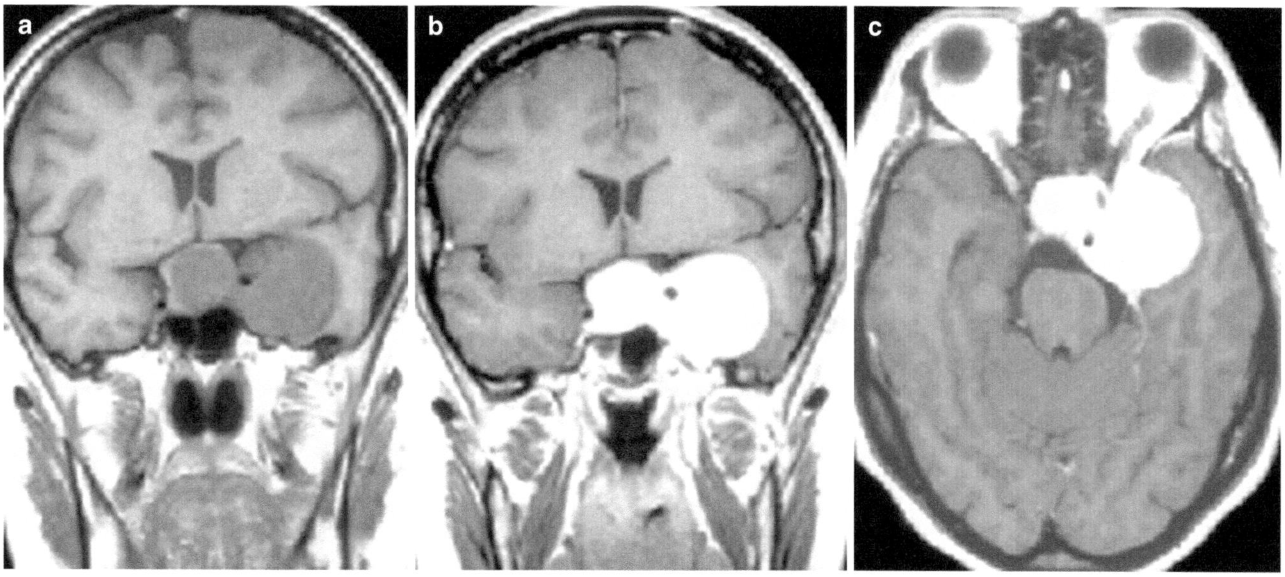

Fig. 15.110 Paraganglioma in the sellar, left laterosellar region. T1-weighted image (**a**) visualizes a hypointense tumor in the left cavernous sinus and sella turcica; compressed adenohypophysis has relatively high MR signal. Post-contrast T1-weighted images (**b**, **c**) show the same level of the contrast enhancement in the paraganglioma and adenohypophysis

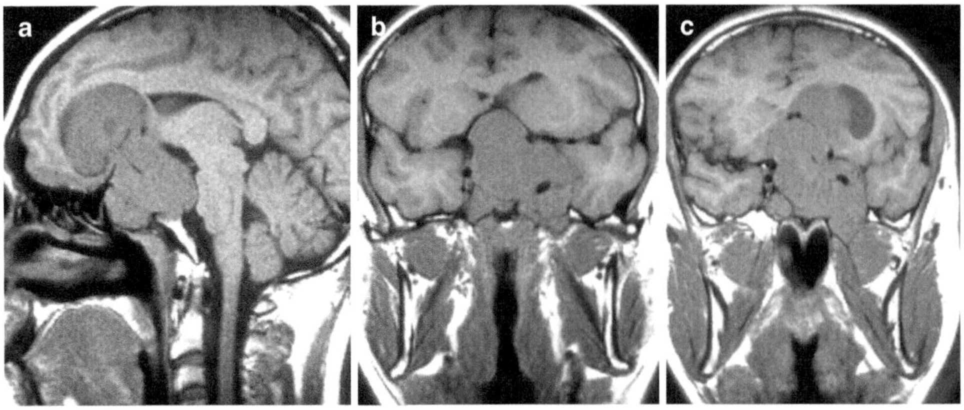

Fig. 15.111 Giant paraganglioma in the chiasmal-sellar area. Left internal carotid artery is surrounded by the tumor. An osseous destruction of the sella turcica and upper clivus is seen. Sagittal T1-weighted image (**a**) shows the upper margin of the tumor which compresses the medial segments of the frontal lobe and the genu of corpus callosum whereas the posterior margin deforms the pons. A laterosellar extending tumor component is well defined on the coronal T1-weighted images (**b**, **c**)

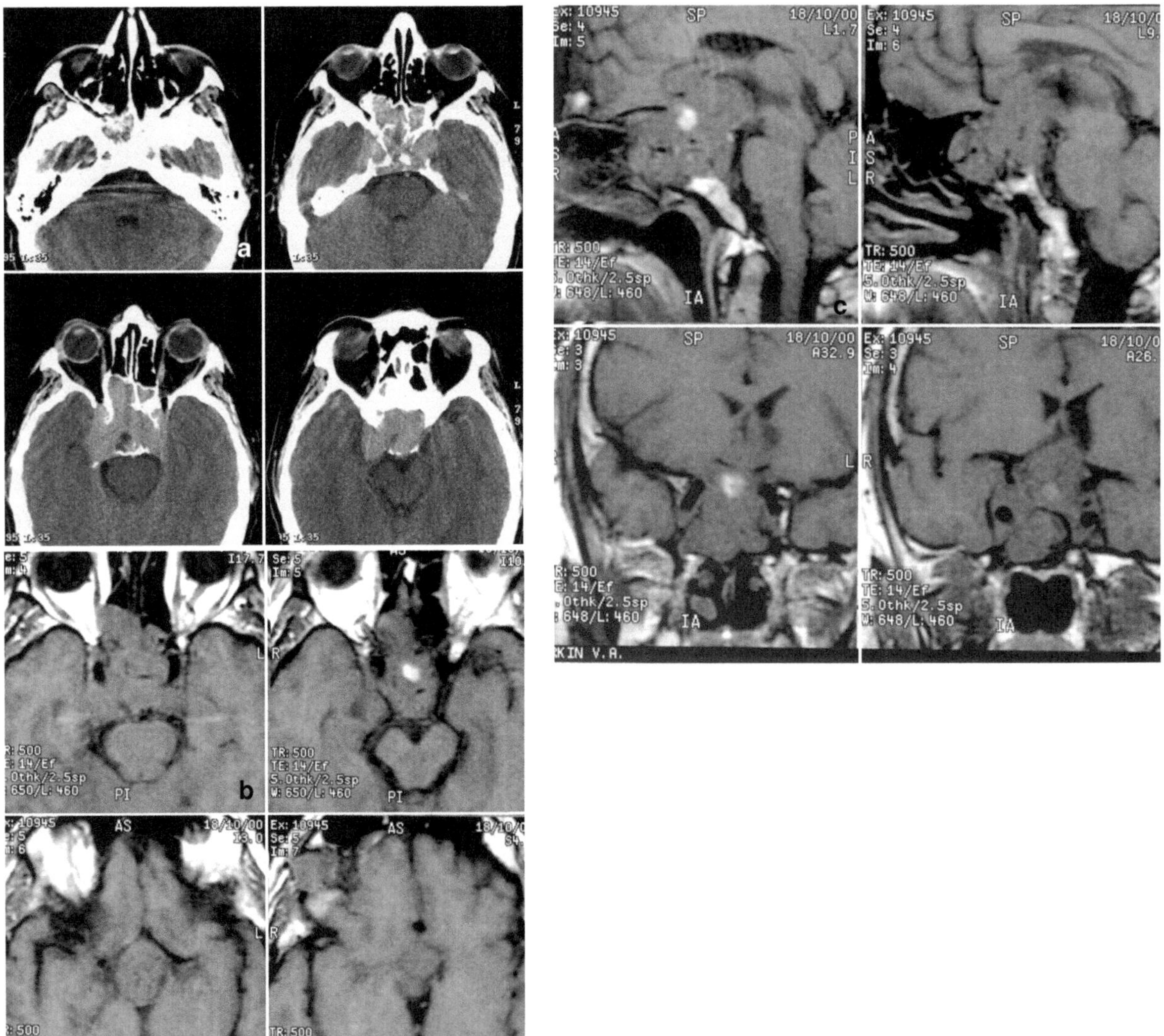

Fig. 15.112 Paraganglioma in the chiasmal-sellar area growing into the sphenoid sinus, ethmoidal bone, and in the laterosellar areas. CE CT scans (**a**), axial, sagittal, and coronal (**b**, **c**) T1-weighted images show a widely extended tumor of the skull base, which is characterized by the strong enhancement on CT. A hyperintense area in the tumor structure on T1-weighted image is explained by intratumoral hemorrhage. Internal carotid arteries are incased by the tumor, but they are not compressed

15.11 Chordomas

Chordomas of the sellar region are rare intracranial tumors, originating from the remnants of primary notochord and accounting for less than 1% of all intracranial tumors. Chordomas are rare in children. About 35–40% of chordomas are found in clivus (the peak of incidence is between 20 and 40 years), 50% of chordomas are located in sacrum (the peak of incidence is between 40 and 60 years, frequently in males), and 15% of cases in the vertebral column. Among intracranial chordomas, the most frequent site is the clivus (near the spheno-occipital synchondrosis), much less frequently, chordomas are encountered in the sellar region or laterally of the pyramid of temporal bone. Sellar and parasellar chordomas account for no more than 30% of all intracranial chordomas. The tumor is prone to multiple relapses, so it is classified as malignant.

These tumors are soft, lobular, gray mass lesions with locally invading growth and necrotic areas on macroscopy. Thick strands of fibrous connective tissue give the mass lesion its lobular structure. Microscopically, the tumor is polymorphic; its cells have different size and shape, often reminiscent of bubbles with small hyperchromatic nuclei and intracytoplasmic vacuoles.

Chordomas of the chiasmal-sellar region are manifested by visual symptoms and pituitary deficiency. When invading the cavernous sinuses, oculomotor signs and signs of the trigeminal nerve involvement occur.

Complete removal of chordoma is possible in rare cases, which is why partial resection with consequent radiation is performed. Radiation with protons beams or linear accelerator therapy is suggested as chordomas are resistant to radiation done with standard protocols. In recent 10 years, CyberKnife is successfully used in the radiation therapy of small skull base chordomas.

Imaging CT and MRI are complementary in neuroimaging of these tumors. CT reveals a soft tissue mass lesion with bone destruction and calcifications (approximately 50% of cases) (Figs. 15.113 and 15.114). On MRI, chordomas are characterized by the variability of signal intensity on T1-weighted images (Sze et al. 1988; Sidorkin 2009). Expansion of the tumor into the bone marrow of the clivus leads to replacement of normal signal of the bone marrow fat by hypointense signal of tumor (Figs. 15.115, 15.116, and 15.117). On T2-weighted images, moderate or marked hyperintense signal may be seen. Septi of fibrous connective tissue appear as hypointense stripes on T2-weighted images, which separate hyperintense lobular areas of a tumor, while calcifications and bone islets appear as hypointense areas (Figs. 15.118 and 15.119). Chordomas are characterized by a low MR signal and high ADC values on diffusion-weighted images. MRI exceeds CT in identification of a tumor expansion and its spatial relationship with brain structures, craniobasal nerves, and vessels. However, destruction of skull base bones and calcifications in the depth of the tumor are better seen on CT. Post-contrast MRI improves neuroimaging of tumor expansion, but may be rather mild (Figs. 15.120 and 15.121). Important differential diagnostic features, typical for the skull base chordomas, are low hemodynamic parameters of the tumor structure. Chordomas show decreased CBV and CBF values on perfusion maps. Mean transit time varies from low to increased (Fig. 15.122). Giant skull base chordomas with extensive bone destruction and enormous enhancing soft tissue component are rare in clinical practice. Tumor extent, high MR signal on T2-weighted images and increased ADC values help making a correct diagnosis in most cases (Fig. 15.123).

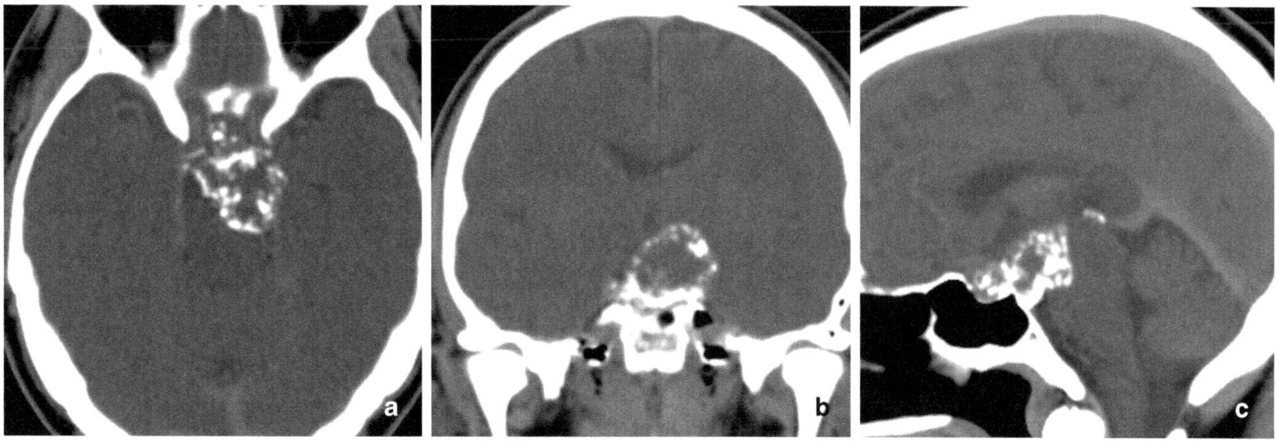

Fig. 15.113 Chordoma of the chiasmal-sellar area. Axial CT scan (**a**) with coronal (**b**) and sagittal reformats (**c**) identify a heterogeneous tumor with multiple small calcifications. A dorsum sella is partially eroded

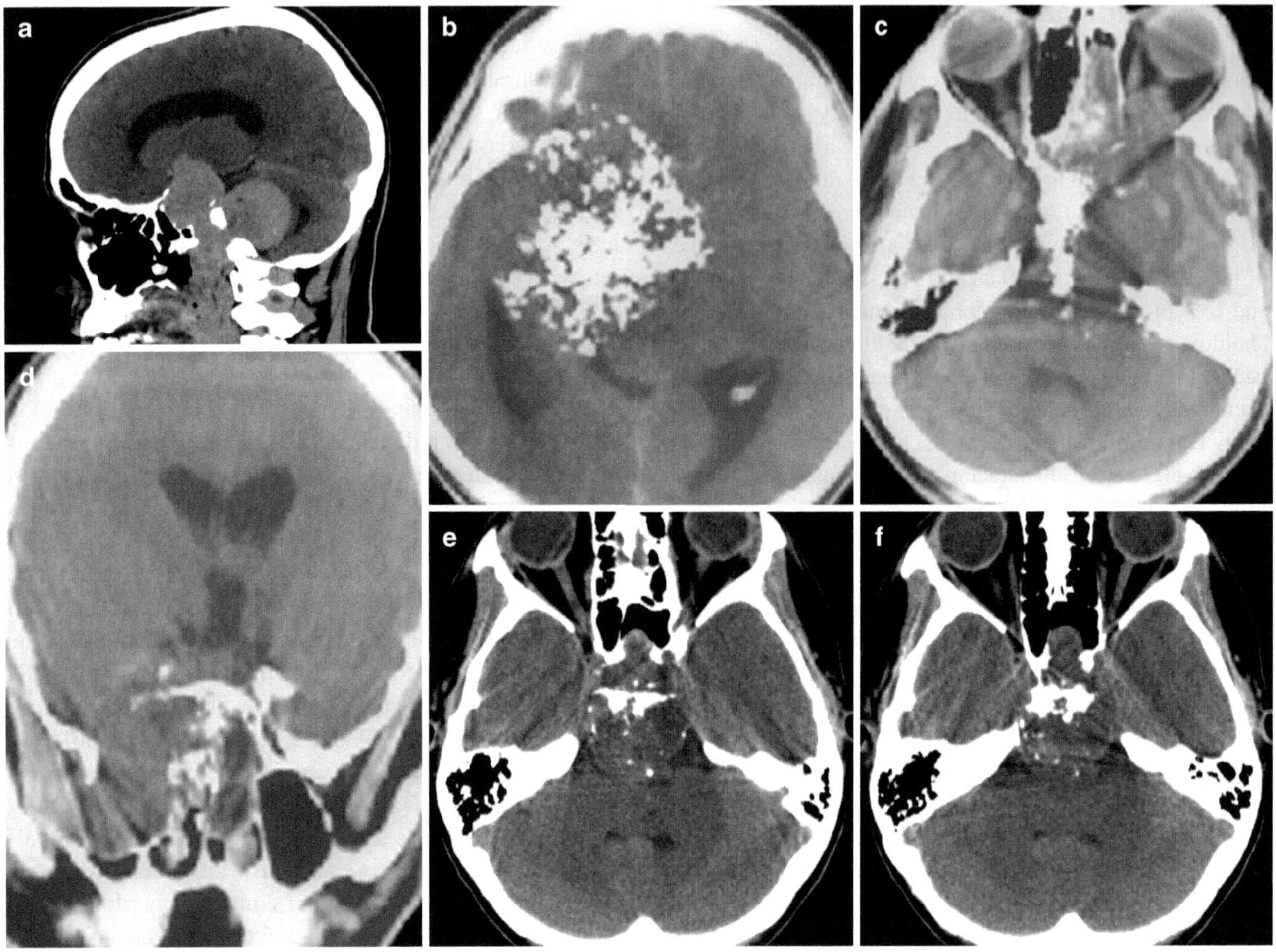

Fig. 15.114 Chordomas in the chiasmal-sellar area. CT-scanning of different patients shows the tumors with various structure and extension. Case 1 (**a**), case 2 (**b**), case 3 (**c**, **d**), case 4 (**e**, **f**)

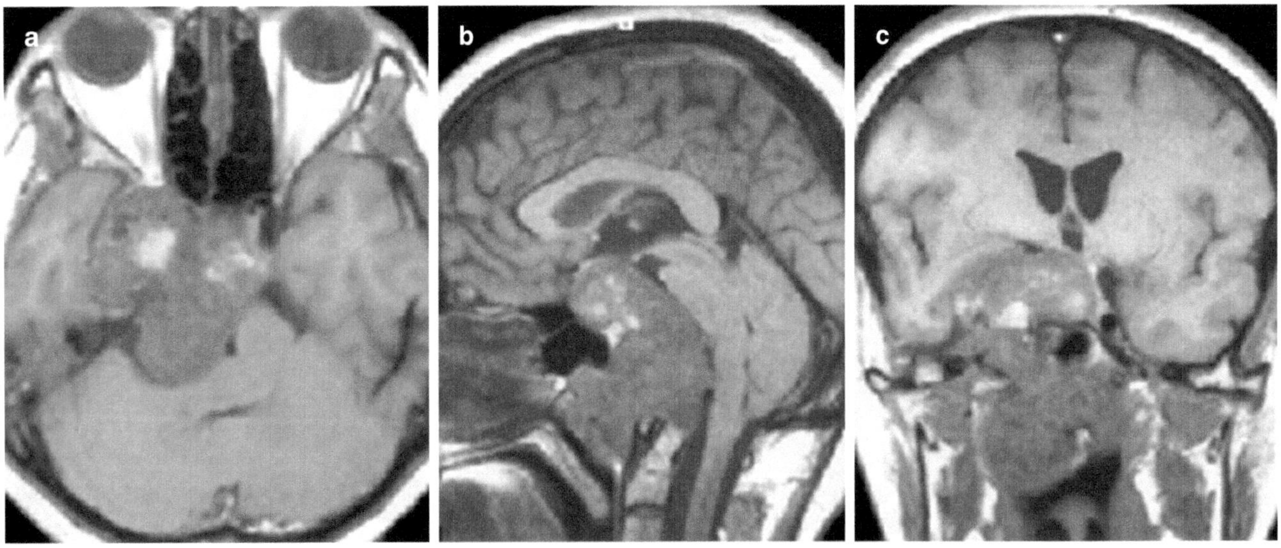

Fig. 15.115 Chordoma of the skull base and chiasmal-sellar area. T1-weighted images (**a**–**c**) reveal a widely extended heterogeneous tumor. A tumor invades the clivus and extends into nasopharynx. Intratumoral hemorrhages have a hyperintense MR-signal

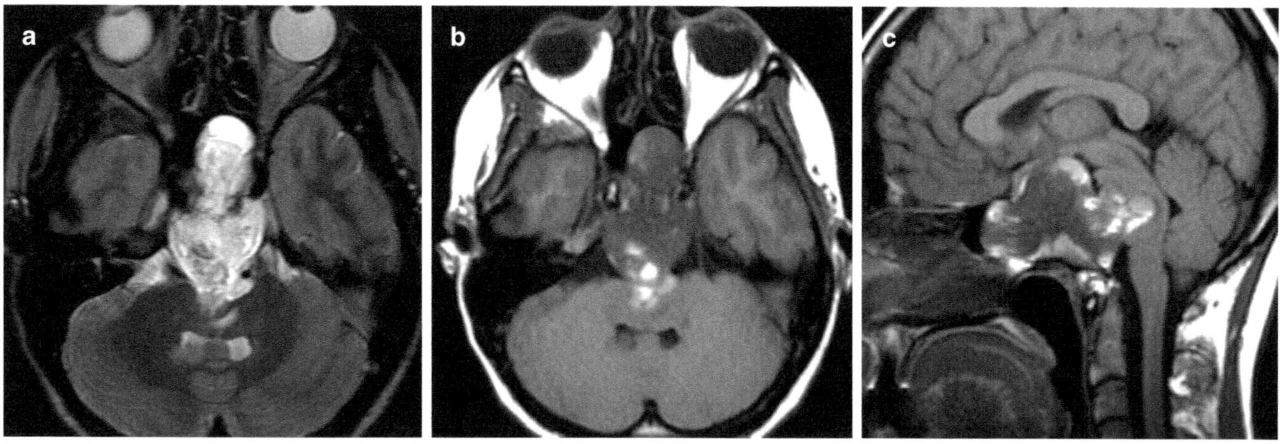

Fig. 15.116 Chordoma of the skull base. T2-weighted (**a**), axial (**b**) and sagittal (**c**) T1-weighted images show a large tumor with hyperintense (hemorrhages) and hypointense (small calcifications) components. Chordoma causes the destruction of the clivus, dorsum sella, invades the body of sphenoid bone, and compress the pons

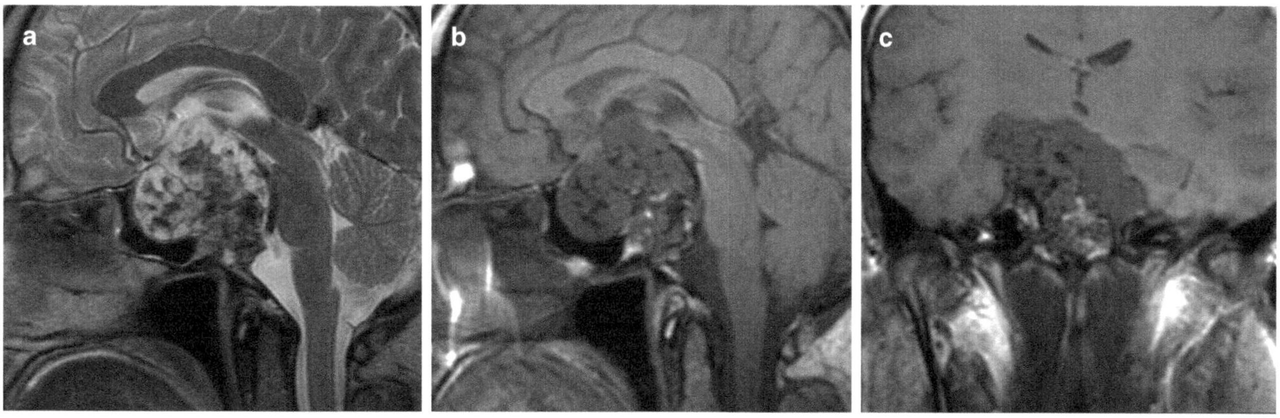

Fig. 15.117 Chordoma of the clivus extending into sphenoid sinus and medial part of the right temporal lobe. Sagittal T2- (**a**), T1-weighted (**b**), and coronal T1-weighted images (**c**) show a heterogeneous tumor with the hypointense on T1 and hyperintense on T2 soft tissue component. Calcifications in the tumor are hypointense in all sequences

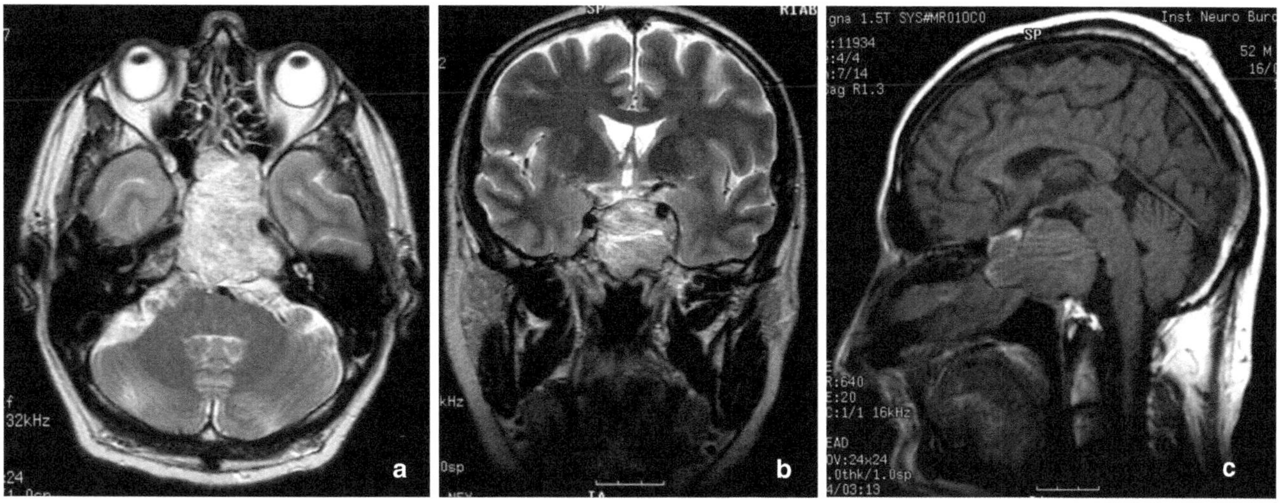

Fig. 15.118 Chordoma of the skull base. T2- (**a**, **b**) and T1-weighted images (**c**) reveal a large tumor, that destroys a sphenoid bone, fills the sphenoid sinus and posterior ethmoidal bone. There is an intracranial tumor component compressing a brainstem. T2-weighted image visualizes multiple septa in the tumor

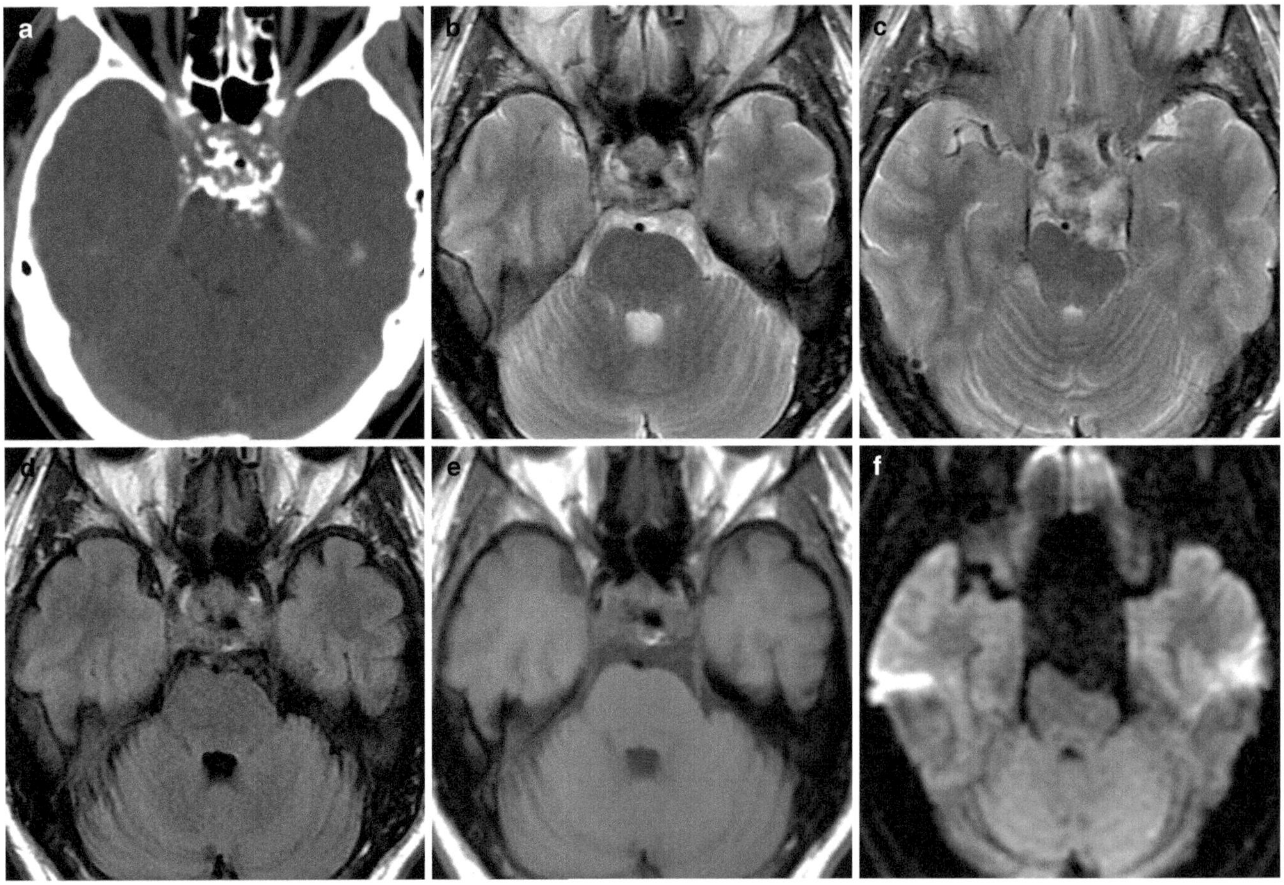

Fig. 15.119 Chordoma of the chiasmal-sellar area. CT scan (**a**) identifies a tumor with calcifications that destroys the sella turcica and clivus. T2-weighted (**b**, **c**), T2-FLAIR (**d**), and T1-weighted (**e**) images show a heterogeneous tumor mainly hypointense due to multiple calcifications. Diffusion-weighted MR image (**f**) shows a decreased signal from chordoma

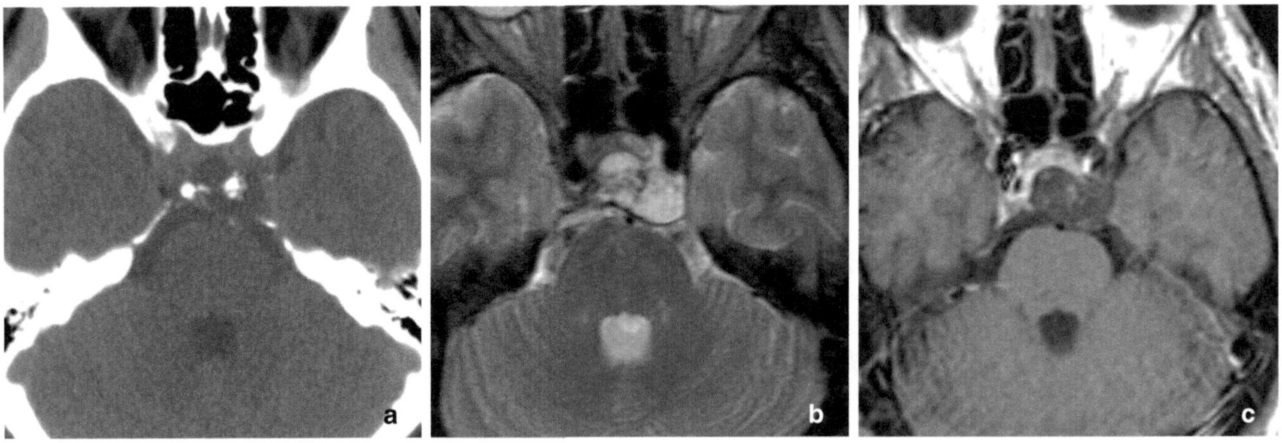

Fig. 15.120 Chordoma of the clivus and sphenoid bone. CT scan (**a**), axial T2-weighted image (**b**) and post-contrast T1-weighted image (**c**) show small calcifications in the tumor and increased MR-signal from the chordoma on T2-weighted image. Contrast enhancement is visualized in the deep part of tumor only

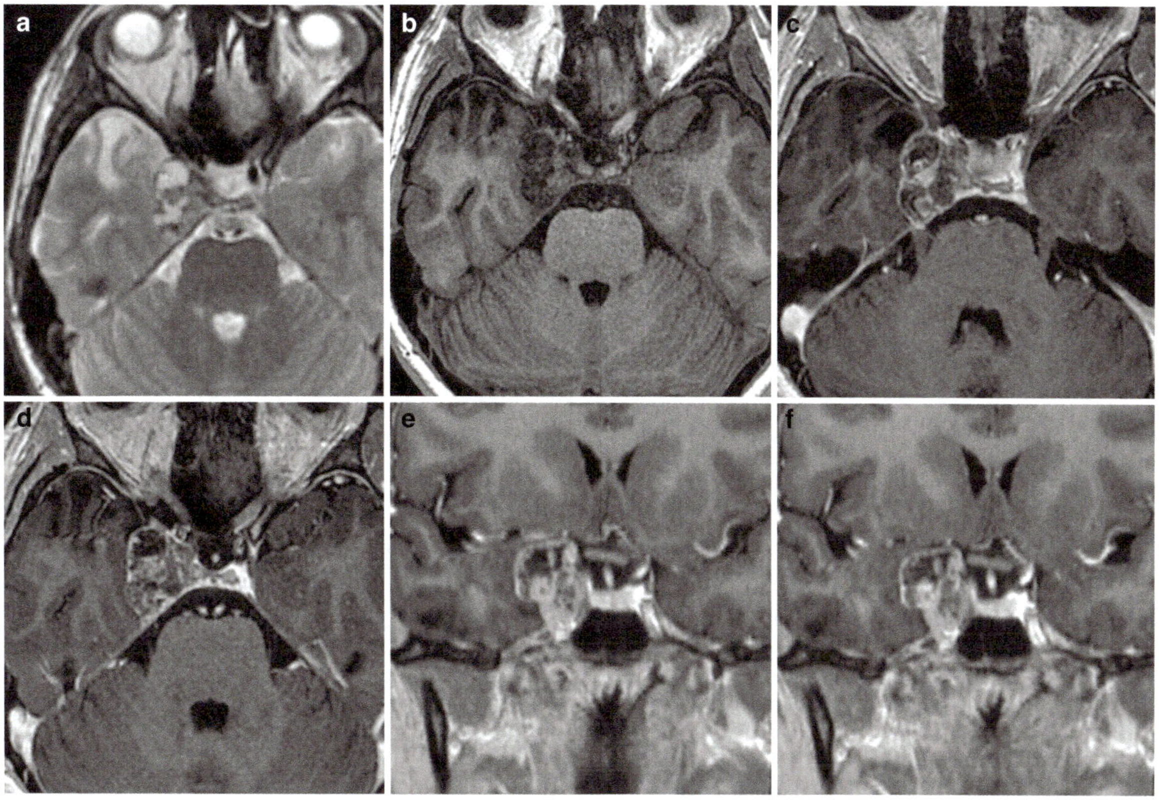

Fig. 15.121 Chordoma of the right laterosellar area with intense heterogeneous enhancement and hypointense areas due to calcifications. T2- (**a**), T1- (**b**), and post-contrast T1-weighted images (**c**–**f**)

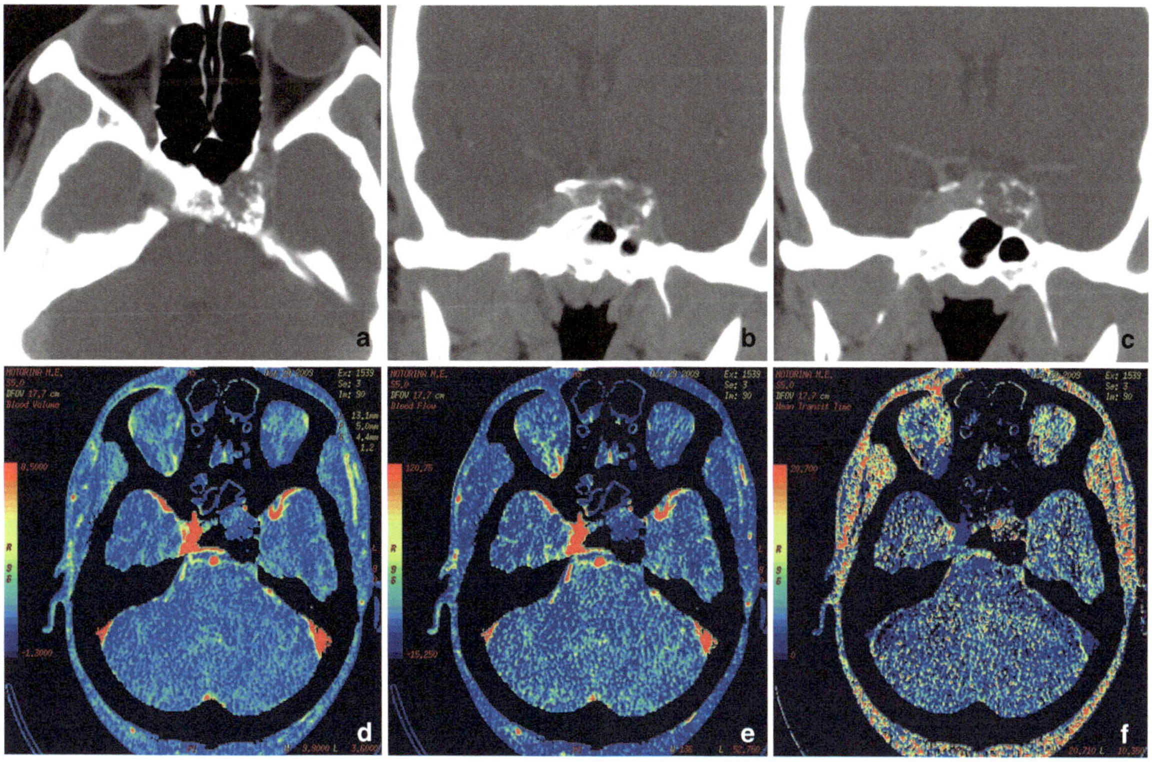

Fig. 15.122 Chordoma in the sellar-laterosellar area. CT scans (**a**–**c**) show a lesion with calcifications destroying the dorsum sellar and the sellar floor on the left. Perfusion parameters in the tumor are lower than in normal brain tissue (CBV—**d**, CBF—**e**), mean transit time is prolonged (MTT—**f**)

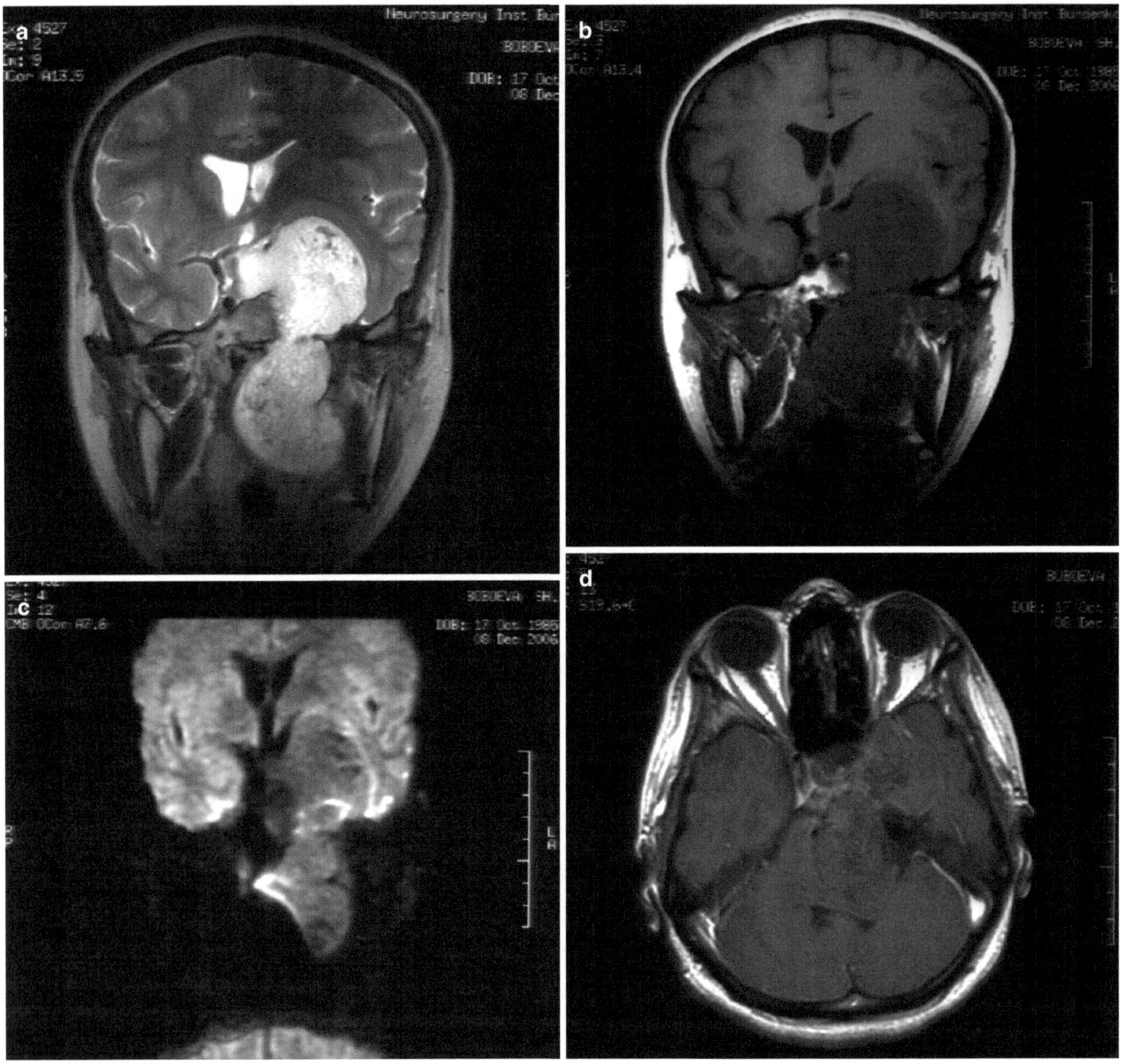

Fig. 15.123 Giant invasive chordoma of the skull base. Coronal T2- (**a**) and T1-weighted images (**b**), post-contrast T1-weighted images (**d**–**f**) demonstrate a large tumor in the middle cranial fossa with the infratentorial growth and brainstem compression, with the expansion into the sella turcica and oropharynges. A tumor is hyperintense on T2-weighted image. A moderate heterogeneous enhancement is revealed. DWI (**c**) shows a low MR-signal from the tumor and high ADC values

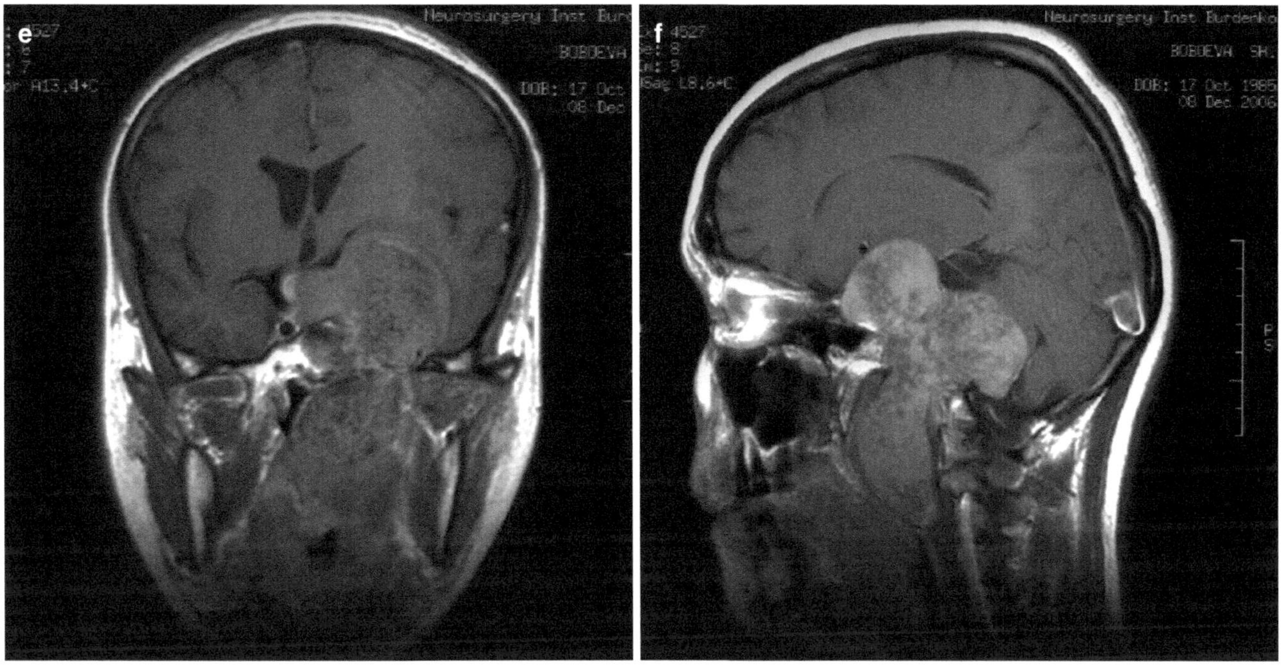

Fig. 15.123 (continued)

Dysembriogenic Tumors and Cysts

16

Contents

Teratomas are nongerminomatous tumors, which arises from multipotential germ cells and are mainly seen in young children predominantly in boys. Teratomas are found in 2–4% of intracranial tumors in children (Osborn et al. 2016).

Teratomas are mass lesions which contain elements of three germinal layers—ectoderm, mesoderm, and endoderm (layers of exfoliated epithelium, sebaceous and sweat glands, hair, crystals of cholesterol, amorphous fat), as well as elements of neural, muscle, and bone tissue. There are three types of teratoma: mature (well differentiated), immature (includes some incompletely differentiated tissue), and teratoma with malignant transformation (Osborn et al. 2016).

Teratomas usually locate at the midline in the sellar-suprasellar region. On CT they have heterogeneous structure with fat, calcifications (sometimes have tooth-like configuration), and soft tissue that enhances (Figs. 16.1 and 16.2).

16.1 Teratoma

On MRI, teratomas have a heterogeneous structure due to calcifications, fat and soft-tissue components, which signal intensity may increase after CE (Liu et al. 2015).

Dermoid cysts are most frequently diagnosed within the age range of 30–50. Dermoid cysts make up approximately <0.5% (Osborn et al. 2016) of all primary intracranial tumors. They are usually located along the medial axis, frequently in the parasellar region, and less frequently in the posterior cranial fossa (Wilms et al. 1991). Dermoids are the lesions which may include the dermal elements such as hair follicles, sweat and sebaceous glands. Slow, expansive growth is typical for these cysts. Besides visual symptoms, headaches, (less frequently) hypopituitarism, cranial neuropathies and diabetes insipidus are typical for suprasellar tumors.

I. Pronin, V. Kornienko, *CT and MRI of Skull Base Lesions*, https://doi.org/10.1007/978-3-319-65957-2_16

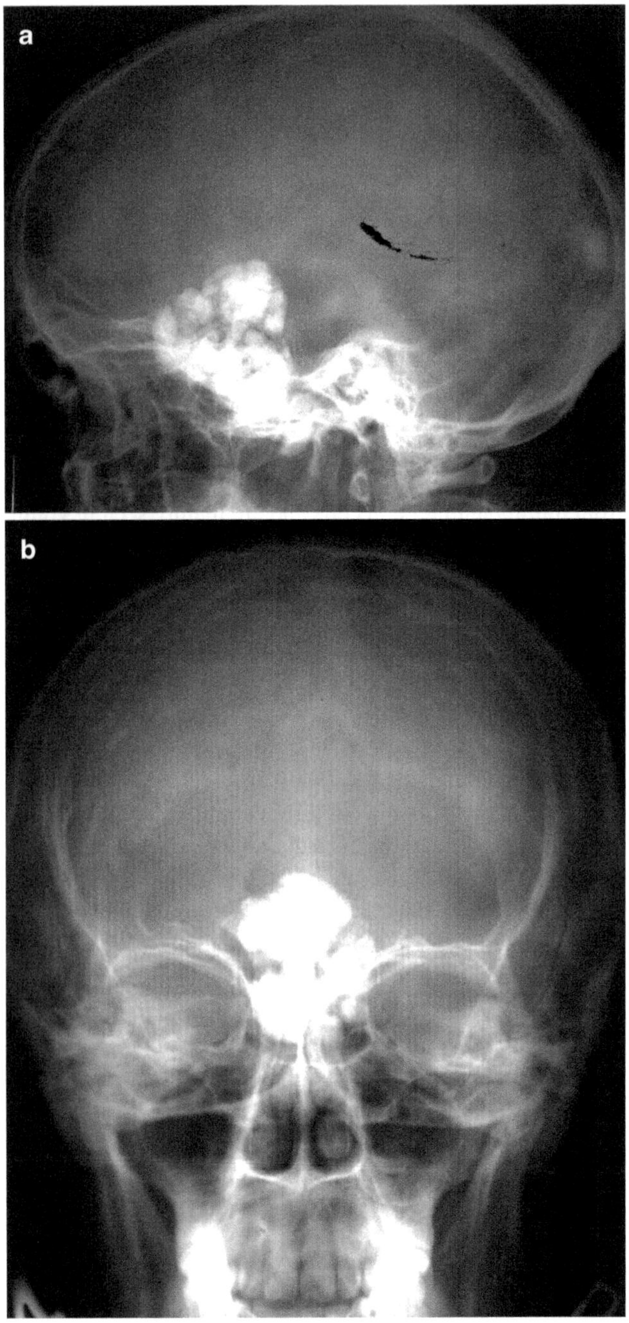

Fig. 16.1 Teratoma in the sellar area in a 5-year-old child. Anterior-posterior (**a**) and lateral (**b**) X-ray scans show an enlarged sella. There are many tooth-like calcifications in the intra-suprasellar area

Imaging On CT, these cysts are characterized by heterogeneous density with calcifications, bony elements, and hypodense fatty inclusions. Dermoid cysts on CT are typically round, are well delineated from brain tissue, and have heterogeneous low density (−20 to −60 HU). Calcifications of the capsule are frequent. Most of the dermoid cysts are presented by a fat component (Figs. 16.3 and 16.4). In cases in which the capsule of dermoid cysts is ruptured small hypodense areas, which represent fat globules, may be seen in the subarachnoid space and the ventricular system with fat-fluid level. After changing patient's head position, displaceability of fat fragments in the ventricles can be estimated (Fig. 16.5). Hyperdense dermoid cysts are rare but possible. Dermoid cysts are typically characterized by increased signal intensity of fat on T1-weighted imaging. On T2-weighted imaging a cyst has variable signal, hypo- or heterogeneously hyperintense (Wilms et al. 1991; Smith et al. 1991). If hair is present in a cyst, then thread-like areas of hypointense signal are seen on MRI (Markus and Kendall 1993). When a cyst ruptures, hyperintense signal of fat-containing lumps is seen in the subarachnoid space and the ventricles (Figs. 16.6, 16.7, and 16.8). MRI should be used with fat suppression sequence. Fat component of dermoid cysts becomes hypointense on T2- and T1-weighted images. Unlike epidermoid cysts, dermoids are usually iso-hypointense on diffusion-weighted MR images. Intravenous CE mildly increases cysts intensity, typically in capsule.

Epidermoid cysts are the congenital benign cysts which arise from inclusion of ectoderm during the neural tube closure (Osborn et al. 2016). Epidermoid cysts are benign and slowly growing lesions, which may have intracranial and intravertebral locations. Epidermoid cysts make up approximately 0.2–1.5% of all primary intracranial tumors. Epidermoids are cysts of adults, usually diagnosed in patients at the aged 20–60 years, and they are mainly located in basal cisterns and laterally. The walls of these cysts are lined with simple, cuboidal squamous epithelium, which cover the external layer of fibrous tissue. The internal part of the cyst is formed from a wax-like material of exfoliated keratin derivate of its wall and of solid cholesterol crystals. In contrast to dermoid cysts, epidermoids do not contain hair follicles and sebaceous glands.

Epidermoid cysts have variably density on CT from −30 HU to that close of the CSF. In 10–25% of them, calcifications are seen within (Tatler and Kendall 1991). Sometimes epidermoid cysts are hyperdense on CT due to hemorrhage, high protein content or deposition of iron-containing pigment (Gualdi et al. 1991). In most cases, epidermoid cysts do not enhance on CT, but exceptions exist. On MRI, these cysts are well identified due to prolonged T1 and T2 relaxation times. The signals are similar to the CSF in the subarachnoid spaces. On T2-FLAIR sequences, epidermoid cysts also demonstrate

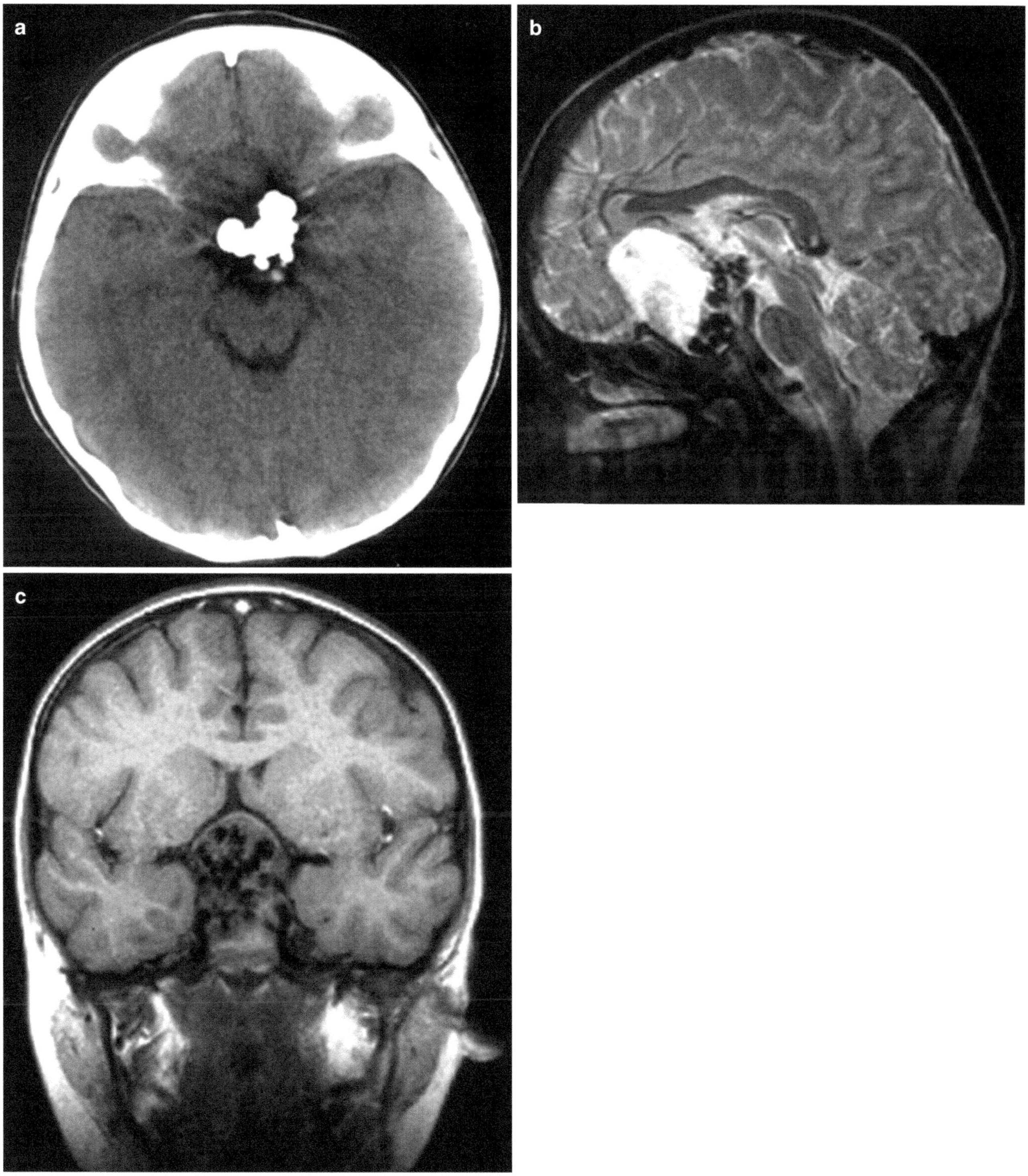

Fig. 16.2 Teratoma in a 5-year-old child (X-ray exam presented in Fig. 16.1). Axial CT scan (**a**) shows a lesion with plenty of calcifications in the sellar-suprasellar area. A tumor is hyperintense on T2-weighted image (**b**) and hypointense on T1-weighted image (**c**) with low signal areas from calcifications

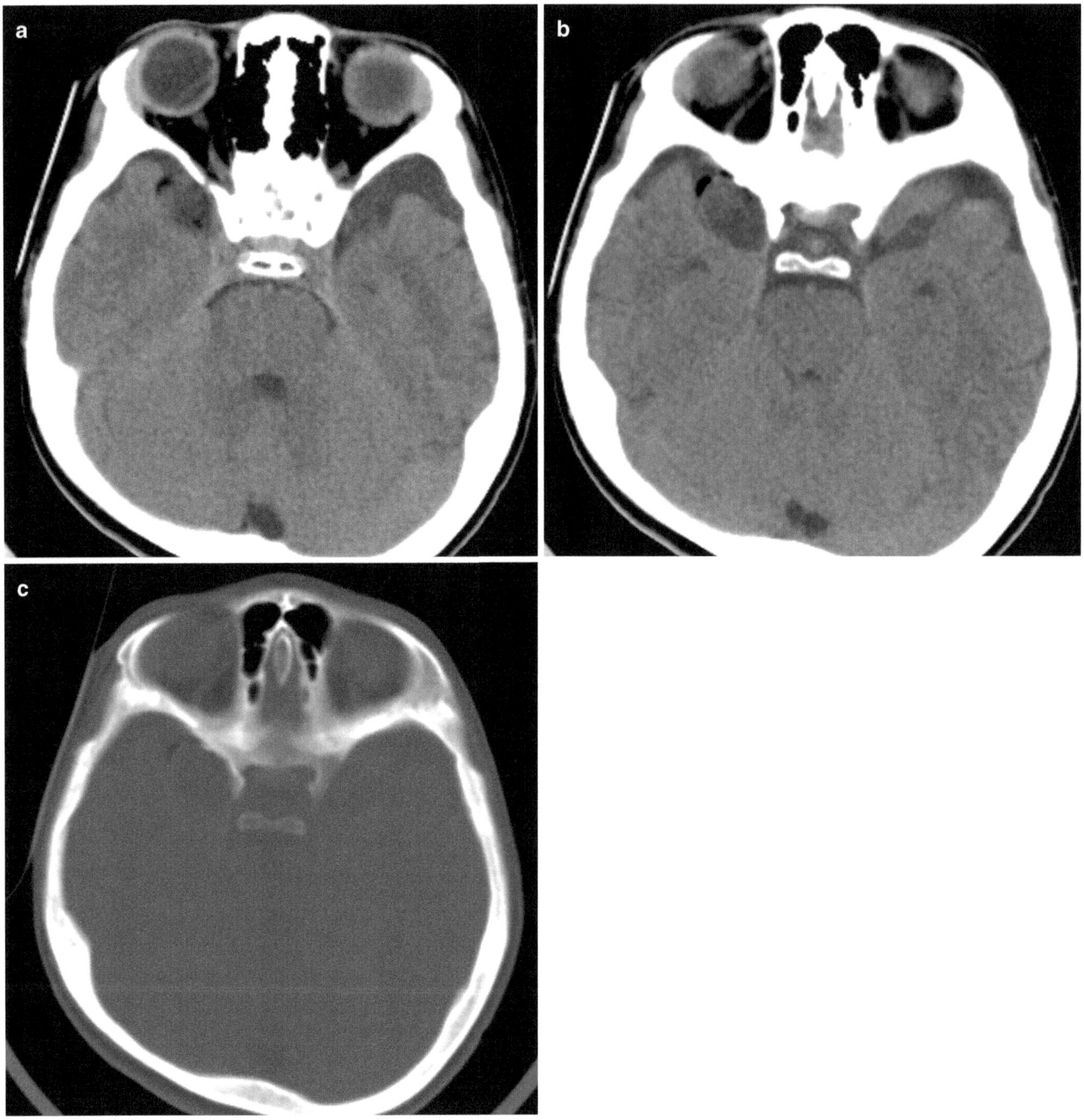

Fig. 16.3 Dermoid of the right parasellar region. Axial CT scans (**a**, **b**) demonstrate a hypodense mass laterally from the anterior clinoid process. There are small areas with negative Hounsfield units (−60H) from fat in the lateral part of the mass. CT scan in bone window mode (**c**) shows the local expansive changes of the clinoid process

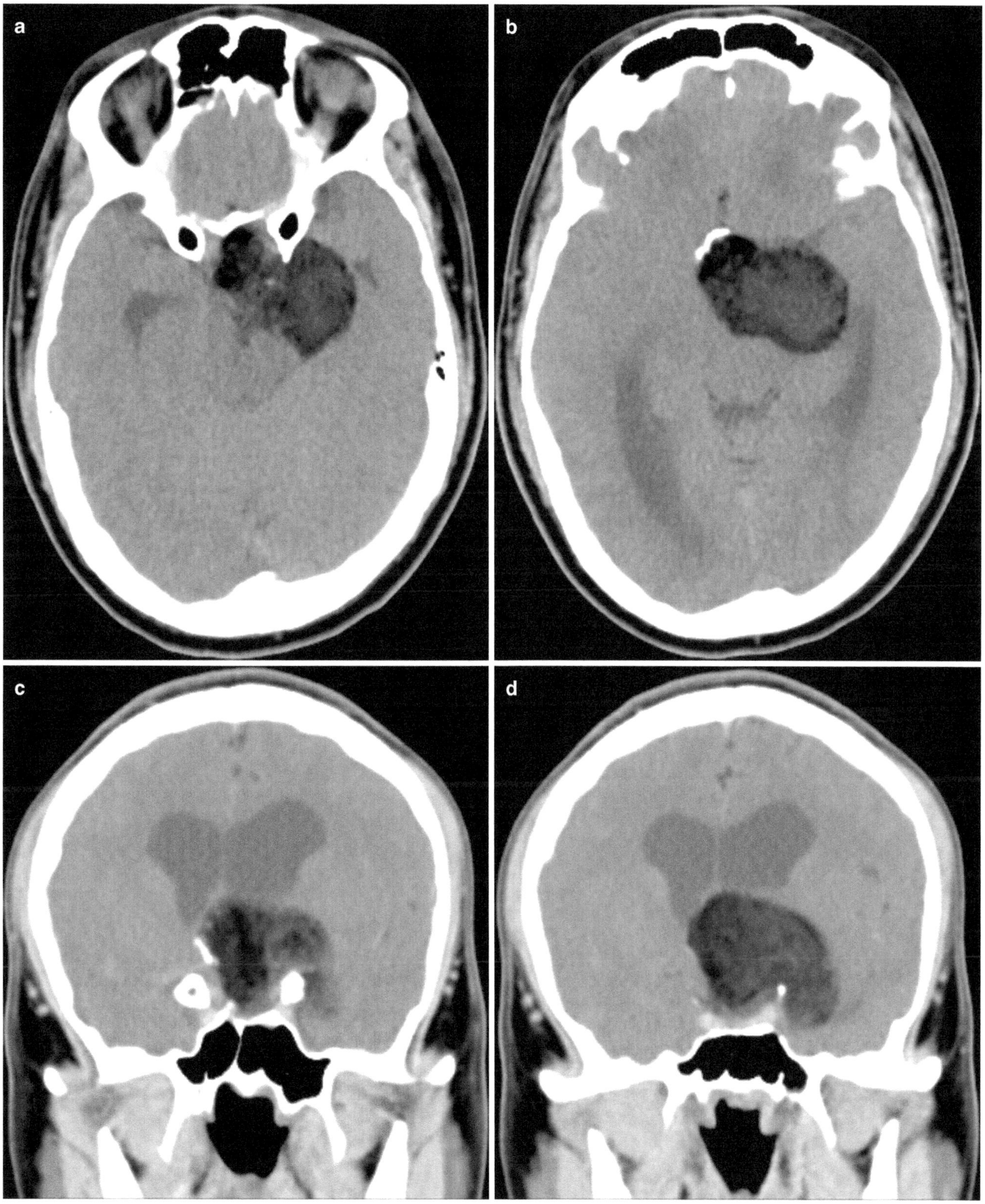

Fig. 16.4 Ruptured dermoid cyst of the suprasellar area. CT scans (**a**–**f**) show a heterogeneous hypointensive relative to the brain lesion. Mixed fatty and calcified areas are in the cyst. Many droplets of fat disseminate in the subarachnoid spaces (**e**, **f**)

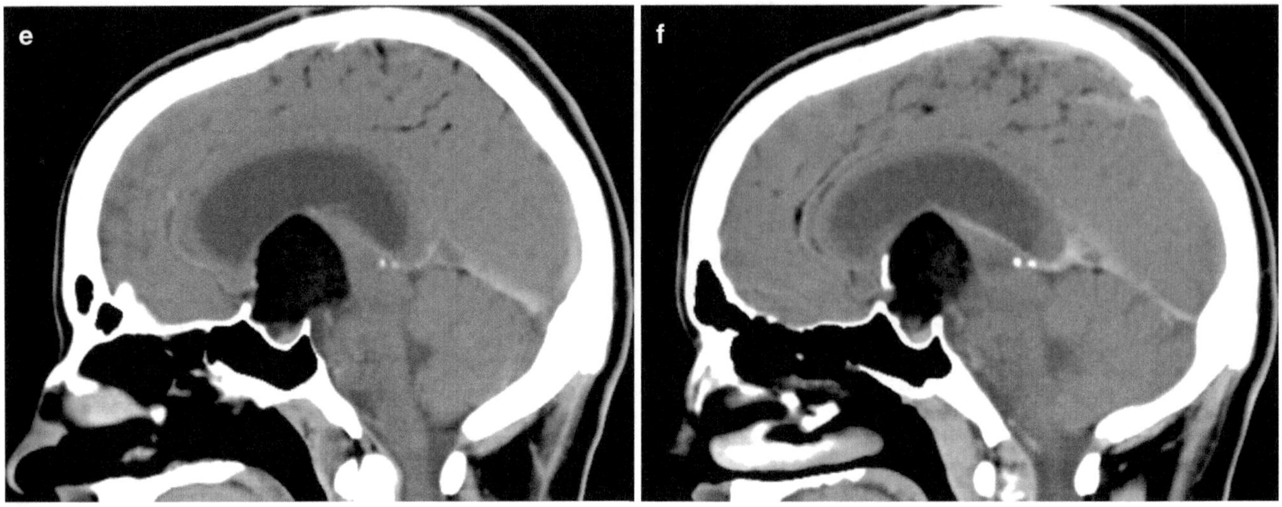

Fig. 16.4 (continiued)

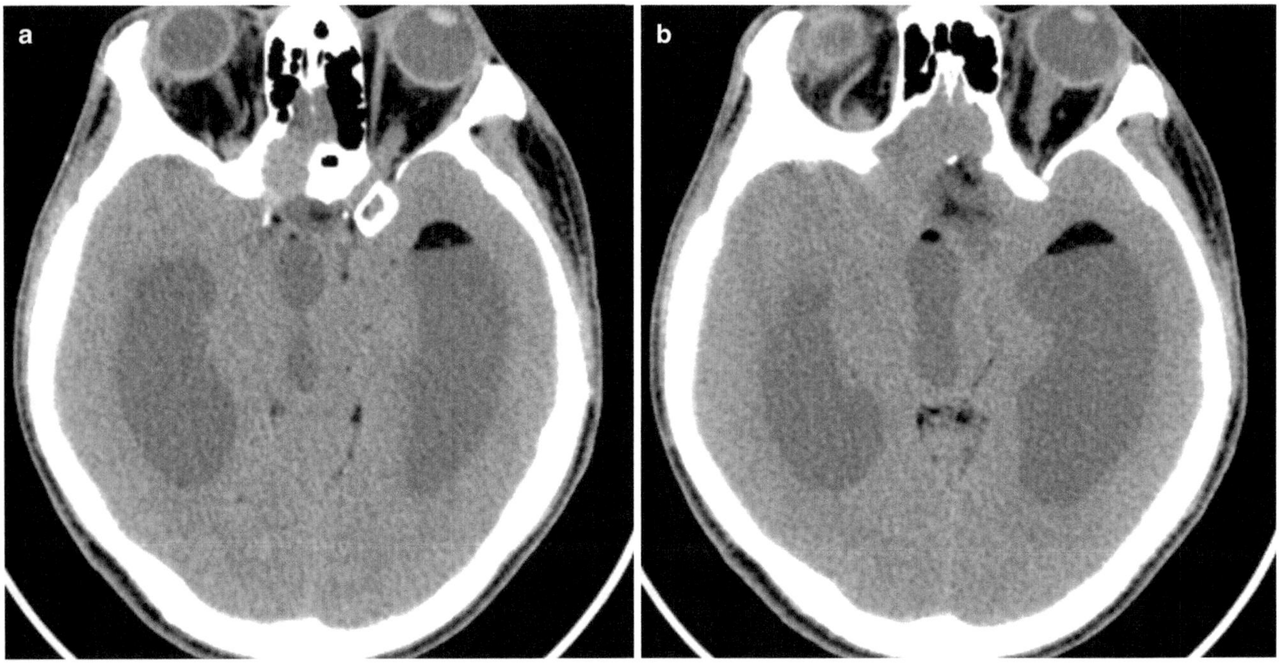

Fig. 16.5 Ruptured dermoid cyst. CT scans show a hypodense mass in the suprasellar region. Fatty areas are in the cyst, fat droplets disseminate to the anterior part of third ventricle, temporal horn of the left lateral ventricle and to the anterior horns of the lateral ventricles (*black areas*, **a–c**). Fatty droplets in the ventricles change their location after head rotation: to the right (**d**) and left (**e**). Fatty inclusions in the cyst and ventricles are hyperintense on T2- (**f**) and especially on T1-weighted images (**g–i**)

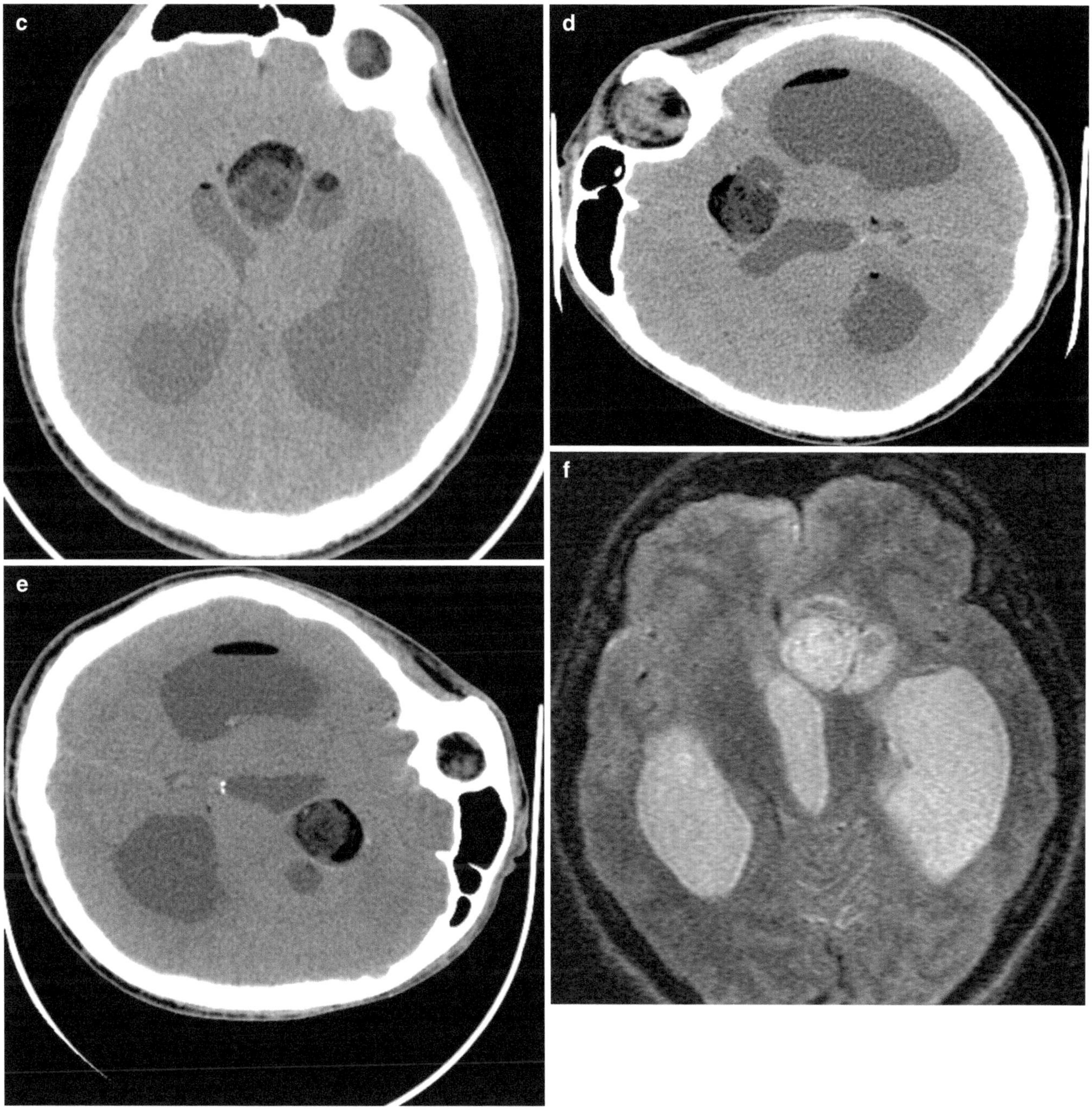

Fig. 16.5 (continued)

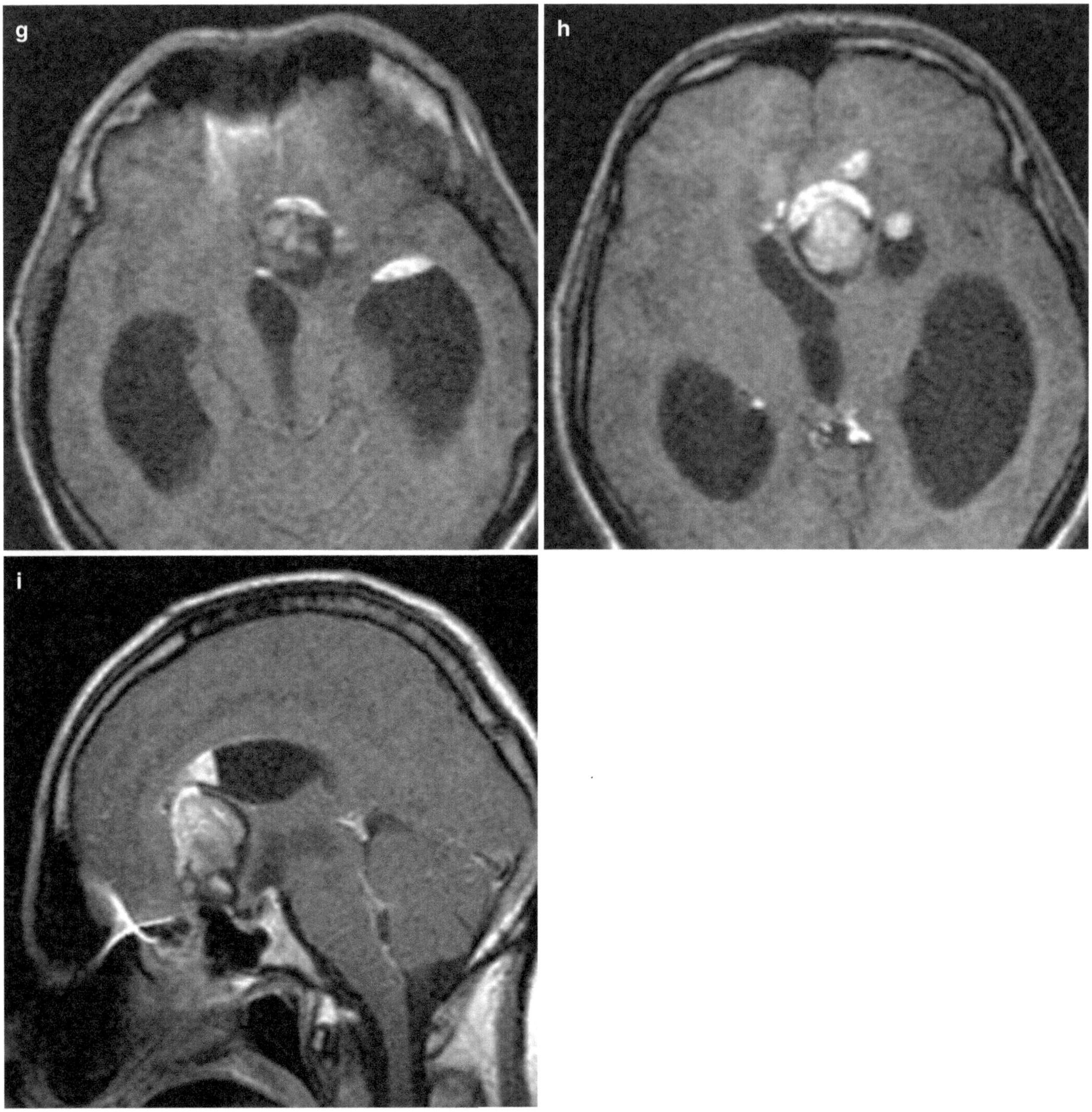

Fig. 16.5 (continued)

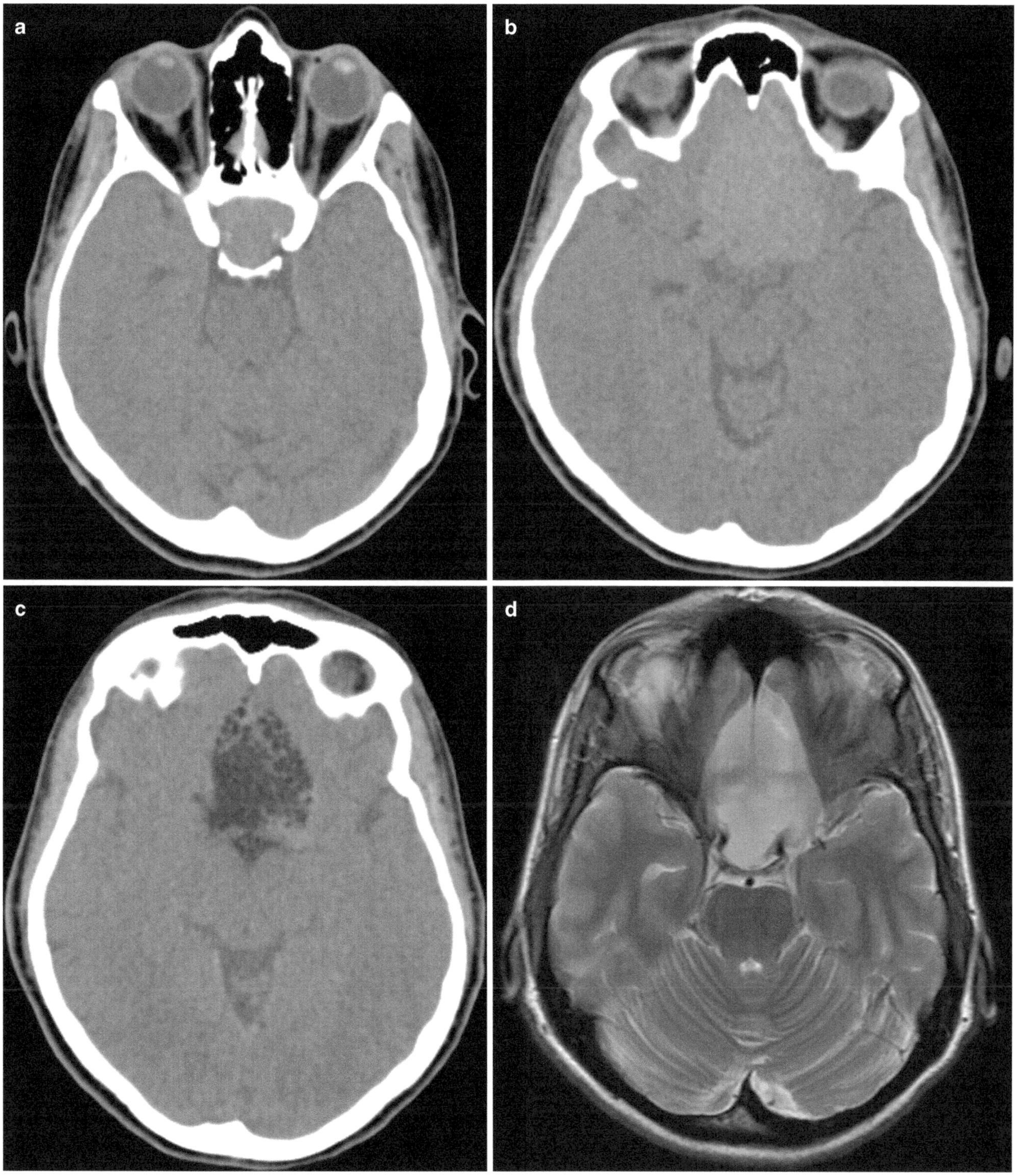

Fig. 16.6 Dermoid cyst of the suprasellar region with extending into the anterior cranial fossa. Axial CT scans (**a–c**) show a mixed hypo- (fat) and hyperdense midline lesion. T2- (**d–f**), T1-weighted images (**g**), T1 with fat suppression (**h**, **i**) show the heterogeneity of the cyst. MRI with fat saturation confirms lipid elements within the cyst. Fatty inclusions are hypointense on SPGR with fat saturation (**j–l**)

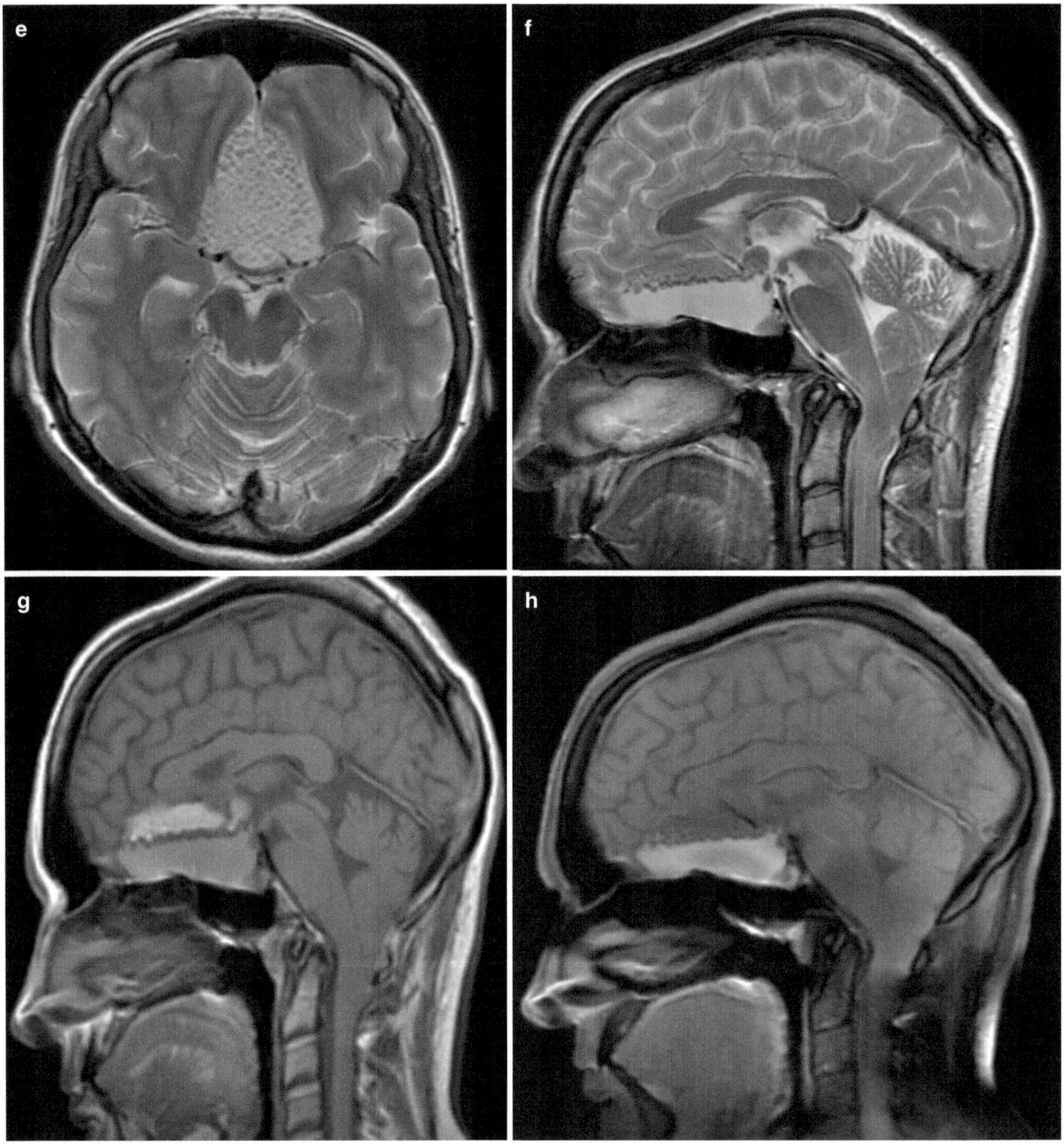

Fig. 16.6 (continued)

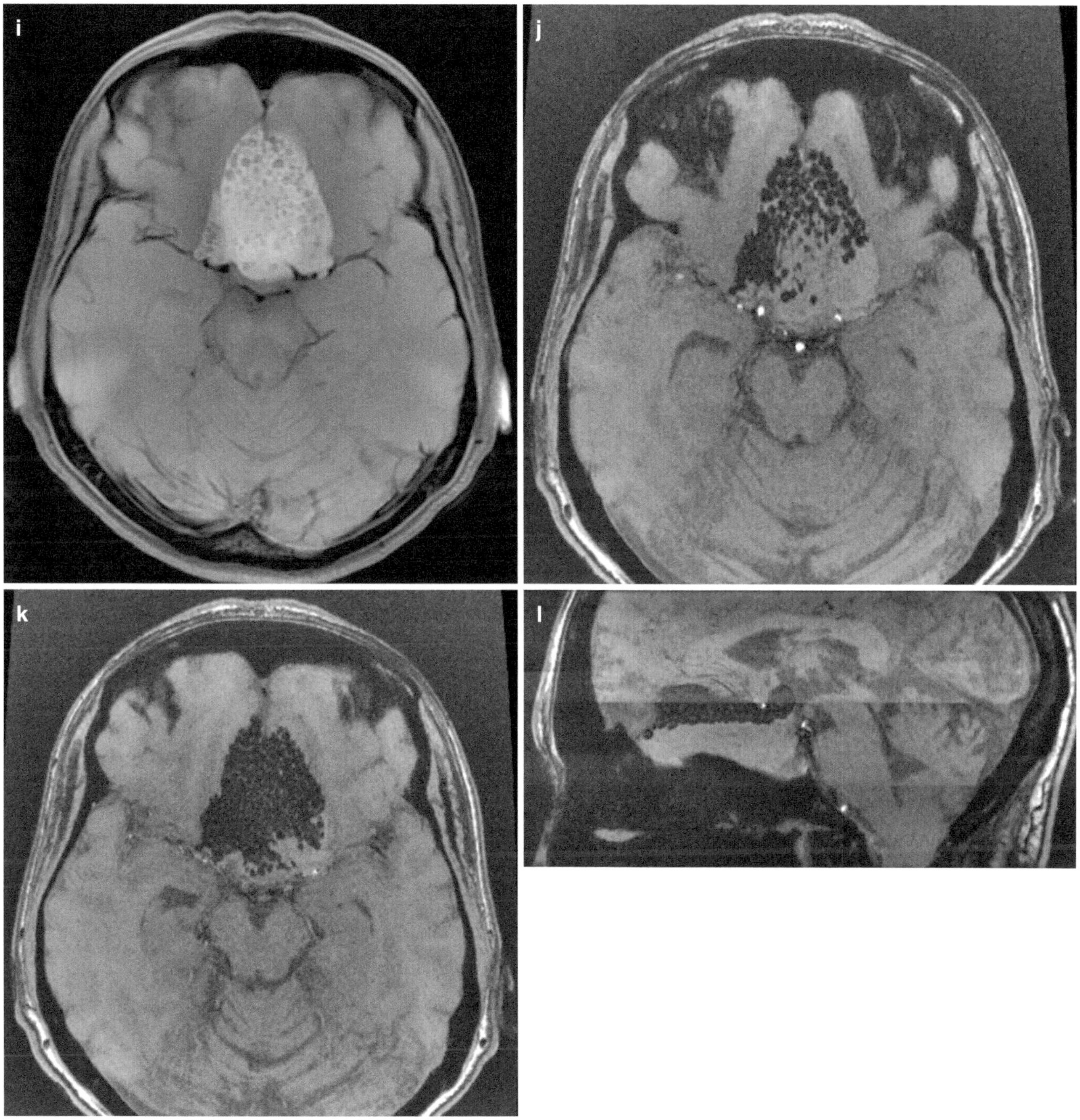

Fig. 16.6 (continued)

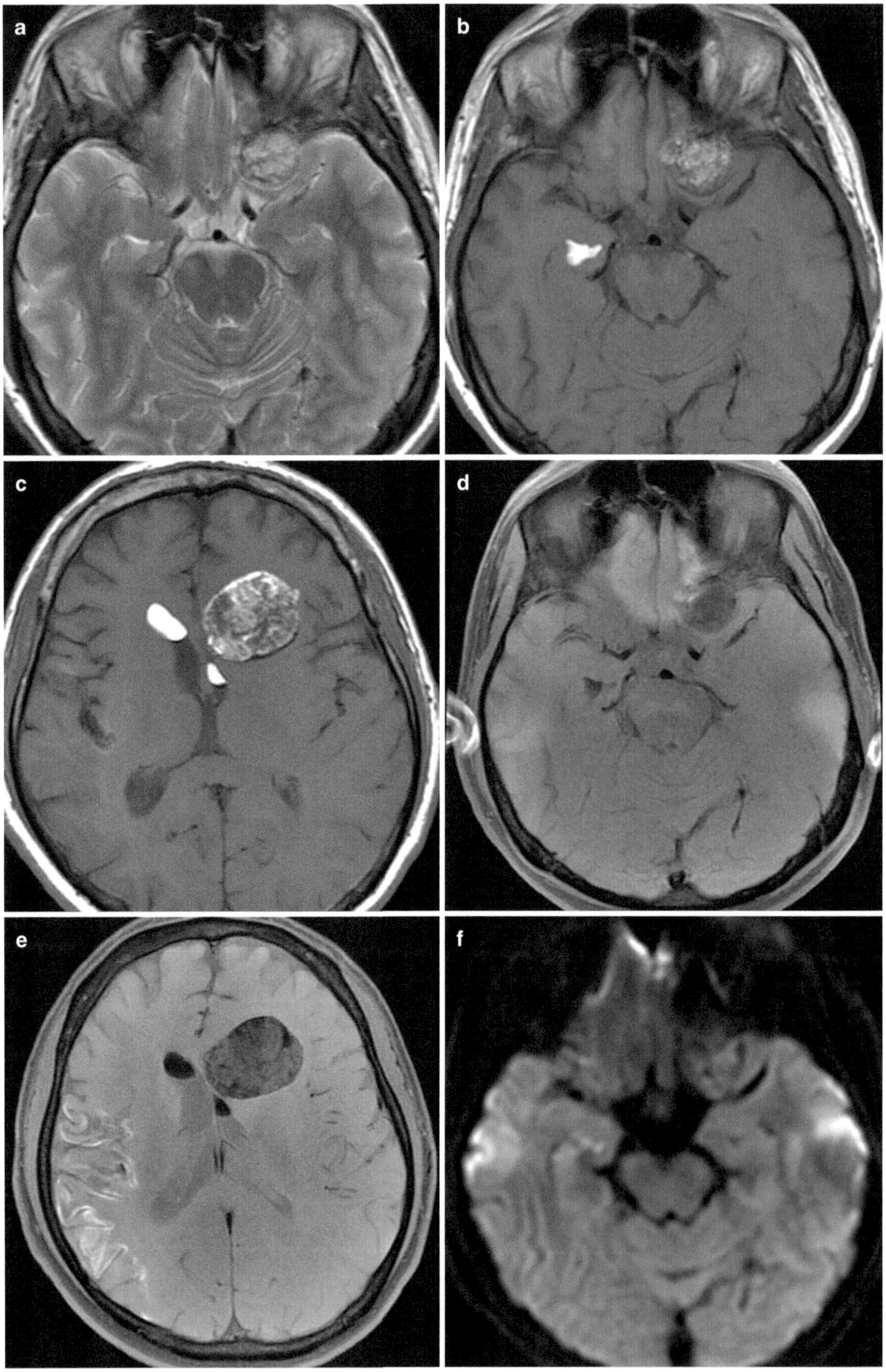

Fig. 16.7 Dermoid cyst over the left anterior clinoid process. Axial T2- (**a**), T1-weighted images (**b**, **c**), T1 + fat-sat (**d**, **e**) reveal a heterogeneous dermoid cyst with fatty content; MR-signal from fat is saturated on T1 + fat-sat. Fatty droplets in the ventricles on T1-weighted images are typical for ruptured dermoid cyst. The dermoid cyst is isointense on DWI (**f**). There is an ischemic area with gyriform hyperintensity related to pseudolaminar necrosis in the right temporal lobe

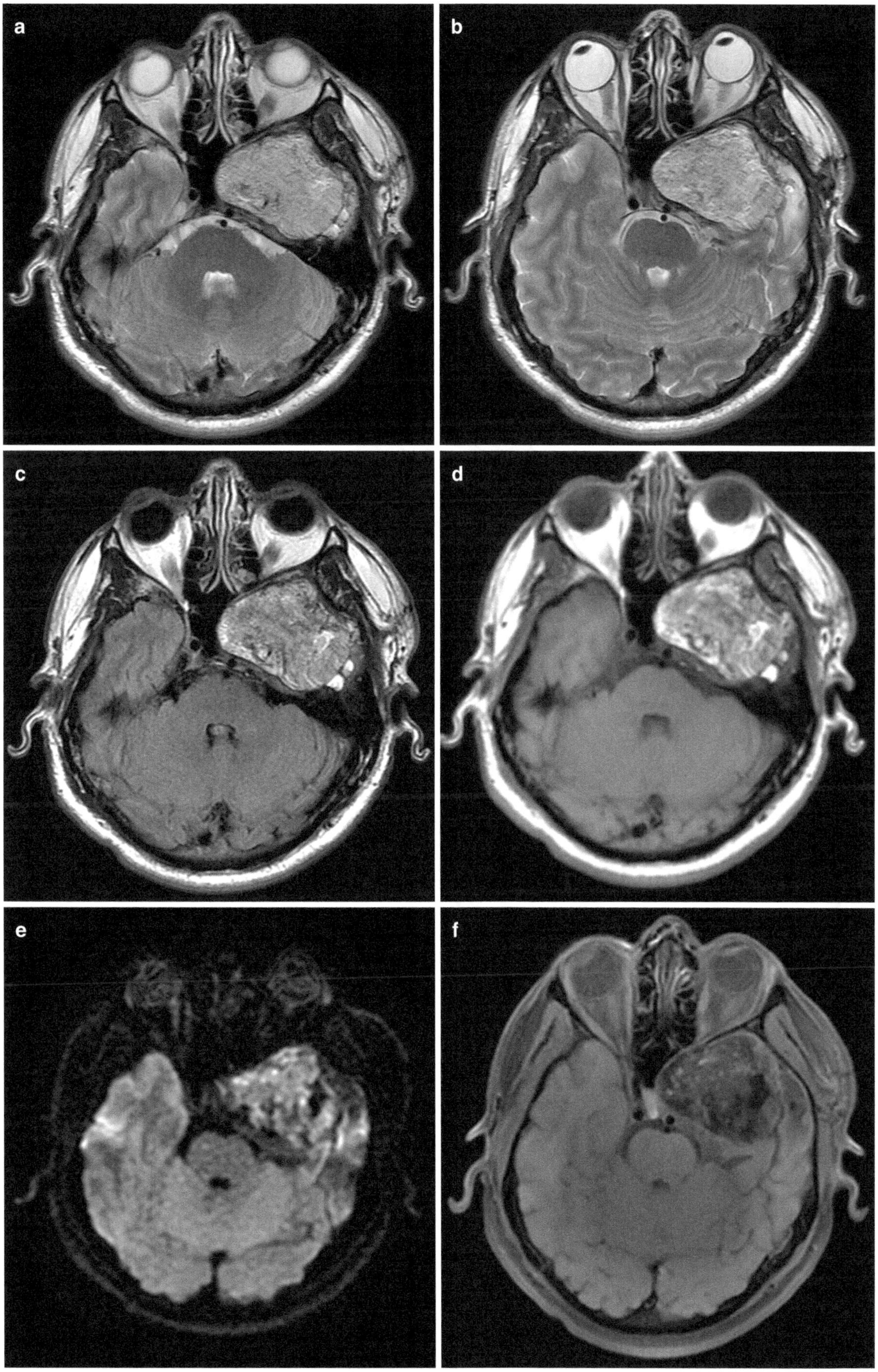

Fig. 16.8 Dermoid cyst of the left parasellar region. T2-weighted images (**a**, **b**), T2-FLAIR (**c**), T1-weighted images (**d**), DWI (**e**) show a large heterogeneous hyperintense cystic lesion. T1 + FS (**f**) show a complete suppression of the fatty mass within the cyst

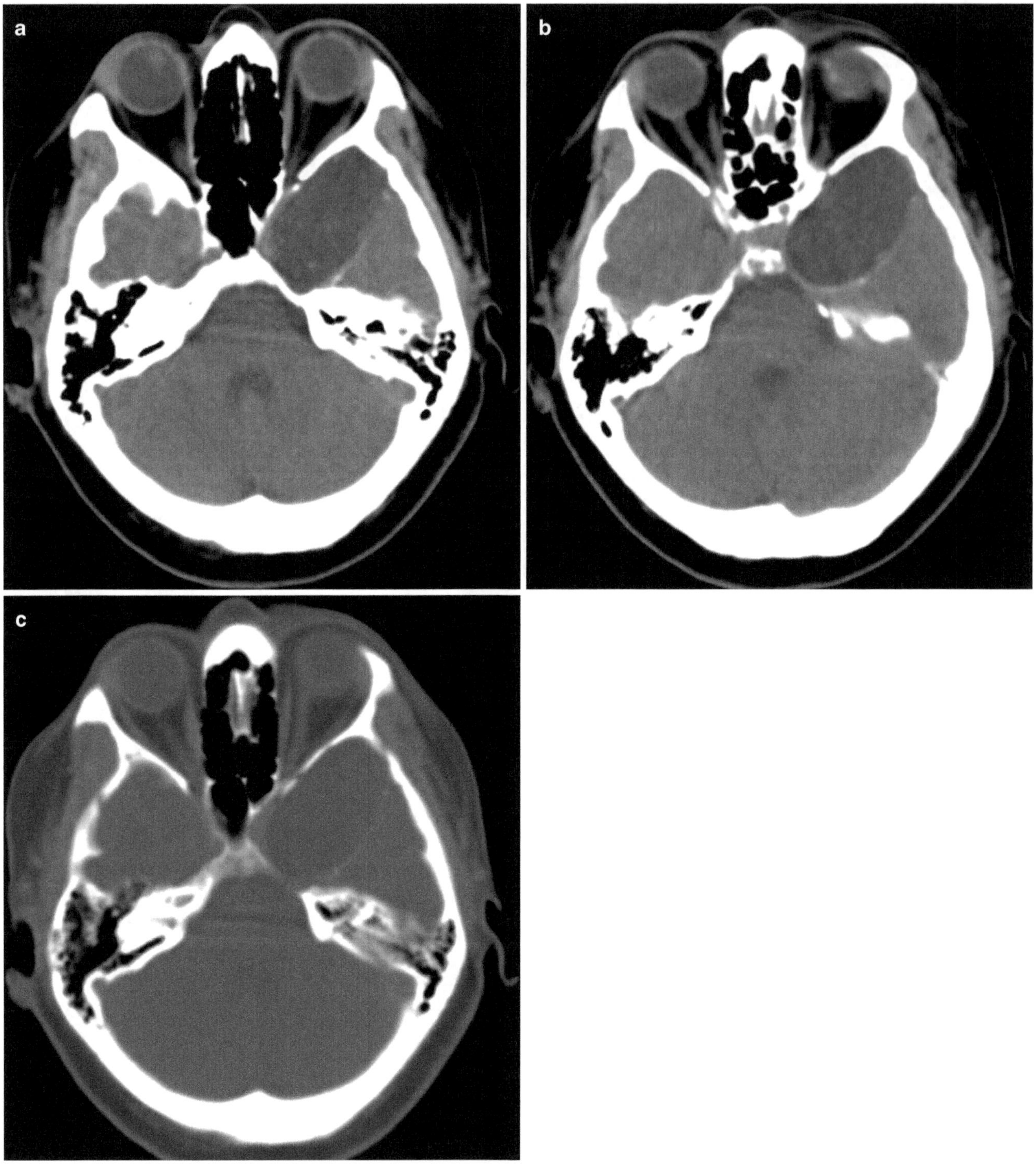

Fig. 16.9 Epidermoid cyst of the left middle cranial fossa. CT scans (**a–c**) show a homogeneous hypodense (0–10H) lesion. Bone CT scan (**c**) demonstrates the remodeled bones of the left middle fossa

hypointense signal, with hyperintense inclusions in their structure (Figs. 16.9, 16.10, and 16.11). Epidermoids are characterized by a scalloped contour and a tendency to encase (without compression) the cranial nerves and blood vessels in the area of its location (Figs. 16.12 and 16.13). There are also cysts that are hyperintense to the CSF on T1-weighted imaging. That is due to high fat content in the cyst (Horowitz et al. 1990; Ren et al. 2012). The cyst capsule is enhanced in about 25% of cases. MRI demonstrates this better than CT. Hyperintense signal on DWI is typical for epidermoid cysts (Fig. 16.14). CT- perfusion study demonstrates absence of blood flow within the cystic lesion.

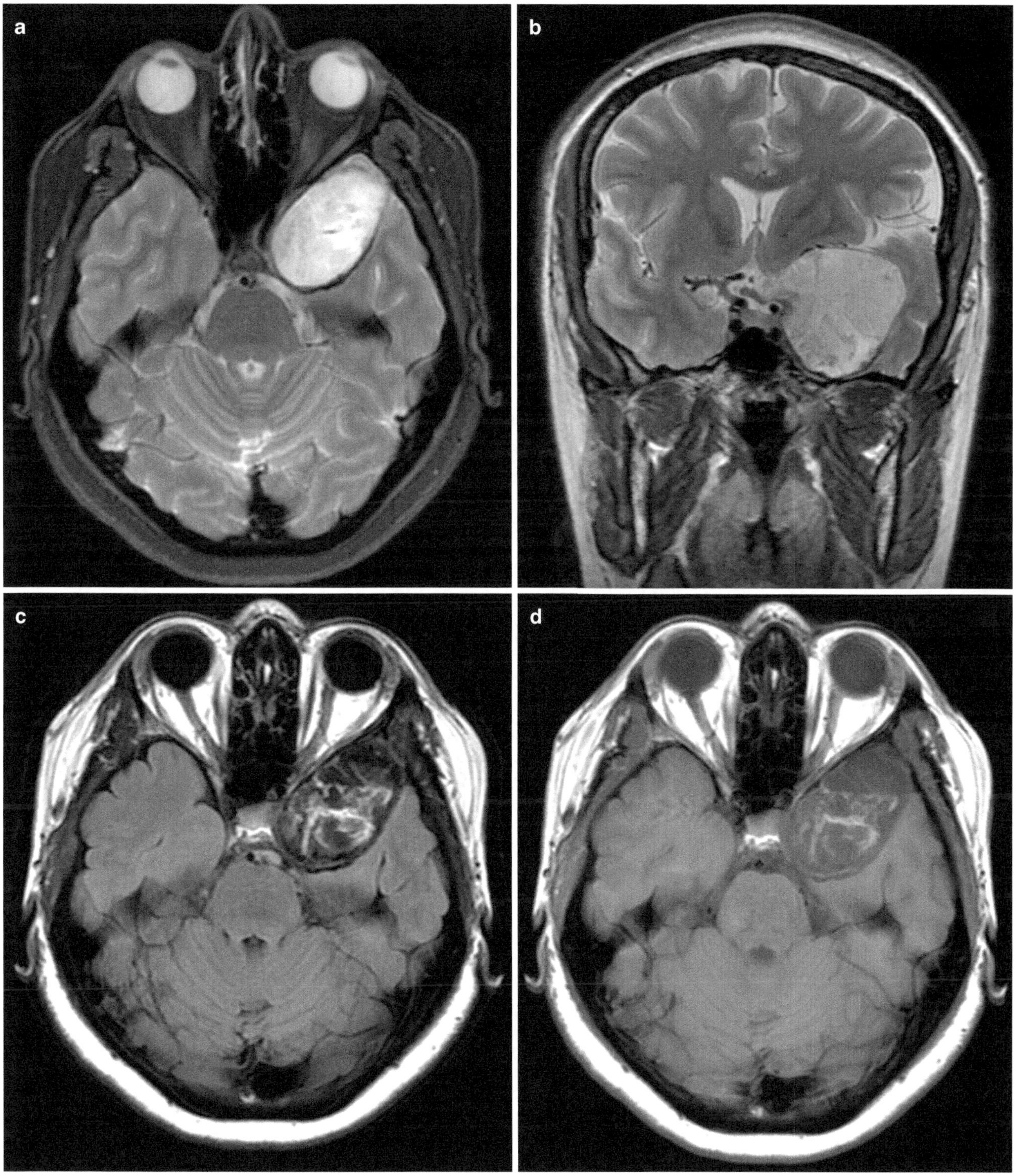

Fig. 16.10 Epidermoid cyst of the left middle fossa (CT presented in Fig. 16.9). T2-weighted (**a**, **b**), T2-FLAIR (**c**), T1-weighted images (**d**) and T1+FS MR (**e**) show a heterogeneous mass without fat component (MR-signal doesn't suppressed on T1 + FS). DWI shows a typical hyperintensity (**f**). The cyst has an increased MR-signal with hypointense (not hemorrhagic) inclusions on SWAN (**g**). Margins of the cyst strongly enhance (**h**, **i**)

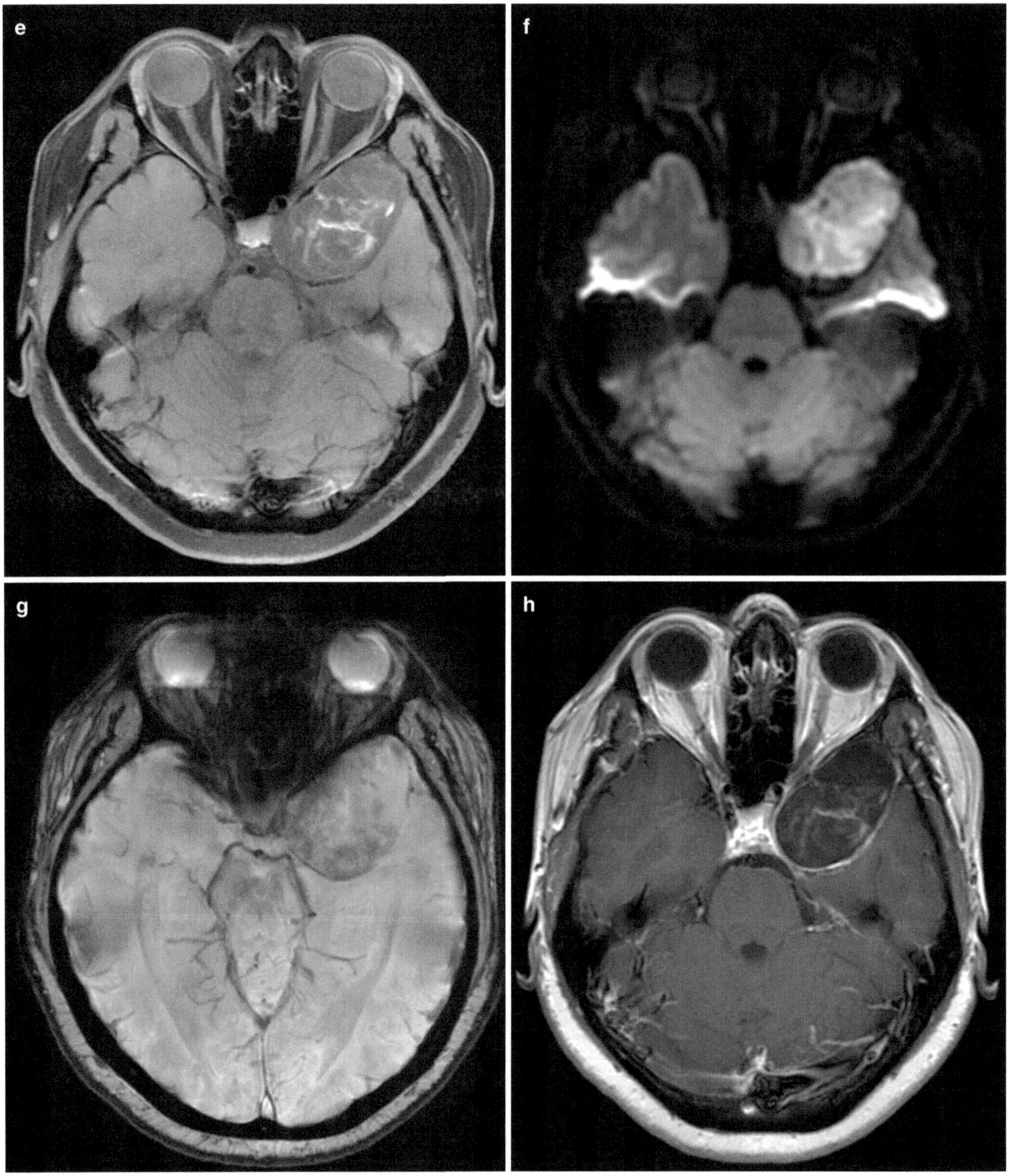

Fig. 16.10 (continued)

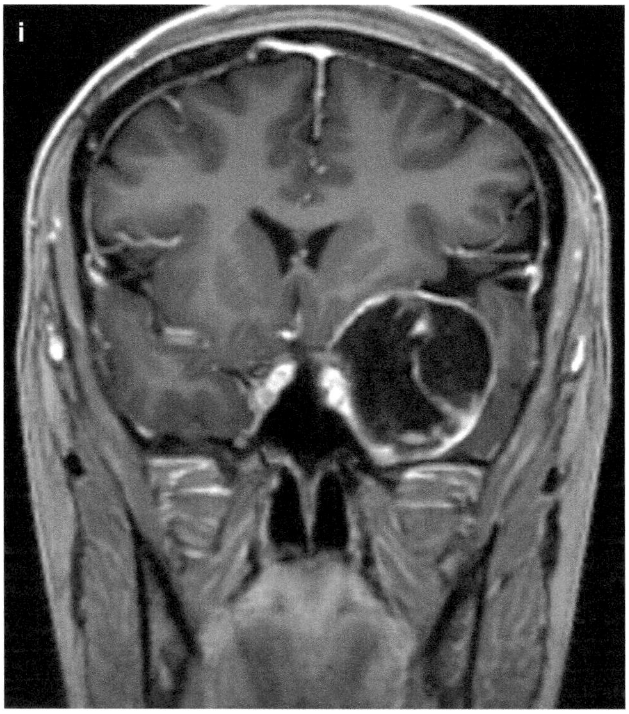

Fig. 16.10 (continued)

16.2 Pituitary Anomalies

The pituitary gland and hypothalamus anomalies frequently coexist with other anomalies of structures located along the medial axis such as those of optic nerves, septum pellucidum, and bones of skull base and palate, etc. (Naidich et al. 1983). Pituitary gland and hypothalamus dysfunction are most often clinically manifested by growth retardation (Hoyt et al. 1970).

The Pituitary Gland Hypoplasia In many cases, routine X-ray exam and CT show the small and flattened sella turcica. The hypoplastic pituitary gland may be smaller than a normal one on CT, but it occupies the usual location. MRI can better visualize the pituitary gland and the pituitary stalk.

The other group of congenital anomalies may be identified only with the help of MRI. Thus, in patients with congenital nanismus, in whom the growth hormone is deficient or other hormonal deficits of adenohypophysis (Fujisawa et al. 1987; Kelly et al. 1988) are found: a small sella turcica, small anterior part of the pituitary gland, absence of normally hyperintensive signal of the posterior part of the pituitary gland, absence of the distal part of the pituitary stalk, or the abnormal hyperintense area in tuber cinereum of the hypothalamus may be identified. In such cases, *ectopic posterior pituitary lobe* is suggested (Fig. 16.15). Almost all patients have a history of complicated or traumatic delivery. It is suggested that the perinatal trauma causes rupture of the pituitary infundibulum and its vascular membrane. That causes isolation of the pituitary gland from the stimulating effects of the hypothalamus; it also causes impairment of its blood supply and decrease of secretion of hormones of the adenohypophysis. The function of the posterior part of pituitary gland usually remains intact. It should be distinguished from lipoma of the floor of the third ventricle. Differentiation of posterior pituitary ectopia from lipoma is possible using the pulse sequence with fat suppression. The signal from the ectopic pituitary posterior gland is not suppressed, while that from a lipoma is. In the latter cases, the hyperintensive signal of neurohypophysis remains in the sella turcica cavity (Fig. 16.16).

Duplication of the pituitary stalk is possible with or without duplication of the pituitary gland. It is usually associated with abnormalities in the tuber cinereum and mammillary bodies, duplication of the basilar artery and widely separated supraclinoid carotid arteries, congenital callosal dysgenesis, Dandy-Walker spectrum. In severe cases, there may be a duplication of the sella turcica (two separated pituitary fossae) (Fig. 16.17).

Pituitary Hyperplasia Pituitary hyperplasia or hypertrophy is a non-tumoral enlarging of the pituitary gland up to 10–15 mm (Fig. 16.18). There are physiologic (in puberty, pregnancy and lactation) and nonphysiologic hyperplasia, which may be associated with a primary hypothyroidism, Cushing disease, Addison disease, Turner syndrome, and Klinefelter syndrome. Nonphysiologic hyperplasia sometimes is seen with some neuroendocrine tumors (Osborn et al. 2016). It also can be observed in intracranial hypotension and dural fistulas.

CT and MRI revealed an enlarged pituitary gland with a homogeneous MR-signal and a mildly convex superior margin on coronal MRI. It should be differentiated from a pituitary adenoma, hypophysitis, metastatic lesions. An enlarged adenohypophysis is homogeneously enhancing using bolus technique.

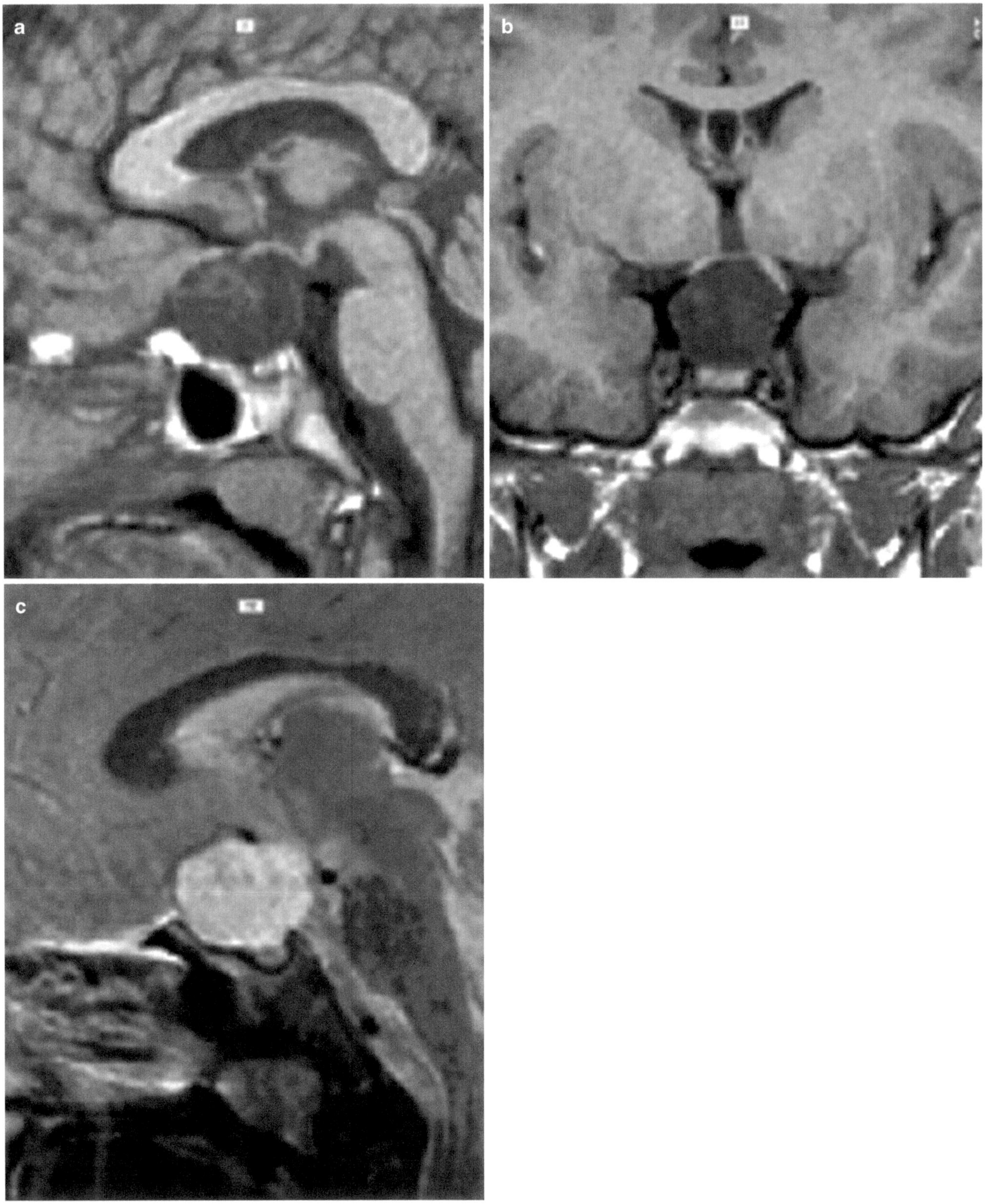

Fig. 16.11 Epidermoid cyst of the suprasellar area. Sagittal, coronal T1-weighted images (**a**, **b**) and sagittal T2-weighted image (**c**) demonstrate a large heterogeneous suprasellar mass, which is hypointense on T1 and hyperintense on T2

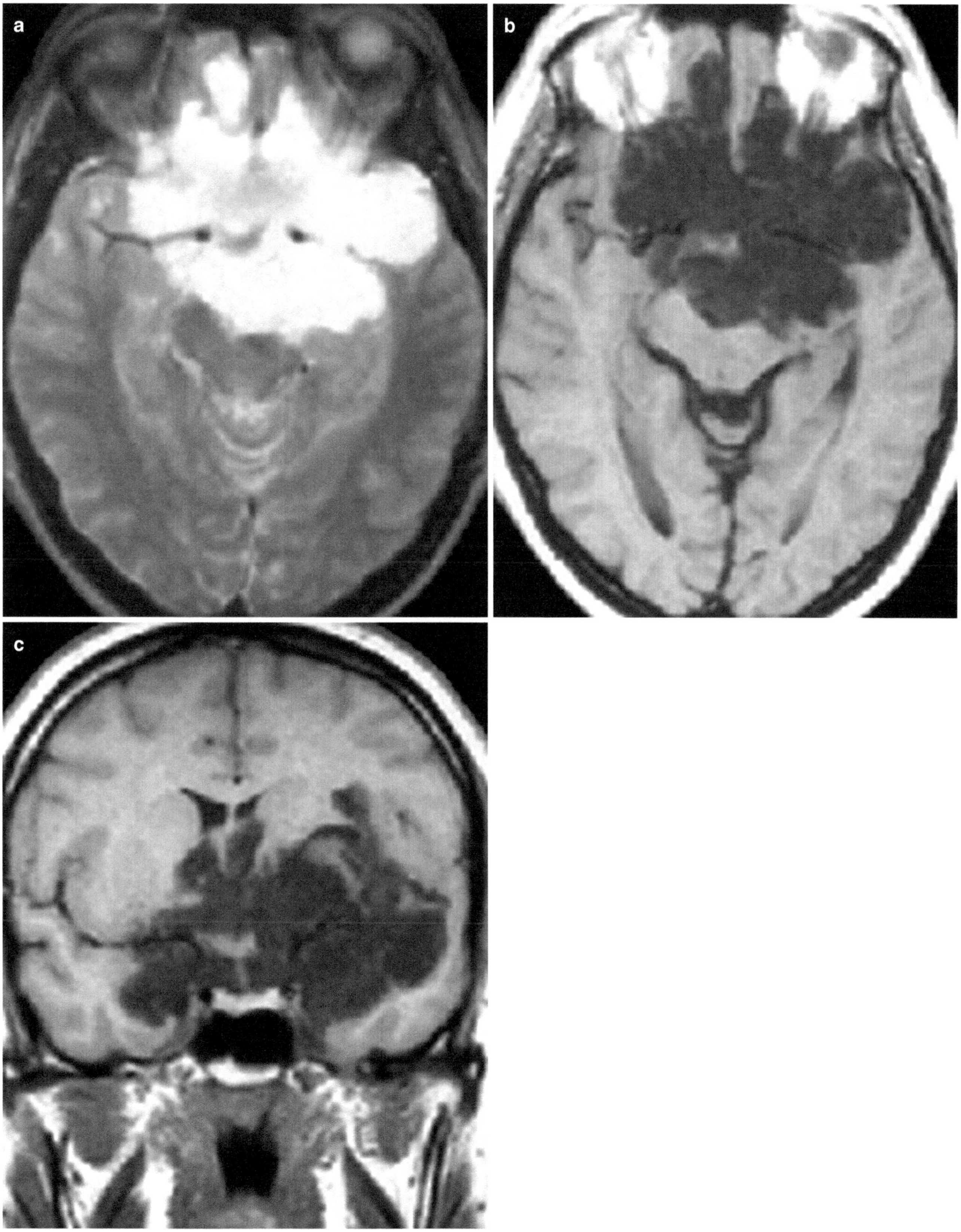

Fig. 16.12 Giant epidermoid cyst of the sellar-parasellar area. T2-weighted image (**a**), axial (**b**) and coronal (**c**) T1-weighted images show an epidermoid cyst with "scalloped" expansion. Epidermoid is slightly hyperintense to CSF. The main arteries of the brain, chiasm, pituitary stalk, pituitary gland are visualized in the central part of cyst

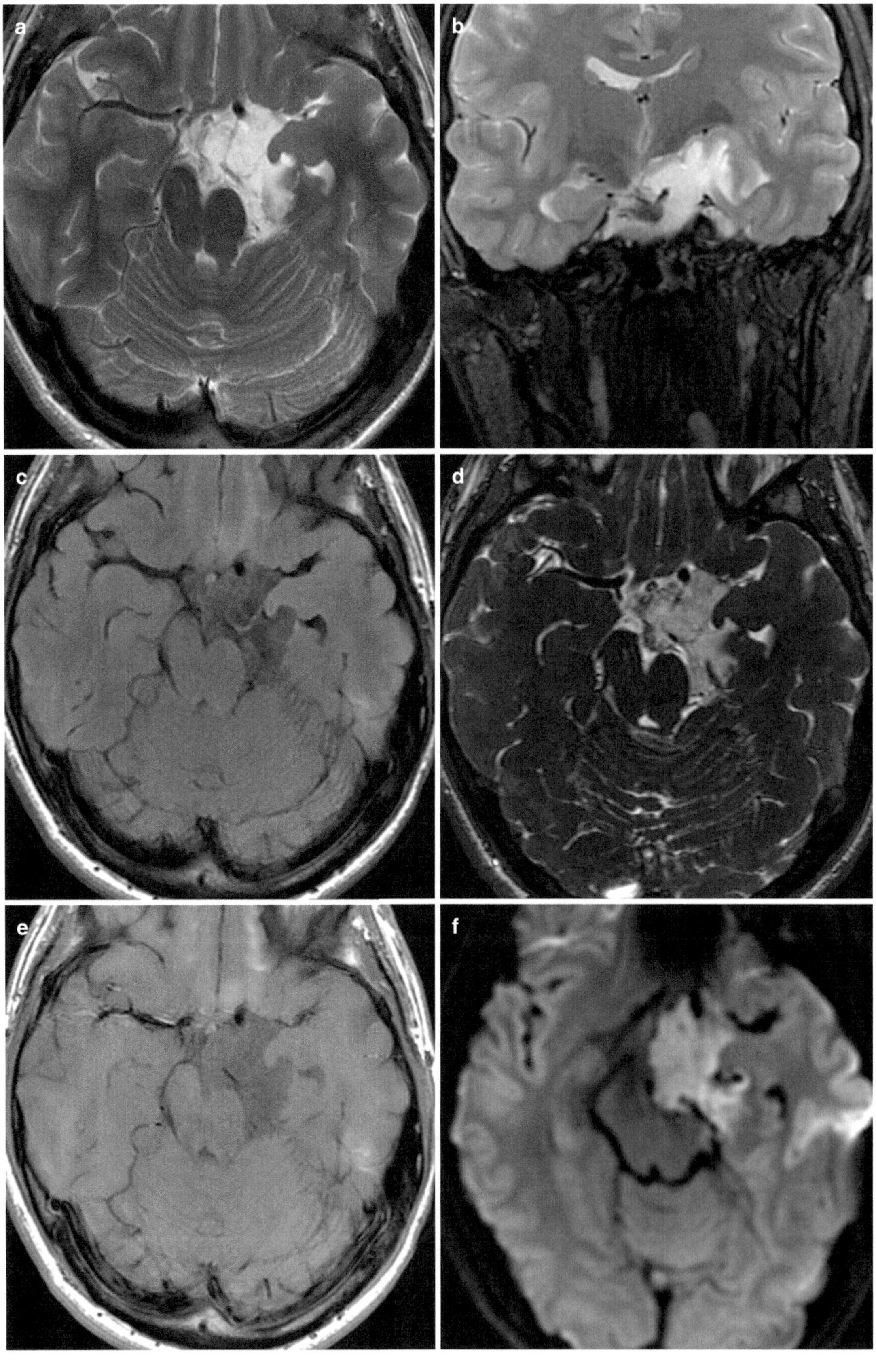

Fig. 16.13 Epidermoid cyst of the suprasellar, interpeduncular, and ambient cisterns. T2-weighted images (**a**, **b**), T2-FLAIR (**c**), FIESTA (**d**), and T1-weighted images (**e**) define a mass lesion with scalloped expansion, which is extended into the suprasellar and brainstem cisterns. The cyst is typically hyperintense on DWI (**f**)

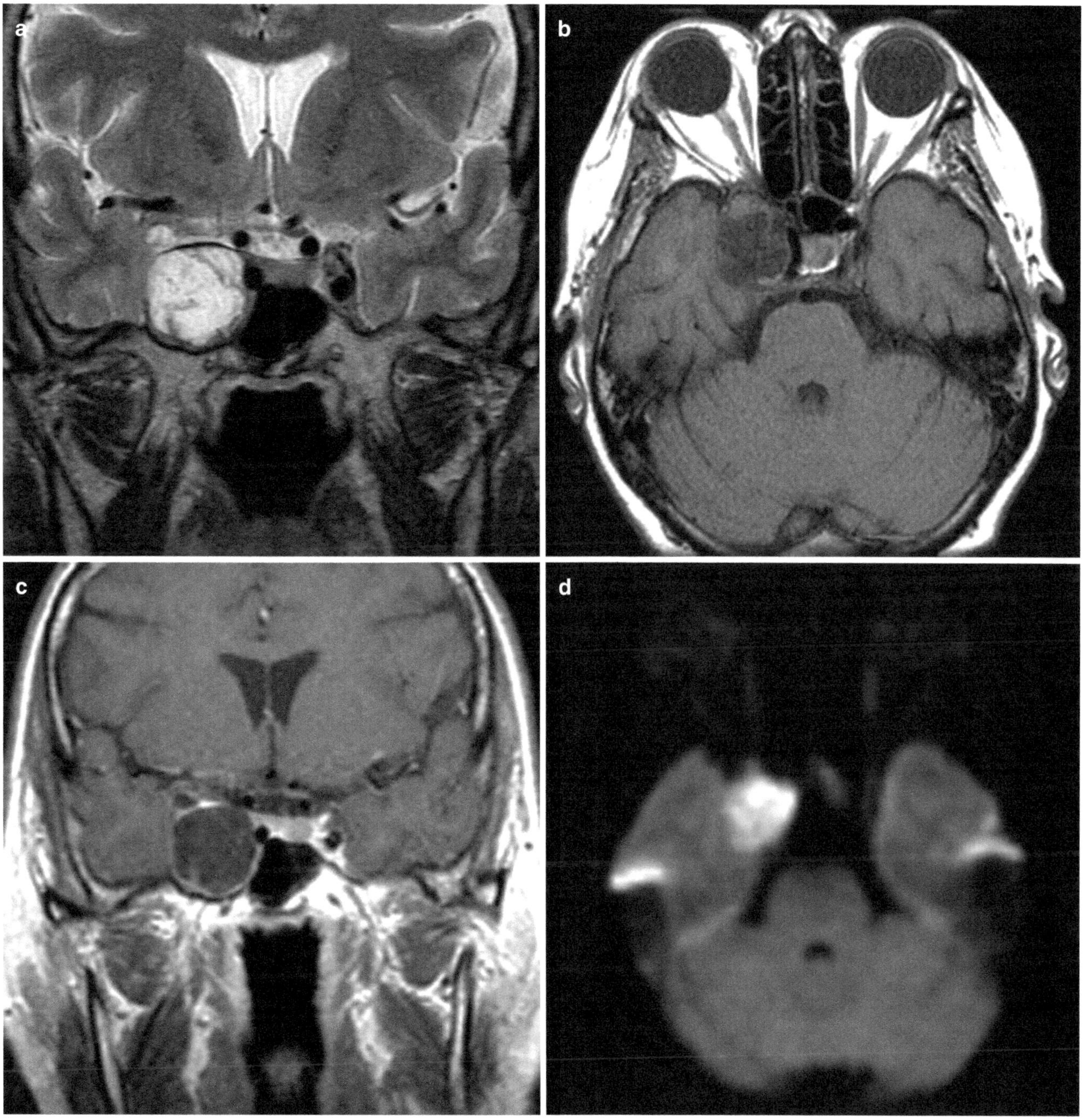

Fig. 16.14 Epidermoid cyst of the right laterosellar area. T2-weighted image (**a**), T1-weighted images before (**b**) and after CE (**c**) show a hyperintense on T2 and hypointense on T1 lesion in the right cavernous sinus. A thin peripheral enhancement is demonstrated at the cyst margins. DWI (**d**) demonstrates the hyperintense MR-signal from the lesion

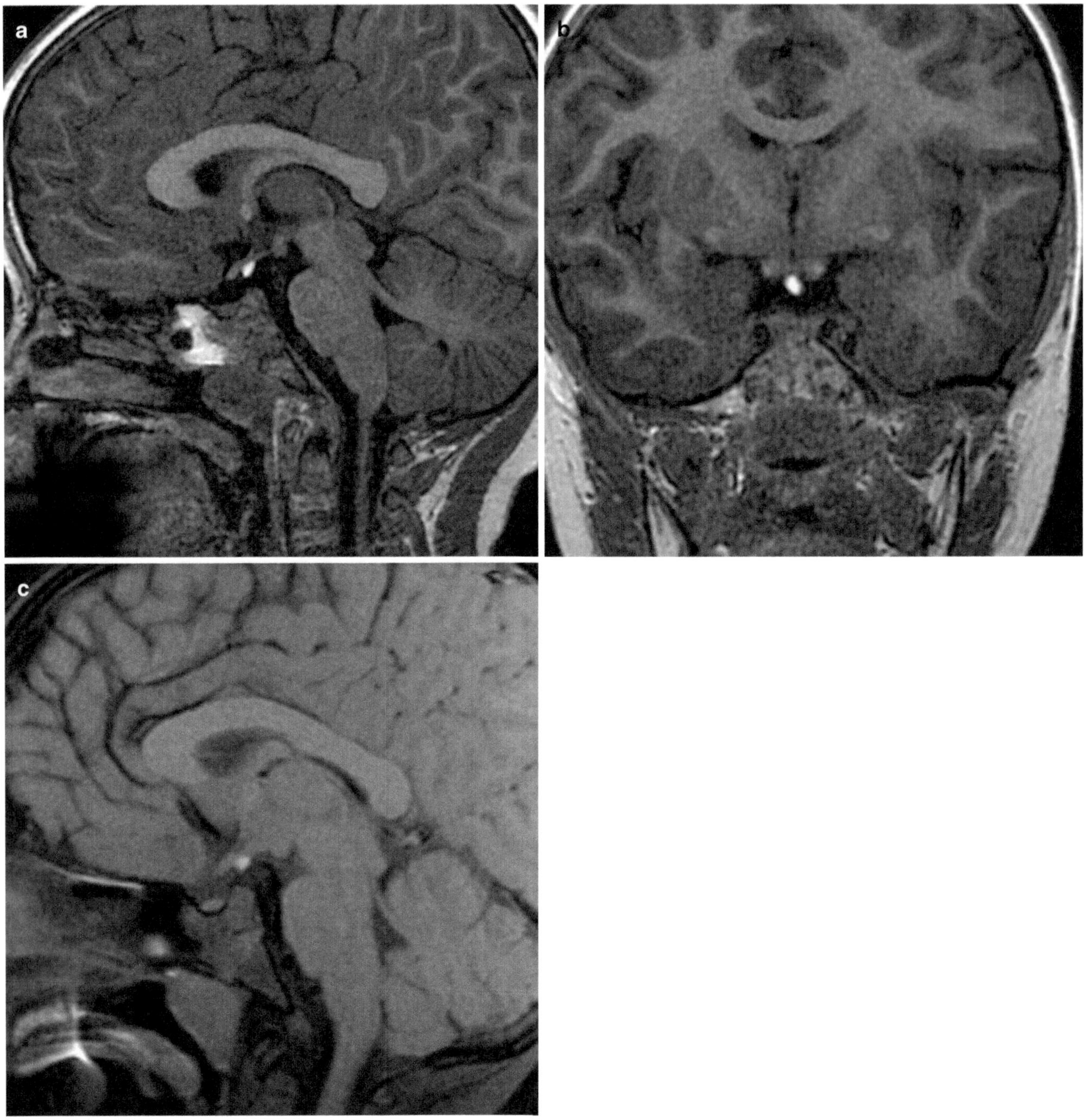

Fig. 16.15 Ectopia of the posterior pituitary gland (a child with dwarfism). Sagittal (**a**) and coronal (**b**) T1-weighted images reveal an ectopic posterior pituitary gland (hyperintensive signal) located at the tuber cinereum area. The anterior pituitary gland is small. The infundibulum is absent. Ectopic pituitary is not suppressed on T1 + fat-sat (**c**). This fact denies the diagnosis of lipoma and confirms an ectopia of posterior pituitary

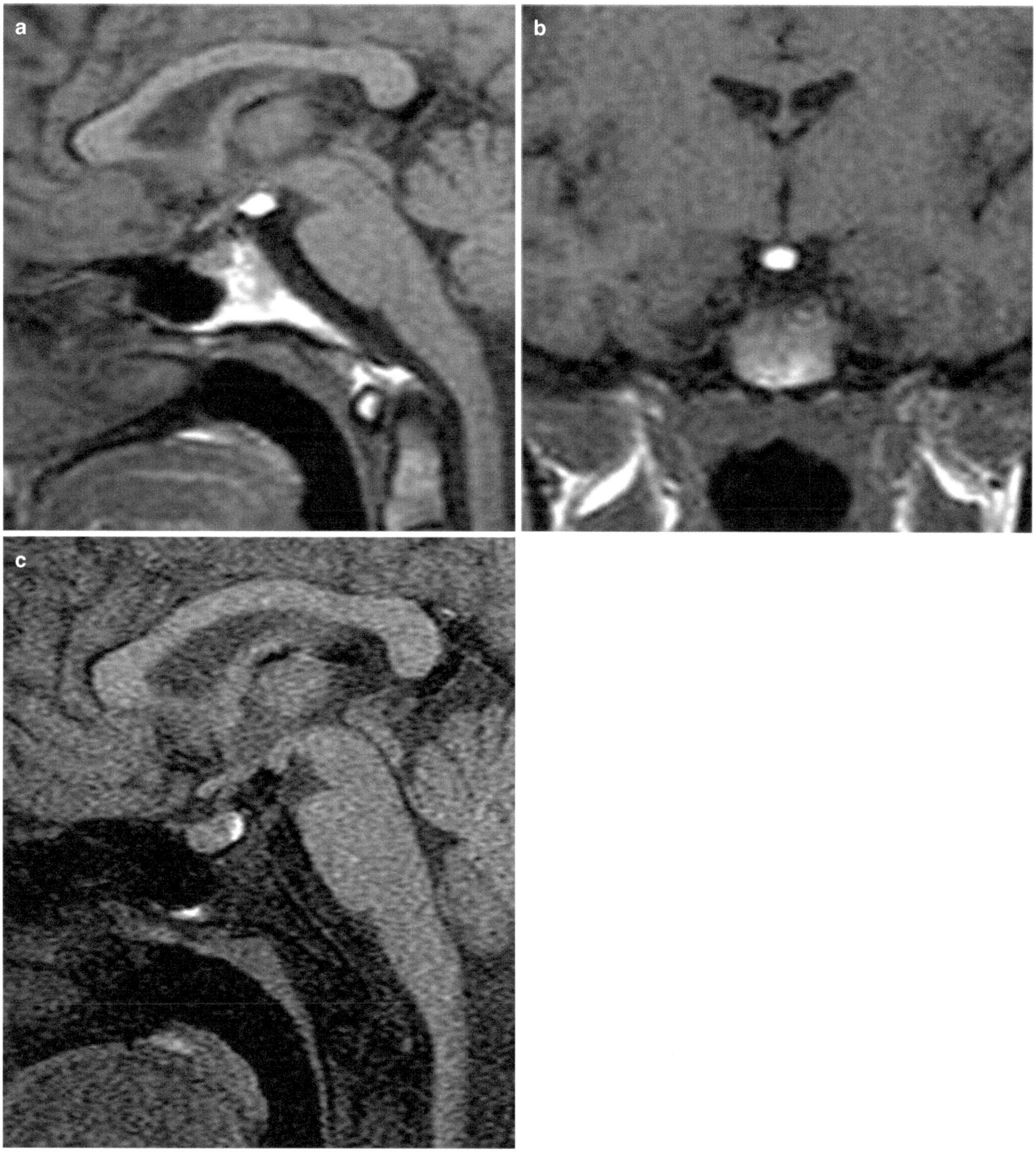

Fig. 16.16 Lipoma of the tuber cinereum area. Sagittal (**a**) and coronal (**b**) T1-weighted images identify a hyperintense small mass at the third ventricle floor area. This small lesion is suppressed with fat saturation (**c**), but posterior pituitary in the sella turcica is not suppressed and remains hyperintensive

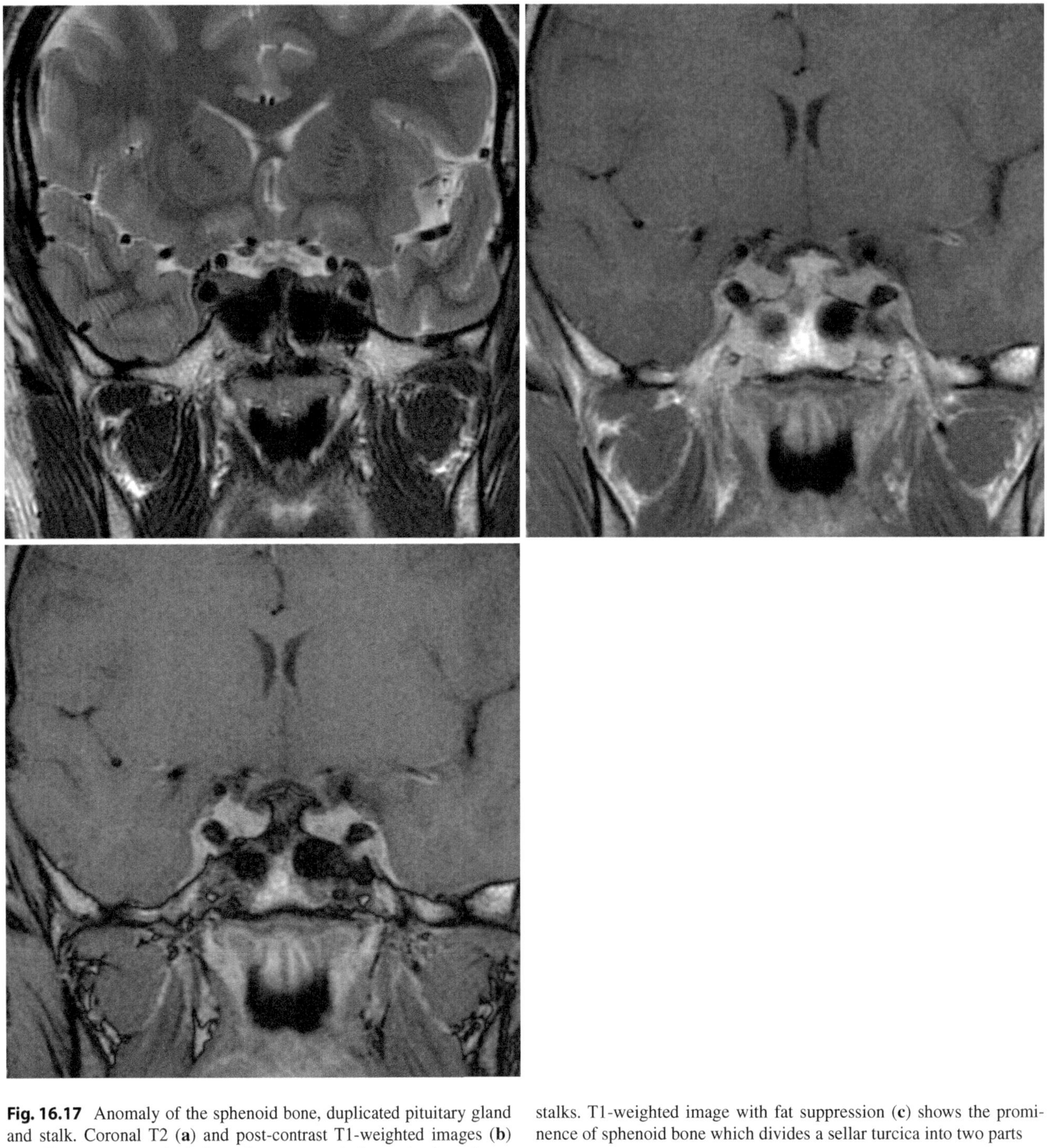

Fig. 16.17 Anomaly of the sphenoid bone, duplicated pituitary gland and stalk. Coronal T2 (**a**) and post-contrast T1-weighted images (**b**) identify two separated pituitary fossae, two pituitary glands and two stalks. T1-weighted image with fat suppression (**c**) shows the prominence of sphenoid bone which divides a sellar turcica into two parts

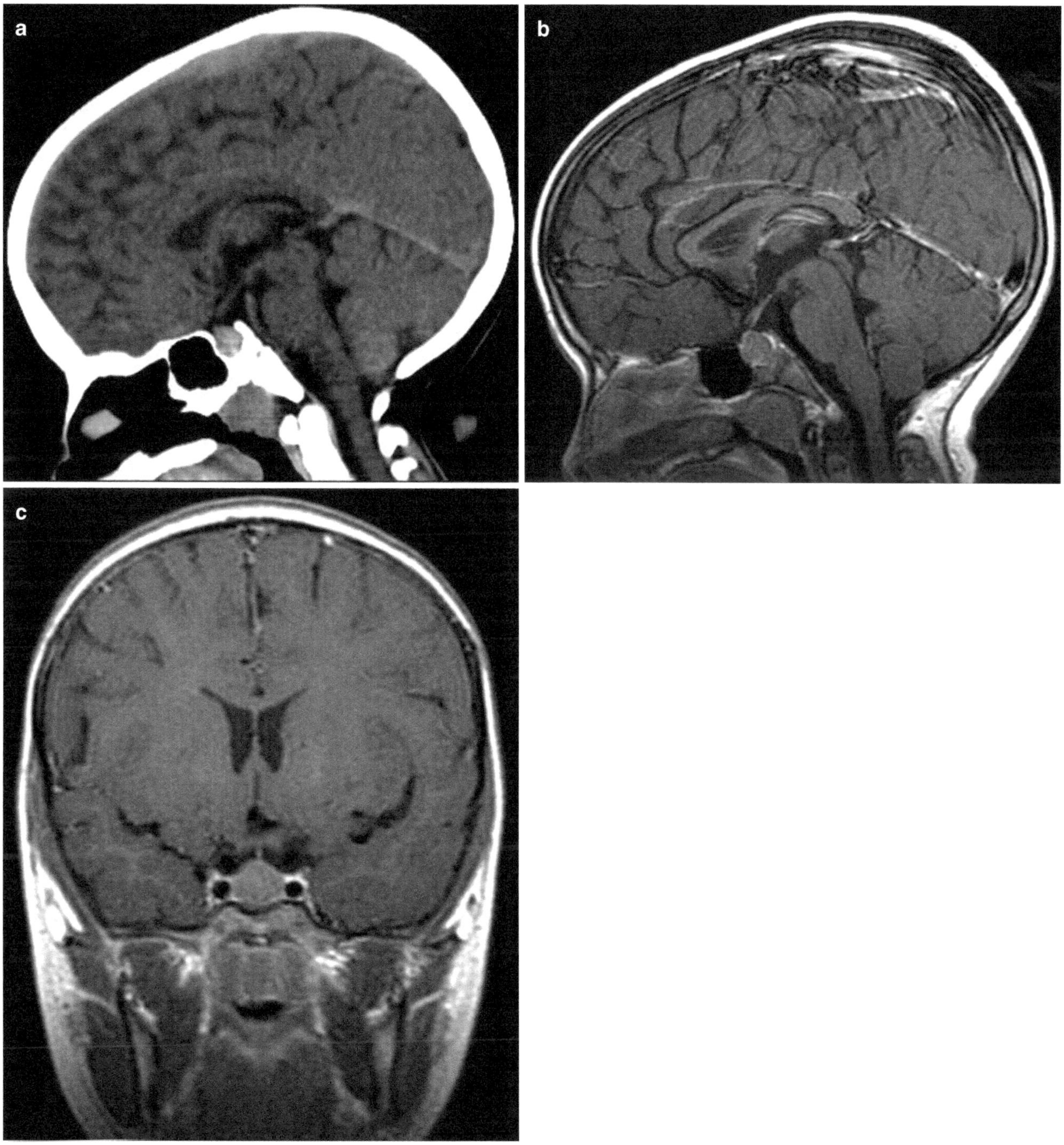

Fig. 16.18 Pituitary hyperplasia in a child with panhypopituitarism, hypothyroidism caused by mutation of the PROP-1 gene. Sagittal CT reformat (**a**), post-contrast sagittal (**b**) and coronal T1-weighted images (**c**) show a uniformly enlarged and homogeneously enhancing pituitary gland

Infectious and Inflammatory Disorders 17

Contents

Infectious disorders of the pituitary are exceptionally rare. There is an opinion that cases of acquired diabetes insipidus may be a result of viral infection of the supraoptic and the paraventricular nuclei of the hypothalamus (Daughaday 1985). Tuberculosis and syphilis that were frequently encountered in the chiasmal-sellar region in the past due to high incidence in the common population are now rare (Fig. 17.1). Even bacterial infections are now rare and become symptomatic only after abscess formation. Nevertheless, two cases of mycotic abscesses of the parasellar region have been followed up in our Institute.

17.1 Pituitary Abscess

Pituitary abscesses are rare. Infection may disseminate into the sella turcica via a hematogenous route or directly from the infected sphenoid or cavernous sinuses (Walia et al. 2010). The following causes of infections in the sella turcica may be seen also: pituitary adenoma, Rathke cleft cyst, and craniopharyngioma (Daningue and Wilson 1977; Selosse et al. 1980; Gupta 1989). The most common clinical manifestations are headaches and visual loss, as abscesses clinically often are similar to hormonally inactive pituitary adenomas. Diagnosis of the abscess of sella turcica is an exceptionally rare occasion.

MRI without CE reveals a mass lesion of the sella turcica indistinguishable from adenoma. After CE, a rim of enhancement is seen on periphery, and the hypointense area remains in the center (Fig. 17.2). The use of DWI allows making the diagnosis of pituitary abscess more specific (Fig. 17.3).

I. Pronin, V. Kornienko, *CT and MRI of Skull Base Lesions*, https://doi.org/10.1007/978-3-319-65957-2_17

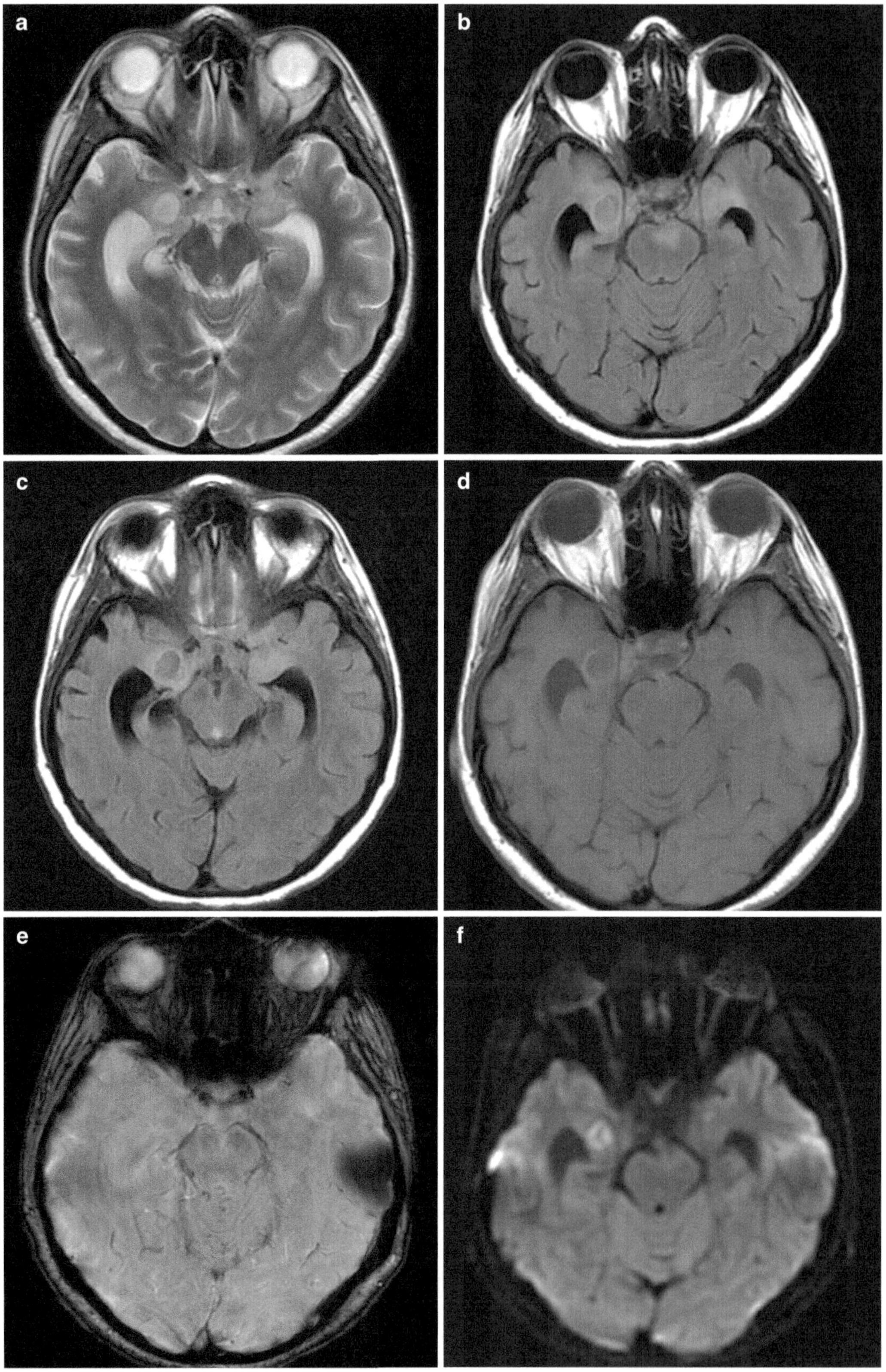

Fig. 17.1 CNS tuberculosis. T2-weighted image (**a**), T2-FLAIR (**b**, **c**), and T1-weighted images (**d**) reveal the heterogeneous hyperintense areas in the sella and laterosellar regions on the both sides. Cystic lesion is visualized in the right temporal region, which correspond to the round nodule with increased MR-signal on DWI (**f**). There is no evidence of hemorrhage in pathological areas on SWAN (**e**). Post-contrast T1-weighted images (**g**, **h**) and T1 + fat-sat (**i**) show multiple lesions in the parasellar areas with peripheral rim enhancement and necrotic centers with low signal

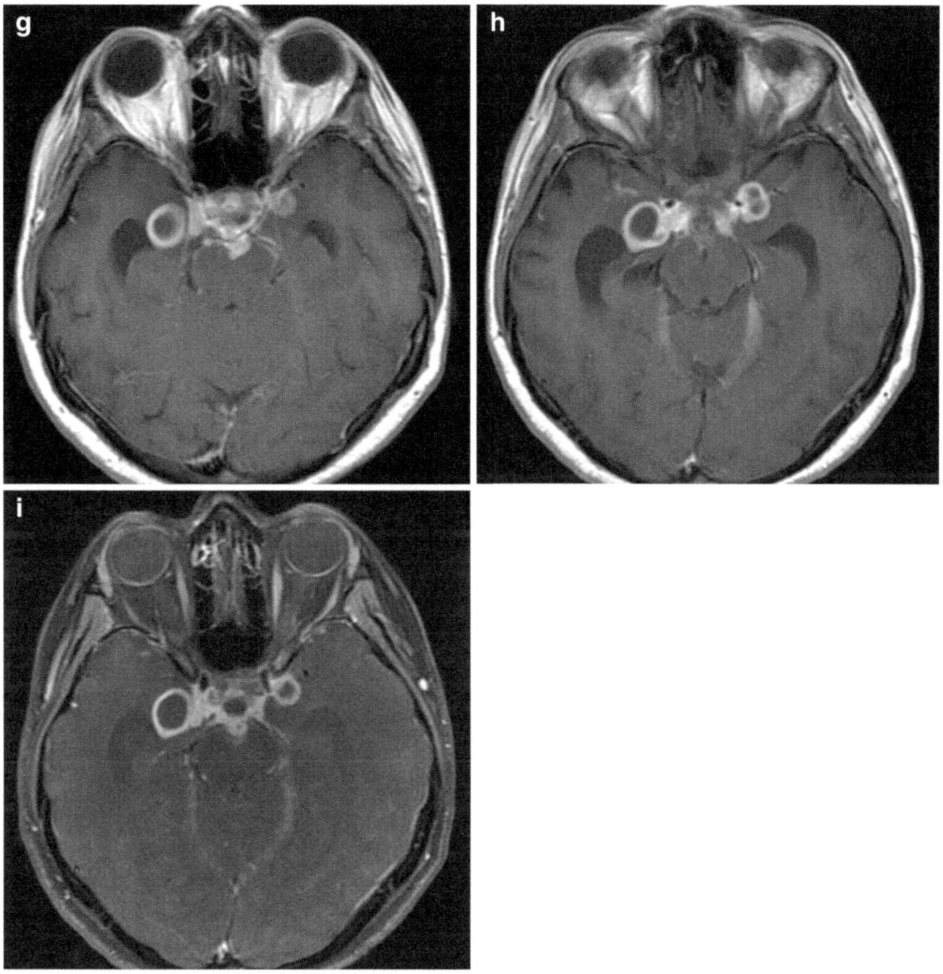

Fig. 17.1 (continued)

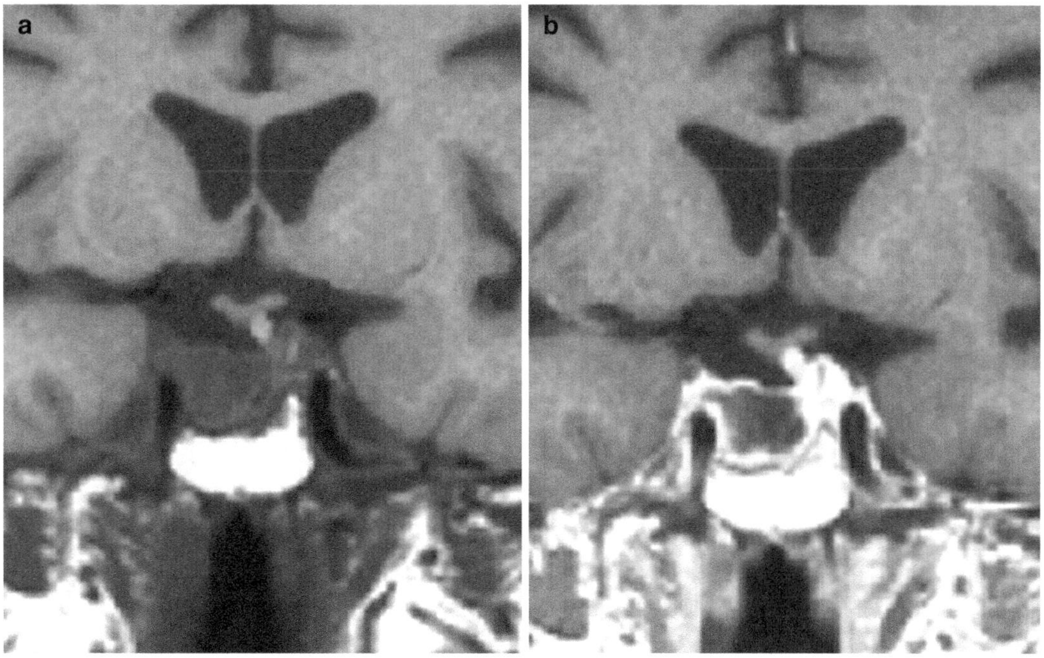

Fig. 17.2 Pituitary abscess. Coronal T1-weighted image (**a**) and post-contrast T1-weighted image (**b**) reveal an intense peripheral rim enhancement with necrotic non-enhanced center of the abscess

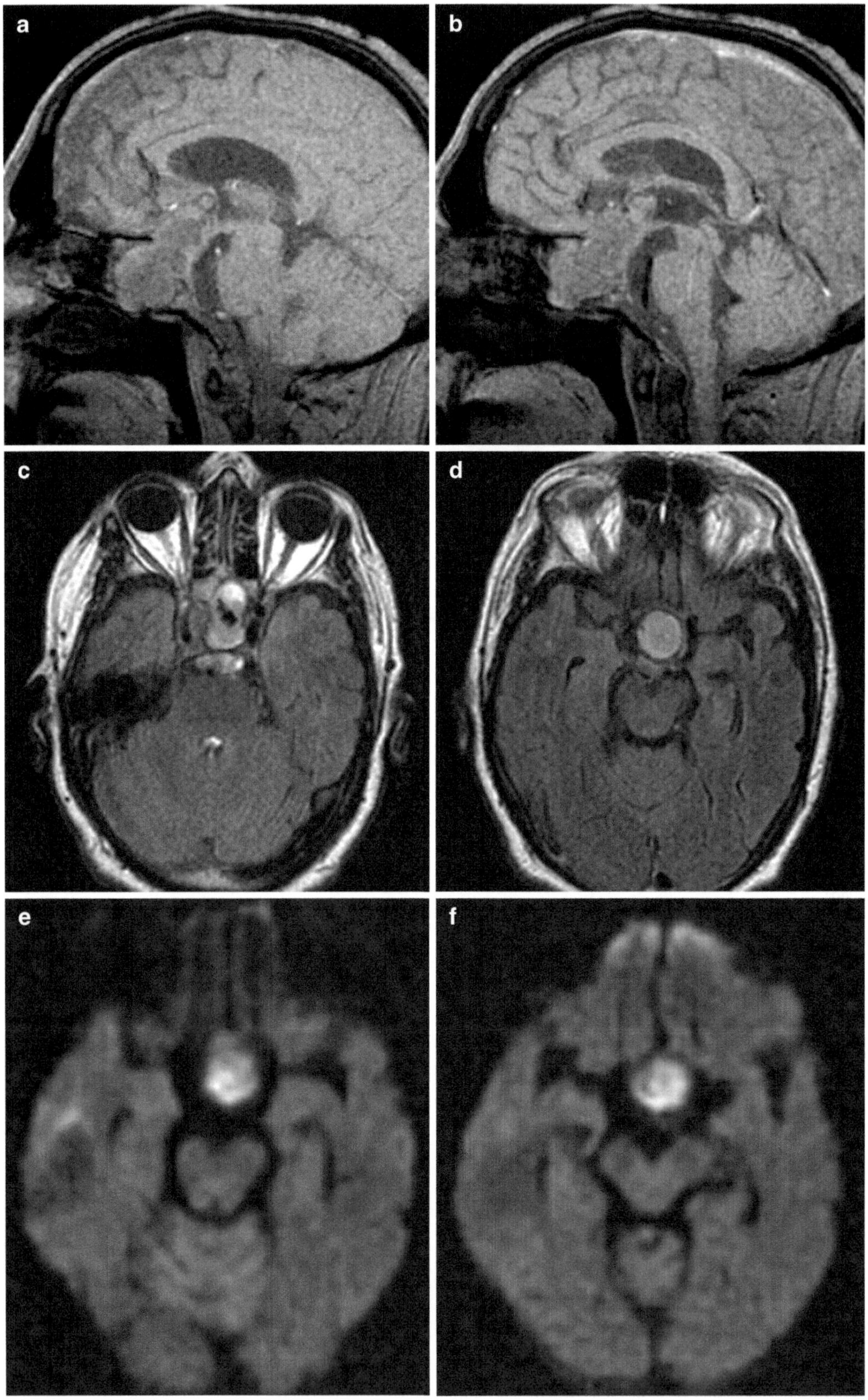

Fig. 17.3 Postsurgical sellar-suprasellar abscess after pituitary adenoma resection. Sagittal T1-weighted images (**a**, **b**) and axial T2-FLAIR (**c**, **d**) show a relatively homogeneous area in the enlarged sella and suprasellar region with the deformation of the third ventricular floor. DWI (**e**, **f**) demonstrates a central diffusion restriction area from the postresection cavity (a purulent content)

17.2 Parasellar Infection

Infection of the suprasellar cistern and the cavernous sinuses is usually a part of a disseminated process and is encountered in cases of intracranial dissemination of the extracranial infection. Brain base meninges and meninges covering the suprasellar cistern are sensitive to tuberculosis and other forms of granulomatous meningitis. Parasitic cysts may also be situated in the cistern, especially cysticercosis. Infection of the cavernous sinuses with their secondary thrombosis is a dangerous complication of periorbital or the other inflammatory disorders (furunculosis, abscesses, etc.). In our practice, we observed formation of an abscess in the temporal region due to an infection of the endovascular balloon installed in the cavity of an arterial aneurysm of the carotid siphon (Fig. 17.4).

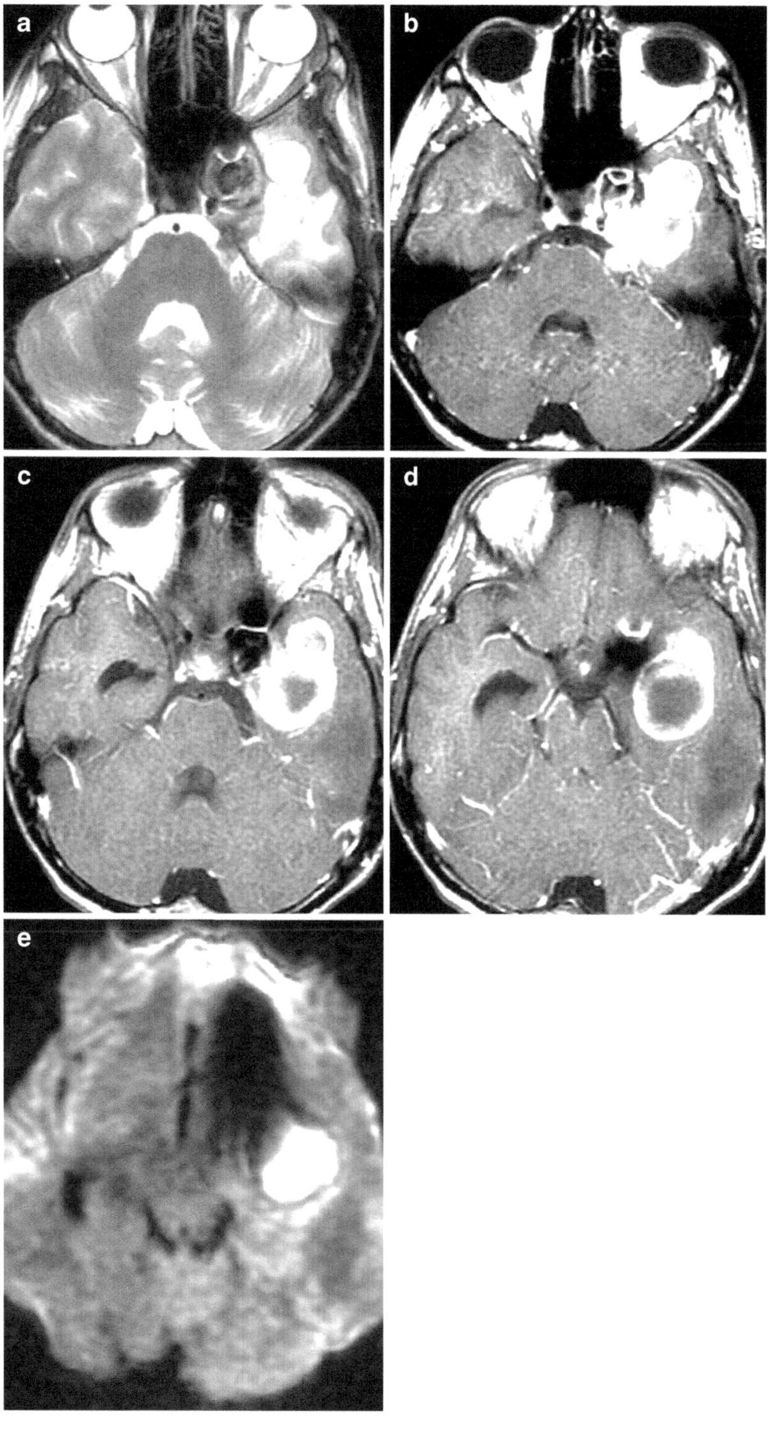

Fig. 17.4 Abscess in the left temporal lobe in combination with the saccular aneurysm of the left internal carotid artery, which is occluded by balloon. T2-weighted (**a**) and post-contrast T1-weighted images (**b**–**d**) reveal an abscess with intense enhancing rim. DWI (**e**, **f**) show an increased signal intensity within the abscess

17.3 Mucocele

Mucocele—is a space-occupying lesion located in the paranasal sinuses (Delfini et al. 1993). If located in the sphenoid sinus the differential diagnosis should be made with tumors of the chiasmal-sellar region. It is seen in children younger than 10 years but may be encountered in adults also. Mucocele is an accumulation of mucus developing after occlusion of a sinus, usually due to inflammatory origin. Trauma or tumor may also be accompanied by secondary mucocele. If the content of mucocele is infected, it is then called mucopyocele (Stankewich 1989).

Mucocele appears as a well-delineated lesion filling the sinus. Frequently it is sphenoid sinus, which may markedly enlarge in size. On CT, mucocele appears as a hypodense structure. On MRI, the signal of mucocele varies. In our observations, mucocele had hyperintense signal on T1- and T2-weighted images, which was probably associated with high protein level and elements of blood products in its content (Figs. 17.5, 17.6, 17.7, and 17.8).

17.4 Lymphocytic Hypophysitis

Lymphocytic inflammation of the pituitary is a rare inflammatory disorder. It is usually seen in the late pregnancy or the postnatal period. It is probably an autoimmune disorder connected with other autoimmune endocrinological disorders such as Hashimoto's thyroiditis. In some cases, circulating autoantibodies to prolactin were revealed. The anterior pituitary lobe and pituitary stalk are affected in hypophysitis. The disorder is characterized by a diffuse infiltration of the adenohypophysis T and B lymphocytes, plasma cells, eosinophils; presence of lymphoid follicles is possible. Widespread fibrosis is observed in the chronic stage of inflammation. Females complain of headache, memory loss, postnatal amenorrhea, lactation impairment, or the combination of the above-mentioned symptoms. The level of pituitary hormones is decreased. It may manifest with symptoms of diabetes insipidus. It occurs in no more than 1–2% of all lesions of sellar area (Osborn et al. 2016).

Imaging CT and MRI demonstrate a diffuse enlargement of the anterior lobe of pituitary gland without any focal changes, the diameter of the pituitary gland can reach 2 cm. The stalk thickening is more pronounced at its lower portion. A marked homogeneous enhancement by affected structures is observed both on CT and MRI (Quencer 1980; Levine et al. 1988). Hypophysitis should be differentiated from pituitary adenoma and abscess.

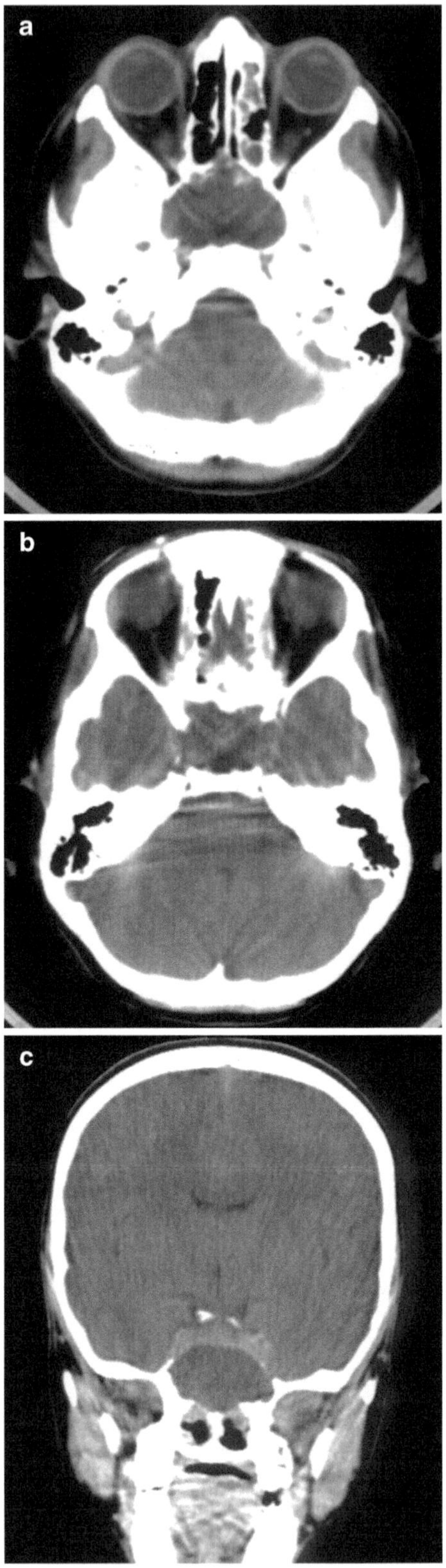

Fig. 17.5 Mucocele of the sphenoid sinus. Axial CT scans (**a**, **b**) and coronal CE CT scan (**c**) show a hypodense lesion in the expanded sphenoid sinus with elevated upward sella turcica

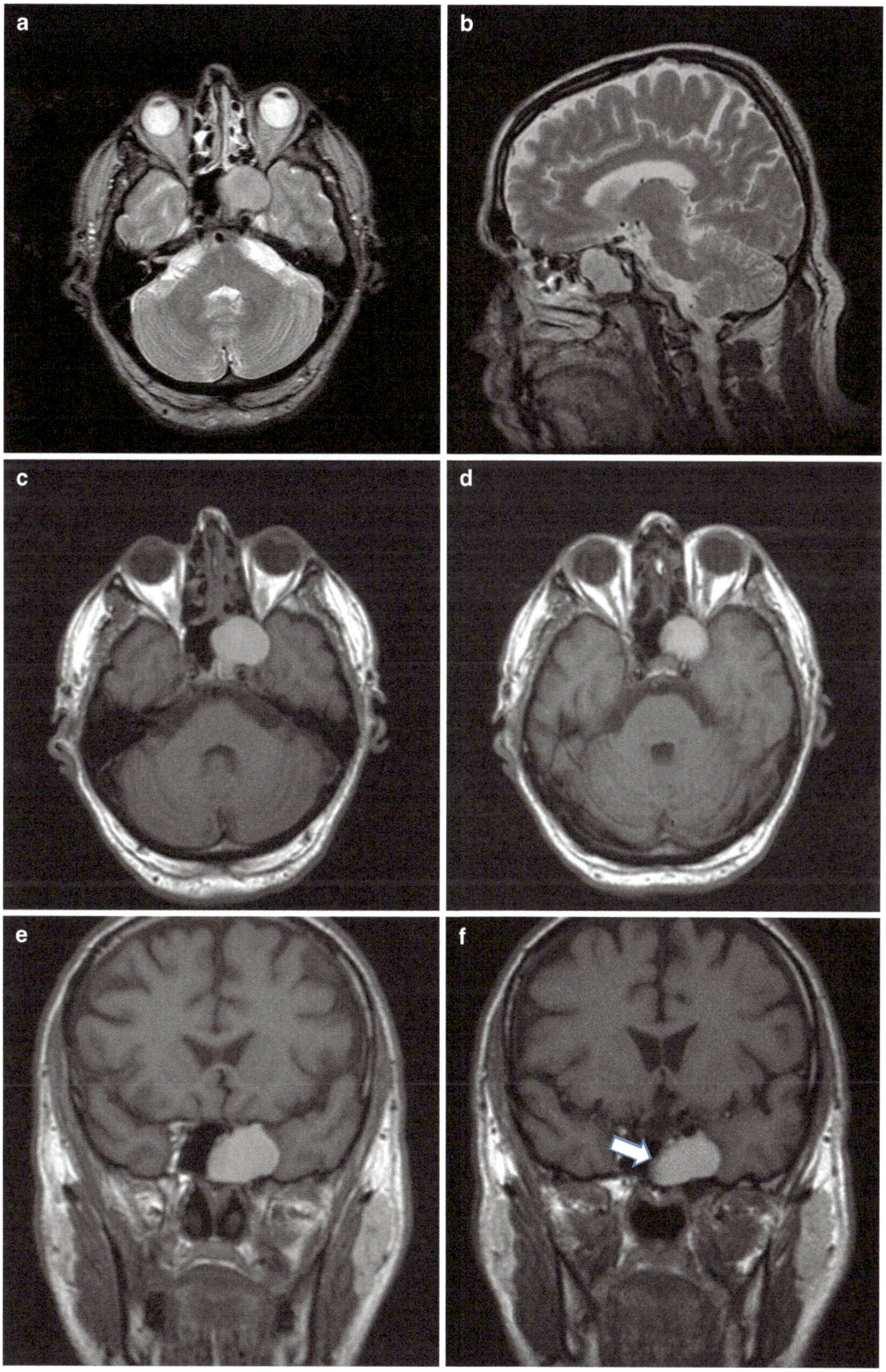

Fig. 17.6 Mucocele in the left part of the sphenoid sinus. T2-weighted images (**a**, **b**), axial (**c**, **d**) and coronal (**e**, **f**) T1-weighted images show an expanded sphenoid sinus with the compression of the left cavernous sinus. Mucocele is characterized by moderate hyperintensity on T2-weighted image and hyperintense signal on T1 due to high protein content. Hypertrophied mucous of the sphenoid sinus has lower signal relative to the mucocele content (*arrow*)

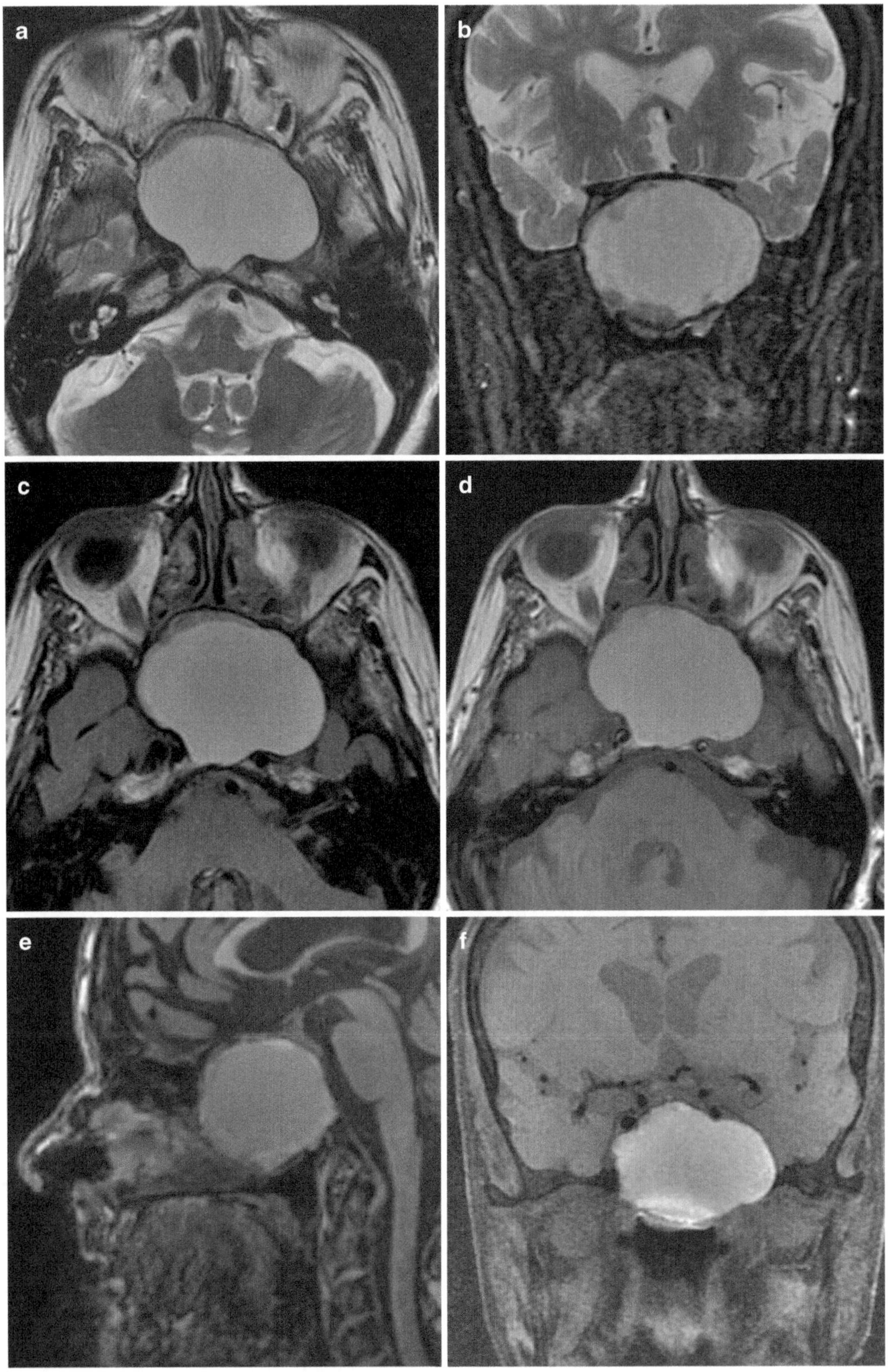

Fig. 17.7 Giant mucocele of the sphenoid sinus. T2-weighted images (**a**, **b**), T2-FLAIR (**c**), T1-weighted images (**d**, **e**) and T1+fat-sat (**f**) show a giant hyperintense cystic lesion in the expanded sinus. Hypertrophied mucous of the sphenoid sinus has lower signal relative to the mucocele content, especially on T2-weighted image. Hyperintensity of the lesion is remaining after fat suppression. DWI (**g**) shows hypointense signal and excludes an abscess or epidermoid cyst. Post-contrast T1-weighted images (**h**, **i**) demonstrate an enhanced hypertrophied mucous within the sphenoid sinus

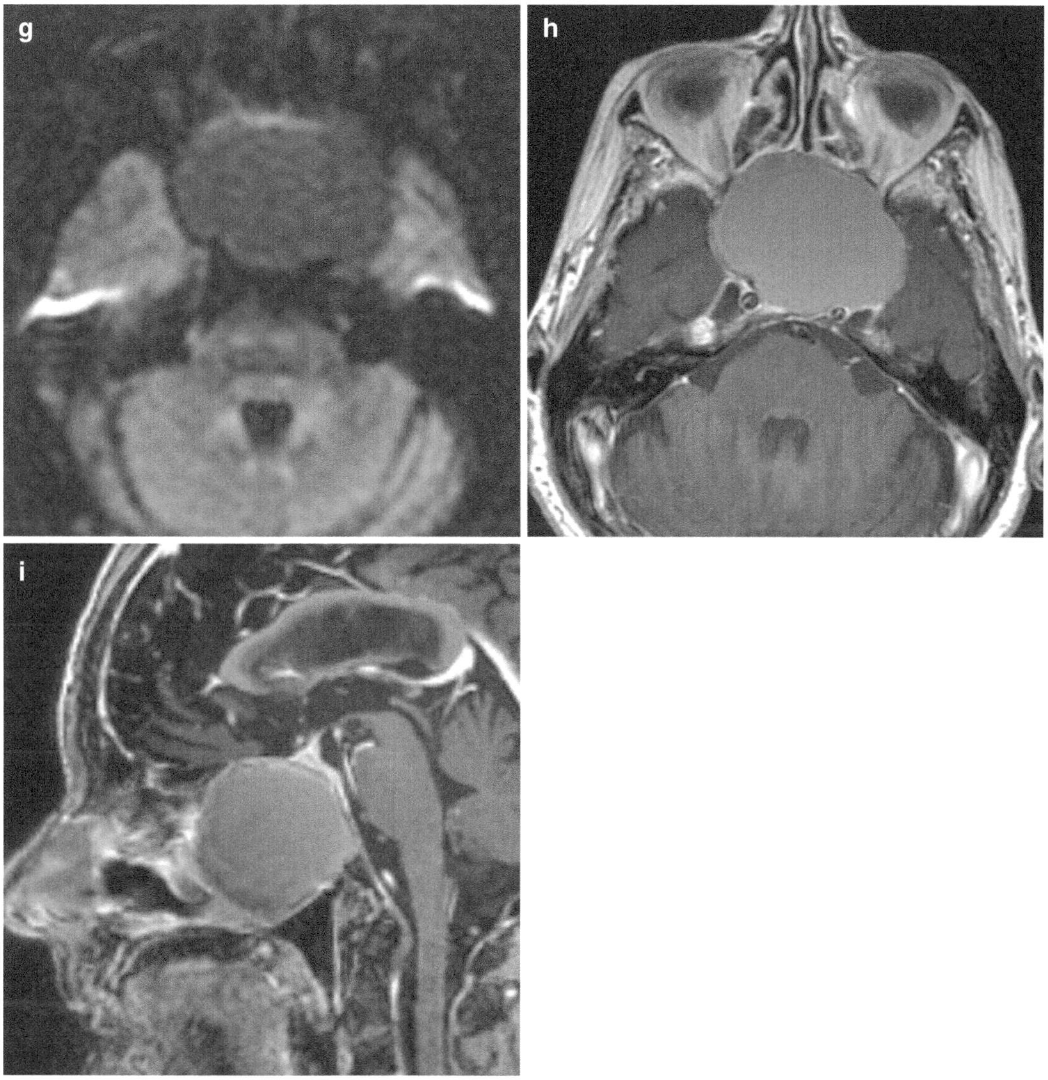

Fig. 17.7 (continued)

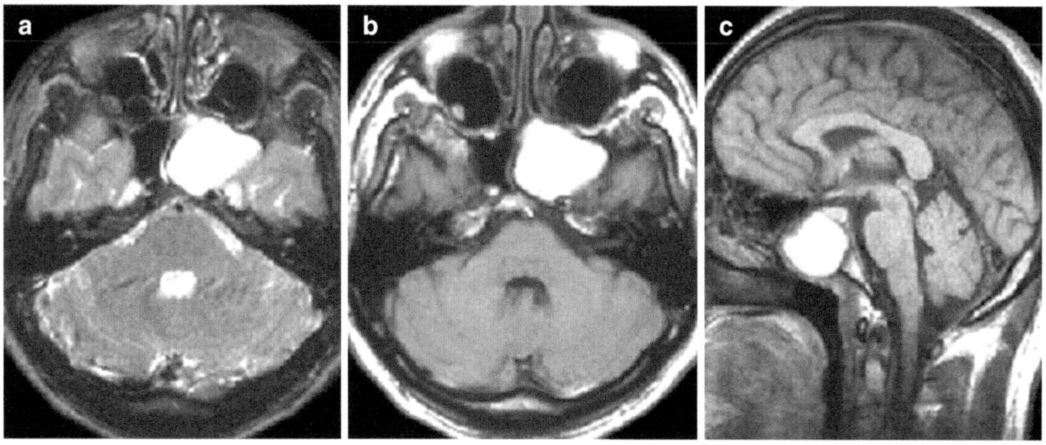

Fig. 17.8 Mucocele of the left part of the sphenoid sinus. Axial T2- (**a**) and T1-weighted images (**b**), sagittal T1 (**c**) show an expanded sphenoid sinus. Mucocele is characterized by the hyperintense signal on T1- and T2-weighted images due to high protein content

17.5 Neurosarcoidosis

Sarcoidosis is a chronic polysystemic inflammatory disorder of unknown etiology. The pulmonary lymphatic nodes are most frequently affected, which are followed by the skin and eyes. CNS involvement is seen in approximately 5% of cases of sarcoidosis. This disorder affects both sexes and may be seen a little bit frequently in females than in males. Any part of the CNS may be involved. Involvement of the hypothalamic–pituitary system is usually manifested by diabetes insipidus, or by deficiency of a single or many other hormones of the anterior part of the pituitary. Clinical manifestations of the disease completely depend on the affected site. The onset is usually painless, but the course is progressive. This disorder usually responds well to steroid treatment.

MRI reveals thickening of infundibulum of the pituitary and the floor of the third ventricle, and thickening and deformation of cranial nerves, leptomeninges (Scott 1993). There are no characteristic features of pathological lesions on MRI, which is why precise differential diagnosis is difficult, unless the systemic sarcoidosis is proven. Multiple disseminated intra-parenchymal and meningeal lesions suggest such a diagnosis. Contrast enhancement is pronounced, predominantly in the leptomeninges (Fig. 17.9).

17.6 Tolosa-Hunt Syndrome

Tolosa-Hunt syndrome is the idiopathic inflammatory disorder of the cavernous sinus. Its clinical manifestations are prominent retro-orbital pain, neuropathies of the third, fourth, and sixth cranial nerves and the first branch of the fifth cranial nerve, with less frequent involvement of the optic nerve and the sympathetic ganglions around the cavernous segment of the internal carotid artery. Symptoms may persist for several days or weeks both, with spontaneous remissions and relapsing. Pathologically the process resembles an orbital pseudotumor (Kline and Hoyt 2001).

Imaging CT usually fails to reveal any changes in this condition (Aron-Rosa et al. 1978) or insignificant changes are found such as asymmetrical enlargement of the cavernous sinuses, CE in the prepontine cistern, or abnormal density of the soft tissues in the orbital apex (Kwan et al. 1987). Enlargement of the cavernous sinus on the affected side is revealed along with MR signal isointense to orbital muscles on T1-weighted imaging and isointense to fat on T2-weighted imaging. The expansion of changes onto the apex of the orbit is seen, which suggests the similarity of this syndrome to orbital pseudotumor in etiology (Yousem et al. 1989). The disorder is responsive to steroid therapy. The differential diagnosis of Tolosa-Hunt syndrome should be made with sarcoidosis, meningioma, lymphoma, metastasis into the cavernous sinus and actinomycosis (Battineni et al. 2007).

17.7 Sheehan Syndrome

It is known that after pregnancy the pituitary gland undergoes marked structural changes. This changes lead to marked decrease of its sensitivity threshold to influence of different pathological factors, such as to ischemia in complicated delivery. As a result, some females develop ischemic necrosis of the adenohypophysis in the early postnatal period, with possible hemorrhage into the necrotic area and the shock-like reaction (Sheehan and Stanford 1961). On MRI, enlargement of the adenohypophysis is revealed, and if a hemorrhage is present, then the picture resembles that of infarction of the pituitary.

17.8 Langerhans Cell Histiocytosis

Langerhans cell histiocytosis is a group of disorders characterized by proliferation of histiocytes (macrophages). Synonyms: histiocytosis X, Hand-Schüller-Christian disease, eosinophilic granuloma, Taratynov disease, Letterer-Siwe disease. This is a rare disease; its incidence in children is 3–4 cases per one million per year, being even rarer in adults. There are single-system (involvement of one organ or organ system) and multi-system (involvement of two or more organs or organ systems) forms of the disease (D'Ambrosio et al. 2008). Single-system disease can occur in a solitary lesion or two or more lesions (multiple), with or without impairment of the function of vital organs.

In cases of a single mass lesion, involvement of cranial vault bones is typical, and in these cases, the hypothalamic–pituitary system is usually not involved. Multifocal granulomatosis is a more aggressive disorder, occurring in childhood. In 25% of cases the classical triad of clinical manifestations is seen: diabetes insipidus, exophthalmos, and foci of lysis of cranial bones (Hand-Schuller-Christian syndrome). In these cases granulomas may be observed in the hypothalamus or in the pituitary stalk. The CNS involvement is usually found if histiocytosis started in other organs and systems. Skull base and cranial vault bones, the posterior fossa structures such as brainstem, and the cerebellar hemispheres are usually affected; the chiasmal-sellar region is much less frequently involved. Granulomatosis in the CNS starts with involvement of the leptomeninges, subarachnoid space with subsequent invasion of the hypothalamus and pituitary gland.

Imaging CT demonstrates thickening and increase of contrast accumulation of the pituitary stalk and at the floor of the third ventricle (Fig. 17.10). On MRI, hyperintensive signal in the hypothalamus on T2-weighted images may be seen and more frequently, thickening of the pituitary stalk is observed (Tien et al. 1990; Maghnie et al. 1992). These changes are better identified in sagittal and

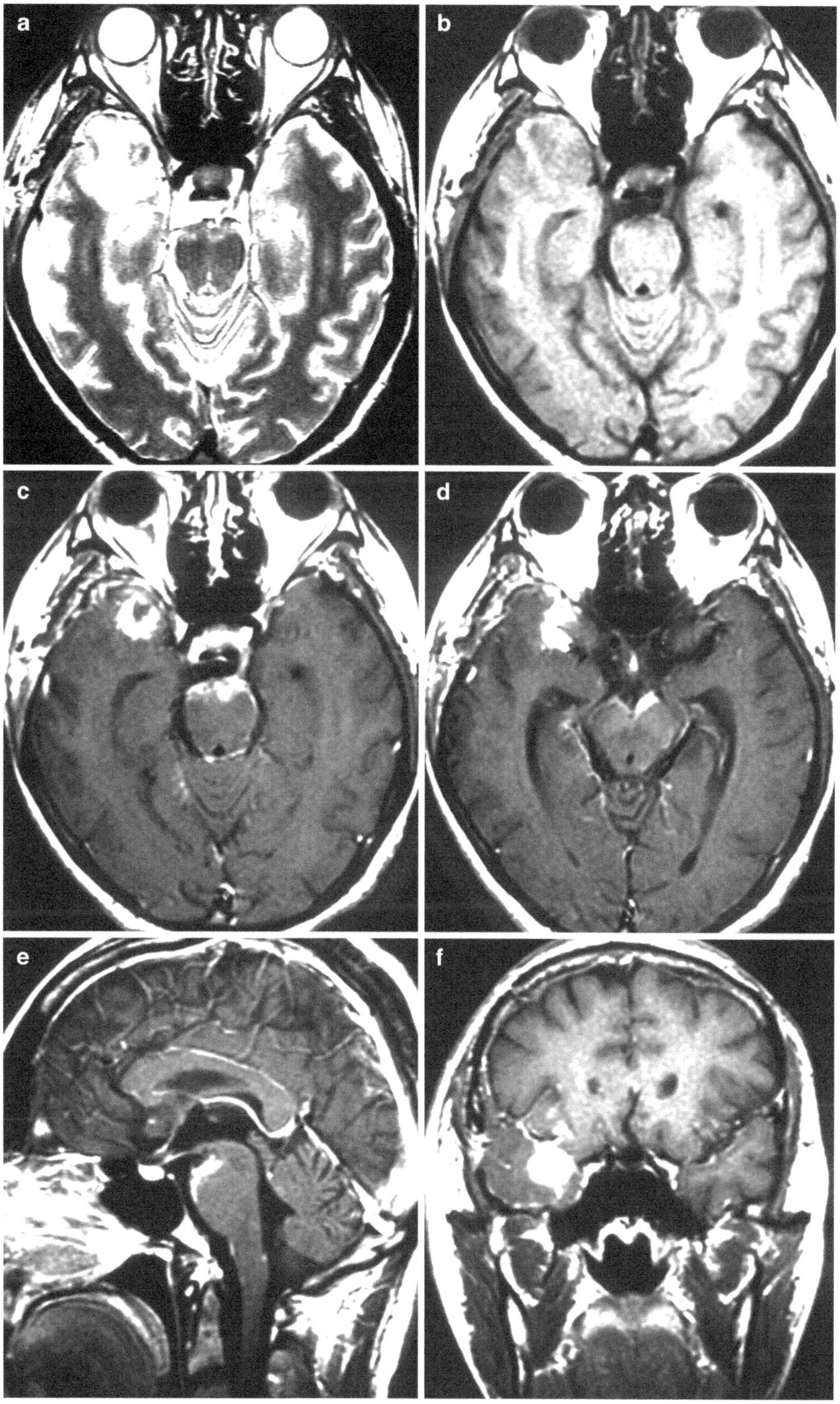

Fig. 17.9 CNS sarcoidosis. T2- (**a**), T1- (**b**), and post-contrast T1-weighted images (**c–f**) reveal an extensive enhancing lesion in the right temporal region, brainstem area, and interpeduncular cistern

coronal planes on MRI (Figs. 17.11 and 17.12), than on CT; however, CT with CE in the coronal plane may also be helpful. Diagnosis is made after biopsy of one of the abnormal areas of bone. In our series of observations of patients with a verified histiocytosis X diagnosis, noteworthy is the case of multifocal brain lesions and involvement of the brain stem mimicking a diffuse glial tumor (Fig. 17.13).

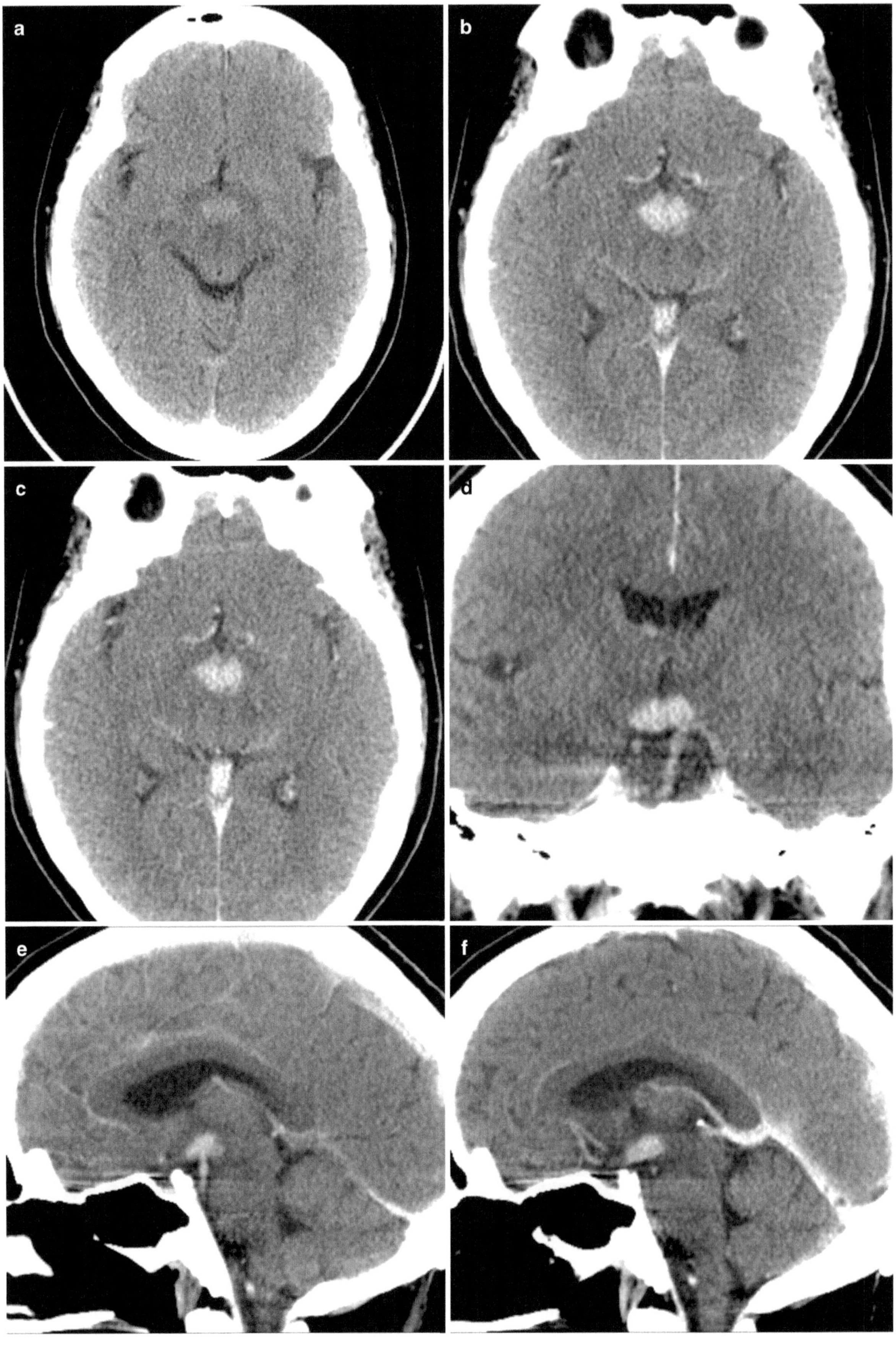

Fig. 17.10 Langerhans cell histiocytosis. NECT (**a**) and CECT (**b–f**) with reformats show a small rounded hyperdense enhancing lesion with a perifocal brain edema in the projection of the third ventricle floor

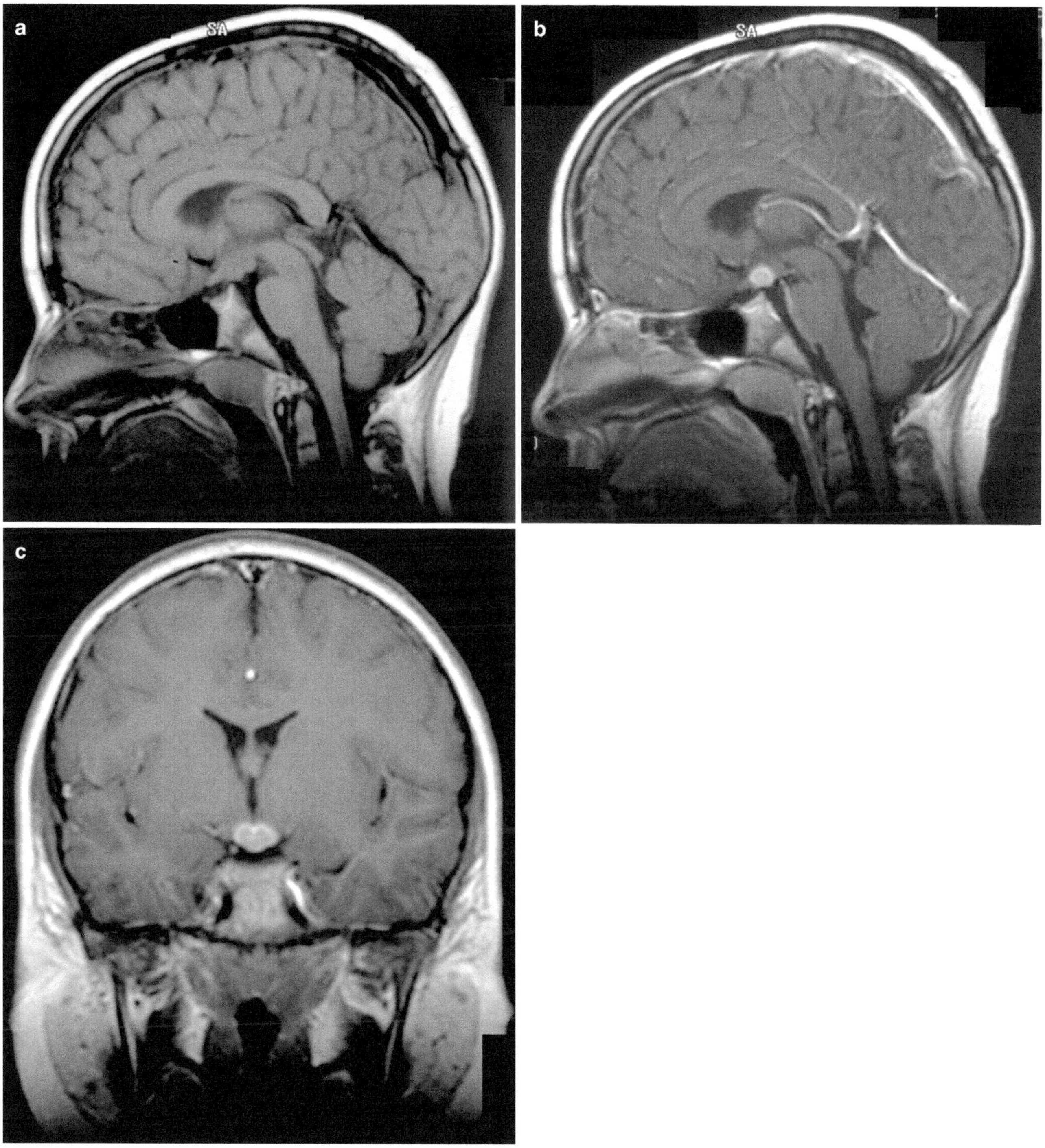

Fig. 17.11 Langerhans cell histiocytosis. Sagittal T1-weighted image (**a**) shows an isointense lesion in the pituitary stalk area and the floor of the third ventricle area. Post-contrast T1-weighted images (**b**, **c**) demonstrate an intense enhancement within the lesion

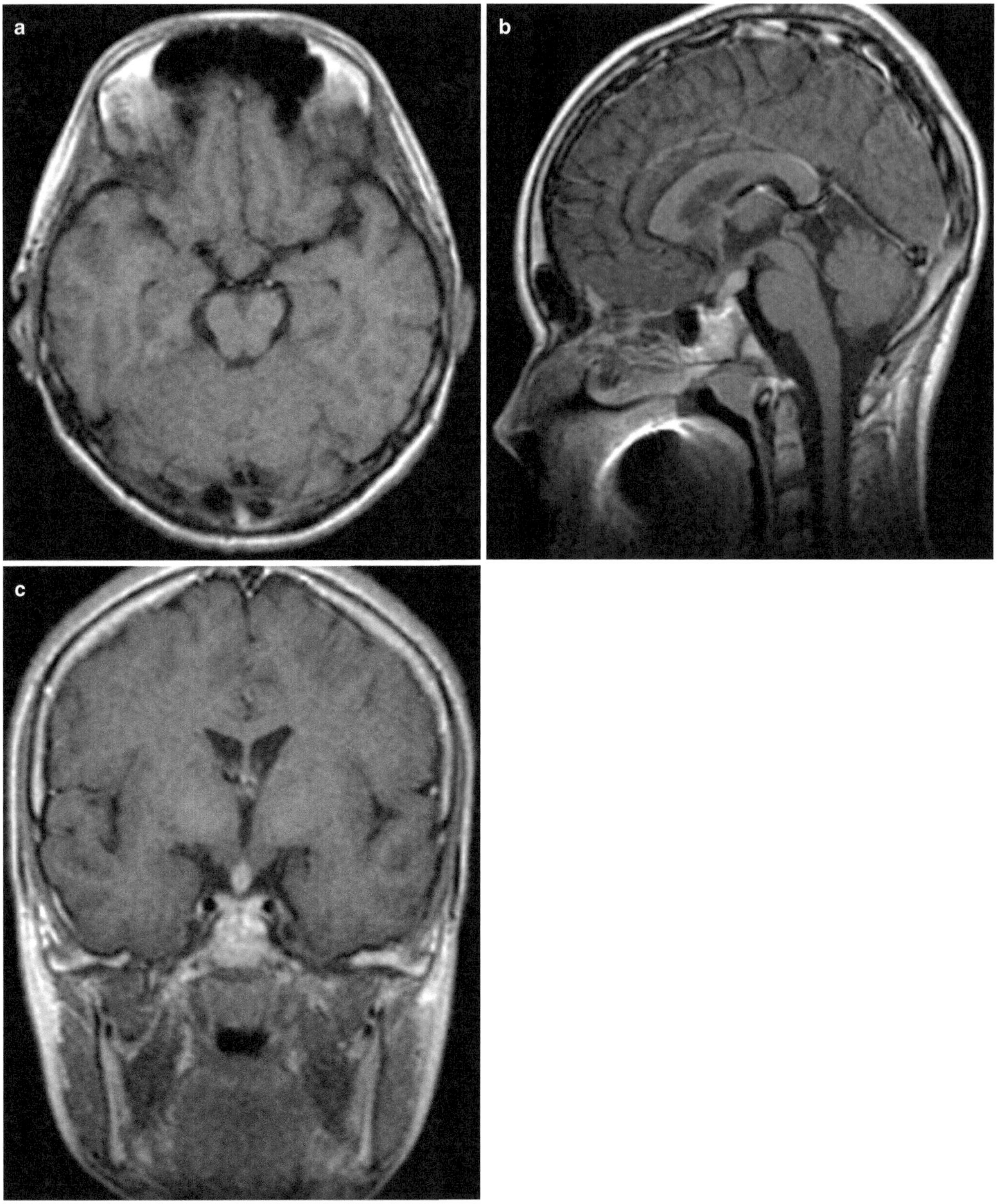

Fig. 17.12 Langerhans cell histiocytosis. Axial T1-weighted image (**a**) and post-contrast sagittal (**b**) and coronal (**c**) T1-weighted images demonstrate an enhancing mass in the pituitary stalk area

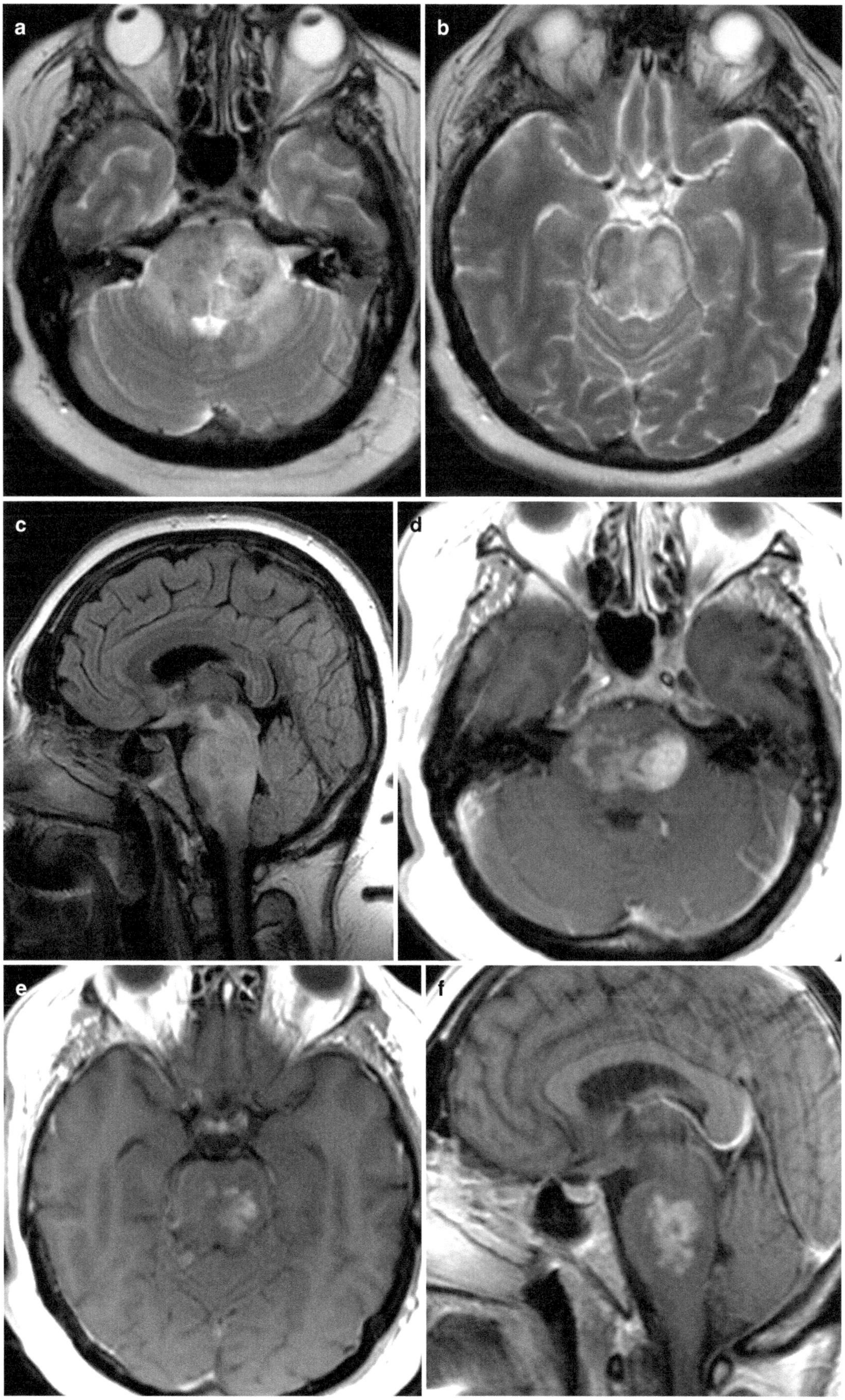

Fig. 17.13 Langerhans cell histiocytosis. T2-weighted images (**a**, **b**), T2-FLAIR (**c**), post-contrast T1-weighted images (**d**–**f**) show a diffuse infiltration of the brainstem by enhancing lesion in a patient with histiocytosis X. This infiltrative lesion mimics a diffuse glioma

18 Congenital and Non-neoplastic Lesions

Contents

18.1 Hamartomas of the Tuber Cinereum

Hamartomas of the tuber cinereum is a rare congenital mass lesion more frequently seen in boys, and is located between the mammillary bodies and pituitary stalk. Hamartoma is not a proper tumor but a congenital non-tumor heterotopia. On histology, a hamartoma consists of accumulations of small and large neurons, astrocytes and oligodendrocytes, which are in correct ratio with tuber cinereum tissue (Matsko and Korshunov 1998). They do not invade the surrounding structures, but may progress slowly, sometimes reaching rather large sizes. The most frequent and early clinical manifestation occurs approximately at the age of 2 years: isosexual precocious puberty. Other signs such as epileptic seizures and behavioral changes occur later when a hamartoma acquires a diameter of about 10 mm (Mittal et al. 2013).

Imaging Neuroimaging in hamartomas is possible only by CT or MRI. On CT, hamartoma is a mass lesion isodense to brain tissue and located in the chiasmal region or in the interpeduncular cistern, clearly delineated by CSF. Intravenous CE does not change its density. Therefore, lesions of up to 1 cm may be missed using the standard CT (Fig. 18.1). On T1-weighted imaging a lesion looks an isointense mass in the tuber cinereum or the mammillary bodies regions, clearly revealed in all the three scanning planes (Fig. 18.2). On T2-weighted and T2-FLAIR images, MR signal varies from isointense to moderately hyperintense. After intravenous CE the signal remains unchanged; this is a differential marker that allows distinguishing hamartoma from, for instance, pilocytic astrocytoma (Figs. 18.3 and 18.4). It is typical for hamartomas that their sizes and invasiveness do not increase on follow-up examination for a long period (except after radiotherapy). In our practice, we observed an area with abnormal contrast enhancement in the hamartoma structure a year after the radiotherapy, which presumably could be due to direct radiation damage to the hamartoma tissue (Fig. 18.5). In patients with hamartomas of the hypothalamus, other

I. Pronin, V. Kornienko, *CT and MRI of Skull Base Lesions*, https://doi.org/10.1007/978-3-319-65957-2_18

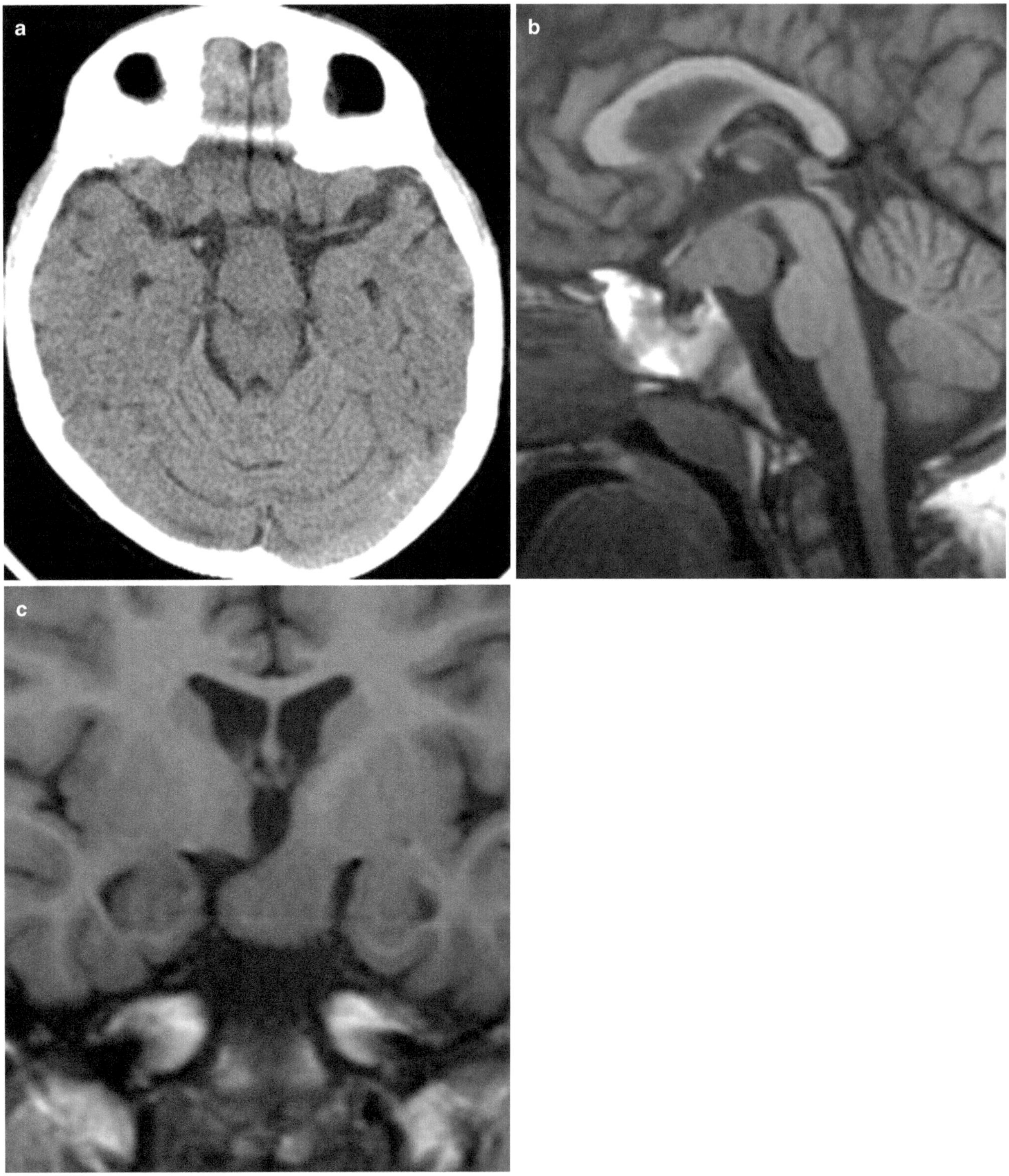

Fig. 18.1 Tuber cinereum hamartoma. CT scan (**a**) shows an isodense mass in the chiasmal and interpeduncular cisterns. Hamartoma is isointense with the brain on sagittal (**b**) and coronal (**c**) T1-weighted images

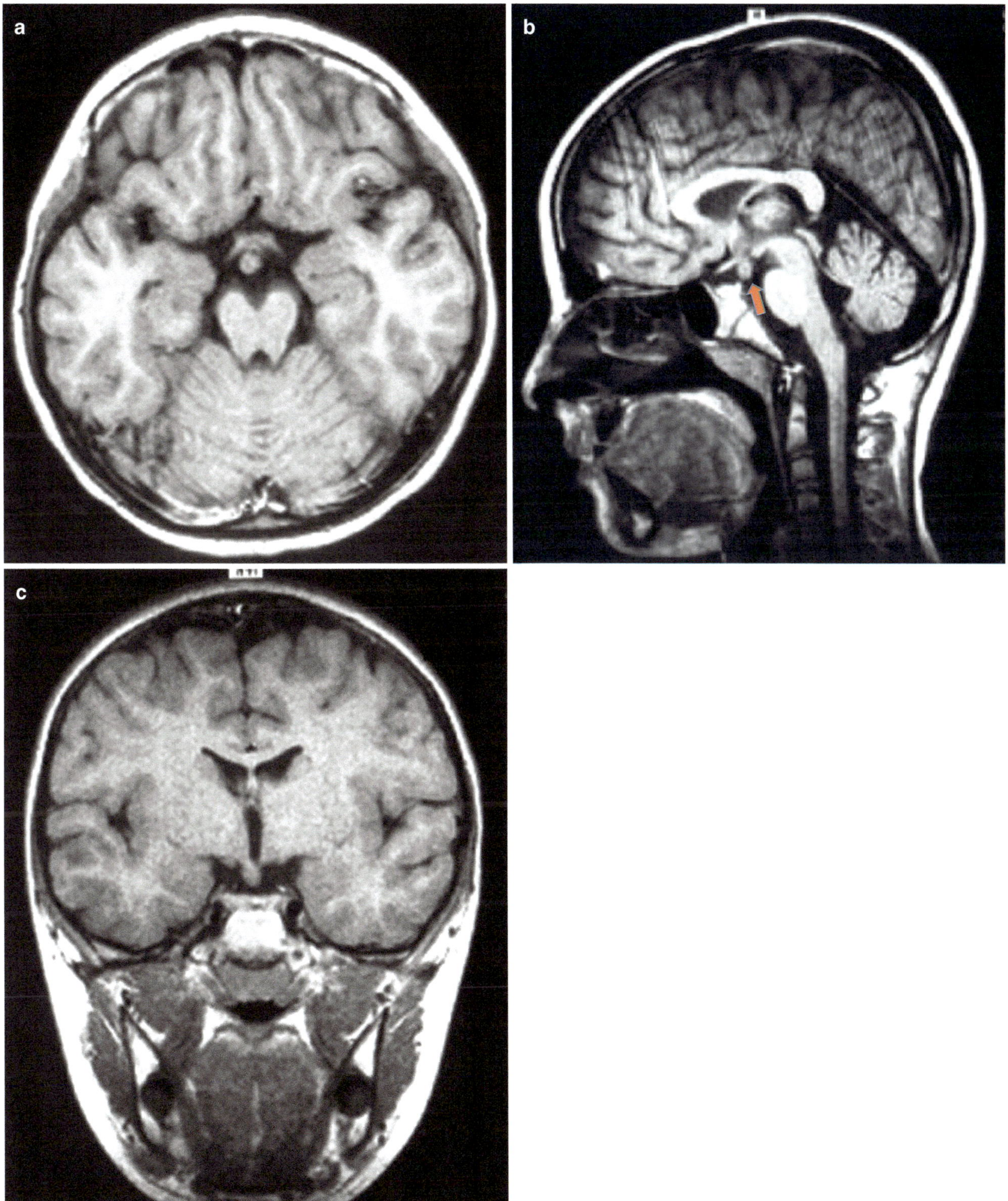

Fig. 18.2 Tuber cinereum microhamartoma (*arrow*). The hamartoma is isointense with gray matter on T1-weighted images (**a**–**c**)

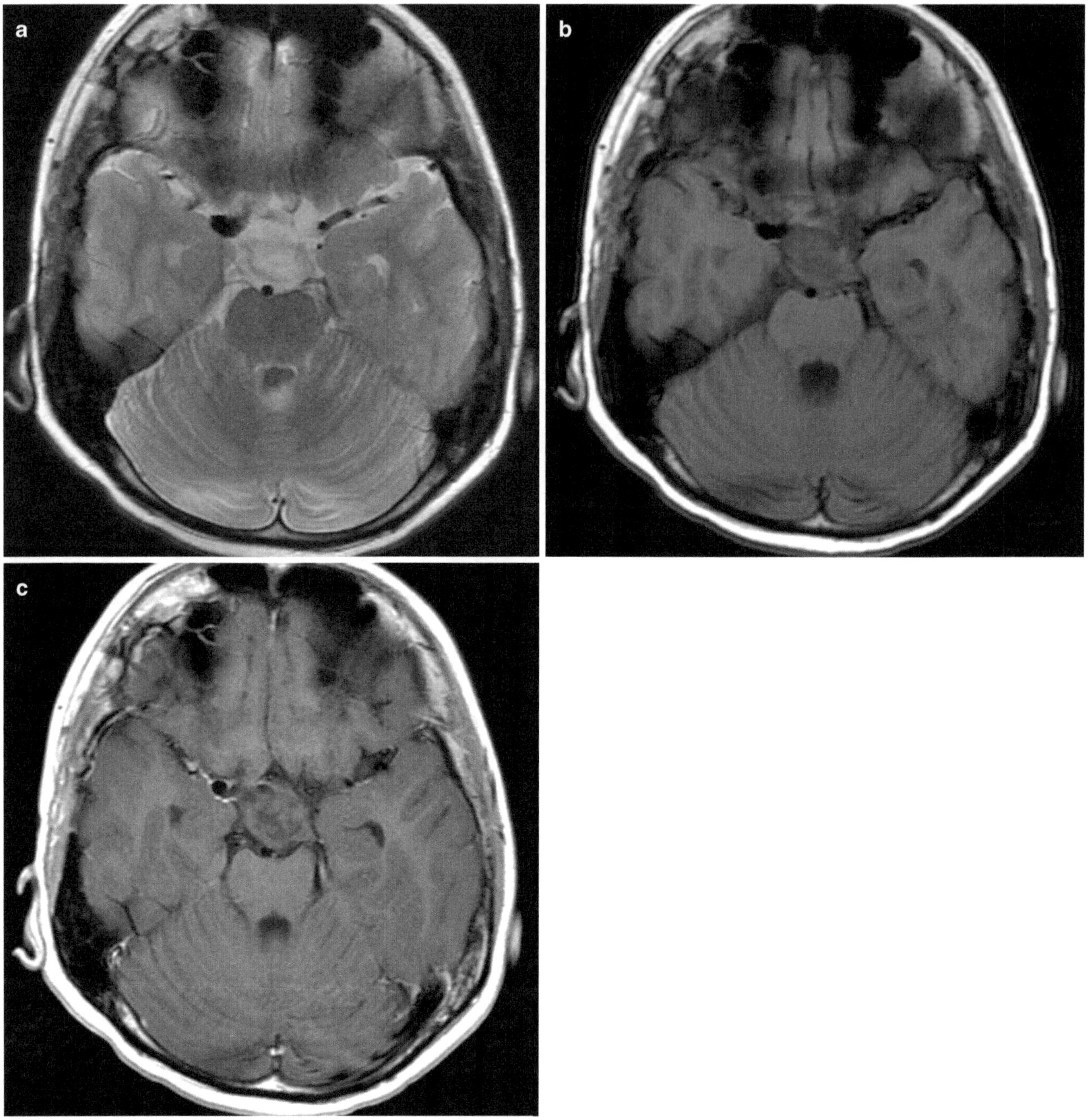

Fig. 18.3 Tuber cinereum hamartoma. T2-weighted (**a**), T1-weighted (**b**), post-contrast T1-weighted images (**c**) show a heterogeneously (hyperintense on T2) relative to the gray matter mass in the suprasellar region. The mass lesion does not enhance

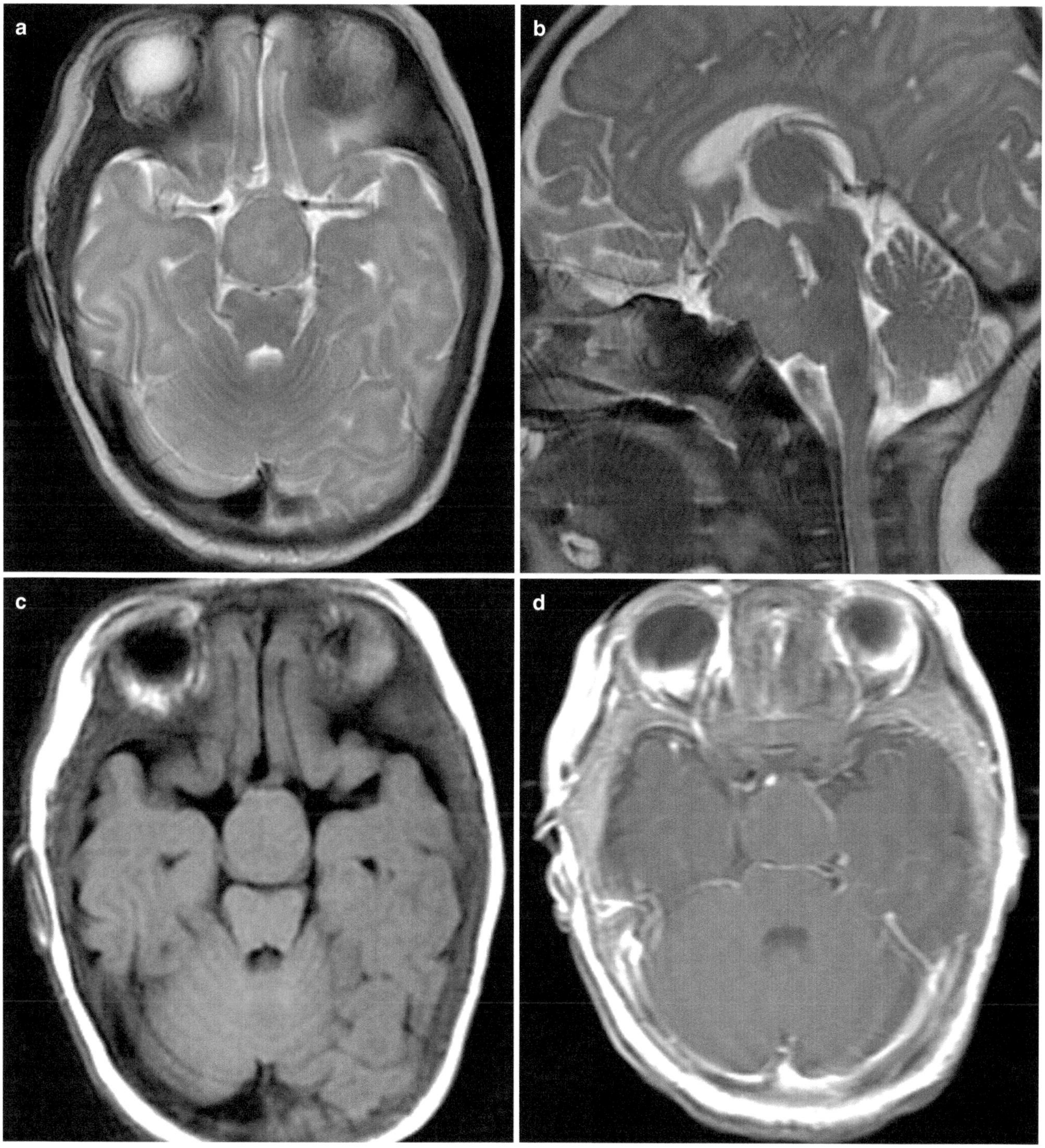

Fig. 18.4 Large tuber cinereum hamartoma (in a 3-year-old child). T2-weighted images (**a**, **b**) and T2-FLAIR (**c**) reveal a large suprasellar mass that is isointense with the gray matter. The mass compresses the brainstem. Post-contrast T1-weighted images (**d**–**f**) show a nonenhancing hamartoma

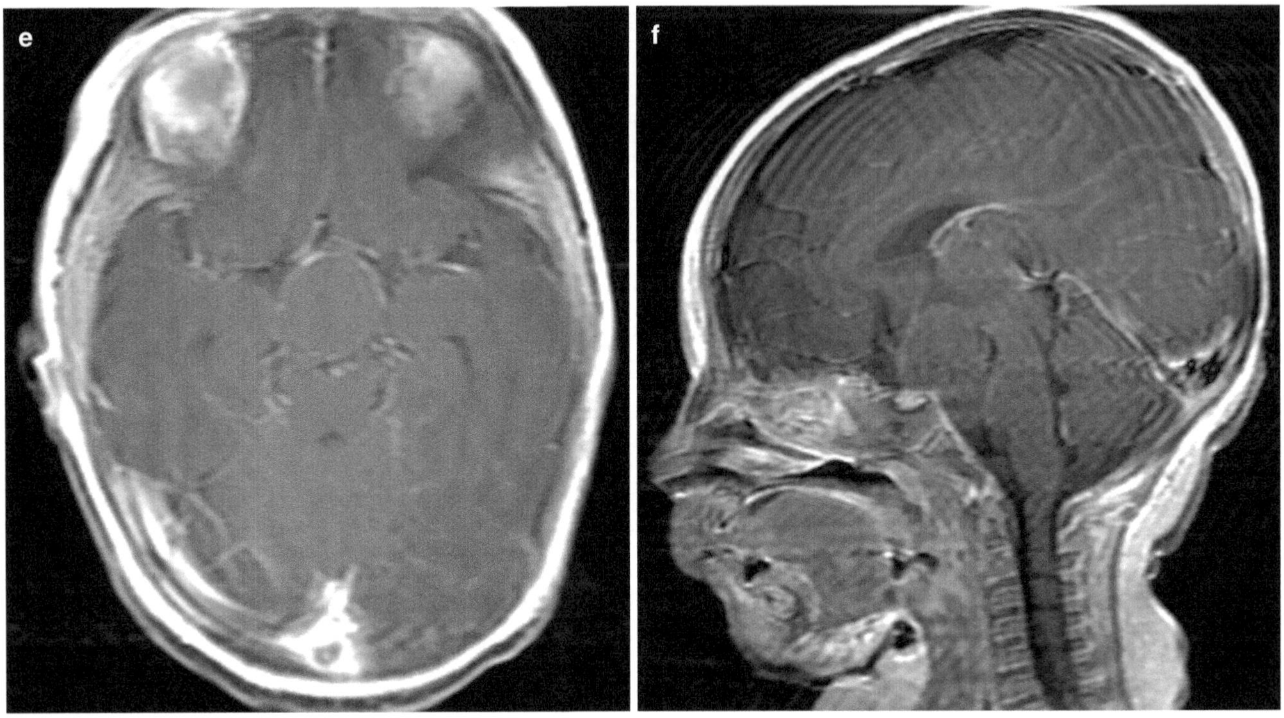

Fig. 18.4 (continued)

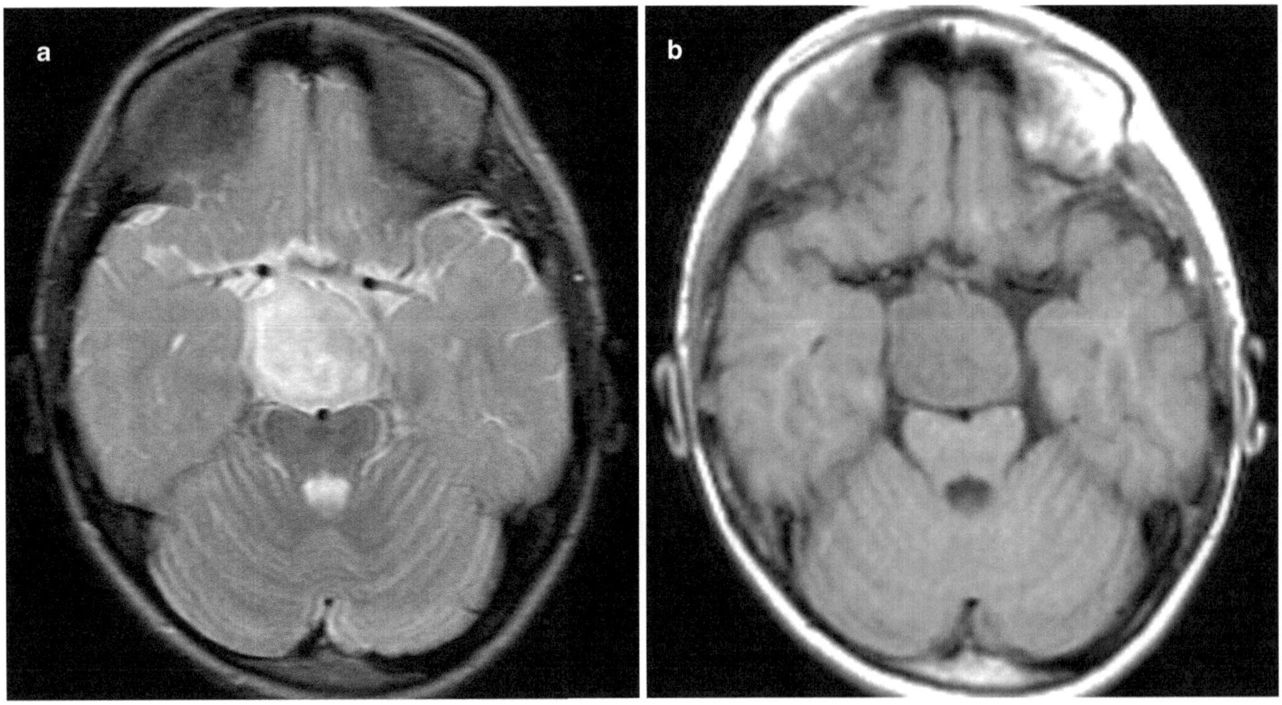

Fig. 18.5 Tuber cinereum hamartoma in a child in a one year after radiation therapy. Axial T2- (**a**), T1-weighted images (**b**) and post-contrast axial (**c**, **d**), sagittal (**e**) and coronal T1-weighted images (**f**) identify a small enhancing area in the hamartoma (*arrow*)

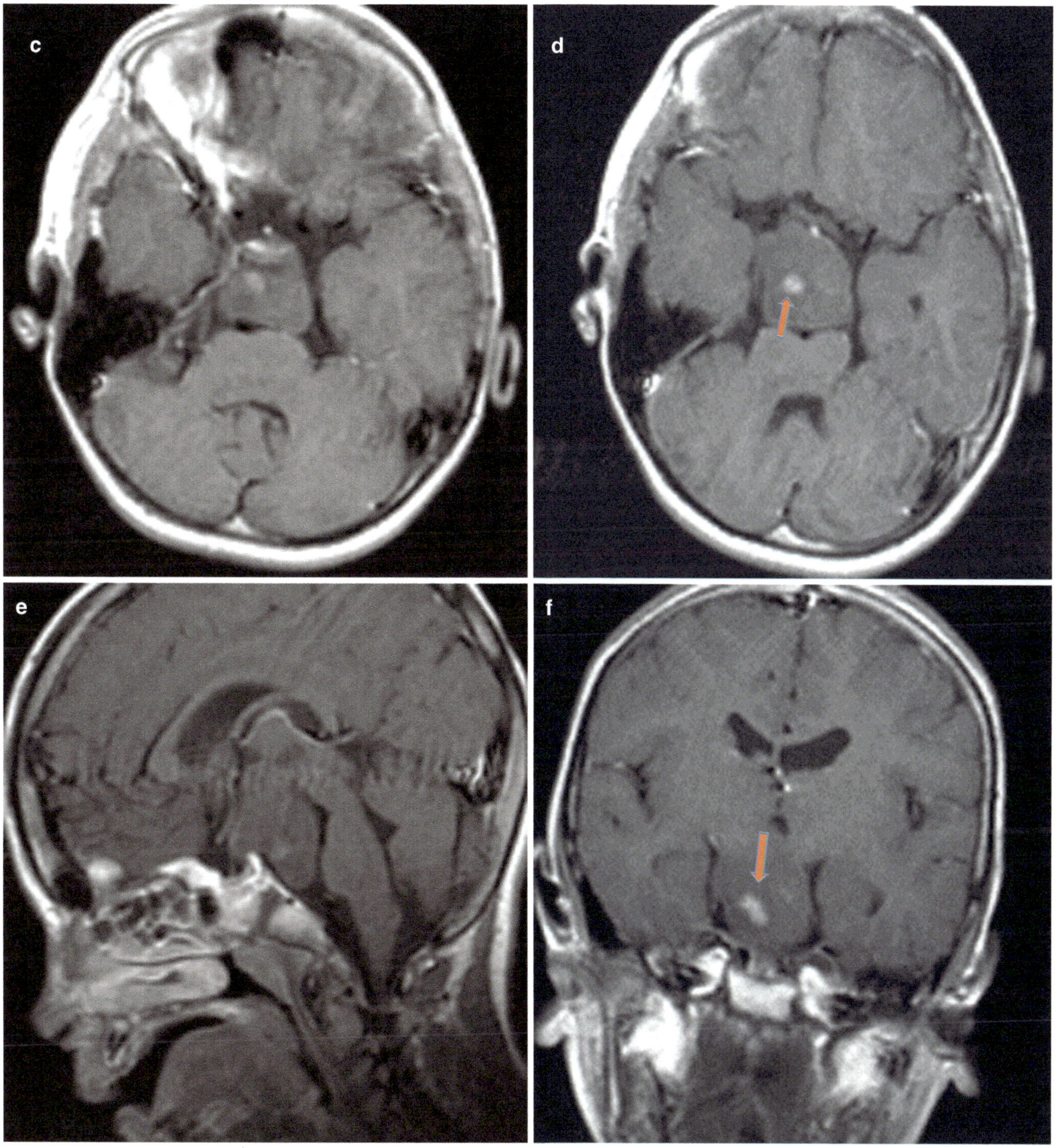

Fig. 18.5 (continued)

cerebral malformations may be revealed: agenesia/hypogenesia of the corpus callosum or cortical disgenesia, which may cause epilepsy (Freeman et al. 2004). Sometimes a lesion may reach such a large size that it causes deformity of the adjacent structures (Fig. 18.6). The differential diagnosis should be made from glioma of the floor of the third ventricle.

18.2 Rathke Cleft Cyst

Rathke cleft cysts (RCC) are non-neoplastic asymptomatic cysts located in the sellar or the intrasuprasellar area (Voelker et al. 1991; Esteves et al. 2015). They are found in less than 1% of primary brain tumors. According to Teramoto et al. (1994) study performed based on 1000 autopsies, asymptomatic Rathke cleft

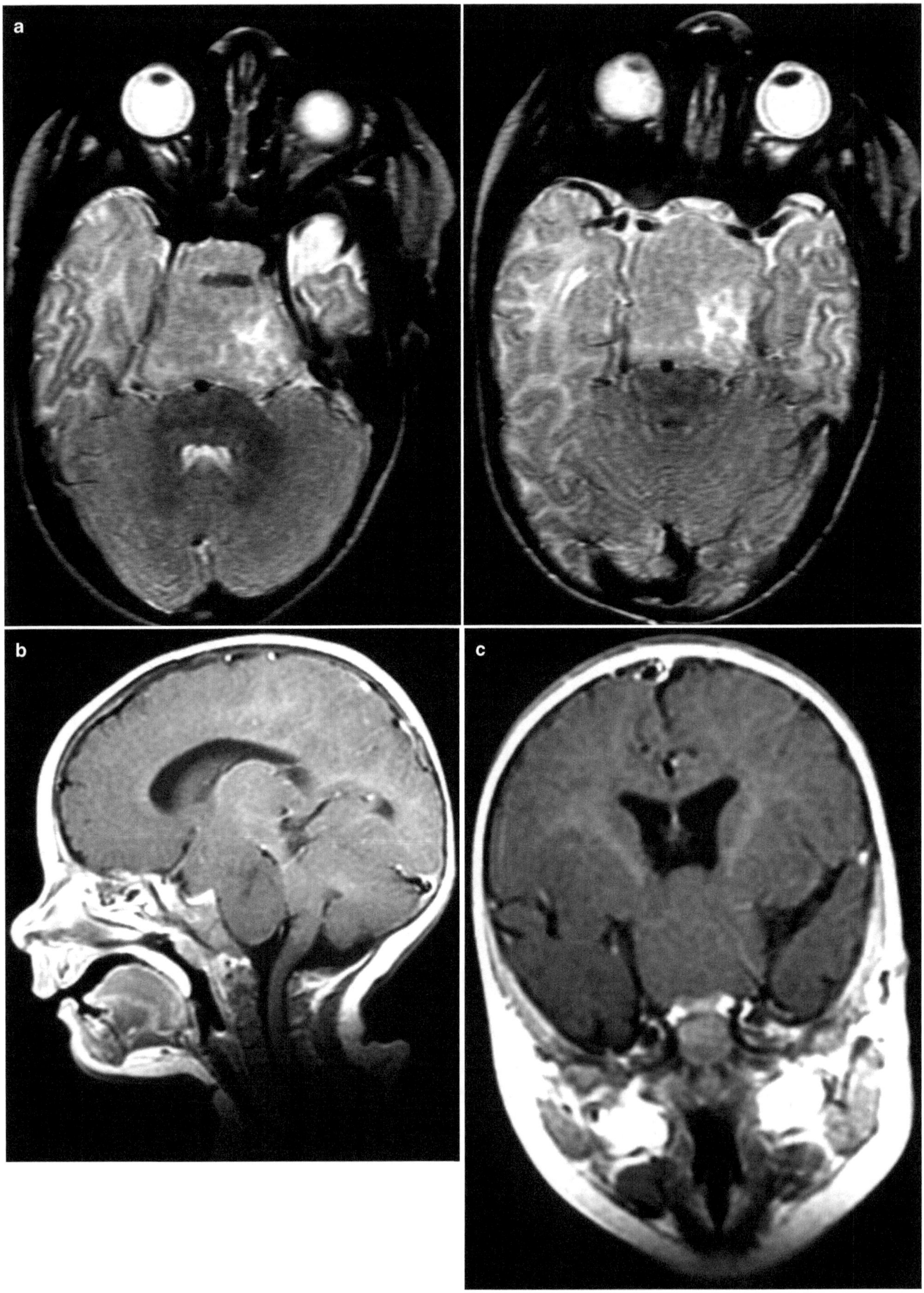

Fig. 18.6 Giant tuber cinereum hamartoma. Axial T2- (**a**), sagittal (**b**), and coronal (**c**) T1-weighted images

cysts were verified in 11.3% of cases. Most of them (87%) were located on the midline and the remainder had an asymmetric localization. Rathke cleft cysts arise from remnants of squamous epithelium of embryonic craniopharyngeal duct (Rathke pouch). Cyst walls are lined by a single layer ciliated cuboidal or columnar epithelium and globlet cells. The cyst contains mucosal or serous fluid. Calcifications of the cyst walls are rarely observed. Cysts are usually located in the central part of the sella turcica and vary in size from several mm to 1–2 cm. RCC may be seen in any age; however, they are more frequent in adults.

Clinically cysts are most often asymptomatic; clinical manifestations appear in those cases when a large cyst compresses the pituitary or the optic chiasm (Kim et al. 2004). They cause headaches, visual loss, various endocrine dysfunctions, including hypopituitarism and diabetes insipidus.

Imaging On CT, round or lobular intra- or suprasellar hypodense mass lesions that do not accumulate contrast medium are seen. On MRI, a round or oval mass lesion is usually seen, which is located between the anterior and the intermediate lobes of the pituitary gland (Figs. 18.7 and 18.8). The signal of such a mass lesion is homogeneous, iso-, or hyperintense on T1-weighted images and iso- or hypointense on T2-weighted images compared with CSF, which allows making the differential diagnosis from craniopharyngiomas (Woo et al. 2000). In cases of intracystic hemorrhages or inflammatory processes the signal becomes heterogeneous. Cysts with mucous fluid are not distinguishable from cystic CPH on MRI—both lesions may be hyperintensive on T1- and T2-weighted images (Ross et al. 1992).

The cyst with serous exudate has identical MR signal characteristics with that of the CSF. The cysts containing exfoliated areas are most difficult entities in terms of the differential diagnosis, as they are difficult to distinguish from solid tumors. However, in contrast to solid tumors these cysts do not enhance (Fig. 18.9).

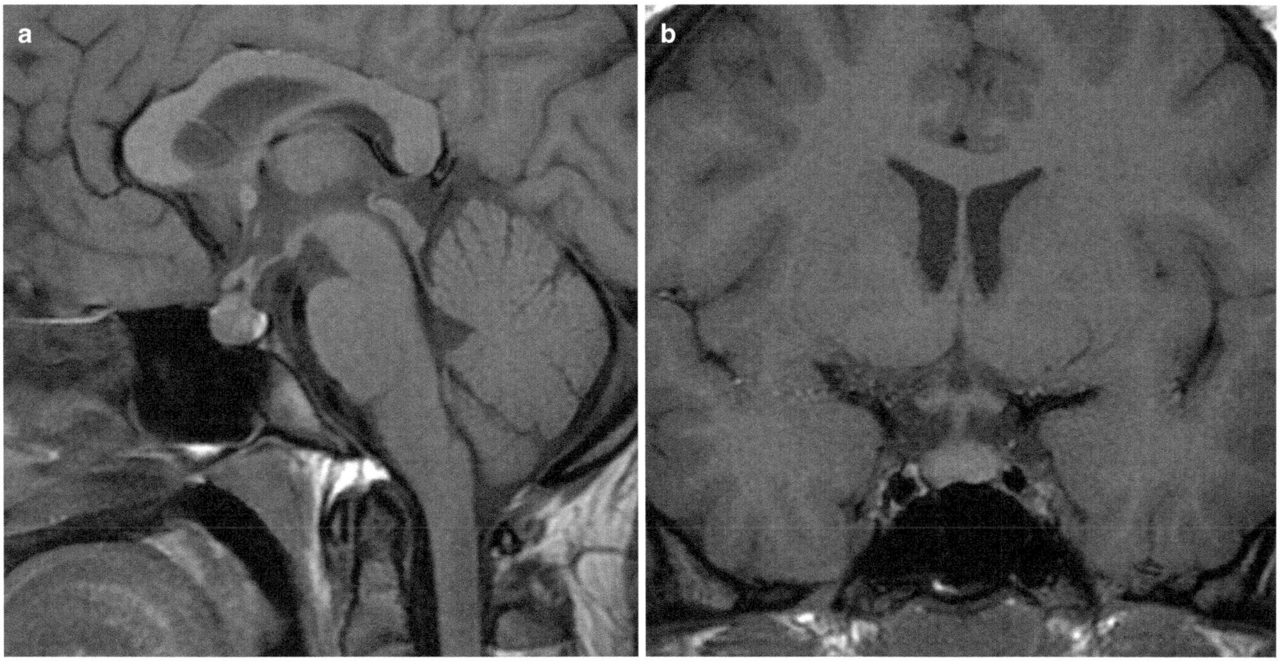

Fig. 18.7 Rathke cleft cyst. Sagittal (**a**), coronal (**b**) T1- and coronal T2-weighted images (**c**) reveal a moderately enlarged adenohypophysis and rounded hypointense on T2 focus within the pituitary gland. Neurohypophysis is typically hyperintense on T1. Post-contrast T1-weighted images (**d**—axial; **e**, **f**—sagittal) show nonenhancing cyst between the adenohypophysis and the neurohypophysis (*arrow*)

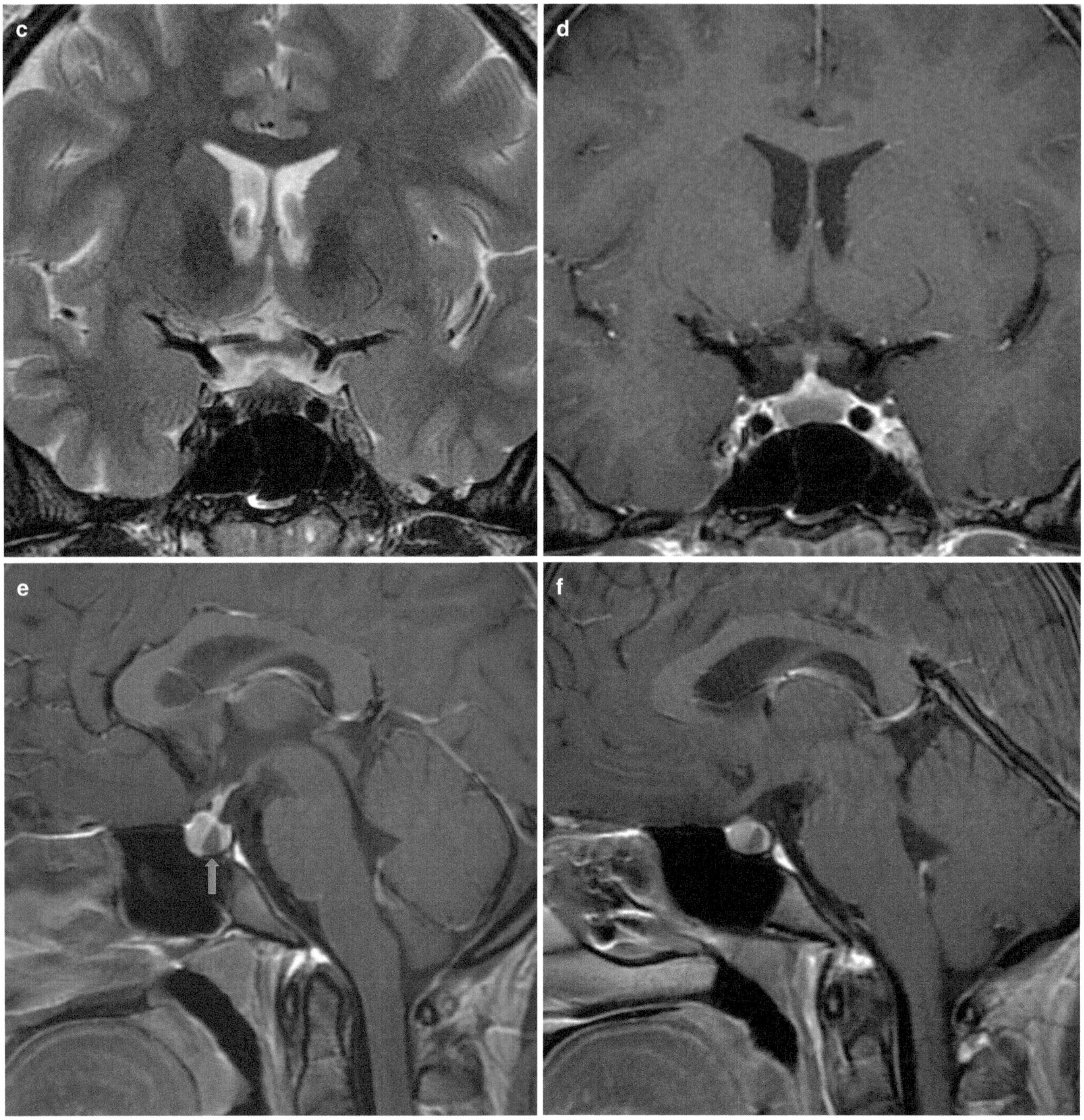

Fig. 18.7 (continued)

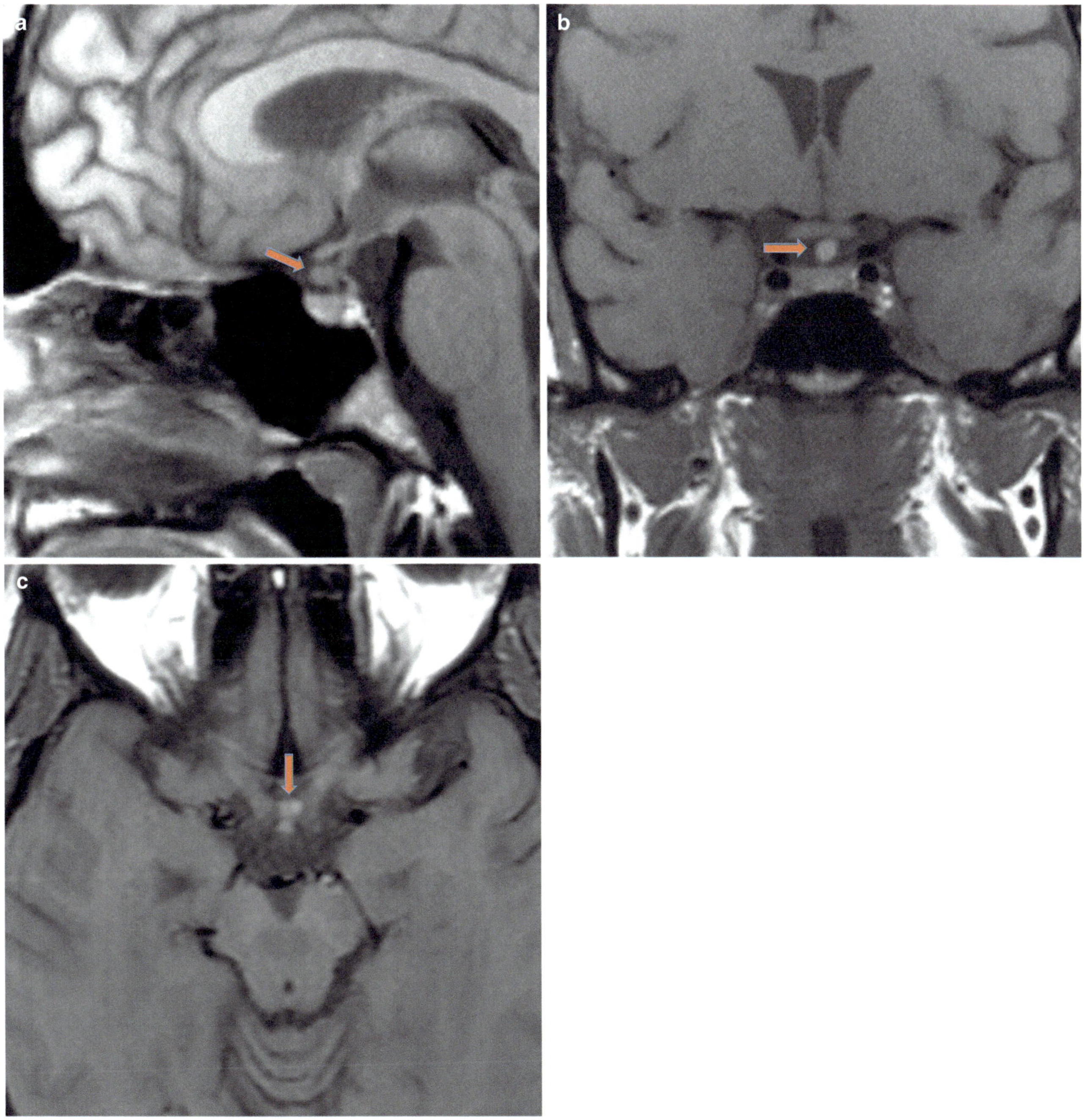

Fig. 18.8 Rathke cleft cyst. Sagittal (**a**), coronal (**b**), and axial (**c**) T1-weighted images reveal a small cyst located anteriorly to the pituitary stalk (*arrows*)

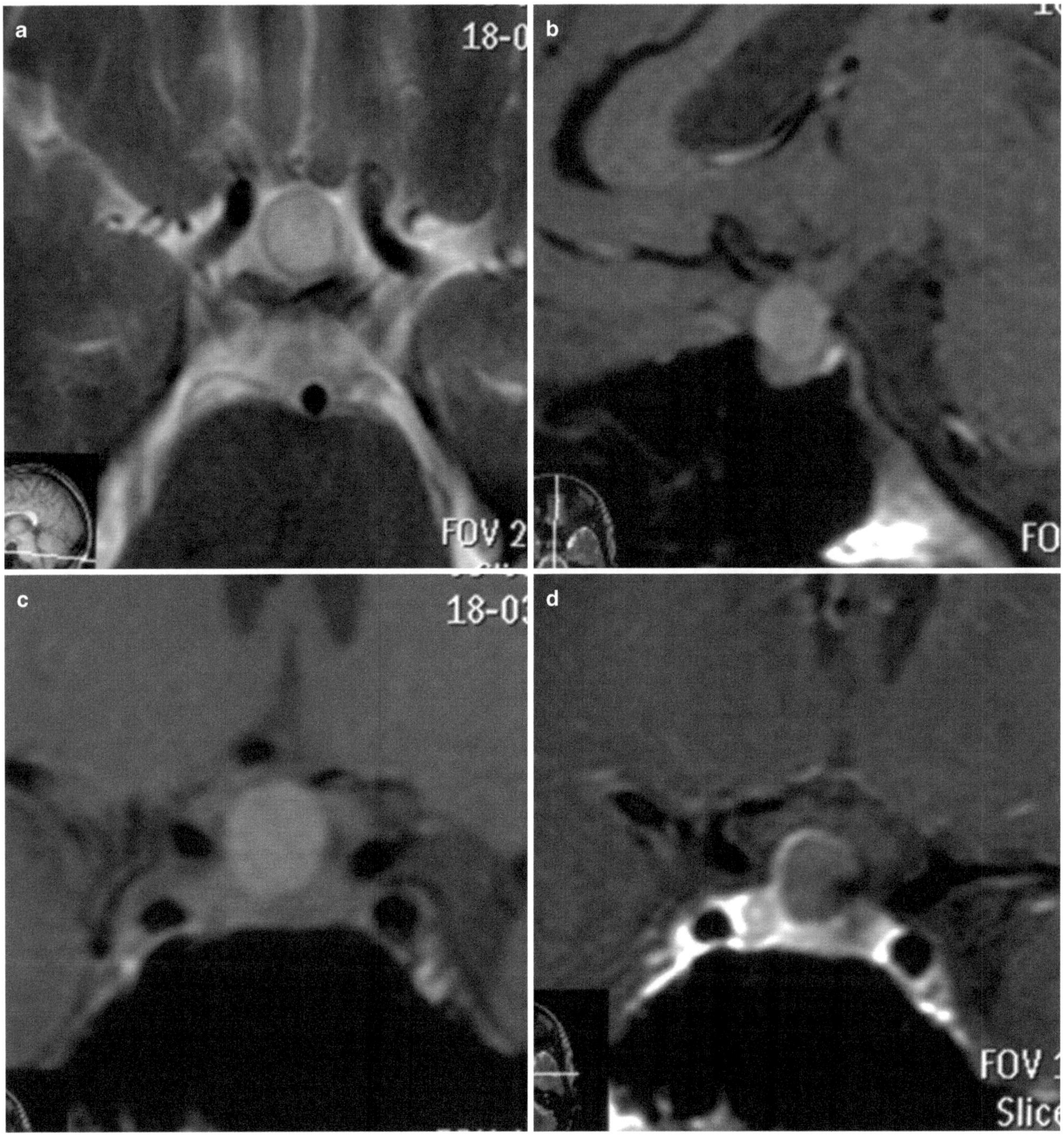

Fig. 18.9 Rathke cleft cyst. Axial T2- (**a**), sagittal (**b**), coronal (**c**) T1-weighted images and post-contrast T1 images (**d–f**) identify a rounded hyperintense nonenhancing suprasellar mass

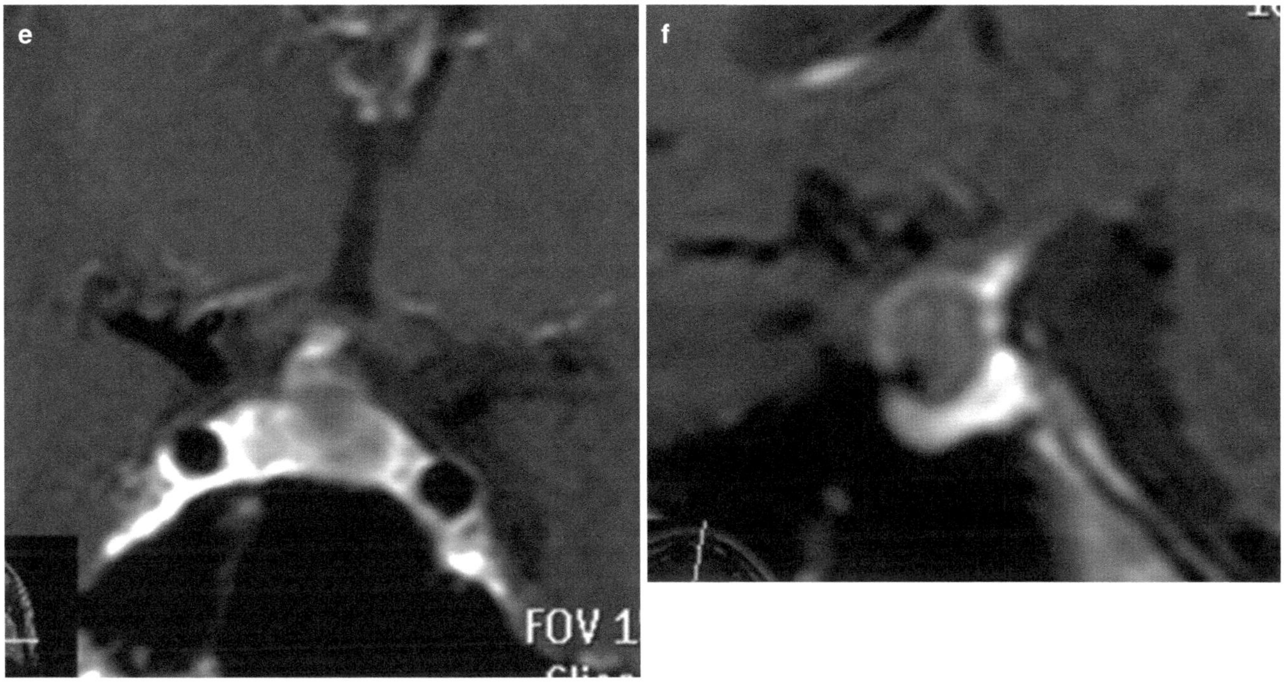

Fig. 18.9 (continued)

18.3 Arachnoid Cysts

Arachnoid cysts are congenital, intraarachnoid extraaxial cysts which are filled with CSF. They are often an occasional finding on CT or MRI in the cranial cavity, but more frequently they are seen in the anterior third of the temporal fossa, making up about 1% of all intracranial nontraumatic mass lesions (Ciricillo et al. 1991). In 10–15% of cases, they are located in the chiasmal-sellar region (Wiener et al. 1987) and more frequently (in 75% of cases) they are found in children (Wester 1992). It is supposed that arachnoid cysts are developmental abnormalities of leptomeninges; however, their precise etiology is unknown. Arachnoid cysts may be small and asymptomatic, but may reach giant sizes and lead to according clinical manifestations (Figs. 18.10 and 18.11). Primary arachnoid cysts are congenital lesions; secondary cysts develop after meningitis, surgery, trauma, etc. An arachnoid scar serves as a wall to a secondary arachnoid cyst. Arachnoid cysts are four folds more common in men than in women; they are usually located within the CSF cisterns enlarging them. Arachnoid cysts comprise no more than 1–2% of all mass lesions of the chiasmal and sellar area.

Imaging On CT a well-delineated and nonenhancing hypodense mass lesion is usually observed. Related expansive bone changes are usually detected, indicating long-term duration of the process (Fig. 18.12). MRI reveals a homogenous and well-delineated area of isointensive signal to CSF in all sequences (Garcia Santos et al. 1993). Changes of signal intensity are absent in the adjacent structures. The suprasellar arachnoid cyst existing for a long time may lead to deformation of the skull base. Cysts in MCF cause deformation of the greater wing of the sphenoid bone can spread into the anterior cranial fossa and clivus area. The walls of cyst do not accumulate contrast medium. Arachnoid cyst is isointense compared to CSF, which makes it different from other cystic mass lesions (epidermoid tumors, CPH). MR myelography may help to identify the borders of a cyst more precisely by differentiating the CSF spaces where signs of pulsation are present. However, imaging of their walls and detection of possible connections to adjacent cisterns is impossible without CT cisternography. MRI is usually sufficient for a diagnosis of arachnoid cysts. The cysts should be primarily differentiated with cholesteatoma, which is characterized by a high MR signal on DW-images, contrary to arachnoid cyst (Figs. 18.13 and 18.14).

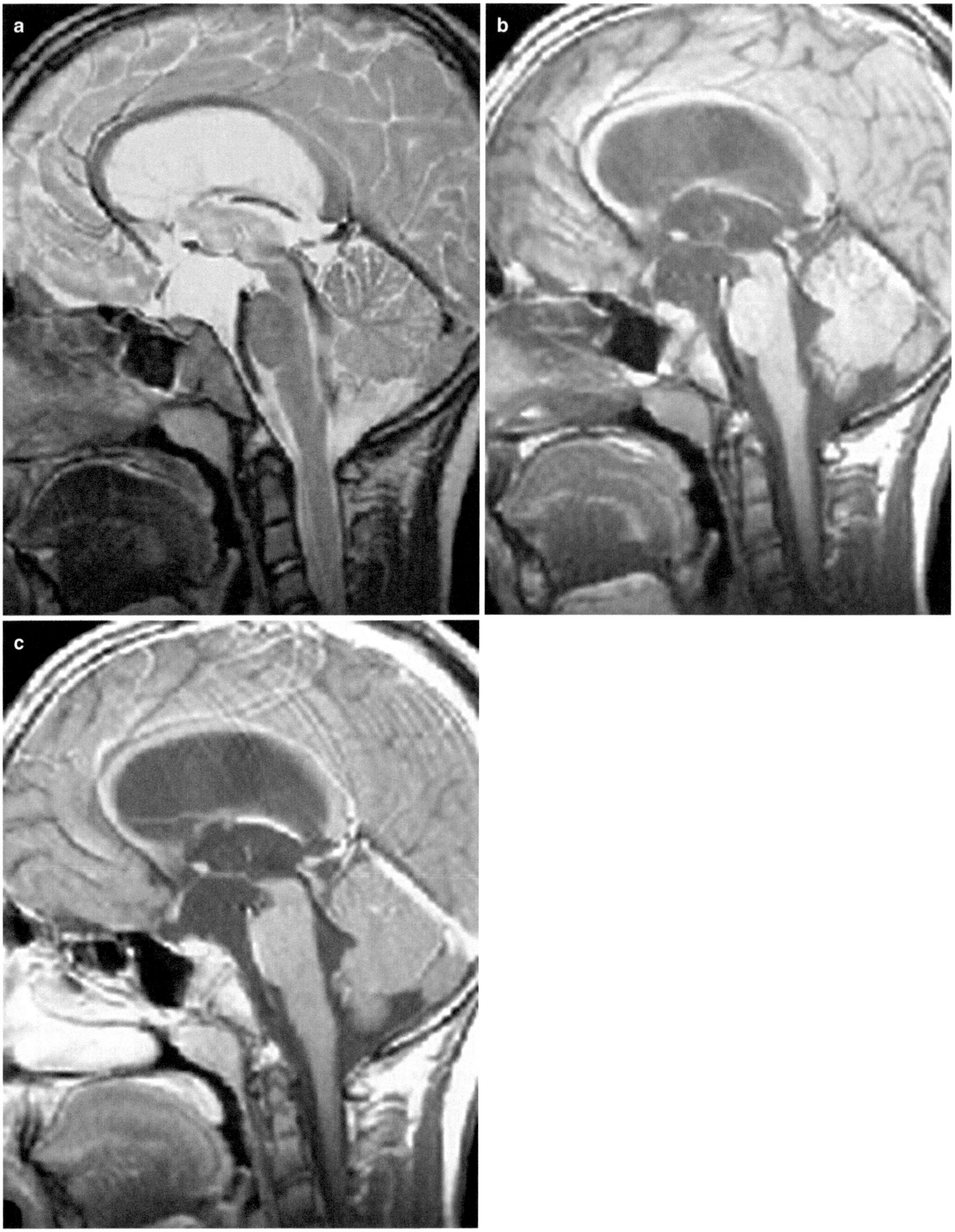

Fig. 18.10 Arachnoid cysts in the suprasellar area. Sagittal T2- (**a**), T1-weighted images (**b**) and post-contrast T1 (**c**) show a nonenhancing suprasellar cyst which is isointense with CSF. The deformation of the third ventricle floor is determined by a cyst

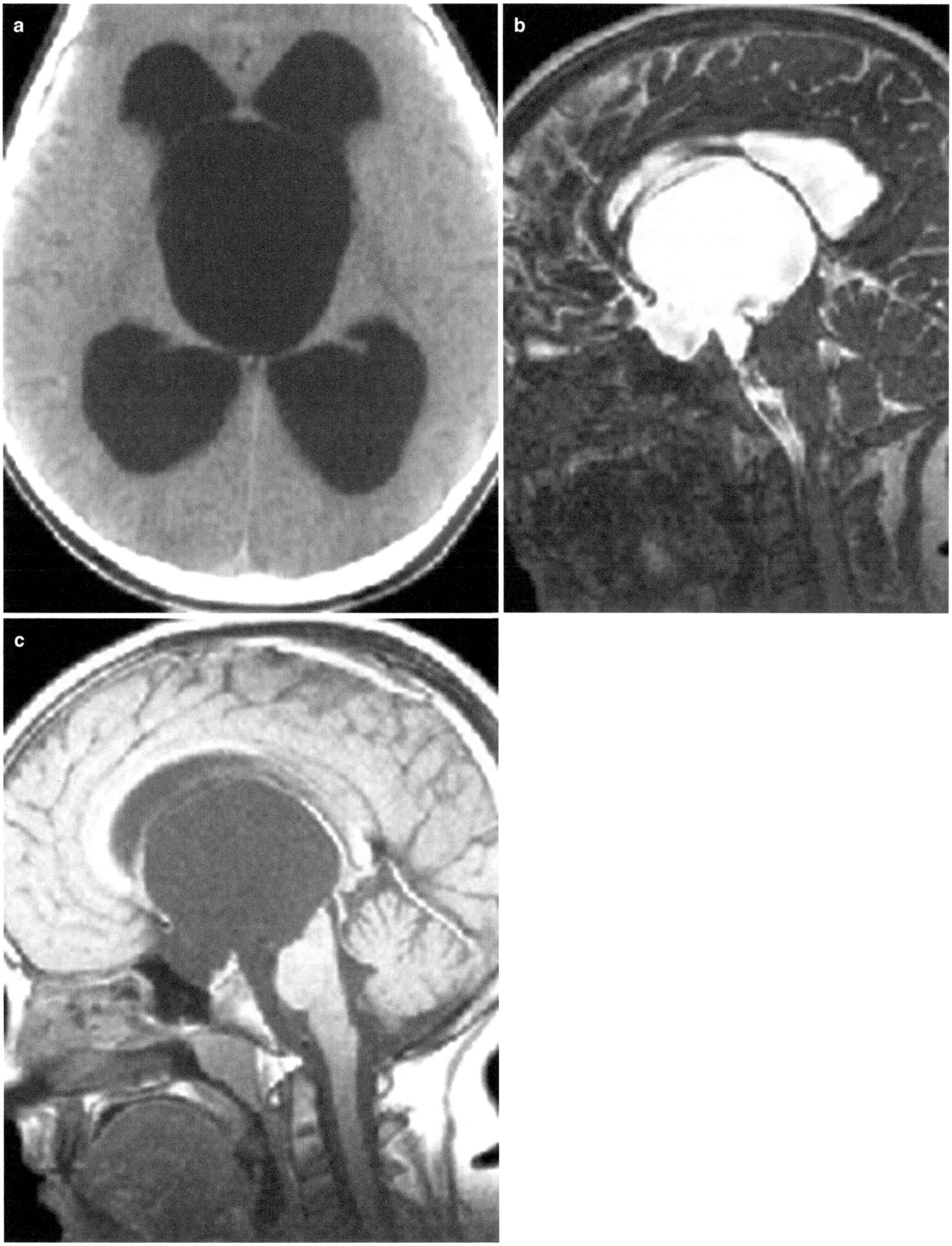

Fig. 18.11 Giant arachnoid cysts of the basal cisterns and the third ventricle causing noncommunicating hydrocephalus. CT scan (**a**), sagittal T2 (**b**) and T1-weighted MR images (**c**) demonstrate an isointensive with CSF cyst

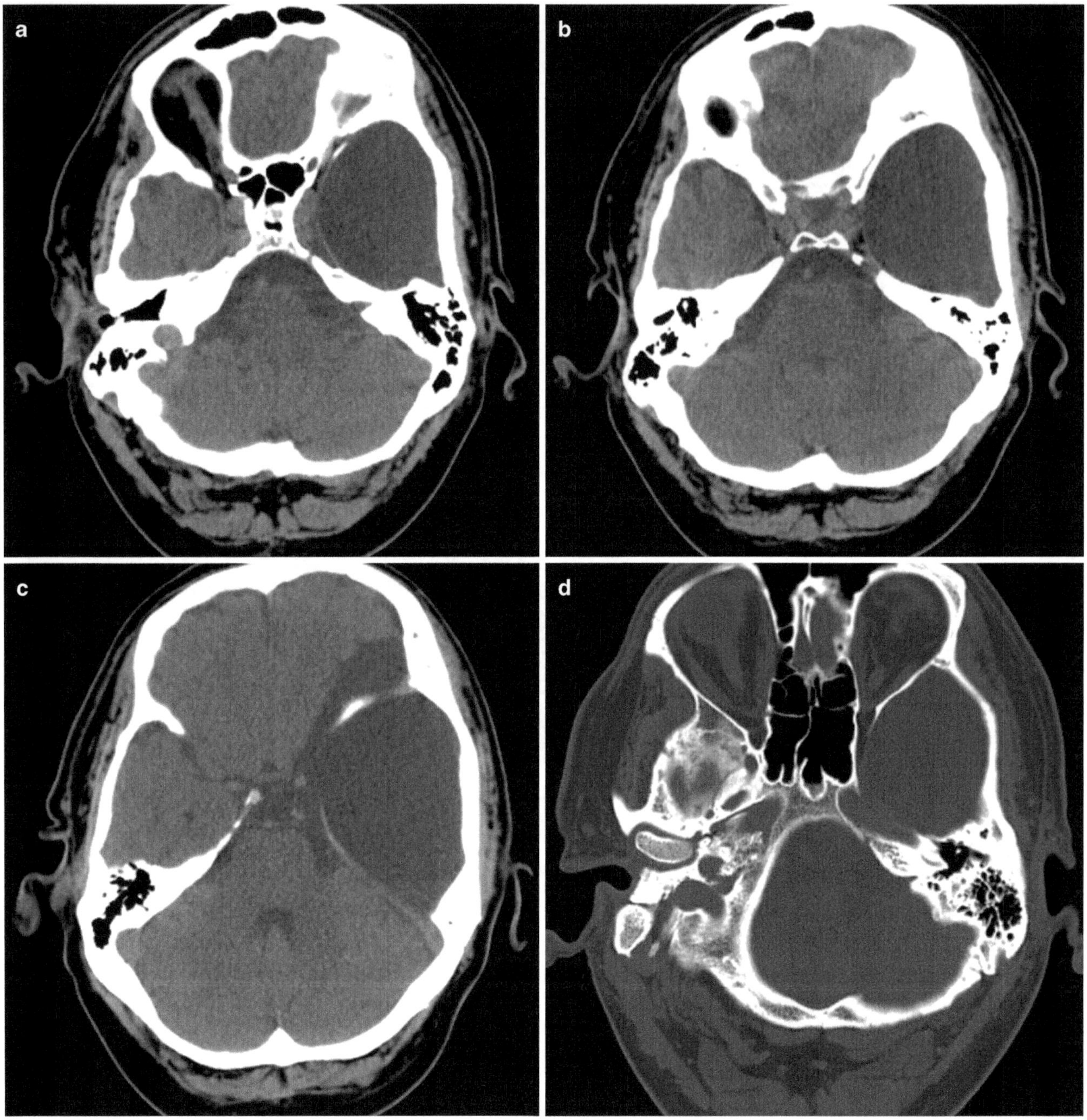

Fig. 18.12 Arachnoid cyst of the left middle cranial fossa. CT scans (**a**–**f**) reveal a hypodense cyst at the base of the middle cranial fossa causing the deformation and thickening of bone structures

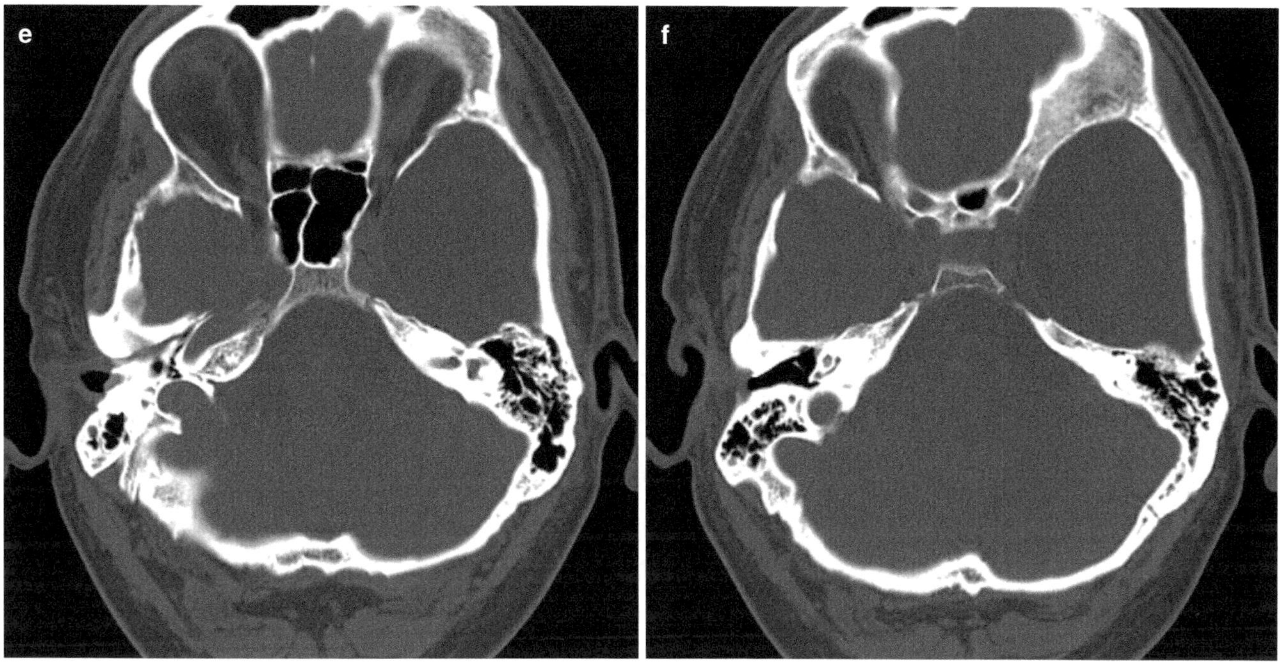

Fig. 18.12 (continued)

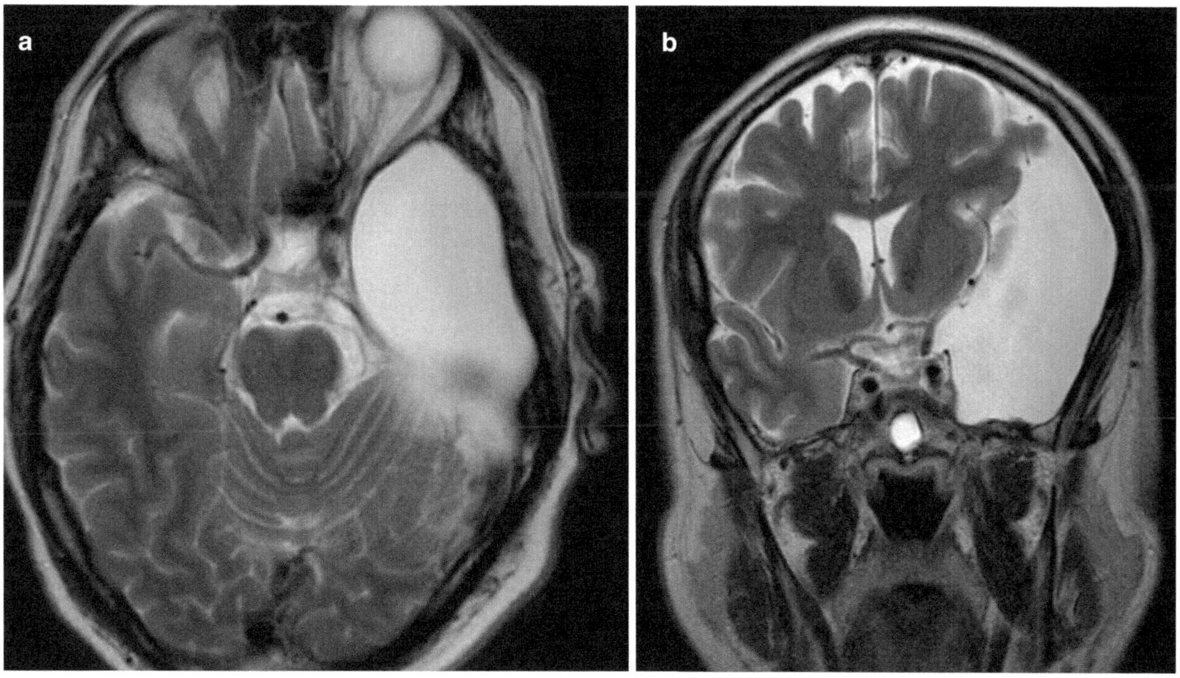

Fig. 18.13 Arachnoid cyst of the left middle cranial fossa (CT presented on Fig. 18.12). T2-weighted images (**a**, **b**), T2-FLAIR (c), DWI (**d**) and post-contrast T1-weighted images (**e**, **f**) reveal a large cyst which compresses and displaces the left temporal lobe. The cyst is isointense with CSF in all sequences, including DWI

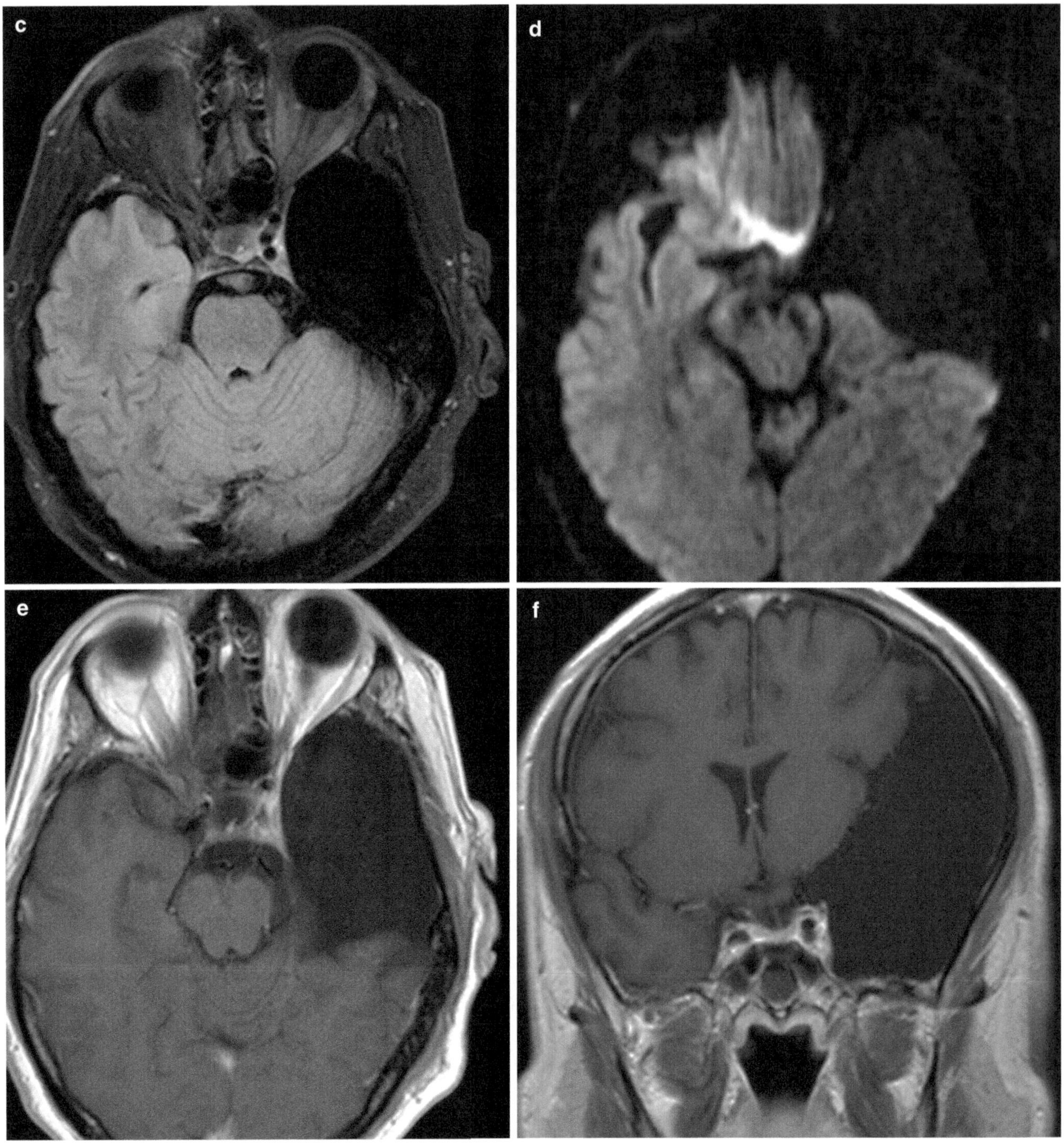

Fig. 18.13 (continued)

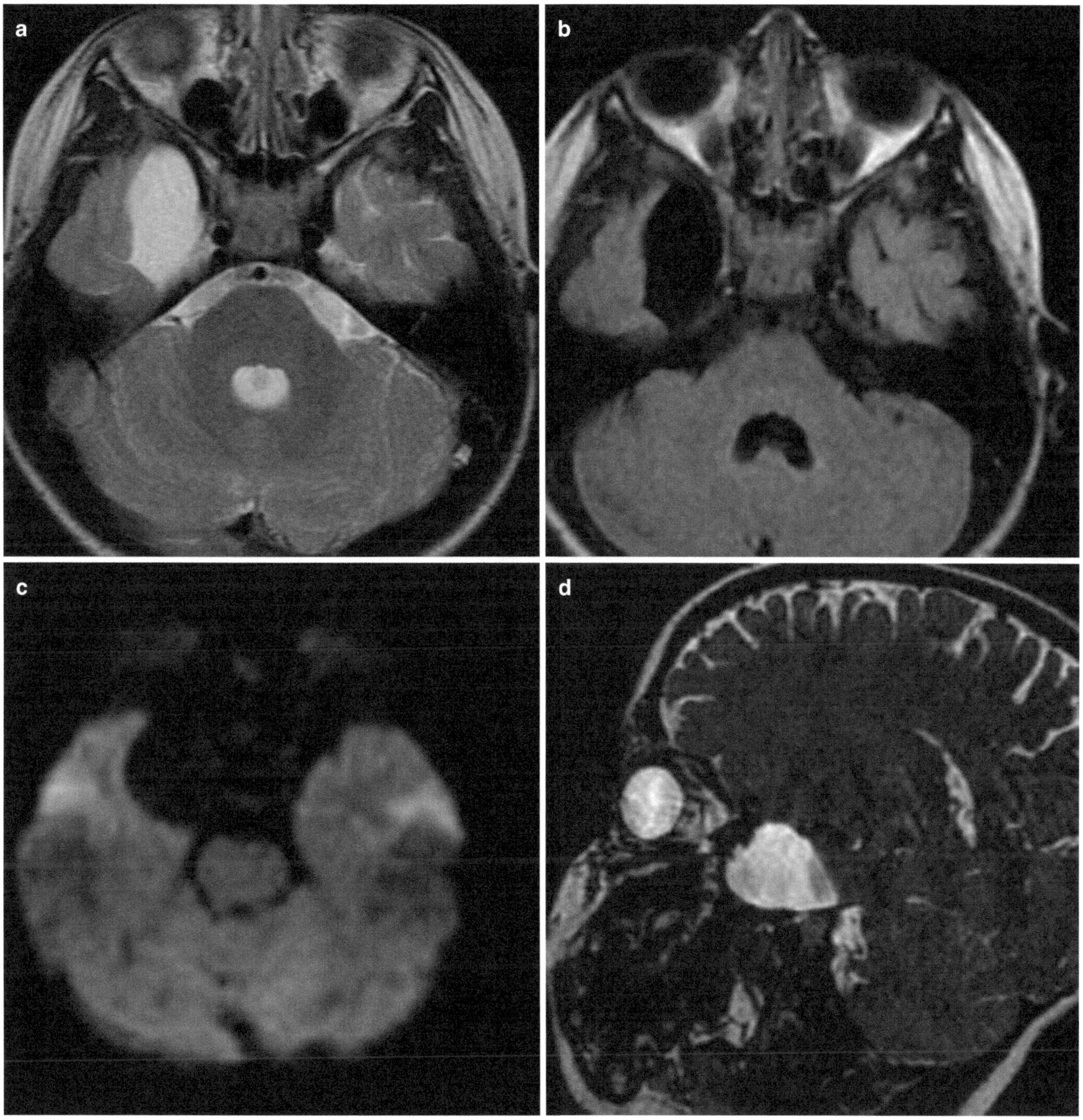

Fig. 18.14 Arachnoid cyst of the left middle cranial fossa. T2-weighted image (**a**) T2-FLAIR (**b**) DWI (c), PSIF-image (**d**), and post-contrast T1-weighted images (**e**, **f**) reveal a nonenhancing cyst in the medial part of middle cranial fossa, which is isointense with the CSF in all sequences, including DWI

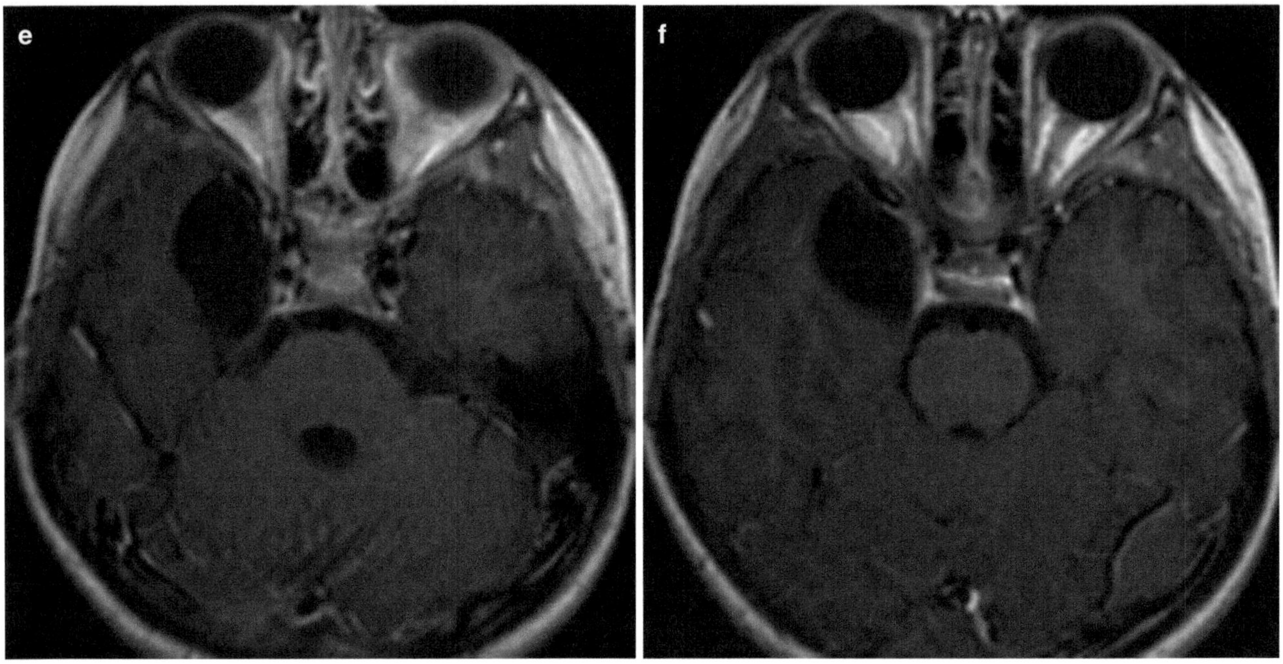

Fig. 18.14 (continued)

18.4 Empty Sella Turcica

The term empty sella turcica in a certain sense is a radiological definition: the sella turcica is always filled with CSF, and contains remnants of the pituitary gland as well as the chiasm and optic nerves from time to time. Dilated subarachnoid space combined with congenital and acquired diaphragm insufficiency is characteristic for the empty sella turcica (Carmel 1985). The term empty sella syndrome stands for a prolapse of the suprasellar cistern into the cavity of the sella turcica and flattening of the pituitary against sellar floor, accompanied by endocrine, neurological, and visual disturbances.

Two variants of the empty sella turcica are distinguished: "complicated" and "non-complicated." The latter does not manifest clinically and usually is an occasional neuroimaging finding. Complicated empty sella turcica manifests with certain clinical signs.

Primary and secondary empty sella turcica are distinguished. Primary empty sella turcica develops due to several physiological or pathological conditions that lead to reduction of the pituitary volume: climax, infarction or necrosis of the pituitary gland, infarction or autolysis of the pituitary adenoma, and rupture of the non-tumor sellar cyst. Primary empty sella turcica is mainly encountered in females after frequent pregnancies or the long-term hormone use.

The most typical clinical manifestations of the primary empty sella turcica are intermittent visual disturbances (changes in the fields of vision, amblyopia, and optic discs abnormalities), combination of refractory arterial hypertension with obesity, reduction of the pituitary-associated sexual function, and the pituitary–suprarenal and the pituitary–thyroid functions, etc.

The secondary empty sella turcica develops after surgical, irradiation or combined treatment of different conditions of sellar-parasellar region due to destruction of the pituitary diaphragm and descending of the suprasellar cisterns into the sella turcica. The clinical picture of secondary complicated sella turcica is variegated and is mainly determined by the syndrome that has taken place before treatment of pituitary adenoma.

The development of empty sella turcica is possible in obstructive hydrocephalus, at the level of the cerebral aqueduct. The enlarging third ventricle prolapses into the bony sella turcica, which is moderately enlarged. The pituitary gland usually flattened against sella floor. The pituitary stalk is often tilted against the dorsum. The optic chiasm can herniate into sella. Similar changes may accompany the growth of a supratentorial brain tumor (Fig. 18.15).

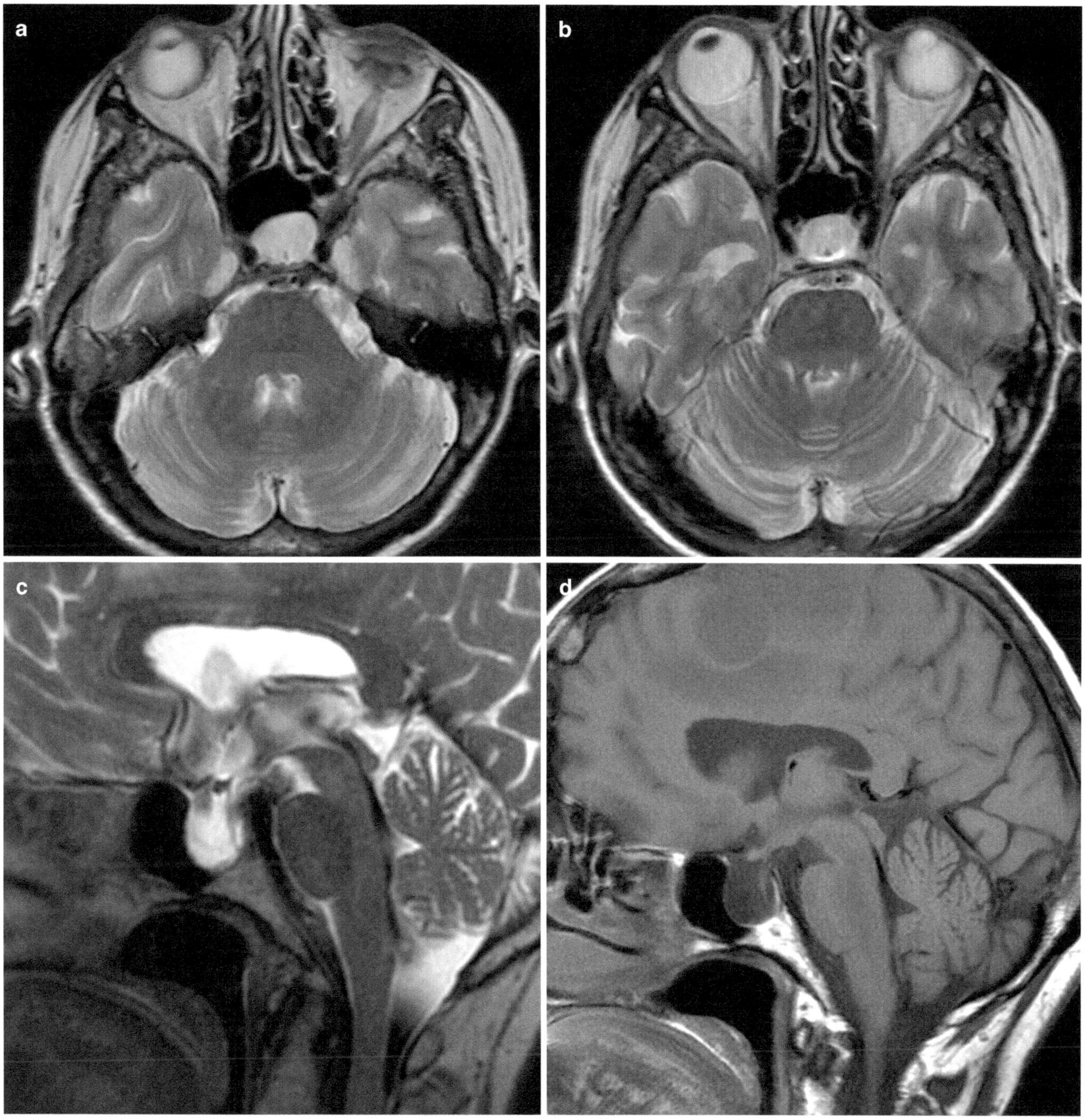

Fig. 18.15 Secondary empty sella turcica. T2-weighted images (**a–c**), T1-weighted image (**d**) and PSIF (**e**, **f**) reveal a moderately enlarged sella turcica with intrasellar CSF signal. A pituitary stalk is at the midline, but tilted posteriorly. A small amount of residual pituitary gland tissue is flattening against the sellar bottom. An optic chiasm is retracted toward the sella. A large intracerebral tumor in the frontal lobe causes the intracranial hypertension with the secondary changes of sella turcica

Fig. 18.15 (continued)

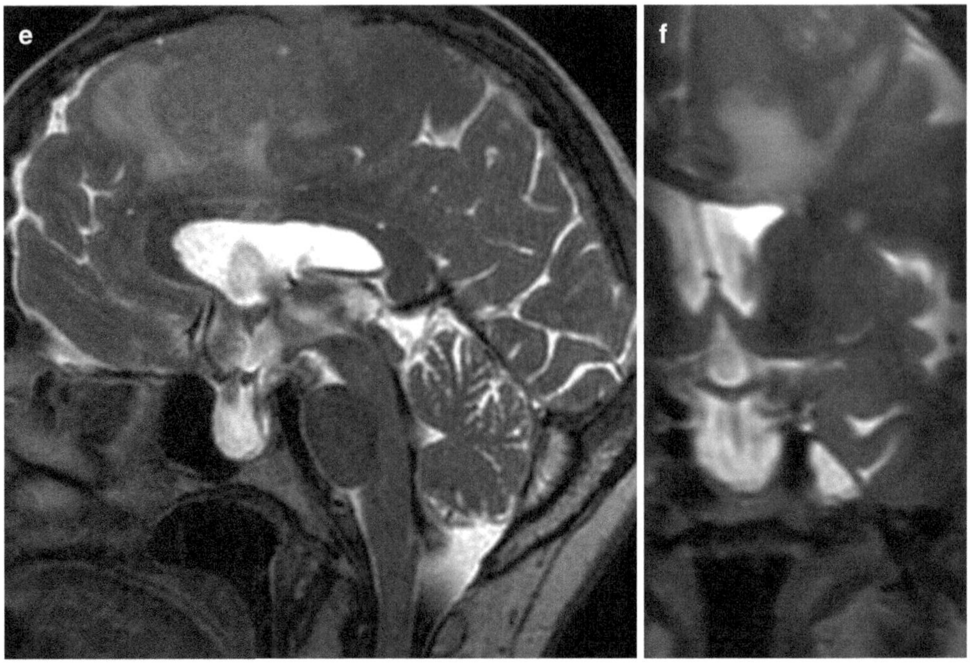

Imaging On CT dilated and deepened sella turcica is usually seen. On rare occasions after reformation in sagittal and coronal planes the pituitary stalk may be visualized within the sella turcica cavity. The density within the sella turcica corresponds to that of CSF. After contrast enhancement, an increase in the density from the cavernous sinuses is observed.

On MRI, changes of the pituitary gland are better seen as gland flattens, or in cases when it acquires a shape of a thin rim that repeats contours of the bottom of sella turcica. Differential diagnosis should be made from sellar cysts. Position of the pituitary stalk is the pivotal sign in these cases. In cases of the empty sella turcica, the stalk is normally positioned; if cysts are present, then the stalk is compressed or displaced. Myelographic sequences with sagittal and coronal planes are advisable to use in order to determine the relationship between suprasellar cerebrospinal fluid spaces and the cavity of the sella turcica (Fig. 18.16).

In complicated cases CT cisternography with water-soluble contrast media is helpful in empty sella turcica diagnosis.

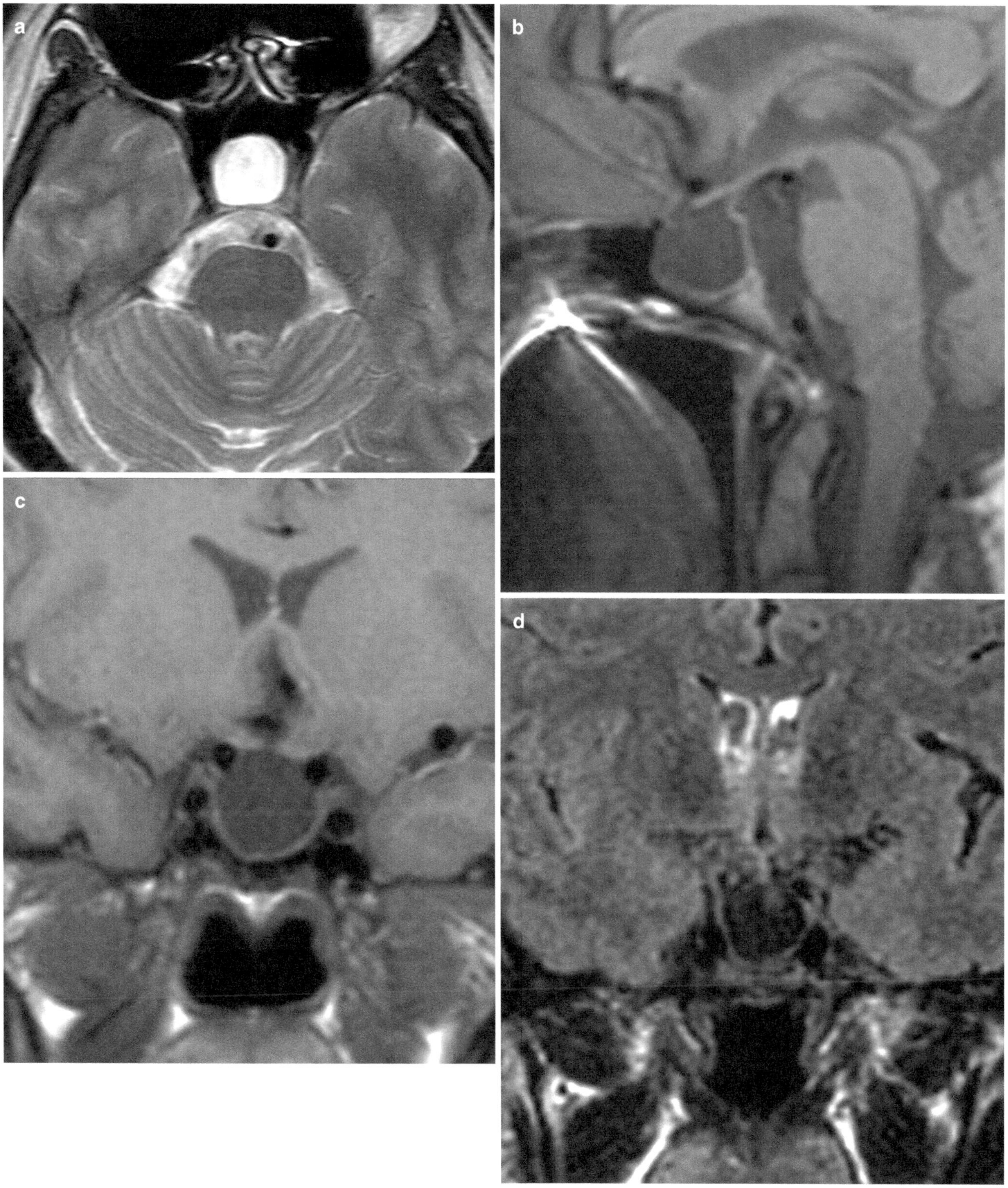

Fig. 18.16 Empty sella turcica. T2-weighted (**a**), T1-weighted images (**b**, **c**) and T2-FLAIR (**d**) show an enlarged sella turcica. Coronal T2-weighted image (**e**) and PSIF (**f**) better visualize an extension of CSF through the wide opening diaphragma sellae. CSF pulsation artifact (a hypointensive area, *arrows*) confirms a connection between the cisterns and sellar area

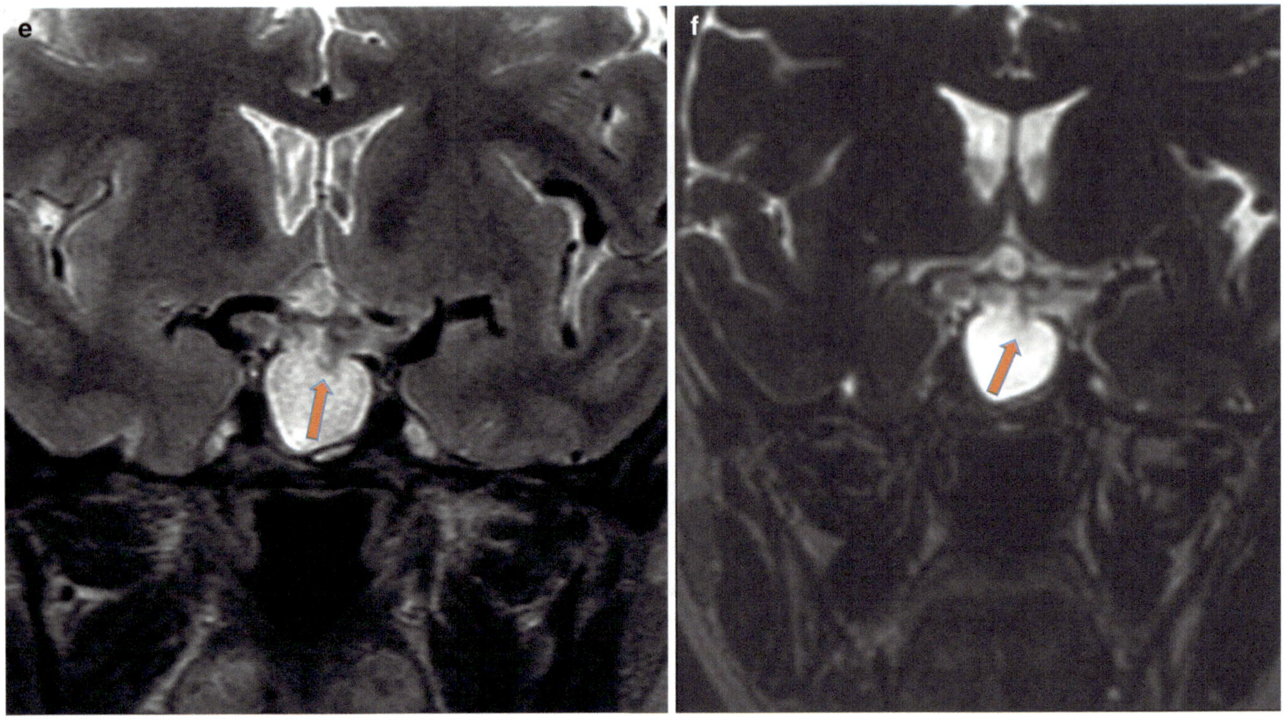

Fig. 18.16 (continued)

19 Saccular Arterial Aneurysm

Content

Saccular arterial aneurysms (SAA) are the space-occupying lesions that can occur in both suprasellar and in parasellar areas. Giant aneurysms located there have clinical manifestations identical to the tumors. Differential diagnosis should be made from tumors of the chiasmal-sellar region. Saccular aneurysms in the chiasmal-sellar region may originate from the cavernous segment of the internal carotid artery as well as from its supraclinoid segment of it. Sometimes aneurysms of the anterior and posterior communicating and basilar arteries may protrude into the suprasellar cistern. Misinterpretation of an aneurysm as a tumor may lead to a surgical accident.

Imaging The main method of diagnosis of vascular pathology is a conventional cerebral angiography. CT and MRI are appropriate to use in prehospital diagnosis. Aneurysms are well delineated and give the so-called "flow voids" effect on T1- and T2-weighted imaging due to rapid blood flow. In addition, rapid blood flow causes marked artifacts on images, which are manifested by multiple shadows in the phase-encoding direction, which are important diagnostic feature them (Fig. 19.1). On T1-weighted images, MR-signal from an aneurysm greatly varies from hypointense (flow-voids) to isointense or even moderately focally hyperintense (an effect of paradoxical signal amplification) due to turbulent flow, saturation effect, and phase dispersion (Osborn et al. 2016). The latter should not be confused with thrombosed SAA, which MR signal on T1-weighted images increases upon formation of methemoglobin in the blood clot (Fig. 19.2). CT or MR angiography may add information about an aneurysm.

It is noteworthy that thrombosis in the cavity of an aneurysm markedly changes its signal characteristics. Thrombi that fill aneurysms usually have laminar structures. They are hyperintensive on T1-weighted images. Thrombosis of an aneurysm may be complete or partial. Hemosiderin deposits may be seen in the adjacent tissues because of old hemorrhage from an aneurysm. These deposits appear as rims of hypointensive signal on T2-weighted images or on gradient

I. Pronin, V. Kornienko, *CT and MRI of Skull Base Lesions*, https://doi.org/10.1007/978-3-319-65957-2_19

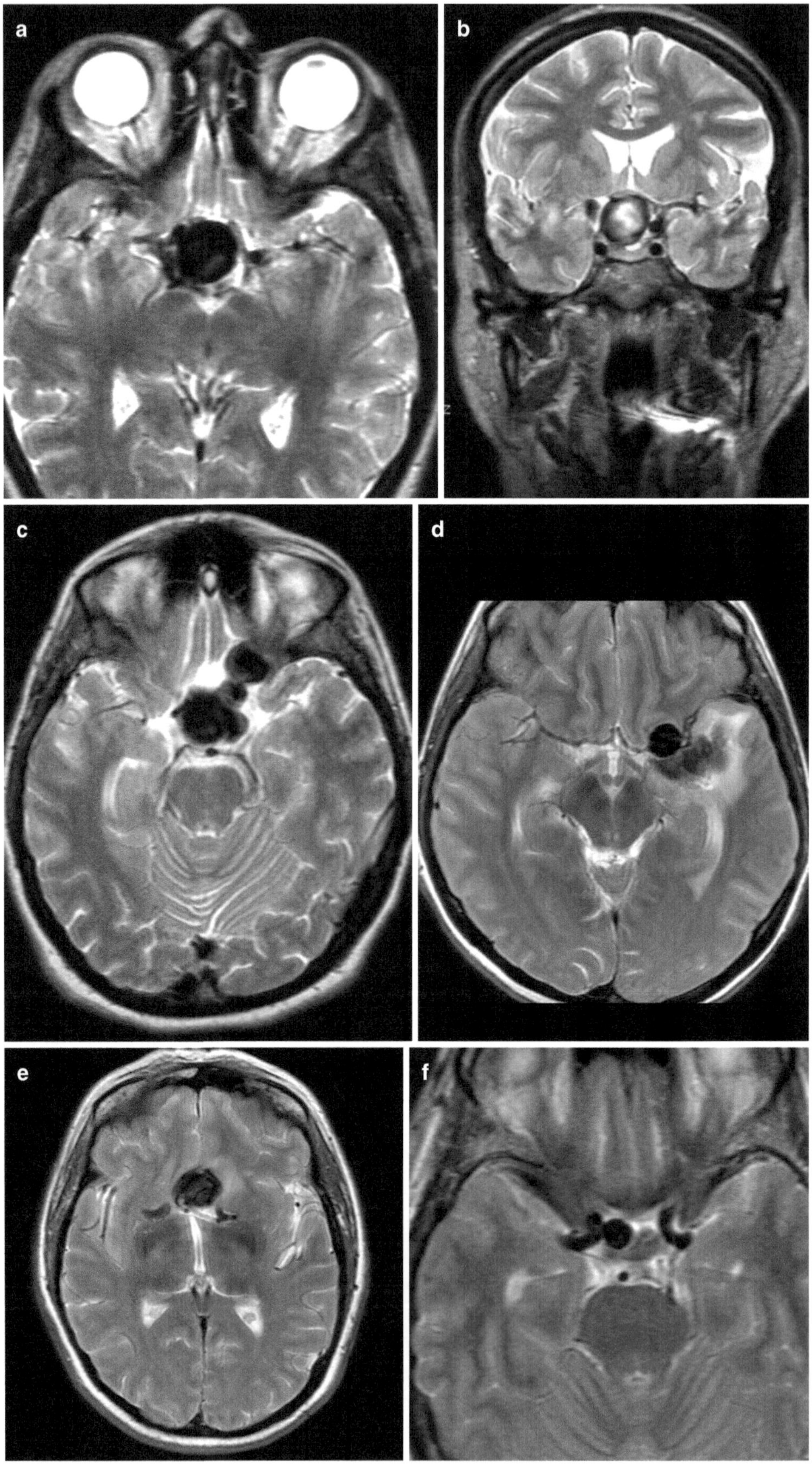

Fig. 19.1 Saccular aneurysms in the chiasmal-sellar region in different patients. T2-weighted images (**a**–**f**) show the arterial aneurysms as rounded hypointense "flow voids" lesions

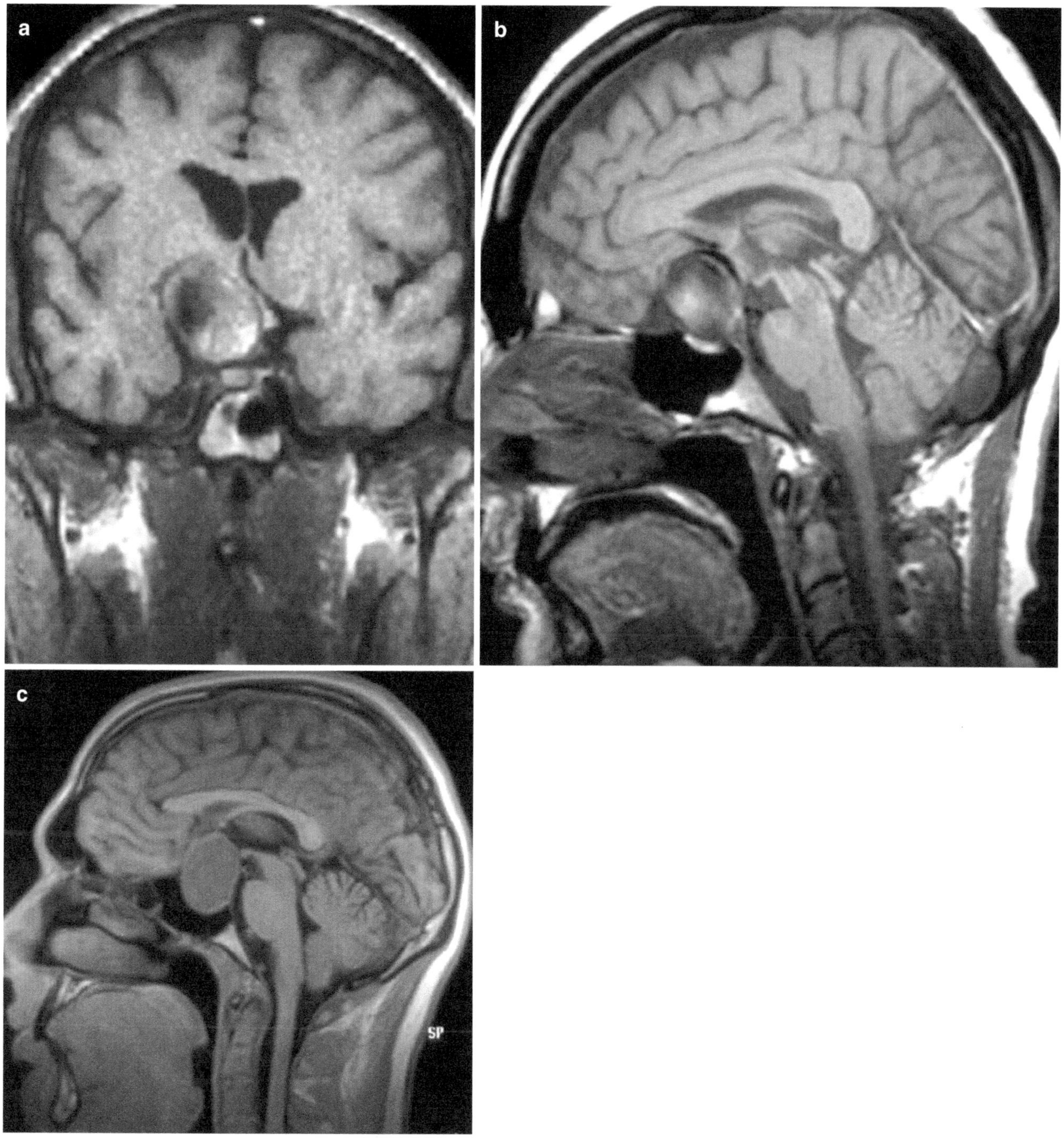

Fig. 19.2 Saccular aneurysms in the chiasmal-sellar region in different patients. T1-weighted images (**a**–**c**) demonstrate a heterogeneous signal from the aneurysms due to turbulent flow inside the lesions

echo images (SWAN, SWI), or perianeurysmal intracerebral hematoma can be diagnosed (Figs. 19.3 and 19.4).

CT before and after CE is less specific than MRI findings are. That is why it is always feasible to add CT-angiography to CT. On CT, SAA appears as a space-occupying lesion with slightly increased density. Giant SAAs may be accompanied by surrounding bone changes. On CE CT, the lumen of the patent aneurysm enhances homogeneously (Fig. 19.5); their contours are smooth and rounded. The use of CT-angiography allows making correct diagnosis in most cases. Additional 2D reformation and 3D reconstruction help distinguish between the functioning and thrombosed parts of SAA (Figs. 19.6 and 19.7). Among new diagnostic techniques, used today in the diagnosis of

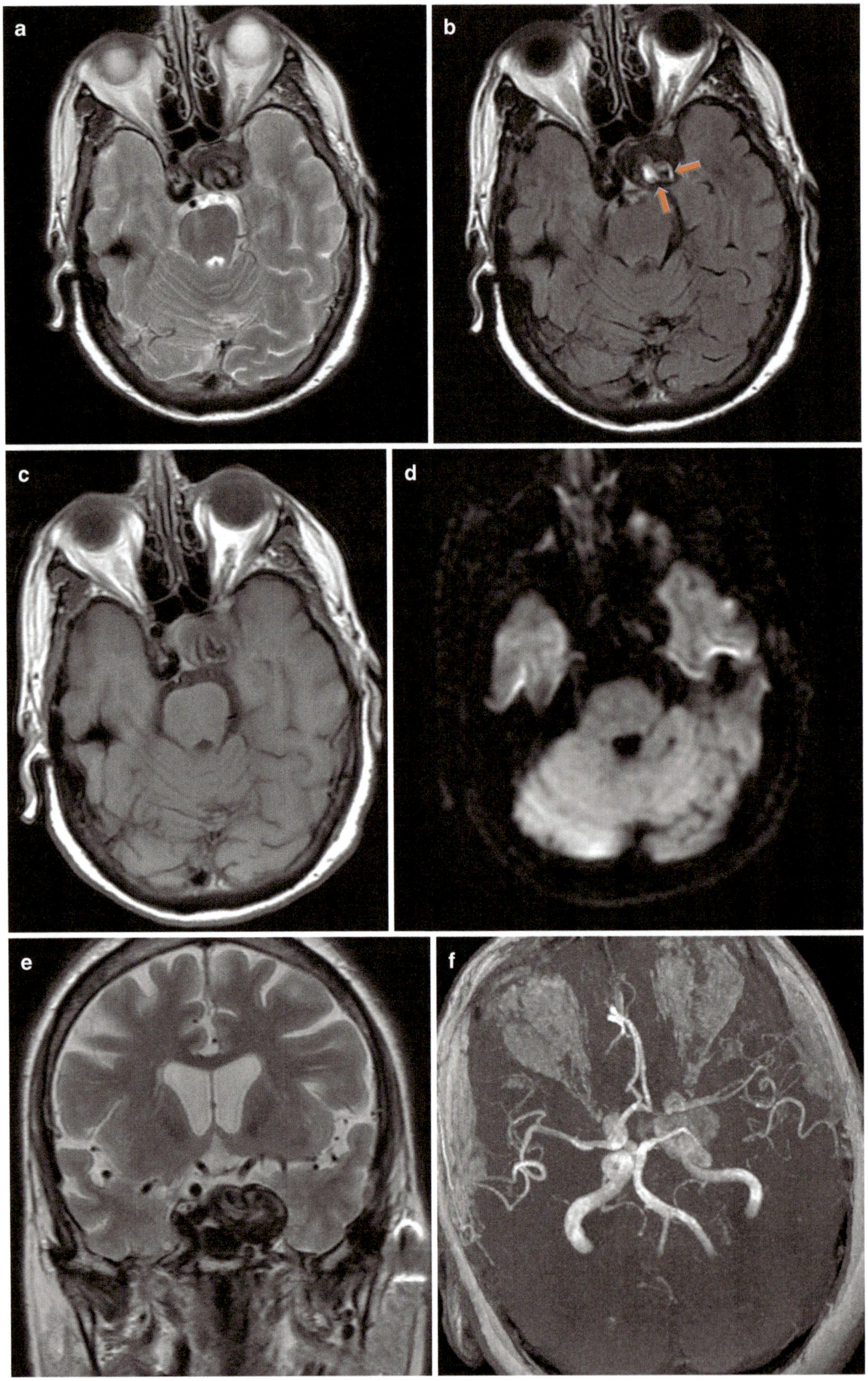

Fig. 19.3 Giant partially thrombosed saccular aneurysm of the left internal carotid artery. T2-weighted images (**a**, **e**), T2-FLAIR (**b**), T1-weighted image (**c**) and DWI (**d**) show a giant aneurysm with mixed signal. An increased signal and pulsation artifacts (turbulent flow) on T2-FLAIR indicate that a functioning part is in the posterior aspect of aneurysm (*arrows*). The anterior part of aneurysm is thrombosed. 3D TOF MRA (**f**) shows the full dimensions of aneurysm (functioning and thrombosed parts)

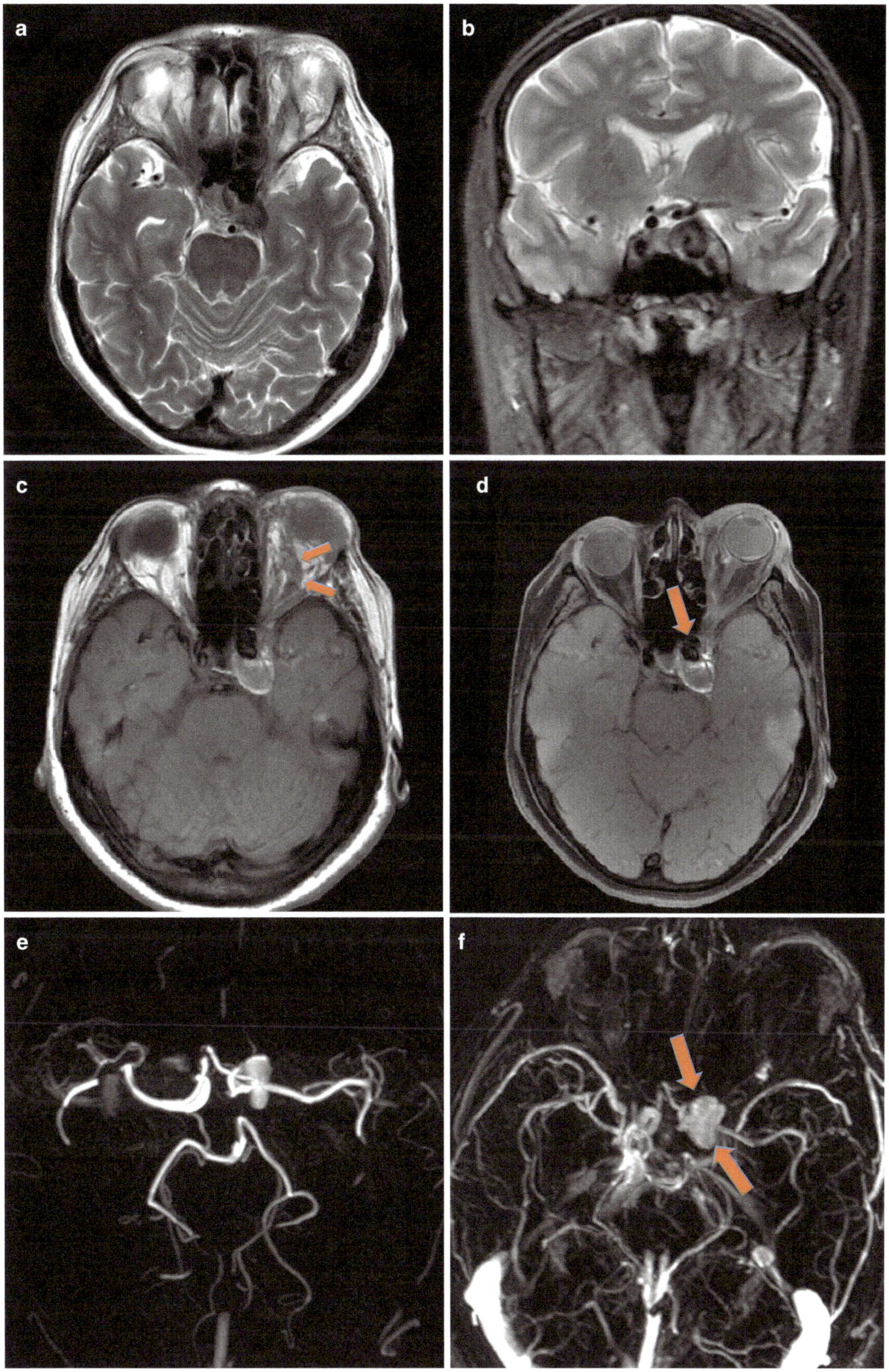

Fig. 19.4 Partially thrombosed saccular aneurysm of the left internal carotid artery. T2 (**a**, **b**), T1 (**c**), T1 + fat-sat (**d**) show a hyperintense on T1-weighted image thrombosed part of aneurysm and hypointense in all sequences a functioning part (*arrows*). A thrombosis of the superior orbital vein is also visualized (*small arrows*, **c**). 3D PC MRA (**e**) and bolus CE dynamic MRA (**f**) clearly show a functioning part of aneurysm (*arrows*)

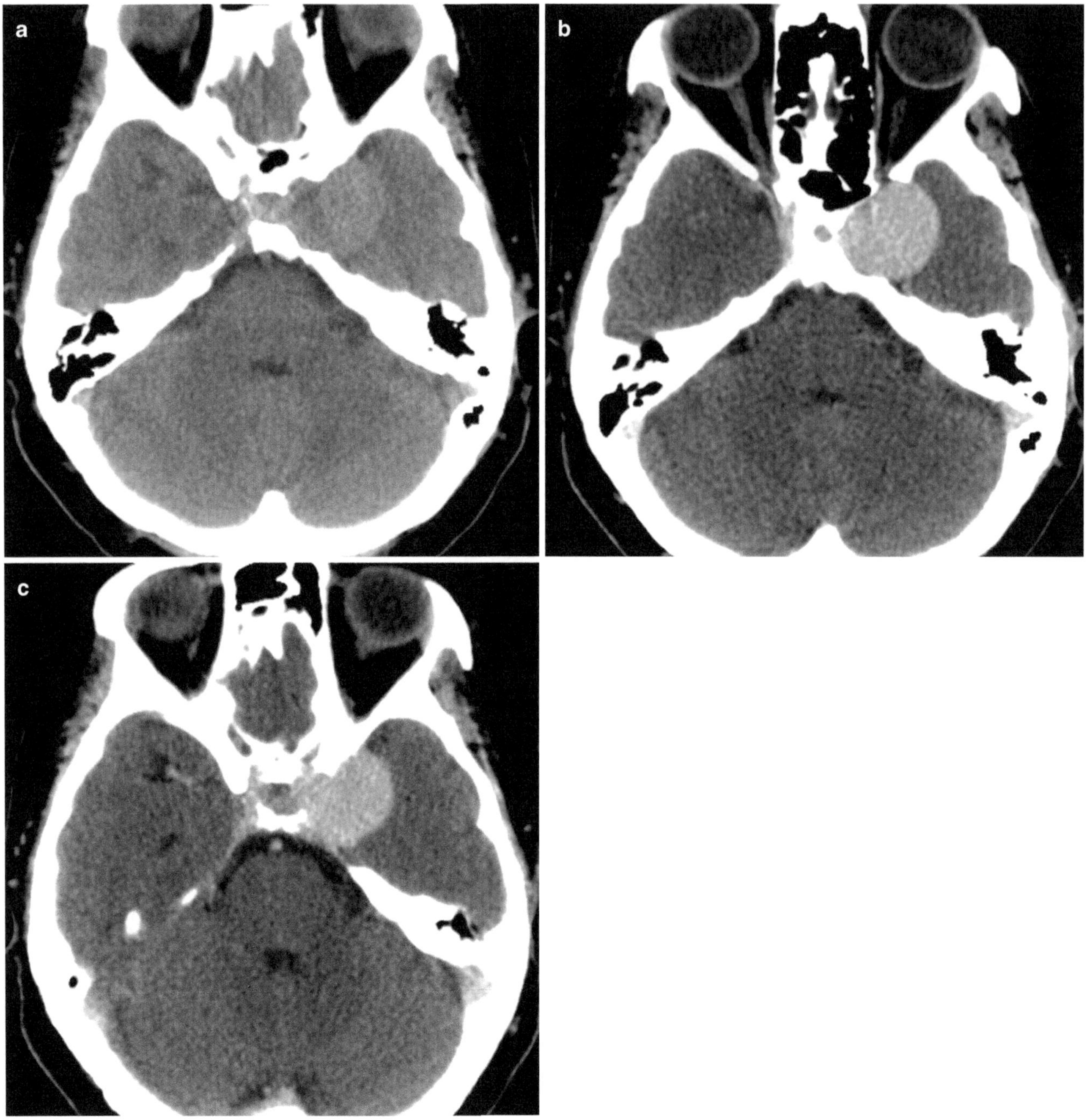

Fig. 19.5 Large saccular aneurysm of the left internal carotid artery. Axial CT scans before (**a**) and after contrast enhancement (**b**, **c**) show an intense and homogeneous enhancement in the lumen of aneurysm

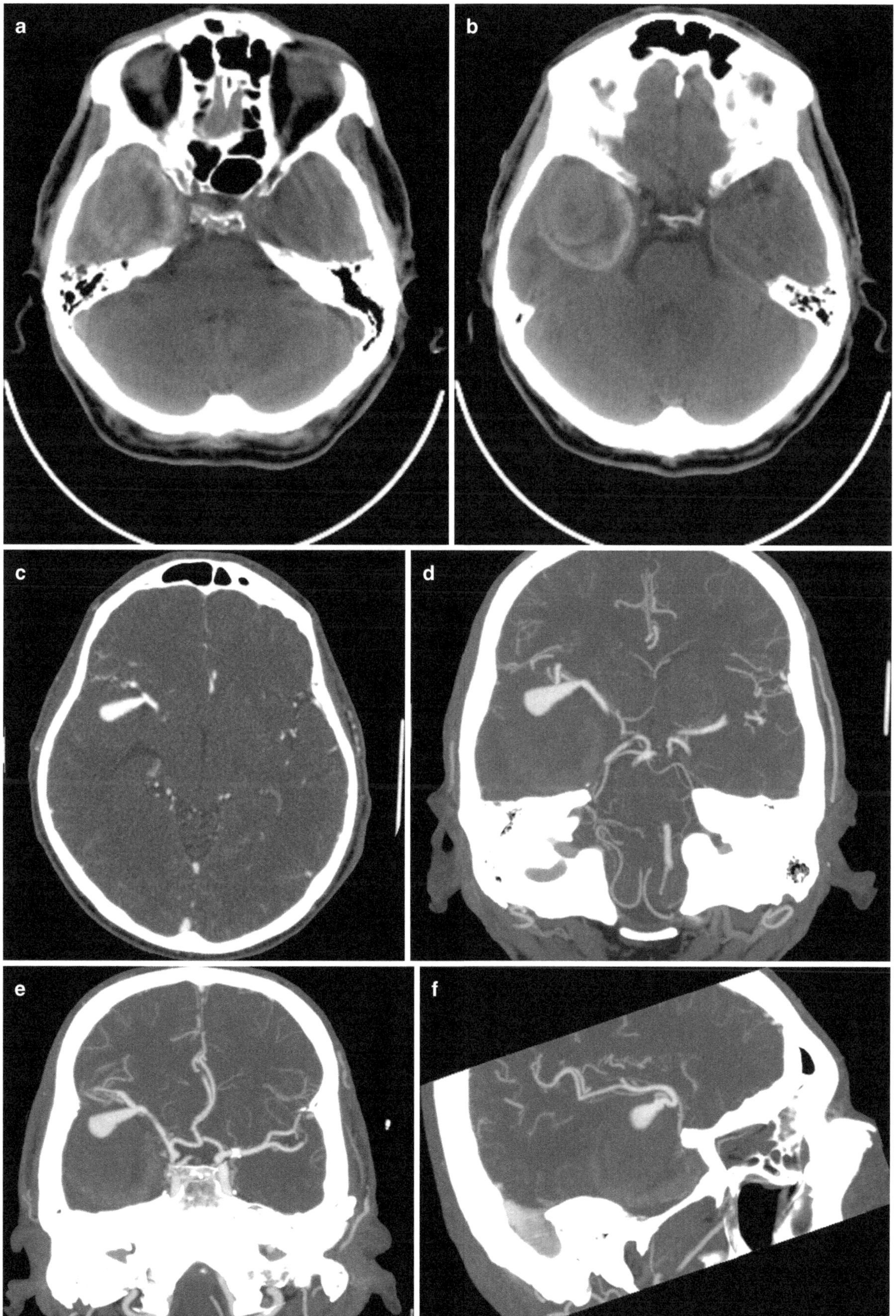

Fig. 19.6 Giant partially thrombosed saccular aneurysm of the right middle cerebral artery. NECT (**a**, **b**) show a heterogeneous lesion in the right middle cranial fossa. CTA with reformations (**c**–**f**) reveal a functioning part of aneurysm of the middle cerebral artery trifurcation placed above the thrombosed part. Right middle cerebral artery is displaced upward

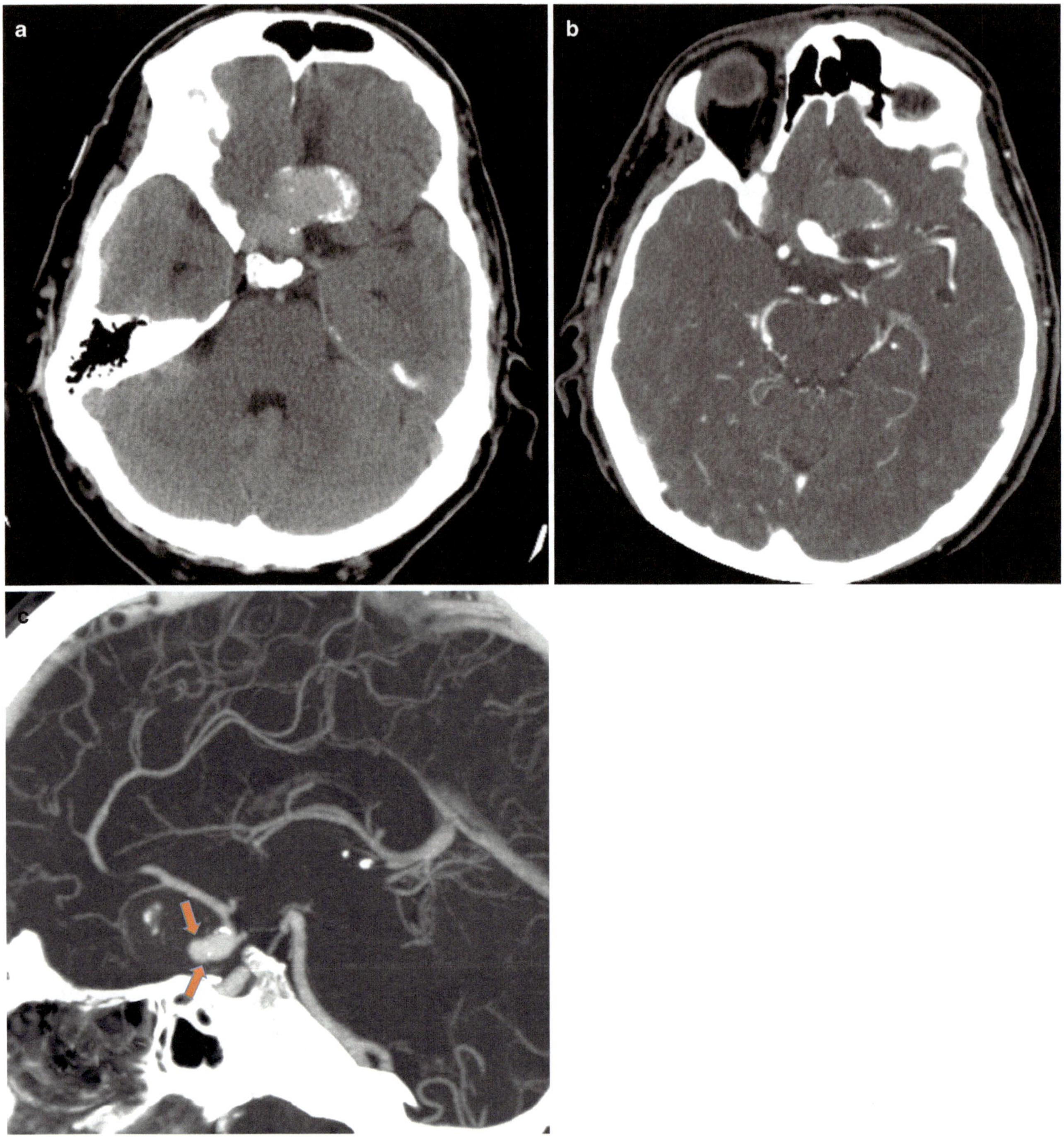

Fig. 19.7 Giant partially thrombosed saccular aneurysm of the anterior cerebral artery—anterior communicating artery. CT scan (**a**, **b**) reveals a hyperdense lesion in the antesellar region. An aneurysm has peripheral calcifications. CTA (**c**–**f**) with reformats shows a small functioning part of the aneurysm of supraclinoid left internal carotid artery (*arrows*)

vascular disorders, bolus MR angiography (TRICKS) and CT-perfusion are noteworthy (Figs. 19.8 and 19.9). The main advantage of these methods is the possibility to dynamically assess the blood flow in the SAA lumen. Quantitative study of blood flow velocity parameters in SAA in a combination with 4D technology is the next stage in a comprehensive evaluation of cerebral vascular disorder.

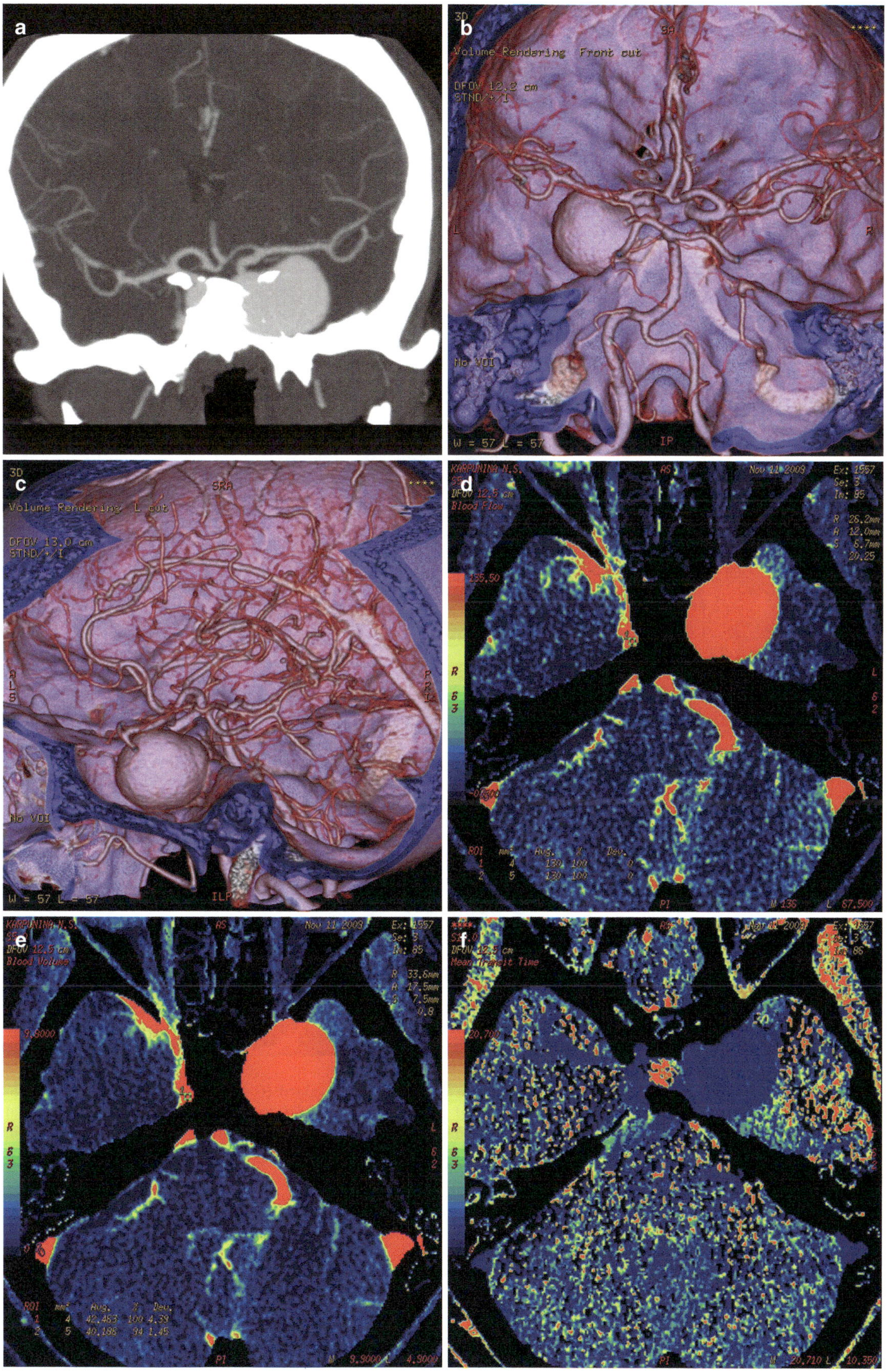

Fig. 19.8 Functioning large saccular aneurysm of the infraclinoid part of internal carotid artery. CTA, coronal reformat (**a**), and 3D (**b**, **c**) show an aneurysm in the left cavernous sinus area. CT-perfusion demonstrates the high level of CBF (**d**), CBV (**e**) and a short MTT (**f**) comparable to the carotid artery flow

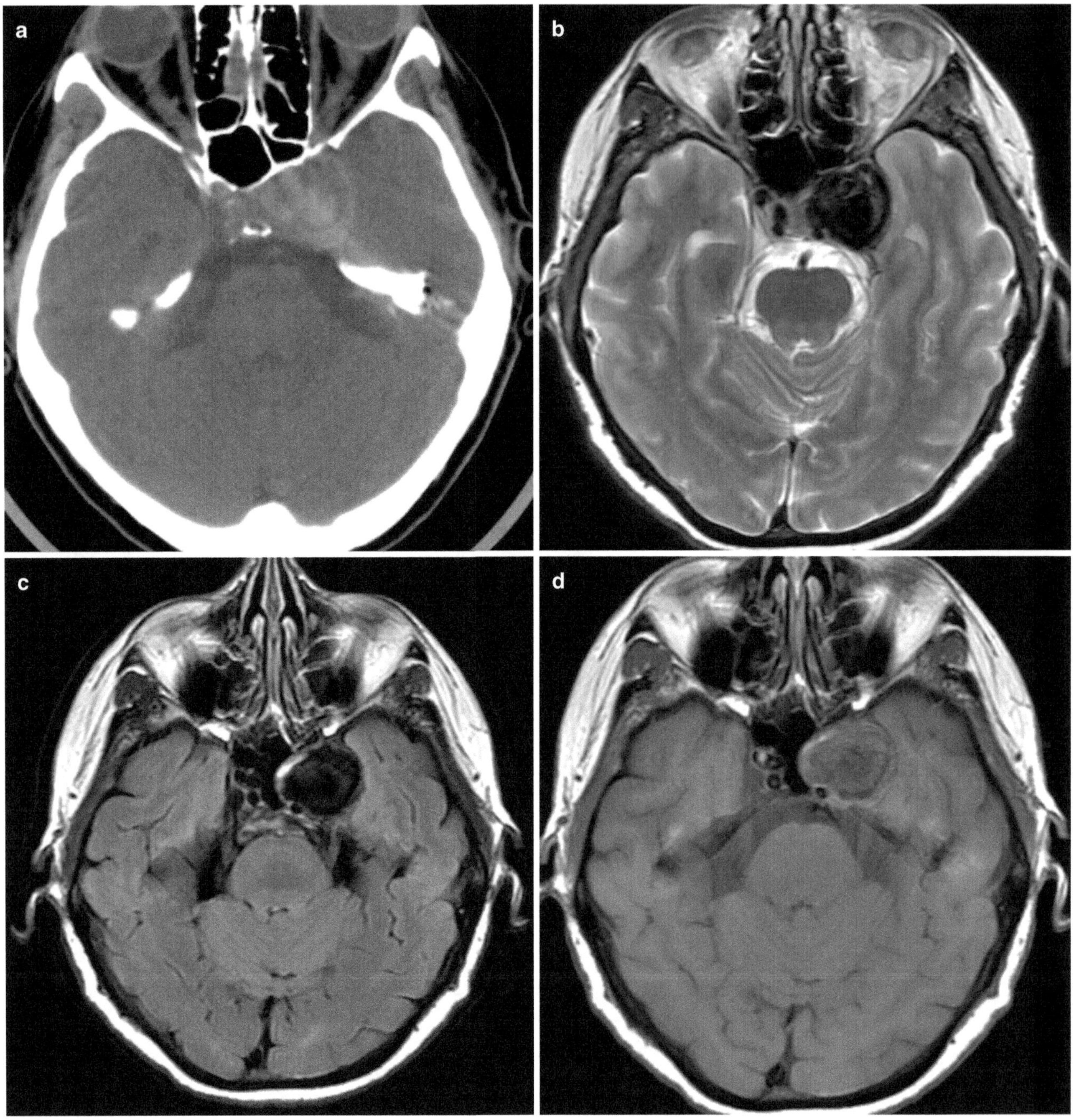

Fig. 19.9 Giant partially thrombosed saccular aneurysm of the supraclinoid part the internal carotid artery. Axial CT scan (**a**), axial T2-weighted image (**b**), T2-FLAIR (**c**), T1-weighted image (**d**), and DWI (**e**) show a moderately hyperdense (on CT) and hypointense (on MRI) rounded lesion in the projection of the left cavernous sinus. Post-contrast T1-weighted (**f**) image demonstrates an enhancement in the lateral wall of the left cavernous sinus. A hypointense signal with artifact from the functioning part of aneurysm is seen (*arrow*). 3D PC MRA (**g**, **h**) and bolus CE dynamic MRA (TRICKS, **i**) clearly visualize a functioning part of aneurysm with irregular shape (*arrows*)

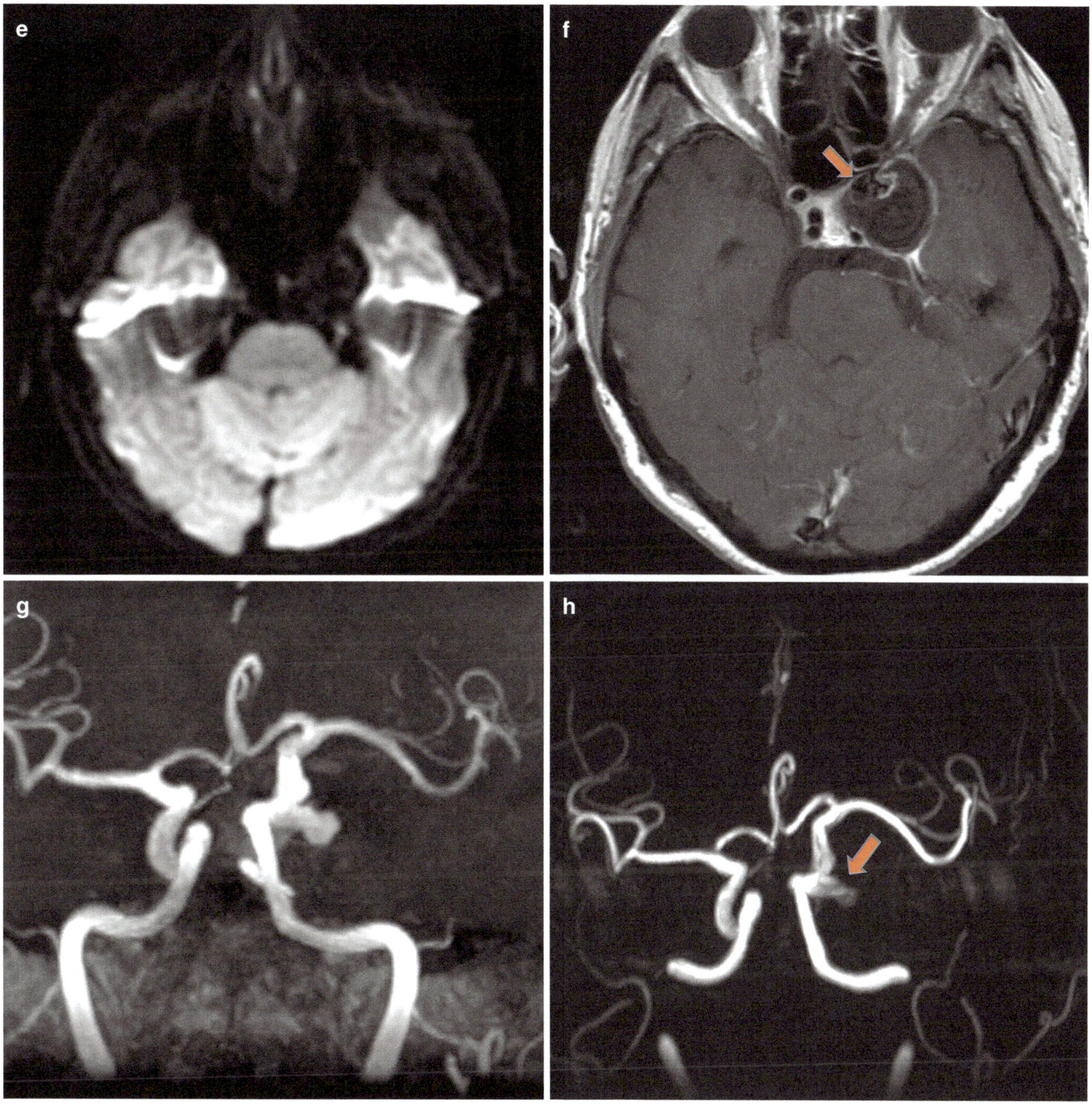

Fig. 19.9 (continued)

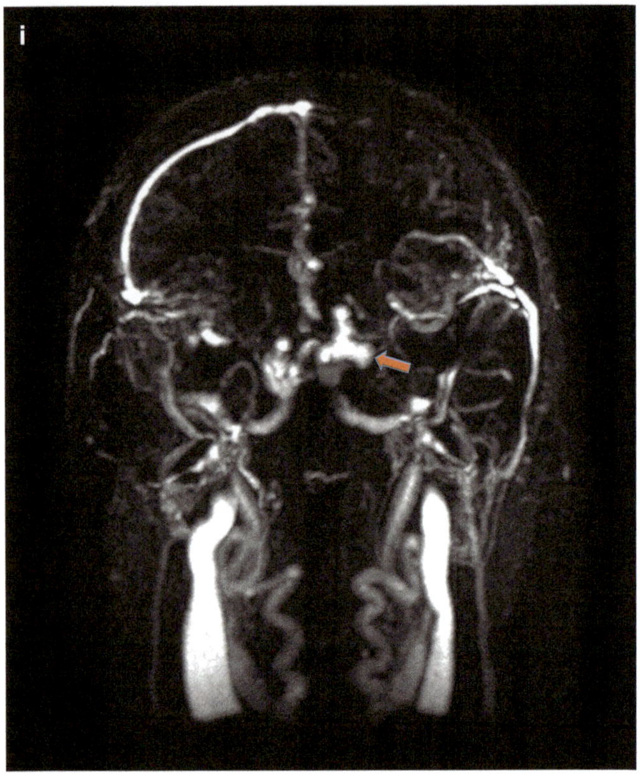

Fig. 19.9 (continued)

19.1 Kissing Carotid Siphons

Kissing carotid siphons (or proximity of siphons) of the carotid arteries is a rare abnormality of the parasellar region, which is characterized by medial displacement of siphons of the internal carotid arteries at the level of the cavernous sinuses with possible compression of adenohypophysis in the sella turcica cavity. Generally, these changes are symmetrical and asymptomatic. A very close proximity of the carotid siphons can cause a symmetrical deformation of the pituitary gland in the form of a lateral compression with predominance of the vertical dimension over the transverse one (Fig. 19.10). On sagittal MRI, it may resemble the sellar pituitary adenoma. This anatomic variant of the internal carotid arteries location should be taken into account when transnasal approach is planned in surgery of the sella turcica cavity to avoid injury to vascular walls.

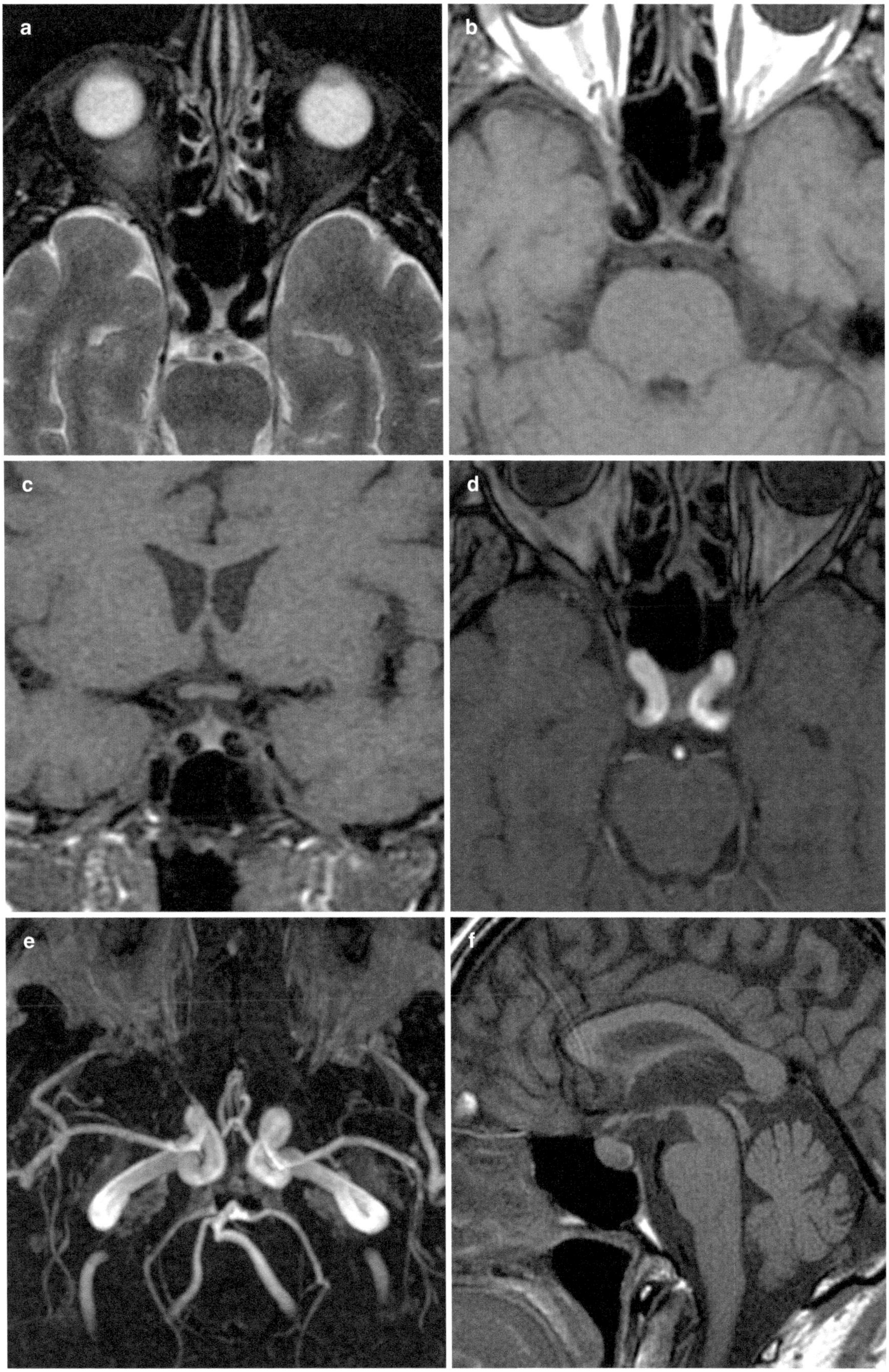

Fig. 19.10 "Kissing" carotid siphons. Axial T2-weighted (**a**), T1-weighted images (**b**, **c**), "raw" data of MRA (**d**), and 3D TOF MRA (**e**) show a very close proximity of the carotid siphons with pituitary gland compression. Sagittal T1 (**f**) reveals an enlargement of the vertical dimension of the adenohypophysis mimicking a sellar tumor in this projection

Presentation of Rare Cases of the Middle Cranial Fossa and Sellar Region Lesions

20

Contents

I. Pronin, V. Kornienko, *CT and MRI of Skull Base Lesions*, https://doi.org/10.1007/978-3-319-65957-2_20

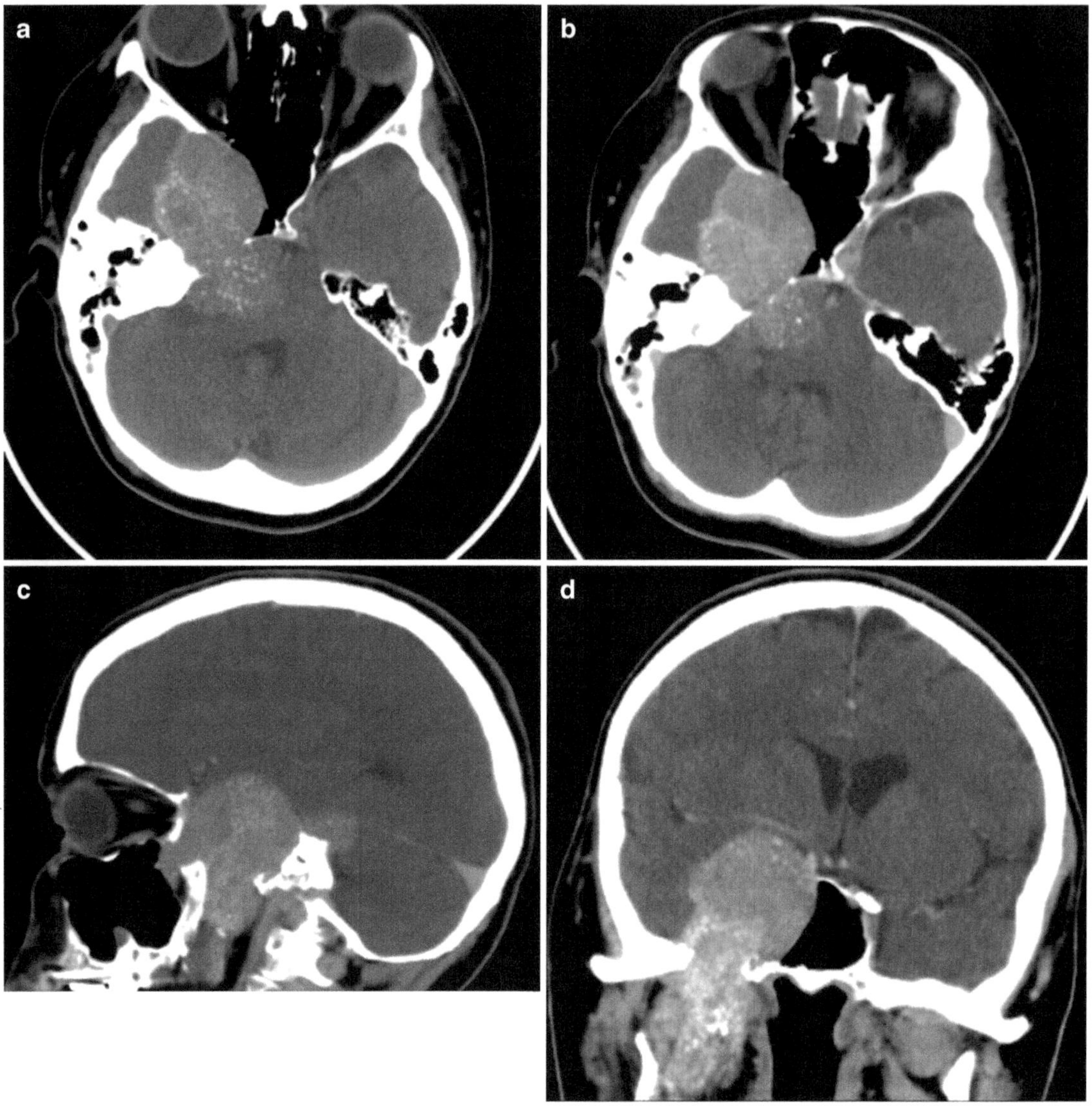

Fig. 20.1 Adenoid cystic cancer (cylindroma) of the right parotid gland. CT scans before (**a**) and after contrast enhancement (**b**–**d**) reveal a tumor with multiple calcifications and inhomogeneous enhancement in the middle cranial fossa. The tumor invades subtentorial and extracranial structures and causes bone destruction. CBF (**e**) is increased heterogeneously in the tumor. T2-weighted image (**f**), T1 (**g**) and post-contrast T1-weighted images (**h**, **i**) show a hypointense on T2-weighted image tumor with multiple microhemorrhages (**i**) and moderate contrast enhancement

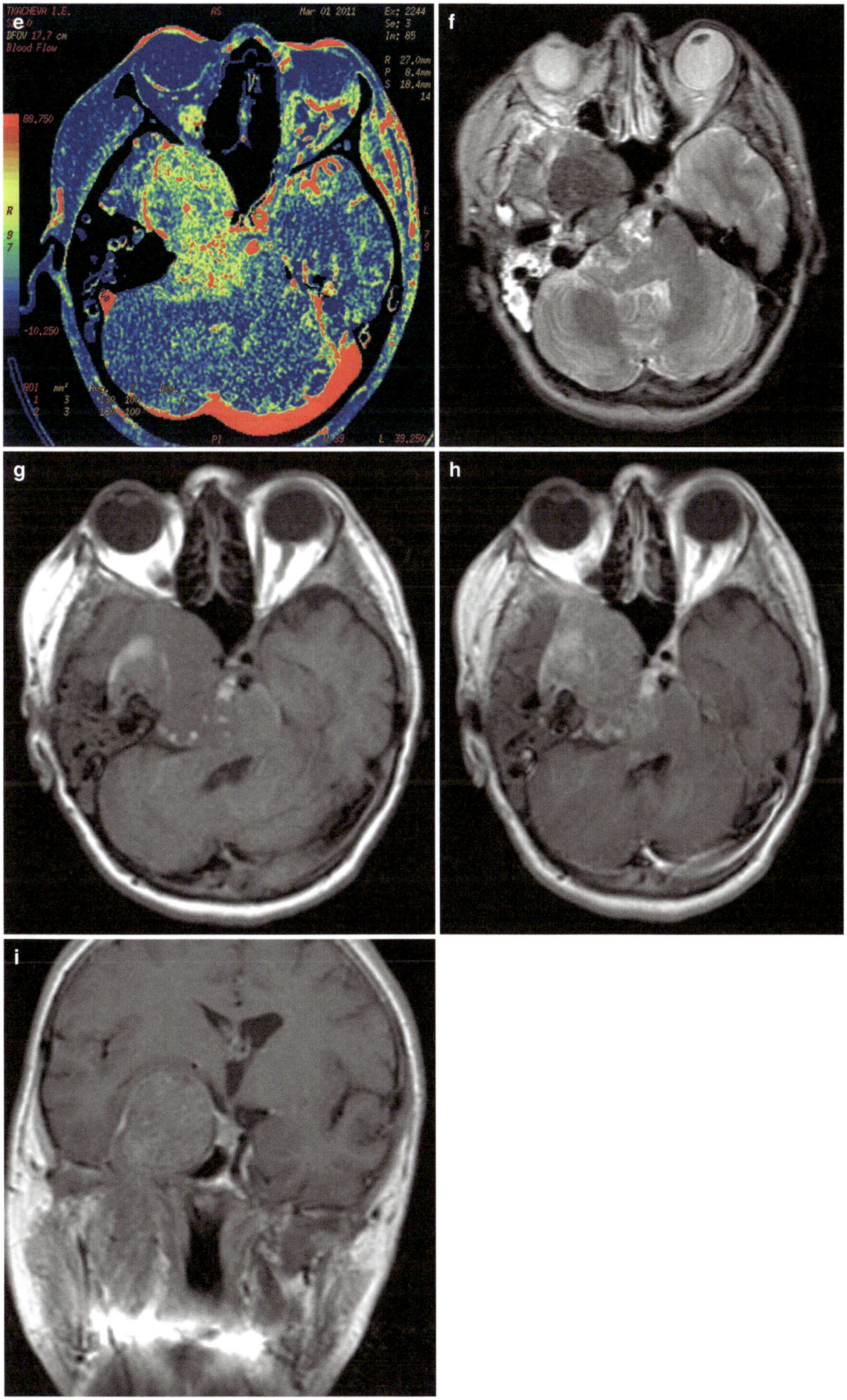

Fig. 20.1 (continued)

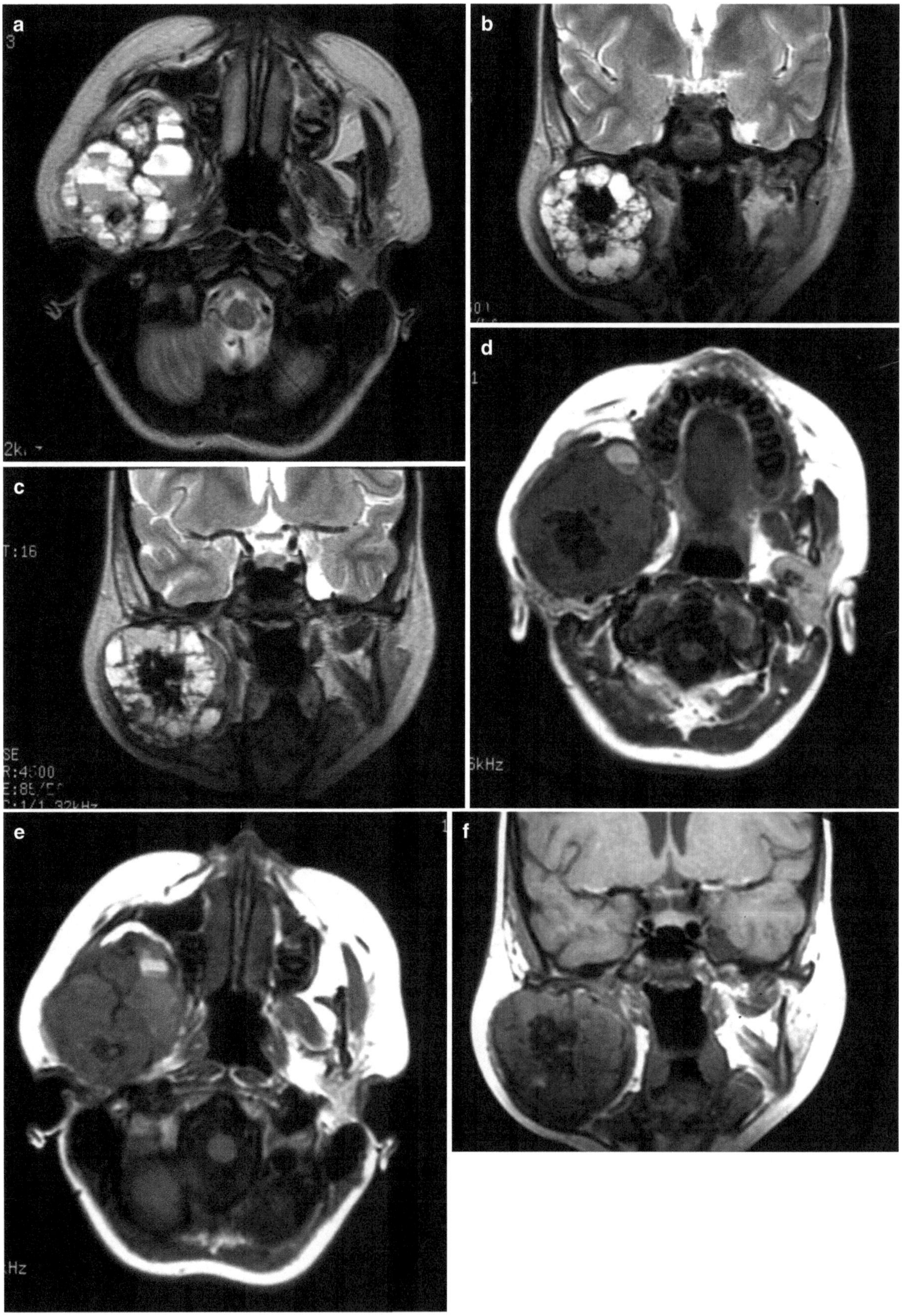

Fig. 20.2 Osteosarcoma in a 11-year-old child. T2- (**a**–**c**) and T1-weighted images (**d**–**f**) show a heterogeneous tumor in the right infratemporal fossa, which consists of many cystic cavities with fluid–fluid level. Soft tissue component of the tumor has hypointense signal on T2-weighted images and isointense on T1-weighted images

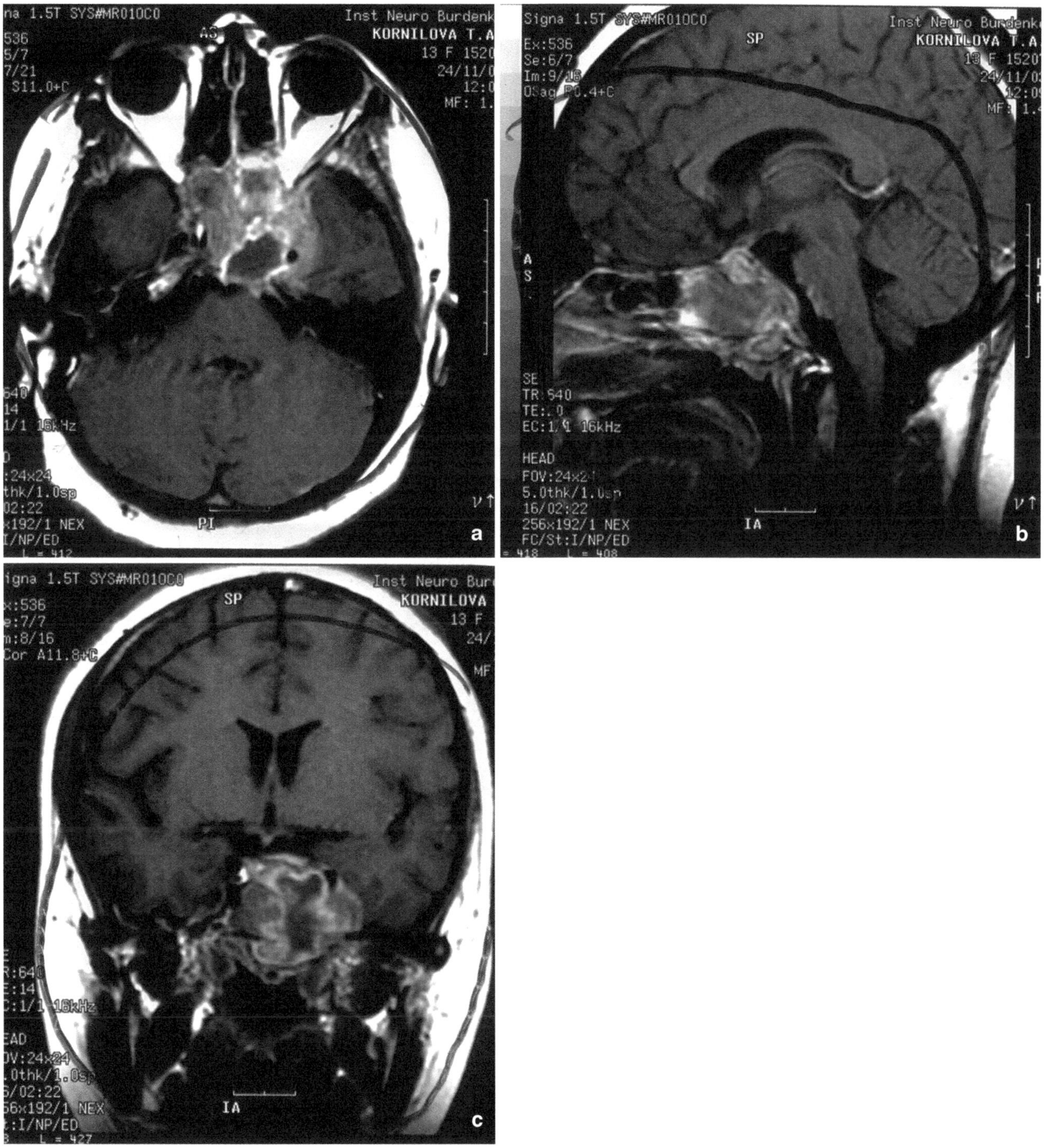

Fig. 20.3 Ewing sarcoma in a 13-year-old child. Post-contrast T1-weighted images (**a**–**c**) reveal a heterogeneously enhancing tumor in the sphenoid bone. The tumor spreads into the medial parts of left middle cranial fossa and into the ethmoid bone. Pituitary gland is shifted upwards and deformed. The tumor invades into the left cavernous sinus and do not compress a lumen of the carotid artery

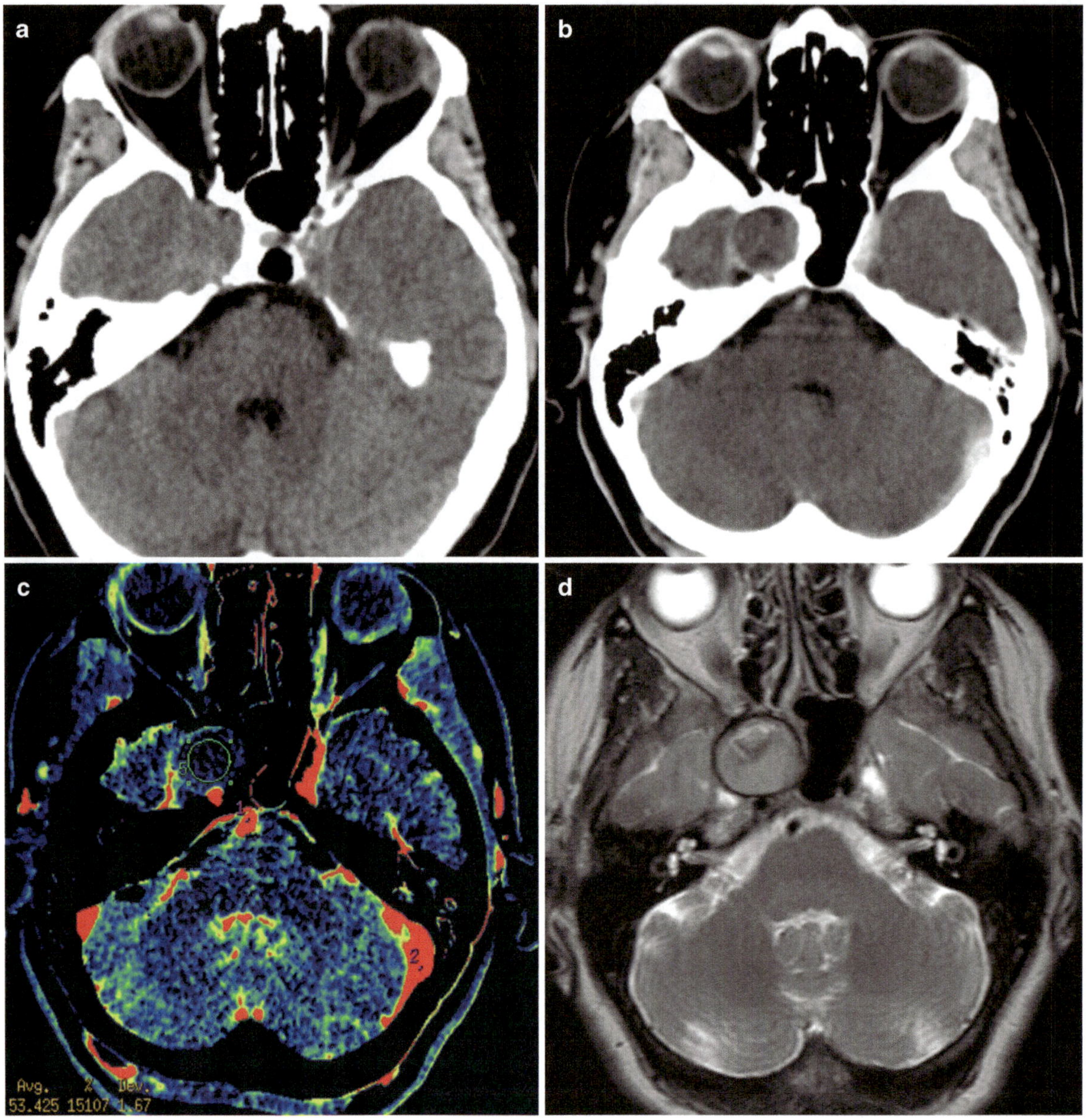

Fig. 20.4 Xanthogranuloma of the right cavernous sinus. CT scans before (**a**) and after contrast enhancement (**b**) show a rounded mass in the right cavernous sinus. Contrast enhancement is visualized in the lateral part of cavernous sinus. There are no areas of increased blood flow in the lesion (CBF–**c**). T2 (**d**), T2-FLAIR (**e**), and T1 (**f**) demonstrate a heterogeneous hyperintense lesion. DWI (**g**) shows a decreased signal. Post-contrast T1-weighted images (**h**, **i**) did not reveal an enhancement in the lesion

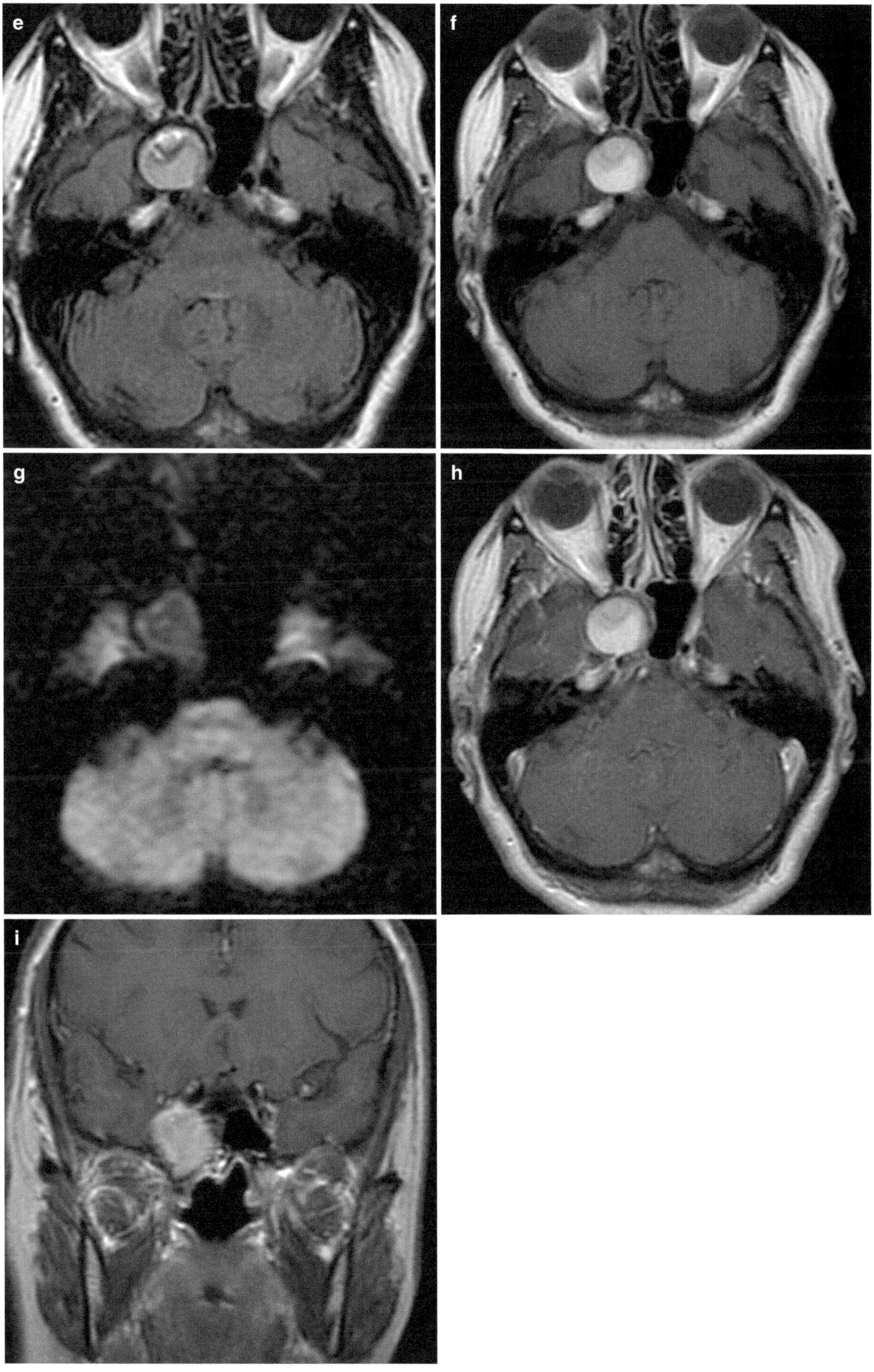

Fig. 20.4 (continued)

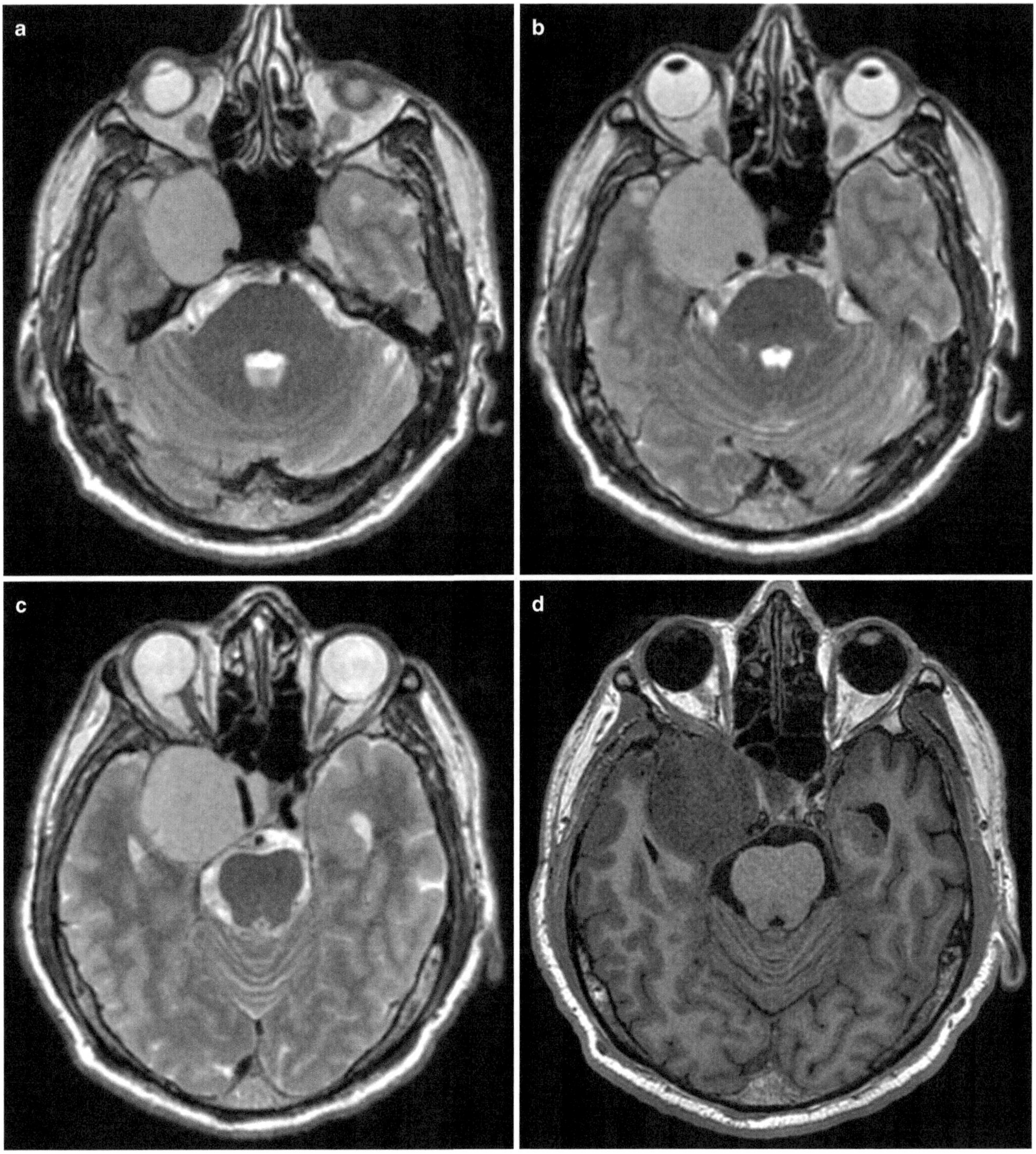

Fig. 20.5 Cavernous hemangioma. T2-weighted images (**a**–**c**), T1-weighted image (**d**) and post-contrast T1-weighted images (**e**, **f**) show a homogeneous tumor in the medial part of middle cranial fossa, which is hyperintense on T2 and hypointense on T1. The tumor homogeneously and intensely enhances. The tumor spreads into the sella turcica and compresses an adenohypophysis. Right internal carotid artery is included into the tumor, but its lumen is not compressed

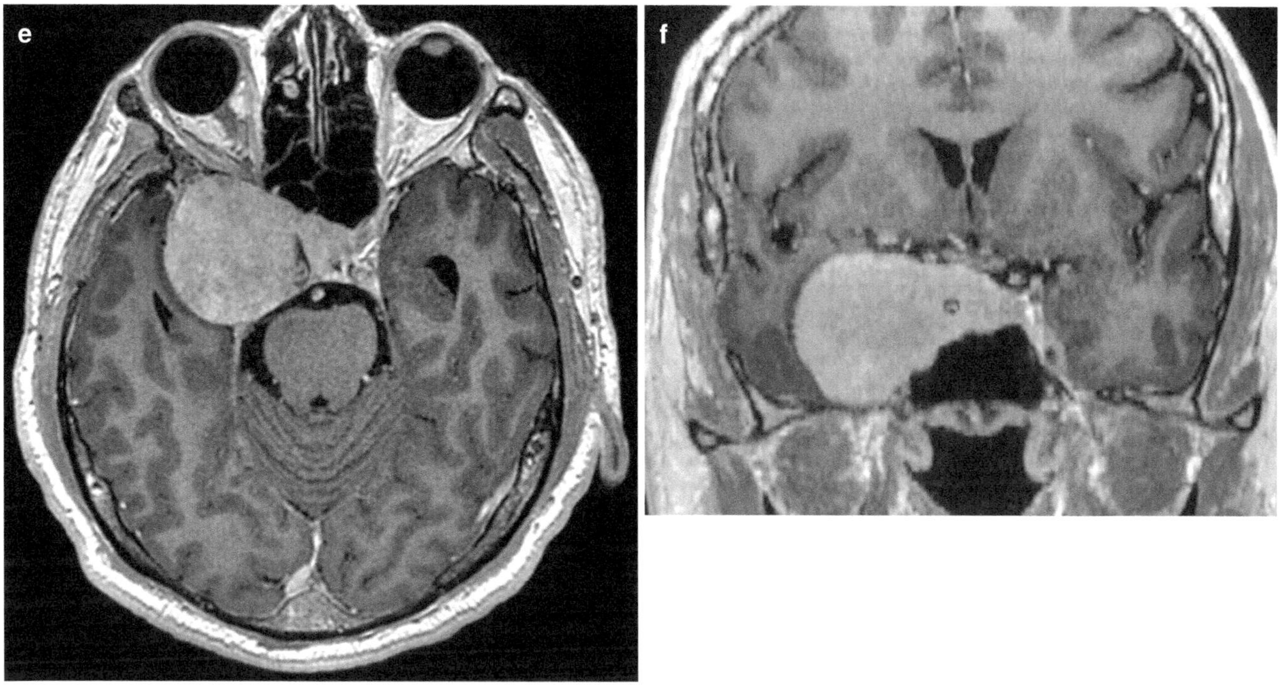

Fig. 20.5 (continued)

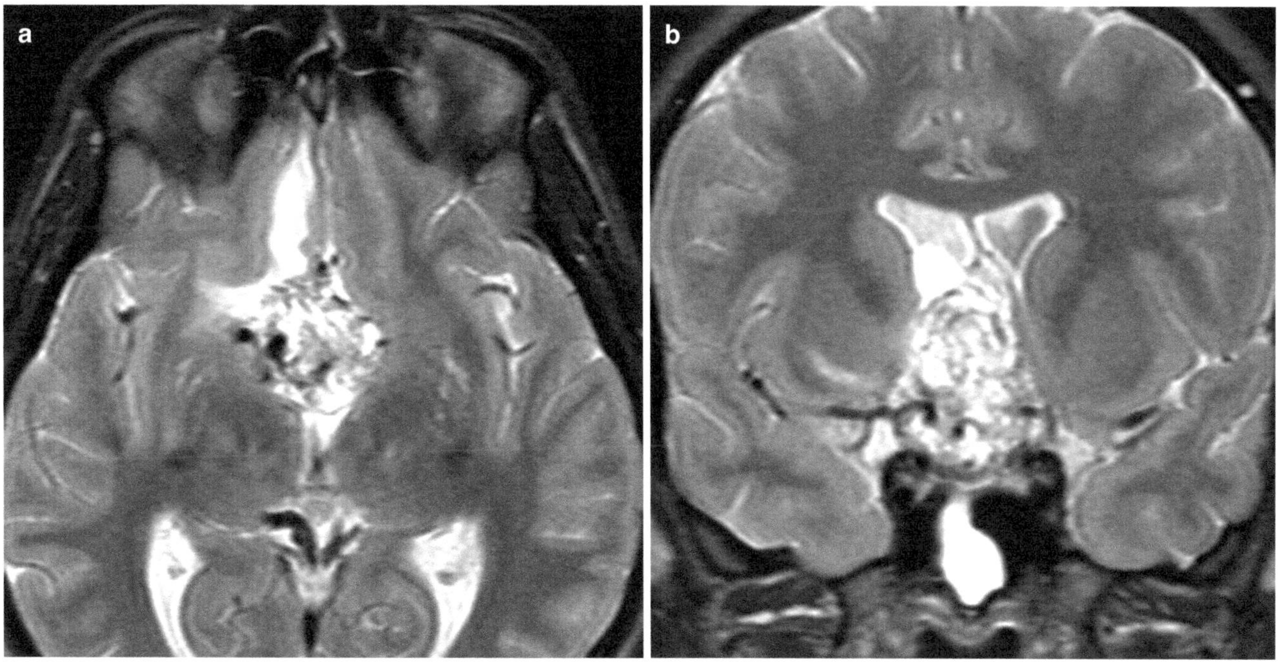

Fig. 20.6 Hemangioblastoma. T2-weighted images (**a**, **b**), T1- (**c**, **d**), and post-contrast T1-weighted images (**e**, **f**) show a heterogeneous suprasellar tumor with prominent flow voids due to large vessels signal. The tumor intensely enhances

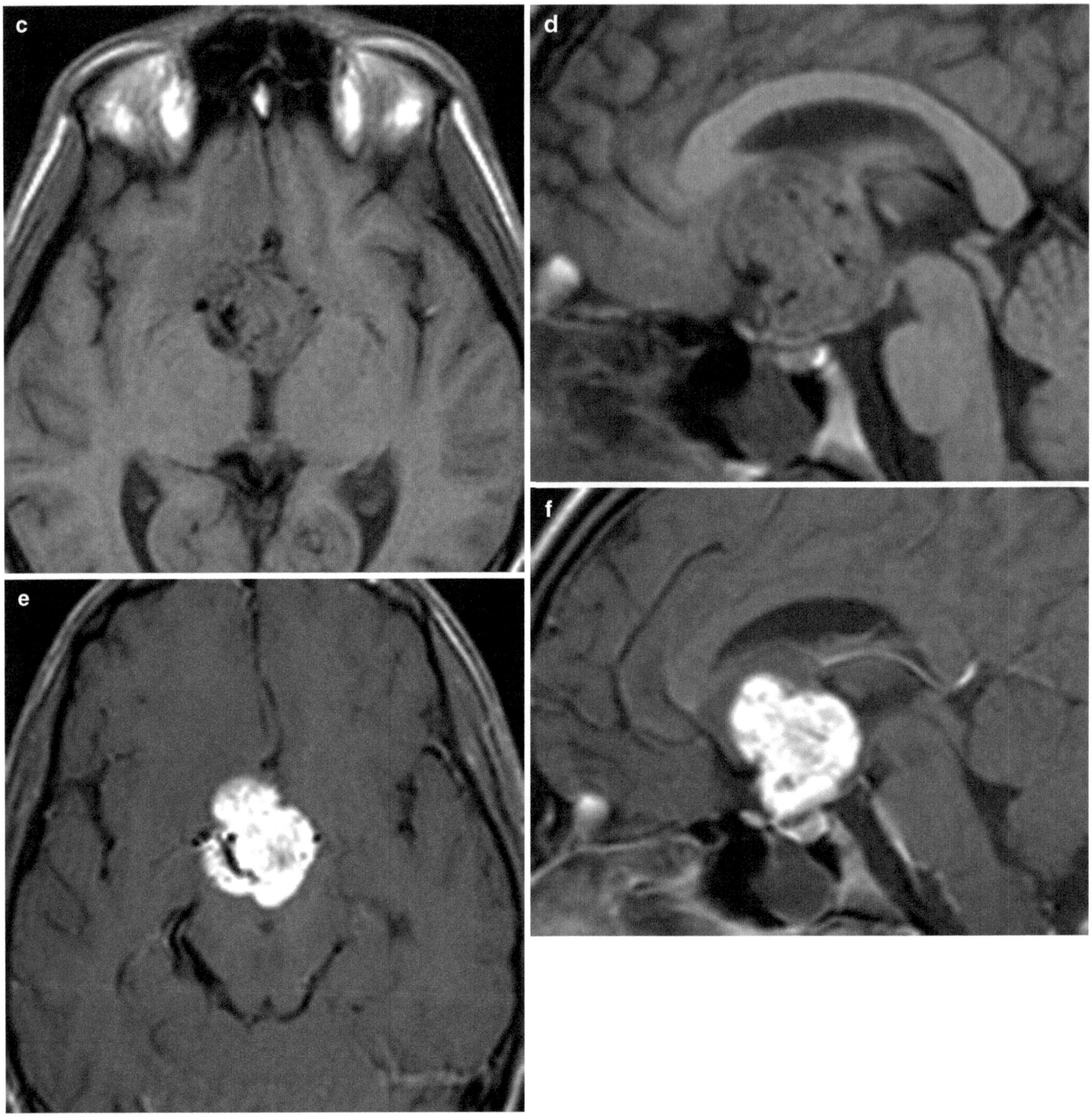

Fig. 20.6 (continued)

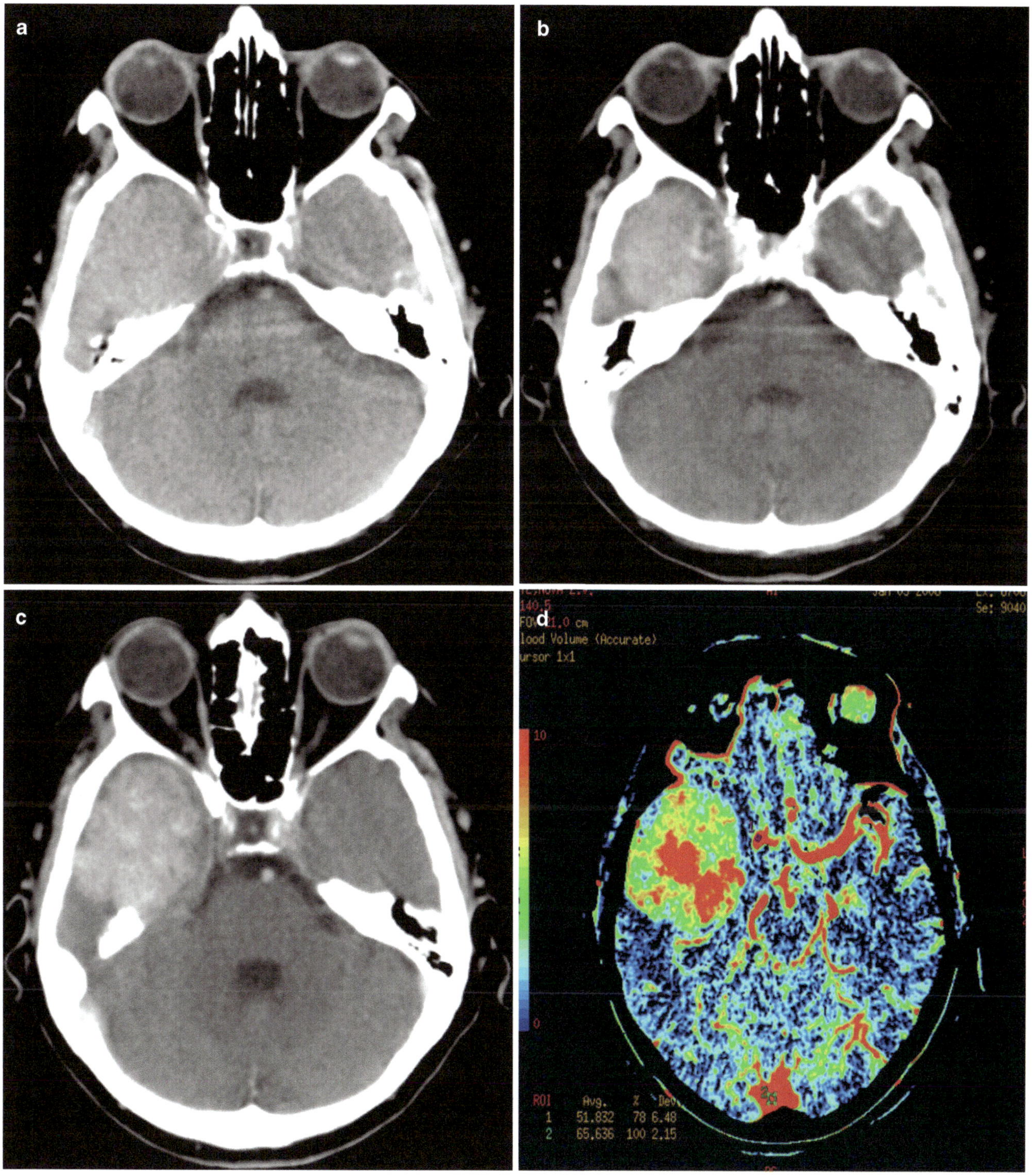

Fig. 20.7 Solitary fibrous tumor (hemangiopericytoma). CT scans before (**a**) and after (**b**, **c**) contrast enhancement show a large enhancing tumor in the middle cranial fossa. Perfusion CT reveals the high blood volume (**d**) and blood flow values in the tumor. The tumor is supplied by the middle meningeal artery and by branches of the middle cerebral artery (DSA, **e**, **f**)

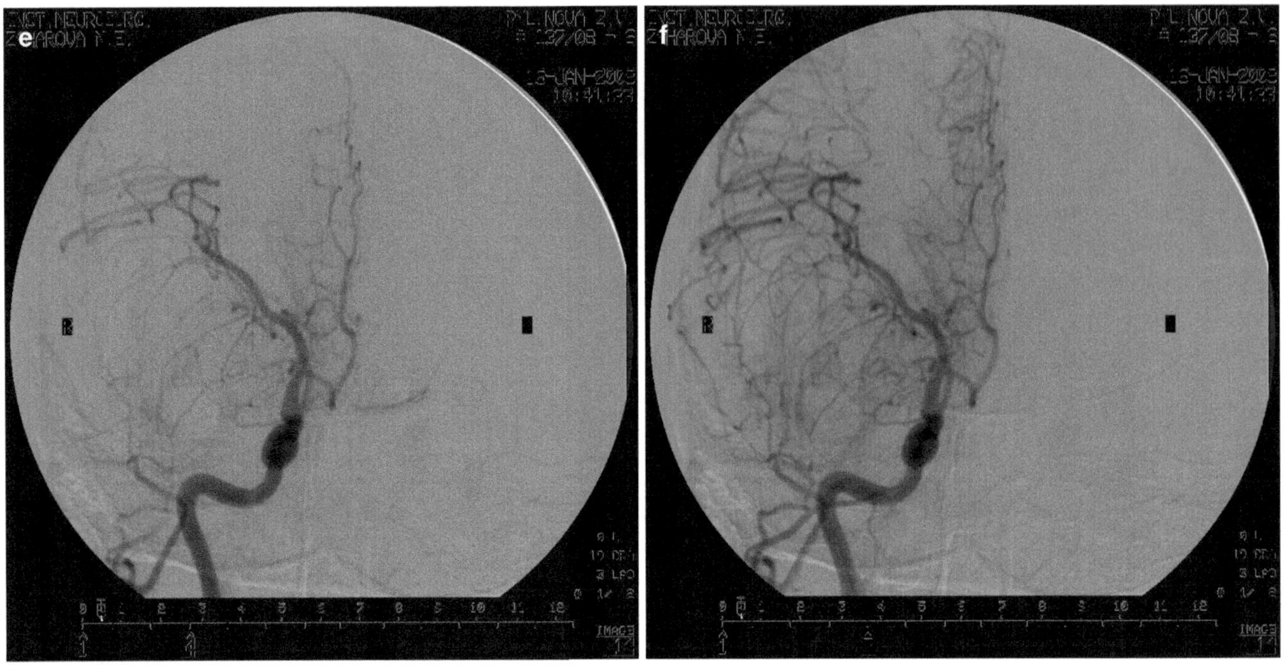

Fig. 20.7 (continued)

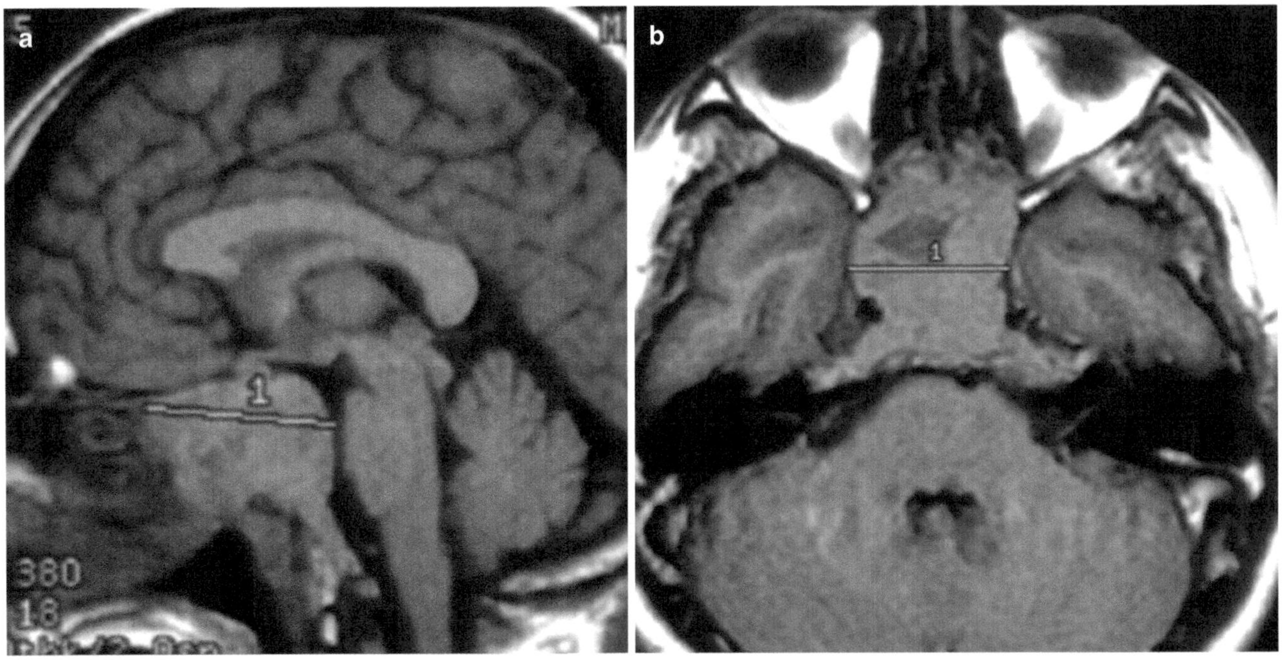

Fig. 20.8 Plasmacytoma of the skull base. T1-weighted (**a**, **b**) and post-contrast T1-weighted images (c, **d**) demonstrate a homogeneous enhancing tumor in the sphenoid bone

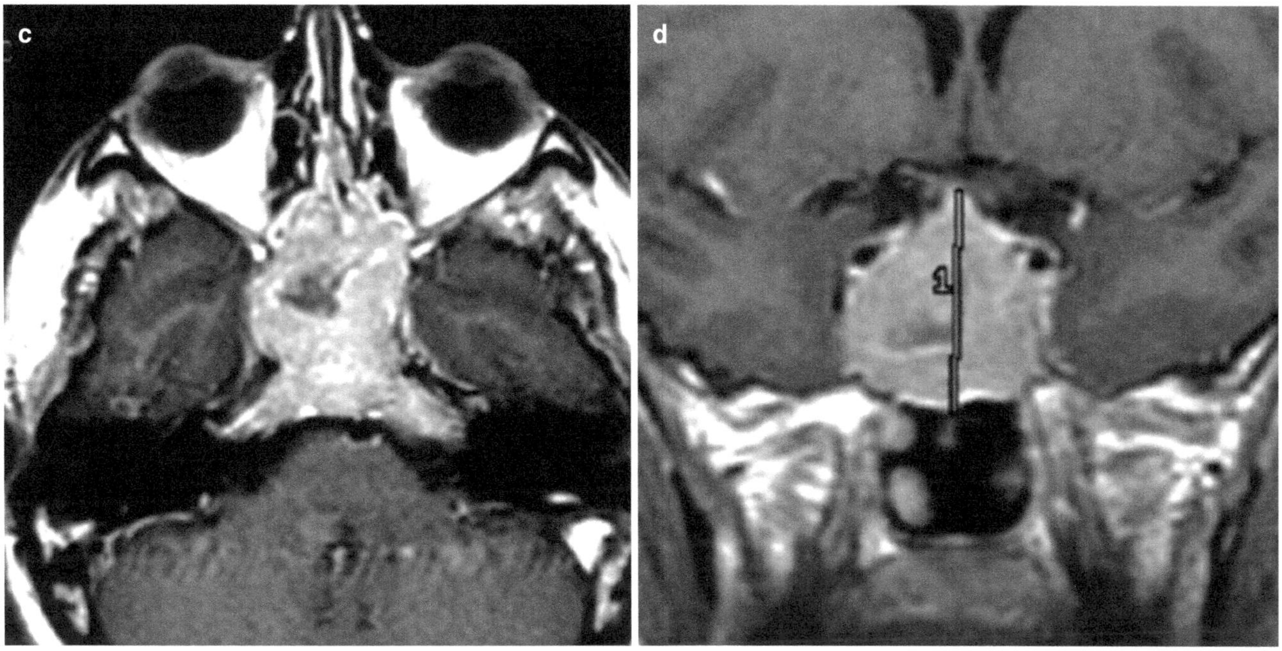

Fig. 20.8 (continued)

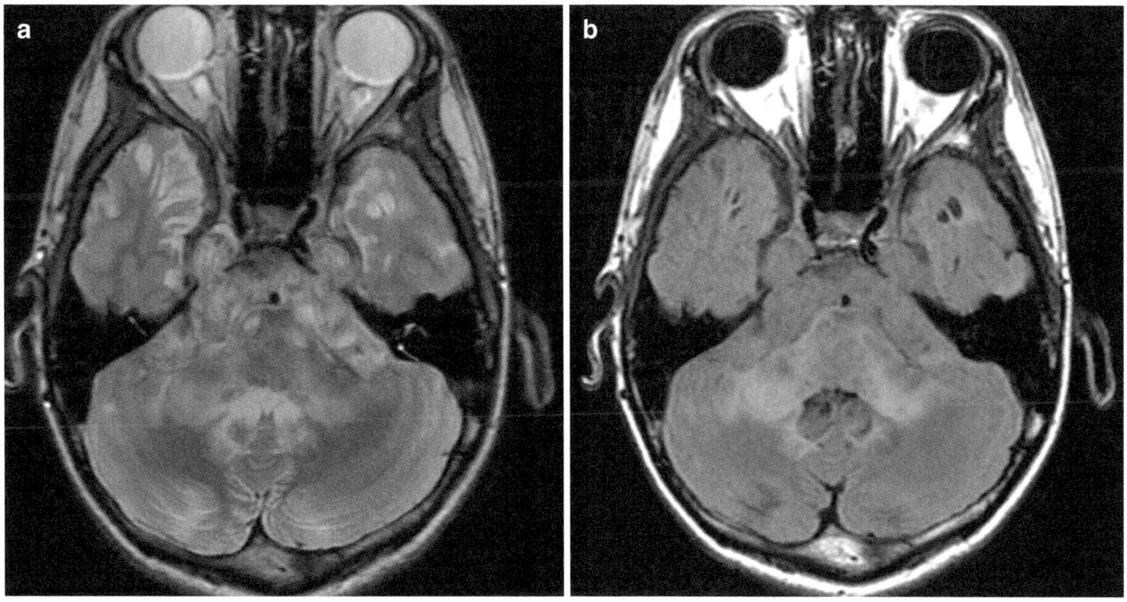

Fig. 20.9 Intracranial subarachnoid fibrosarcoma. T2-weighted image (**a**), T2-FLAIR (**b**), T1-weighted (**c**), and post-contrast T1-weighted images (**d–f**) show an extensive diffuse dural-based intensively enhancing mass in the basal cisterns, over the brainstem and over the right cerebral hemisphere. Contrast enhancement is also marked on CT (**g**). Perfusion study demonstrates a moderately increased blood flow (CBF–**i**) and low blood volume (CBV) in the tumor

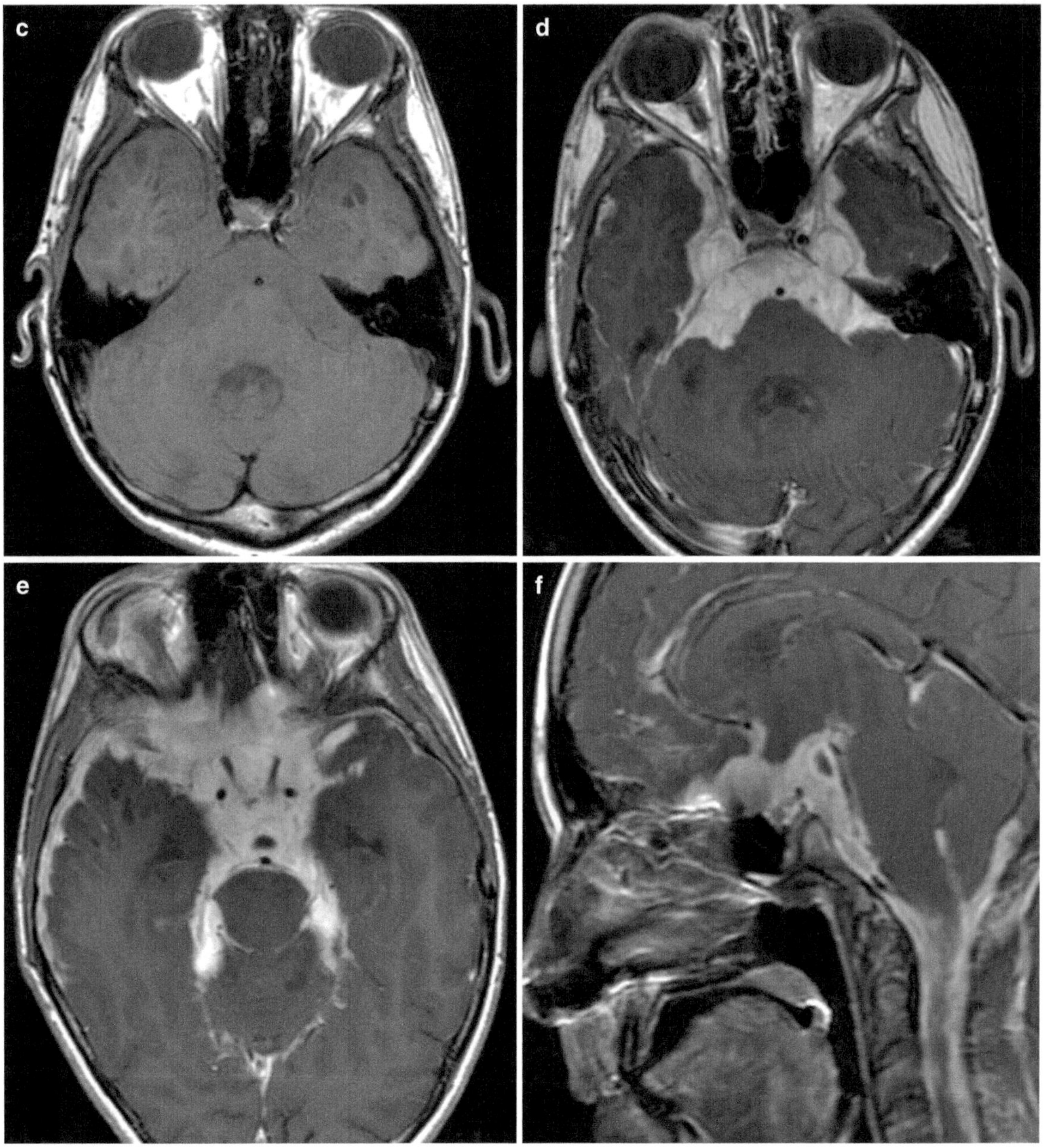

Fig. 20.9 (continued)

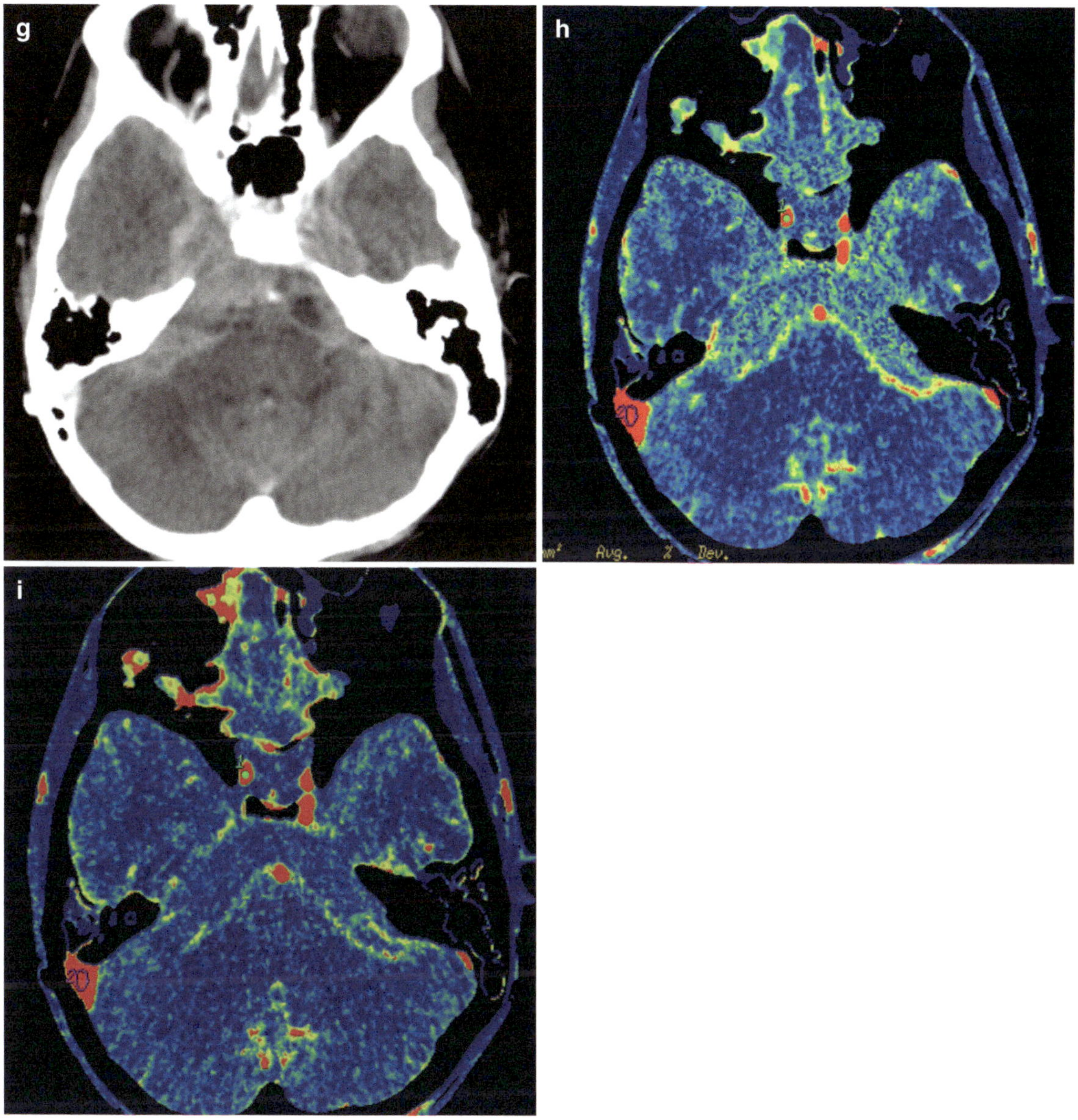

Fig. 20.9 (continued)

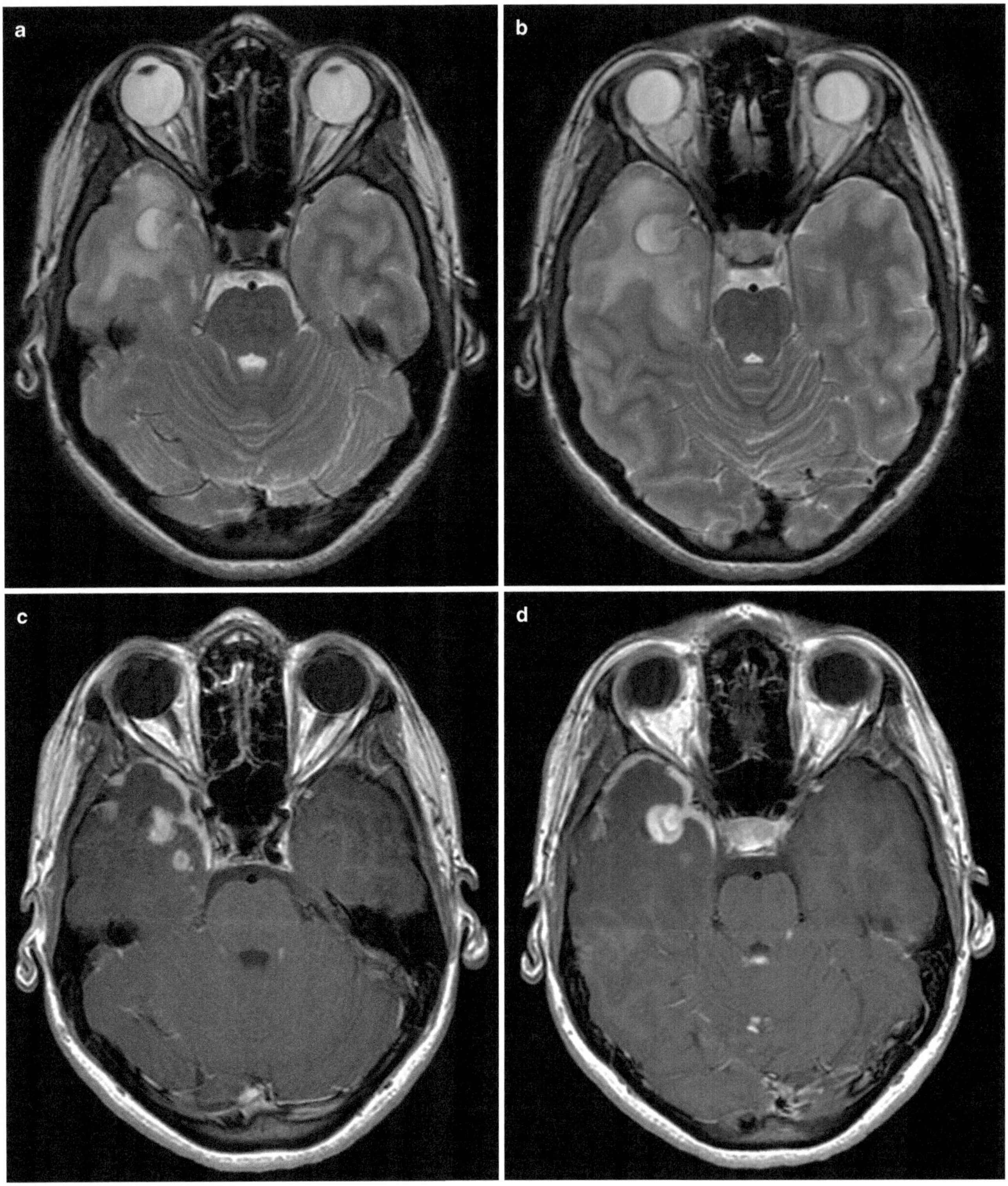

Fig. 20.10 Pilocytic astrocytoma of the right temporal region. T2-weighted images (**a**, **b**) and post-contrast T1-weighted images (**c**–**f**) show an extended intensively enhancing mass in the right temporal lobe which is involving the subarachnoid convexital spaces and chiasmal cisterns. T1 + fat sat (**e**, **f**) is better for imaging of the infiltrative lesion spreading

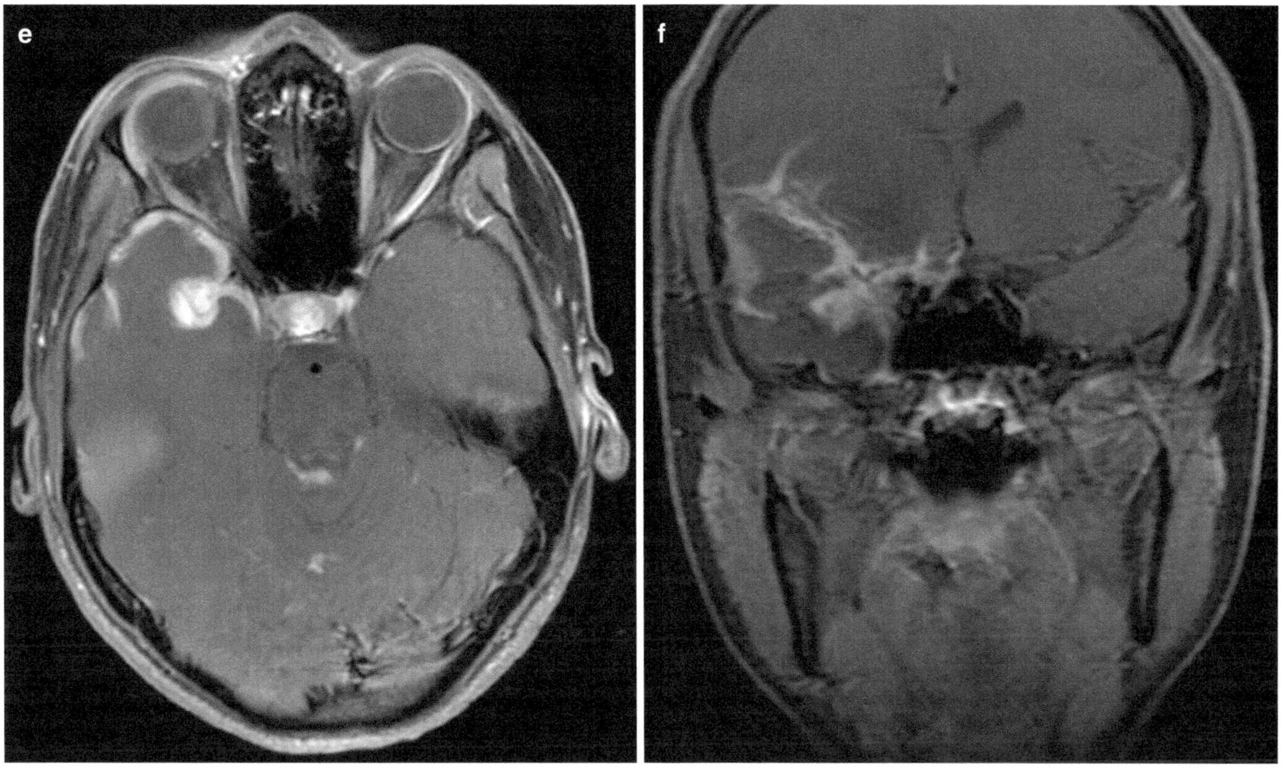

Fig. 20.10 (continued)

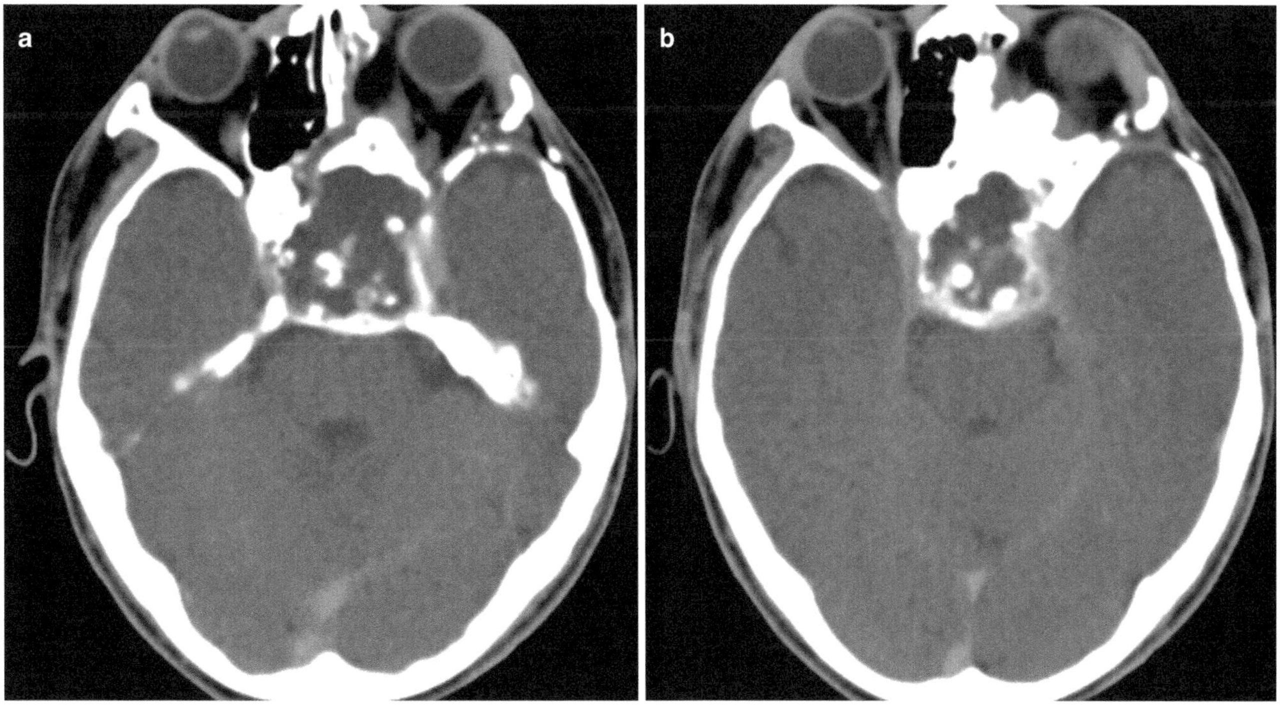

Fig. 20.11 Ossifying fibroma of the skull base. Axial (**a**, **b**) and coronal (**c**–**f**) CT scans demonstrate a large heterogeneous tumor of the sphenoid bone with the lytic center and a hyperdense rim. There are calcifications in the central part of the tumor. The extent of the bone changes of the skull base is better visualized in "bone window" mode

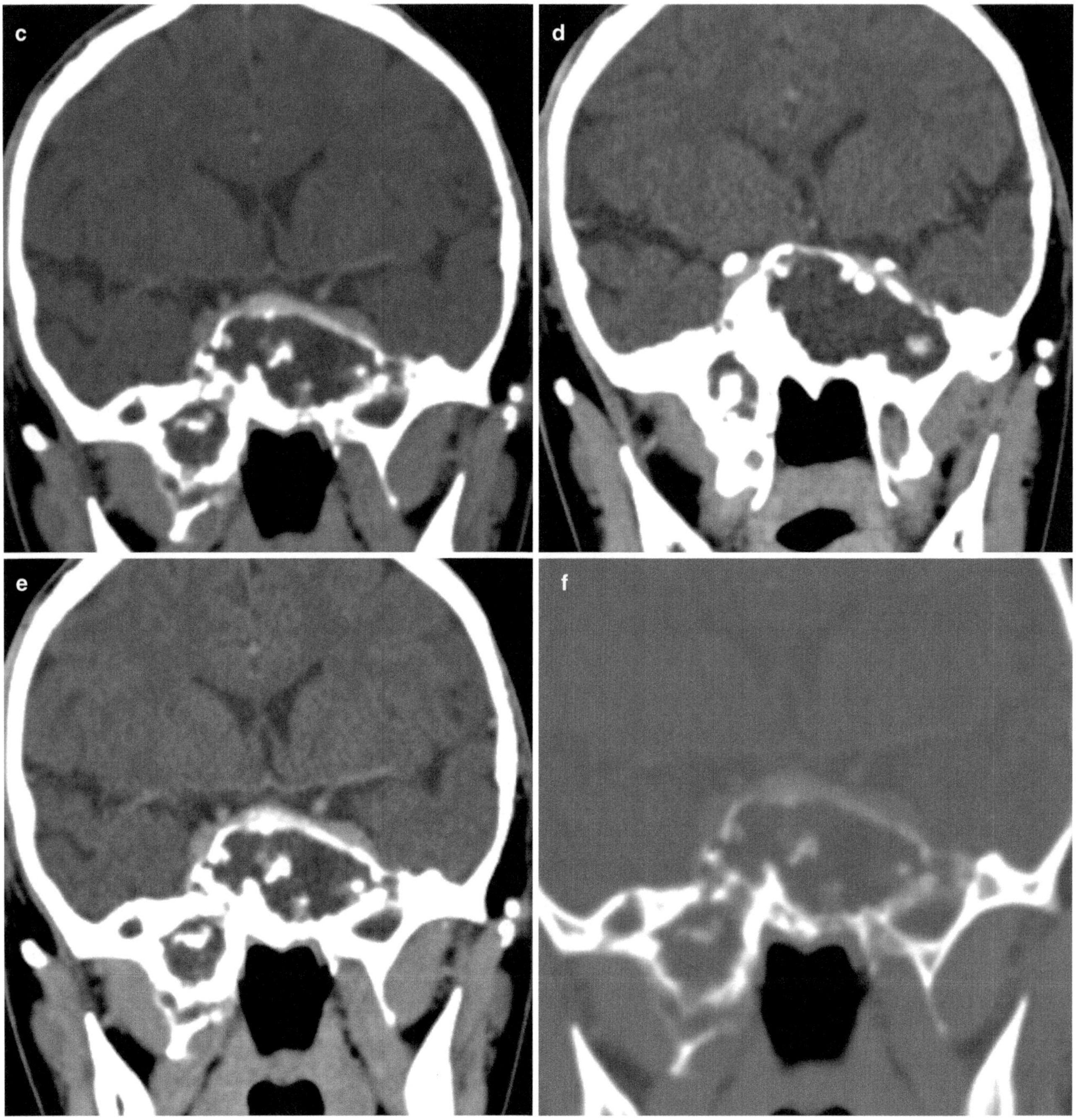

Fig. 20.11 (continued)

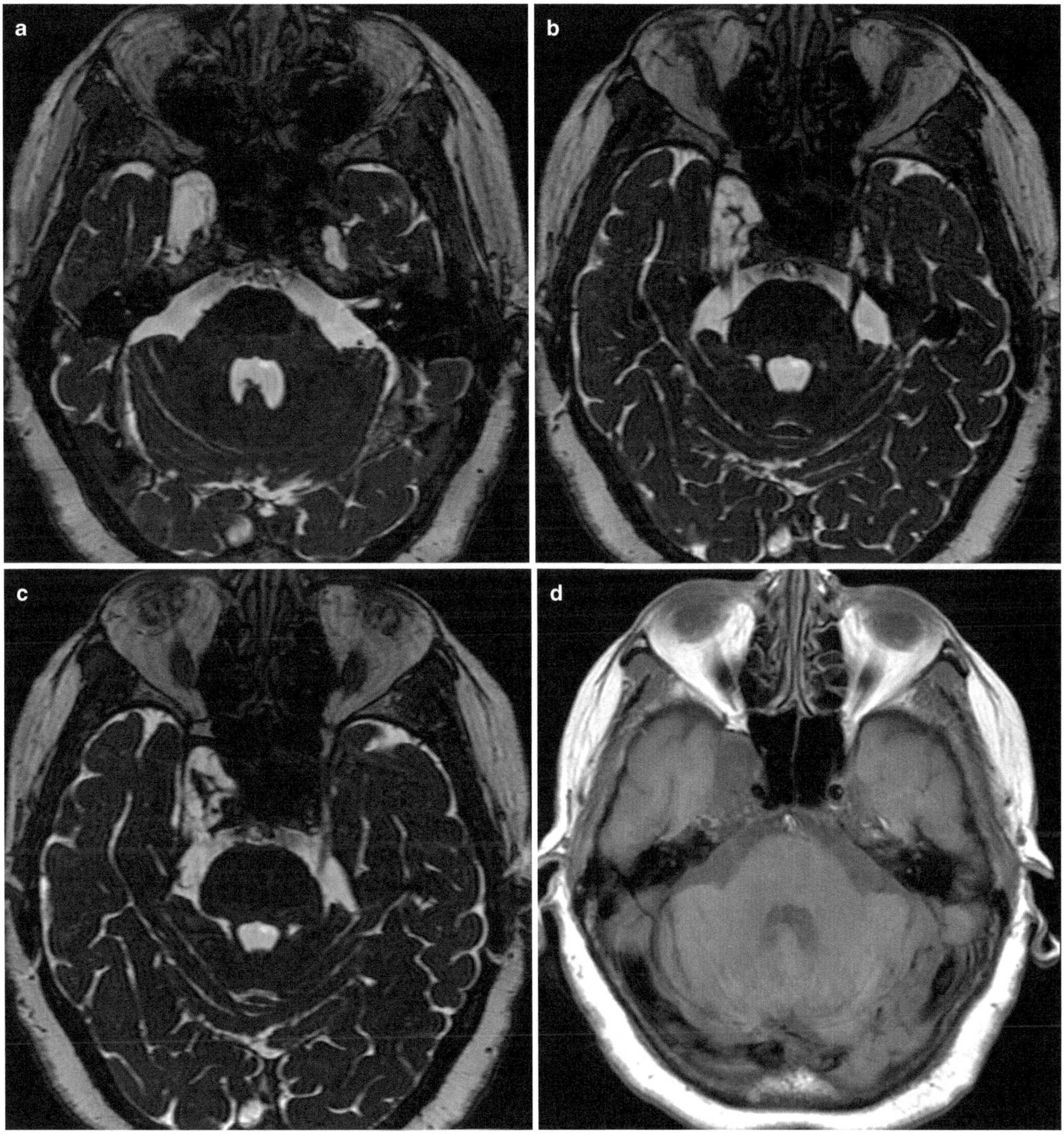

Fig. 20.12 Meningocele of the cavernous sinus. T2 (FIESTA) (**a–c**), T1-weighted image (**d**) and post-contrast T1-weighted images (**e–h**) show a CSF-like cystic lesion with the internal connective tissue septa in the right cavernous sinus. The cavernous sinus is expanded. The defect of the dura (*arrows*) is visualized in the area of the entrance of the trigeminal nerve into trigeminal cave. Post-contrast T1-weighted images demonstrate an enhancement in the compressed right cavernous sinus, which is defined the margins of meningocele. T1-weighted image (**h**) and FIESTA (**i**) supplement with information about a defect of dura and lesion size

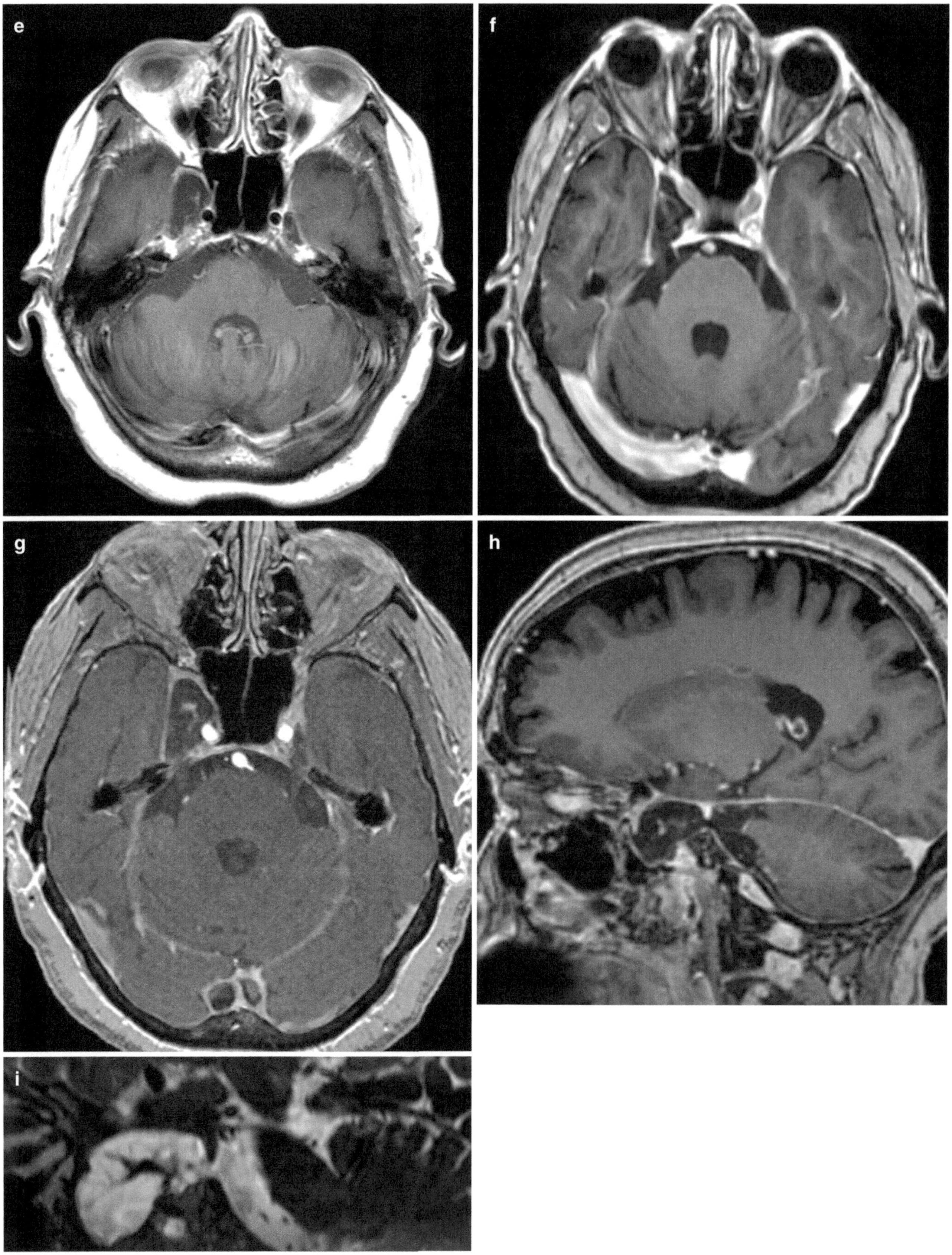

Fig. 20.12 (continued)

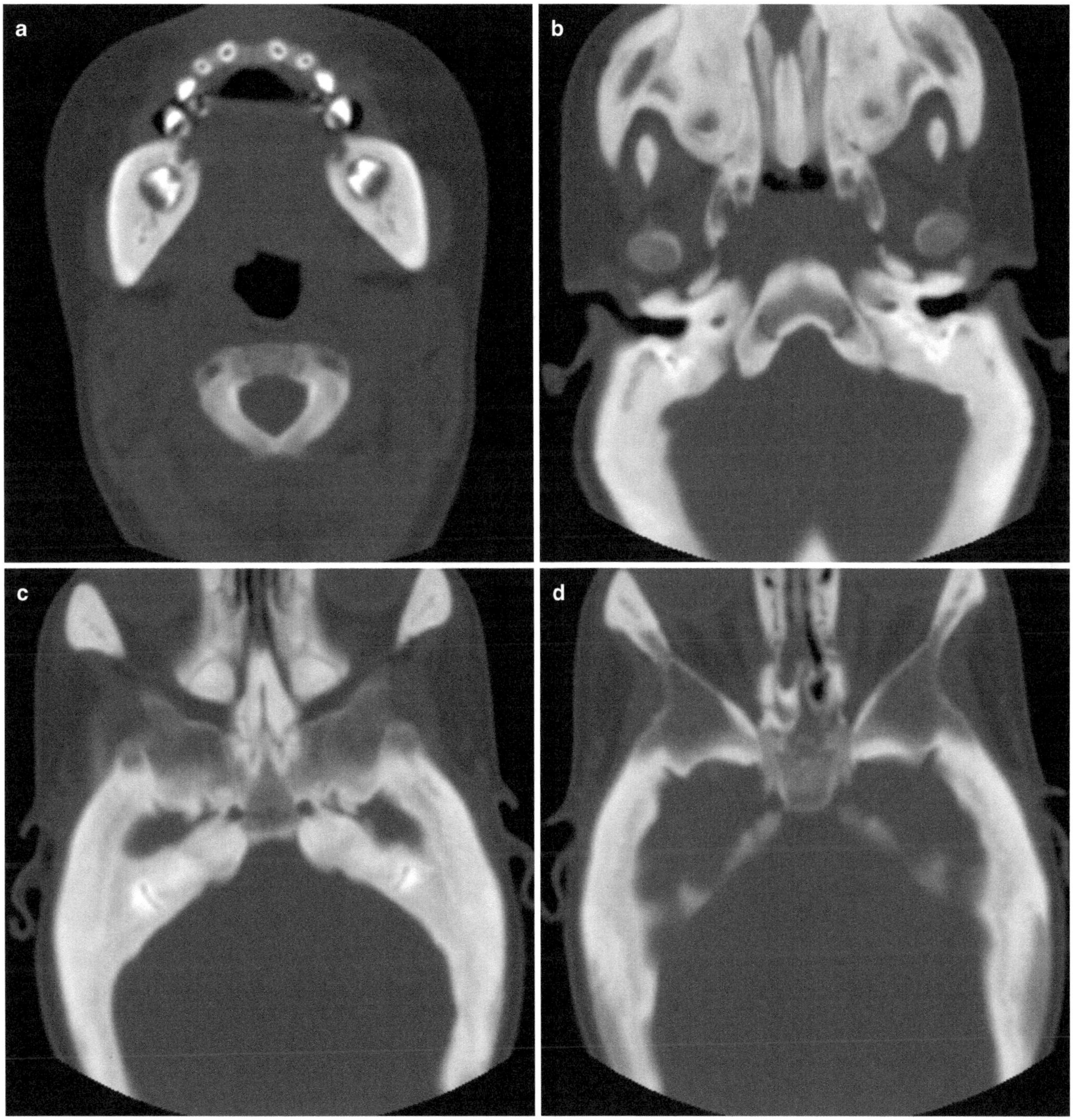

Fig. 20.13 Craniometaphyseal dysplasia (Pyle disease), a 2.5-year-old child. Axial CT scans (**a**–**d**) show a diffuse thickened calvaria, facial and skull base bones, dolichocephalic deformation of the skull vault. The floor of the cranial cavity is smoothed; cranial canals and foramina are narrowed. The differentiation between the diploe and cortical bone is absent. T2-weighted images (**e**, **f**) and T1-weighted images (**g**–**i**) show the deformation of the skull and brain. The bones of the cranial vault and base are hypointense on MRI. The diagnosis was confirmed by genetic analysis and detection of changes in the metaphysis of the long tubular bones

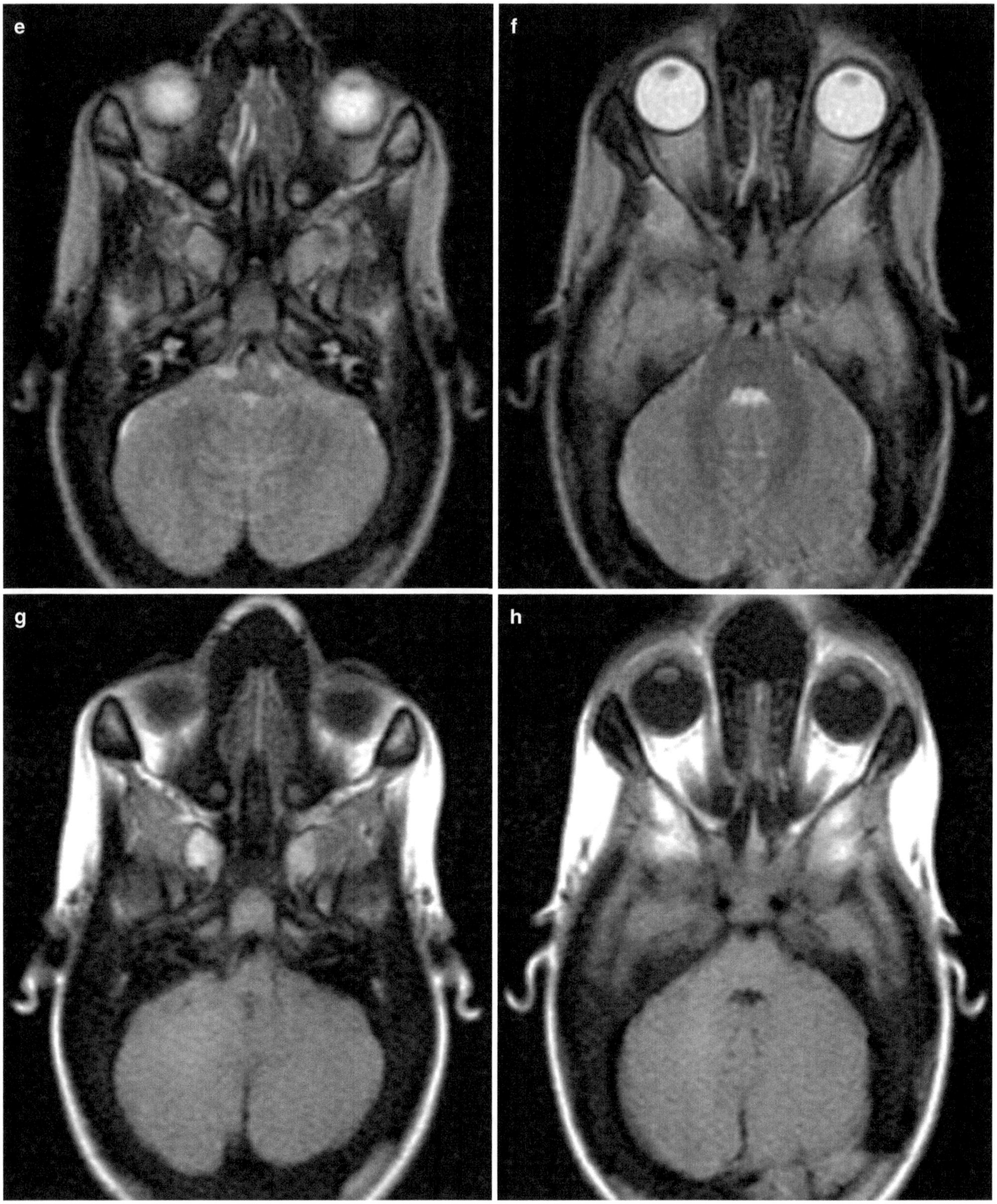

Fig. 20.13 (continued)

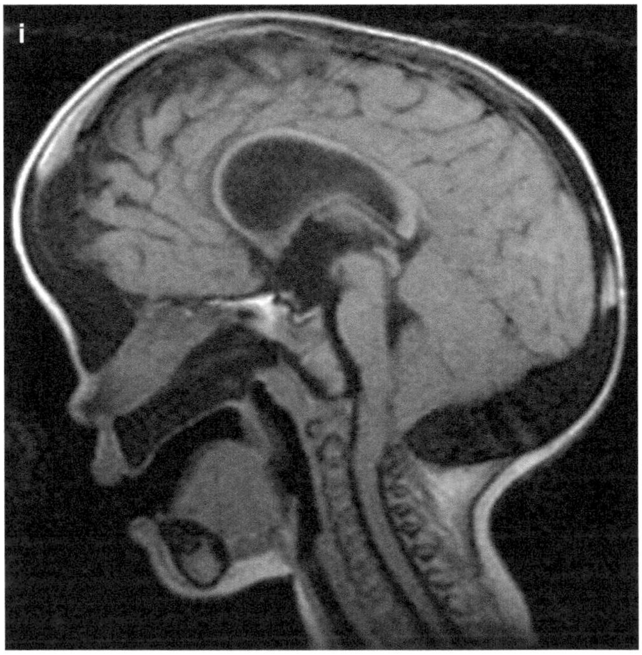

Fig. 20.13 (continued)

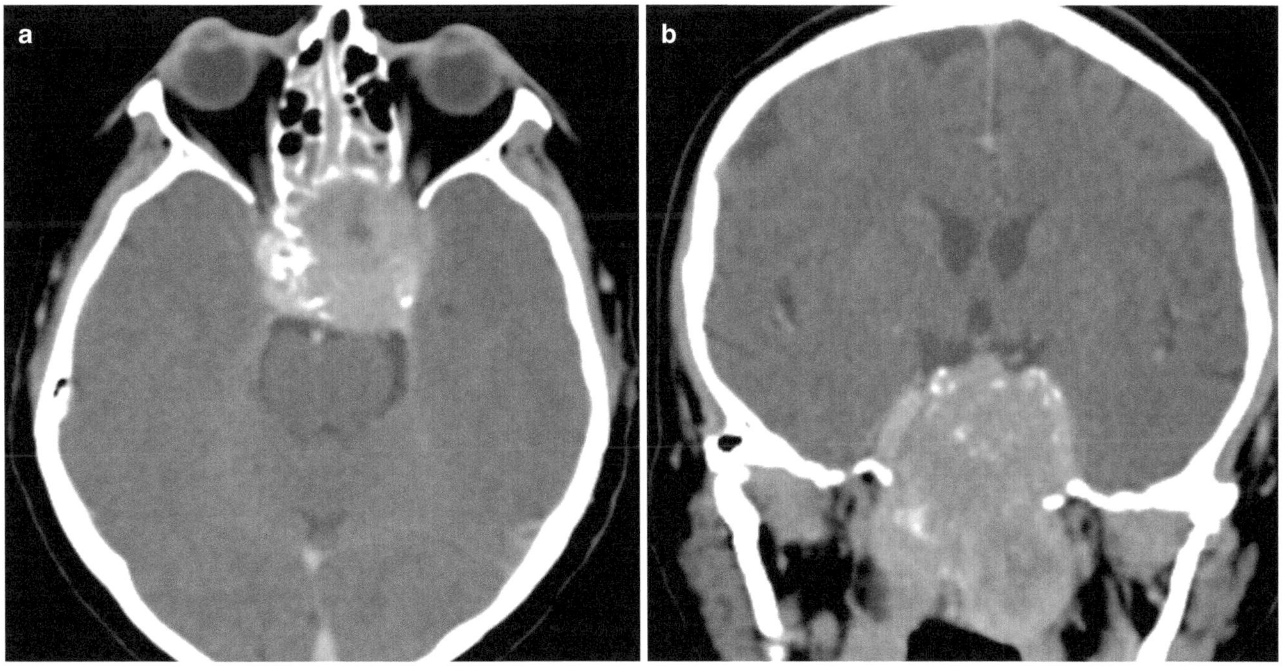

Fig. 20.14 Aspergillosis of the sphenoid sinus. CECT scans (**a**–**c**) detect a large intensively enhancing lesion, which almost completely destroys the sphenoid bone and extended into the nasopharynx. T1- (**d**) and T2-weighted images (**e**, **f**) reveal a moderate hyperintensity on T1 and hypointensity on T2. In the anterior part of the lesion there is a small postsurgical cavity. A diffuse enhancement on T1-weighted images (**g**, **h**) is as prominent, as on CT. Histopathologic specimen (**i**)

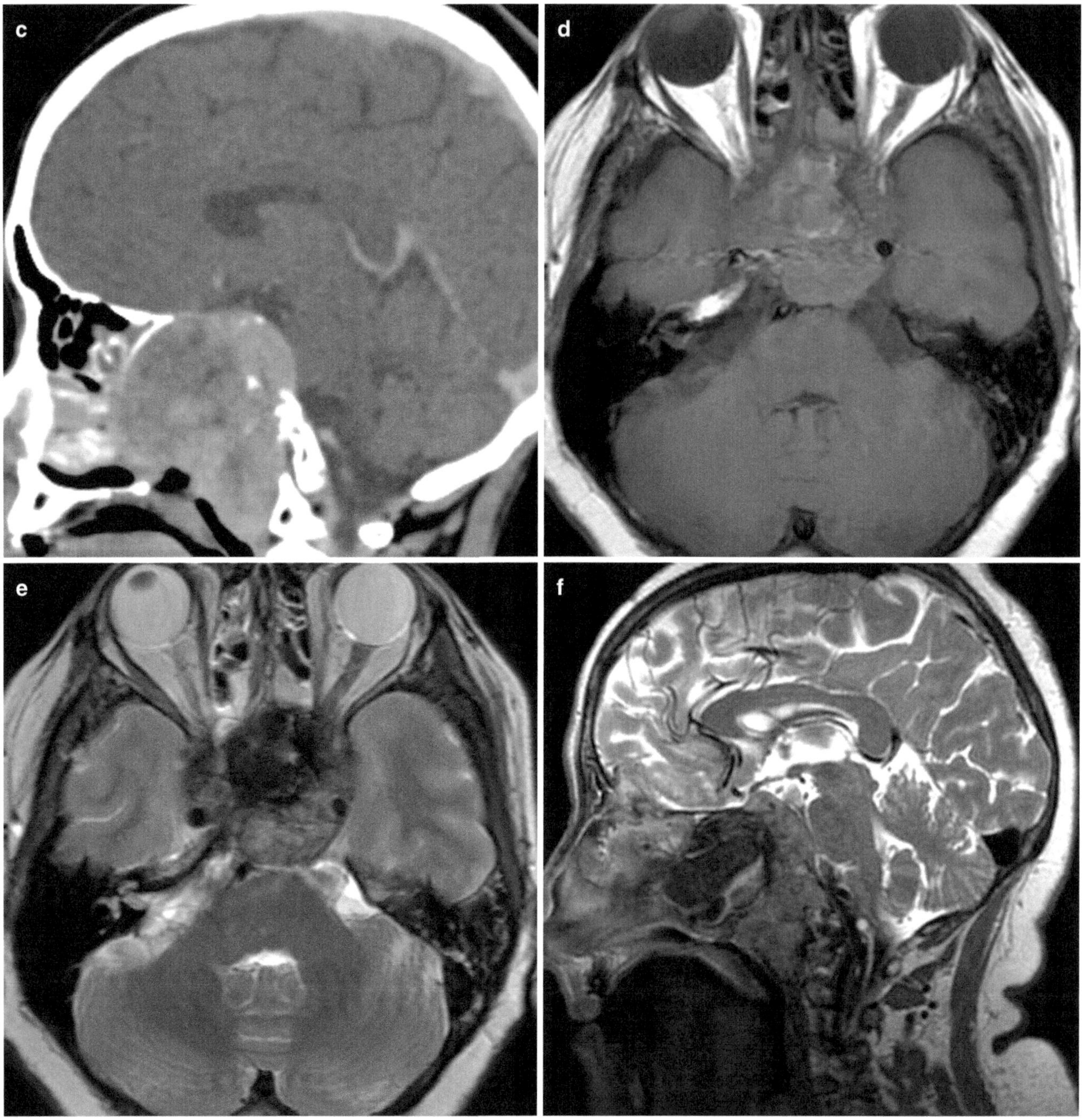

Fig. 20.14 (continued)

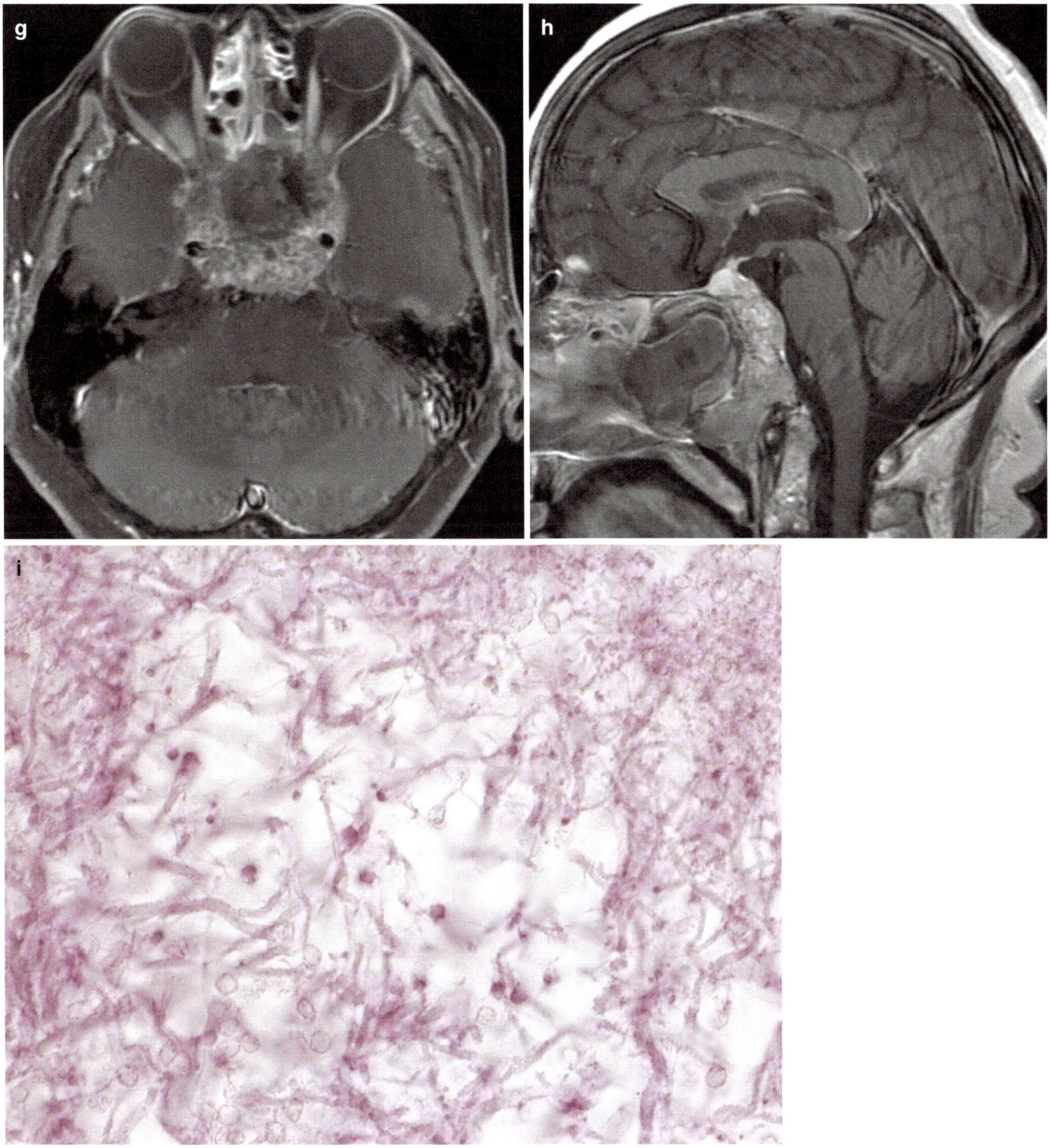

Fig. 20.14 (continued)

Part IV

Posterior Cranial Fossa and Skull Base Lesions

21 Introduction to Posterior Cranial Fossa and Skull Base Lesions

Posterior Cranial Fossa (PCF) is an area limited by the tentorium cerebelli from above (hence the second name—subtentorial region) and the foramen magnum from below. Lateral walls are the petrous pyramids of the temporal bones, the sphenoid bone is in front, and the occipital bone is below and behind. Cerebral structures located within these anatomical limits include the brainstem (pons and medulla oblongata) and the cerebellum, between which lies the 4th ventricle. Cerebrospinal fluid spaces in the posterior cranial fossa are often called basal cisterns. The most significant are anterior and lateral pontine and medullary cisterns, cerebellopontine cistern, ambient cistern, etc. Distal parts of vertebral arteries with posterior inferior cerebellar arteries arising from them, almost the entire basilar artery with its main branches (anterior inferior cerebellar and superior cerebellar arteries, etc.) are located in the subtentorial region. This is to be recalled that the apex of the basilar artery and its branches, posterior cerebral arteries, are located above the tentorium, i.e. supratentorially. The most important venous structures of the PCF base include transverse, sigmoid, occipital and inferior petrosal sinuses and jugular vein bulb. It is appropriate to recall and remind the anatomical bone canals and foramina through which cranial nerves enter the cranial cavity: *porus acusticus internus*, through which *a. labyrinthi, n. facialis (VII), n. vestibulocochlearis (VIII), n. intermedius (XIII)* pass; *foramen jugulare*, through which n. *glossopharyngeus (IX), n. vagus (X), n. accessorius Willisii (XI), v. jugularis interna* pass. This portion of the jugular foramen is also sometimes called *pars vascularis*. The medulla oblongata with meninges, *aa. vertebrales, plexus venosi vertebrales interna, n. accessorius* pass through the foramen magnum; *n. hypoglossus (XII)* passes through *canalis hypoglossi*.

In this chapter we focus your attention only on disorders that affect mainly the base of the posterior cranial fossa, its bone structures and meninges. We will pay less attention to the description of lesions and tumors of neuroepithelial and other origin, such as gliomas, ependymomas, medulloblastomas, etc. The reader can find detailed information on intra-axial space-occupying lesions in our earlier publications (Kornienko and Pronin 2009).

Particular interest will be focused on basal space-occupying lesions, which are often located at extradural and sometimes extracranial sites.

The base of the posterior cranial fossa and its bone structures can contain both neoplastic lesions (most frequently extraaxial or extracranial lesions growing in this area, less common metastases and intracerebral tumors originating from the adjacent brain structures) and a number of non-neoplastic pathologies that primarily include a group of congenital bone diseases, vascular disorders (arterial aneurysms, AVMs, and other vascular malformations), inflammatory and other lesions.

Depending on the age, there is a certain pattern in the distribution of histological types of tumors occurring in this anatomical region. In adults, for example, extraaxial tumors predominate in the posterior fossa: schwannomas (7.2%) and meningiomas (5%), epidermoid cysts (0.2–1.8%) and metastases (Kornienko and Pronin 2009). In children, intraaxial neoplasms are the most commonly diagnosed, with subtentorial tumors comprising from 50 to 55% of all childhood brain tumors (Russell and Rubinstein 1989; Osborn 2004a, b). An exception is patients aged less than one year old, in whom supratentorial tumors predominate. It should also be noted that the highest proportion of tumors in the posterior fossa in children occur between the ages of 2–5 years old (>60%). In the second decade, a tendency to a decrease in the number of subtentorial tumors and an increase in supratentorial neoplasms is noted.

By incidence, space-occupying lesions in adults can be distributed as follows: schwannomas, meningiomas, metastases, epidermoid cysts, arachnoid cysts, lipomas, saccular arterial aneurysms, and arteriovenous malformations.

Clinically, lesions of the posterior cranial fossa base are characterized by involvement of the cranial nerves, as all of them, except for I, II, and III pairs of nerves, are located in the subtentorial structures, and, starting with VII nerve, pass

I. Pronin, V. Kornienko, *CT and MRI of Skull Base Lesions*, https://doi.org/10.1007/978-3-319-65957-2_21

through the foramina in the skull base. In cases with large intracranial expansion the signs of intracranial hypertension can be detected.

In order to describe disorders of the PCF base and improved readability of a rather large material we chose mixed arrangement of subsections based on both tumor's histology and anatomical sites of lesions. We have distinguished the following anatomic areas: petrous pyramid of the temporal bone and cerebellopontine angle, clivus and craniovertebral junction. This version of description of pathologies (along with subject index), in our opinion, will allow readers to quickly and efficiently find the information and use it in their clinical practice.

Among anatomical structures of the posterior cranial fossa, the petrous apex is a special note, since, despite its small anatomical size, a rather large group of abnormal processes develop in this area. These can be neoplastic lesions requiring surgical treatment (e.g., tumors or inflammatory purulent complications) or processes that are not subject to surgery, but often mimic tumors, leading to misdiagnosis in a number of cases and inadequate subsequent care and even surgery. The only diagnostic imaging methods such as CT and MRI including advanced technologies of neuroimaging play a major role in the interpretation of changes detected between the tumors and non-tumor lesions.

22 Congenital Abnormalities and Disorders

Contents

22.1 Impaired Pneumatization of the Petrous Pyramid

Pneumatization of the paranasal sinuses and mastoid cells is achieved by a sacciform protrusion of the nasal mucosa and middle ear mucosa into the compact bone. Development of the temporal bone pneumatization begins at the age of 4–5 months and completes by 5–6 years of life (the first period). It is most pronounced in mastoid cells, the latter are formed by confluence of mastoid surfaces of the petrous and squamous portions of the temporal bone, therefore, one of the mentioned parts can be sometimes hypopneumatized. Pneumatization process occurs simultaneously with the replacement of diploic bone by compact one, which is mainly completed at the age of 8–12 years old (the second period). Concomitant middle ear inflammations during child development lead to the formation of different types of mastoid pneumatization. Subsequently, peripheral groups of cells develop and periantral cavities diminish. Pneumatization is very intense in the vertical direction and in the depth of the mastoid. By the end of the second period, the growth is basically completed, and differentiation of the cell structure begins. The third period (13–16 years of age) is not accompanied by an extension of the total pneumatization area, and only reorganization of the cellular structure occurs due to thickening of the bone walls; diploic mastoid cells are gradually replaced by a more compact bone. As a rcsult of such a complex development process, variability of mastoid types is very high, and asymmetry is observed in at least 25% of children. Studies conducted by Haynes et al. (1988) and Hasso et al. (1988) showed that there are two basic types (limited and generalized) and four subtypes (cellular-diploic, cellular-compact, bullous diploic, and bullous-compact) of pneumatization.

Despite the fact that the petrous apex is presented primarily by compact bone, its partial pneumatization is observed in about 30% of adult population, which has various

I. Pronin, V. Kornienko, *CT and MRI of Skull Base Lesions*, https://doi.org/10.1007/978-3-319-65957-2_22

radiological manifestations depending on a degree of aeration indicated above. In approximately 5% of cases, formation of pneumatic cavities at the projection of the apex is asymmetrical, creating certain diagnostic difficulties.

Imaging CT is the method of choice, clearly visualizing the extent of pneumatization of the petrous apex and mastoid cells by typically low (air) density (Schuknecht et al. 1986). At the same time, integrity and structure of the cortical surfaces of the temporal bone, bordering the pneumatized cavity, can be easily estimated. However, in order to obtain this information, thin spiral scanning need to be applied with subsequent display of CT findings with bone window. The most frequent is a symmetrical hyperpneumatization of temporal bones, while asymmetrical changes are less frequent (Fig. 22.1).

The greatest difficulties in petrous apex MRI assessment occur due to asymmetric contents of the fatty bone marrow, which is appeared as a limited area with a high MR signal on T1-weighted images and a moderately high signal on T2-weighted images. Sometimes misinterpretation of MRI findings may lead to misdiagnosis and even wrong treatment (for example, in cases when radiotherapy is considered for a "suspected" tumor, etc.). In doubtful cases with the presence of residual bone marrow in the projection of the pyramid, techniques with suppression of MR signal from fat should be used (disappearance of hyperintense signal is noted) or a CT study to exclude bone-destructive changes in this area should be performed (Fig. 22.2). In addition, one shouldn't forget about clinical symptoms that are presented in cases with tumors and typically absent in many cases with abnormal pneumatization and fatty bone marrow. In some cases overtreatment can be avoided by using dynamic MRI or CT follow-up. No changes in MR signal and CT density, as well as an absence of bone destruction, suggests the benign nature of processes at the projection of the petrous apex.

22.2 Dysembryogenic Tumors and Cysts

Cholesteatoma (epidermoid cyst, EC) (from the Greek: chole + stear, steatos—fat; oma—tumor) is a space-occupying lesion surrounded by a capsule that typically develops in the middle ear, usually accompanied by chronic tympanic or epitympanic inflammation. It represents accumulation of keratin, cholesterol crystals, and desquamated keratinized epithelium. The term "cholesteatoma" was introduced in 1838 by the German pathologist J. Muller, who pointed to its content of cholesterol.

Cholesteatoma, or epidermoid, accounts for 4–9% of all cases among disorders of the petrous pyramid. Etiology and pathogenesis are not completely understood. Cholesteatoma is believed to be a consequence of growth of the external auditory meatus epidermis into the tympanic cavity through a marginal perforation in the tympanic membrane.

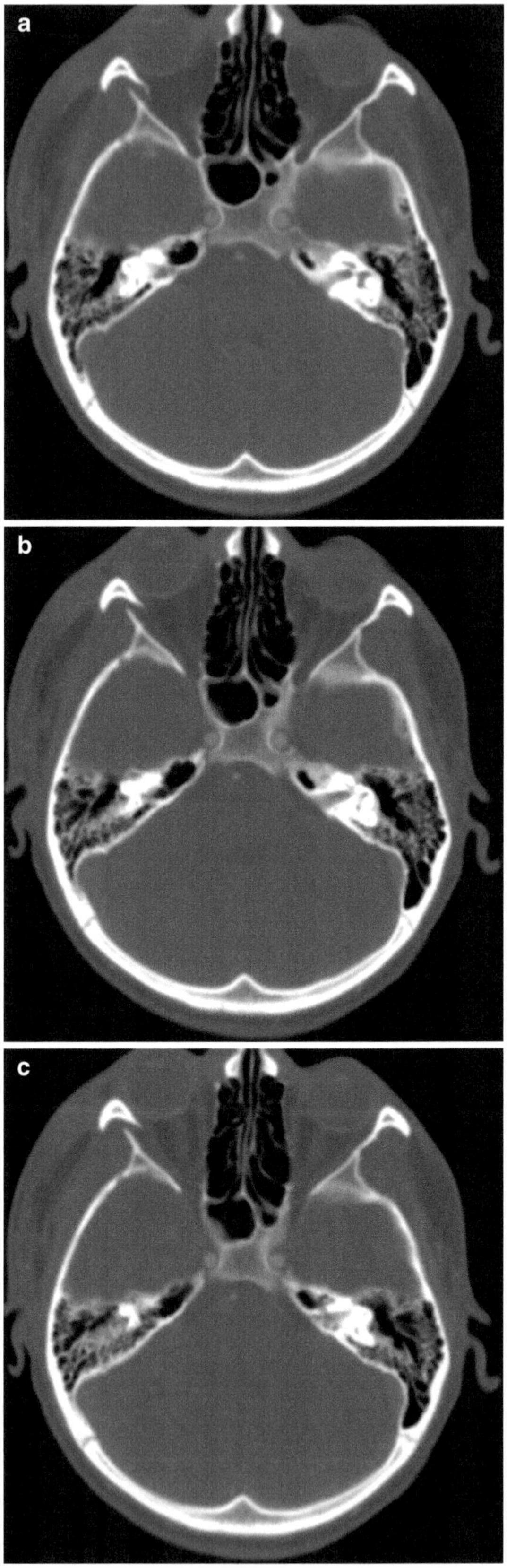

Fig. 22.1 Hyperpneumatization of the apex of the temporal bone. On CT scans in the 'bone window' mode (**a–c**) an asymmetric pneumatization of the temporal bone apex (D > S) is defined. It is also presented an increased pneumatization of mastoid process cells from both sides

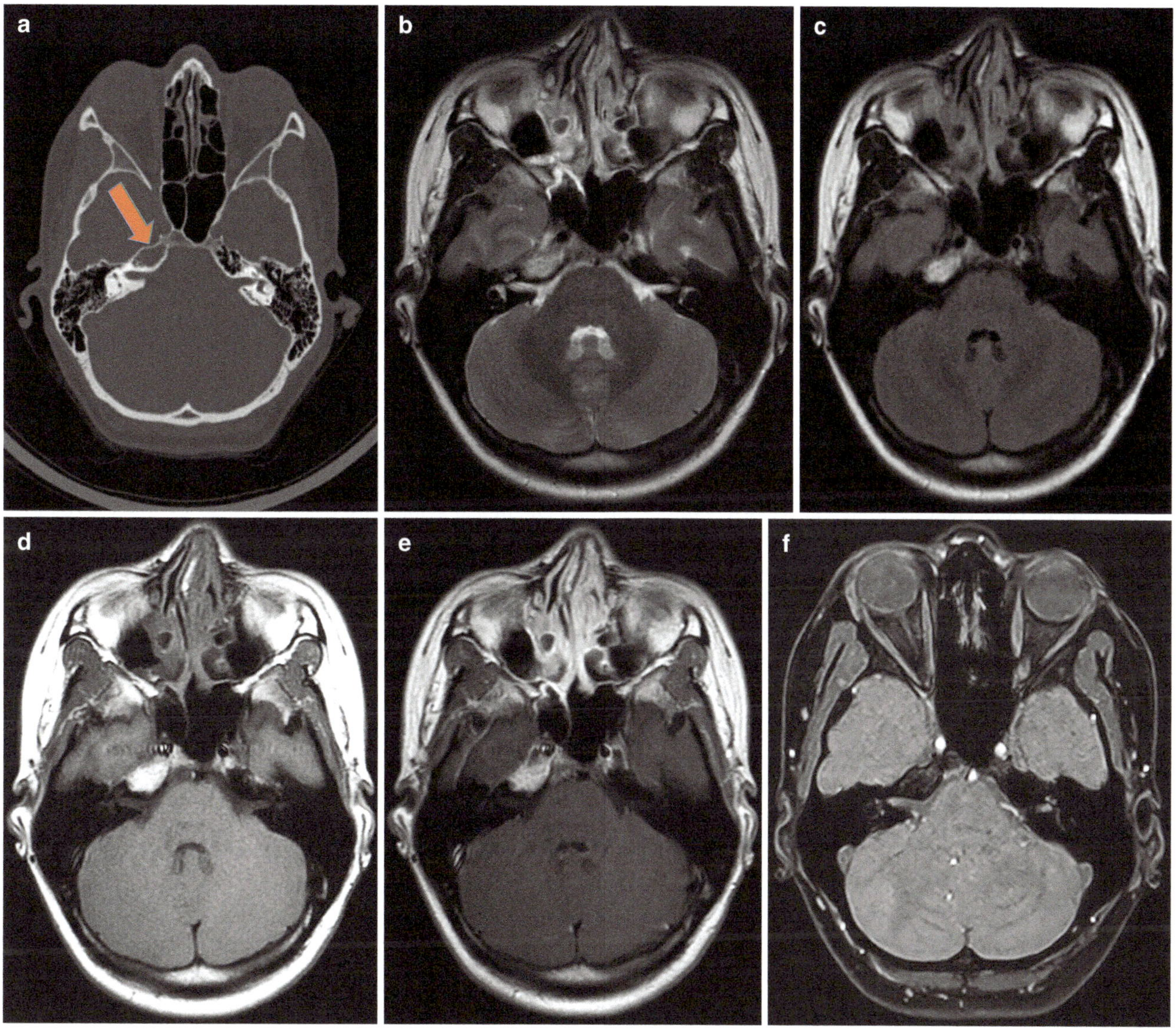

Fig. 22.2 Asymmetric pneumatization of the apex of the temporal bone. On CT scan (**a**) in the "bone window" mode an asymmetric pneumatization of the temporal bone apex is defined with opacification on the right (*arrow*). MR imaging with using T2 (**b**), T2-FLAIR (**c**), T1 before (**d**) and after (**e**) contrast enhancement demonstrated hyperintense MR-signal from the right temporal bone apex. T1-weighted MR image with Fat-Sat (**f**) shows disappearance of high signal from the apex

Desquamation of keratinized squamous cells and their accumulation in the middle ear cavity leads to the formation of a compact mass. Exerting pressure on the bone tissue, growing into it (chemical components of cholesteatoma and its decay products contribute to this process), this lesion destroys the bone structure. According to literature, epidermoid cysts are found in 3 patients per 100.000 children and in about 9 cases per 100.000 adults. ECs in the internal ear cavity are usually diagnosed in patients under 50 years old, while other sites are commonly identified between the ages of 40–70 years old.

These are the following types of cholesteatoma:

- *Acquired cholesteatoma* usually occurs as a result of inflammation in the middle ear and Eustachian tube dysfunction. Accumulation of keratin residues inside the middle ear can cause conductive hearing loss or chronic ear suppuration (chronic otorrhea).

1. Primary acquired cholesteatoma occurs as a result of formation of a saccular cavity (pouch) in the eardrum and negative pressure inside the middle ear. Once the pouch becomes too deep and keratin elimination from the fold is impossible, its residues begin to accumulate. It amounts up to 80% of the inner ear cholesteatomas. It is usually located at the projection of pars flaccida of the tympanic membrane.
2. Secondary acquired cholesteatoma (up to 18% of inner ear cholesteatomas) develops because of ingrowth of squamous cells from edges of the tympanic membrane rupture. This rupture most often occurs as a result of an infectious process.

- *Congenital cholesteatoma* is usually found in children and generally develops from embryonic epithelial residues. It can be located anywhere in the temporal bone: inner ear, mastoid process, petrous apex, squamous part of the temporal bone and even in the external auditory canal. Such type of lesion, but located in other cranial bones or intracranially and extraaxially, is also called an epidermoid cyst. Congenital cholesteatomas constitute only 2% of all inner ear cholesteatomas.

There are publications which also describe cholesteatomas located in the tympanic cavity, depending on the location in relation to the tympanic membrane: cholesteatomas of pars flaccida and pars tensa. Lesions with rare localization form a separate group: mural cholesteatomas and cholesteatomas of the external auditory meatus (Barath 2011.

For a long time cholesteatoma can persist without any specific symptoms, however, most patients complain of dull, nagging, bursting, pressing, or shooting ear pain; headache, dizziness are also possible due to labyrinthitis (Darrouzet et al. 2002). Discharge from the ear is usually scarce, with putrid smell. Whitish curdy lumps can be found in purulent discharge. In case of purulent otitis exacerbation, cholesteatoma undergoes purulent decay, which often leads to an erosion or a fistula of the semicircular canal and vertigo, facial nerve palsy, labyrinthitis, subperiosteal abscess development (often with a periodically closing fistula), meningitis, thrombophlebitis of the sigmoid sinus, cerebellum or brain abscess and even otogenic sepsis (Melero et al. 2000).

Congenital and acquired cholesteatomas behave aggressively, destroying adjacent bones and being located near vitally (brainstem, internal carotid artery, jugular bulb, middle and posterior fossa) and functionally (cochlea, labyrinth, facial nerve) important structures.

Imaging CT with high spatial resolution is considered as the method of choice, which allows to demonstrate soft-tissue component and bone-destructive changes in the petrous pyramid with high sensitivity. However, CT specificity is relatively low due to the fact that both granulomatous masses and cholesterol granulomas or even a tumor may have similar diagnostic signs. In most cases, CT shows areas of bone destruction with well-defined contours in the pyramid of temporal bone anteriorly to the jugular bulb and medially to the tympanic membrane. Bone erosion is observed in 80–96% of cholesteatomas, with greater frequency in children. Cholesteatomas themselves have hypodense characteristics. They do not enhance, which is considered as one of the diagnostic signs inherent to this lesion. In the presence of calcified fragments in the capsule, the latter have a higher density (Figs. 22.3 and 22.4).

The typical MR-feature of cholesteatoma is a marked signal increase from its mass on DWI-sequences. ADC maps demonstrate a moderately pronounced increase in the apparent diffusion coefficient. On T2-weighted images cysts are hyperintense and indistinguishable from inflammatory changes. On T1-weighted images cholesteatomas are hypointense. On T2-FLAIR scans, the lesion is characterized by a moderate MR-signal with hyperintense inclusions. Contrast enhancement on MRI studies in most cases is not observed. In rare cases, slight contrast enhancement of the cholesteatoma capsule can be visualized. The method of choice for cholesteatoma diagnosis is DWI MRI. The lesions smaller than 1 cm are readily visualized during the study (Figs. 22.5, 22.6, 22.7, 22.8 and 22.9).

In case of intracranial location, multiple tumor "sleeves" invading the subarachnoid spaces are noted. The symptom of scalloped borders is a typical radiological feature. Cholesteatoma masses "softly" compress the adjacent brain structures (brainstem, middle cerebellar peduncle) with minimal clinical symptoms, despite a relatively large size of the cyst in most cases at the moment of primary diagnosis.

Another important indication for using diffusion-weighted sequences in the diagnosis of cholesteatoma is postoperative follow-up. Majority of cholesteatoma's residues are easily identified as areas with a high MRI signal (Fig. 22.10).

Differential Diagnosis Arachnoid cyst, cystic schwannoma of VII nerve, inflammatory changes, tympanic paraganglioma, cholesterol granuloma, hemangioma of VII nerve, squamous cell carcinoma of the inner ear.

Dermoid Cyst (dermoid) is a form of dysembryogenic mass lesions that are characterized by the presence of epithelial elements with separate dermal components (hair, etc.) in their structure. They usually have a cystic structure with clearly defined outer boundaries. In case of location on the midline, a combination with other malformations, such as dermal sinus, is possible. They consist of less than 1% of all neoplasms of the posterior fossa.

Imaging Dermoid cysts on CT are often hypodense due to the cystic component and high content of fat elements within the cyst. CT density can reach −60–80 HU in the areas with the highest fat content. In cystic portion, the density decreases not so markedly, but its values in the cyst are higher than those of CSF in the ventricles. Calcifications are usually located in the cyst wall and observed in approximately 15% of cases.

Dermoid cysts)are hyperintense on T1-weighted images and iso- or hyperintense on T2-weighted MR images. Sometimes contrast enhancement in the capsule can be observed. However, because of the initially high MR-signal on T1-weighted sequences, enhancement of the cyst walls is not so obvious. In such cases, it is advisable to use Fat-Sat technique, so that MR signal from fat is suppressed, and accumulation of contrast agent can be estimated more accurately. On diffusion-weighted sequences, unlike epidermoids, dermoid cysts tend to show no signs of diffusion restriction and have isointense characteristics on DWI MR. In case

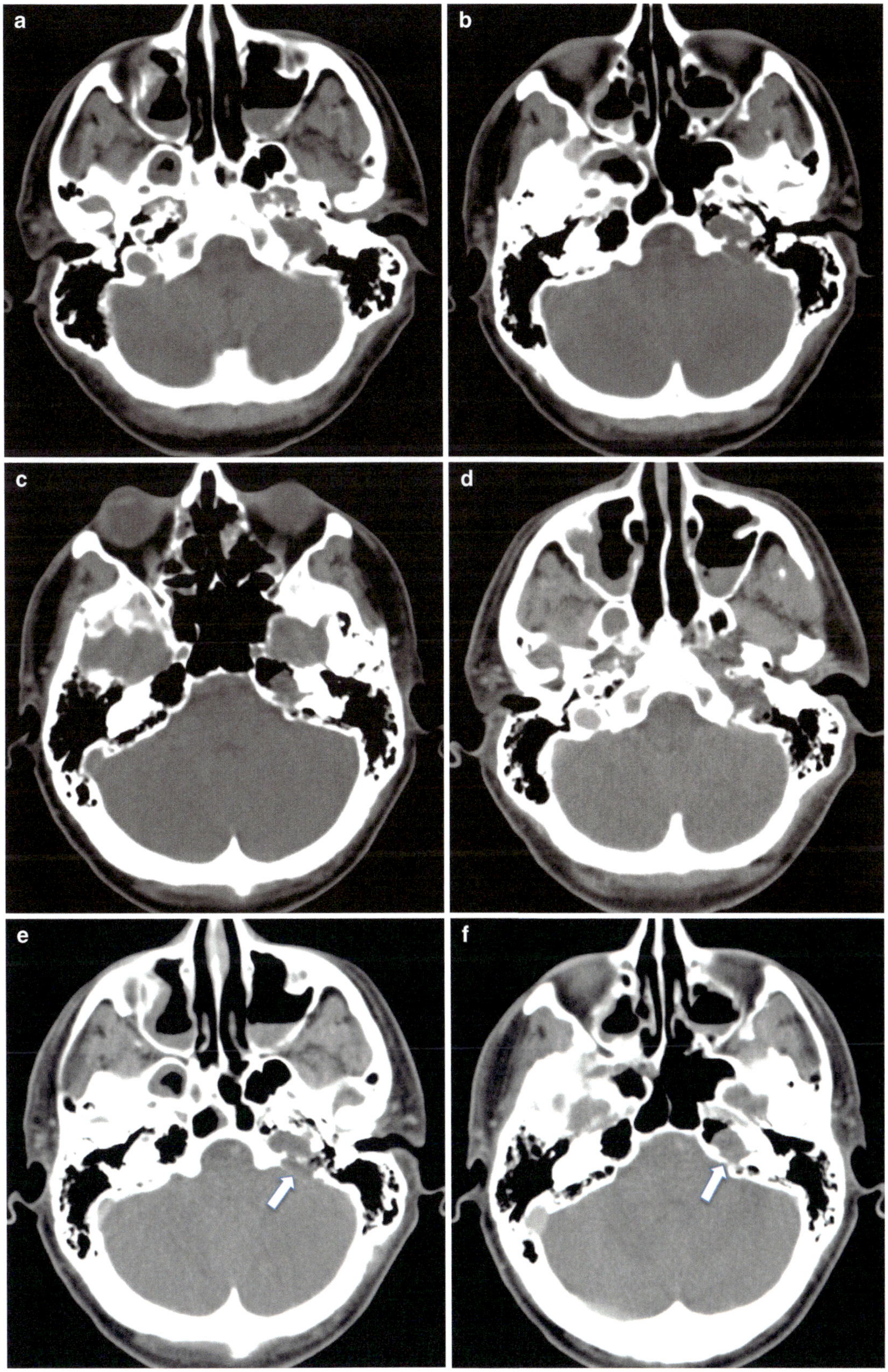

Fig. 22.3 Cholesteatoma of the temporal bone pyramid (*left side*). On CT scans before (**a–c**) and after (**d–f**) contrast enhancement on the background of hyperpneumatization of the both pyramids there is a slightly hypodense lesion which causes bone destruction (*arrows*). The front pole of the cyst is clearly visible on the background of air in the projection of the apex. The medial contour is clearly outlined by the enhanced dura (**g**, **h**). Coronal CT scan (**i**) confirms the location of the cysts in the projection of the bone structures

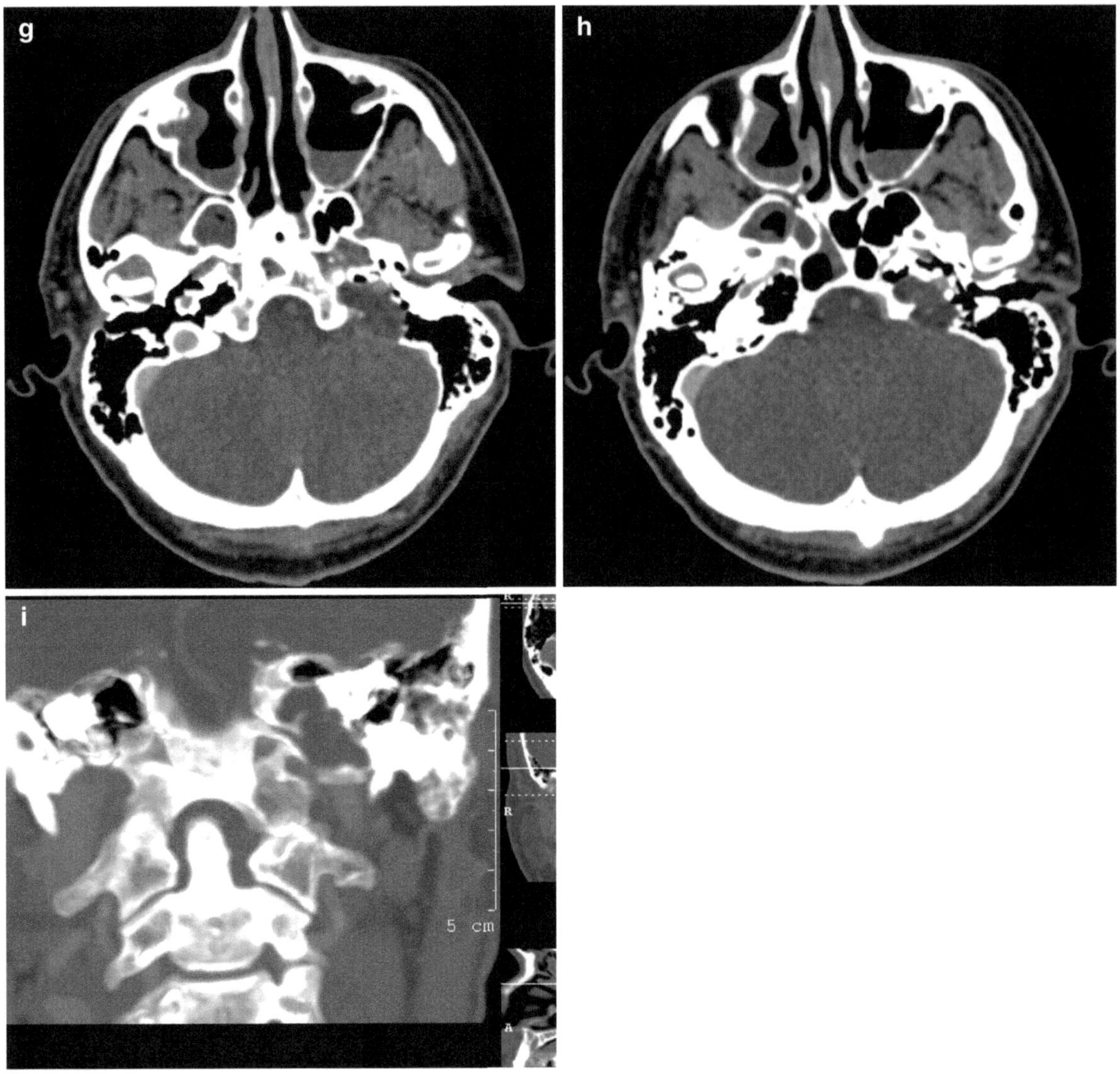

Fig. 22.3 (continued)

Fig. 22.4 Cholesteatoma. The lateral CT-topogram (**a**) shows a ring-like area in the occipital bone. CECT scans in axial (**b**), coronal (**c**, **d**), and sagittal (**e**) projections demonstrate an oval expansile hypodense lesion in the area where the occipital bone transforms into the base of the temporal bone pyramid. It is clearly demonstrated the relationship cyst and the right transverse sinus. CT scan in the "bone window" mode (**f**) and 3D reconstruction (**g**, **h**) show a clear outlined of the bone destruction area. The cyst on T2- (**i**), T2-FLAIR (**j**), and T1-weighted (**k**) MR images has fairly homogeneous signal features. Hyperintense MR signal on the DWI (**l**) is typical for cholesteatoma

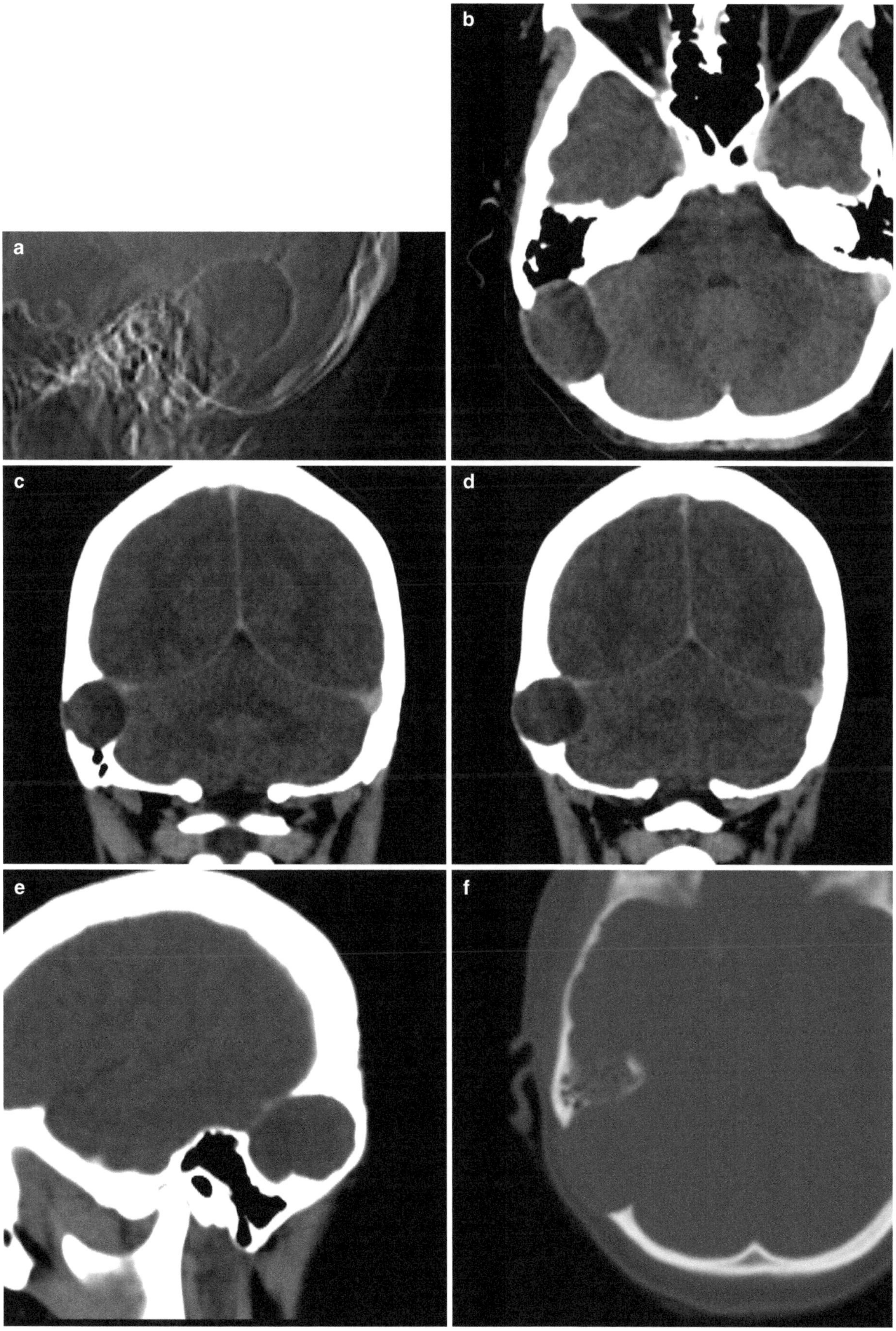
a
b
c
d
e
f

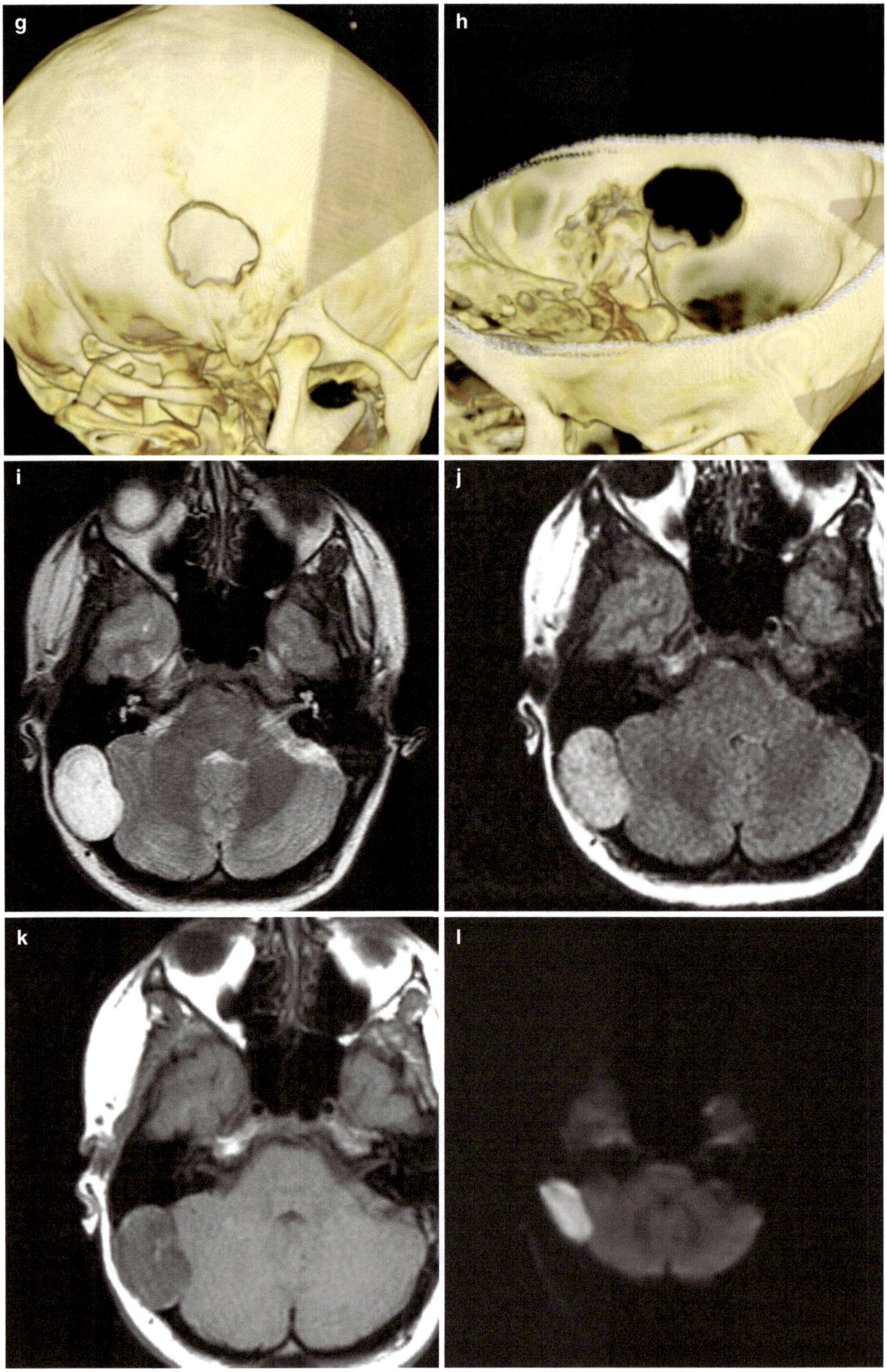

Fig. 22.4 (continued)

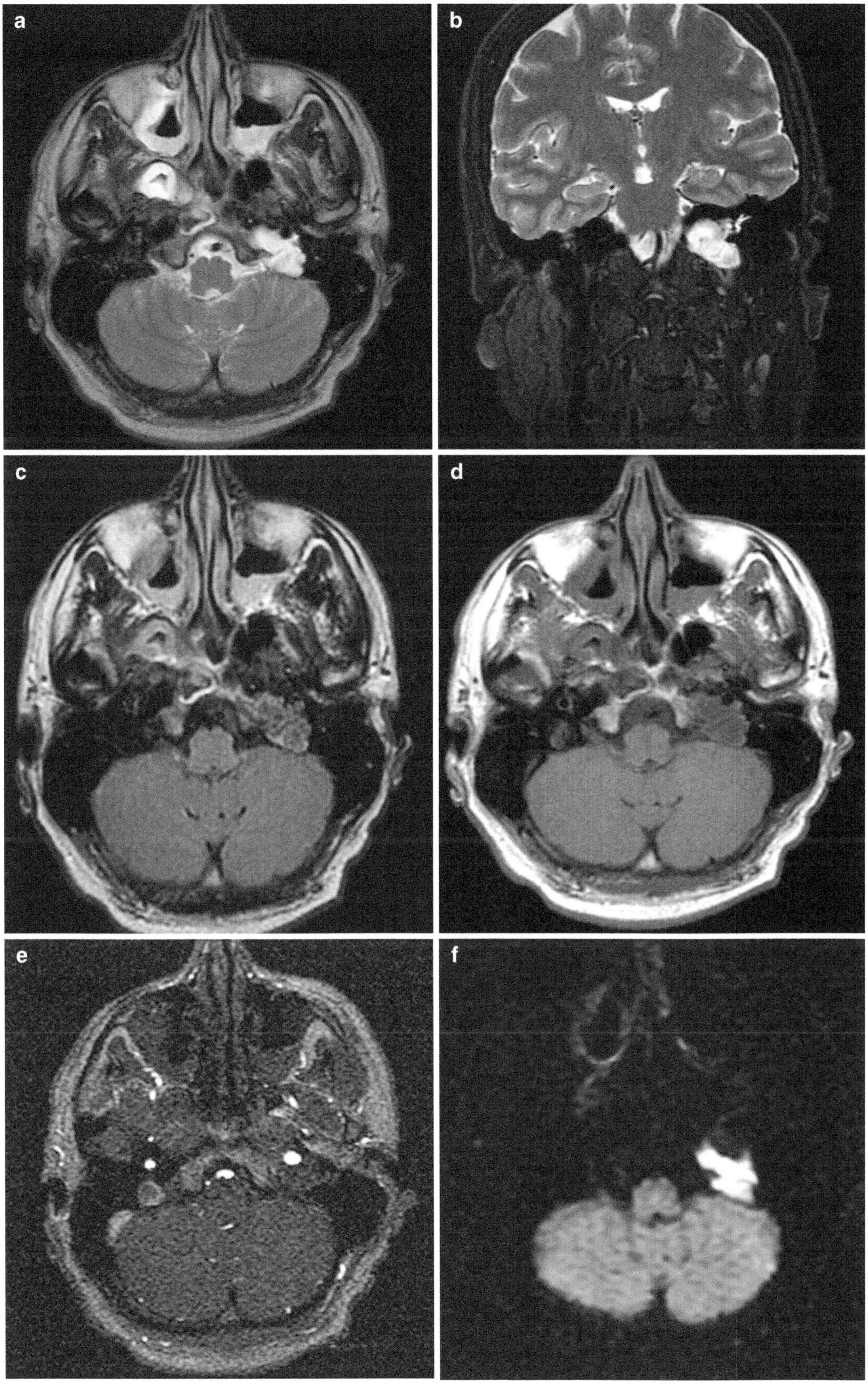

Fig. 22.5 Cholesteatoma of the petrous apex on the left. On T2-weighted (**a**, **b**) and T2-FLAIR (**c**) MR images an expansile lesion that occupies the left petrous apex is visualized. It has well-defined contour with multiple eversions. The MR-signal on T1-weighted image is slightly hypointense (**d**). There is a close vicinity to the internal carotid artery on MR-angiogram (**e**). The main characteristic of cholesteatoma is bright signal on DWI (**f**)

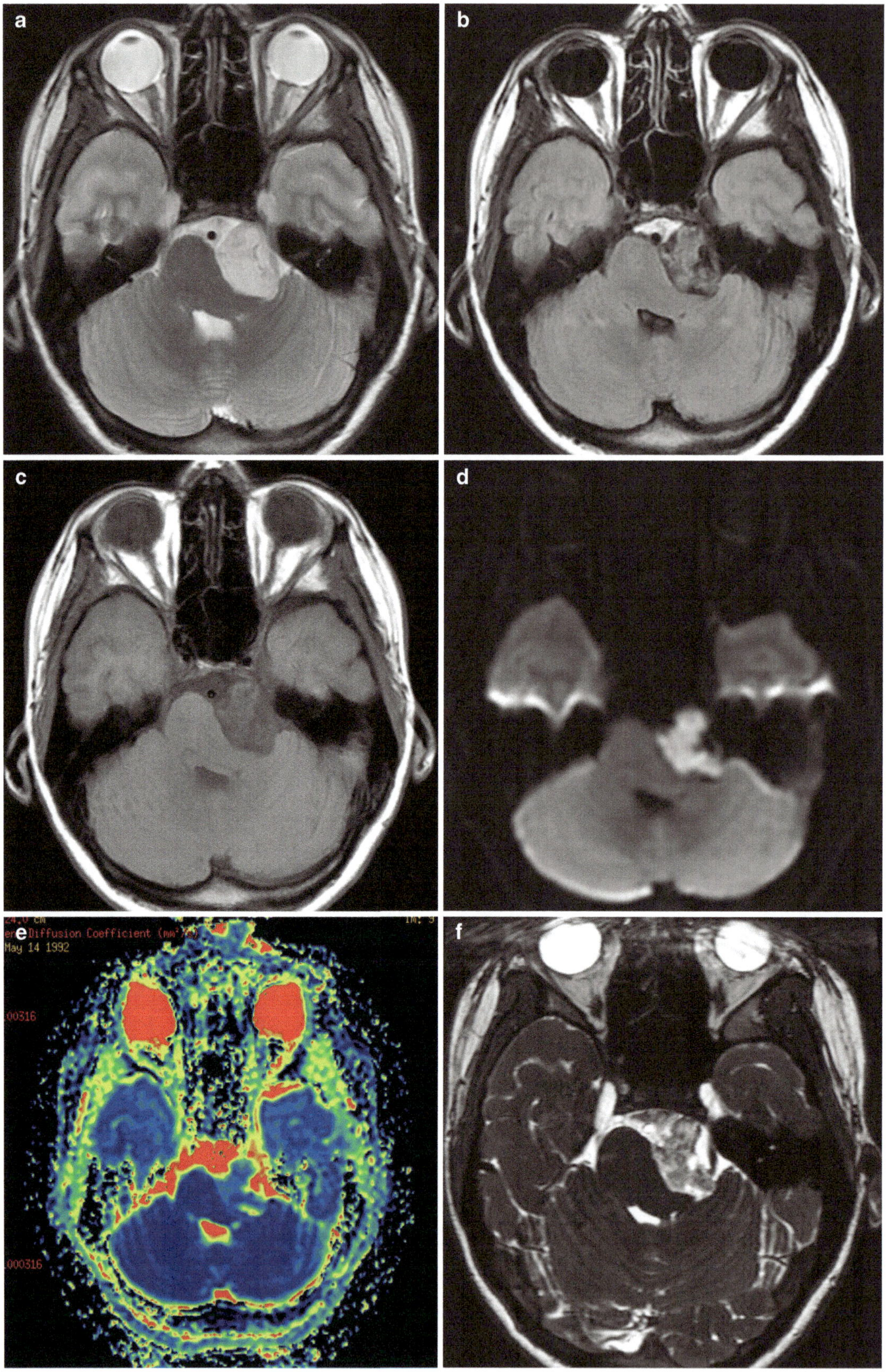

Fig. 22.6 Cholesteatoma of the left petroclival region. Axial T2- (**a**), T2-FLAIR- (**b**), and T1- (**c**) weighted images demonstrate a lesion with increased signal on T2, heterogeneous isointensity on T2-FLAIR and heterogeneously hypointense on T1. On diffusion-weighted image a lesion has hyperintense MR-signal (**d**). ADC values is slightly increased (**e**). Using FIESTA program can improve delineation of the cysts from the cerebrospinal fluid spaces of the brain base (**f**)

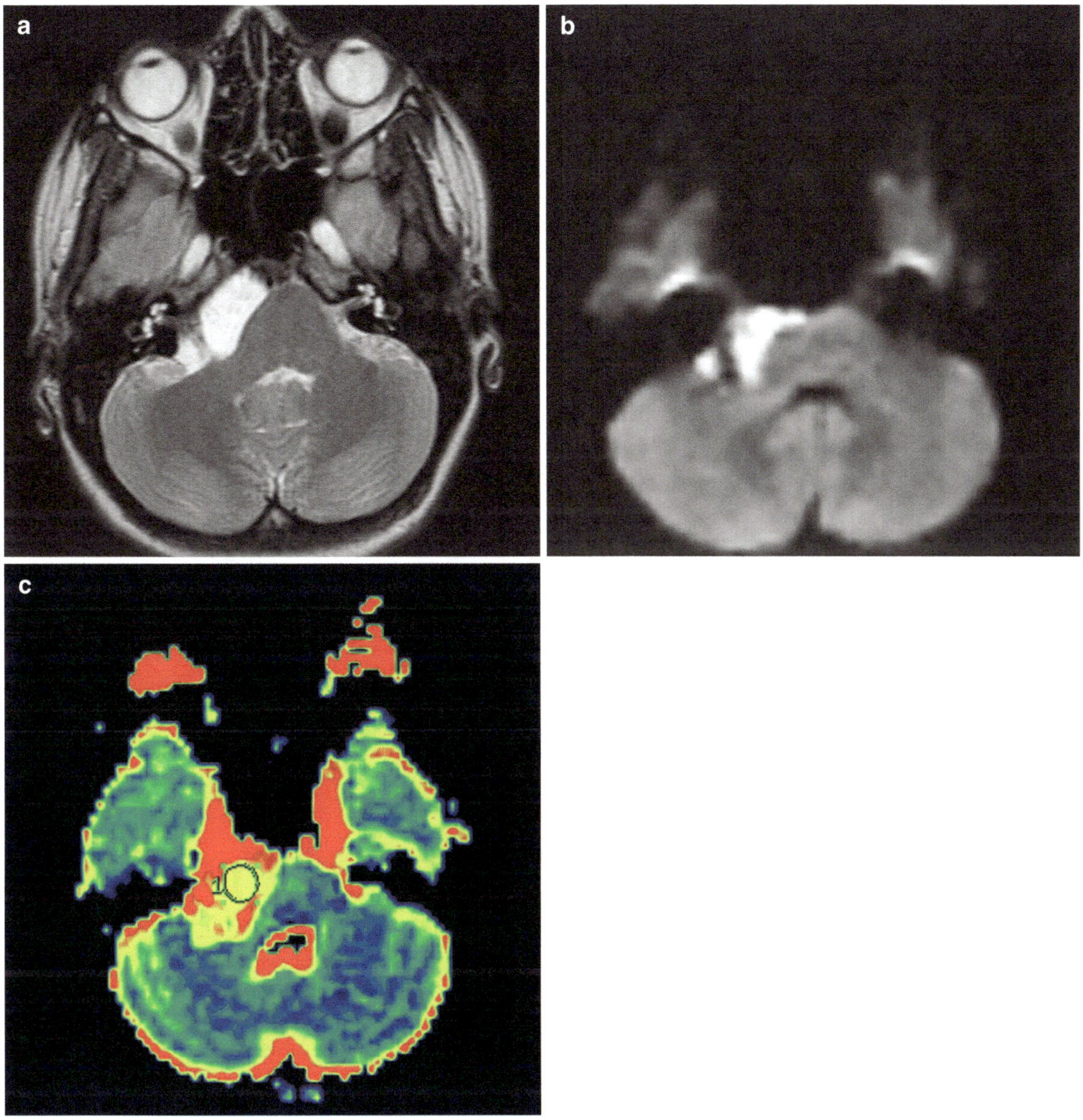

Fig. 22.7 Cholesteatoma of the right cerebello-pontine angle. MR imaging in T2 (**a**) and DWI (**b**) sequences shows a hyperintense_mass lesion. The cyst has hyperintense MR-signal on diffusion-weighted image and elevated ADC values on ADC-map (**c**)

of infected dermoid cyst (e.g., via a corresponding dermal sinus), MR-signal on diffusion-weighted sequences can be increased, creating difficulties in the differential diagnosis with epidermoid cyst and abscess (Fig. 22.11). Sometimes dermoid cysts are represented mainly by cystic component with high protein content, which leads to increased density on CT and a decreased MR-signal on T2-weighted images and an increased signal on T1-weighted scans*)* (Fig. 22.12).

Lipomas of the posterior fossa account of approximately 10% of all intracranial lipomas. They are most frequently localized in the cerebellopontine angle (Cohen and Powers 1992). The tumor belongs to dysembrygenic lesions (together with epidermoids, dermoids, and teratoma).

Imaging CT features are typical for all lipomas: they are hypodense compared to the CSF (usually lipomas have density up to −40–80 HU). Sometimes small or large calcifications can be visualized in the structure or on the periphery of lipomas (Dalley et al. 1986). Unlike dermoid cysts, lipomas mainly consist of adipose tissue (a combination with fibrous elements is possible) without a cystic component.

On T1-weighted images lipomas are characterized by a high signal, while on T2-weighted sequences MR-signal can vary, but often is moderately hyperintense. It is useful to apply a fat signal suppression technique for confirming the diagnosis (Figs. 22.13, 22.14 and 22.15).

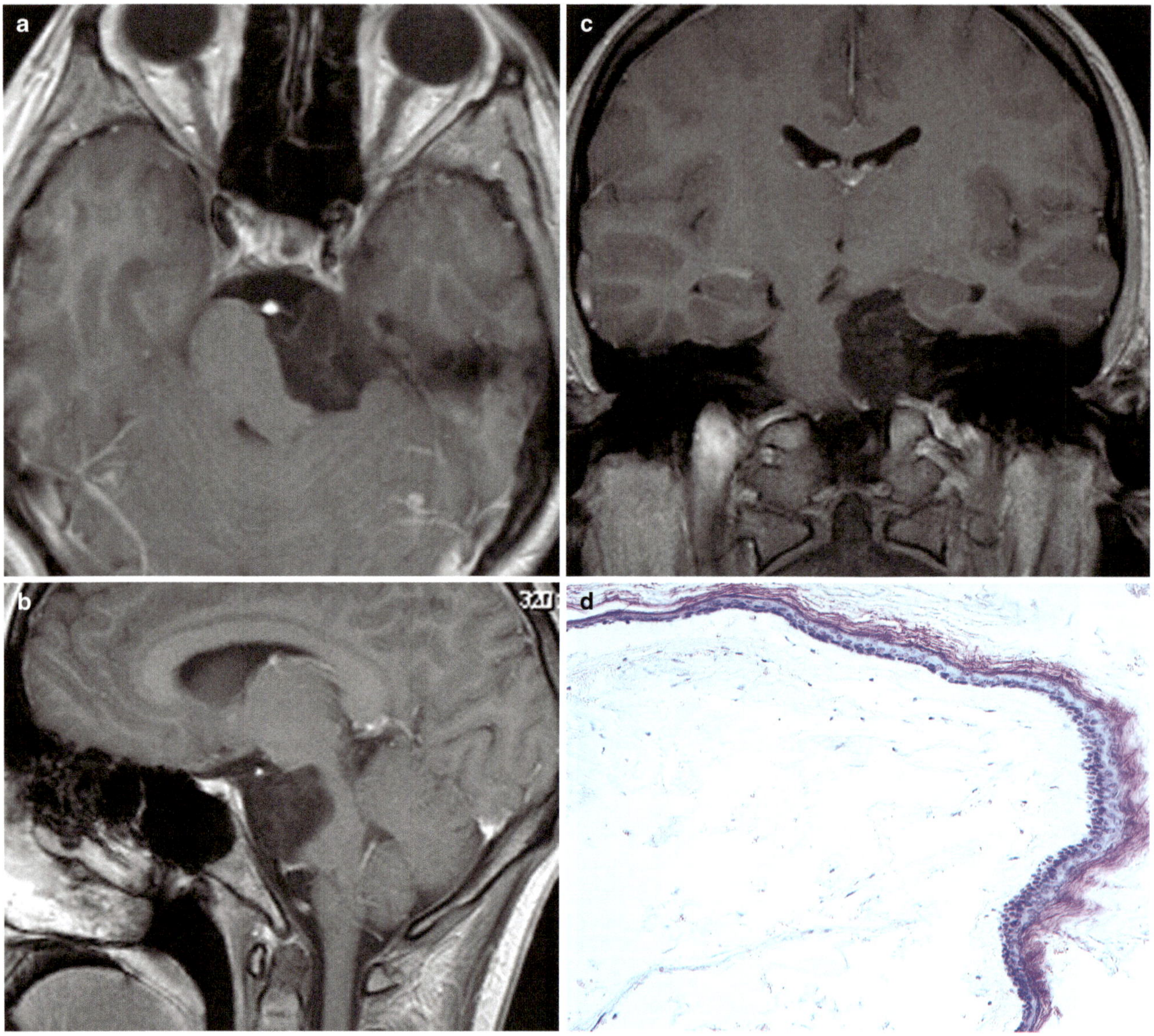

Fig. 22.8 Cholesteatoma of the left petroclival region. On post-contrast MR images in axial (**a**), sagittal (**b**), and coronal (**c**) projections a hypointense mass lesion without signs of a contrast agent accumulation. Histologic specimen of the cholesteatoma wall (**d**)

Differential Diagnosis subacute cerebellar hematoma (high MR signal on Fat-Sat T1-weighted sequences), teratoma, schwannoma, meningioma.

Teratomas are rare dysembryogenic tumors that occur mainly in the posterior part of the 3rd ventricle and pineal region, they amount to 15% of all tumors at this location in children of all ages. Teratomas are very rarely diagnosed in the posterior fossa (less than 1%).

Teratomas may be both mature and malignant. Mature teratomas are characterized by the presence of differentiated tissues (epithelium, cartilage, muscle, etc.) arranged in the form of organoid structures, such as cysts lined up by squamous (or other) epithelium. Malignant forms are represented by tissues originating from all germ layers.

Imaging Diagnosis of the tumors is based on the complex use of CT and MR imaging, where features are varied and reflect the variability of tumor components. Cartilage and calcified fragments have a high density on CT and a decreased signal on MR images (especially on T2-weighted sequences). On the contrary, fatty inclusions are presented by areas with low density and a high signal on T1-weighted MR-images (Fig. 22.16). Formation of cysts is typical for teratomas. With giant tumors, hydrocephalus of the ventricular system can develop. Malignant tumors, for example, teratoblastomas, are characterized by rapid and aggressive growth, marked contrast enhancement, while maintaining the heterogeneity of the tumor structure (Fig. 22.17).

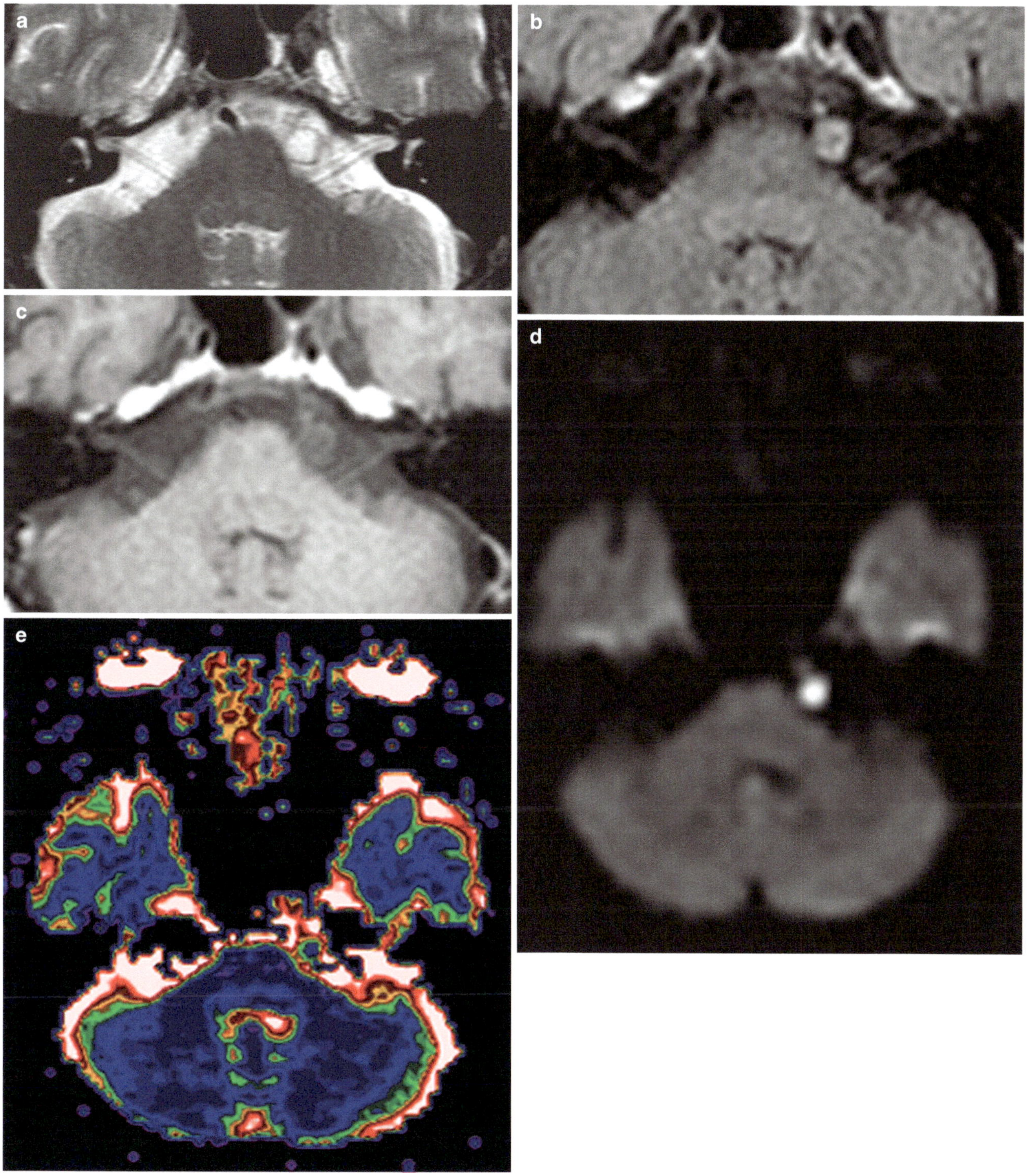

Fig. 22.9 Microcholesteatoma cyst of the lateral pons cistern on the left. Axial T2- (**a**), T2-FLAIR- (**b**), and T1- (**c**) weighted images reveal a small rounded lesion that is hyperintense on T2 and T2-FLAIR and hypointense on T1. A high MR signal on the DWI (**d**) and a moderate increase in ACD (**e**) values are typical features of the cholesteatoma

Effusion In rare cases, pneumatic cells of the petrous apex can be filled with inflammatory effusion primarily caused by inflammation in the middle ear with occlusion of the connecting duct between the middle ear cavity and cells of this area. It is found in less than 1% of all diagnostic brain studies (Crabtree 1983).

Imaging On CT, at the projection of the petrous apex, a portion with decreased density is observed without concomitant bone-destructive changes. In bone window scanning, bone trabeculae separating the individual cells can be seen. This is the main differential diagnostic criterion for suspected inflammatory process (apexitis).

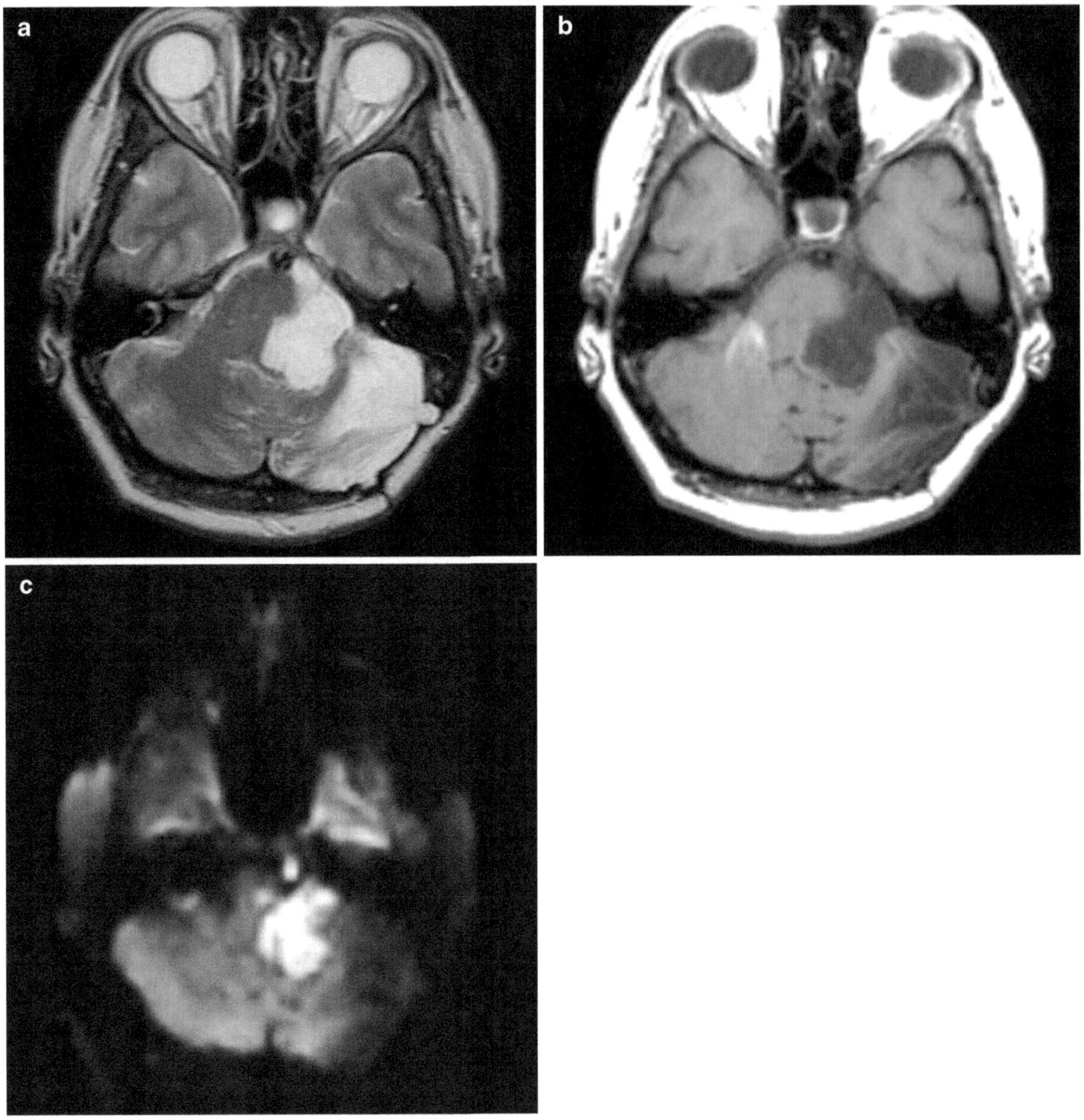

Fig. 22.10 Cholesteatoma of the left cerebello-pontine angle after the partial surgical resection. MR images in T2 (**a**) and T1 (**b**) modes do not allow to determine the radicality of the surgical resection due to the same intensity of the MR signal from the postoperative cavity and the remnants of the lesion. Diffusion-weighted image (**c**) shows a hyperintense MR-signal from the cholesteatoma

MRI demonstrates an area of increased MR-signal on T2-weighted sequences, the signal on T1-weighted sequences can be intermediate due to differences in effusion viscosity and presence of protein components (Fig. 22.18). Additionally, local inflammatory changes in the tympanic cavity can be detected. Contrast enhancement is not typical for this type of pathology.

Mucocele Mucocele represents a cystic enlargement usually of one of the paranasal sinuses. A mucocele capsule is formed from the inflamed mucosa of the paranasal sinuses, turning it into a closed pouch. The cyst contains bright, grayish-yellow or amber, viscous, odorless mucus, sometimes a dense protein mass in the form of a soft jelly. The mucus consists of the mucin, cholesterol, and fat. A microscopic examination indicates the presence of squamous and ciliated epithelium, leukocytes (neutrophils). The mucus is almost always sterile in bacteriological tests. In case of the development of complications with a purulent component, the process is regarded as pyocele.

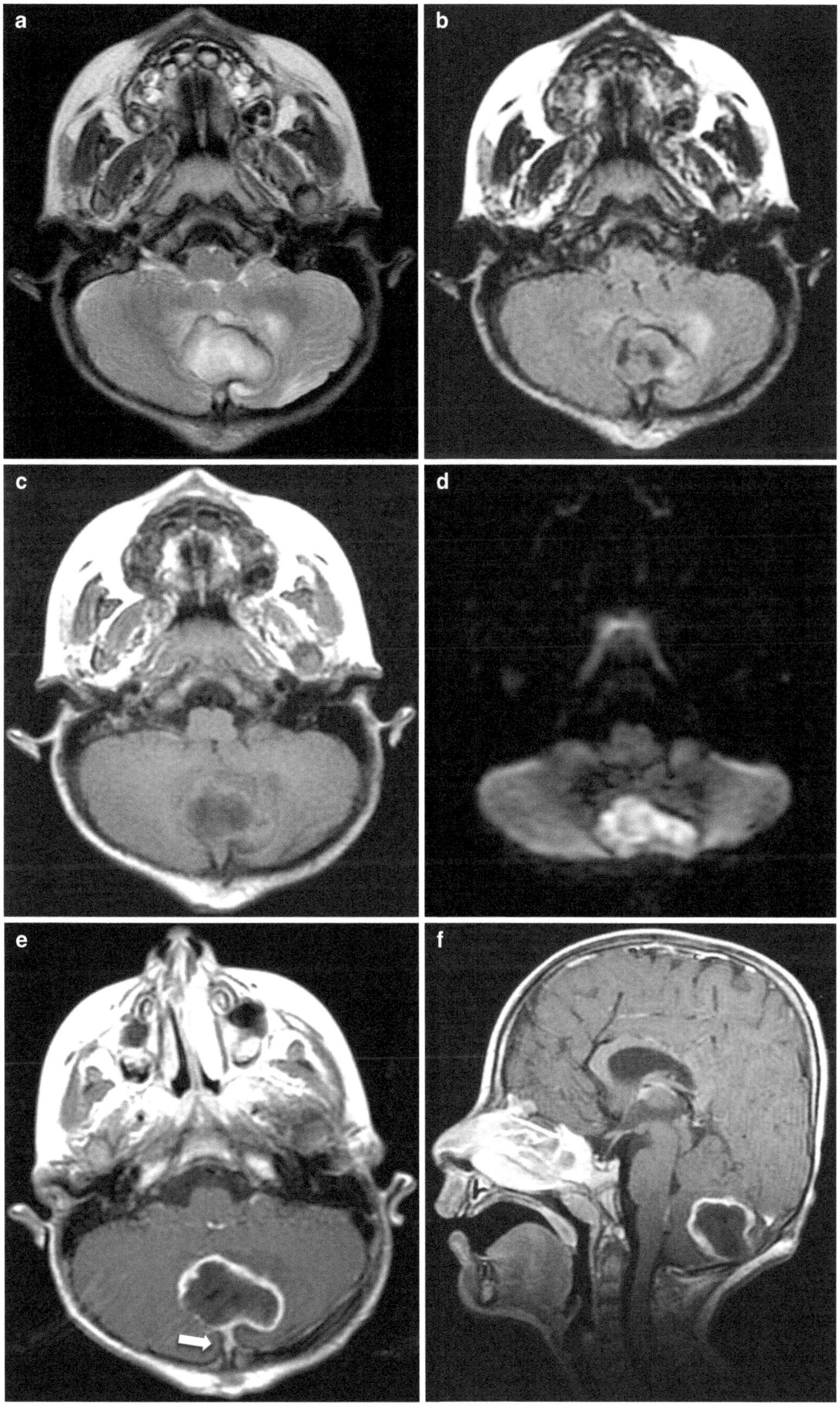

Fig. 22.11 Dermoid cyst of the posterior cranial fossa (superinfected) in a 3 years old child. MRI with using T2- (**a**), T2-FLAIR- (**b**), and T1- (**c**) weighted images reveal a heterogeneous mass located along the midline, which has a hyperintense signal from the center and hypointense rim. There is a perifocal edema around the lesion. The diffusion-weighted image (**d**) shows a high signal. After i/v contrast enhancement, a thick capsule with relatively even contours (**e**, **f**) became clearly defined. There is a dermal sinus in the occipital region (*arrow*)

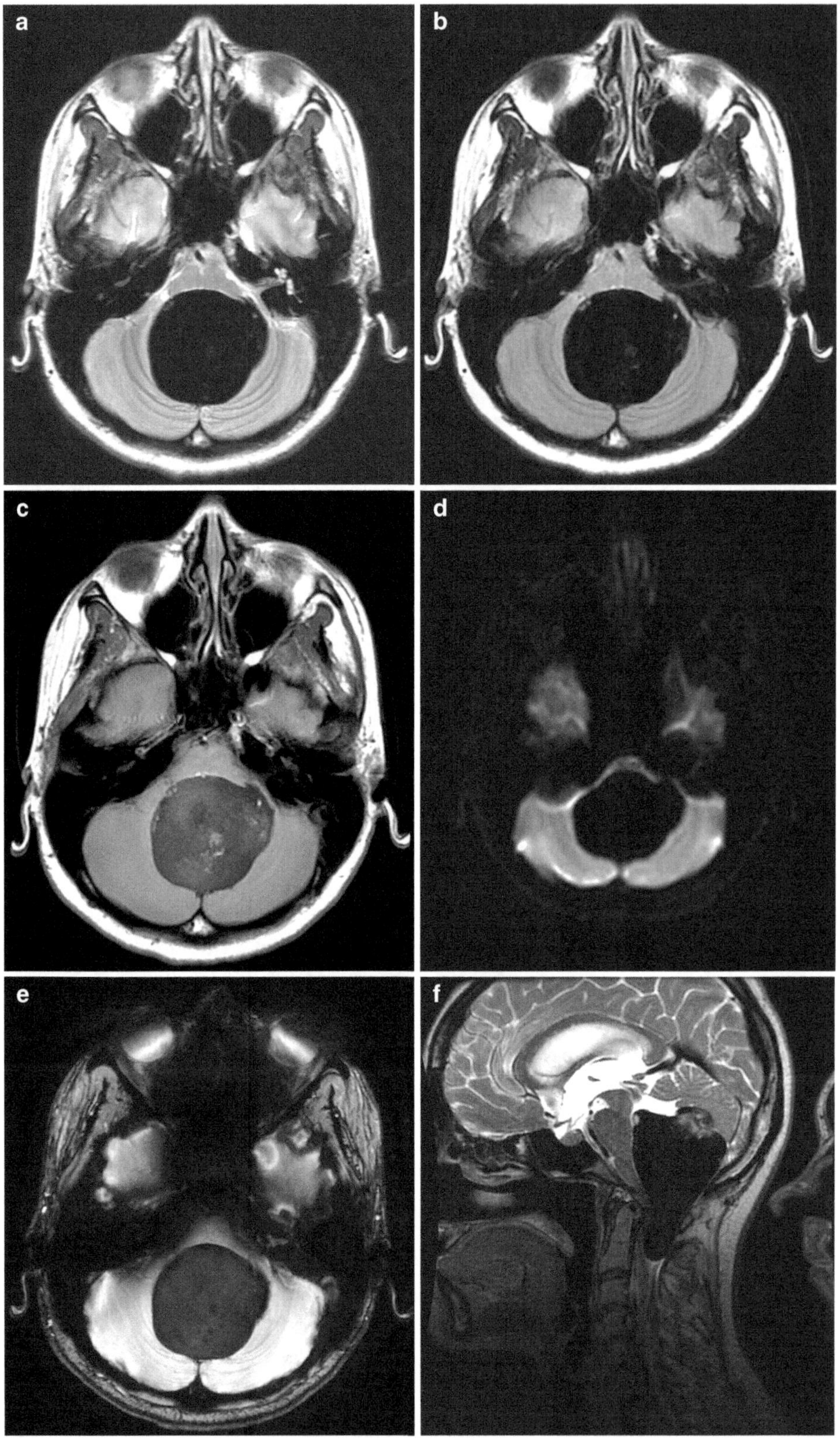

Fig. 22.12 Dermoid cyst of the posterior fossa. Axial T2- (**a**), T2-FLAIR- (**b**), T1- (**c**), DWI- (**d**), and SWAN- (**e**) weighted MR images demonstrate a large totally hypointense lesion in projection of lower aspects of 4th ventricle. There are few hyperintense on T1 inclusions within the lesion. Series sagittal MR images in T2- (**f**), T1- (**g**), and T1 with Fas-Sat (**h**) sequences show a strongly hypointense on T2 and heterogeneously iso-hyperintense on T1 MR images mass with extension into the spinal canal. The saturation of hyperintense MR-signal from fat tissue on T1 MRI with Fat-Sat technology can be seen. ASL MRI perfusion (**i**) demonstrates an absence of blood flow within the lesion ("negative" perfusion). On CT scans (**j**, **l**) the lesion has a hyperdense features with small calcified and fatty inclusions. (**k**) view of the lesion during surgery

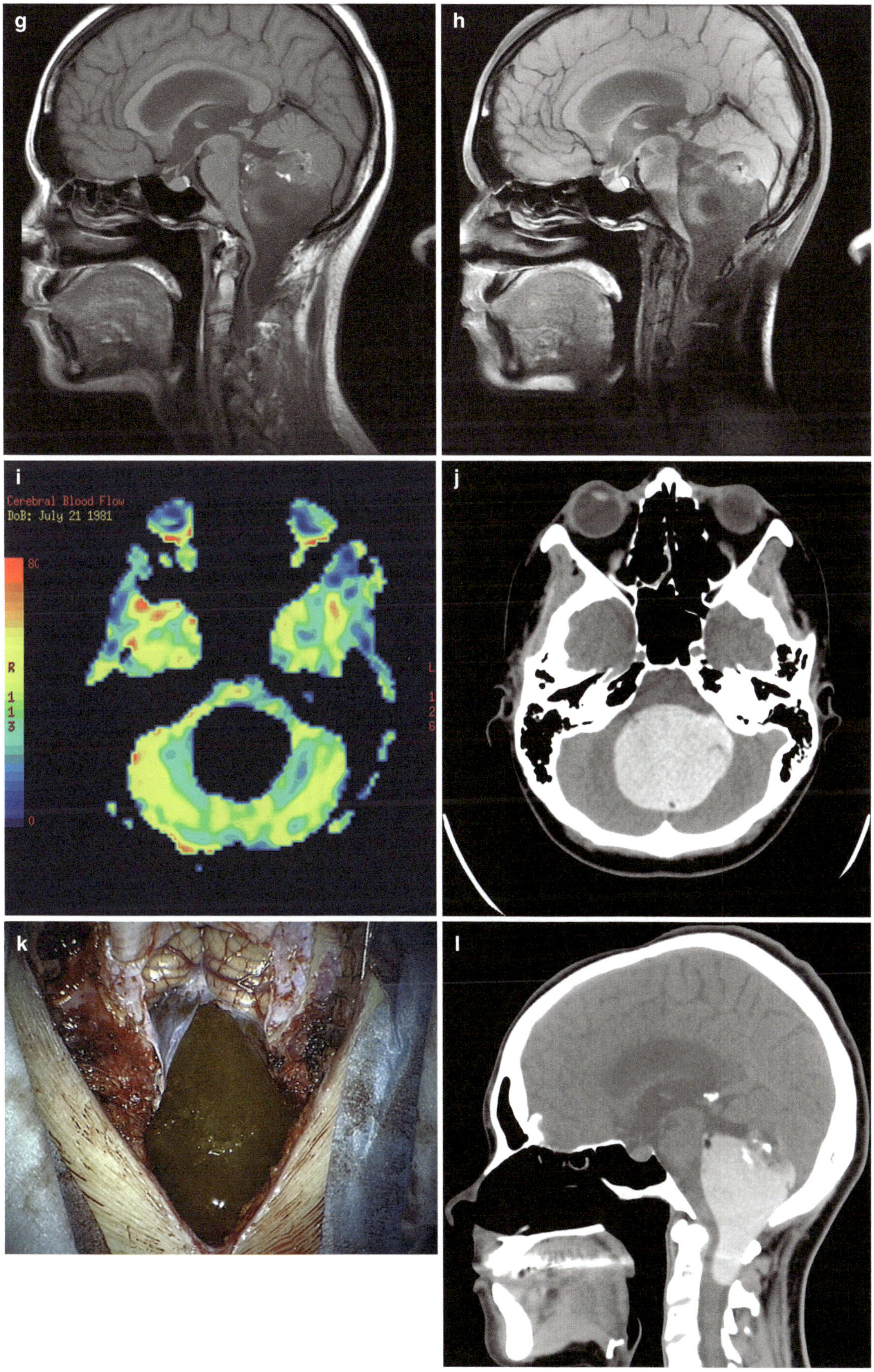

Fig. 22.12 (continued)

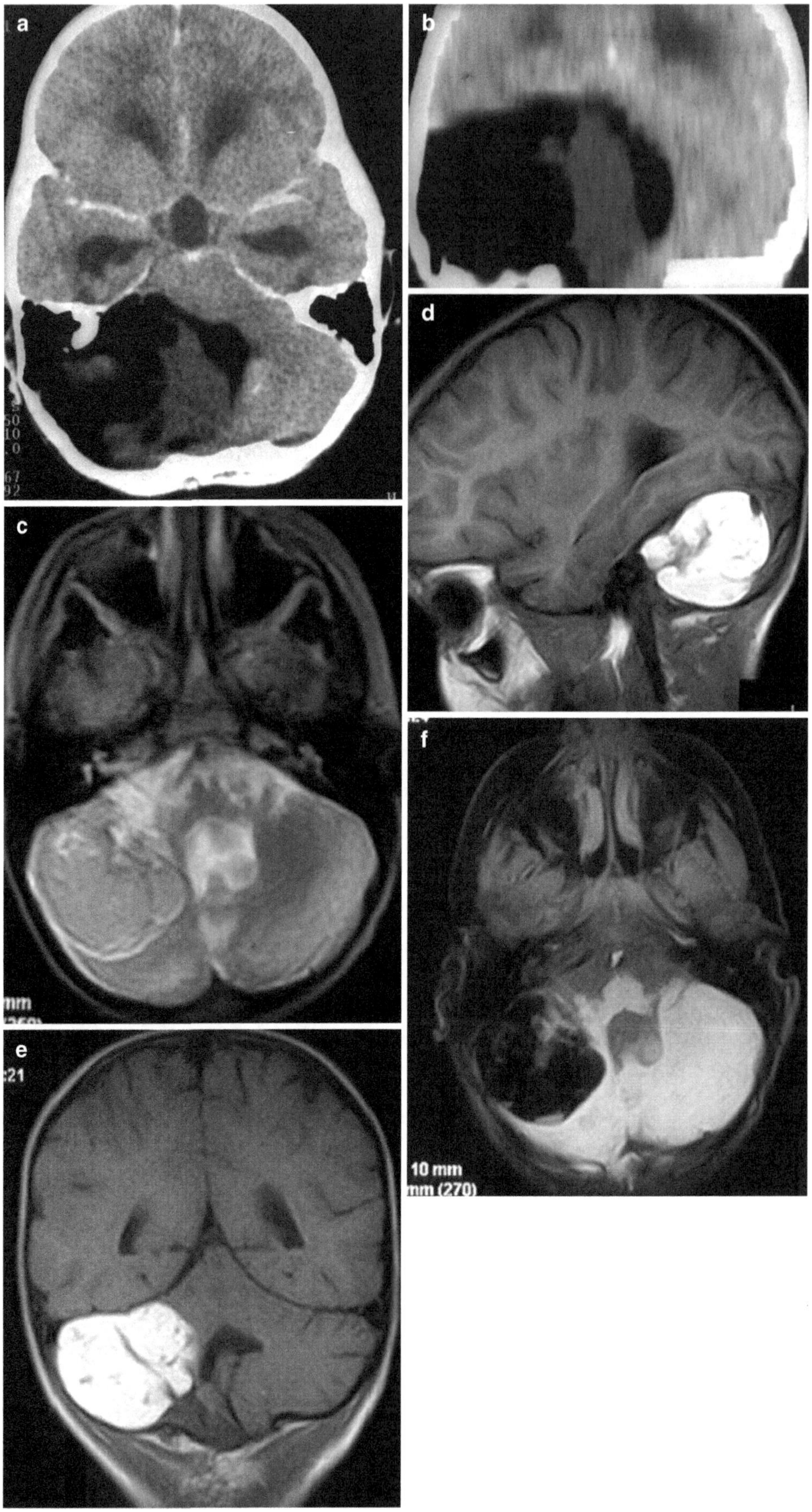

Fig. 22.13 Lipoma of the posterior cranial fossa. CT imaging in axial (**a**) and coronal (**b**) projections reveals a large hypodense lesion with heterogeneous structure that occupies the right half of posterior cranial fossa. T2- (**c**), T1- (**d**, **e**), and T1 + Fat-Sat (**f**)-weighted images show the lesion that has prominent hyperintense MR-signal in T1 and isointense to brain on T2. Fat suppression technology completely decreases the signal intensity from the lipoma

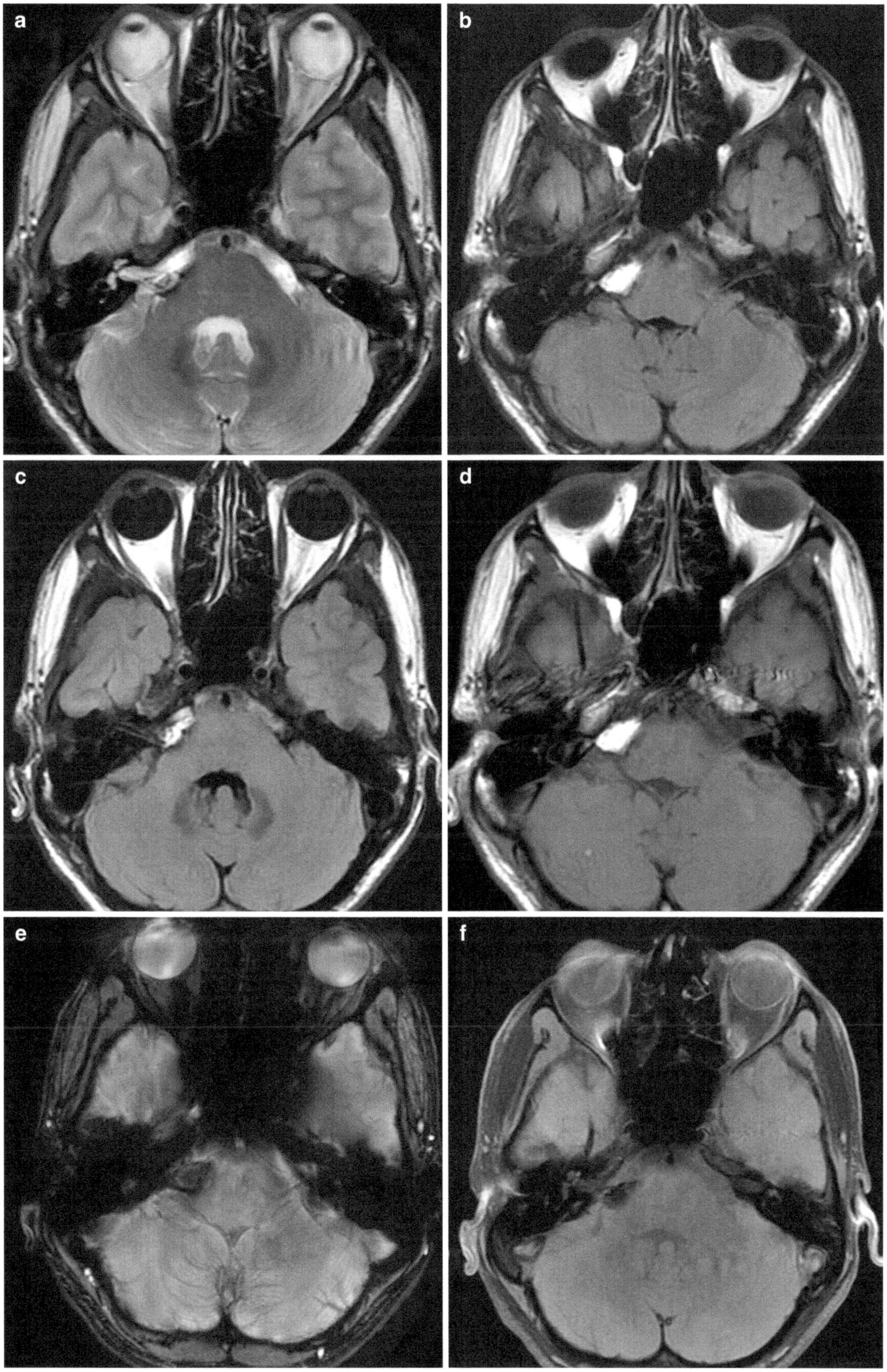

Fig. 22.14 Lipoma of the right cerebello-pontine angle. Axial T2- (**a**), T2-FLAIR- (**b**, **c**), and T1- (**d**) weighted images demonstrate a small hyperintense lesion in the projection of the cerebello-pontine angle. Hypointense band due to chemical shift artifact is identified in the T2-scan (**a**) on the border with brain stem. In SWAN sequence (**e**) the lipoma has hypointense MR-signal. Fat suppression technology completely decreases the signal intensity from the lipoma (**f**)

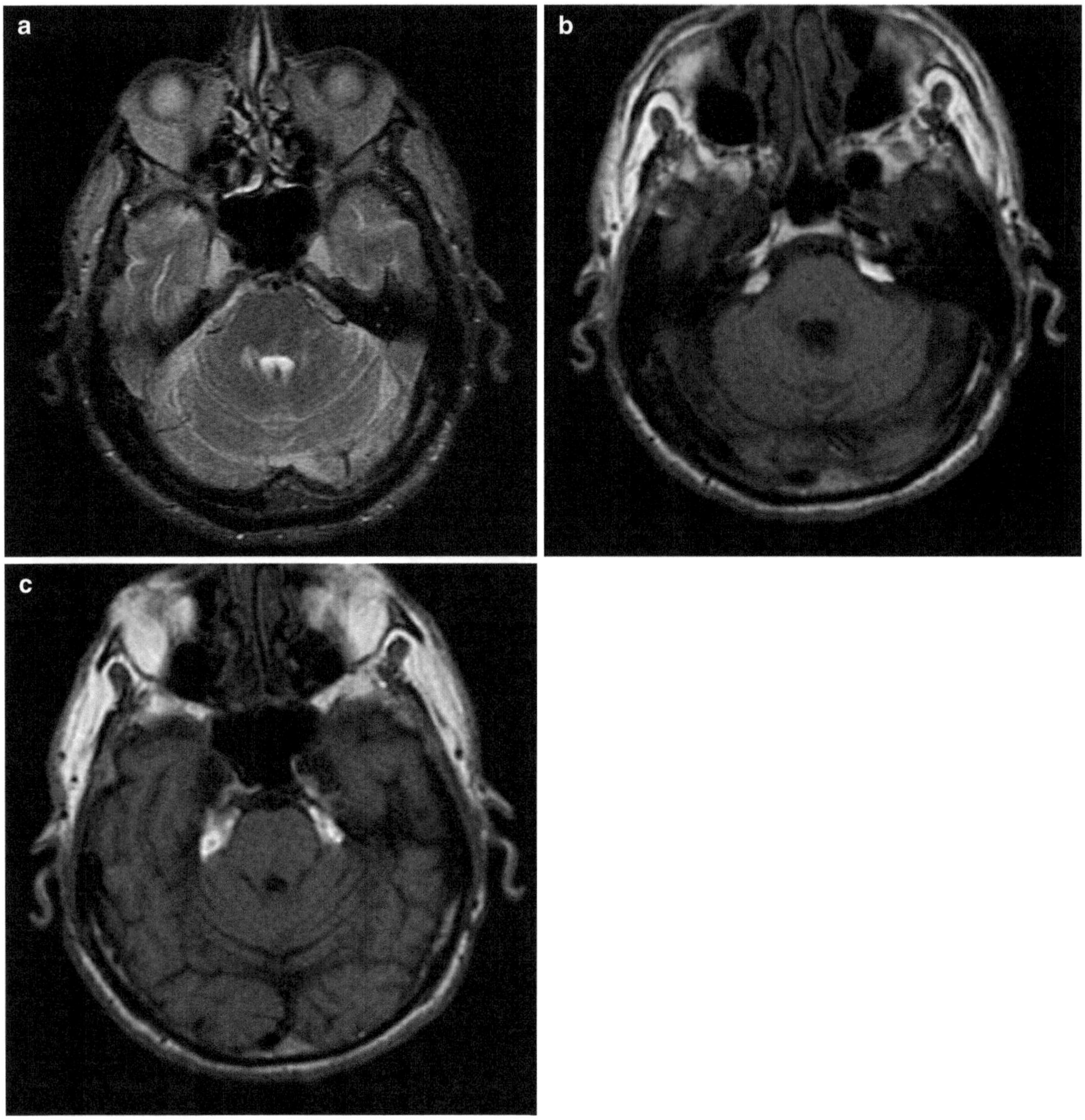

Fig. 22.15 MR imaging after the surgery concerning neurovascular conflict from both sides. The areas with MR-signal typical for adipose tissues on T2- (**a**) and T1- (**b**, **c**) weighted images are identified in the projection of the lateral cisterns of the pons. In this case fat tissue was used as a protector between the root of trigeminal nerve and the branches of the superior cerebellar arteries

The mechanism of mucocele development: occlusion of the excretory duct entry of the paranasal cavity causes excessive accumulation of continuously produced mucoid non-inflammatory fluid. There comes a point when the fluid doesn't fit the cell and begins to press on the mucosa and bone walls of the cavity. Due to constant pressure sinus walls begin to atrophy, get thinned and partially resorbed. The sinus cavity becomes enlarged.

Location the mucocele within the petrous apex is extremely rare. Unlike cholesterol granuloma, it does not contain blood lysis products. Like other lesions of the petrous apex, mucocele can clinically manifest by hearing loss, positional vertigo, headache, and facial spasms.

Imaging On CT, there is an increase in the petrous apex volume with the presence of the cavity (area of decreased density) limited by thin bony walls. Bony septa in the mucocele cavity are absent, but there is no evidence of bone destruction. Contrast media is not accumulated within said cystic cavity.

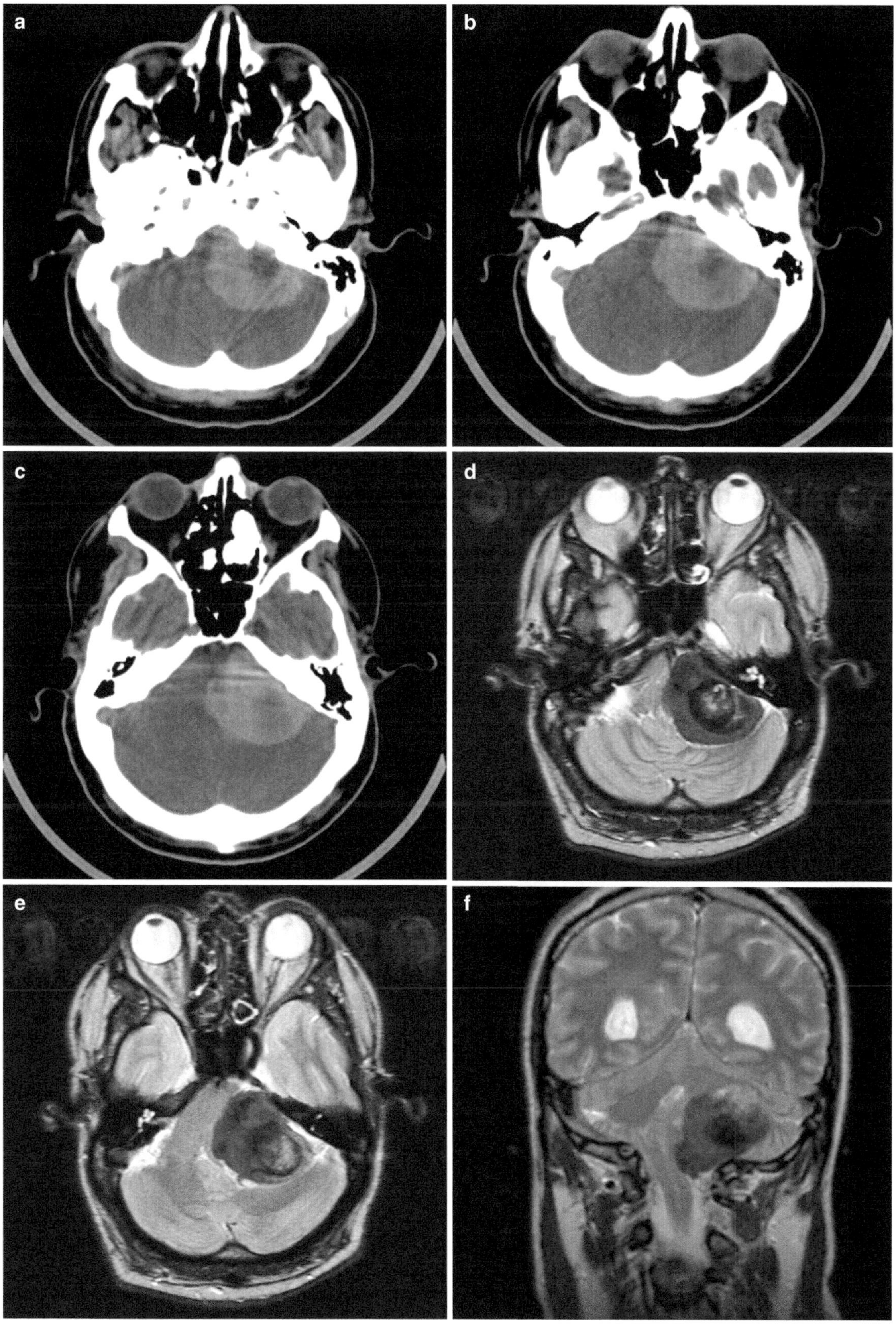

Fig. 22.16 Teratoma of the left cerebello-pontine angle. Axial NECT scans (**a–c**) reveal a hyperdense oval lesion with hypodense center that occupies the lateral aspects of the posterior cranial fossa. MR imaging using T2 (**d–f**)-weighted images shows the heterogeneous hypointense signal from the lesion. Coronal scan demonstrates the brain stem displacement. There is no perifocal edema. On T1-weighted images (**g–i**), the teratoma is characterized by the predominantly high MR-signal

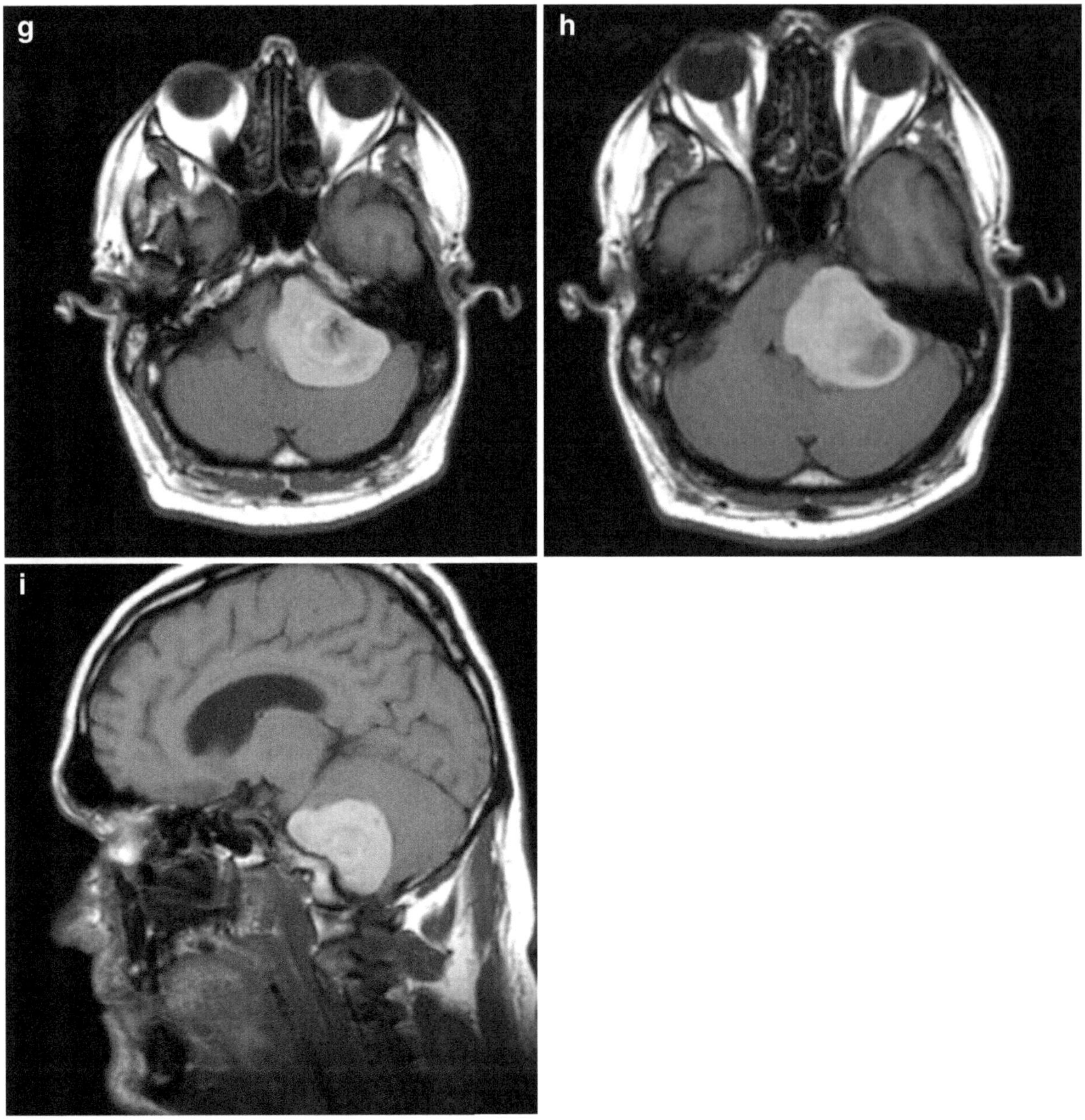

Fig. 22.16 (continued)

On MRI, mucocele contents have a hyperintense MR-signal on T2-weighted images. On T1-weighted images, a moderately pronounced increase in the MR-signal from the protein component is possible. On DWI, there are no signs of restricted diffusion (MR-signal is not increased, in contrast to pyocele and abscess). Contrast enhancement is not typical for mucocele (Fig. 22.19).

Differential Diagnosis Cholesteatoma (high signal on DWI MR), cystic schwannoma of V nerve (tumor capsule enhancement, a dumbbell form with growth along the root of the trigeminal nerve), chondrosarcoma (marked bone destruction and heterogeneous contrast enhancement).

Petrous Apex Cephalocele Cephalocele is a prolapse of meninges (+CSF) from the lateral aspects of the Meckel's cavity into the petrous apex (Gray et al. 1995). Etiological factors include acquired and congenital changes (Moore 2001). The clinical signs of this disorder include, in the first place, trigeminal neuralgia due to trigeminal nerve displacement and deformation.

Imaging MRI and CT can show both a uni- and bilateral cystic lesion with smooth walls and no signs of bone invasion, which has a relationship with the lateral parts of the Meckel's cavity and extends from there to the petrous apex (Klein et al. 1989). Multiplane MRI with the use of myelo-

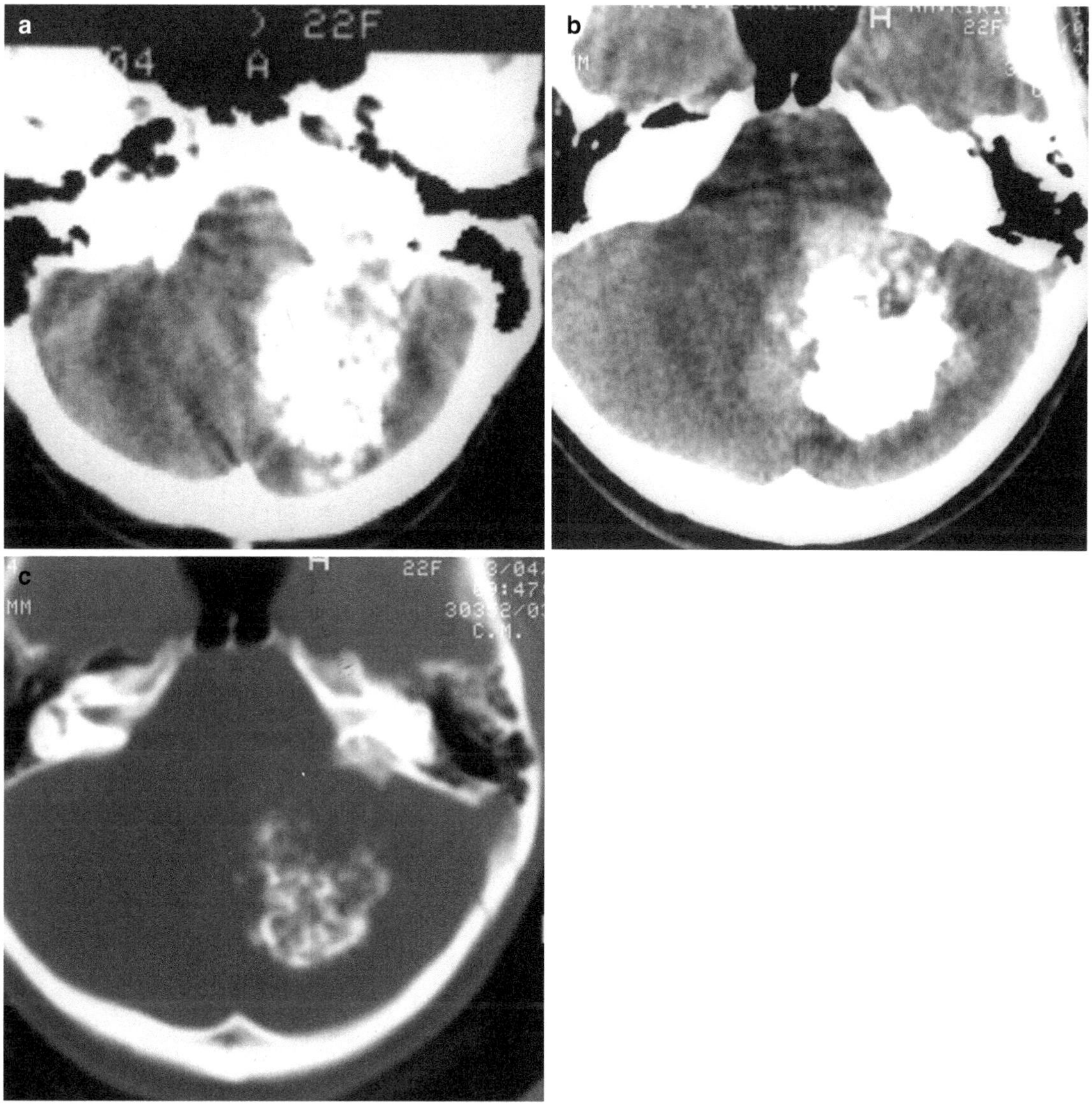

Fig. 22.17 Teratoblastoma of left cerebellar hemisphere. Axial CT scans (**a**, **b**, **c**) reveal a hyperdense tumor due to calcifications in its structure

graphic sequences is better for visualizing the relationship between cerebrospinal fluid spaces (e.g., Meckel's cavity) and the lesion (Figs. 22.20 and 22.21).

It is believed that CT cisternography is also a useful method for identification of the cerebrospinal fluid spaces with cephalocele located at this site.

The main feature that distinguishes cephalocele from inflammatory changes at the projection of the apex is eccentricity of localization of the lesion center closer to the Meckel's cavity, and not vice versa, at the projection of apical bone structures, like in cases with inflammation. In rare cases MRI can identify a prolapse of the adjacent temporal lobe part.

***Arachnoid cyst** of the petrous apex* is a very rare disorder diagnosed within the petrous apex. Its etiology is still unknown. Some authors attribute its occurrence at such an unusual site to a birth defect, others consider multifactorial etiology with a combination of inflammatory, traumatic causes and local defects in formation of the arachnoid membrane (Rock 1986). The diagnosis is confirmed by finding a cyst with radiographic signs indistinguishable from those of cerebrospinal fluid, with its walls being lined up with the arachnoid membrane and collagen.

Imaging CT and MRI visualize a cystic lesion without any evidence of bone destruction. On CT images, symptoms of

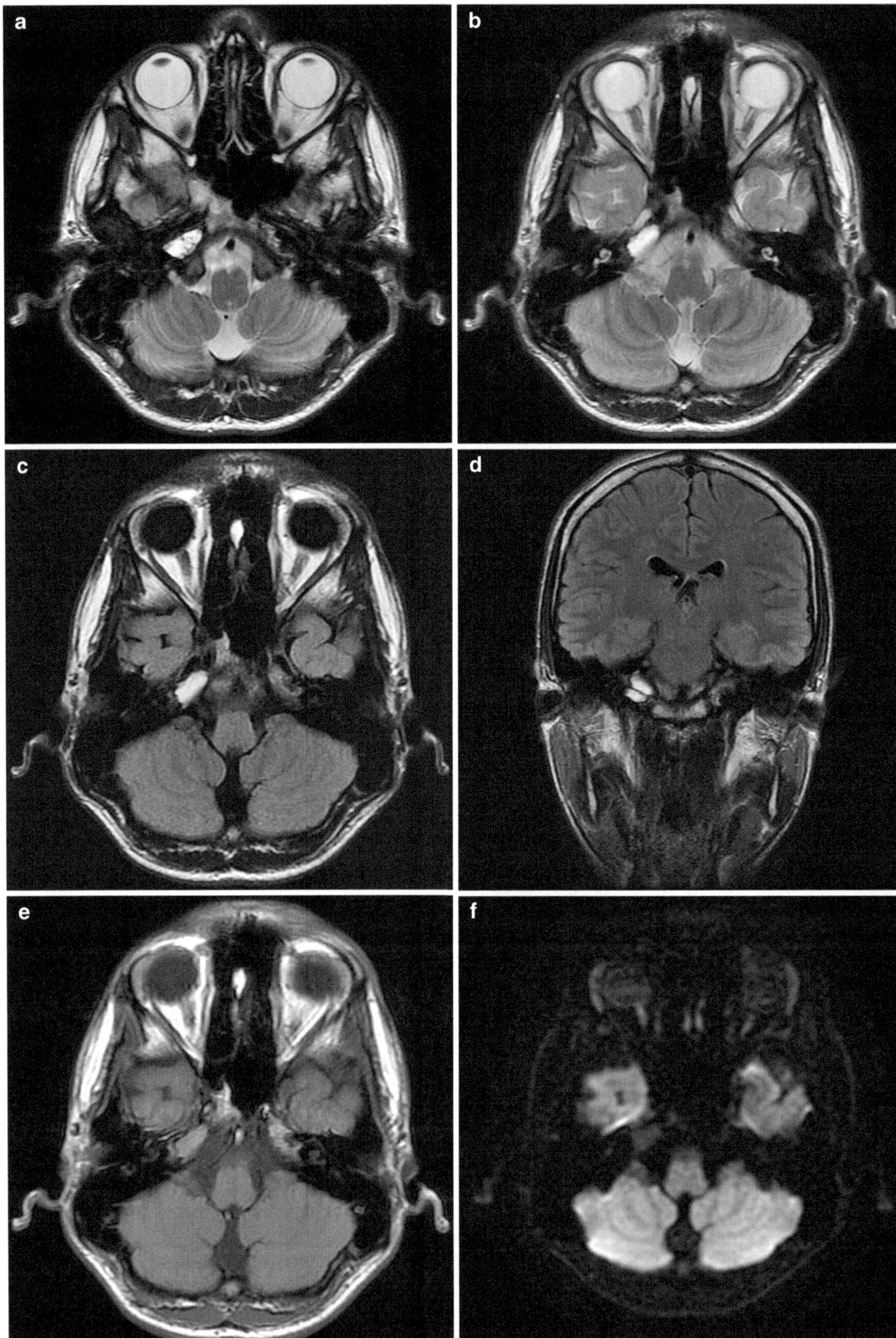

Fig. 22.18 Effusion. MR imaging using T2- (**a**, **b**) and T2-FLAIR- (**c**, **d**) weighted images reveal an area of hyperintense MR-signal in the projection of the pyramid apex of the right temporal bone. On T1-weighted image (**e**) the lesion has a slightly hyperintense signal compared to brain. There is no restriction diffusion within the exudate area on DWI (**f**)

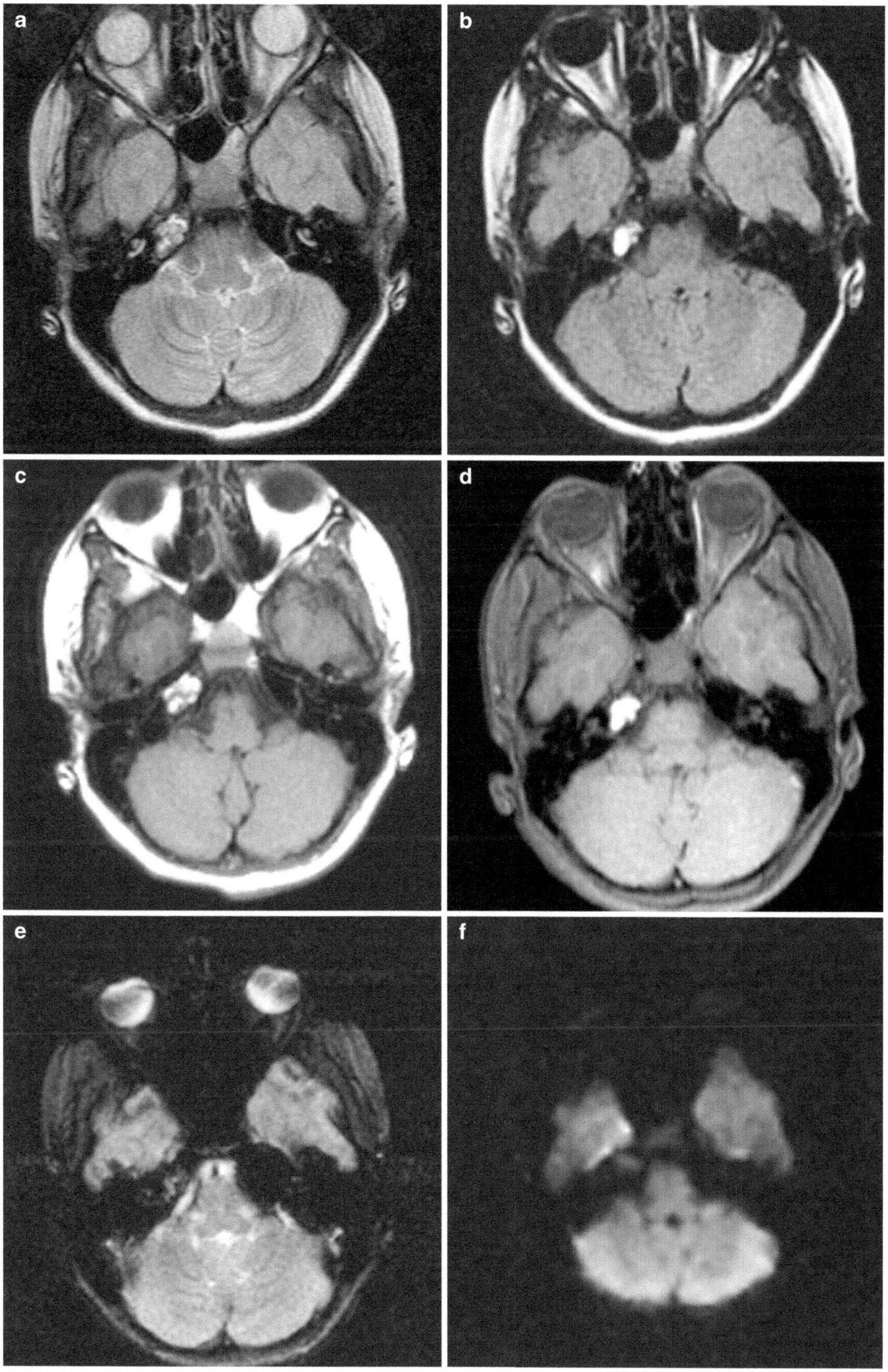

Fig. 22.19 Mucocele of the right pyramid apex. MRI using T2- (**a**), T2-FLAIR- (**b**), T1- (**c**), and T1 + Fat-Sat (**d**)-weighted images define the area of hyperintense MR-signal in the projection of the pyramid apex of the right temporal bone. T1-weighted image with suppression of fat excludes the presence of fat component in this area. MR-signal is slightly increased (**e**) on GRE image. Diffusion-weighted MRI (**f**) does not reveal diffusion restriction within the mucocele area

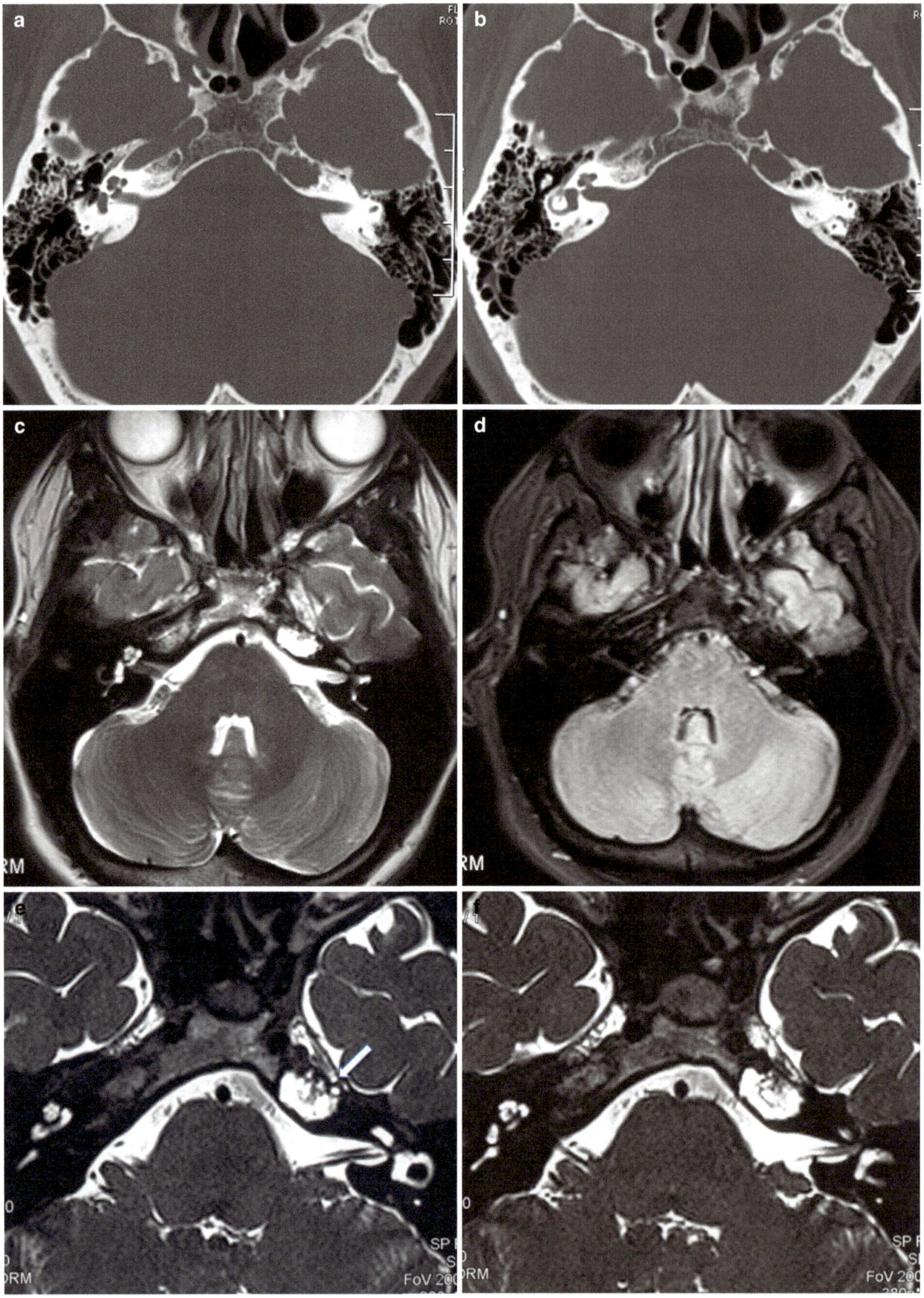

Fig. 22.20 Meningocele of the left pyramid apex of temporal bone. Axial CT scans (**a**, **b**) reveal an expansile lesion with irregular shape in the projection of the left apex of the temporal bone pyramid. MRI shows the hyperintense MR-signal on T2-weighted image (**c**), low signal on T2-FLAIR (**d**) image in accordance with the signal characteristics from CSF in the basal cisterns. FIESTA sequence demonstrates a small defect (*arrows*) in the posterior wall of Meckel's cavity, prolapse of meninges and cerebrospinal fluid spaces into the cavity of pyramid apex (**e–i**)

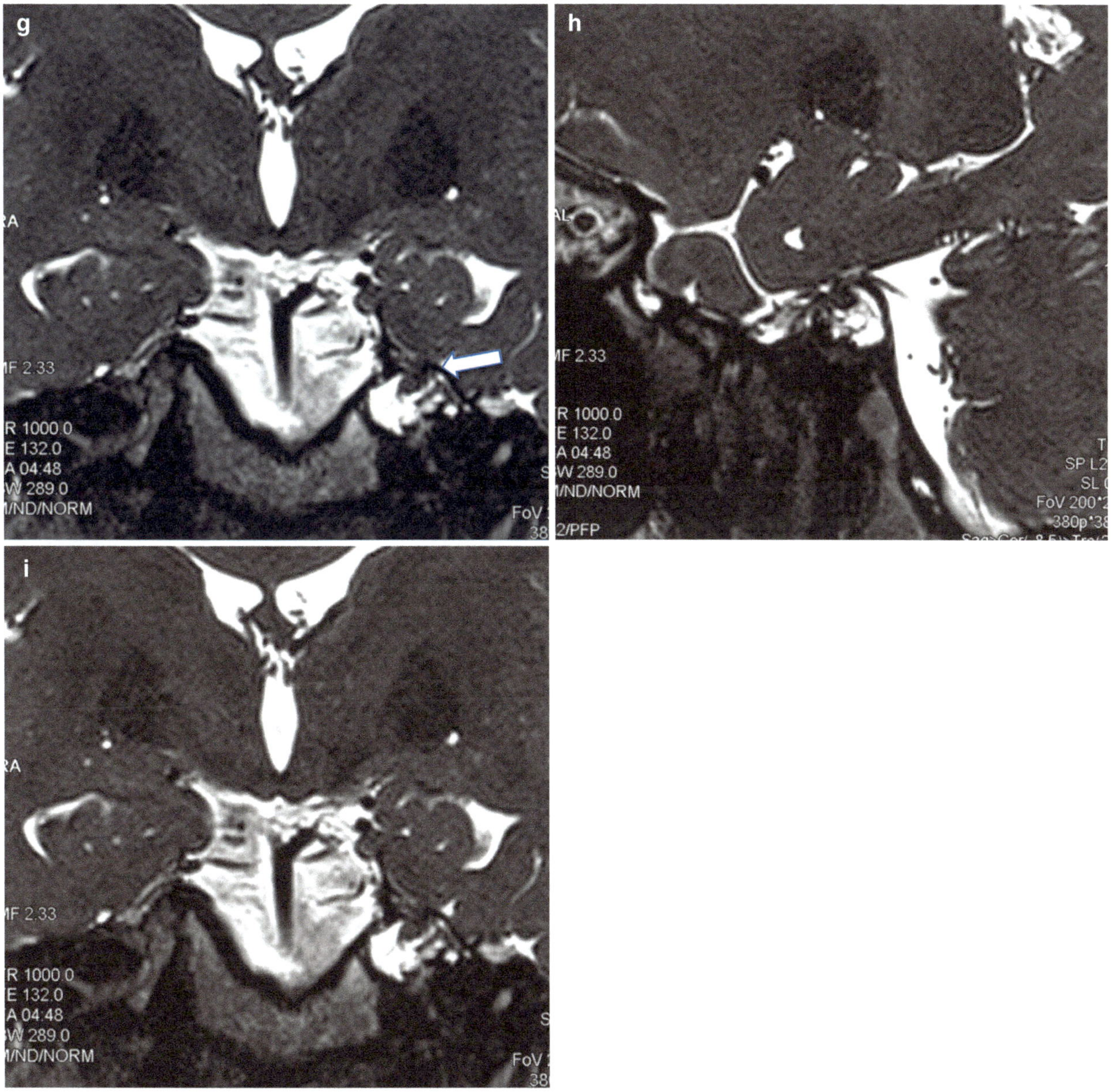

Fig. 22.20 (continued)

contents do not change density, nor MR-signal characteristics (Figs. 22.22, 22.23, 22.24, and 22.25).

Asymmetry and Dehiscence of the Jugular Vein Bulb It may be completely absent, or can be very pronounced, have a large size and reach the internal carotid artery trunk anteriorly, the facial nerve laterally, lead to a narrowing of the infralabyrinthine space and reach infralabyrinthine ampullar portion of the posterior semicircular canal. It may be located between the vestibule and the posterior cranial fossa or surround the vestibular aqueduct and reach the petrous ridge, being located between the lateral sinus outside and the internal acoustic meatus inside. This group of anatomical variations can also include a high riding jugular bulb and unilateral hypoplasia of the jugular vein with signs of narrowing of the bone ring on the side of hypoplasia. In an anatomical study on temporal bone blocks, an atypical high riding jugular bulb was found in 3.5–7% of samples (Katsuta and Rhoton 1997). At the same time, this is one of the most common types of vascular abnormalities in the structure of the pyramid, manifested by a jugular bulb spread to the middle ear with a prolapse of the sigmoid (jugular) plate. This type of disorder can be determined even by otoscopy. It is more common on the right side.

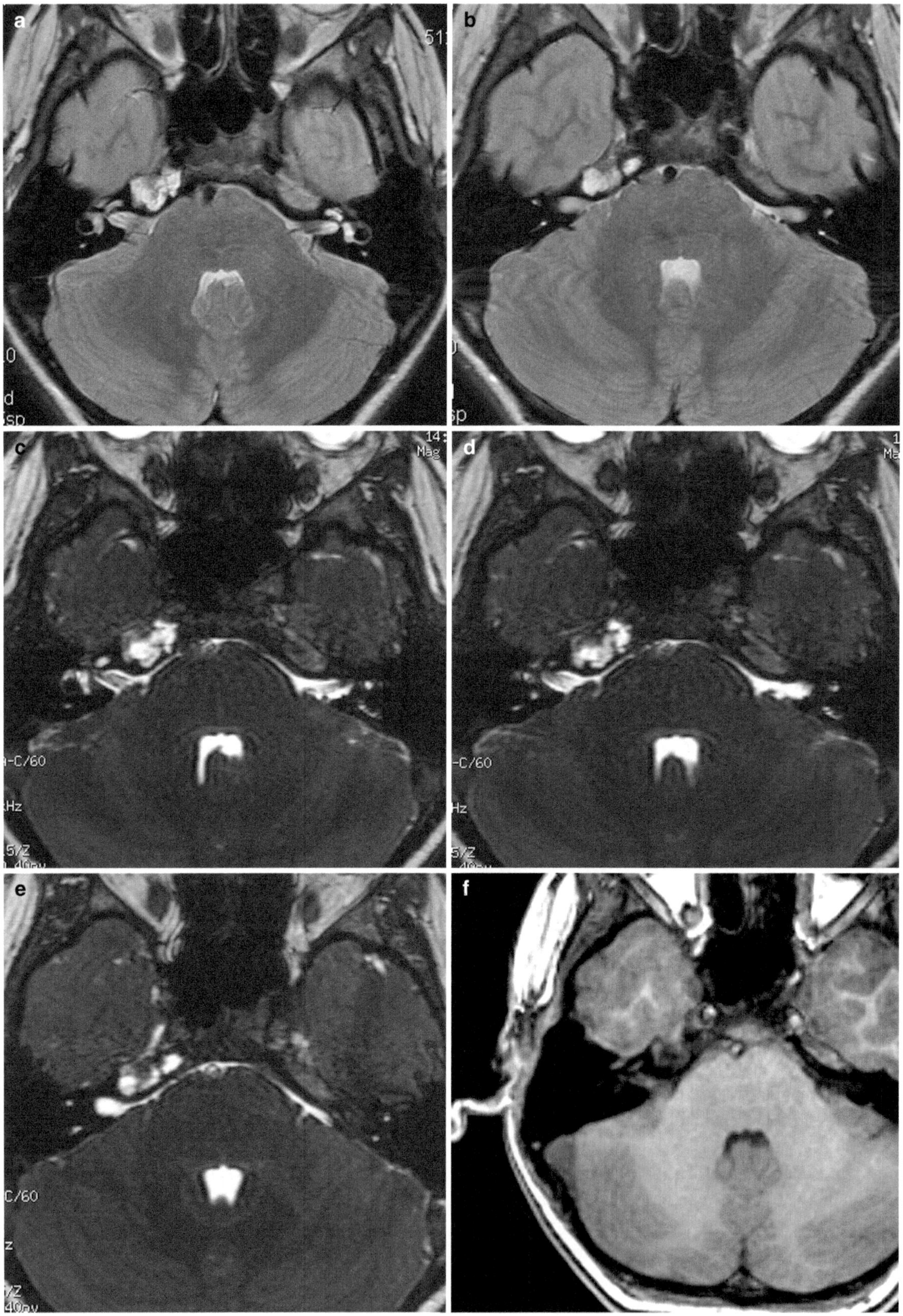

Fig. 22.21 Meningocele of the right pyramid apex of temporal bone. MR imaging with the use of T2 (**a**, **b**) and FIESTA sequence (**c**–**e**) demonstrates a lesion with a high MR-signal corresponding to the cerebrospinal fluid in the projection of the apex of the right pyramid. The defect of meninges in the posterior parts of Meckel's cavity and the prolapse of brain tissue into the meningocele cavity are visualized. T1-weighted images (**g**–**i**) show a local herniation of the brain tissue more distinctly (*arrows*)

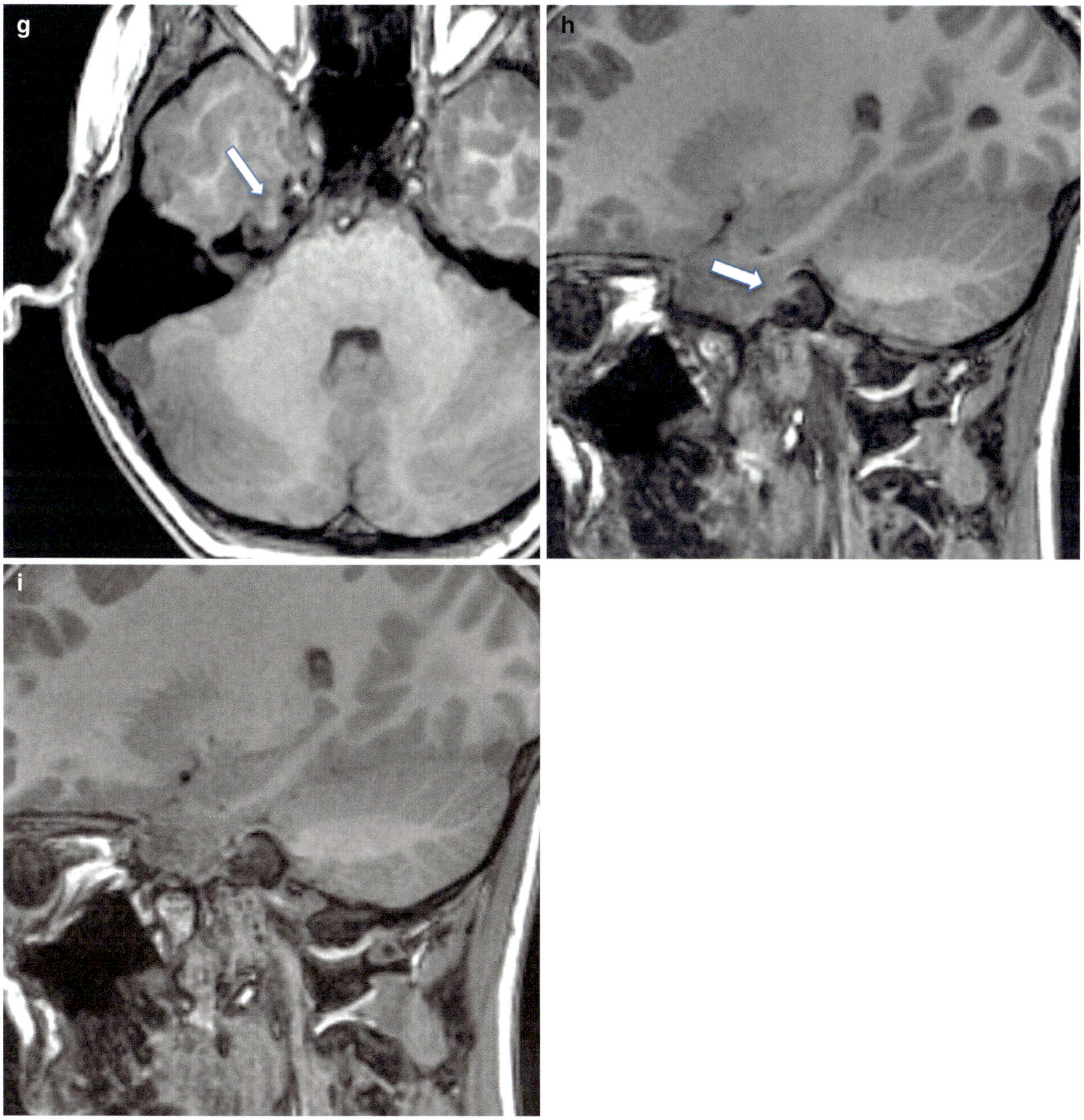

Fig. 22.21 (continued)

bone excavation are present, which suggests a prolonged cystic process (Lee et al. 1979). An MR-signal in all pulse sequences is identical to that of the cerebrospinal fluid in the cisterns of the skull base. There is no abnormal enhancement within the arachnoid cyst following the intravenous contrast agents administration. *The differential diagnosis* is carried out with all apical cystic lesions, especially with effusion, mucocele, cephalocele, and cholesteatoma.

Arachnoid cysts of the cerebellopontine angle are rare, sometimes they are visualized in conjunction with cysts of the other (sub- and supratentorial) brain areas. Clinical manifestations of these cysts depend on their size. They grow slowly (like all arachnoid cysts), so their symptoms are milder than those of tumors. Arachnoid cysts can sometimes extend into the middle cranial fossa with a brain aqueduct deformation, leading to obstructive hydrocephalus.

Imaging On CT and MRI, contours of cysts are well-defined, smooth, without any perifocal edema. Their density on CT and MR relaxation properties are similar to those of CSF on all modes and sequences. Unlike tumors, after administration of the contrast agent, cystic walls and their

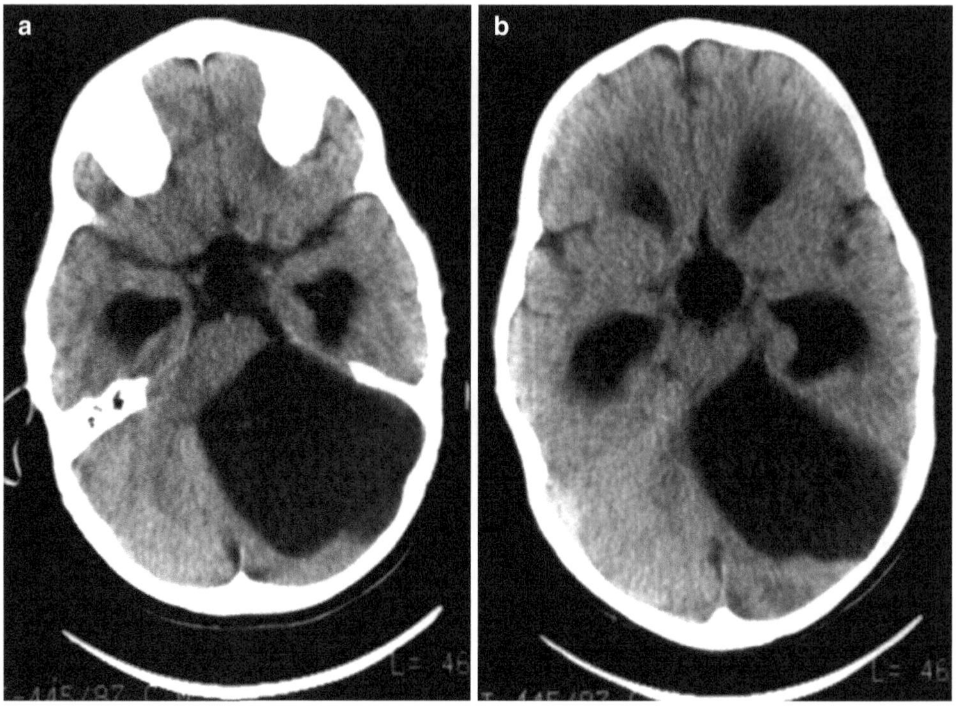

Fig. 22.22 Arachnoid cyst of left half of the posterior cranial fossa. Axial NECT scans (**a**, **b**) define a large isodense with cerebrospinal fluid lesion in the lateral part of the posterior cranial fossa. The brain stem and the cerebellar vermis are deformed. Lateral and the third ventricles are enlarged due to compression of brain aqueduct

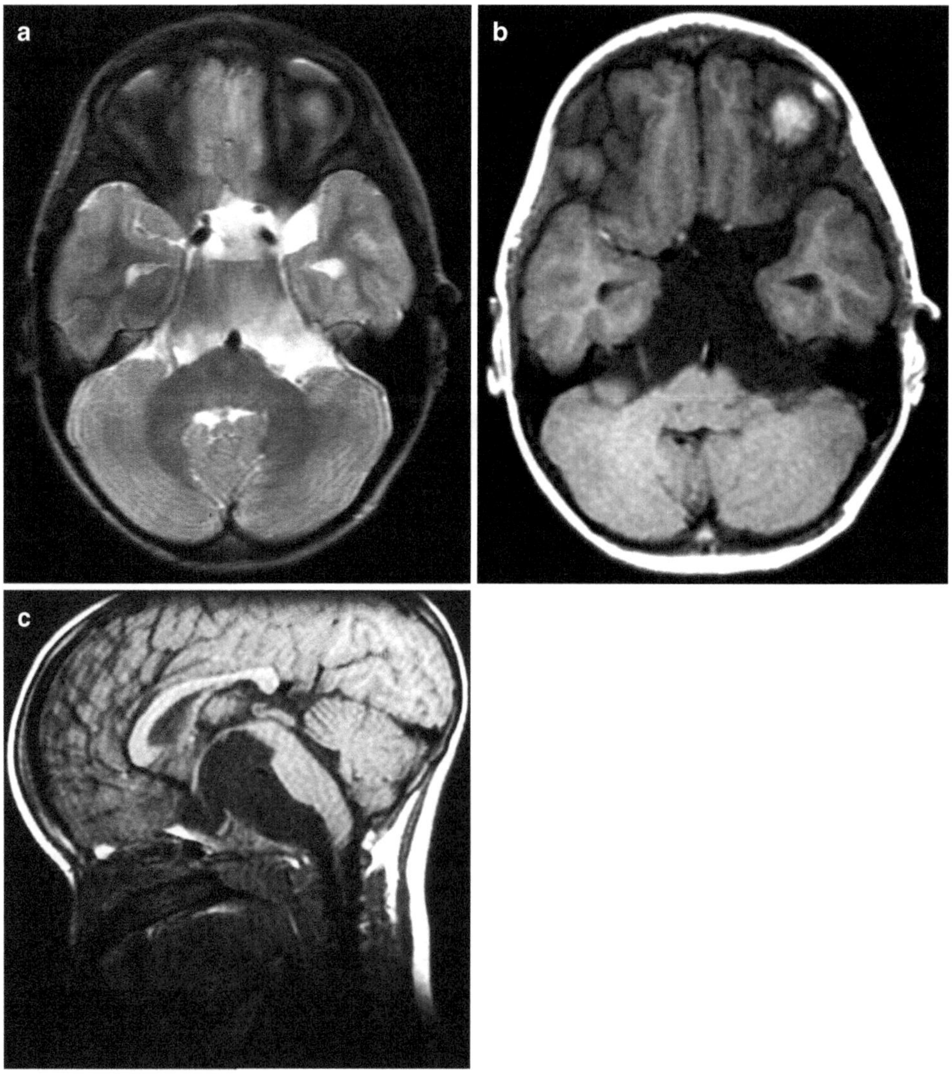

Fig. 22.23 Arachnoid cyst of the basal cisterns. Axial T2- (**a**) and T1- (**b**, **c**) weighted images show a large isointense to CSF lesion that dislocates the pons posteriorly and causes of arch-like displacement of floor of the 3rd ventricle

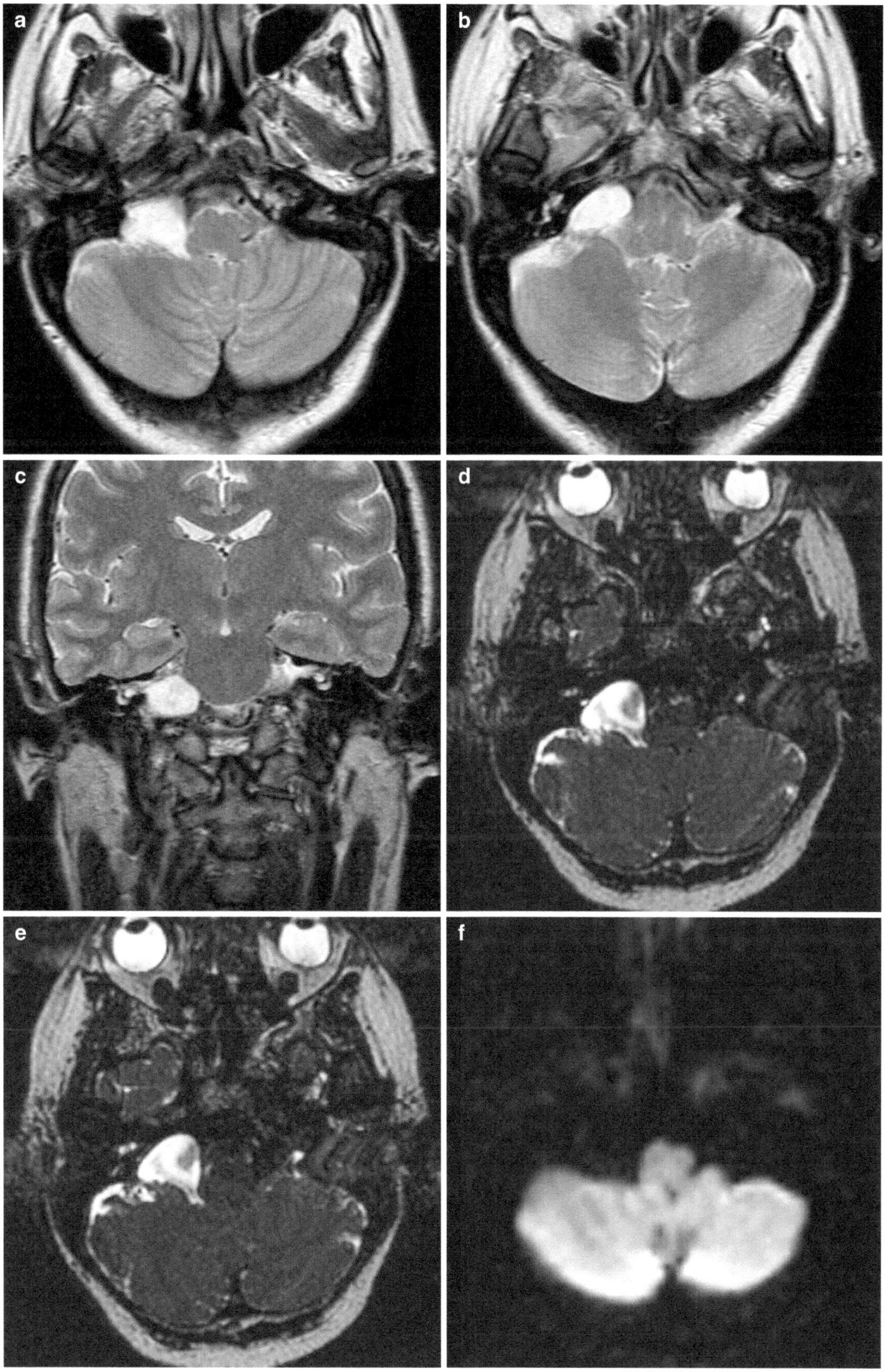

Fig. 22.24 Arachnoid cyst of the right cerebello-pontine angle. Axial and coronal T2- (**a**, **b**, **c**) and PSIF- (**d**, **e**) weighted images show a hyperintense lesion that has identical features to the CSF. There is no restricted diffusion on diffusion-weighted image, cyst is characterized by low MR-signal intensity (**f**)

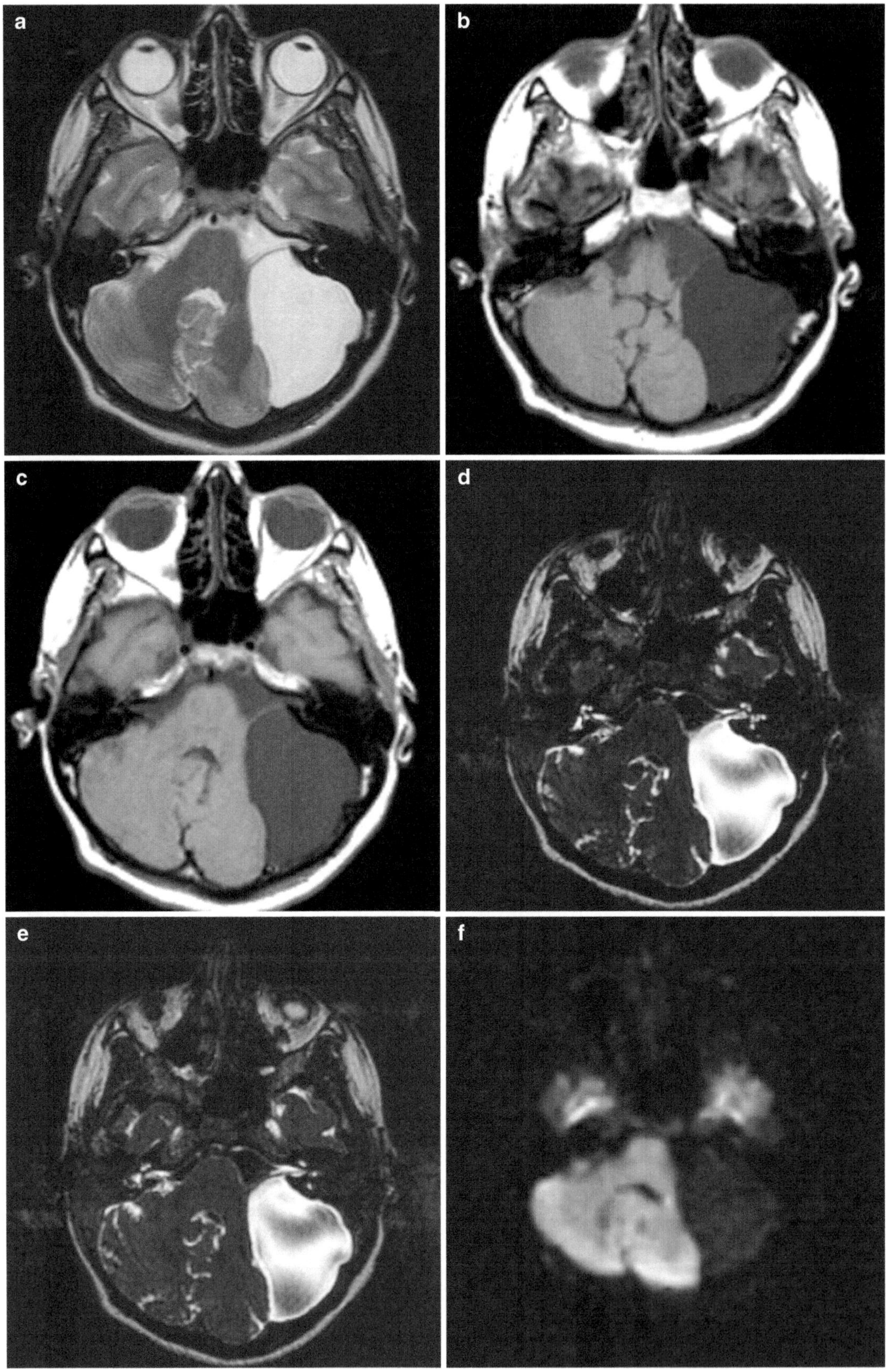

Fig. 22.25 Arachnoid cyst of the left half of posterior fossa. Axial T2- (**a**), T1- (**b**, **c**), and PSIF- (**d**, **e**) weighted images show a large cystic lesion that has identical features to the CSF. PSIF sequence demonstrates the cyst separation from the basal cisterns where low MR-signal due to pulsation of CSF is visualized. There is no restricted diffusion on diffusion-weighted image (**f**), cyst is characterized by low MR-signal intensity

It should be noted that asymmetry of jugular bulbs, often diagnosed with direct venography, routine CT studies or MR venography, is a variant that should be regarded as normal (the right one is usually larger) rather than abnormality. This is associated with a wide dural sinus and jugular vein itself on the relevant side. An important additional diagnostic criterion in favor of normal variant is absence of defects in the surrounding bony structures. As a rule, abnormal deformation in the jugular bulb area is clinically asymptomatic, but in some cases, such changes may be accompanied by pulsating tingling, headaches, unilateral hearing loss. This pathology is often regarded as so-called diagnostic "findings" discovered when examining patients for other reasons.

Imaging In case of simple anatomical asymmetry, CT reveals a unilateral increase of the jugular foramen, without surrounding bone erosions. A high riding enlarged jugular bulb is distinguished by a marked expansion of the roof of the jugular bulb upwards, sometimes up to the internal auditory canal. This is the main diagnostic feature of this "abnormality." Following standard contrast enhancement (more specific than bolus mode), a concomitant filling of the sigmoid sinus, jugular bulb and internal jugular vein itself with the absence of filling defects within their lumen is observed (Caldemeyer et al. 1997) (Fig. 22.26).

Sometimes, together with enlargement of the jugular bulb ("bulging bulb") and expansion of the jugular foramen, lysis

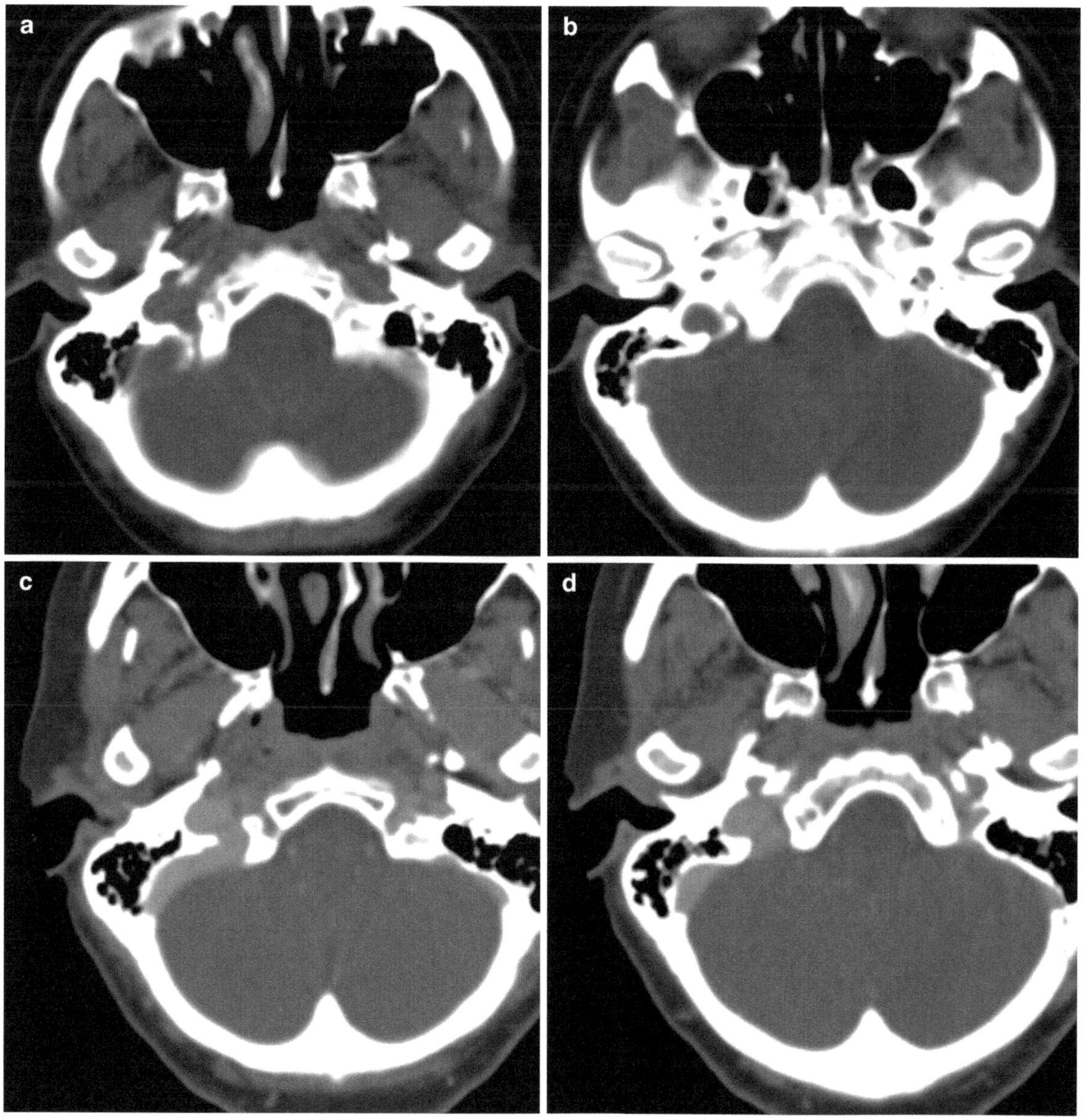

Fig. 22.26 Dilatation of the right jugular vein foramen. On series of NECT scans (**a**, **b**) the increase in size of right jugular vein foramen is visualized. The left jugular vein foramen is narrowed. CT angiography (**c**–**f**) reveals the uniform filling with contrast agent the dilated jugular bulb on the right. CT-perfusion study (CBF (**g**), CBV (**h**), MTT (**i**)) confirms the hemodynamics characteristics of venous flow in the right jugular vein bulb

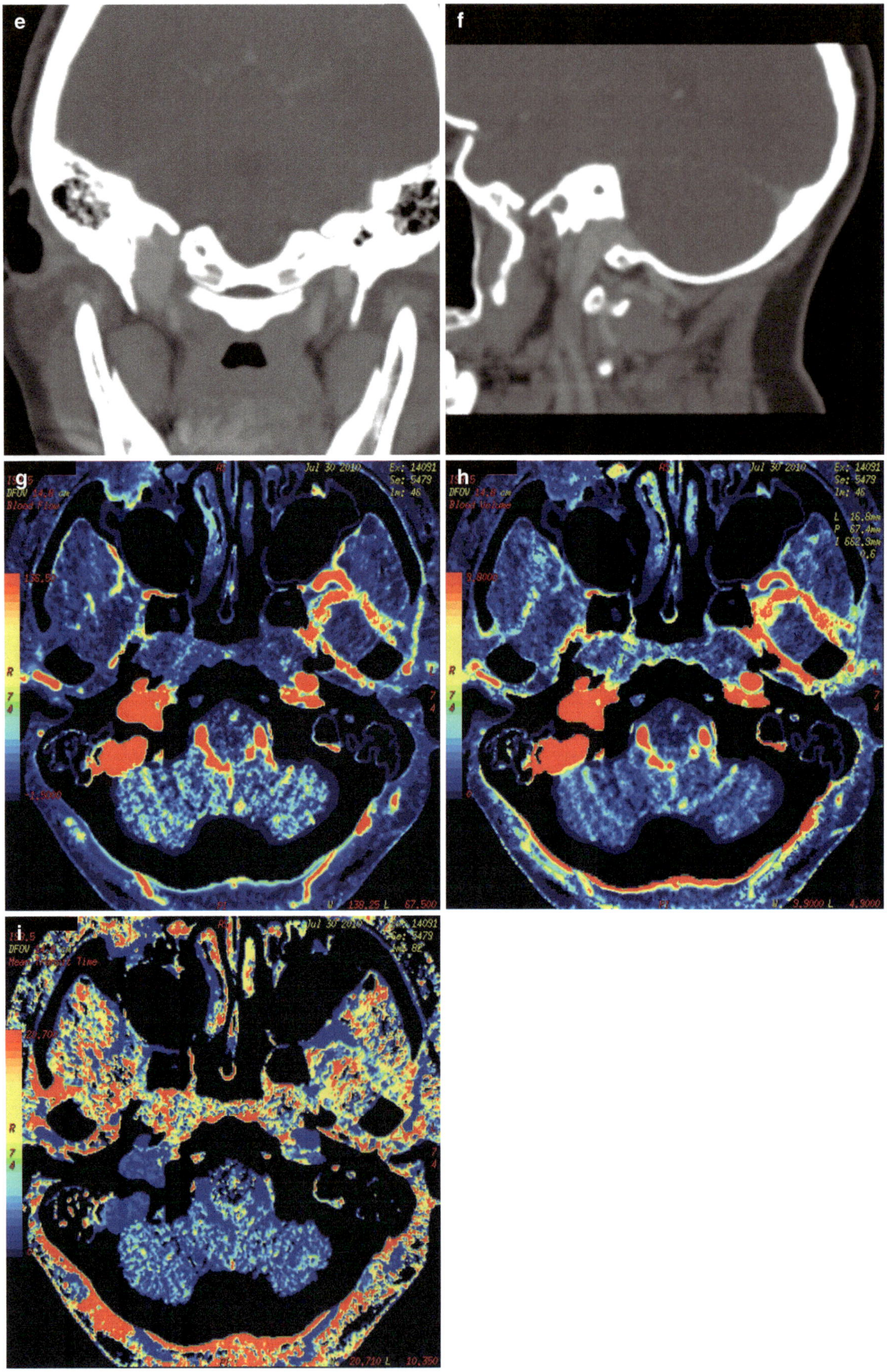

Fig. 22.26 (continued)

of one bony walls with possible partial prolapse into posterior inferior aspects of the tympanic cavity can be observed on CT. An absence of bone destruction of the remaining foramen walls and homogeneous contrast enhancement rules out any other origin of bone changes.

MRI usually demonstrates a heterogeneous MR-signal on standard T1- and T2-weighted sequences with signs of blood flow turbulence at the projection of the jugular foramen within the jugular vein (Fig. 22.27).

A useful method for identification of "abnormality" (or a normal variant) is MR-venography with 2D TOF or 3D PC sequences, which do not differentiate MR-signal differences from the jugular vein. Homogeneous contrast enhancement within the venous system also supports vascular and non-neoplastic origin of the detected asymmetry.

Differential Diagnosis Jugular vein diverticulum, paraganglioma (accompanied by destructive changes of the bone, abundant vasculature on angiography), jugular foramen schwannoma (filling defect on CT-angiography, contrast-enhanced lesion on T1-weighted Fat-Sat sequences), meningioma (sclerotic or hyperostotic bone changes along the jugular foramen contrast enhancement reveals a dural "tail").

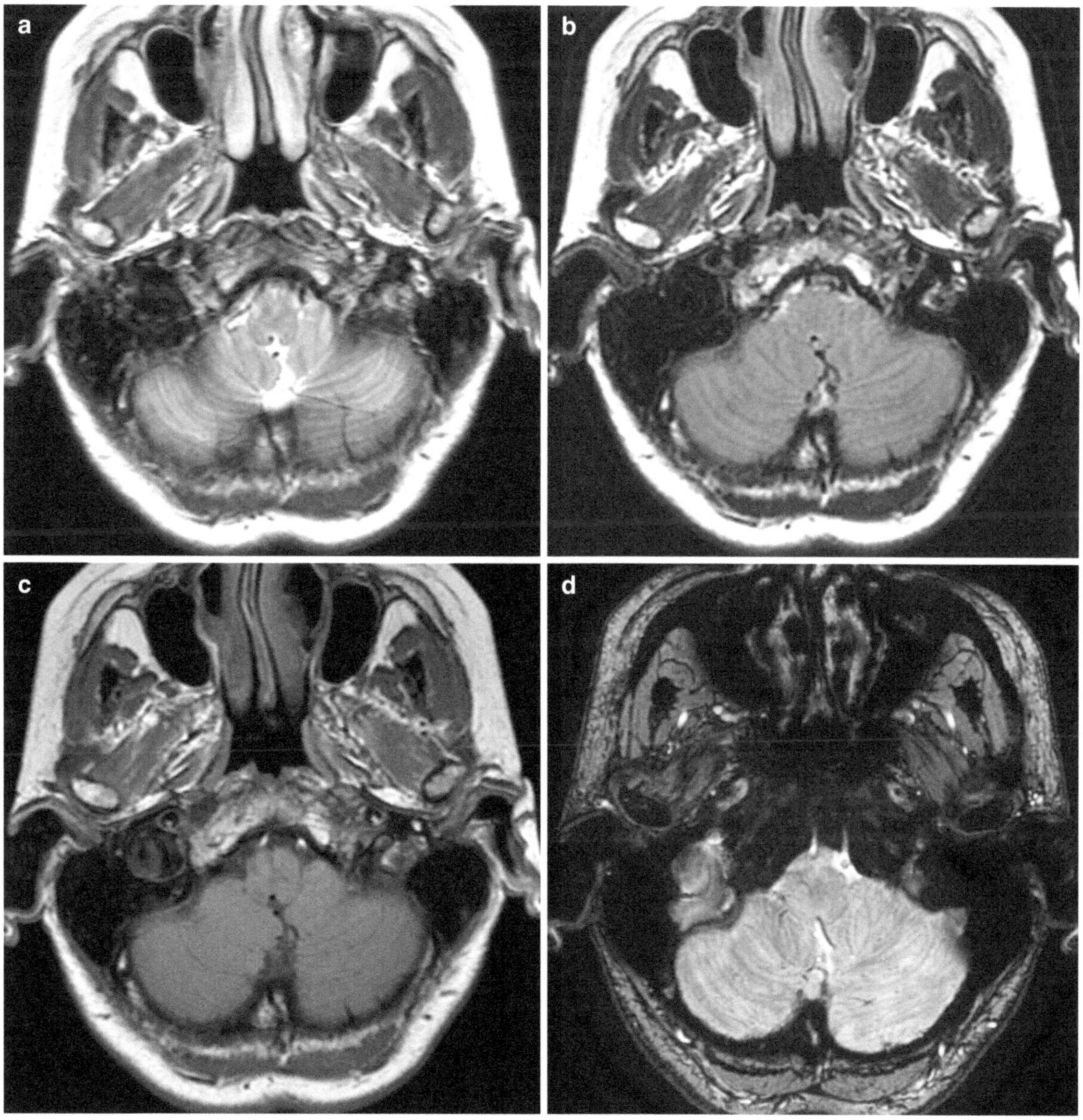

Fig. 22.27 Dilatation of the right jugular vein foramen (CT data were presented in Fig. 22.26). On T2- (**a**), T2-FLAIR- (**b**), T1- (**c**), and SWAN- (**d**) weighted MR images the asymmetrical increase in size of right jugular vein foramen is revealed. Within the dilated jugular bulb the artifact from hyperpulsation and fast flow is visible. MR-angiography (**e**) demonstrates the typical location of internal carotid artery regarding jugular vein. Contrast-enhanced images (**f–h**) show a heterogeneous and hyperintense MR-signal in projection of increased jugular bulb. Coronal T2-weighted image (**i**) demonstrates a dilated right internal jugular vein

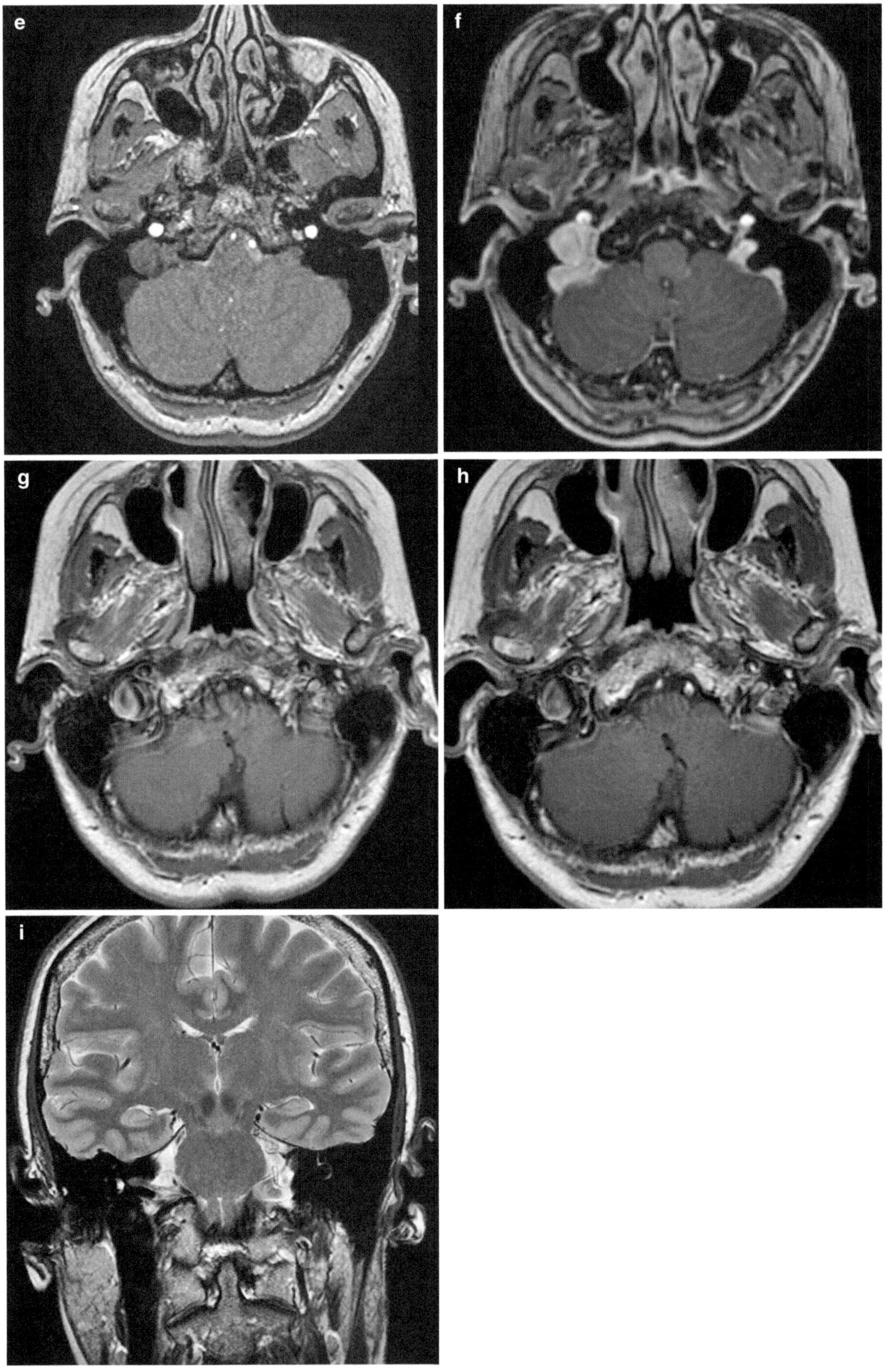

Fig. 22.27 (continued)

Jugular vein bulb diverticulum is a separate type of deformation of the jugular bulb, which often occurs as a post-traumatic complication. Morphologically it appears as a saccular protrusion of the cranial parts of the bulb. The sigmoid plate remains intact. It occurs more frequently on the left side. It is usually asymptomatic, but may cause dizziness, unilateral pulsating tingling (Presutti et al. 1991; Bilgen et al. 2003).

Imaging CT scans reveal inversion of the jugular bulb, which finger-like prolapses into bones upwards, may have a little neck; cortical bone of the adjacent structures is intact. It enhances on post-contrast scans concurrently with other venous structures.

On T2-weighted MR images this variant often cannot be visualized because of its small size and low MR signal from the flowing blood. Sometimes due to turbulence an increased signal occurs on T1-weighted images. Contrast agent fills the diverticulum cavity, as well as the jugular bulb and vein (Schmerber et al. 2002). In case of suspected diverticulum, contrast-enhanced 3D TOF MR angiography with subsequent multi-plane reformation at the pyramid level may be useful.

Differential Diagnosis Dural fistula (there is arterial inflow from dural meningeal blood vessels), cholesteatoma (high MR signal on DWI), paraganglioma (bone destruction, etc.).

22.3 Acquired Disorders

22.3.1 Tumor-like Lesion

Cholesterol granuloma (xanthogranuloma) belongs to one of the most frequent pathologies encountered within the pyramid apex (about 60% of cases). It develops mainly at the projection of the pneumatized part of the apex, the reason for its formation is inadequate ventilation of pneumatic cells or bone marrow hyperplasia (Jackler et al. 2003). Repeated cycles of cell obstruction in combination with bleeding and formation of cholesterol crystals result in the formation of a granuloma. This lesion usually reaches a large size at the time of initial diagnosis. Histopathologically, the granuloma has a thin capsule without typical characteristics of chronic subdural hematoma. The typical feature is the presence of cholesterol crystals in different proportions in the cystic component. After surgical removal it appears as a cystic lesion with brown liquid component (Griffin 1987).

Imaging CT study reveals an expansively growing cystic mass lesion at the projection of the pyramid apex with a smooth inner contour formed by thinned bones. If sufficiently large, there are areas of bone lysis. In this area, CT with contrast enhancement can visualize a weakly enhanced thin capsule (Fig. 22.28).

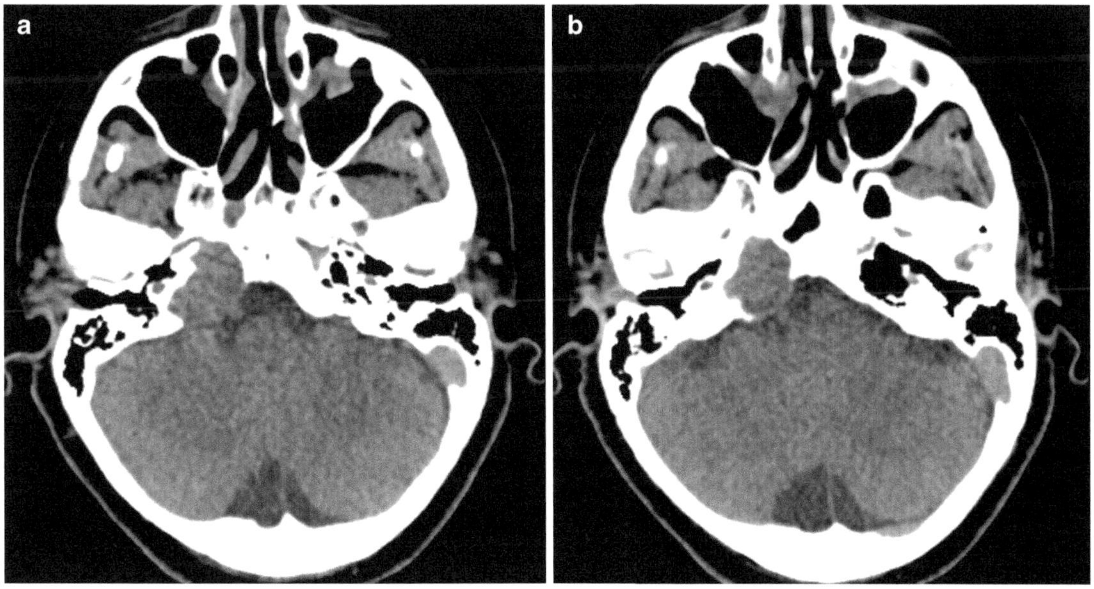

Fig. 22.28 Xanthogranuloma of the right apex of temporal bone pyramid. Axial CT scans in standard (**a**, **b**) and bone window (**c**, **d**) mode demonstrate an expansile lesion in projection of right pyramid apex with fairly clear contours. On T2-weighted (**e**) image the lesion has heterogeneous and hypointense MR-signal. T1-weighted images (**f**, **g**) show a high signal from the lesion, that doesn't change on T1-Fat-Sat images (**h**, **i**)

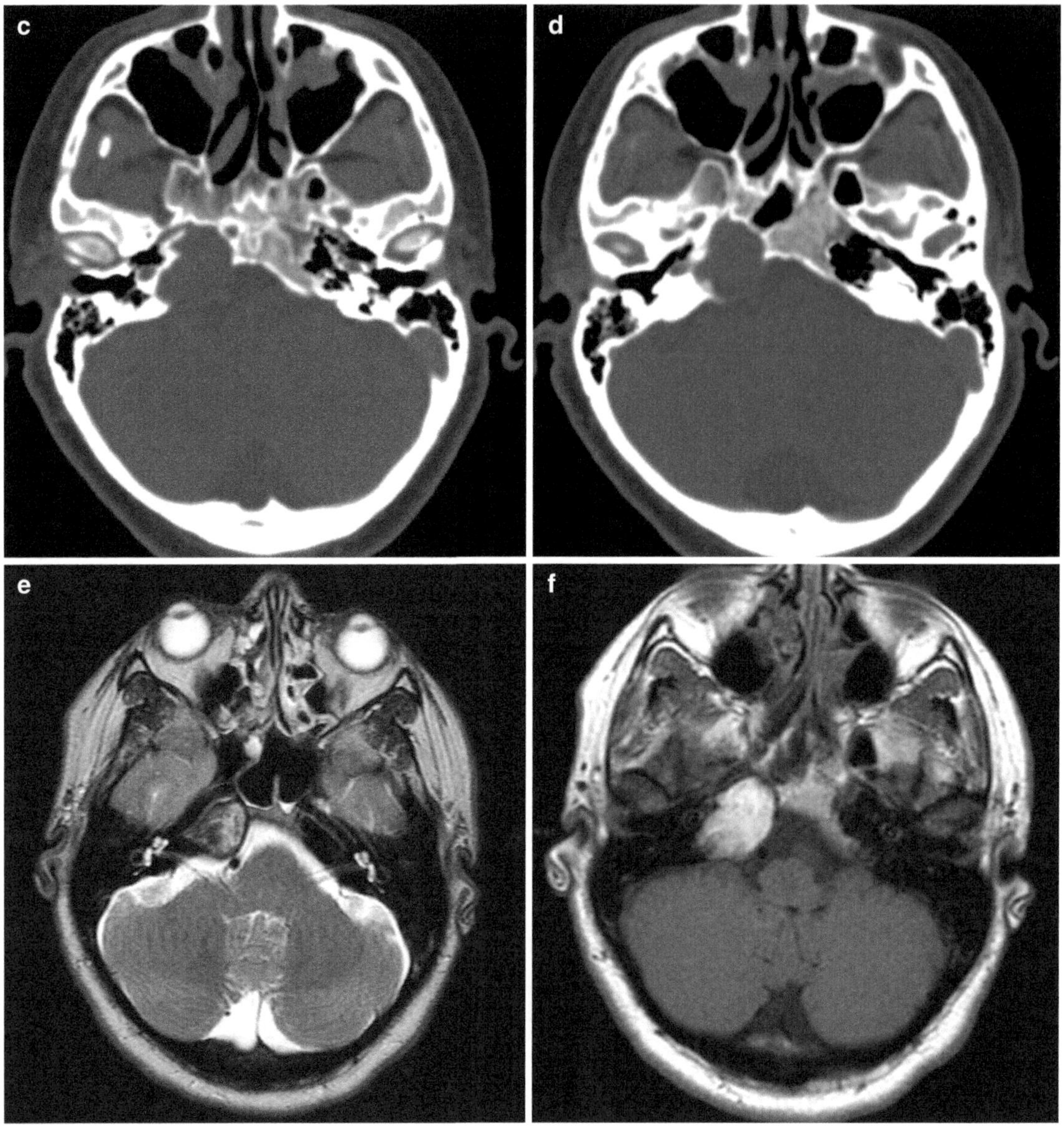

Fig. 22.28 (continued)

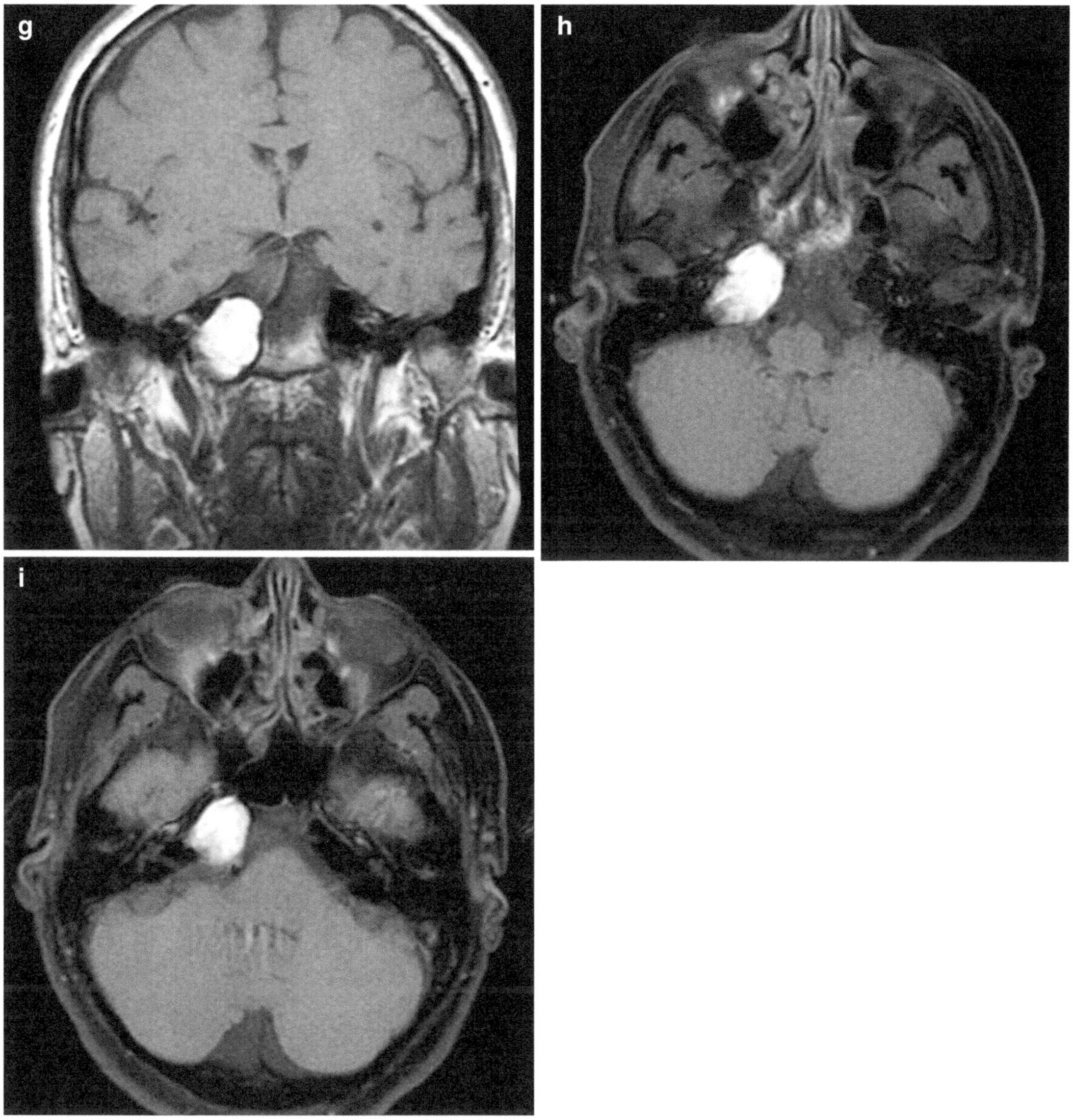

Fig. 22.28 (continued)

On MRI, cholesterol granuloma has a high MR-signal on T1- and T2-weighted images, which makes it similar to subacute or chronic hematoma by MRI manifestations and distinguishes from other cystic lesions frequently encountered in the temporal bone (Martin et al. 1989). On DW-images, granuloma has a hypointense MR-signal that distinguishes it from cholesteatoma.

Proton MR-spectroscopy detects a high lipid-lactate complex in cystic contents of granuloma. Contrast enhancement is observed only in the capsule, cystic contents not being contrast-enhanced (Fig. 22.29). In case of subtotal surgical removal, granuloma remotely (due to its slow growth) recurs within a few years (Fig. 22.30). According to Greenberg (1988), MRI was a more sensitive and specific method in assessment of cholesterol granuloma status in all pre- and postoperative cases.

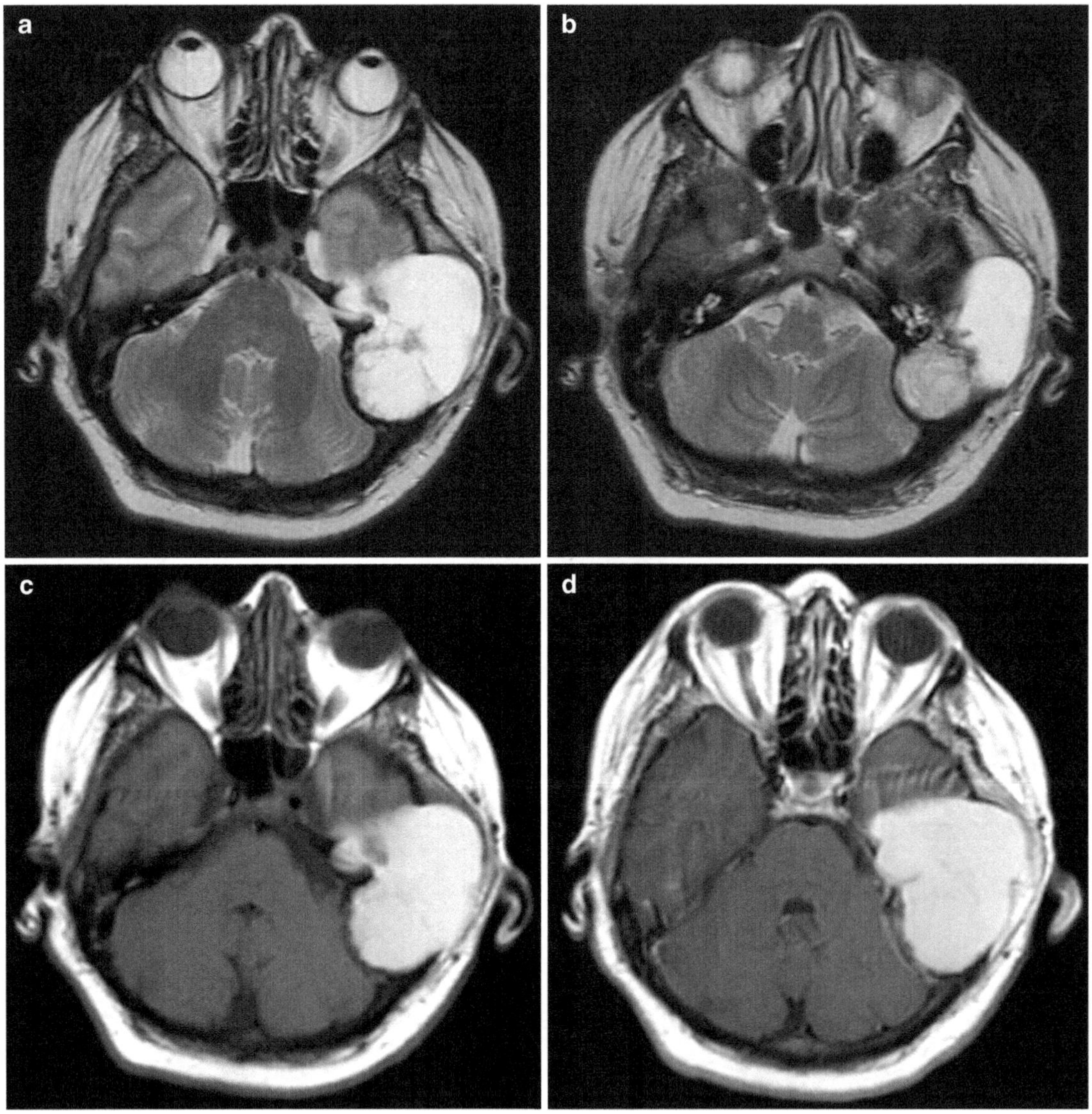

Fig. 22.29 Giant xanthogranuloma of the left temporal bone pyramid. Axial and coronal T2- (**a**, **b**) and T1- (**c**–**e**) weighted MR images show an expansile lesion in projection of left pyramid with heterogeneous hyperintense signal on T2 and homogeneously hyperintense signal on T1 with fairly clear contours. On DWI (**f**) the lesion has a slightly hypointense compared to brain MR-signal. Histologic specimen (**g**) demonstrate the presence of cholesterol crystals in the xanthogranuloma

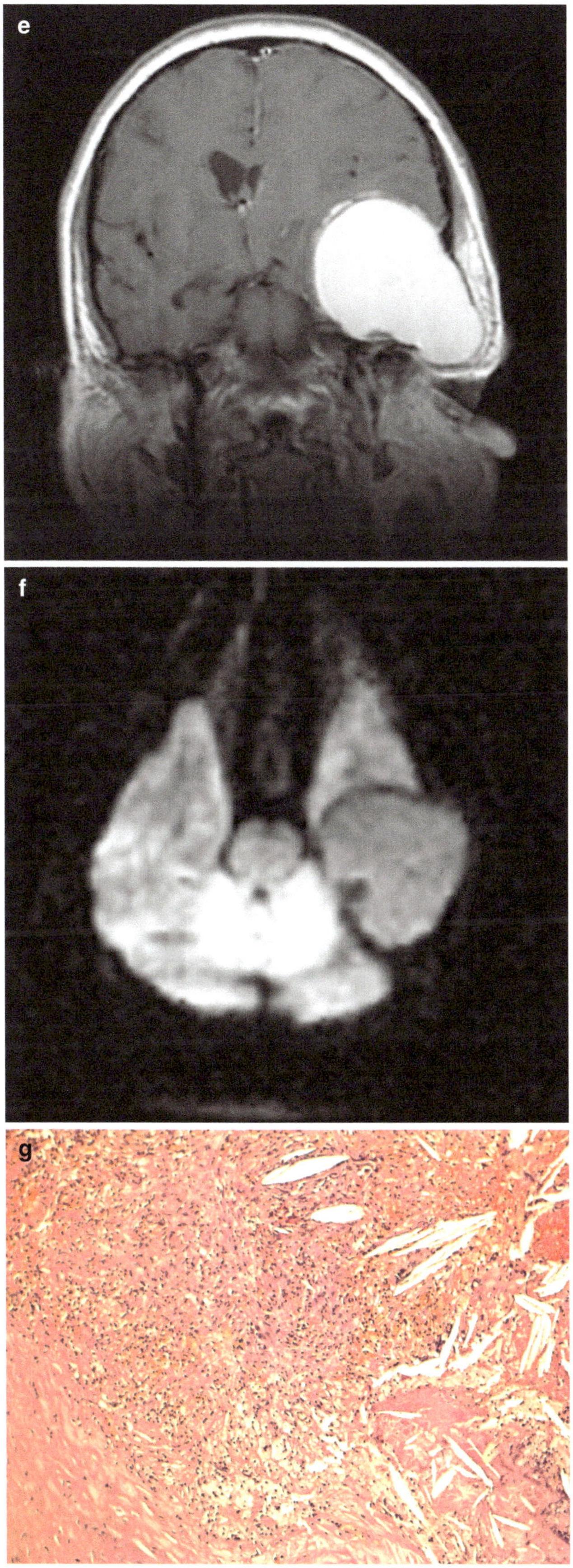

Fig. 22.29 (continued)

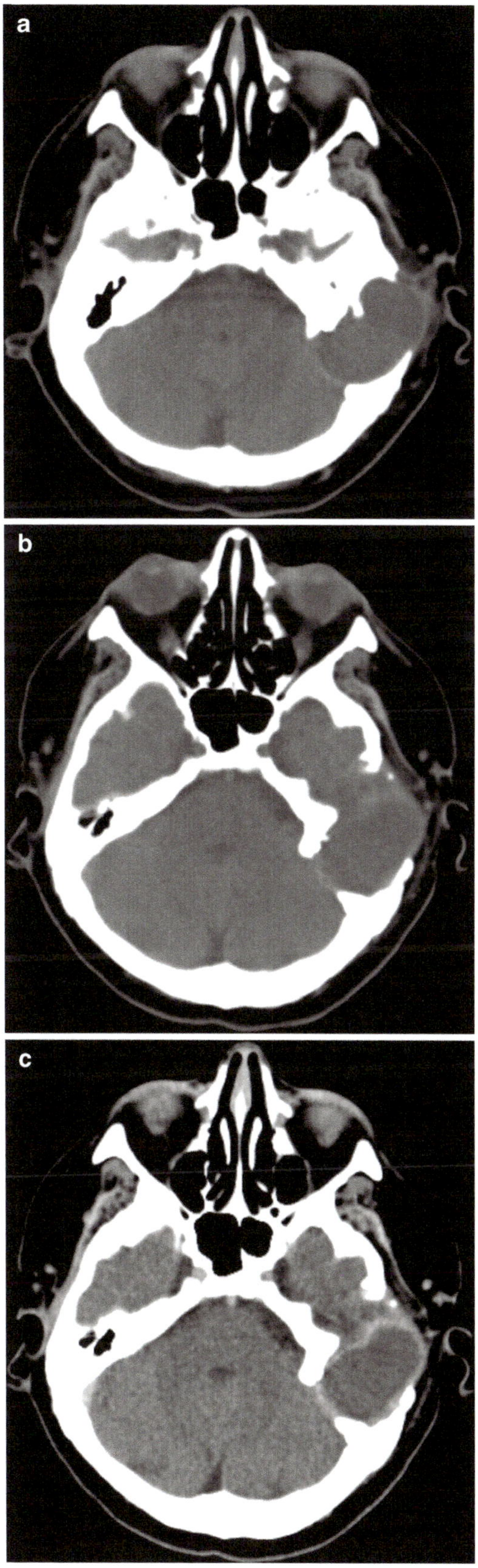

Fig. 22.30 Xanthogranuloma of the left temporal bone pyramid. Axial CT scans before (**a**, **b**) and after (**c**) contrast enhancement demonstrate an expansile lesion in projection of left pyramid apex with enhanced capsule (the same patients that was presented on Fig. 22.29, 6 years after subtotal resection)

23 Benign Tumors

Meningiomas of the posterior cranial fossa constitute about 9–10% of all intracranial meningiomas. These are slow-growing benign tumors, due to which they usually grow large, severely displacing brain structures (including the brainstem), dislocating and/or overgrowing the main arteries of the skull base and the caudal cranial nerves. All this leads to a development of neurological deficit. Tumors with this localization are mainly diagnosed in patients aged 31–60 years old (more than in 70% of cases), 3–4.5 folds more often in women than in men. The site of original growth for most PCF meningiomas is the dura covering various parts of the clivus, posterior surface of the pyramid, including the jugular foramen region. Less frequently meningiomas grow from the dura lining up the inner surface of the occipital bone and the region of the confluence of sinuses. According to data of Burdenko National Center of Neurosurgery, out of 202 verified PCF meningiomas, tumors with petroclival localization (64%) were most often identified, followed by tumors attached to the posterior surface of the pyramid (31%). Meningiomas of the foramen magnum and jugular foramen comprised 3 and 1.5% of cases, respectively.

Majority of PCF meningiomas, according to the WHO 2016 criteria, are classified as benign tumors (90–93%). Stage II and III of malignancy is typical for a small percentage of tumors (less than 10%).

Imaging On standard CT scans the tumor is usually isodense or slightly hyperdense relative to the brain and is poorly distinguished from the latter. Exceptions are calcified meningiomas, which usually represent psammomatous tumor type (Figs. 23.1 and 23.2). After contrast enhancement, meningiomas become hyperdense in most cases. However, even with large sizes, neoplasms exhibit a high degree of contrast homogeneity. This tumor is characterized by a wide attachment to the medial surface of the pyramid, clivus or occipital bone. On CT, in some cases, local hyperostosis in meningioma matrix is clearly visualized (Figs. 23.3 and 23.4). Bone destruction is a less frequent feature occurring in PCF meningiomas. CT angiography (Fig. 23.5) and direct angiography

I. Pronin, V. Kornienko, *CT and MRI of Skull Base Lesions*, https://doi.org/10.1007/978-3-319-65957-2_23

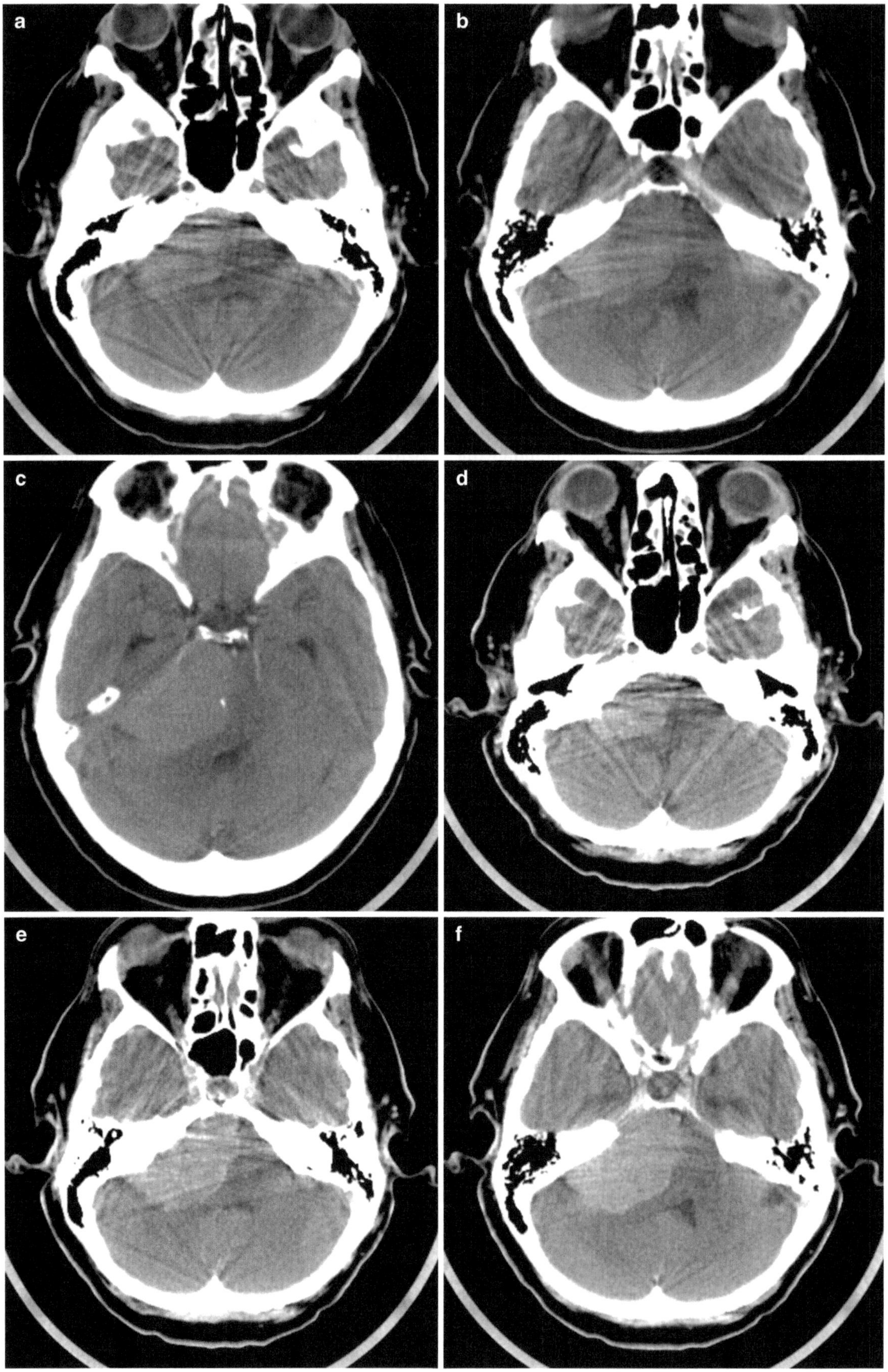

Fig. 23.1 Meningioma of the right petroclival region and cerebellopontine angle. On axial CT scans before (**a–c**) and after (**d–f**) contrast enhancement a large homogeneously strongly enhanced tumor is visualized. Tumor causes the brain stem dislocation

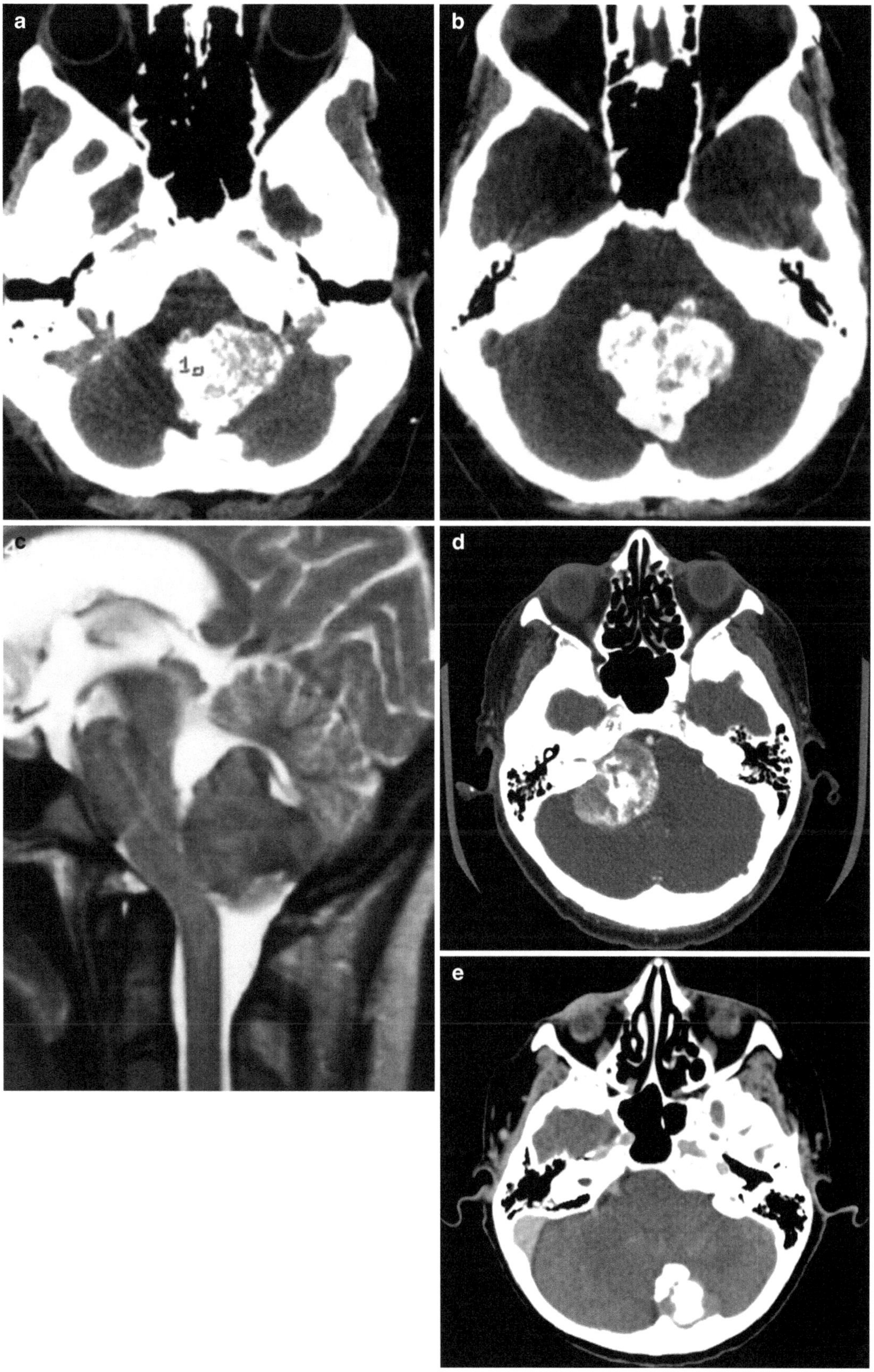

Fig. 23.2 Meningiomas of posterior cranial fossa with massive calcifications (different patients). Case 1. Axial NECT scans (**a**, **b**) demonstrate a large calcified tumor with attachment in projection of sinus confluens. On T2-weighted sagittal MR-image (**c**) meningioma characterized by low MR-signal. Case 2. Psammomatous meningioma of the right cerebellopontine angle (**d**). Case 3. Calcified meningioma of the sinus confluens. Axial CECT scan (**e**) shows a hyperdense lesion with peripheral enhanced soft-tissue component

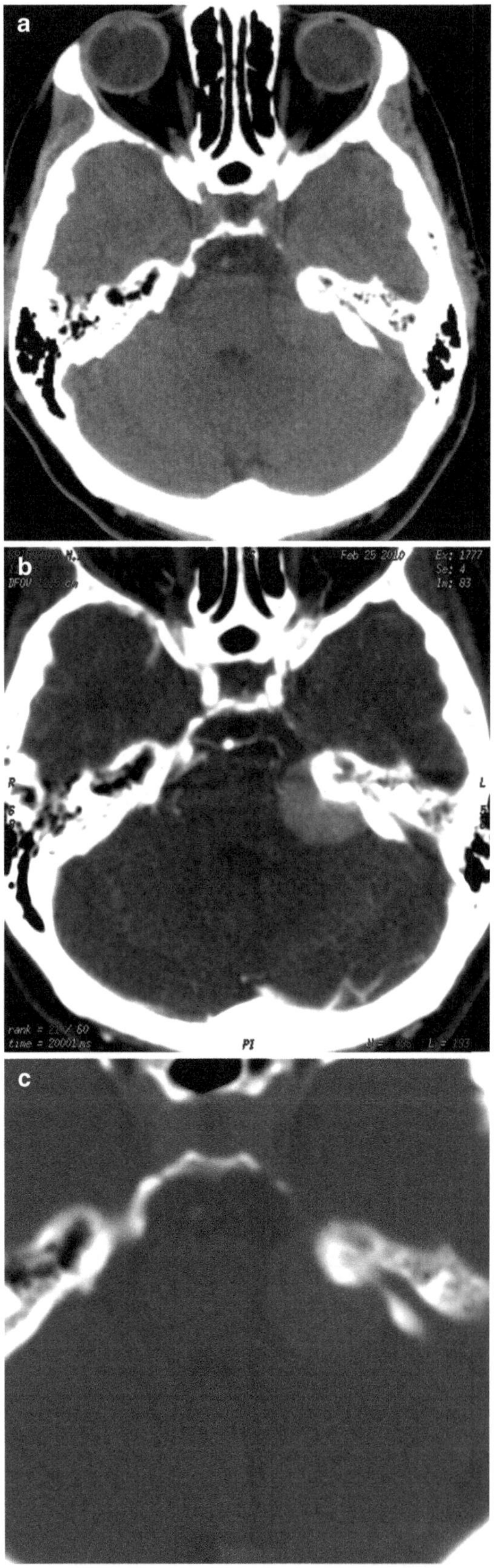

Fig. 23.3 Meningioma of the left cerebellopontine angle. Axial CT scans before (**a**) and after (**b**, **c**) contrast enhancement demonstrate a soft-tissue lesion with local hyperostosis in projection of meningioma matrix. Tumor is characterized by strong and homogeneous contrast enhancement

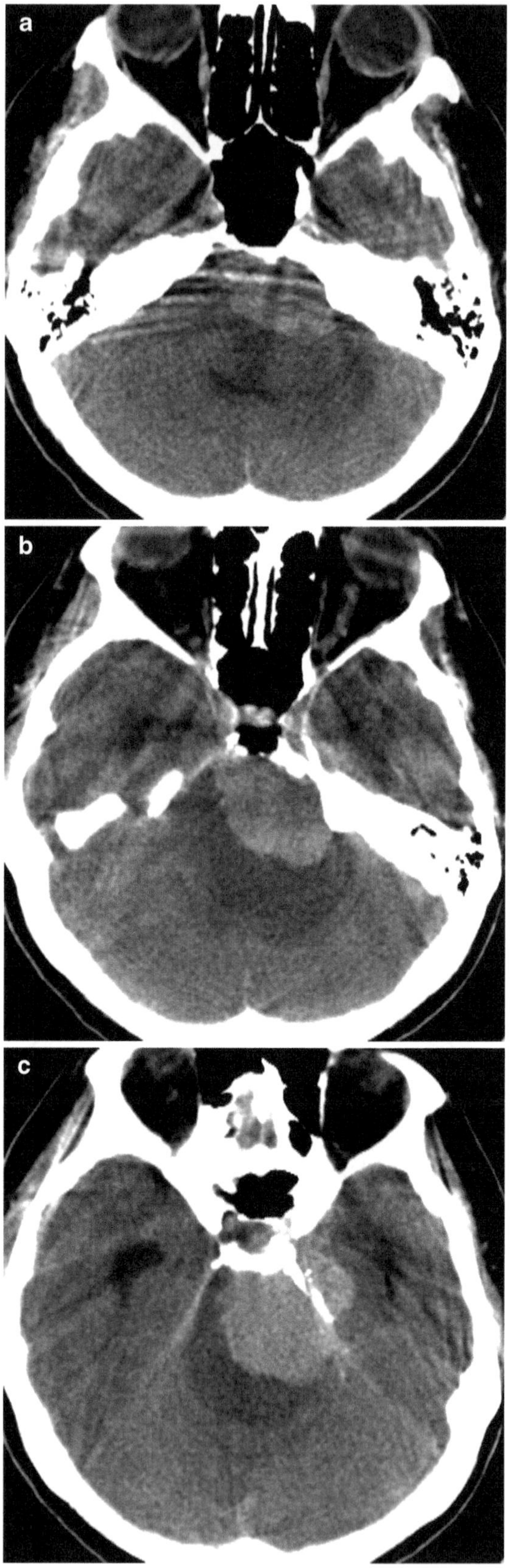

Fig. 23.4 Meningioma of the left petroclival region. On axial CT scans before (**a**) and after (**b**, **c**) contrast enhancement a large homogeneously strongly enhanced tumor is visualized. Tumor causes the brain stem edema and dislocation. There is the extent of the tumor into supratentorial region. Calcified tentorium in the meningioma matrix can be seen

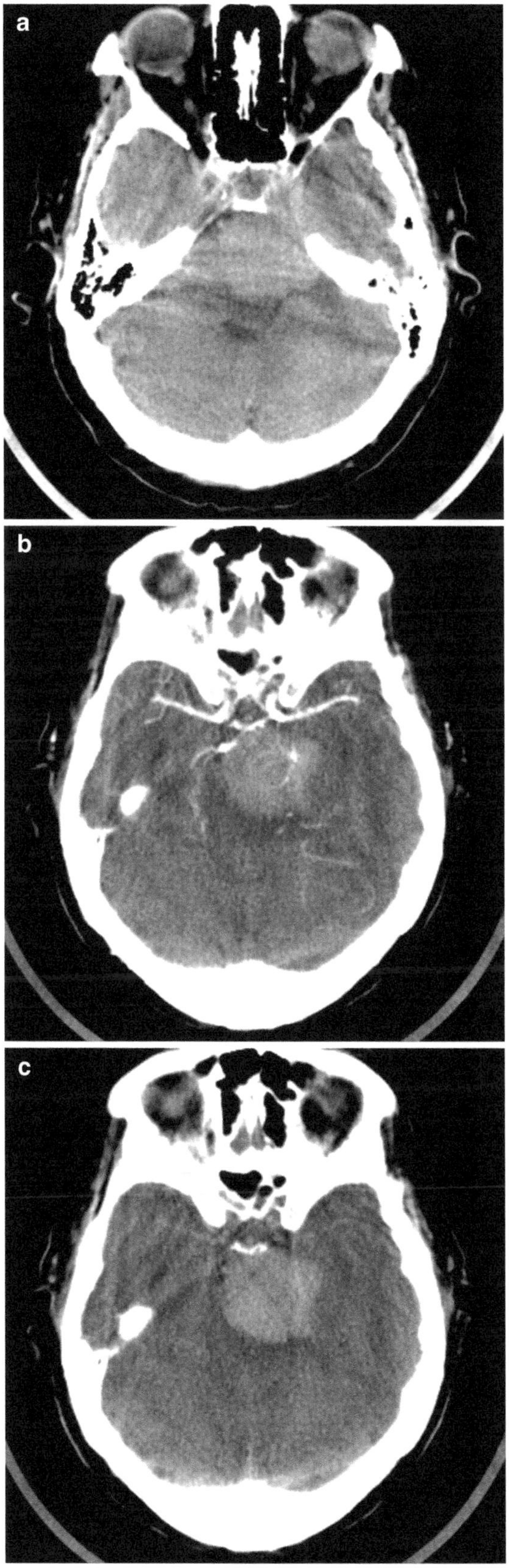

Fig. 23.5 Meningioma of the left petroclival region. On axial NECT scan (**a**) a large slightly hyperdense tumor is visible. Tumor causes the brain stem edema and dislocation. CT-angiography (**b**) as well as contrast enhanced CT scan (**c**) demonstrates a prominent enhancement and meningioma matrix vessels

(Fig. 23.6) are useful in determining the degree of meningioma blood supply and dislocation (or overgrowing) of the large arteries (basilar artery, carotid siphon in case of antegrade growth).

On perfusion CT studies, meningiomas are divided into three main forms depending on hemodynamic types, which correlate well with the results of direct cerebral angiography. We identified the following hemodynamic tumor types: I type—low CBV values (2.5–5 ml/100 g), CBF (25–30 ml/100 g/min) in the absence or minimally expressed tumor vasculature on angiography; type II—a moderate increase in CBV, CBF (up to 10–11 ml /100 g and 70–80 ml/100 g/min, respectively) with a moderate vascular spot in the capillary phase of angiography; type III—a pronounced increase in meningioma hemodynamics (CBV up to 21–24 ml/100 g, CBF up to 110–125 ml/100 g/min) in the presence of a highly vascularized tumor on angiograms (Fig. 23.7). Knowledge of these perfusion characteristics of meningiomas allows to plan the surgical approaches and assessing the risk of intraoperative bleeding. Another very important diagnostic finding, typical for meningiomas, is a vascular tumor matrix. It is well visualized on CT-perfusion images in the shape of diverging rays or a thickened base. Planning a surgical approach on account of meningioma matrix characteristics is necessary for complete surgical removal and prevention of the intra- and postoperative complications.

On T1-weighted MR images, meningiomas in the majority of cases (60%) are visualized as mass lesions, isointense in relation to the brain tissue, located in the lateral parts of the posterior cranial fossa. In other cases, meningiomas have hypointense MT-characteristics. On T2-weighted sequences, this tumor may have a variable MR signal from hypointense, more typical for psammomatous and fibroblastic types of meningiomas, to moderately hyperintense, characterizing meningothelial tumors (Fig. 23.8). Calcified tumor portions are visualized on MRI considerably worse than on CT. Large tumors cause marked compression of the brainstem. In contrast to CT, MRI better identifies concomitant changes (edema, ischemia) in the compressed brainstem (Fig. 23.9).

Most meningiomas (~100%) intensively and homogeneously enhance (Figs. 23.10 and 23.11). In our series, only a few fully calcified meningiomas showed no contrast enhancement. A characteristic feature of meningeal tumors on a post-contrast MR-series is the presence of a "dural tail," representing accumulation of the contrast agent along the tumor edge extending on the infiltrated (or reactively changed) dura (Fig. 23.12).

A CSF cleft (a hyperintense thin rim along the contour of the tumor) on T2-weighted sequence is the second characteristic of meningiomas, which reflects extraaxial location of tumors. If the picture on standard T2-weighted images is unconvincing, the use of myelographic sequence with thinner slices is possible.

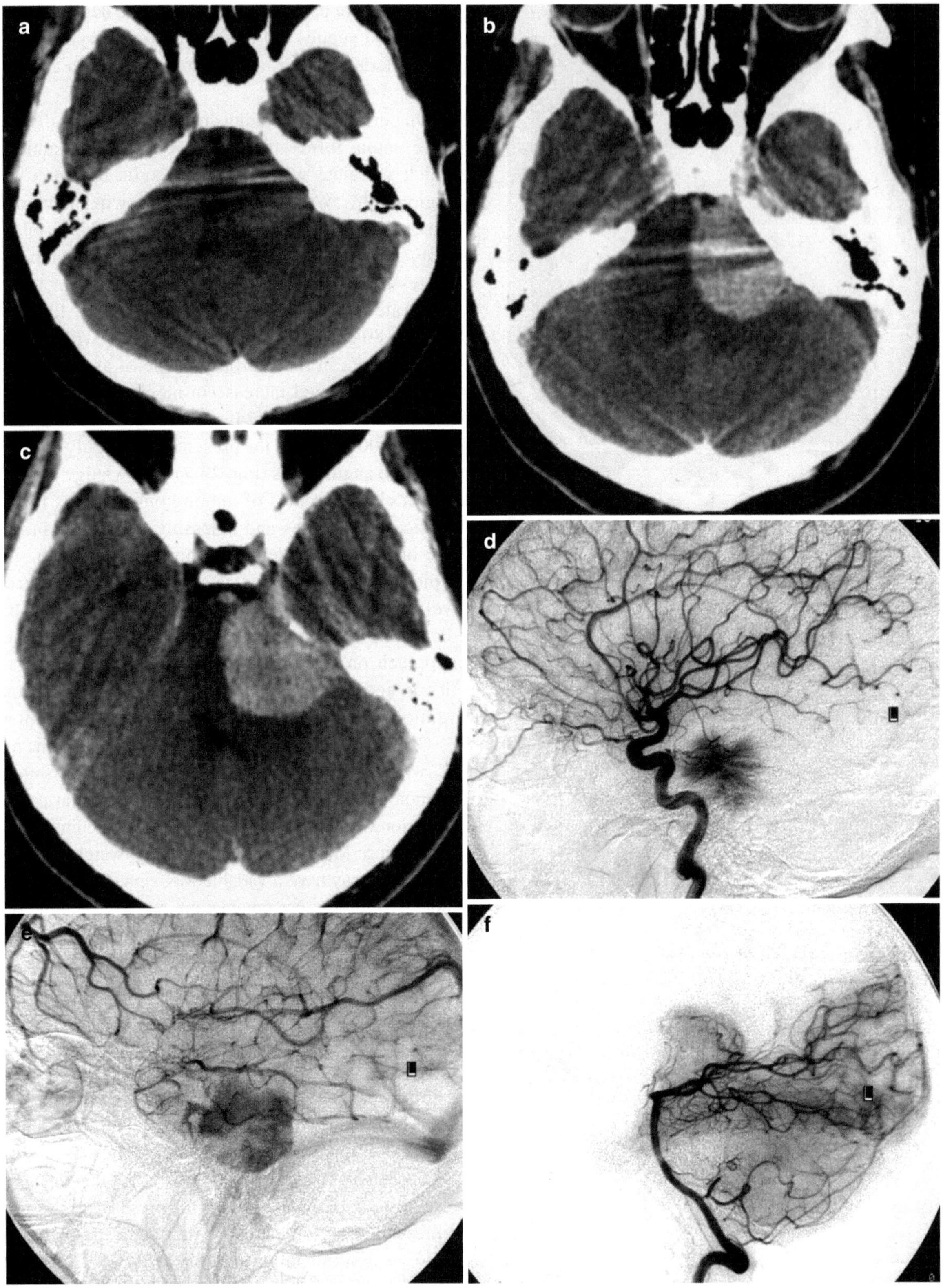

Fig. 23.6 Meningioma of the left petroclival and cerebellopontine angle region. On axial CT scans before (**a**) and after (**b**, **c**) contrast enhancement a large homogeneously strongly enhanced tumor is visualized. Tumor causes the brain stem dislocation. DSA (**d–f**) reveals the abundant blood supply of the meningioma from short meningeal branches of ICA. On the lateral angiogram of the vertebral artery territory the avascular area on the tumor location can be seen (**f**)

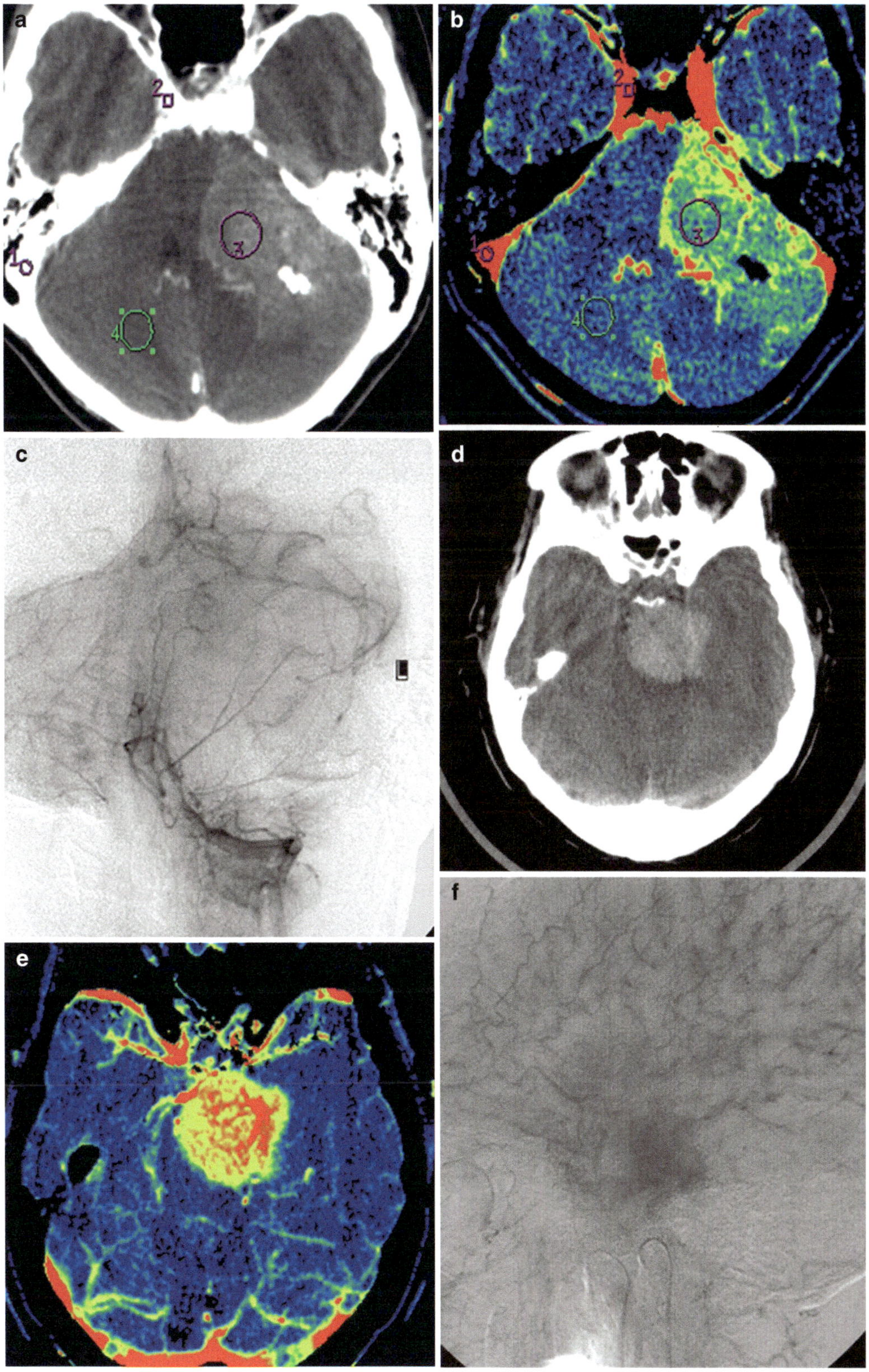

Fig. 23.7 Different patterns of meningioma hemodynamics and blood supply. Type I: meningioma with low perfusion and low blood supply (CT scan (**a**), CT-perfusion CBF map-(**b**), DSA-capillary phase (**c**)). Type II: meningioma with medium values of elevated perfusion and capillary spot on DSA (CT scan (**d**), CT-perfusion CBF map (**e**), DSA-capillary phase (**f**)). Type III: meningioma with high values of elevated perfusion and prominent capillary spot (abundant vasculature) on DSA (CT scan (**g**), CT-perfusion CBF map (**h**), DSA-capillary phase (**i**))

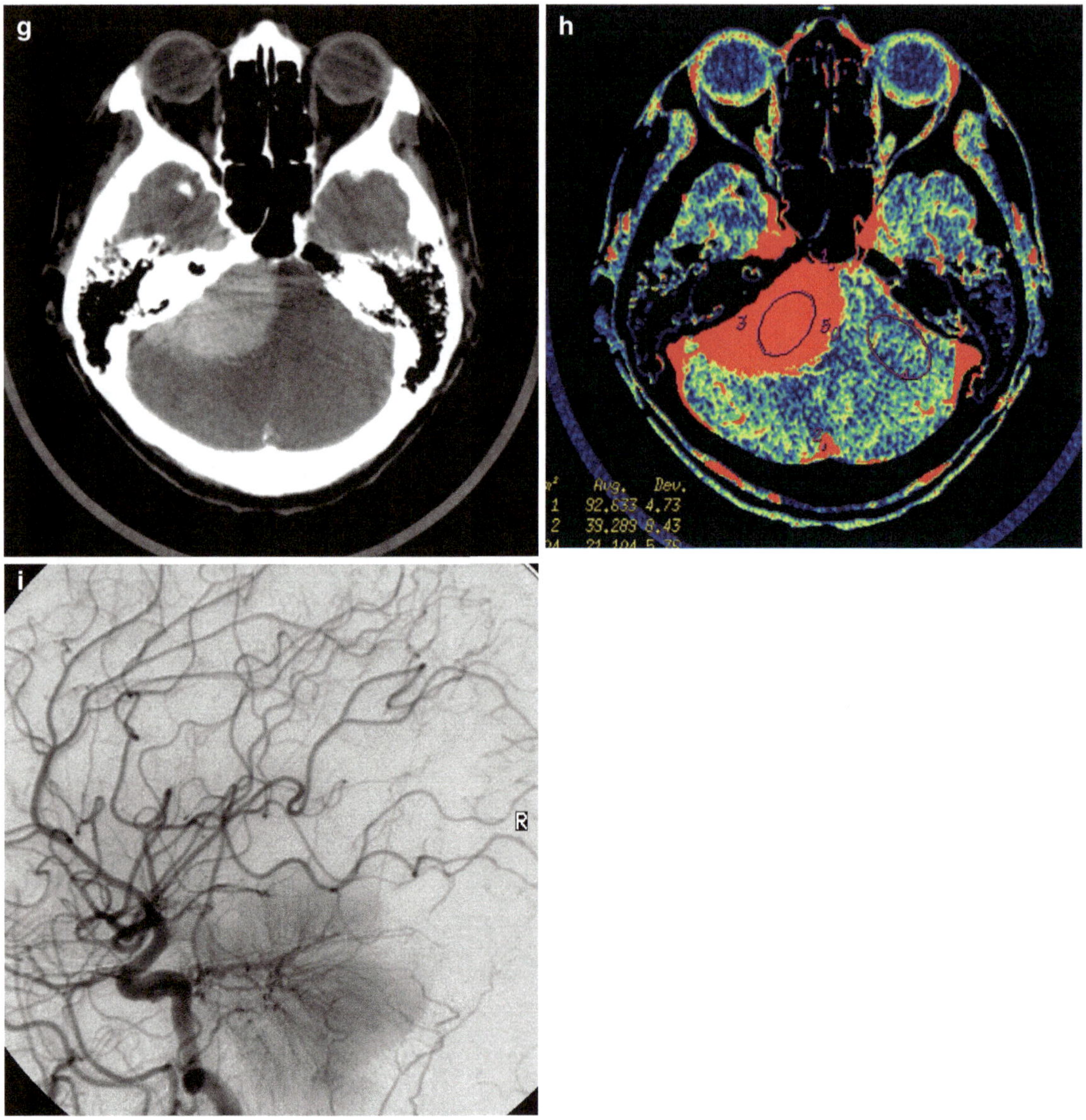

Fig. 23.7 (continued)

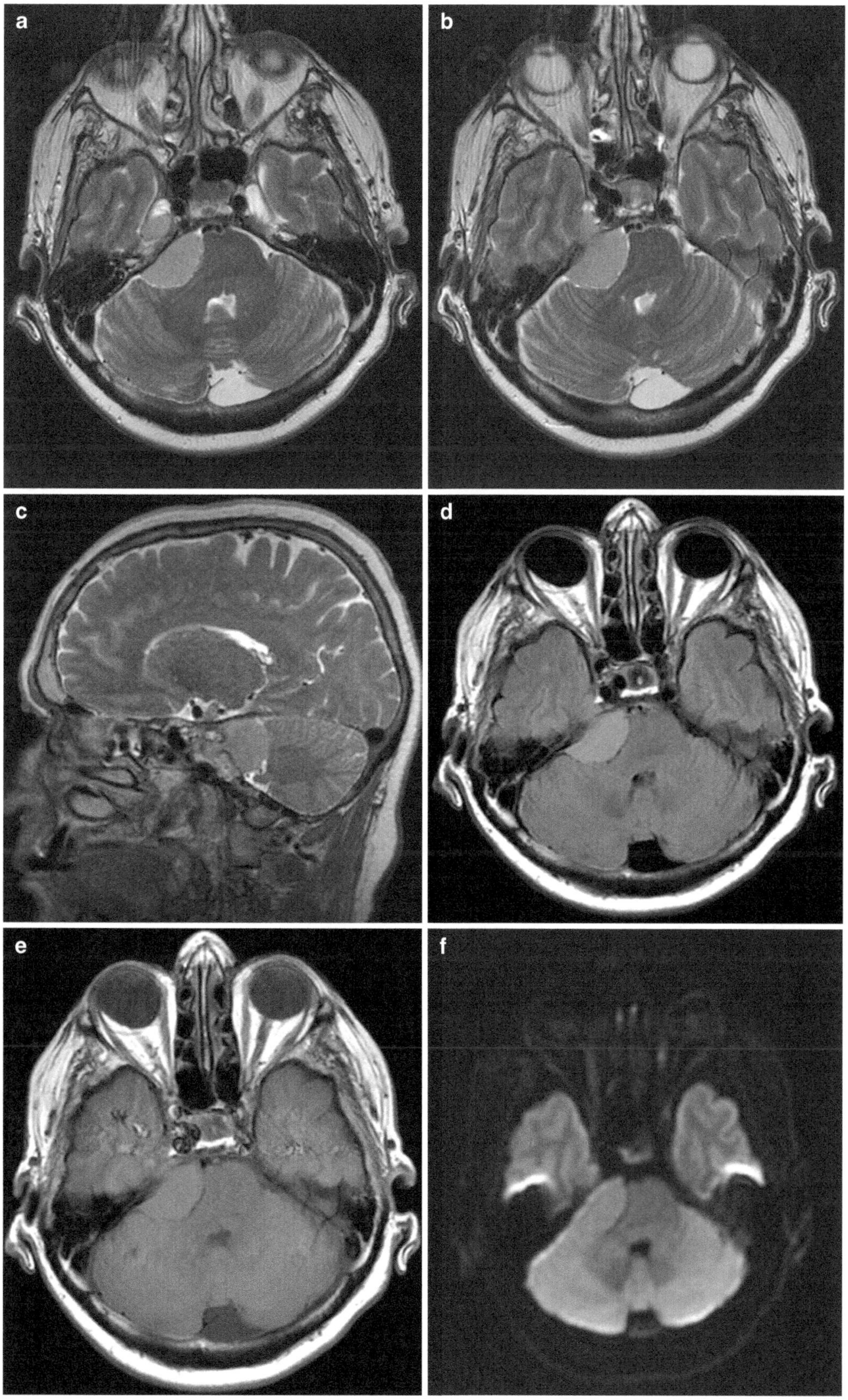

Fig. 23.8 Meningioma of the right petroclival and cerebellopontine angle region. Axial and sagittal T2- (**a**, **b**, **c**), T2-FLAIR (**d**) and T1- (**e**) weighted MR-images show a solid lesion in projection of the right petroclival and cerebellopontine angle region with extension into Meckel's cavity. Tumor has homogeneous hyperintense signal on T2 and T2-FLAIR images. There is isointense signal on T1 and DWI (**f**)

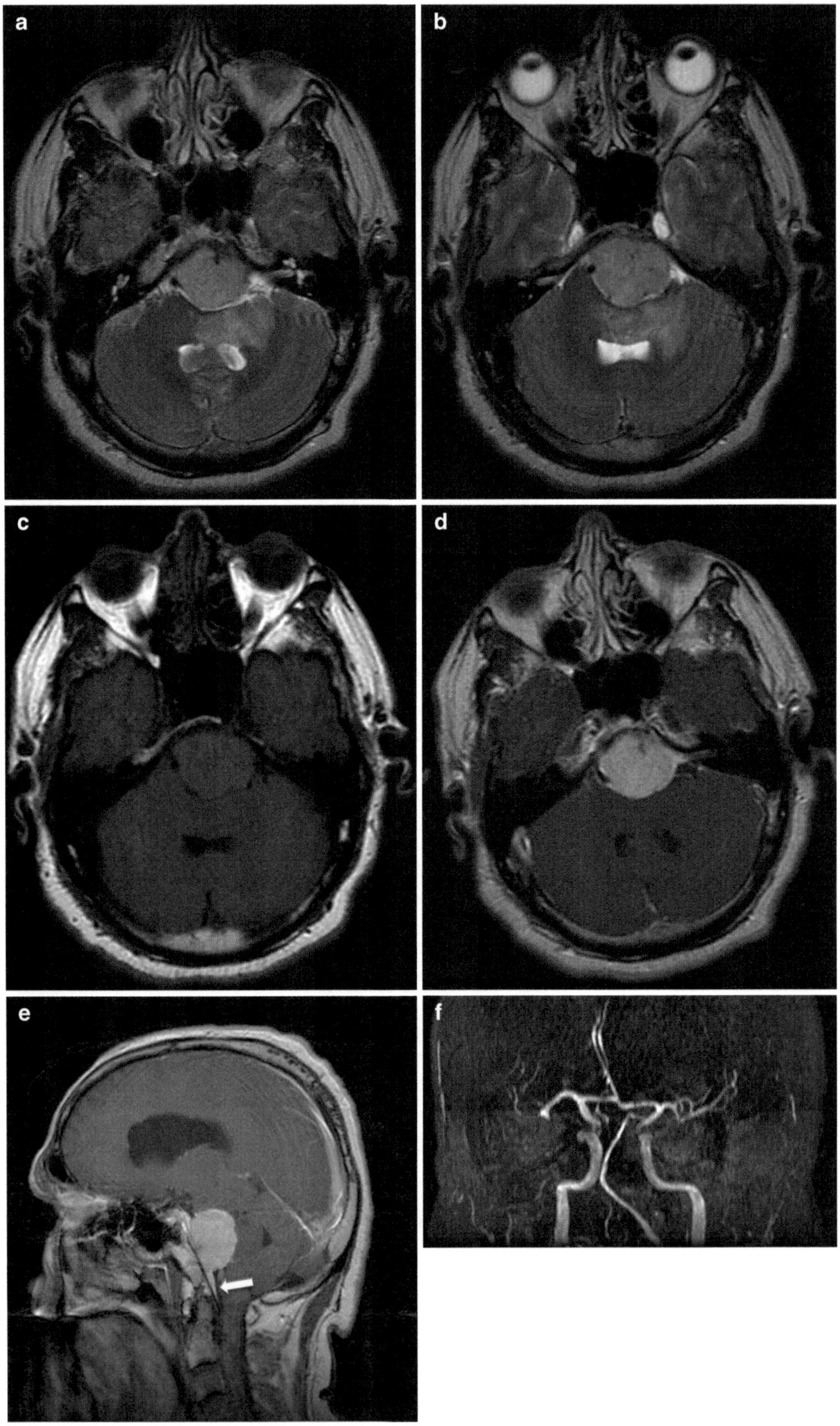

Fig. 23.9 Meningioma of the clivus. Axial T2- (**a**, **b**), T1- before (**c**) and after (**d**, **e**) contrast enhancement MR-images show a solid with homogeneous structure and strongly enhanced tumor with wide attachment to the clivus. Tumor leads to dislocation and edema of the pons. There is "dural tail" sign (*arrow*). 3D TOF MR-angiography reveals the vertebral artery displacement on the right (**f**)

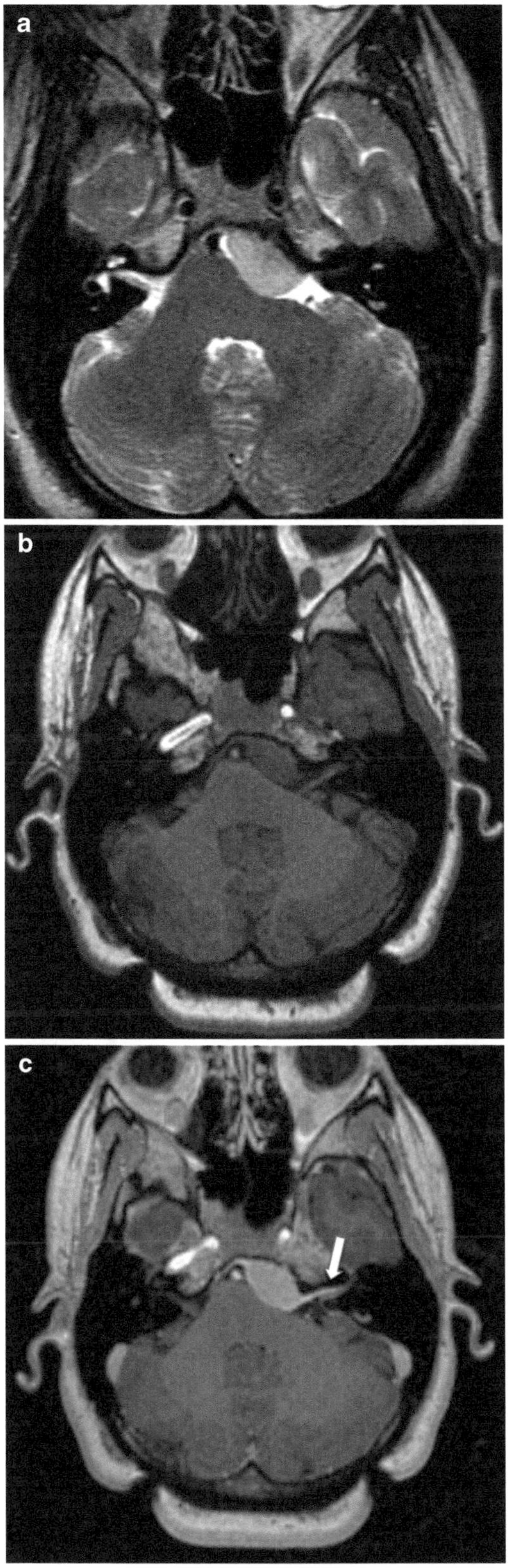

Fig. 23.10 Small meningioma of the left petroclival region. Axial T2- (**a**) and T1- (**b**) weighted MR-images show a solid lesion in projection of the left petroclival area with wide attachment to the clivus and apex of the pyramid surface. Tumor is characterized by the homogeneous and prominent enhancement (**c**). There is "dural tail" sign (*arrow*) with extension into the porus acusticus interior

Petroclival meningiomas typically grow from the apex of the pyramid to the clivus area (or vice versa), resulting in a severe dislocation of the brainstem. Contrast enhancement allows visualizing the tumor spread into the cavernous sinus and medial parts of MCF (Figs. 23.13 and 23.14).

Cerebellopontine angle meningioma (up to 10–15% of all lesions of this location and takes second place in frequency after vestibular schwannomas) is not characterized by penetration of tumor masses into the internal auditory meatus with subsequent expansion of the latter. Such manifestations can be visualized only with large tumors, but this is an exception rather than a rule (Figs. 23.15 and 23.16).

On DWI, meningiomas are distinguished by certain heterogeneity of MR signal changes and ADC with a tendency to distinction between benign, atypical, and anaplastic forms (ADC values of 0.83 ± 0.11; 0.91 ± 0.16 and 0.97 ± 0.19 respectively). In general, meningiomas have a higher MR signal on DWI and lower ADC than vestibular schwannomas (Fig. 23.17).

Jugular foramen meningioma grows from the dura lining up the edge of the jugular foramen or arachnoid cells growing along the initial segments of the cranial nerves in the jugular foramen. This meningioma can occlude the jugular vein and dural sinuses, leading to sinus thrombosis (Korshunov 2019). According to statistic data, they comprise 5% of the posterior fossa meningiomas. If the tumor grows upwards and laterally, it can invade into the middle ear and mastoid, in case of lateral growth it affects the pyramid at the site of the mastoid segment of VIIth nerve, in case of anterior and medial growth, it spreads into the apex of the pyramid and ICA canal. Initial clinical manifestations are associated with involvement of IX–XI nerves. Patients can experience pulsating tingling; subsequently, involvement of the VII–VIII pairs of cranial nerves is possible (MacDonald et al. 2004).

CT scans often detect sclerotic bone changes around the jugular foramen. The tumor has a moderately increased density on non-enhanced slices, sometimes with calcifications at the projection of matrix. Meningioma intensively accumulates contrast agent, becoming hyperdense. A hypo- and isointense lesions on T1- and T2-weighted MR-sequences tend to spread along the dura and dural spaces, rarer into the area of basal cisterns. They may have an extracranial component. Enhanced "dural tail" is clearly visualized using intravenous contrast enhancement. The size of meningioma is best assessed on a series of postcontrast images with fat suppression technique (Fig. 23.18).

Foramen magnum meningioma is relatively rare among PCF meningiomas (no more than 10%). Low tumor location within the posterior cranial fossa near foramen magnum leads to earlier, than in meningiomas of other sites, occurrence of clinical symptoms associated with compression of the medulla oblongata and impairment of CSF circulation spaces between the brain and spinal cord (Roberti 2001).

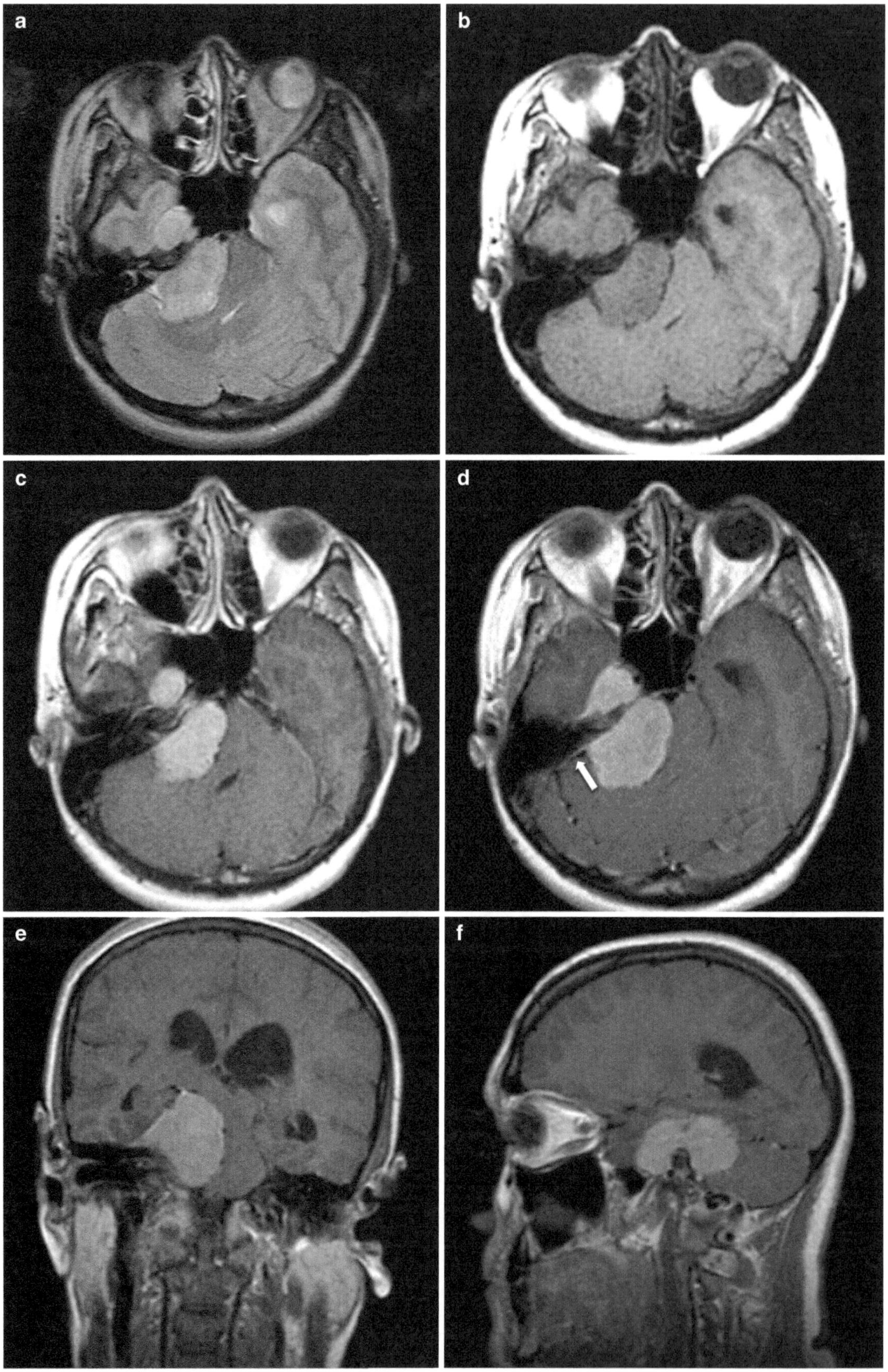

Fig. 23.11 Meningioma of the right petroclival and cerebellopontine angle region. Axial T2- (**a**) and T1- (**b**) weighted MR-images demonstrate a solid lesion in projection of the right petroclival and cerebellopontine angle region with extension into Meckel's cavity and cavernous sinus. Tumor is characterized by the homogeneous and prominent contrast enhancement (**c**–**f**). There is "dural tail" sign (*arrow*) along the pyramid with extension even into the internal acoustic meatus (**d**)

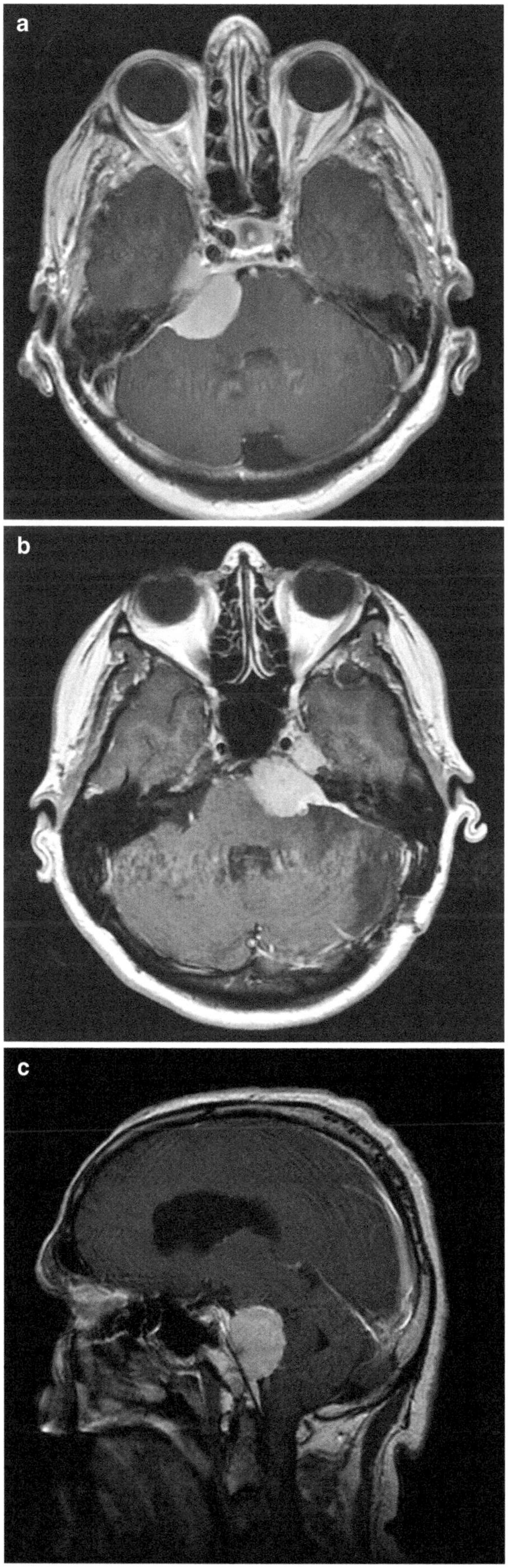

Fig. 23.12 Different meningiomas of petroclical region with "dural tail" sign. MR-imaging with contrast enhancement (**a–c**)

The tumor more often grows at the anterior and antero-lateral surface of the foramen magnum and has both intracranial and intravertebral components (Figs. 23.19 and 23.20). A kidney shape with the convex posterior contour is typical. CT and MRI tumor findings are identical to those of other meningiomas. Contrast enhancement is a mandatory attribute of preoperative diagnosis (Fig. 23.21) and postoperative follow-up. New possibilities in visualization of blood supply sources of foramen magnum meningiomas appeared with the use of 3.0 T scanners, especially with new high-resolution MR angiographic techniques (Fig. 23.22).

PCF convex meningiomas are rare tumors in comparison with supratentorial meningiomas. Small-size tumors are seen on CT scans only if they have a size greater than 2 cm or there are calcifications in the tumor's stroma. Only on post-enhanced images the meningioma contours and its dimensions can be determined. MRI is a more accurate method for visualization of the small tumors. However, intravenous contrast enhancement provides a more reliable diagnosis in this case, too. In general, the objective of diagnosis is to determine extraaxial meningioma location (undistinguishable from supratentorial lesions) and the relationship with the major venous sinuses (most often transverse sinus, rarely sigmoid sinus). With this purpose, it is advisable to use angiography techniques, such as 2D TOF with contrast enhancement. The use of perfusion techniques helps assess the blood supply of meningioma (usually determined as perfusion types I and II) and better plan a surgical approach to the neoplasm (Fig. 23.23).

Differential Diagnosis Vestibular schwannoma and trigeminal nerve schwannoma, neurosarcoidosis, plasmacytoma (causes destruction of bone structures, moderately hypointense signal on T2), chordoma (located on the midline, causes destruction of the clivus, has bony inclusions, a higher signal on T2), metastases (destroy the bone tissue due to the rapid growth, heterogeneously enhance, often with surrounding brain edema), lymphoma (a rapidly growing tumor with severe clinical signs, causes the development of an extensive peritumoral edema, has a high MR-signal on DWI, "dural tail" sign is atypical), hemangioblastoma (high degree of contrast enhancement, lumpy contour, perifocal edema, high CT-perfusion values, wide attachment to the bones of the skull base is atypical).

Cranial Nerve Schwannomas Schwannoma (neuroma, neurinoma, neurilemmoma) is a benign tumor, which originates from the Schwann cells of the cranial and spinal nerves. There are two types of histological pattern of schwannomas—Antony A and Antony B. Antony A is characterized by the presence of elongated bipolar cells with indistinct borders and elongated nuclei. These cells form palisade-like structures, presented by rows of nuclei arranged parallel to each other, which alternate with cellular areas of fibrous structure. An isolated Antony A structure is more common in

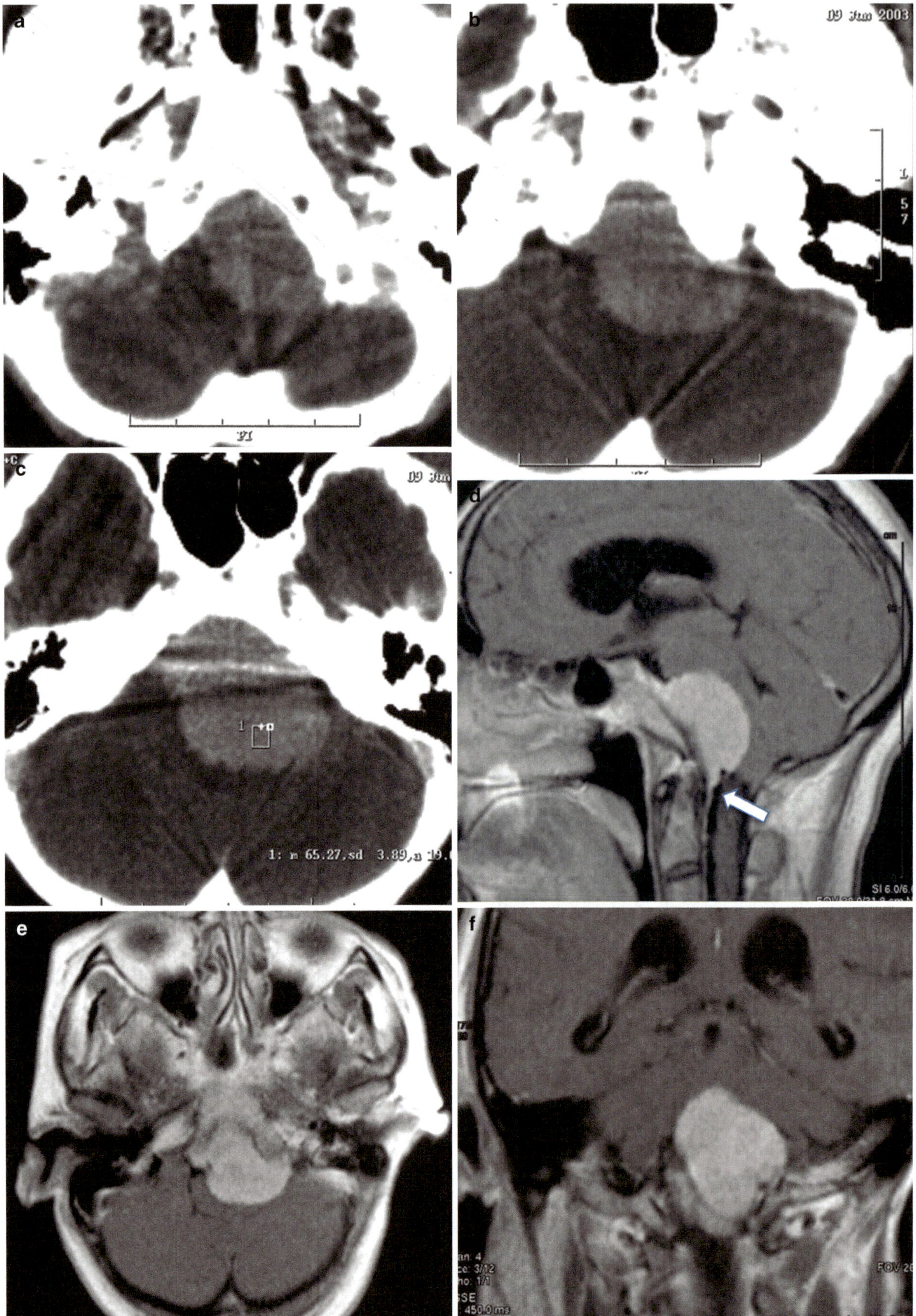

Fig. 23.13 Petroclival meningioma. Axial CECT-scans revealed a large tumor that has intense contrast enhancement (**a**–**c**). On enhanced MRI (**d**–**f**) the tumor is characterized by a strong enhancement, a wide base, attaching to the dura in the clivus region. There is "dural tail" sign (*arrow*) along the clivus

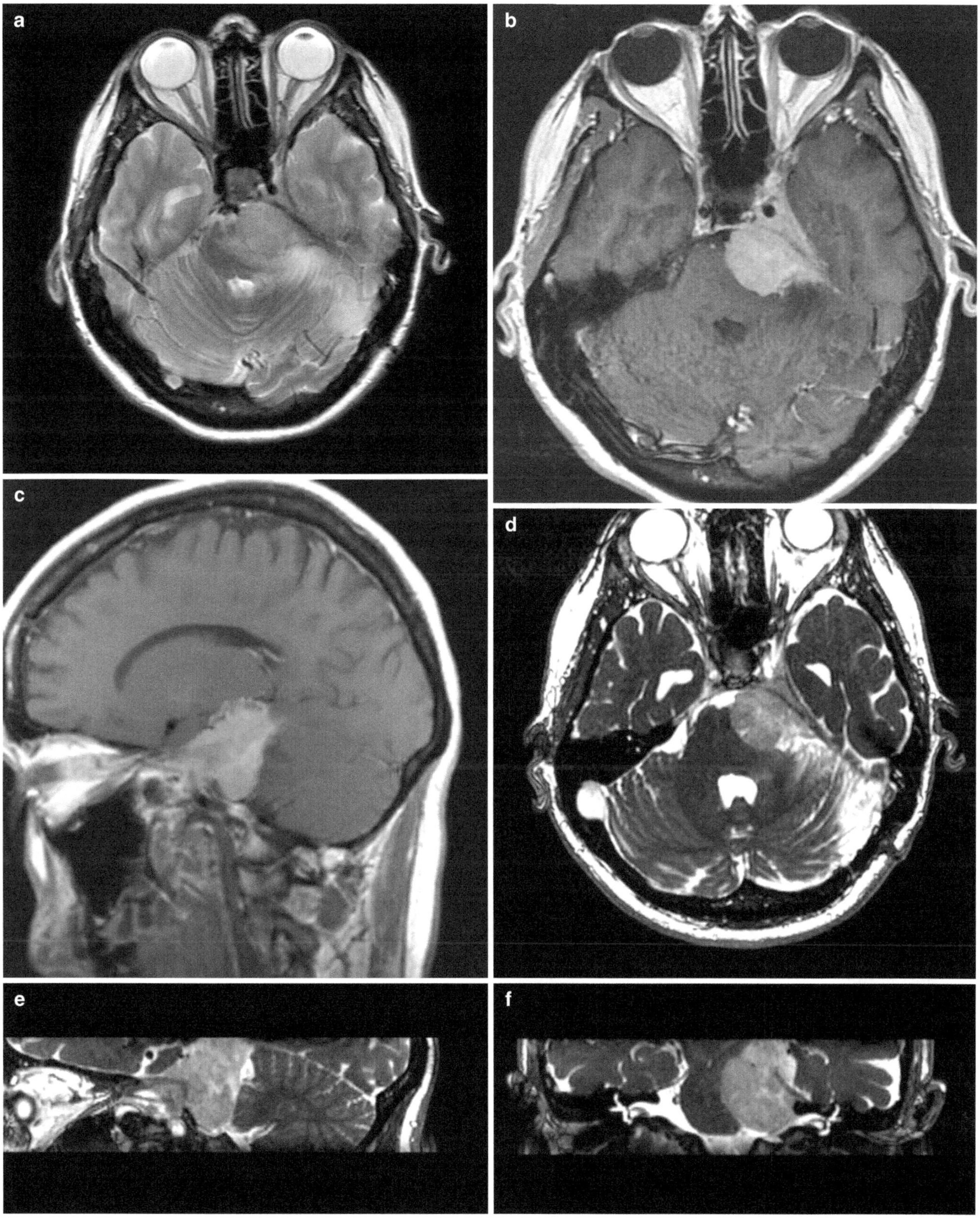

Fig. 23.14 Petroclival meningioma (partial tumor's resection). There is a slightly hyperintense to the pons on T2-weighted image (**a**) petroclival tumor with prominent and homogeneous contrast enhancement on T1-weighted images (**b**, **c**). Tumor extends into the left Meckel's cavity and cavernous sinus. Meningioma has a hyperintense MR-signal on MR-myelography images (FIESTA: **d**–**f**) with better demarcation with brain stem compared to T2-WI. The brainstem is compressed and swollen

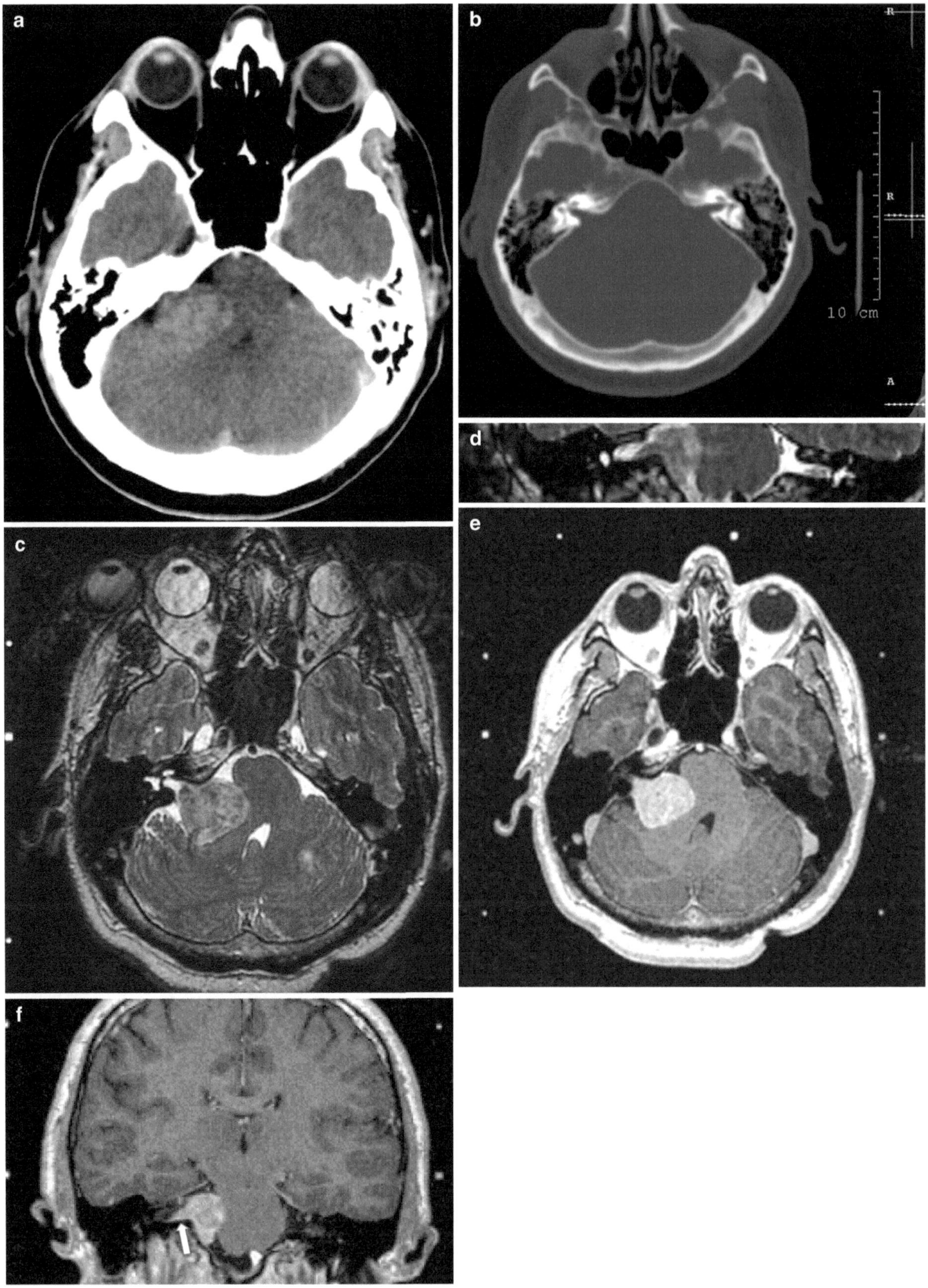

Fig. 23.15 Meningioma of the right cerebellopontine angle. Axial CECT scans with using of bone window mode (**a**, **b**) revealed a solid tumor in the projection of the cerebellopontine angle without an extension in the bony canal of internal acoustic meatus. There is an extension of the meningioma into the internal acoustic meatus (*arrow*) on T2-weighted MRI (FIESTA: (**c**, **d**)) and T1-weighted postenhanced MR-images (**e**, **f**)

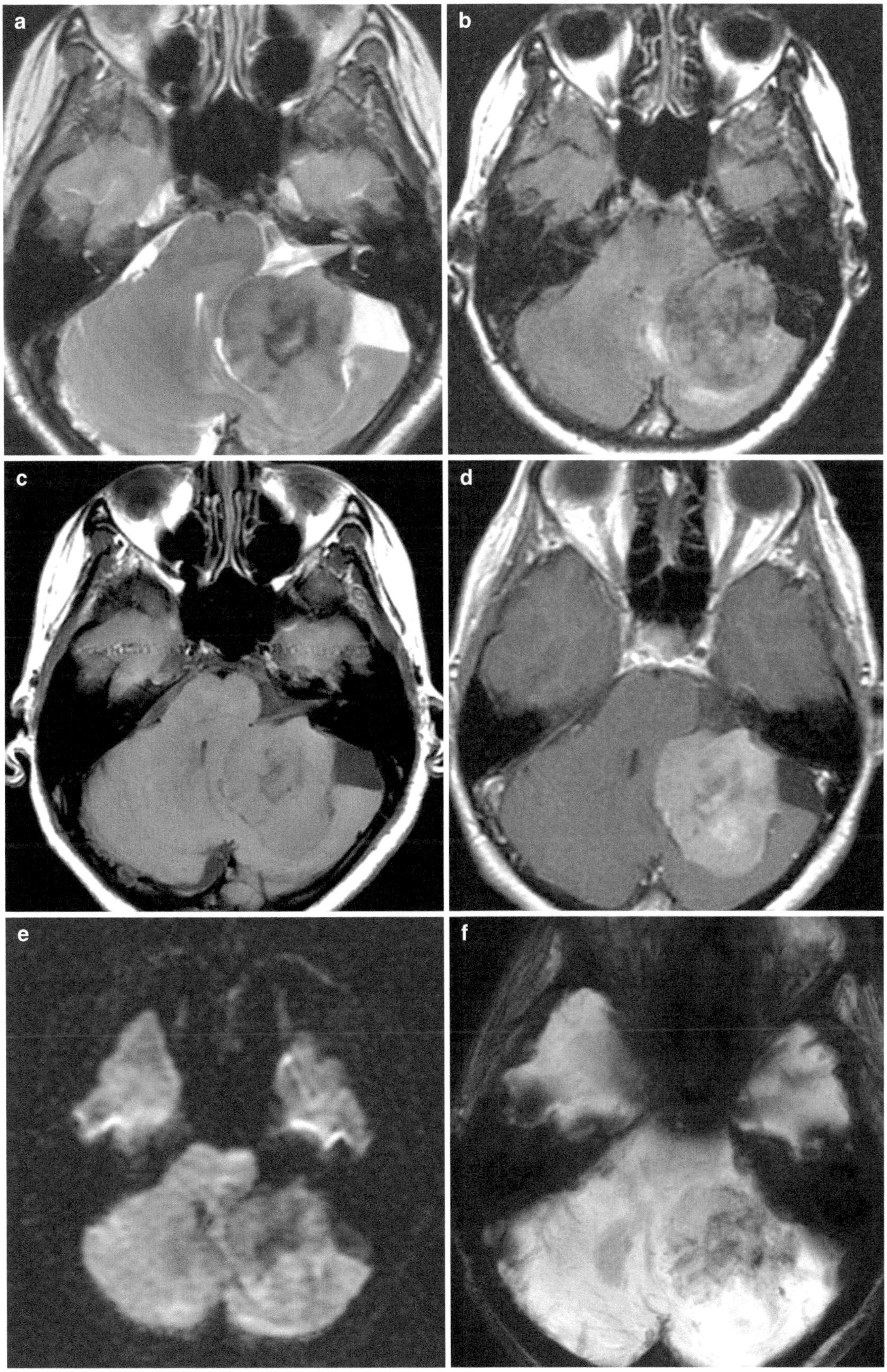

Fig. 23.16 Giant meningioma of the left cerebellopontine angle. On T2- (**a**) and T2-FLAIR (**b**) MRI a large solid hypointense tumor is visible. Tumor has an isointense MR-signal on T1-weighted image (**c**) and is characterized by prominent contrast enhancement (**d**). On DWI (**e**) meningioma is predominantly iso-hypointense. There are multiple hypointense areas in the tumor's structure on SWAN (**f**) due to calcifications

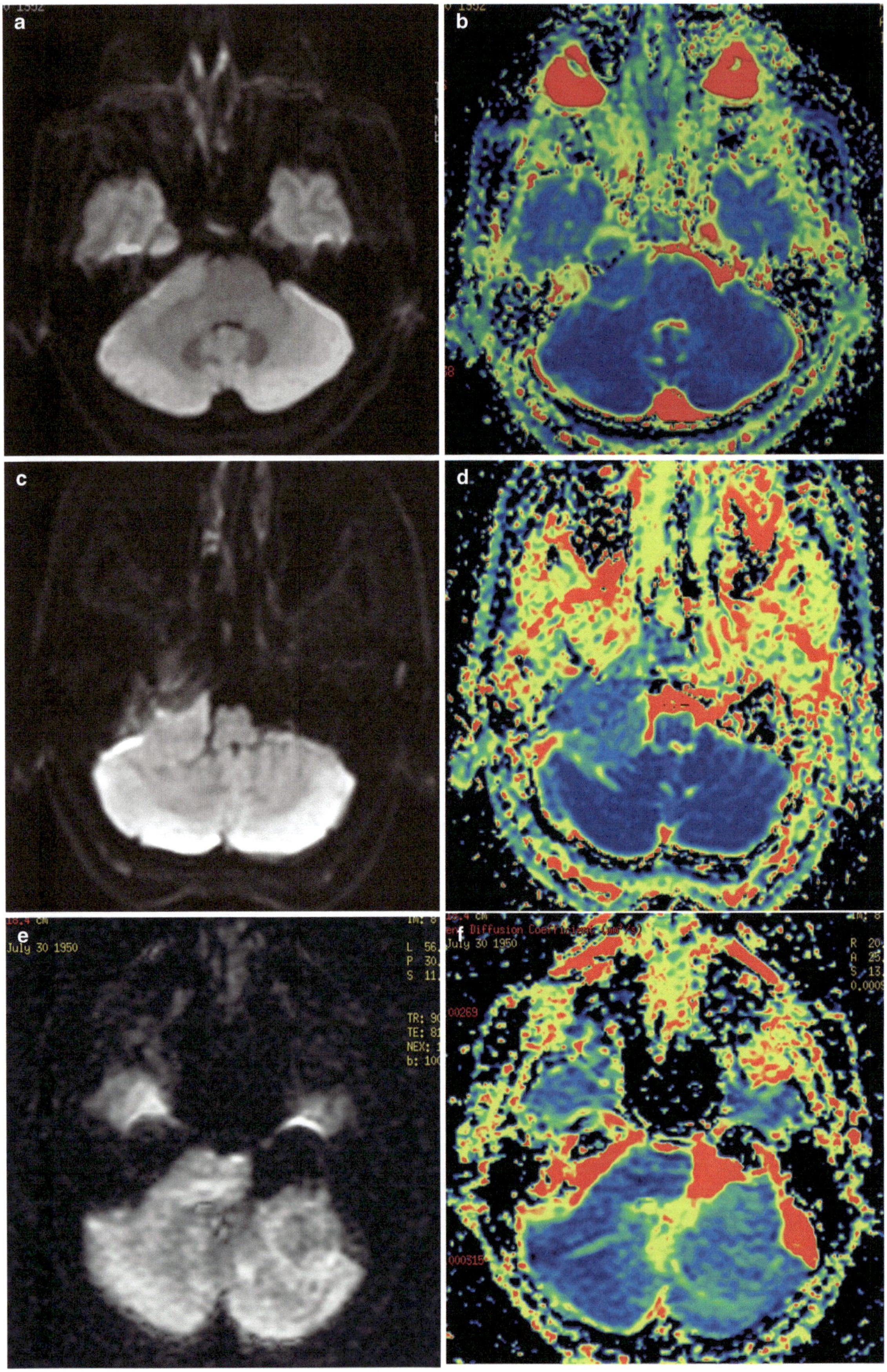

Fig. 23.17 Meningiomas of the petroclival region (different patients, case № 1 (**a**, **b**), case № 2 (c, **d**), case № 3 (**e**, **f**)). Meningiomas are characterized by iso-hyperintense MR-signal on DWI (**a**, **c**, **e**) and quite similar to brain ADC values (ADC maps (**b**, **d**, **f**))

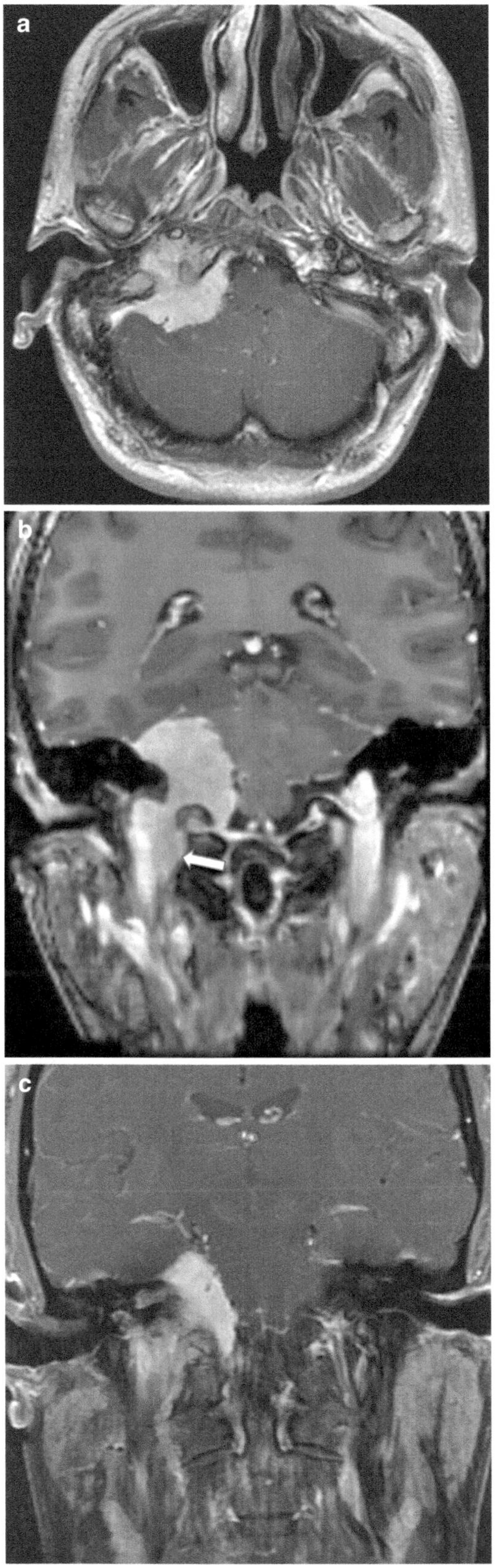

Fig. 23.18 Meningioma of the cerebellopontine angle with an invasion of the jugular foramen. Contrast enhanced MRI (**a**–**c**) demonstrates an enhanced tumor that penetrates into the lumen of the jugular foramen and then extracranially along the jugular vein (*arrow*)

spinal schwannomas. Antony B type is characterized by the reticular structure with loosely arranged cells with lymphocyte-like nuclei. Intracranial schwannomas are usually characterized by a combination of these types of microscopic tumor structure.

While schwannoma is one of the most common tumors of the cerebellopontine angle and PCF in general, neurofibroma is a tumor that histopathologically differs from schwannoma by a large amount of collagen, its intracranial localization is diagnosed much less frequently. The most frequent neurofibroma location is spinal and peripheral nerves, especially in a combination with neurofibromatosis type II. Neurofibromas usually occur at the projection of the orbit and the middle cranial fossa. In the latter case, this is a so-called plexiform neurofibroma type (for NF I type). The cerebellopontine angle is an extremely rare localization for neurofibromas.

Macroscopically, schwannoma is a rounded, sometimes lobular lesion with a marked connective tissue capsule. In some schwannomas, a large number of vessels are determined, often with thickened, hyalinized walls, sometimes even venous lacunae are observed. If the tumor is localized in the subtentorial area, it often originates from the root of the auditory nerve (vestibular portion), lying in the cerebellopontine angle, rarer from the root of fifth nerve (in the area of Gasser's ganglion) and very rarely from the roots of the facial, glossopharyngeal and vagus nerves (usually in neurofibromatosis type II). In pediatric clinical practice, schwannomas account for about 2% of tumors of the subtentorial area, usually in patients with neurofibromatosis. Typically, schwannomas originate from the vestibular portion of the VIIIth nerve, however, sensorineural hearing loss is the leading clinical symptom. Symptoms of involvement of the vestibular portion occur later.

There are three stages of vestibular schwannoma:

Stage 1—the tumor size does not exceed 2–2.5 cm, with symptoms of impairment of hearing and vestibular system: unilateral deafness and loss of vestibular function on the same side, as well as taste loss, light facial nerve palsy;

Stage 2—the tumor has a size of 3–4 cm (looks like a walnut), symptoms at this stage are more pronounced due to the pressure on the brainstem, multiple spontaneous nystagmus, impaired balance and coordination;

Stage 3—the tumor size is of 5–6 cm (a chicken egg), its clinical manifestations are caused by a sharp compression of brain structures: severe nystagmus, hydrocephalus causes psychiatric disturbances, visual impairment may occur due to compression of the optic nerves.

Clinical signs of vestibular schwannoma consists of three main groups of symptoms—symptoms of involvement of cranial nerves, brainstem symptoms, and cerebellar disturbances. The auditory nerve impairment is observed in 95% of cases, but the first signs of the disease usually include tinnitus observed in 60% of patients, and hearing loss, first in high pitches. Signs of vestibular nerve impairment are

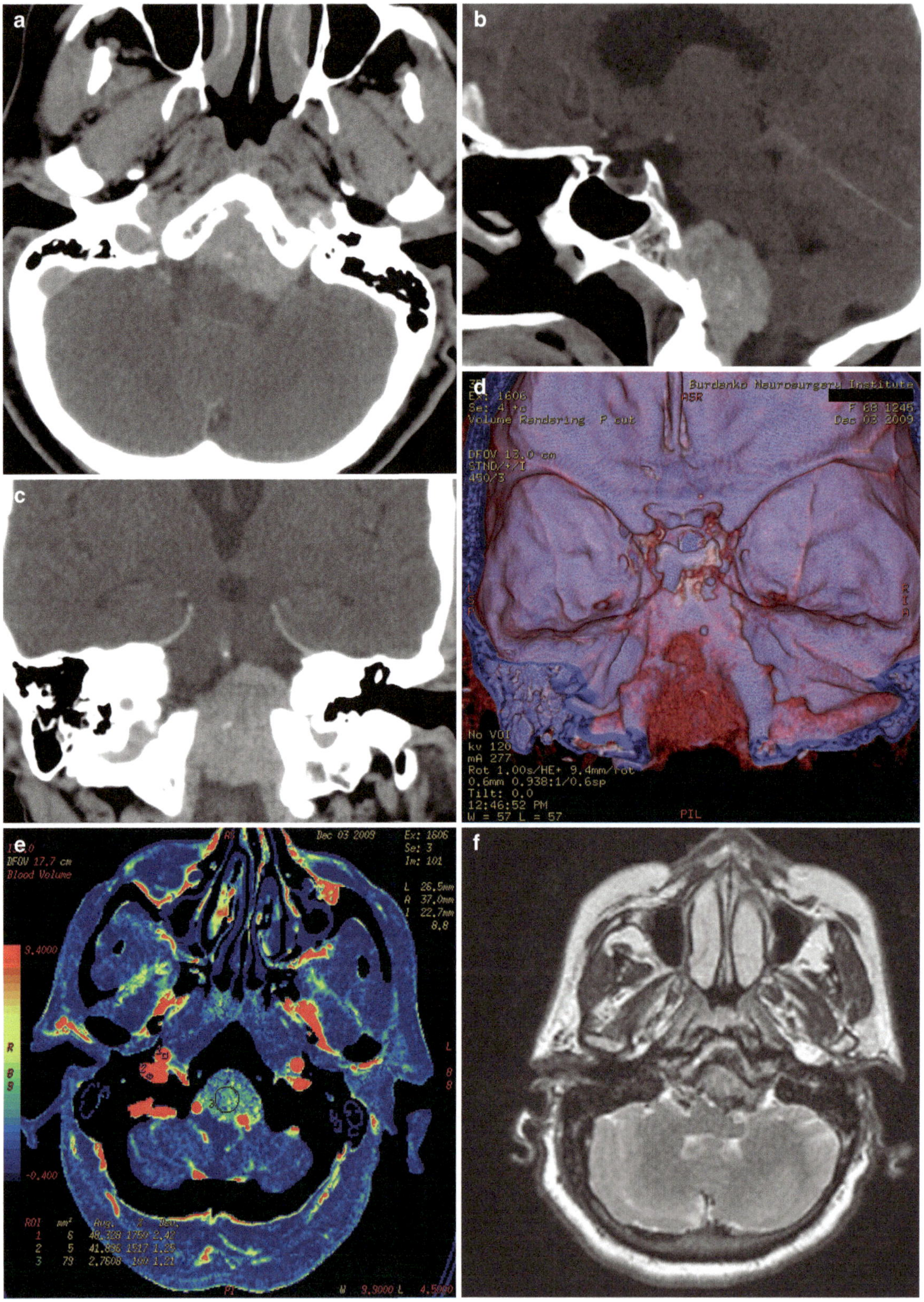

Fig. 23.19 Meningioma of the foramen Magnum. Contrast enhanced CT scans (**a**–**c**) revealed a solid enhancing tumor with focal clivus destruction area. Tumor has homogeneous structure and enhancement. 3D CT reconstruction (**d**) visualizes well the region of bone's destruction. On CT-perfusion study ((**e**), CBV) meningioma is characterized by elevated blood volume parameters. T2-weighted MRI (**f**, **g**) and T1-weighted images after contrast enhancement (**h**, **i**) demonstrate clearly the meningioma's location and solid structure, compression of the brainstem and the symptom of "dural tail"

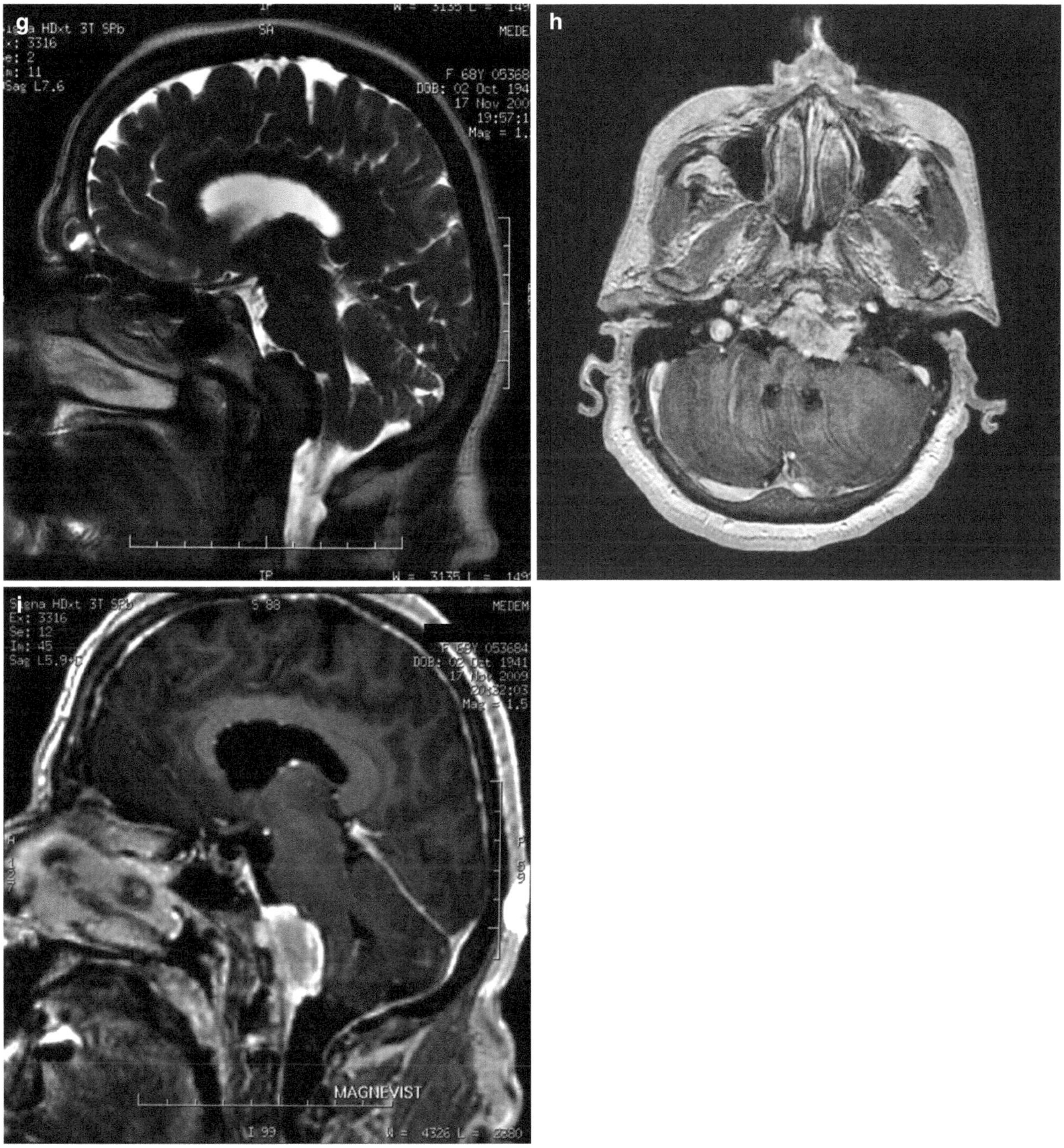

Fig. 23.19 (continued)

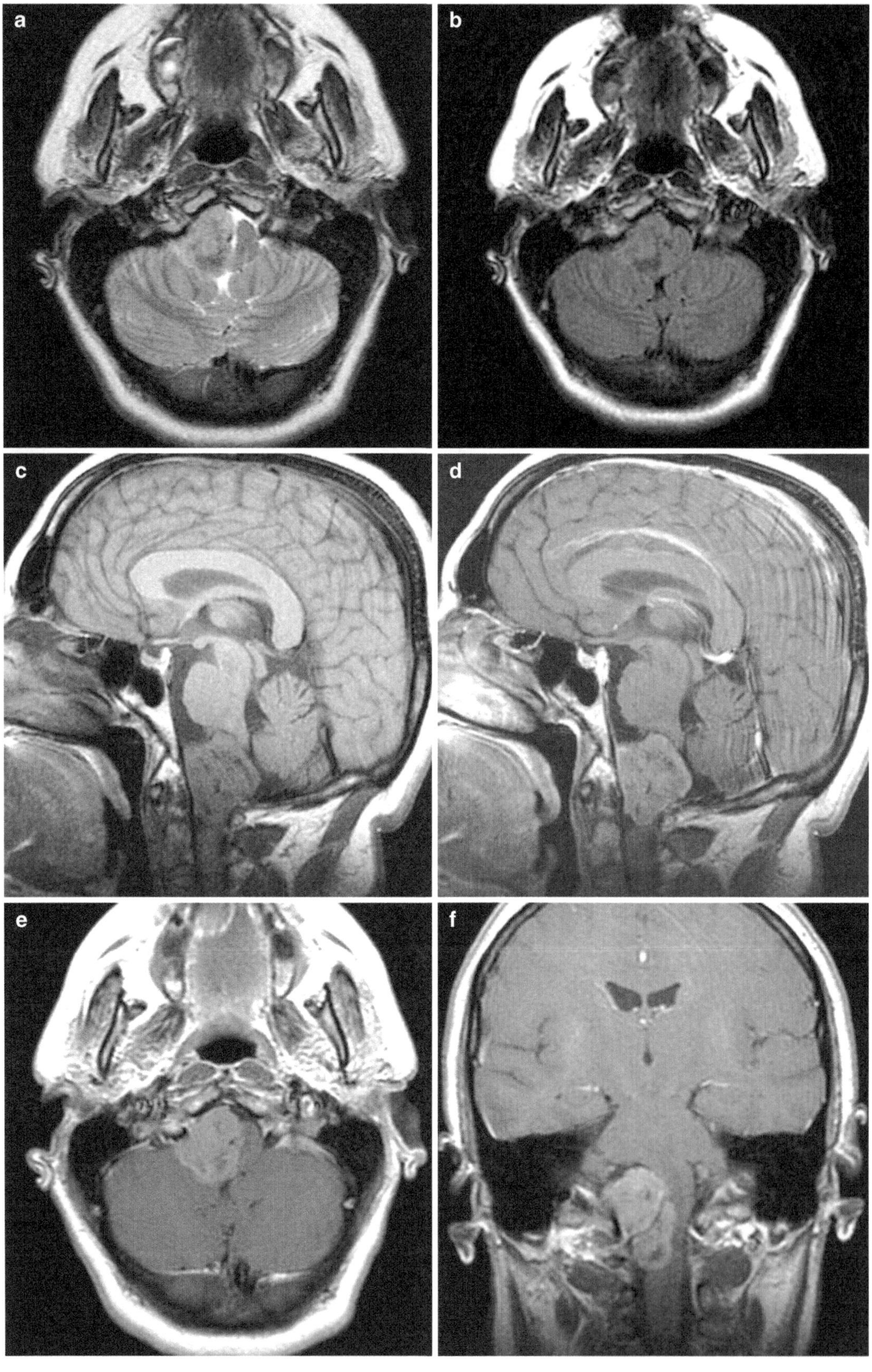

Fig. 23.20 Meningioma of the foramen Magnum. T2- (**a**), T2-FLAIR- (**b**) and T1- (**c**) weighted MR images show an isointense to brain solid tumor in the projection of craniocervical junction on the right. Tumor causes of significant dislocation of the brainstem. There is an intense contrast enhancement of the meningioma's stroma (**d–f**) on T1-weighted MRI

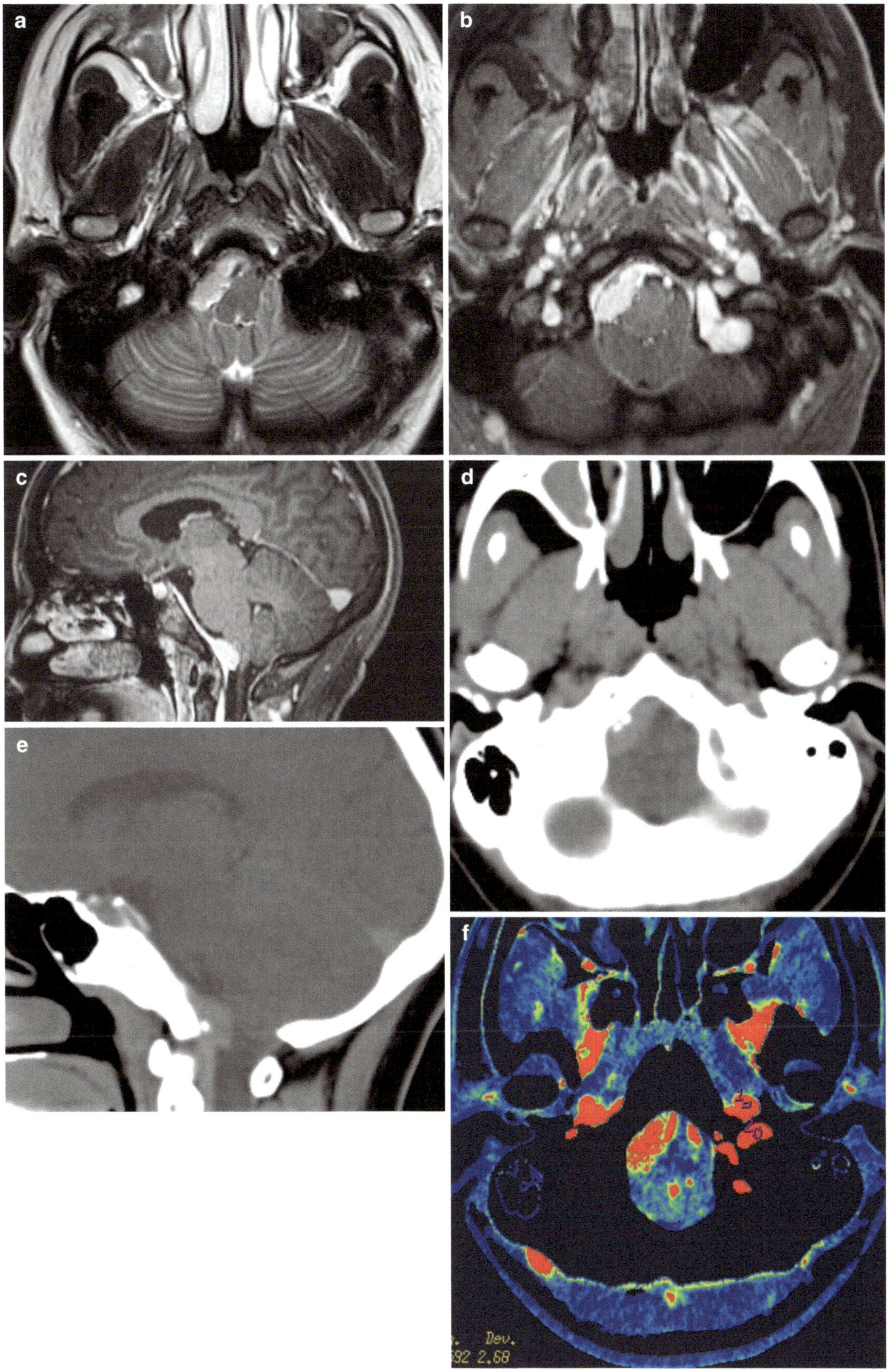

Fig. 23.21 A small meningioma of the foramen magnum on the right. On T2-weighted MR image (**a**) and postenhanced T1-weighted images (**b**, **c**) a small flat-shaped meningioma in the right half of the foramen magnum can be seen. The brainstem is partially compressed. The tumor is significantly enhanced (**b**, **c**). There are microcalcificates in the meningioma matrix on enhanced CT scans (**d**, **e**), these are not visible on MRI. CBV map shows an elevation of perfusion parameters in meningioma (**f**)

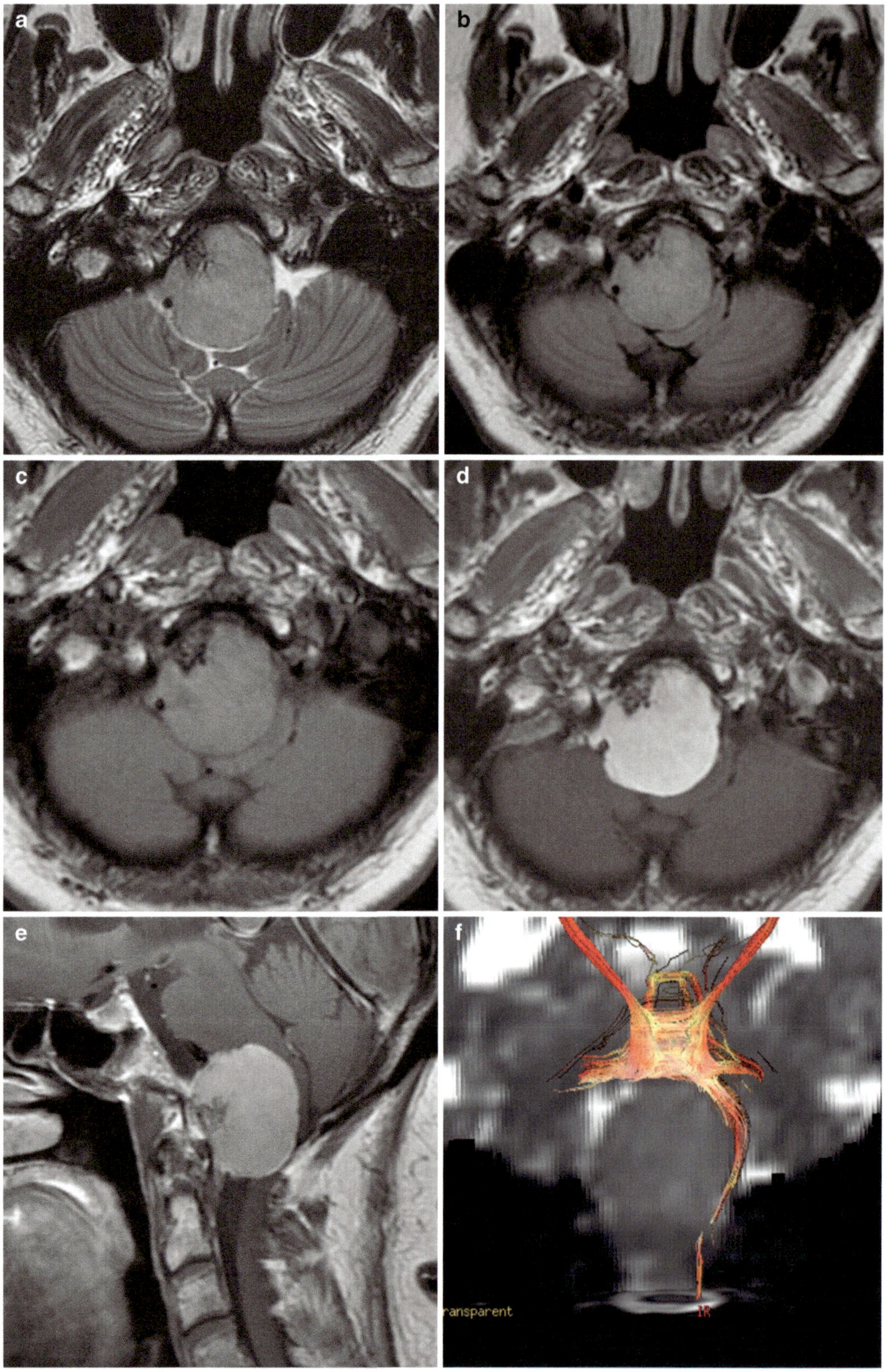

Fig. 23.22 Meningioma of the foramen magnum. T2- (**a**), T2-FLAIR- (**b**), and T1- (**c**) weighted MR images show an isointense to brain solid tumor in the projection of craniocervical junction on the right. Tumor causes of significant dislocation of the brainstem. There is an intense contrast enhancement of the meningioma's stroma (**d**, **e**) on T1-weighted MRI and hypointense central area due to matrix's calcification. MR-tractography (**f**) reveals the dislocation of cortico-spinal tract on the left. High resolution 3D TOF MR-angiography (**g**–**i**) demonstrates the blood supply of the meningioma from two branches of right vertebral artery. On enhanced CT scans a meningioma is characterized by strong and homogeneous contrast enhancement (**j**–**m**). Calcification in the matrix meningioma can be clearly seen on CT than on MRI. Perfusion studies with using CT (CBV map (**n**)) and ASL MRI (CBF map (**o**)) confirmed the high level of meningioma hemodynamics

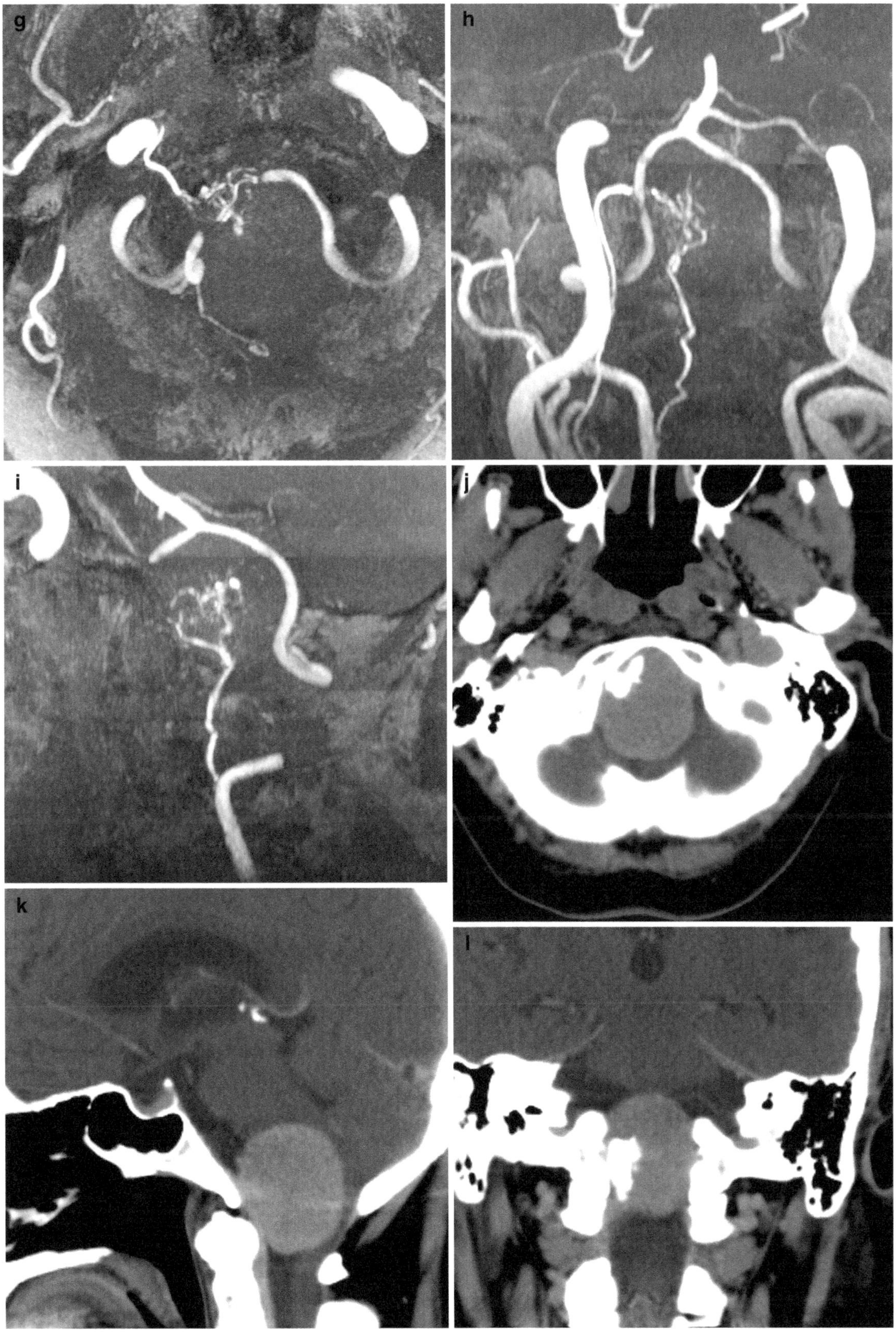

Fig. 23.22 (continued)

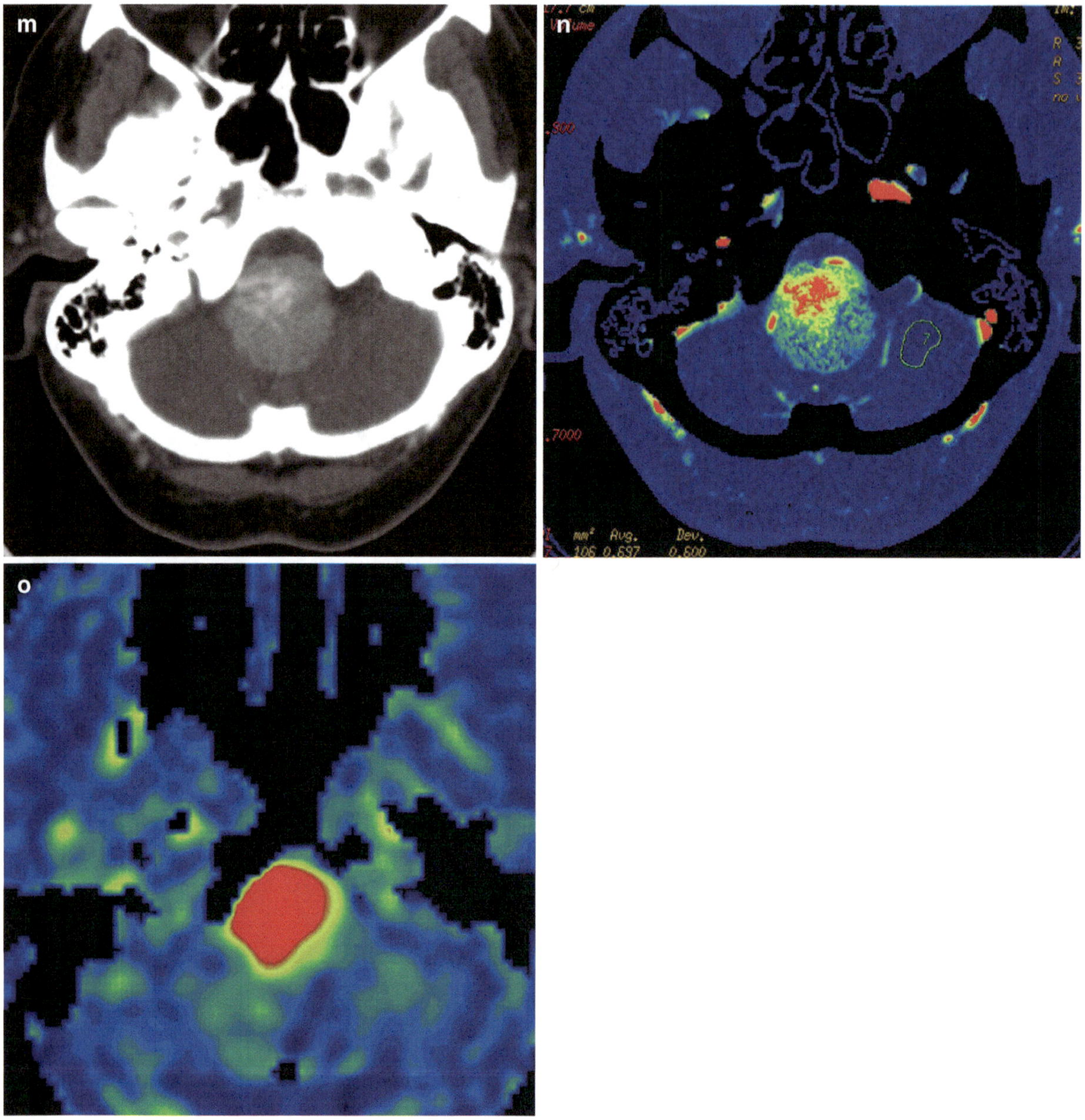

Fig. 23.22 (continued)

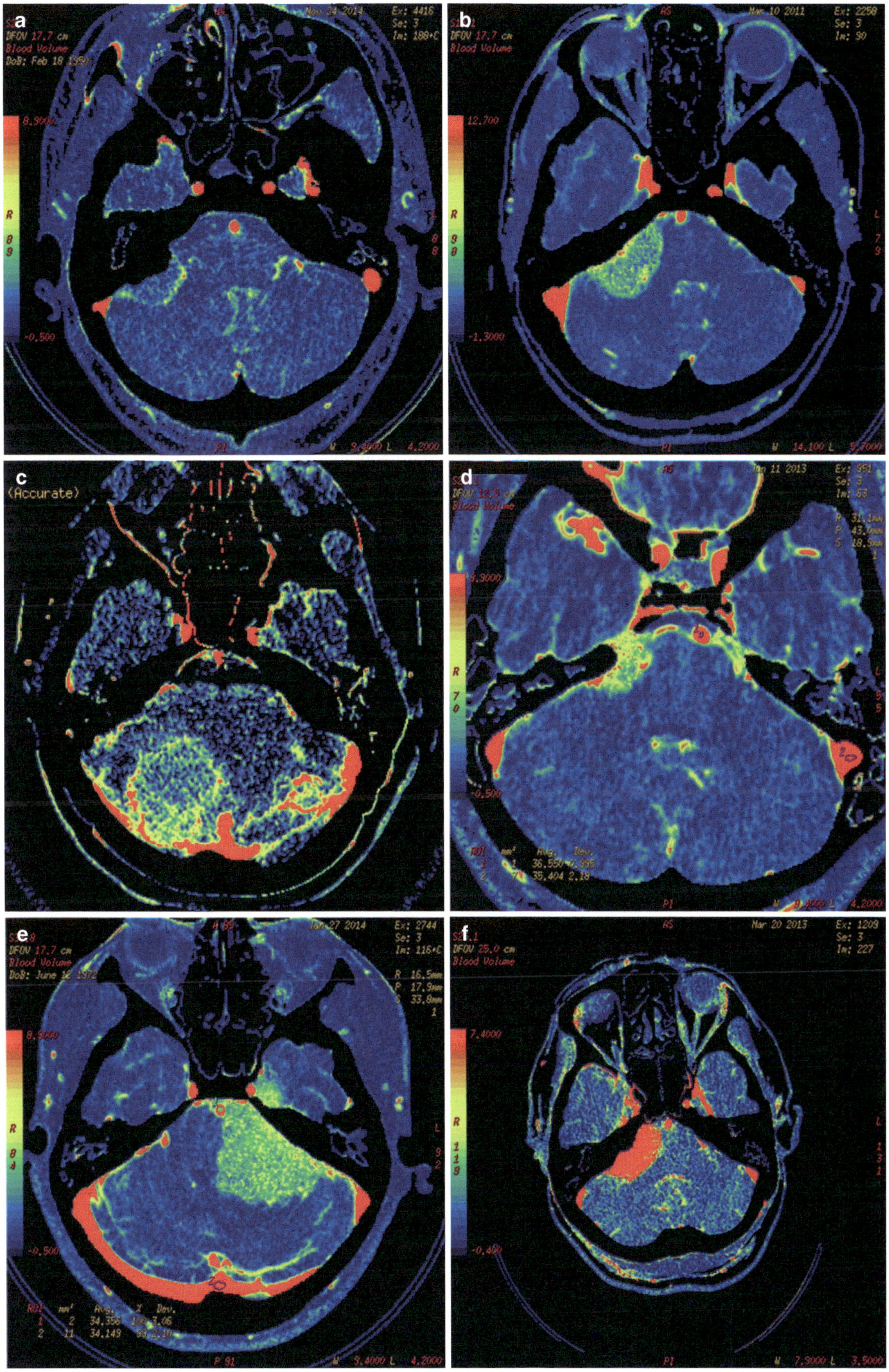

Fig. 23.23 Different patterns of meningioma's perfusion (different patients): from low to high perfusion. CBV maps (**a**–**f**)

observed in 60% of patients and are periodically manifested with a sense of instability with sudden turning of the head or body, i.e. "dizziness" mostly characterizes the impairment of statokinetic balance, while true vestibular (systemic) dizziness is rare in schwannomas. Spontaneous horizontal nystagmus at early stages of the disease is detected approximately in 30% of patients. Development of the disease eventually leads to a complete loss of vestibulocochlear nerve function, which is manifested by deafness and loss of vestibular excitability on the affected side. Development of vestibular schwannoma leads to the significant impact on the facial nerve, which is closest to VIIIth nerve. Symptoms of trigeminal nerve involvement have been reported in 15% of patients with tumors growing outside the internal auditory canal (intracranially), which is indicative for schwannomas larger than 2 cm. The clinical symptoms of the involvement of IX, X, XII nerves appear much later and only in cases with large tumors (larger than 4 cm). These patients have hypoesthesia and taste disturbance on the back third of the tongue, hypoesthesia of the mucous of the upper pharynx, asymmetry of the soft palate, dysphonia and atrophy of a half of the tongue on the side of the tumor. Symptoms of brainstem and cerebellum involvement can be identified.

By their localization, *vestibular schwannomas* are divided into three main categories:

1. Intracanalicular—located within the internal auditory meatus (Fig. 23.24);
2. Intra- and extracanalicular—grow both into the inner ear canal and the cerebellopontine cistern (Figs. 23.25 and 23.26).
3. Extracanalicular schwannomas originate from the part of the nerve that runs in the cerebellopontine cistern.

Tumors grow slowly (2–10 mm per year), have a capsule (Fig. 23.27). They account for almost 80% of the cerebellopontine angle tumors, and in 4–5% of cases they are bilateral (Charabi et al. 1995). They occur in about 8–10% of all intracranial tumors. Tumors usually develop after the age of 30. Multiple lesions are observed in neurofibromatosis type II. Schwannomas more often occur in women. Schwannomas are benign tumors, their malignization is rare.

Imaging On CT, schwannomas smaller than 1 cm are difficult to detect. Even large tumors on CT scans without contrast enhancement have the density close to that of the brain tissue (Figs. 23.28 and 23.29). The cystic portion of schwannoma is characterized by low density. An important component of schwannoma CT-diagnosis is an analysis of the images obtained in bone-window mode: in most cases, the tumor causes enlargement of the internal auditory canal (Fig. 23.30). Following contrast enhancement, an increase in the tumor density from mild to severe is observed. In these conditions, the structure of the neoplasm and mass effect on the adjacent brain structures are better determined (Fig. 23.31). Large vestibular schwannomas or bilateral tumors can cause the development of hydrocephalus of the third and lateral ventricles.

On MRI, the tumor has a typically hypointense signal on T1-weighted images and hyperintense signal on T2-weighted sequences (Curati et al. 1986). Most vestibular schwannomas follow the direction of the internal auditory canal, with the minor part of the tumor, located in it, comprising its smaller portion. Tumor in such cases appears as a "hanging drop." Its contour is generally smooth, there is so-called "CSF cleft" detected along its periphery. The deformation and compression of cerebellum and brainstem depend on the size of the tumor (Figs. 23.32 and 23.33). Small vestibular schwannomas (usually Antony A histologic subtype) homogeneously accumulate contrast agent. Areas of heterogeneity, including regions due to cyst formation, are typical for large-sized schwannomas, usually larger than 3 cm, of Antony B subtype or mixed Antony A and B type (Fig. 23.34). All schwannomas intensively and heterogeneously accumulate contrast media in more than 70% of cases.

On DWI, schwannomas have an iso- or hypointense MR-signal compared with the surrounding brain tissue and are characterized by relatively high ADC values due to wide intercellular spaces and high water content (Fig. 23.35). In most of CT-perfusion studies, schwannomas demonstrate a moderate and heterogeneous elevation of CBV and, to a lesser extent of CBF. MTT values are higher compared with those of meningiomas (Fig. 23.36). MR-spectroscopy detects an increase in myo-inositol peak (3.55 ppm), while alanine peak (typical for meningiomas) is absent in schwannomas (Fig. 23.37). Development of the new MR pulse sequences, in particular SWI, SWAN and others, allowed to visualize changes in the structure of the tumor, which had previously never been diagnosed. Almost all schwannomas greater than 2 cm show microhemorrhages in the tumor's stroma. They have hypointense MR-signal on SWI sequences. Perhaps, this phenomenon explains the fact of the cystic cavities occurrence within schwannomas, unlike, for example, within meningiomas (Fig. 23.38). Bolus enhancement and dynamic MR scanning (TRICKS, etc.) helps assess the degree of macroscopic tumor blood supply that previously could be assessed only by direct cerebral angiography (Fig. 23.39). Multiple brain lesions (multiple schwannomas, multiple neurofibromas, etc.) are observed mostly in range of neurofibromatosis type II (Fig. 23.40).

Schwannomas of Vth nerve, located in the posterior cranial fossa, develop from a cisternal portion of the trigeminal nerve root, occupy the area of the cerebellopontine angle and lateral pontine cistern. Giant vestibular schwannomas grow into the Meckel's cavity and along the course of the trigeminal nerve root, acquiring a dumbbell shape. Onset of

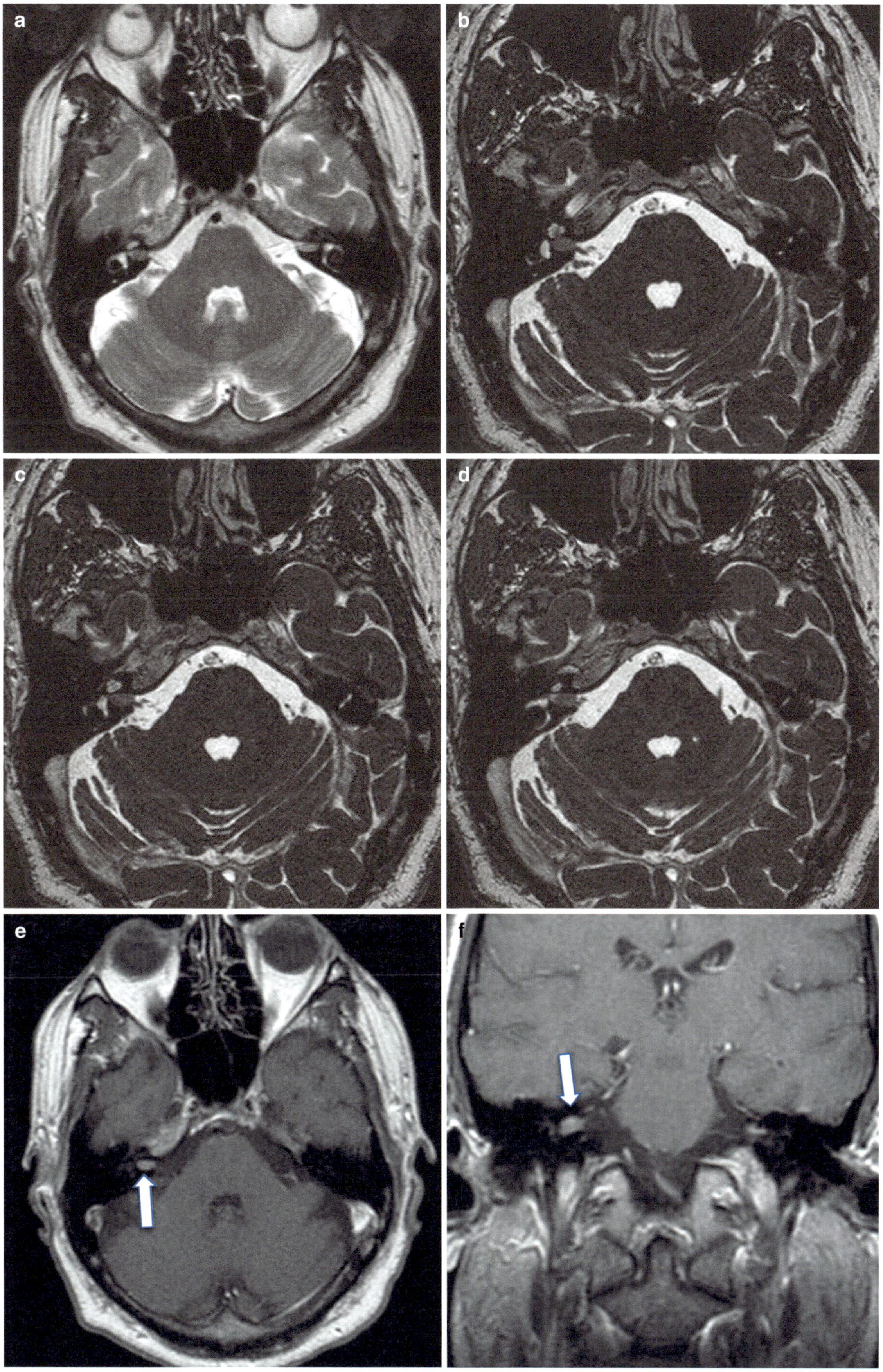

Fig. 23.24 Micro-schwannoma of the right vestibulocochlear nerve. There is an intracanalicular tumor on T2 (a), FIESTA (**b**–**d**) and T1 after contrast enhancement (**e**, **f**) MR images. This lesion shows a moderate enhancement (*arrows*)

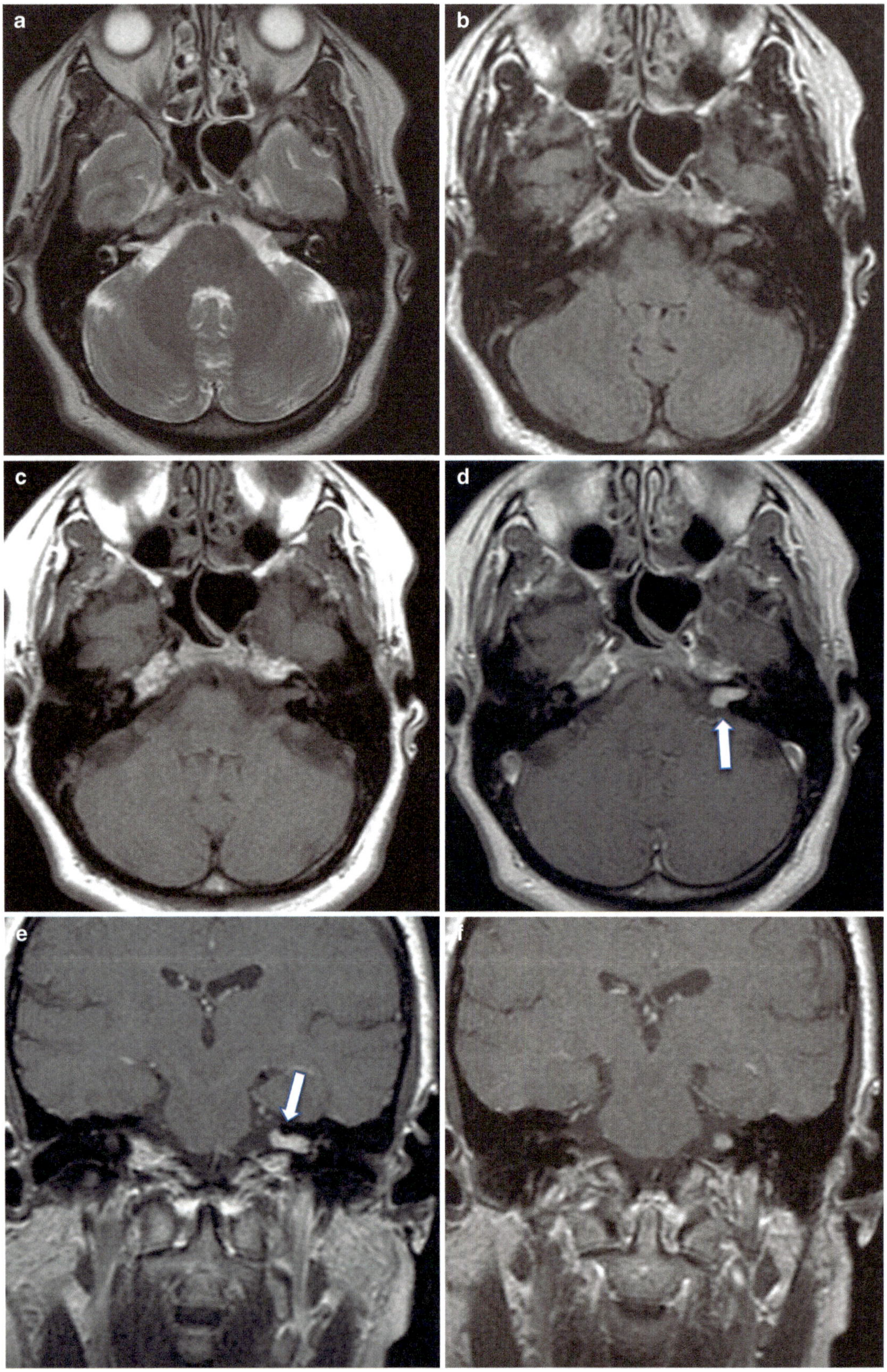

Fig. 23.25 Micro-schwannoma of the left vestibulocochlear nerve. There is an intra- extracanalicular tumor on T2- (a), T2-FLAIR- (**b**), T1 before (**c**) and after (**d**–**f**) contrast enhancement MR images. This lesion demonstrates a moderate enhancement (*arrows*) that allows to better visualize this lesion

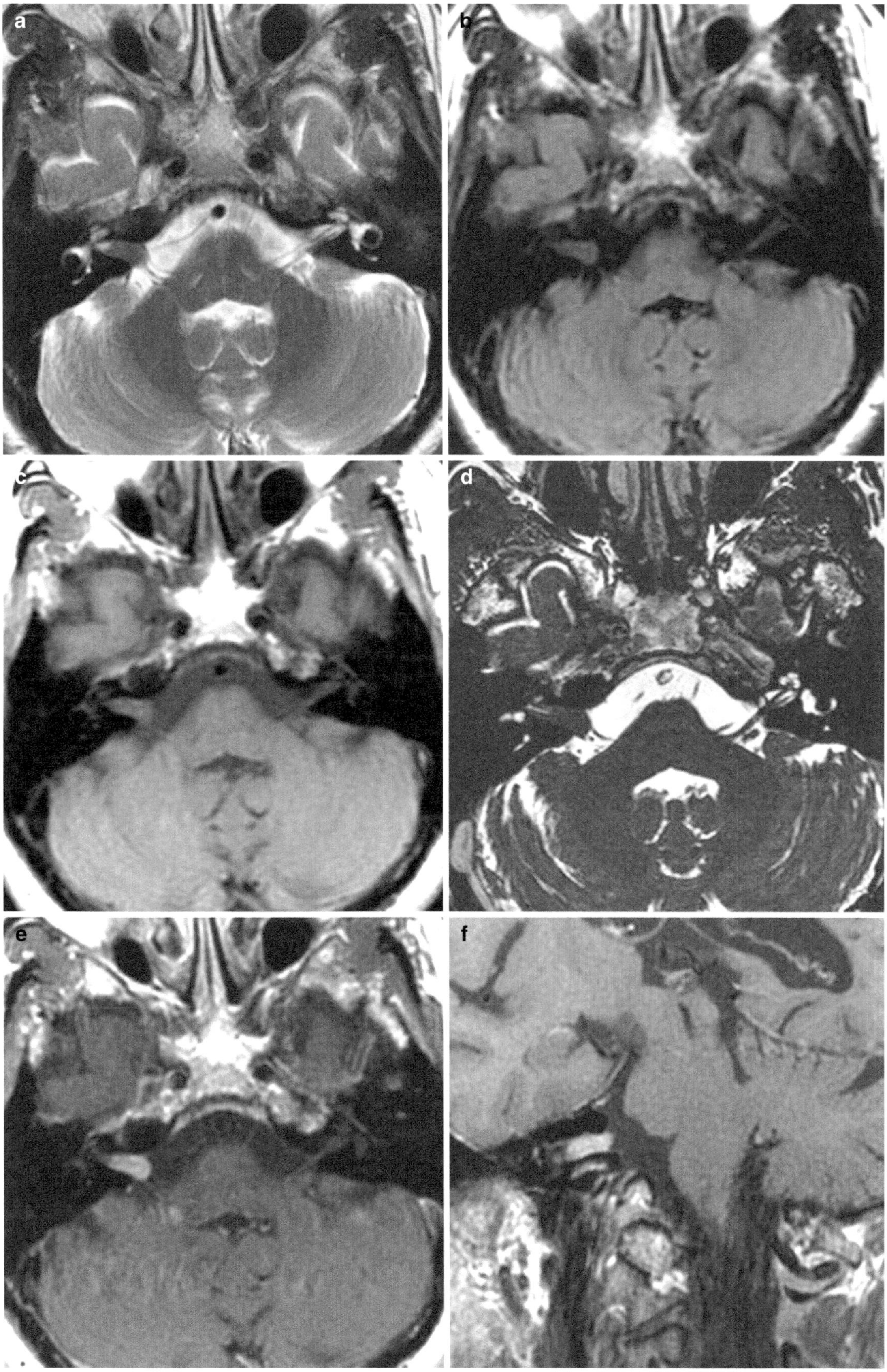

Fig. 23.26 Micro-schwannoma of the right vestibulocochlear nerve. This small tumor can be clearly seen with all MR-sequences but especially with using contrast enhancement. T2 (a), T2-FLAIR (**b**), T1 (**c**), FIESTA (**d**) and T1 after (**e**, **f**) contrast enhancement

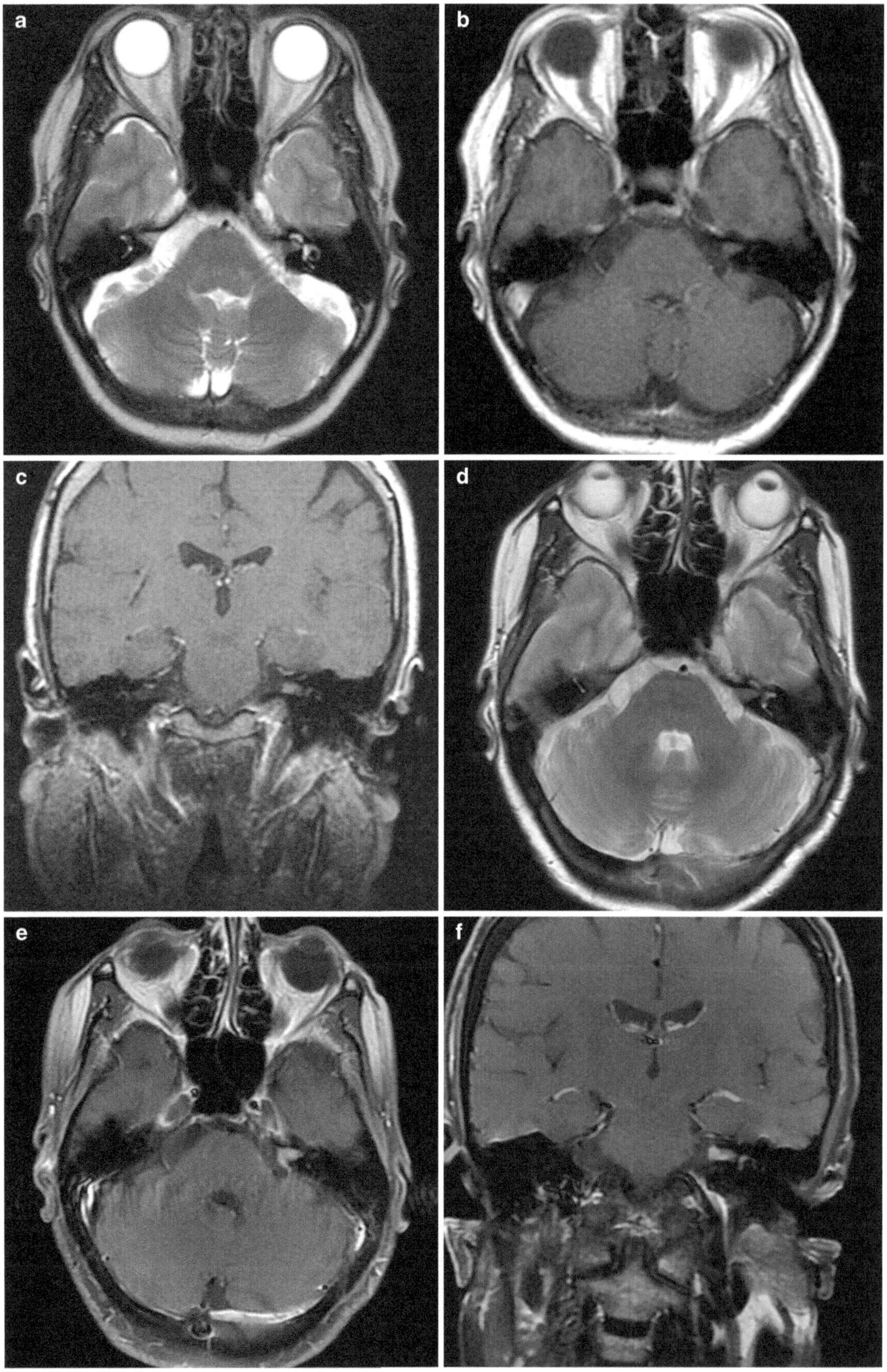

Fig. 23.27 Micro-schwannoma of the left vestibulocochlear nerve. Dynamic MRI (one and half year) revealed a slow growth of a lesion during this period of time. Initial MRI: T2- (**a**), enhanced T1- (**b**, **c**) weighted MR images. Follow-up MRI: T2- (**d**), enhanced T1- (**e**, **f**) weighted MR images

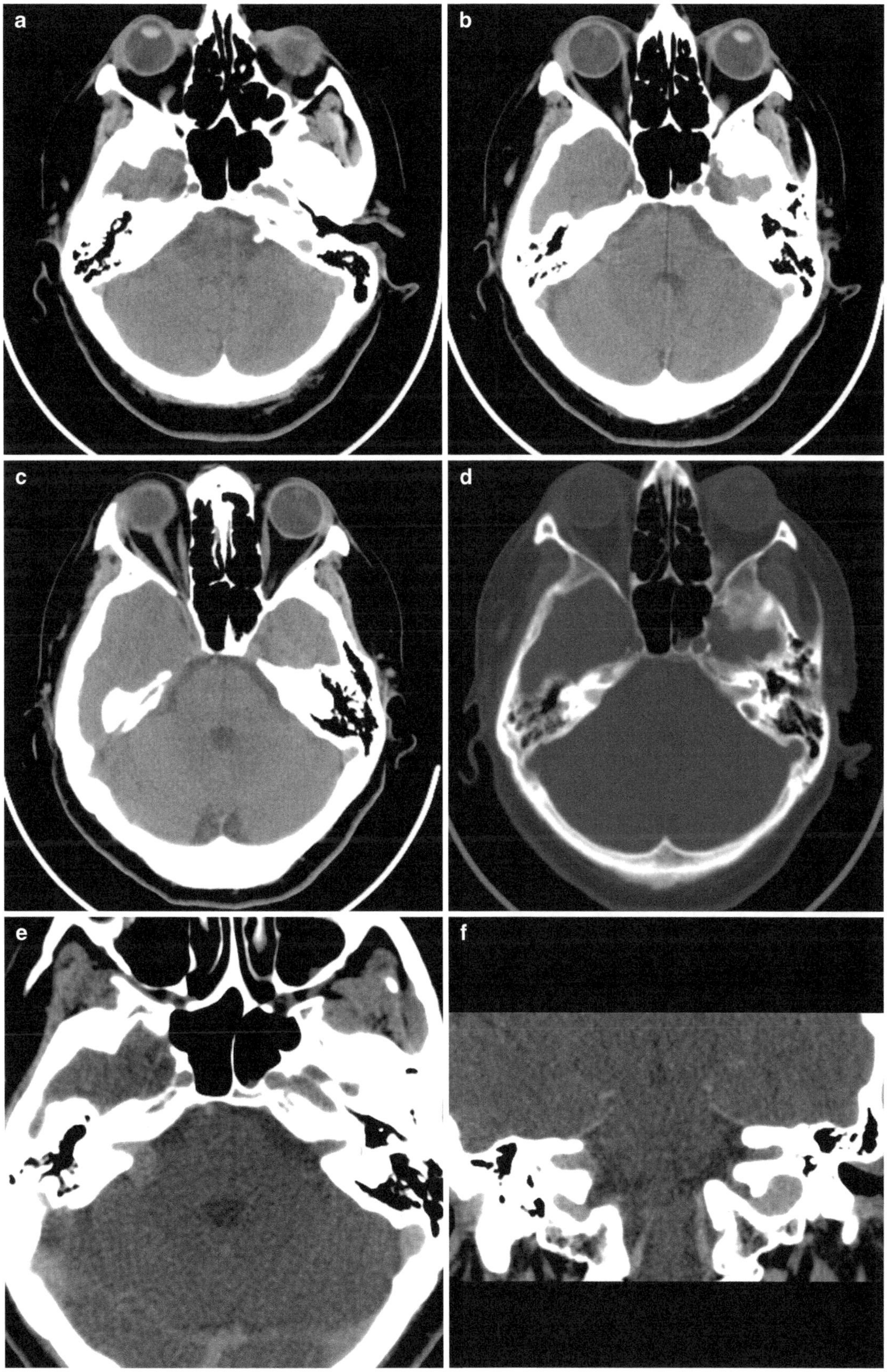

Fig. 23.28 Schwannoma of the right vestibulocochlear nerve. Axial NECT scans (**a**–**c**) don't show any changes of density in the projection of cerebellopontine angle. CT in "bone window" mode doesn't find evident asymmetry of internal acoustic meatus's size (**d**). Small extra-intracanalicular tumor is visible only after intravenous contrast enhancement (**e**, **f**)

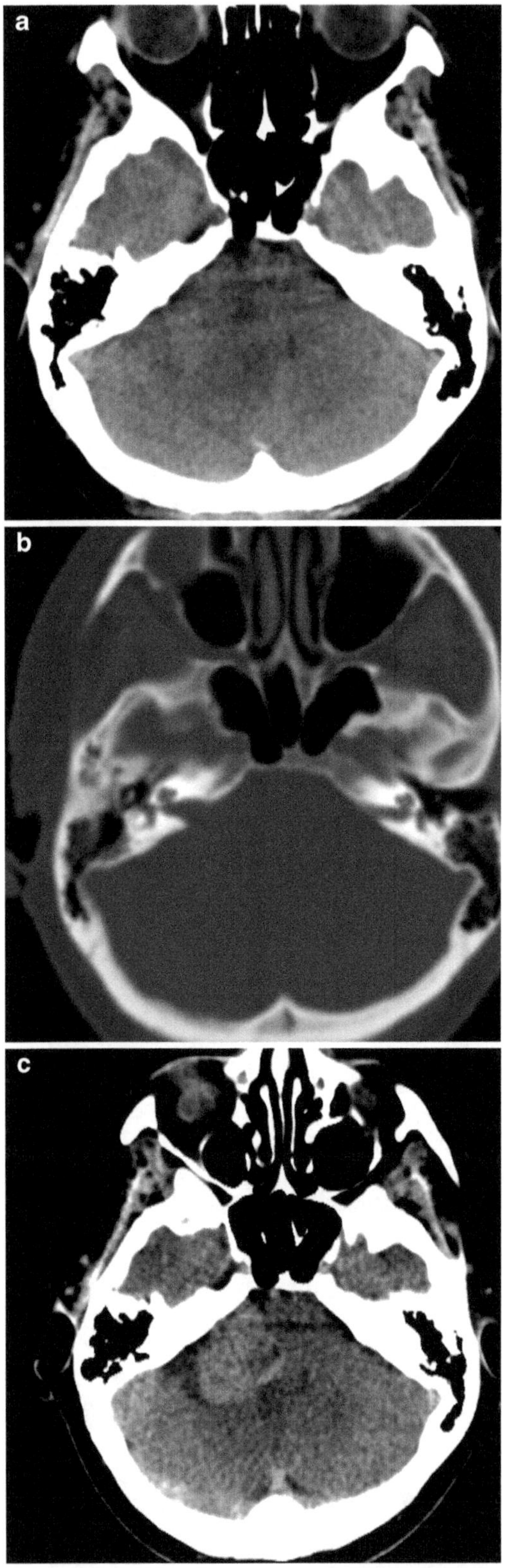

Fig. 23.29 Large schwannoma of the right vestibulocochlear nerve. Axial NECT scan (**a**) show uncertain changes of density in lateral aspects of the posterior fossa and cerebello-pontine angle on the right. There is a dislocation and compression of IVth ventricle. In "bone window" mode (**b**) the widening of the right internal acoustic meatus can be seen. The tumor is characterized by a significant contrast enhancement (**c**) and fairly clearly visible on postenhanced CT scan

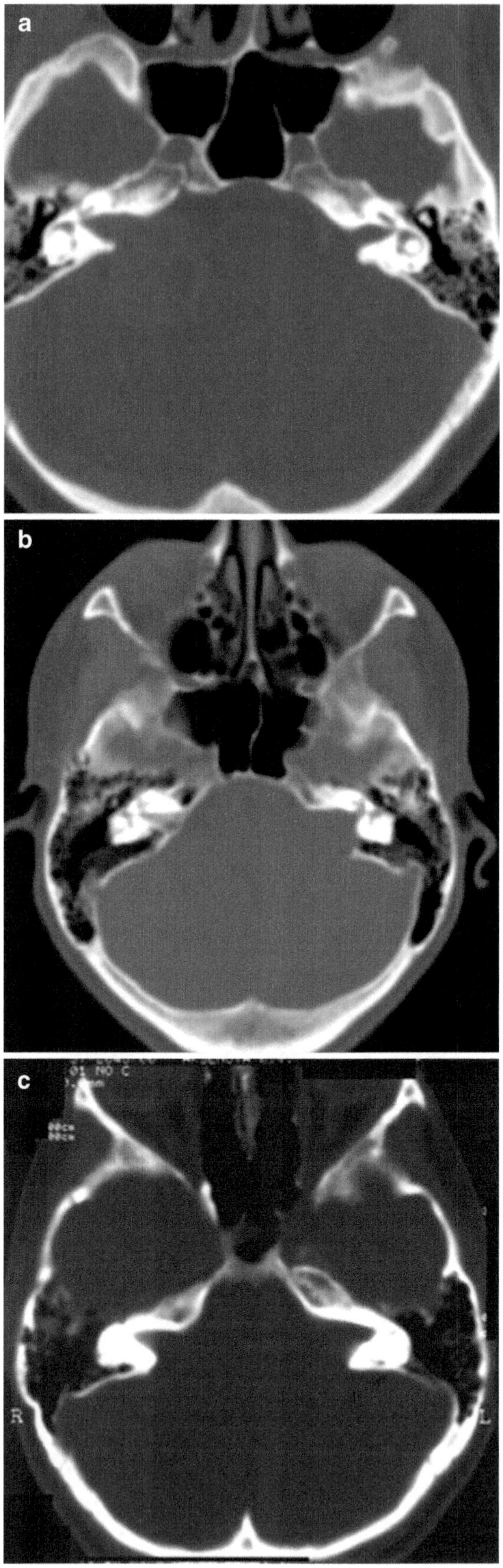

Fig. 23.30 Variants of the internal acoustic meatus's widening in cases of vestibulocochlear nerve's schwannomas. (**a**) the right side tumor, (**b**) the left side tumor, (**c**) both side tumors

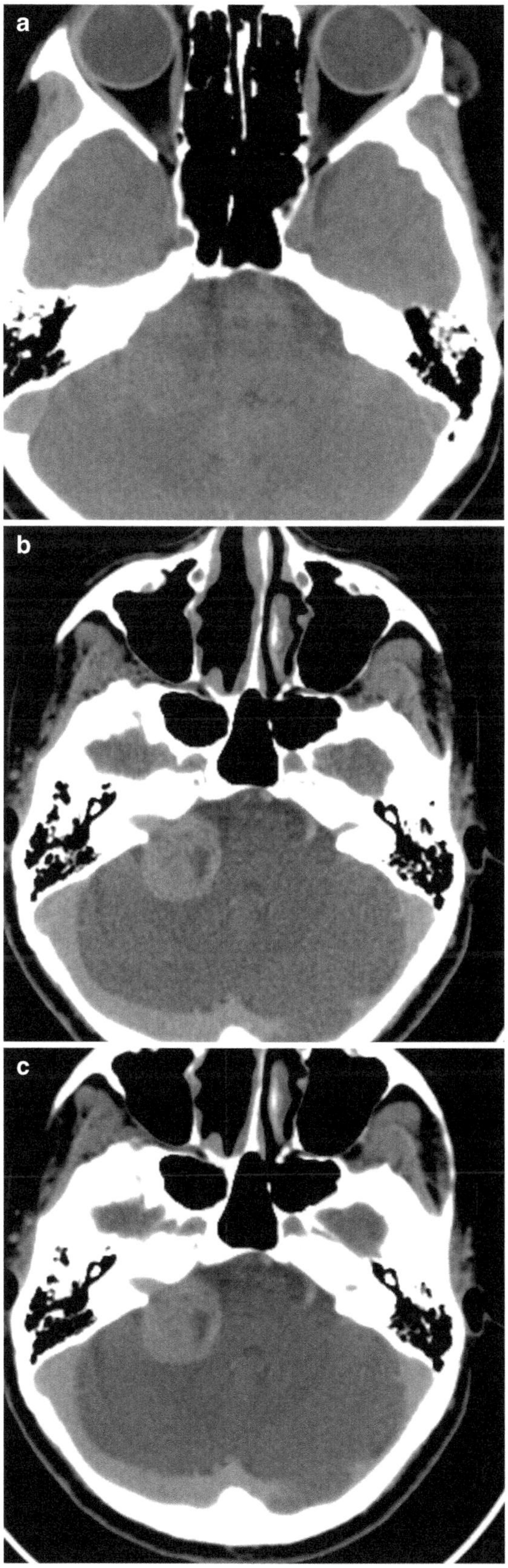

Fig. 23.31 Schwannoma of the right vestibulocochlear nerve. NECT scan (**a**) doesn't identify the tumor in cerebellopontine angle on the right due to its isodensity (**a**). The tumor is characterized by prominent enhancement and clearly depicts on postenhanced CT scans (**b**, **c**)

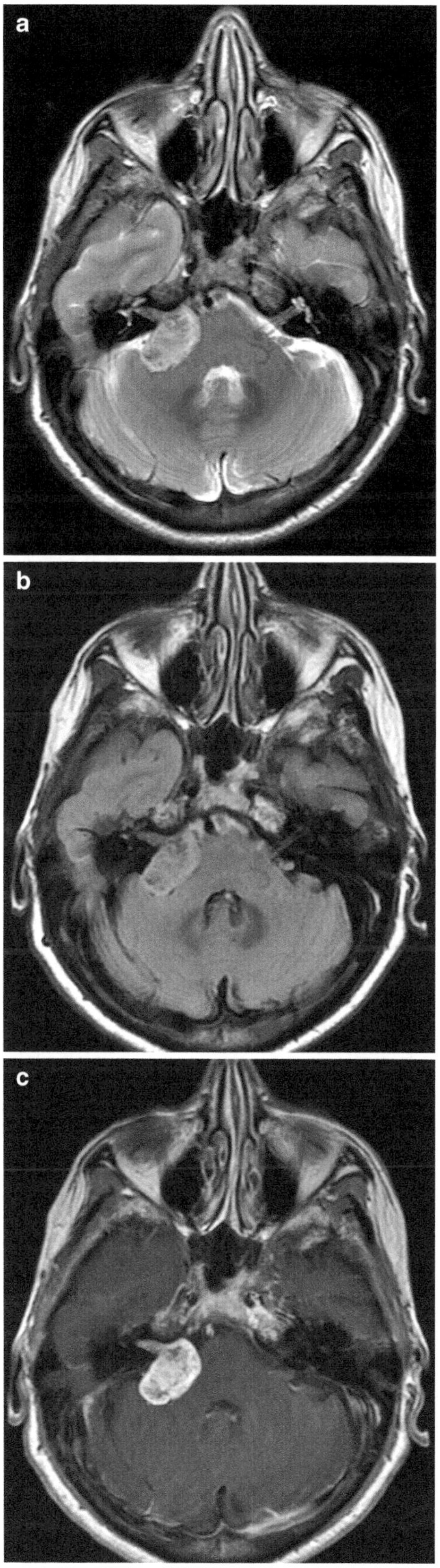

Fig. 23.32 Schwannoma of the right vestibulocochlear nerve. The tumor has a hyperintense MR-signal on T2- (**a**), T2-FLAIR- (**b**) weighted MRI. Heterogeneity of lesion's structure and its internal acoustic meatus's expansion are better visible after contrast enhancement (**c**)

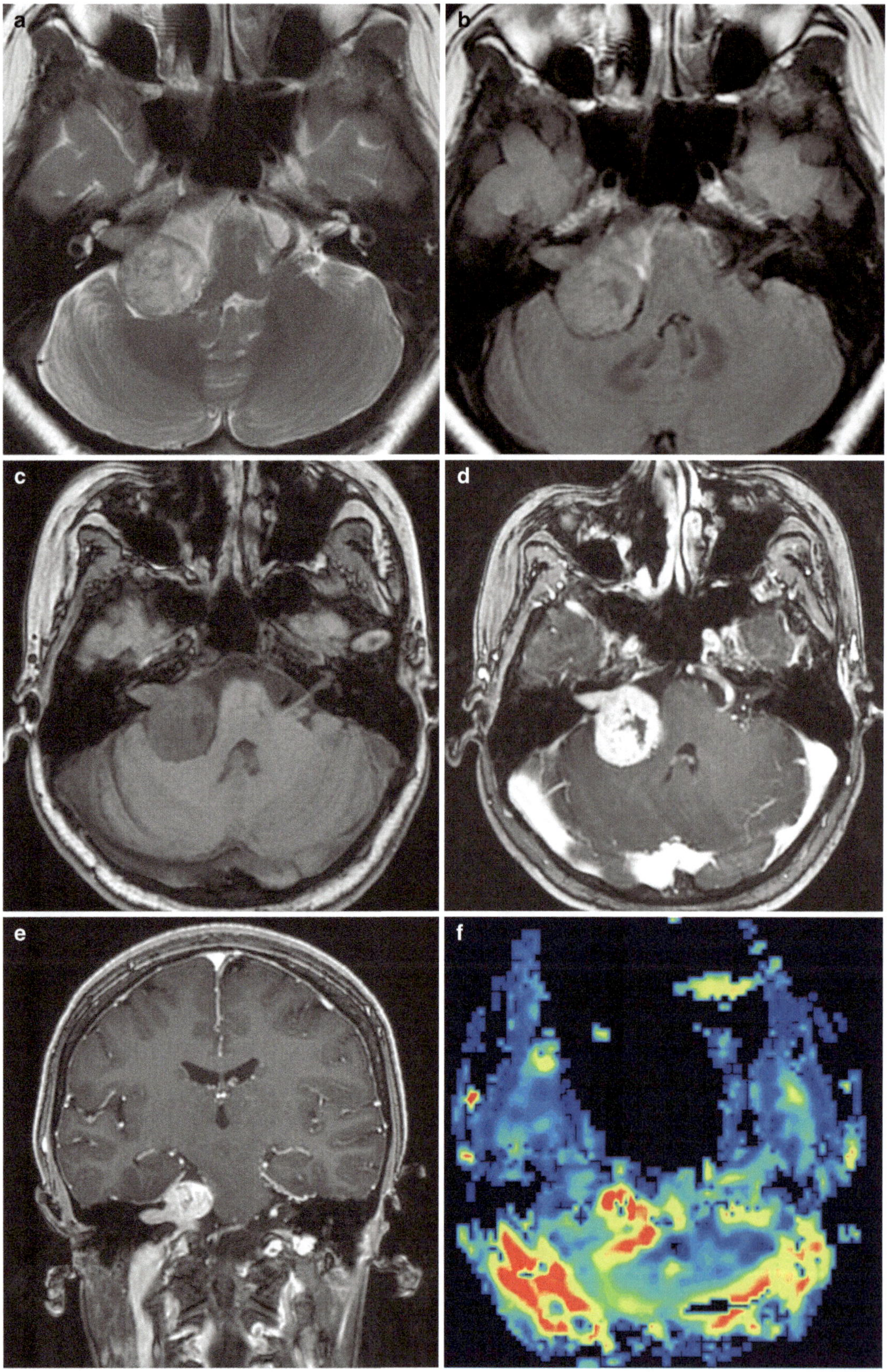

Fig. 23.33 Large schwannoma of right vestibulocochlear nerve. The tumor has a slightly hyperintense MR-signal on T2- (a), T2-FLAIR- (**b**) weighted MRI and hypointense signal on T1-WI (**c**). Tumor is characterized by prominent contrast enhancement and clearly depicts on postenhanced MR scans (**d**, **e**). Dynamic susceptibility enhanced MR-perfusion study shows an elevation of perfusion values (rCBV map (**f**))

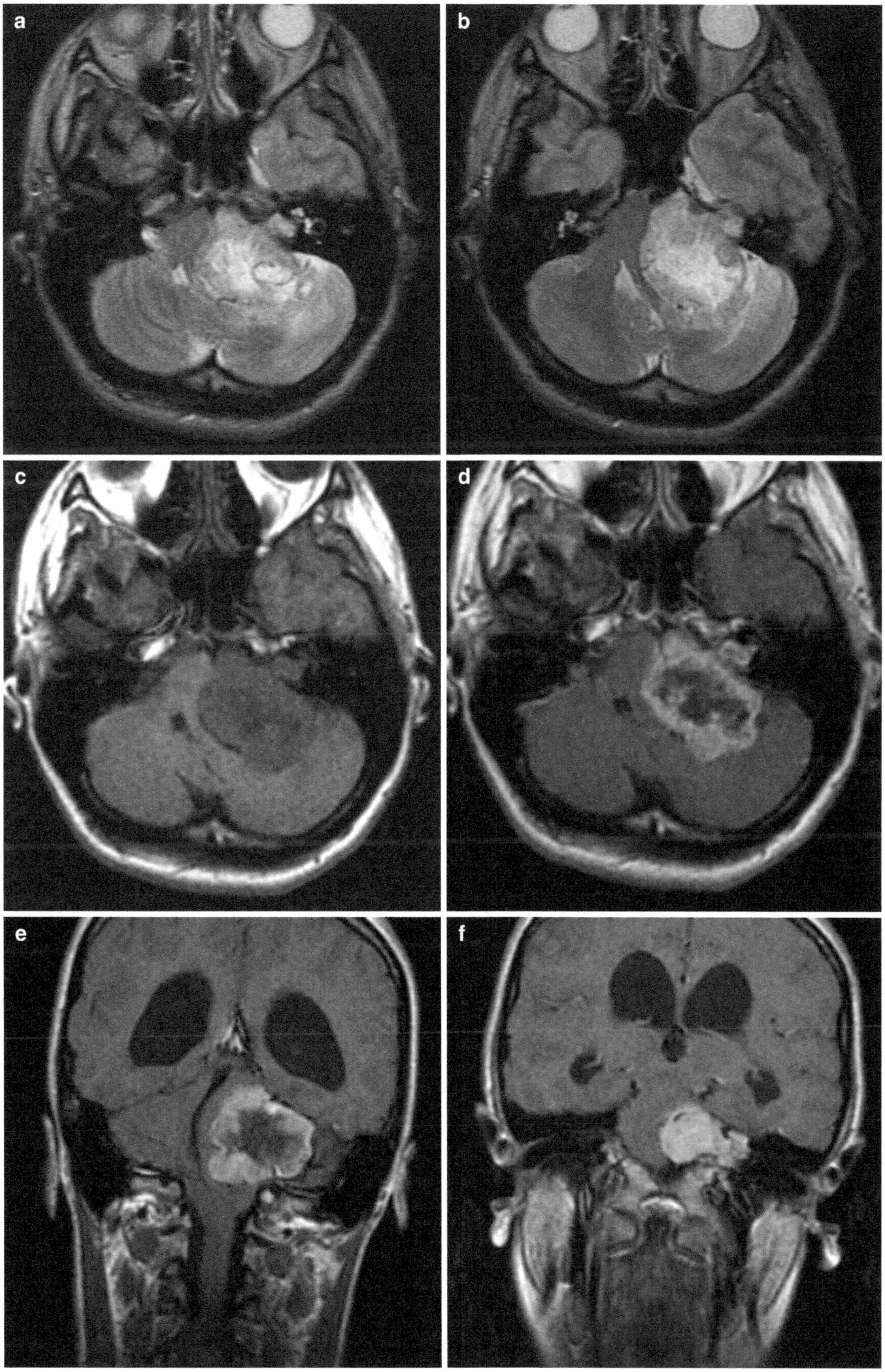

Fig. 23.34 Giant schwannoma of the left vestibulocochlear nerve. Axial T2- (**a**, **b**), T1 before (**c**) and T1 (**d**–**f**) after contrast enhancement MR images reveal a large heterogeneous lesion in projection of left cerebellopontine angle with perifocal edema. On postenhanced MR images a tumor is characterized by prominent peripheral enhancement with necrotic nonenhanced center

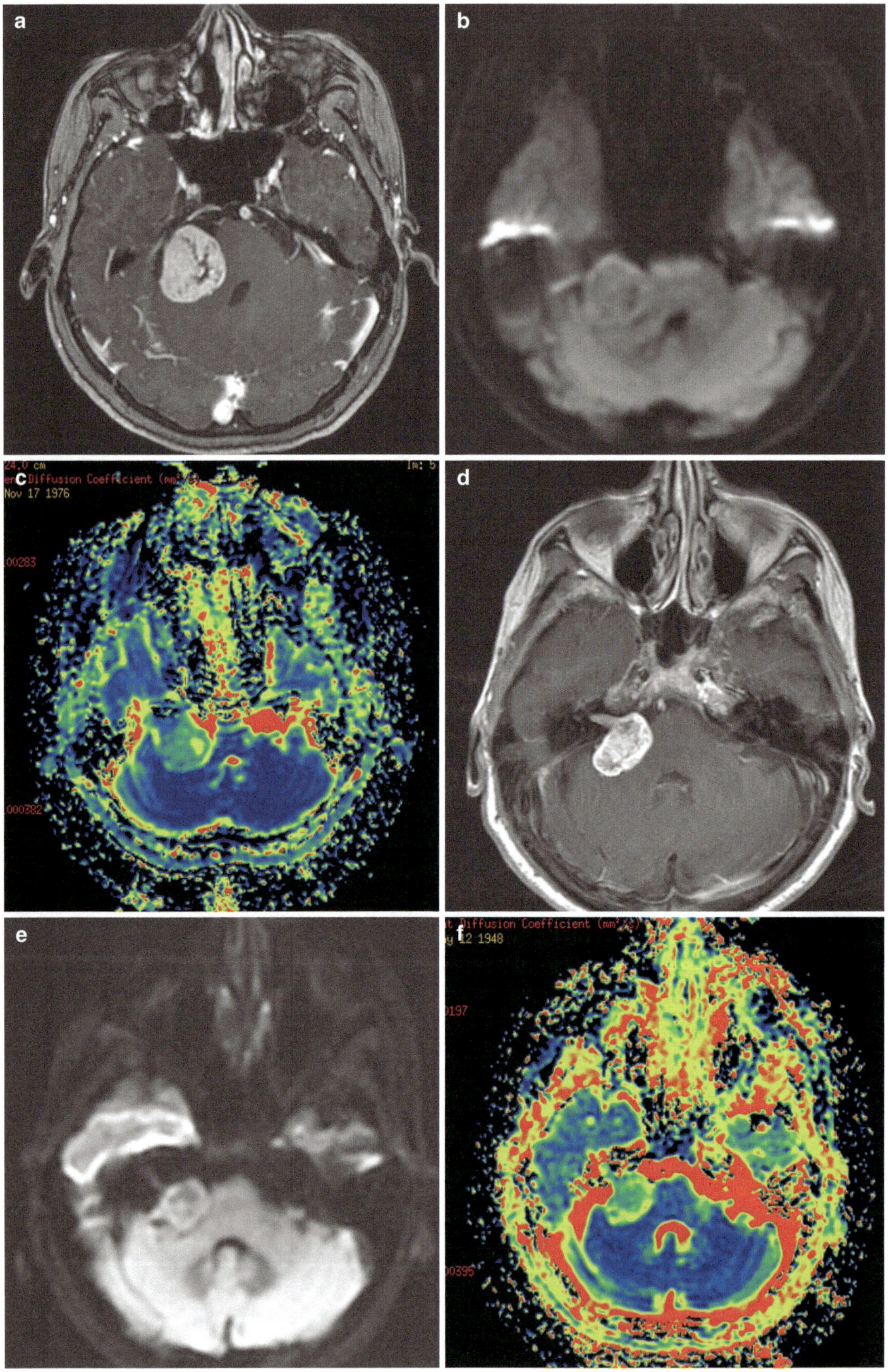

Fig. 23.35 Schwannoma of the right vestibulocochlear nerve (two different cases). Case 1. Axial contrast enhanced T1-weighted MR image (**a**) demonstrates a strongly enhanced tumor, that has isointense MR-signal on DWI (**b**) and increased ADC values on ADC map (**c**). Case 2. Enhanced tumor (**d**) of the right cerebellopontine angle has a heterogeneous iso-hypointense signal on DWI (**e**) and high values of ADC (**f**)

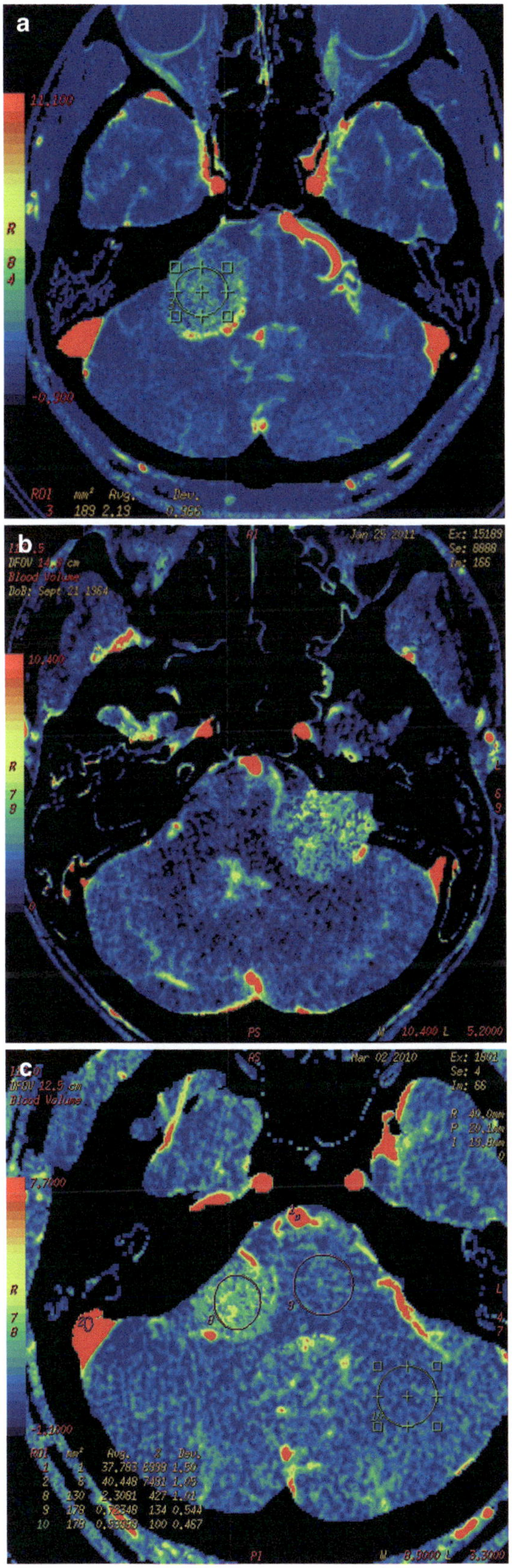

Fig. 23.36 Different patterns of CBV maps in vestibulocochlear nerve's schwannomas (different cases). CT-perfusion studies (**a**–**c**) show a moderate increased values of cerebral blood volume (CBV) in the tumor's structure

manifestations of the disease makes it possible to differentiate them from VIIIth nerve schwannomas. In general, in the majority of cases modern neuroimaging techniques can easily visualize the tumor relationship to the root of the trigeminal nerve and its spreading into the medial parts of the middle cranial fossa. CT and MRI features of vestibular schwannomas do not differ from those of VIIIth nerve tumors. Contrast enhancement facilitates a more precise delineation of the tumor mass from the surrounding brain substance. Multiplanar imaging is an important component of the complete neoplasm topography assessment. The use of MR-sequences with high spatial resolution and myelography-like techniques improves the visualization of the surrounding brain tissue, shifted cranial nerves and large arteries. Difficulties in tumor assessment usually arise when schwannomas become large (5–6 cm) and cause local bone changes in the petrous apex and even the clivus. Nevertheless, the effect of schwannoma on the bone structure is expansive, not destructive, which is better confirmed by CT than MRI (Figs. 23.41 and 23.42).

Schwannomas (neurinomas) of the facial nerve develop from VIIth nerve sheathes and can be located both at its intracranial and extracranial segments. This type of schwannomas is quite rare, accounting for less than 1% of all tumors of the temporal bone, but causes facial nerve palsy in approximately 50% of cases. The tumor is more common in women aged 20–40 years old, grows slowly, can reach large sizes, thus causing considerable destruction of the temporal bone (Phillips et al. 2002).

Depending on the initial localization, there are schwannomas of the labyrinth, tympanic and mastoidal segments of the nerve. The latter is more common. Its earliest and often the only clinical manifestation is facial nerve palsy, persisting for several years. Hearing is typically intact or slightly reduced.

A labyrinthine segment schwannoma is clinically manifested via paresis of the facial nerve with neurosensory or mixed hearing loss (Liu et al. 2001).

First clinical signs of schwannomas of the tympanic segment of the facial nerve are often auditory disorders: a conductive or mixed hearing loss, noise, congestion and heaviness in the ear. These symptoms may precede the appearance of VII nerve palsy for several years.

Imaging Mastoidal type of schwannoma's localization is observed on CT as an extended mastoid portion of the facial nerve canal. Sometimes there are destructive changes in the mastoid, destruction of the lower back wall of the external auditory canal with tumor invasion into its lumen in the form of a circular nodule with well-defined and smooth contours.

On CT, the labyrinthine segment schwannoma is a space-occupying lesion, which causes a significant enlargement of the labyrinthine segment of the facial nerve canal, and leads

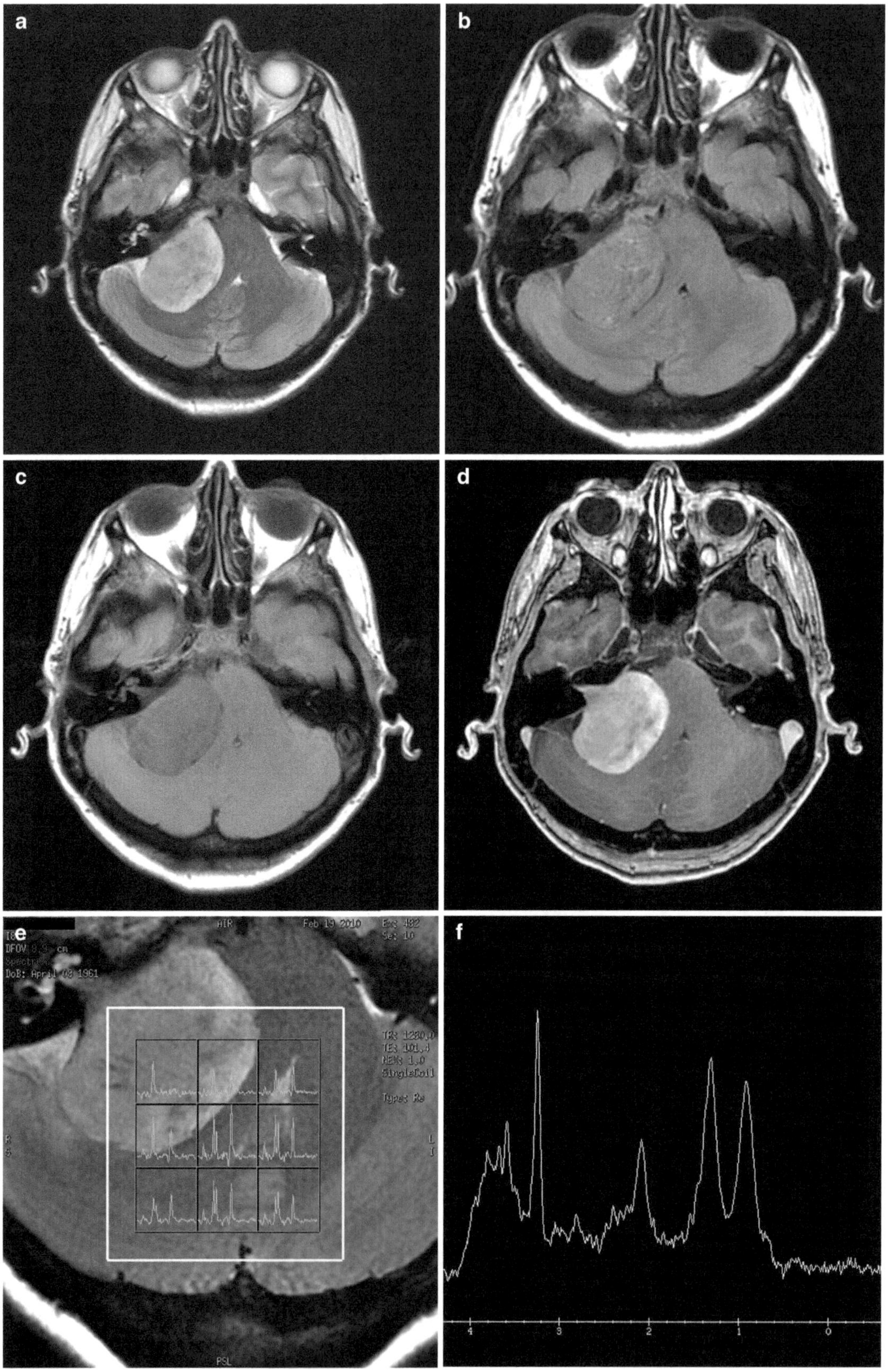

Fig. 23.37 Giant schwannoma of the right vestibulocochlear nerve. MR imaging using T2- (**a**), T2-FLAIR (**b**) and T1- (**c**) weighted images visualizes a large tumor in projection of the right cerebellopontine angle that has a homogeneous hyperintense signal on T2 and hypointense signal on T1. Tumor is characterized by prominent and atypically (for such size of the schwannoma) homogeneous contrast enhancement and extension into internal acoustic meatus (**d**). H1 MR spectroscopy (**e**, **f**) revealed the increased myo-inositol peak, low peak of NAA and high peaks of choline and lipid-lactate complex

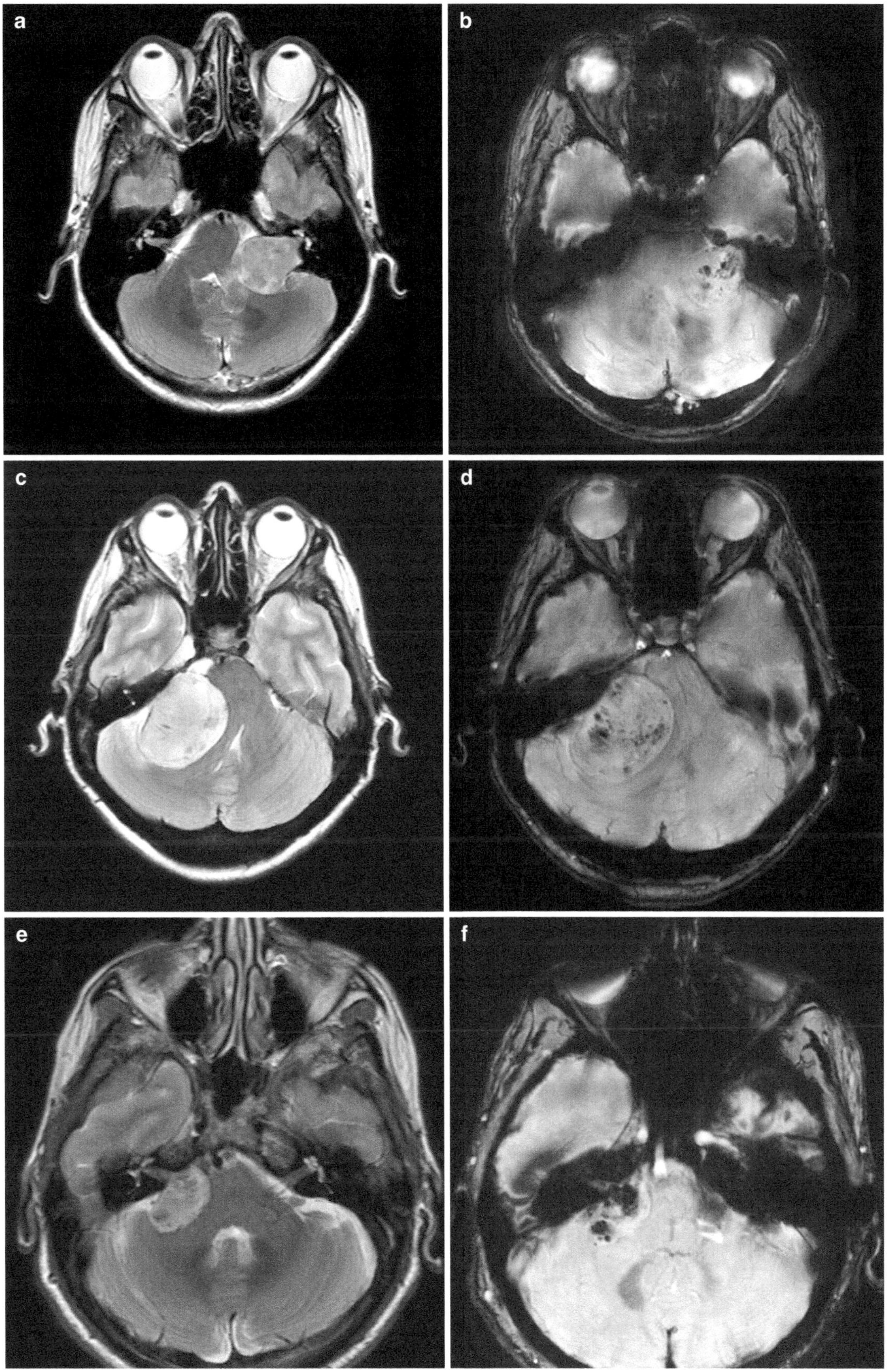

Fig. 23.38 Schwannomas of vestibulocochlear nerve (different patients). Case 1. (**a**, **b**), case 2 (**c**, **d**), and case 3 (**e**, **f**). On T2-weighted MR images (**a**, **c**, **e**) tumors with different size and heterogeneous hyperintense MR-signal are depicted. There are multiple hypointense spots (intratumoral hemorrhages) in the each tumor's stroma on SWAN (**b**, **d**, **f**) MRI

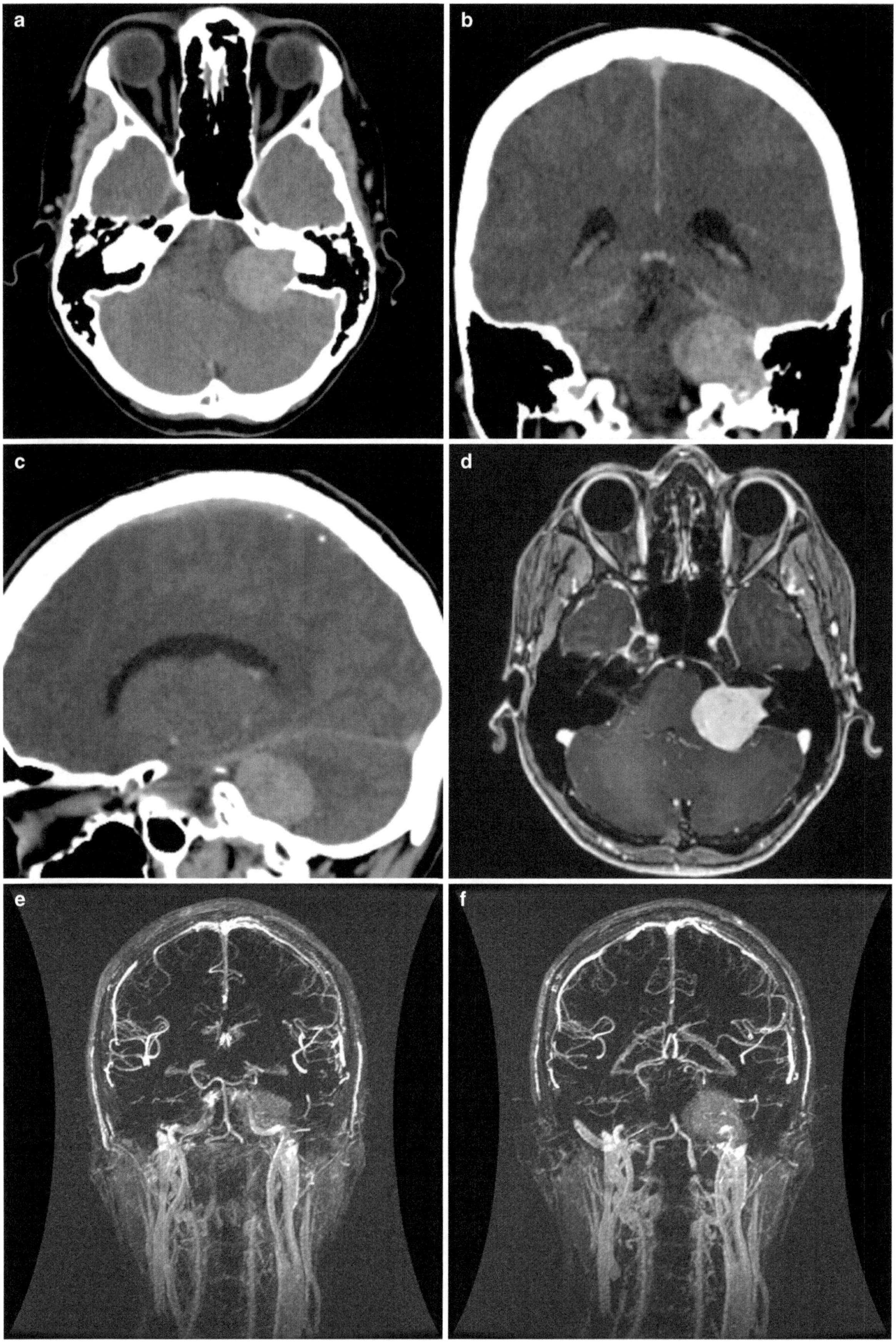
a
b
c
d
e
f

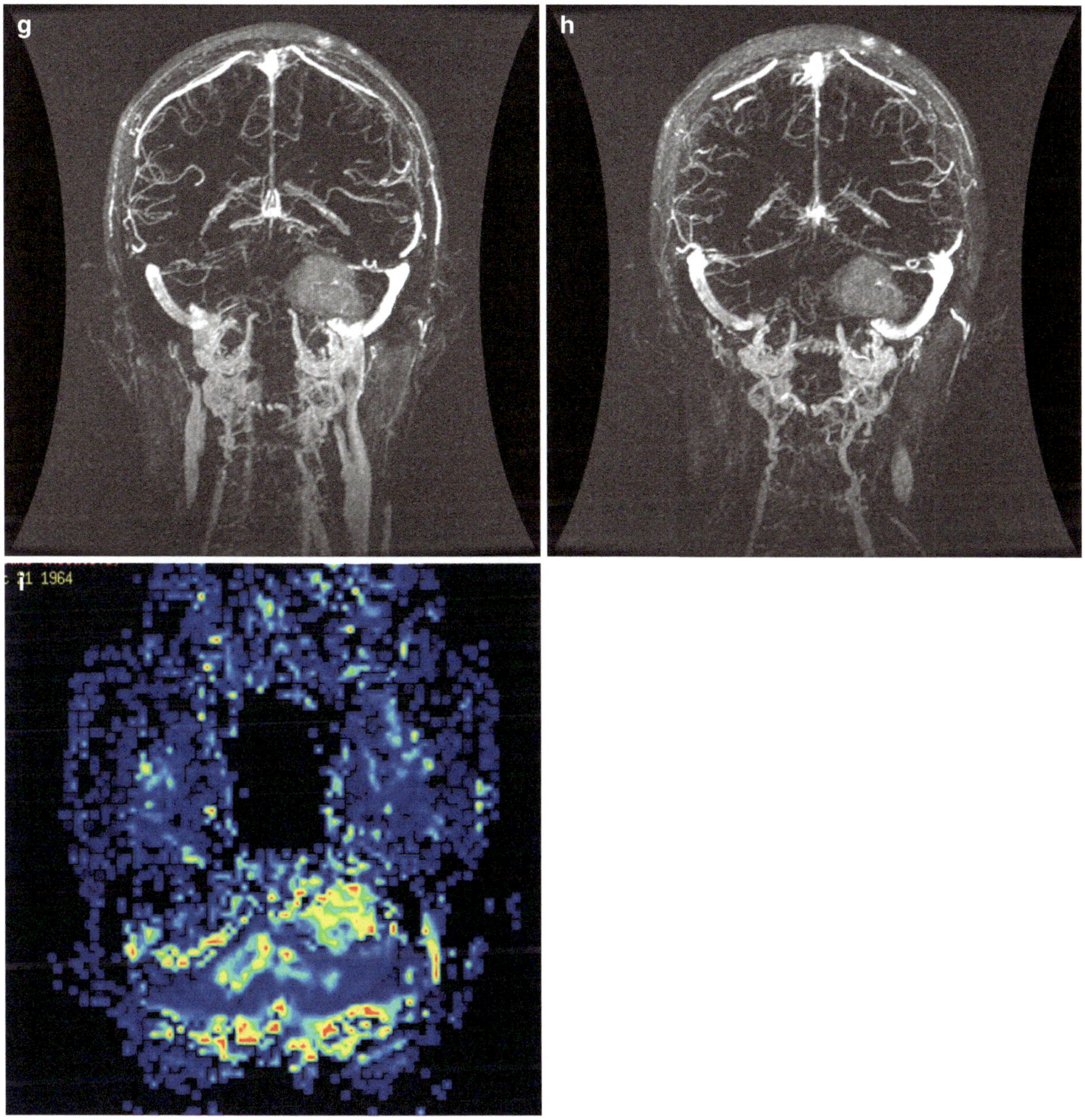

Fig. 23.39 (continued)

Fig. 23.39 Schwannoma of the left vestibulocochlear nerve. Series of contrast enhanced CT scans (**a**–**c**) demonstrates a homogeneously enhanced tumor in projection of left cerebello-pontine angle with extension into internal acoustic meatus. On MRI (**d**) a tumor has strong contrast enhancement as well. On TRICKS series (**e**–**h**) tumor is characterized by relatively fast and prominent contrast enhancement. The relationship between lesion and blood vessels of the posterior cranial fossa can be estimated. MR-perfusion study (**i**) shows a moderate increased rCBV values

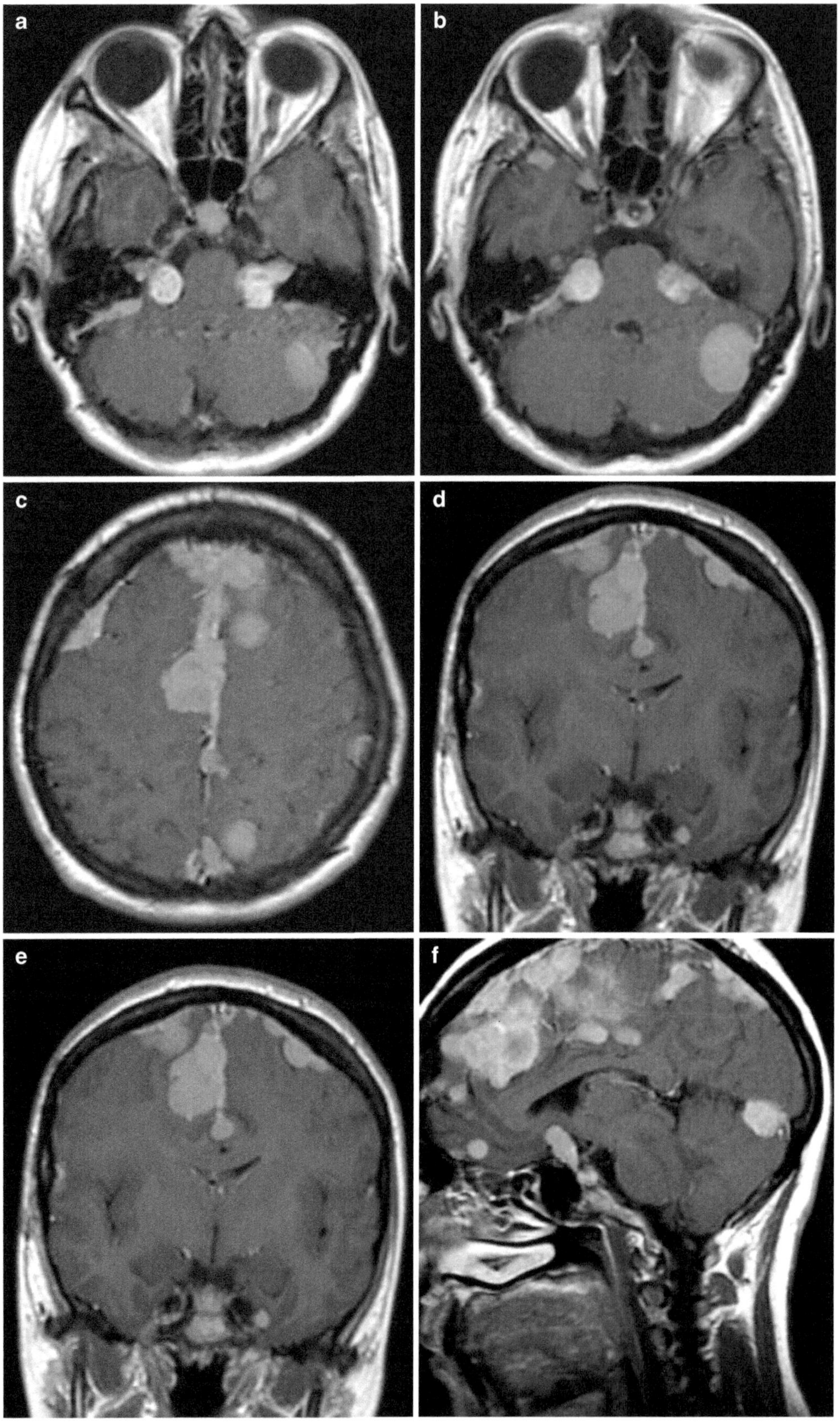

Fig. 23.40 Neurofibromatosis, type II. Bilateral acoustic schwannomas and multiple meningiomas of intracerebral location. Axial (**a–c**), coronal (**d**, **e**), and sagittal (**f**) MR images after contrast enhancement show bilateral acoustic schwannomas and multiple extraaxial tumors with sub- and supratentorial location that resembles meningiomas

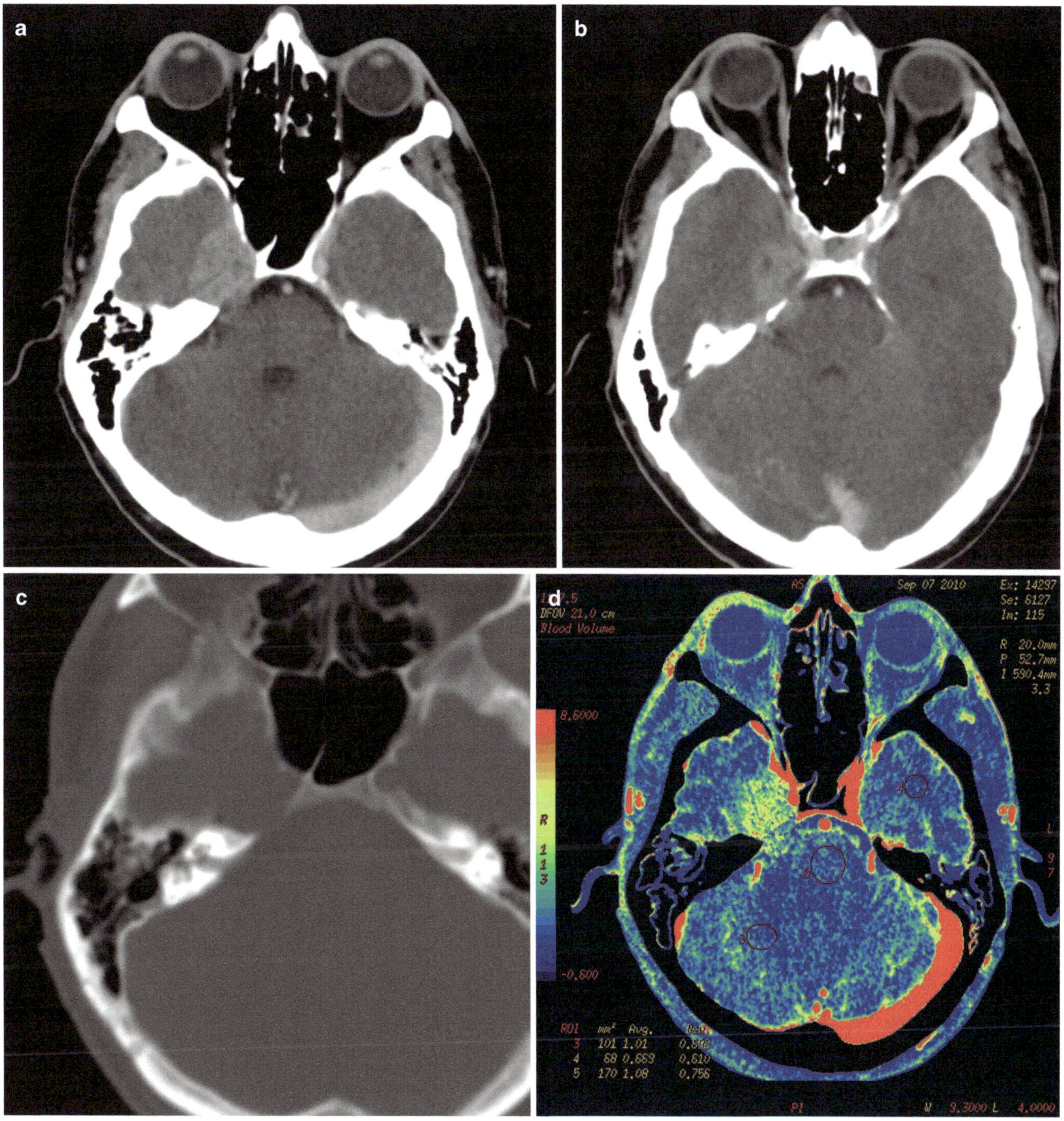

Fig. 23.41 Schwannoma of the trigeminal nerve. Axial CECT scans (**a**, **b**) in standard and "bone window" modes (**c**) demonstrate a solid hyperdense enhancing tumor in the projection of right Meckel's cavity and cavernous sinus. There is a focal of bone excavation of right petrous apex. There is a moderate increasing of CBV in tumor's stroma on CT-perfusion study (**d**)

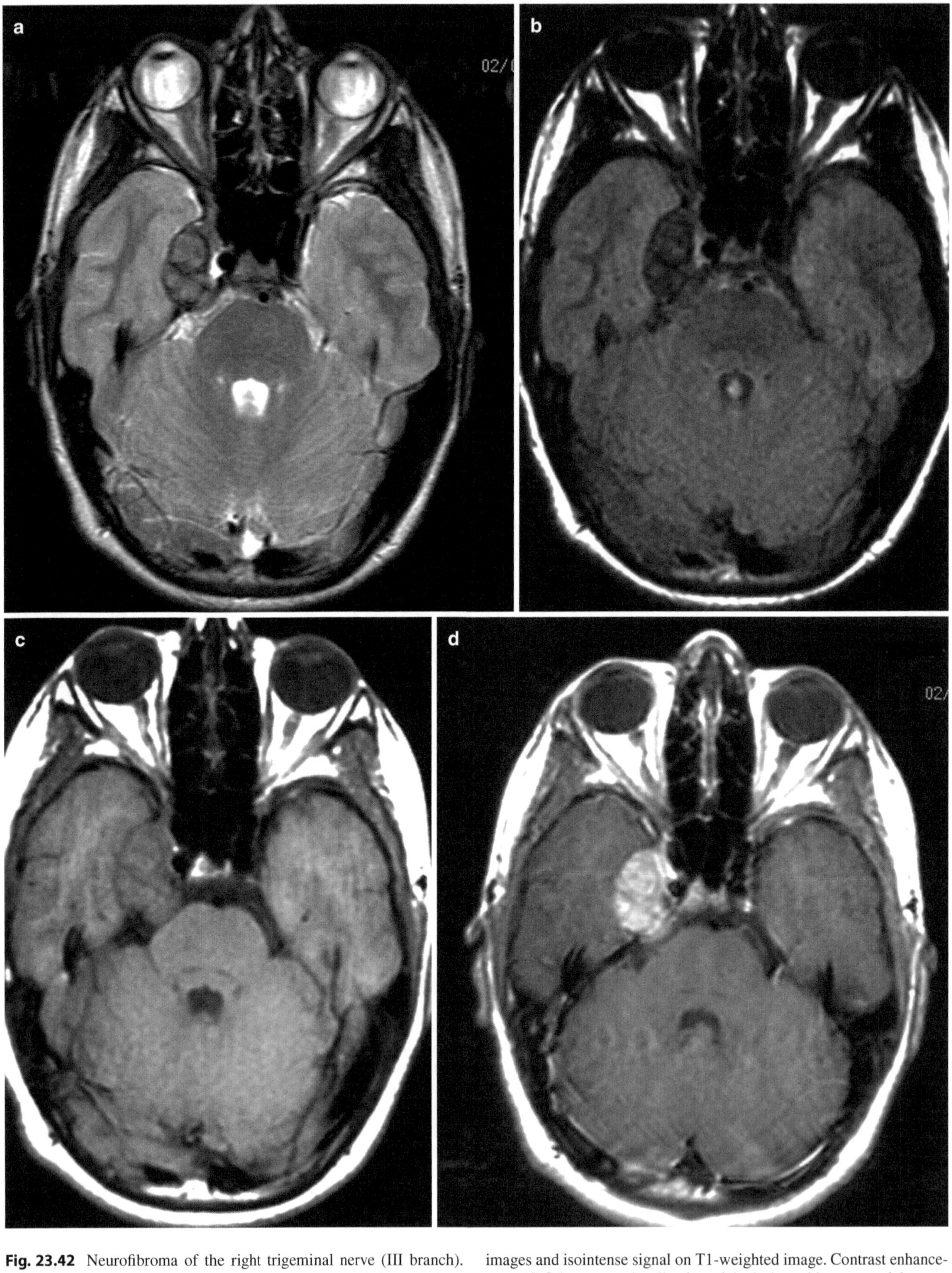

Fig. 23.42 Neurofibroma of the right trigeminal nerve (III branch). Axial T2- (**a**), T2-FLAIR- (**b**), and T1- (**c**) weighted MR images show solid heterogeneous tumor in projection of right Meckel's cavity. Neurofibroma has hypointense signal on T2- and T2-FLAIR-weighted images and isointense signal on T1-weighted image. Contrast enhancement (**d–f**) improves visualization of the lesion with extracranial extension through the foramen ovale

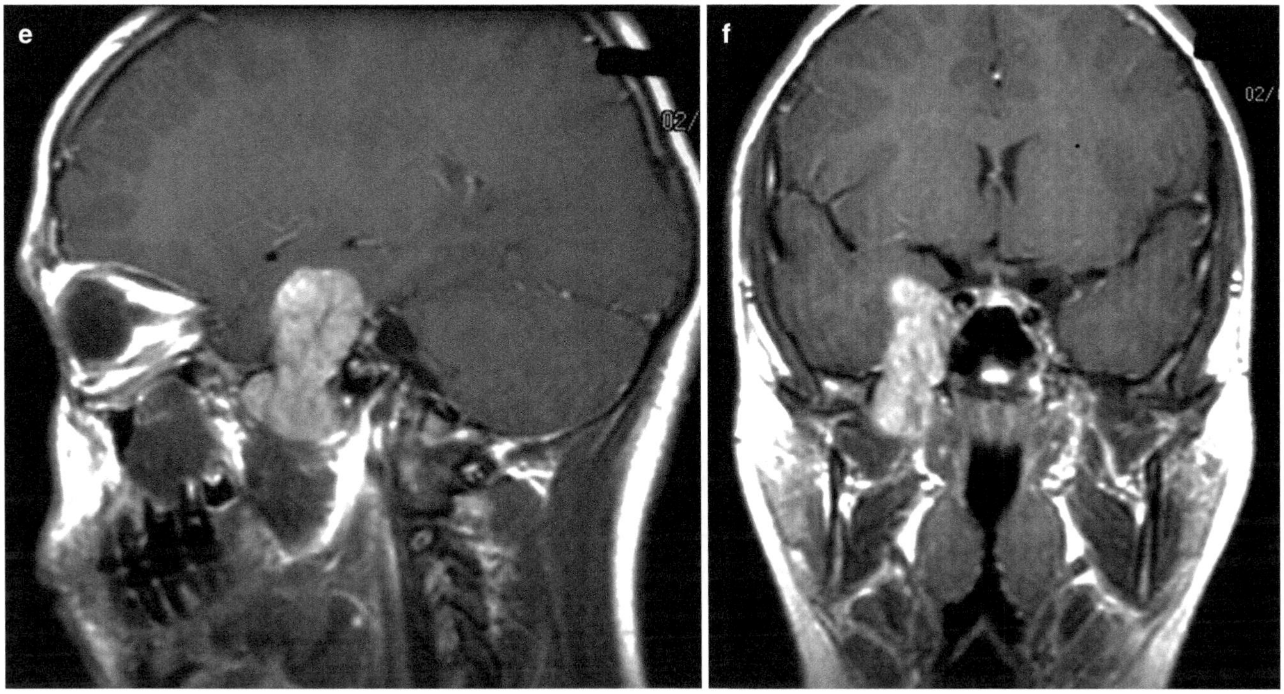

Fig. 23.42 (continued)

to destruction of the anterio-superior edge of the pyramid in the geniculate ganglion fossa (Chung et al. 1998). Osseous destruction of facial nerve canal walls can be associated with partial erosion of the auditory bones and their lateral displacement. In some cases, there is destruction of the labyrinthine capsule at the level of the cochlea and semicircular canals, which indicates the presence of a mass lesion in the tympanic cavity. Large tumors cause an extensive bone destruction of the upper wall of the pyramid and can form large intracranial soft-tissue components (Figs. 23.43 and 23.44).

On MRI, even small tumors are visualized. They have isointense signal on T1-weighted sequences and a moderately hyperintense signal on T2-weighted MR-scans. The tumor quite intensely accumulates contrast agent and can be better visualized on T1-weighted sequences using Fat-Sat technique. In case of intracranial growth, tumor can invade the internal auditory canal with destruction of its floor and the upper wall. A cystic component of the tumor is clearly seen after intravenous contrast enhancement. Sagittal MR-slices are the best in the visualization of schwannoma spreading along the bony canal at the projection of the pyramid, and coronal scans are useful in assessing schwannoma growth into the middle cranial fossa (Figs. 23.45 and 23.46).

Schwannomas of IX, X, and XI cranial nerves, unrelated to neurofibromatosis type II, account for up to 2.5% of tumors. Combining these schwannomas into the so-called group of "jugular foramen schwannomas" is fully justified, since identification of the source of tumor growth within this anatomic area is quite difficult, and sometimes impossible for objective reasons. Clinical signs: the disease can manifest as a vestibular schwannoma with the development of neurosensory hearing loss (90%), hemifacial spasm, hoarseness of voice, aspiration (in case of involvement of the recurrent nerve, branch of Xth cranial nerve), pulsating tingling, neuropathy of IX–XI nerves.

CT scans show an enlarged jugular foramen with thin sclerotic margins. In case of extracranial growth, schwannomas grow into the nasopharyngeal carotid space; if growing upwards, it is spreading along the course of IX–XI nerves towards the brainstem. Coronal CT imaging may show an amputation of the lateral jugular tubercle "bird's beak." Tumors typically intensively accumulate contrast agent (Fig. 23.47).

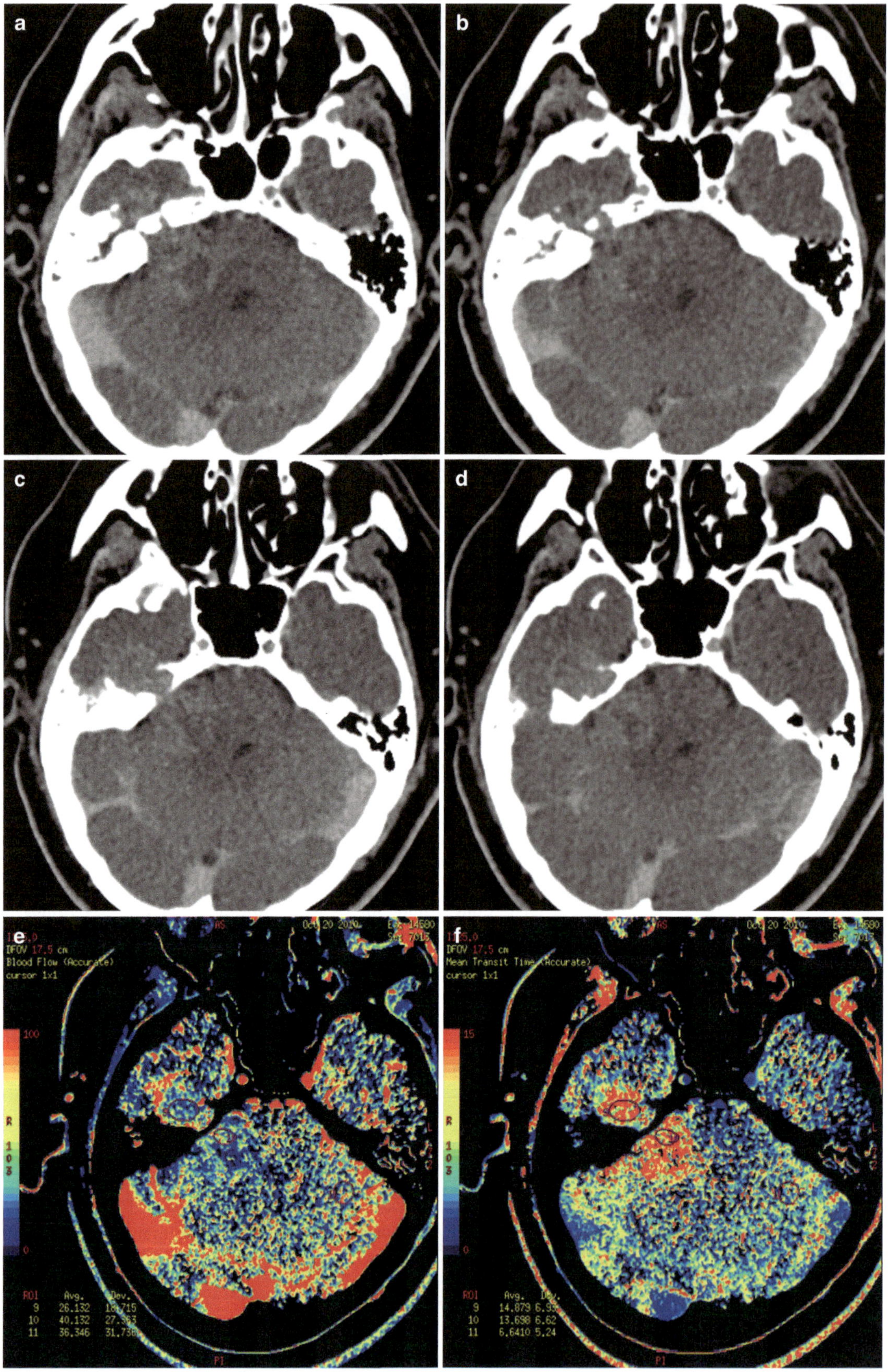

Fig. 23.43 Schwannoma of the right facial nerve. Axial CECT scans (**a**–**d**) reveal heterogeneously enhancing tumor with supra- and infratentorial extension. There is a focal pyramid bone destruction. CT-perfusion study demonstrates typical hemodynamics features of schwannomas: low CBF values (**e**) and prominent prolongation of MTT (**f**)

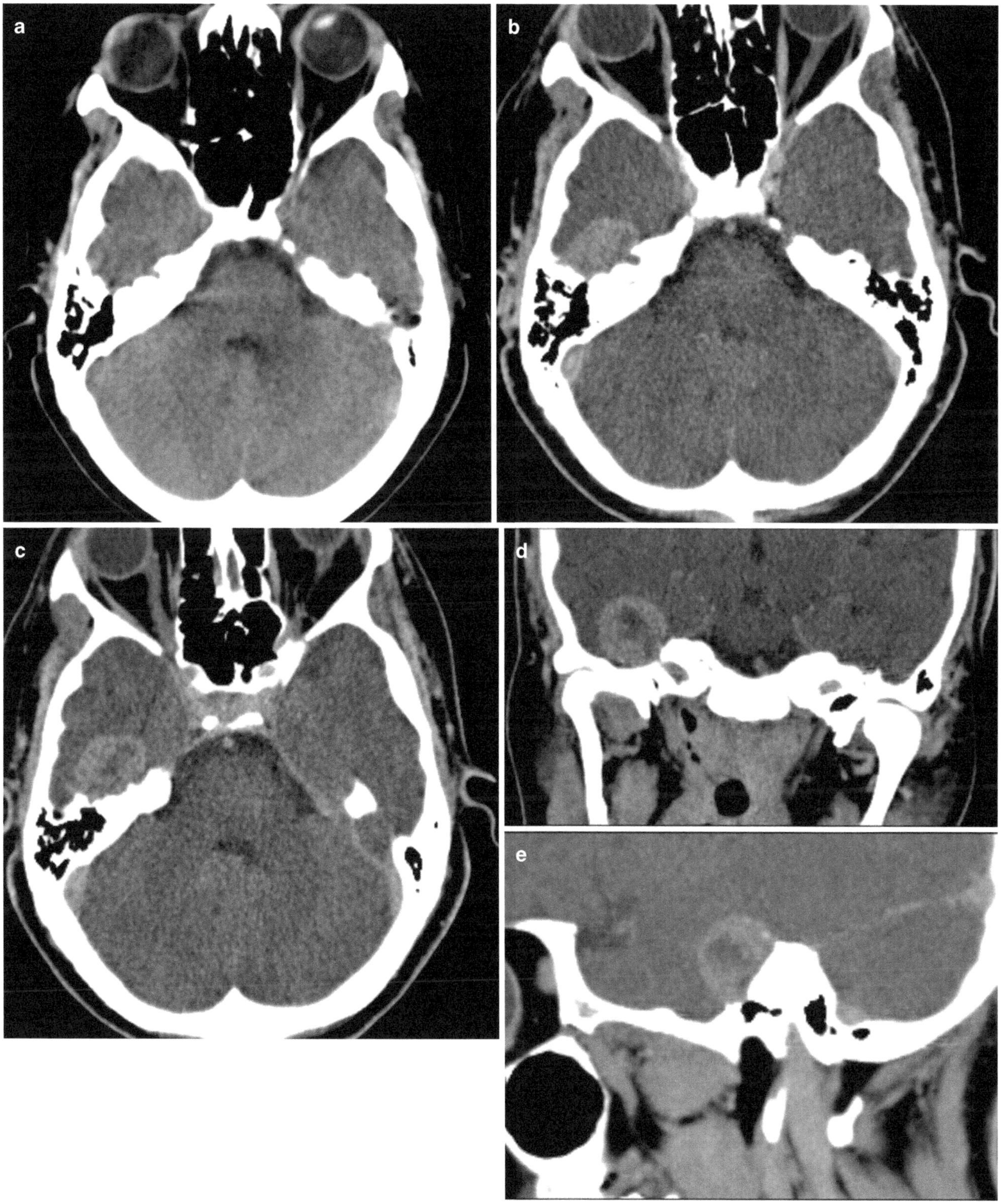

Fig. 23.44 Schwannoma of the right VIIth cranial nerve. Axial CECT scans (**a**–**e**) show a heterogeneously enhancing tumor on the base of middle cerebral fossa with a focal roof of temporal bone destruction. CT-perfusion study demonstrates typical hemodynamics features of schwannomas: low CBF (**f**), intermediate elevated CBV (**g**) values and prominent prolongation of MTT (**h**). Permeability parameter also increased (**i**)

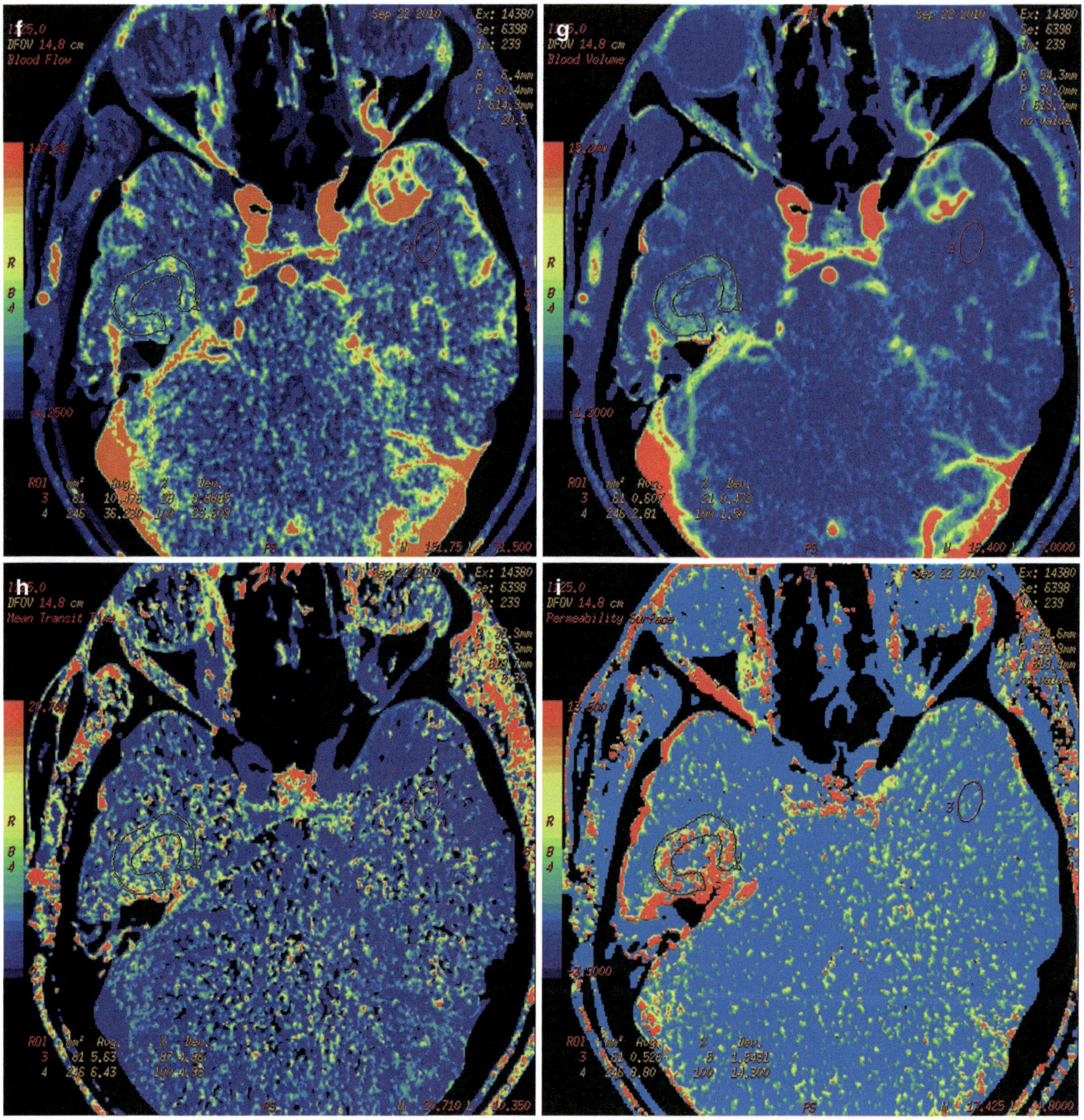

Fig. 23.44 (continued)

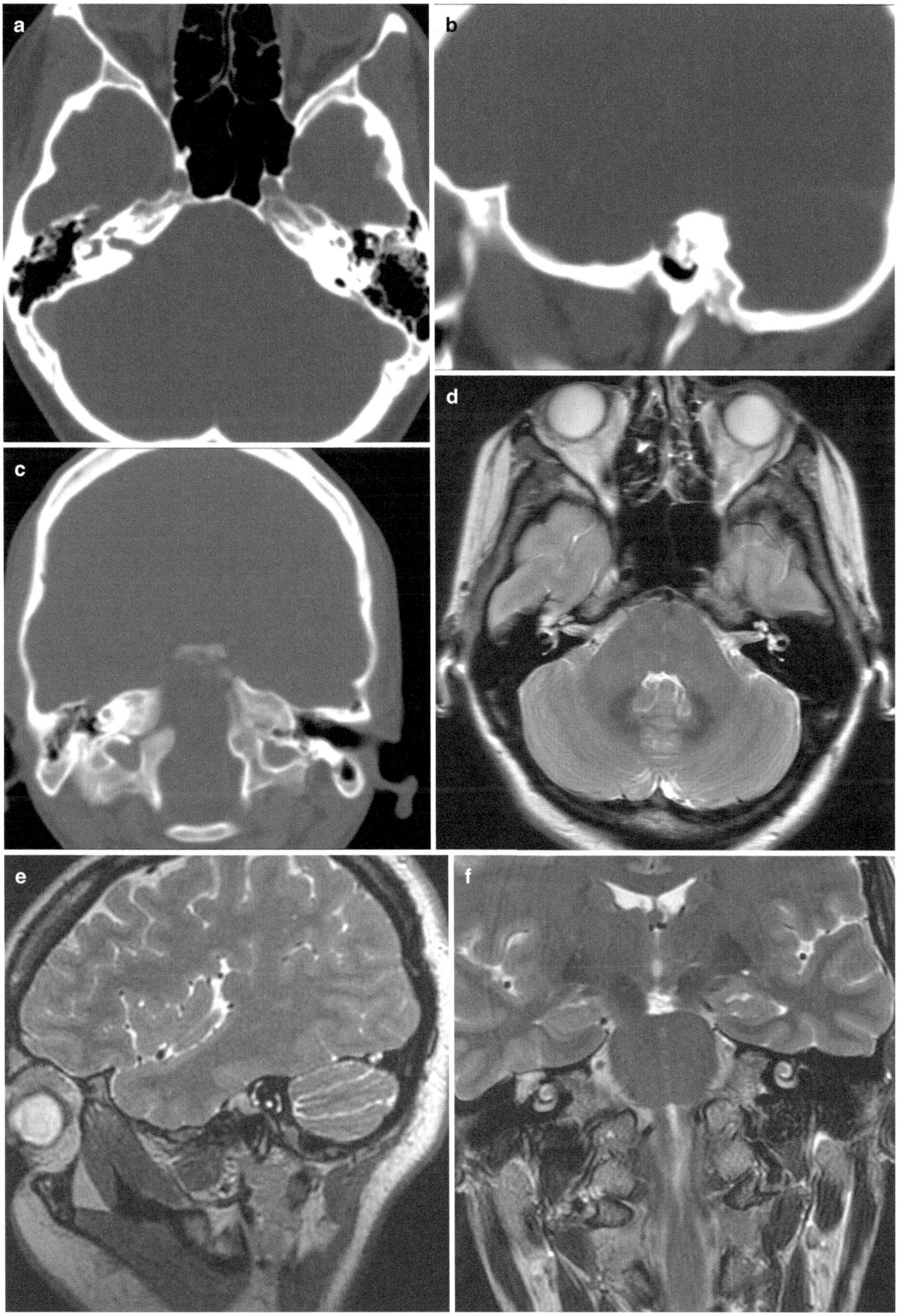

Fig. 23.45 Schwannoma of the right facial nerve. Axial (**a**), coronal (**b**), and sagittal (**c**) CECT scans demonstrate a small enhancing lesion in the projection of facial nerve ganglion, causing focal pyramid bone destruction. On T2-weighted MR-images a lesion has hyperintense MR-signal (**d**–**g**). Contrast enhancement, especially with Fat-Sat technique, improves the visualization of the lesion (**h**–**l**)

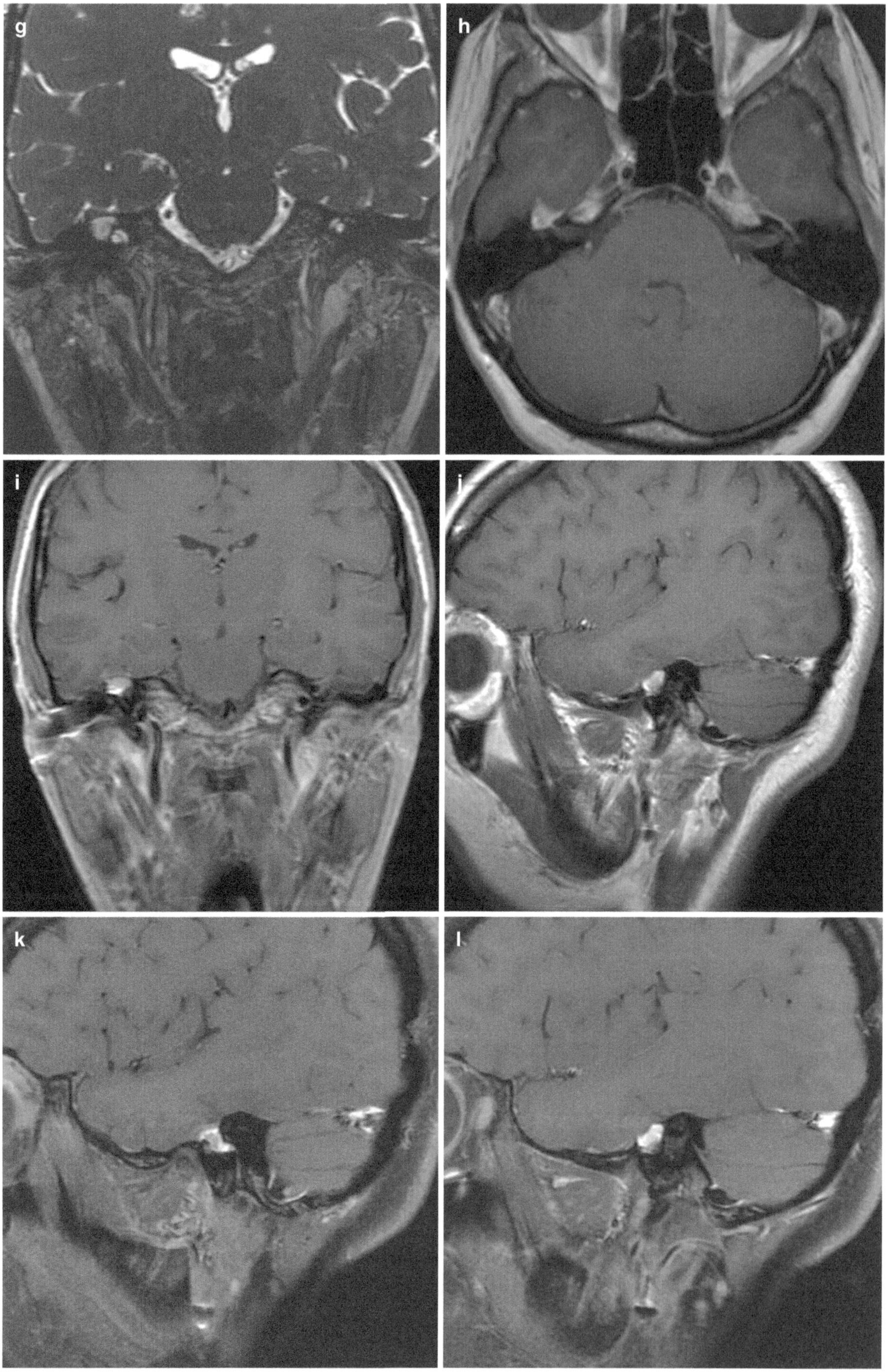

Fig. 23.45 (continued)

On T1-weighted MR-sequences, the tumors usually have hypointense MR-signal, on T2-weighted images MR signal is typically hyperintense. In majority of the cases tumor's stroma is uniform, nevertheless tumor is characterized by prominent contrast enhancement. In large-size tumors cysts may be present (25%) (Fig. 23.48).

Schwannomas of XIIth cranial nerve typically grow along its root into the homonymic bony canal in the occipital bone. CT and MRI characteristics are identical with all schwannomas (Figs. 23.49, 23.50 and 23.51). This type of schwannomas are extremely rare. Also, tumors of C1 root with growth in the cranial cavity can be rarely visualized (Fig. 23.52).

MRI undoubtedly plays a major role in assessing the growth dynamics of PCF schwannomas previously treated by radiosurgery (by "Gamma Knife" or "Cyber Knife," etc.). This method allows not only to evaluate the tumor's dimensions before and after the treatment, but also to visualize appearance of necrotic and cystic changes in the schwannoma's tissue, developing in response to radiation damage. T2-weighted and T2-FLAIR MR-sequences are the modalities of choice in the assessment of the adjacent brain stem for early verification of post-radiation complications (edema, acute radiation necrosis). In case of brain stem hyperintensity adjacent to schwannoma, it is always advisable to use intravenous contrast enhancement. This allows differentiating post-radiation brain edema (nonenhanced) from radiation necrosis (peripheral enhancement). CT is a less sensitive method for a complex evaluation of post-radiation changes both within the schwannoma and the brainstem structures. Nevertheless, if CT-perfusion studies are used as a monitoring of treatment efficacy, negative blood flow can be much earlier (comparing to MR-perfusion) identified in the neoplasm structure as the treatment response. In general, this effect occurs within the first months after radiosurgery. A reduction of schwannoma's size in the response to radiation therapy in most cases is detected only by the end of the first year after the treatment (Fig. 23.53).

Differential Diagnosis With all space-occupying lesions of the lateral parts of the posterior cranial fossa.

First of all, this is meningioma (accompanied by hyperostotic bone changes, dural tail, growth along the meninges), followed by paraganglioma (high perfusion values, mottled

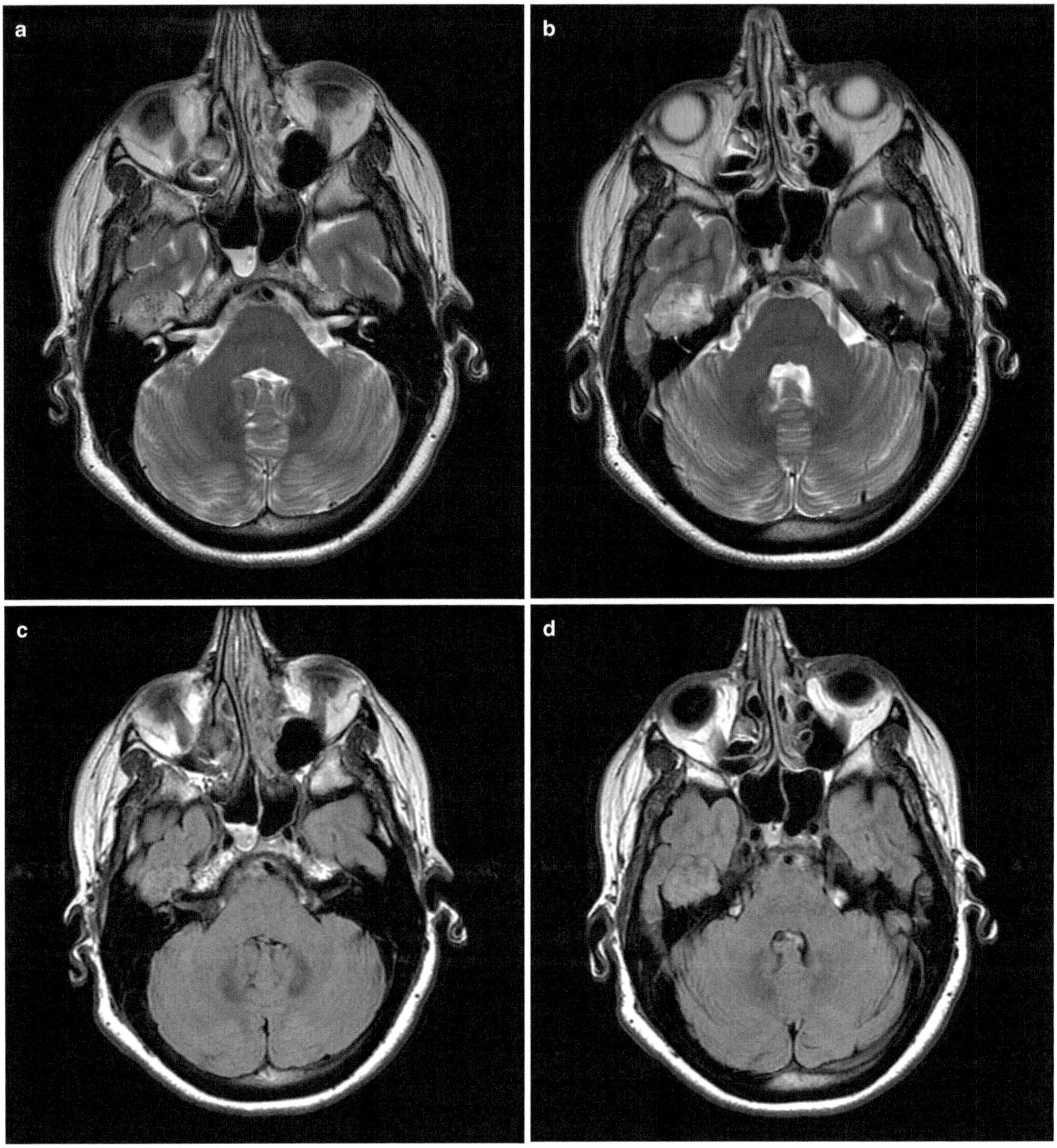

Fig. 23.46 Schwannoma of the right VIIth cranial nerve. Axial T2- (**a**, **b**), T2-FLAIR (**c**, **d**), as well as coronal T2- (**e**, **f**)) weighted MR-images demonstrate a heterogeneous and hyperintense (on T2) solid lesion in the projection of the middle cranial fossa base and the roof of temporal bone pyramid. Tumor is characterized by prominent contrast enhancement improving the visualization of lesion extension (**g**–**i**)

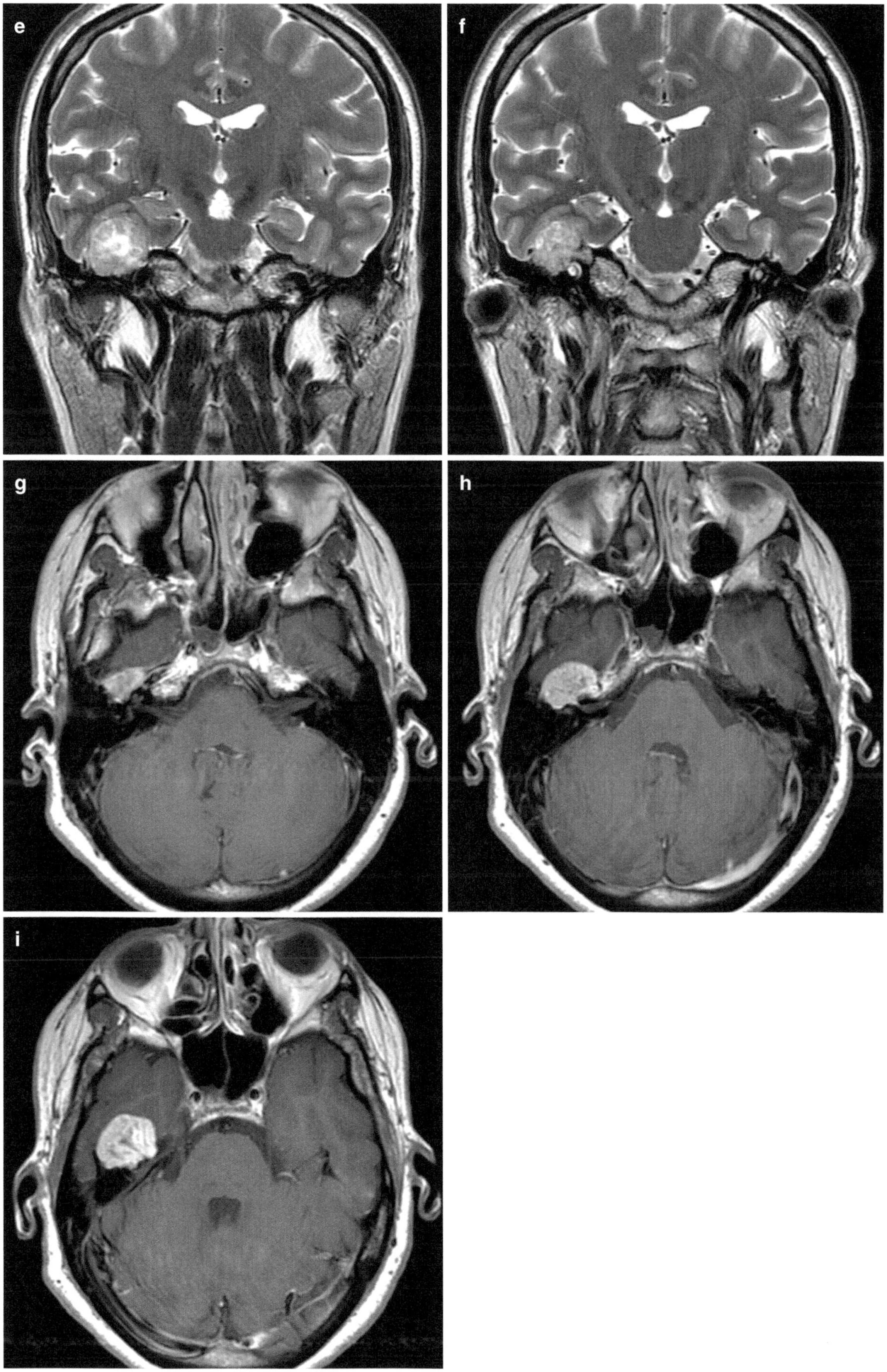

Fig. 23.46 (continued)

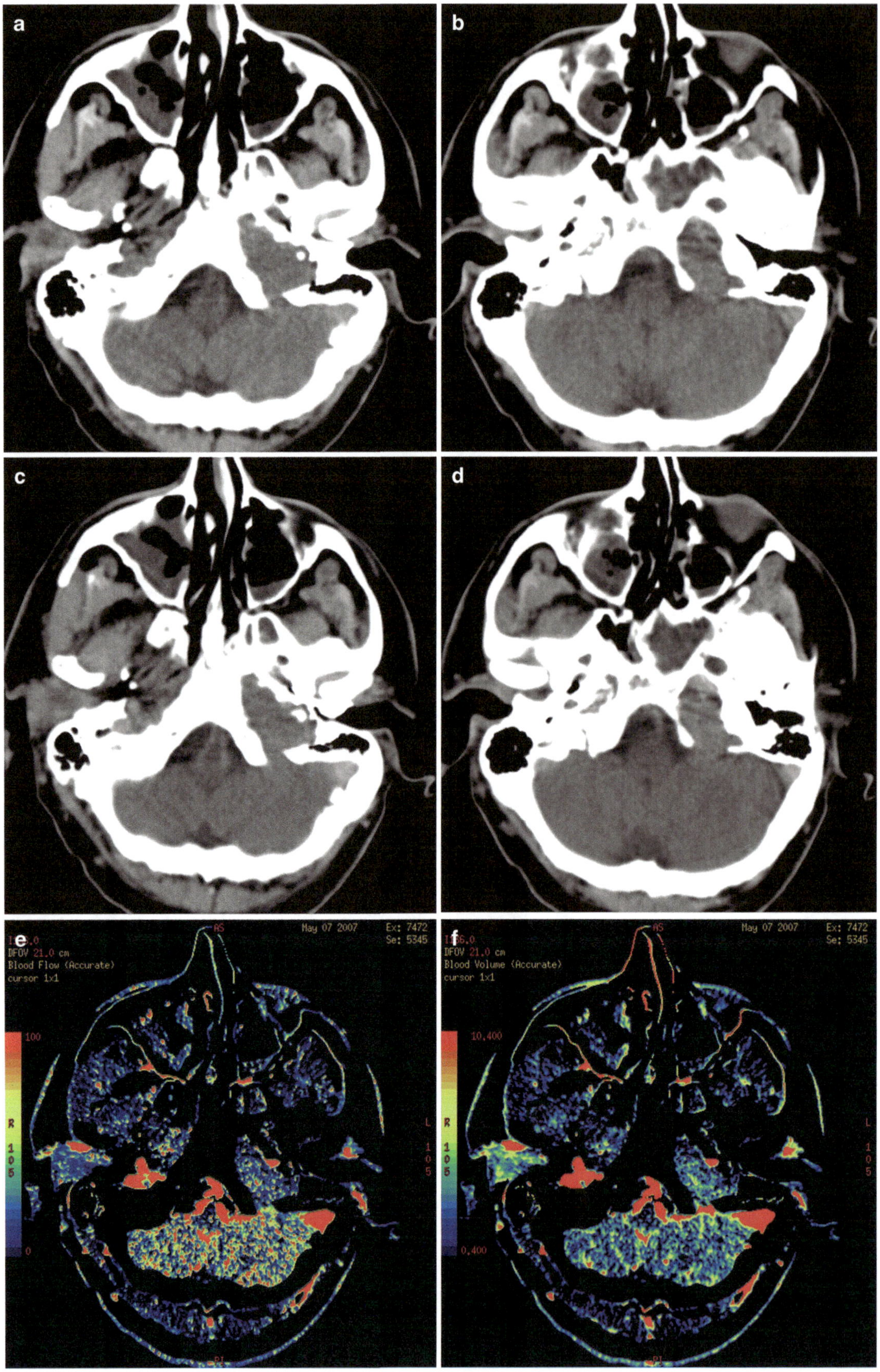

Fig. 23.47 Schwannoma of the left jugular vein foramen. Axial CT scans before (**a**, **b**) and after (**c**, **d**) contrast enhancement demonstrate initially isodense and slightly enhancing tumor in projection of jugular foramen causing the focal bone excavation. CT-perfusion study demonstrates typical hemodynamics features of schwannomas: low CBF (**e**) and intermediate elevated CBV (**f**) values

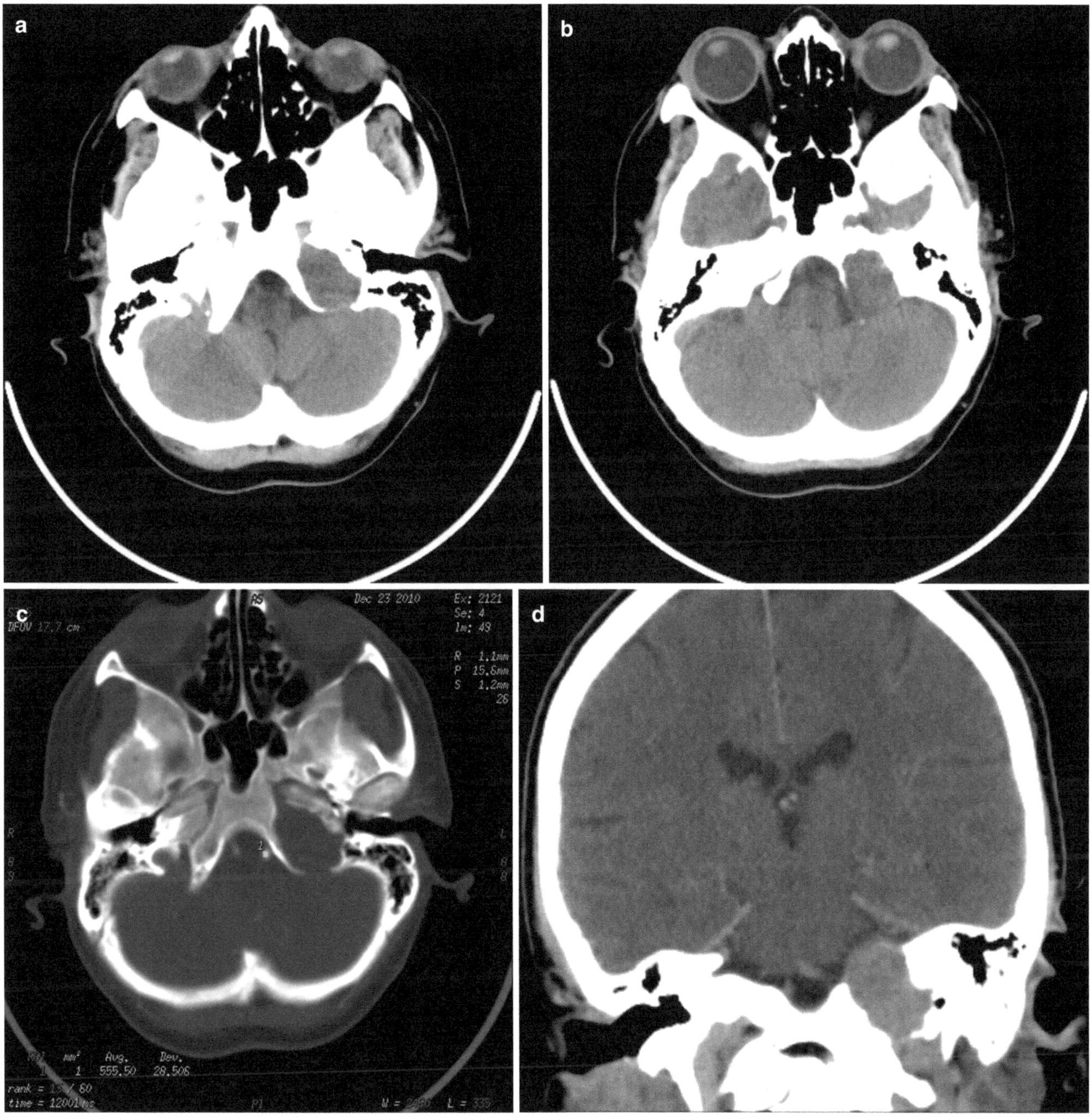

Fig. 23.48 Schwannoma of the left jugular vein foramen. Series of CT scans before (**a**, **b**) and after (**d**, **e**) contrast enhancement demonstrates initially isodense and intermediate enhancing tumor in projection of jugular foramen causing the focal bone excavation (**c**). CT-perfusion study reveals low CBF (**f**) values in the lesion. Tumor is characterized by hyperintense MR-signal on T2-weighted images (**g**, **h**) and prominent contrast enhancement improving the visualization of lesion extension (**i**–**l**)

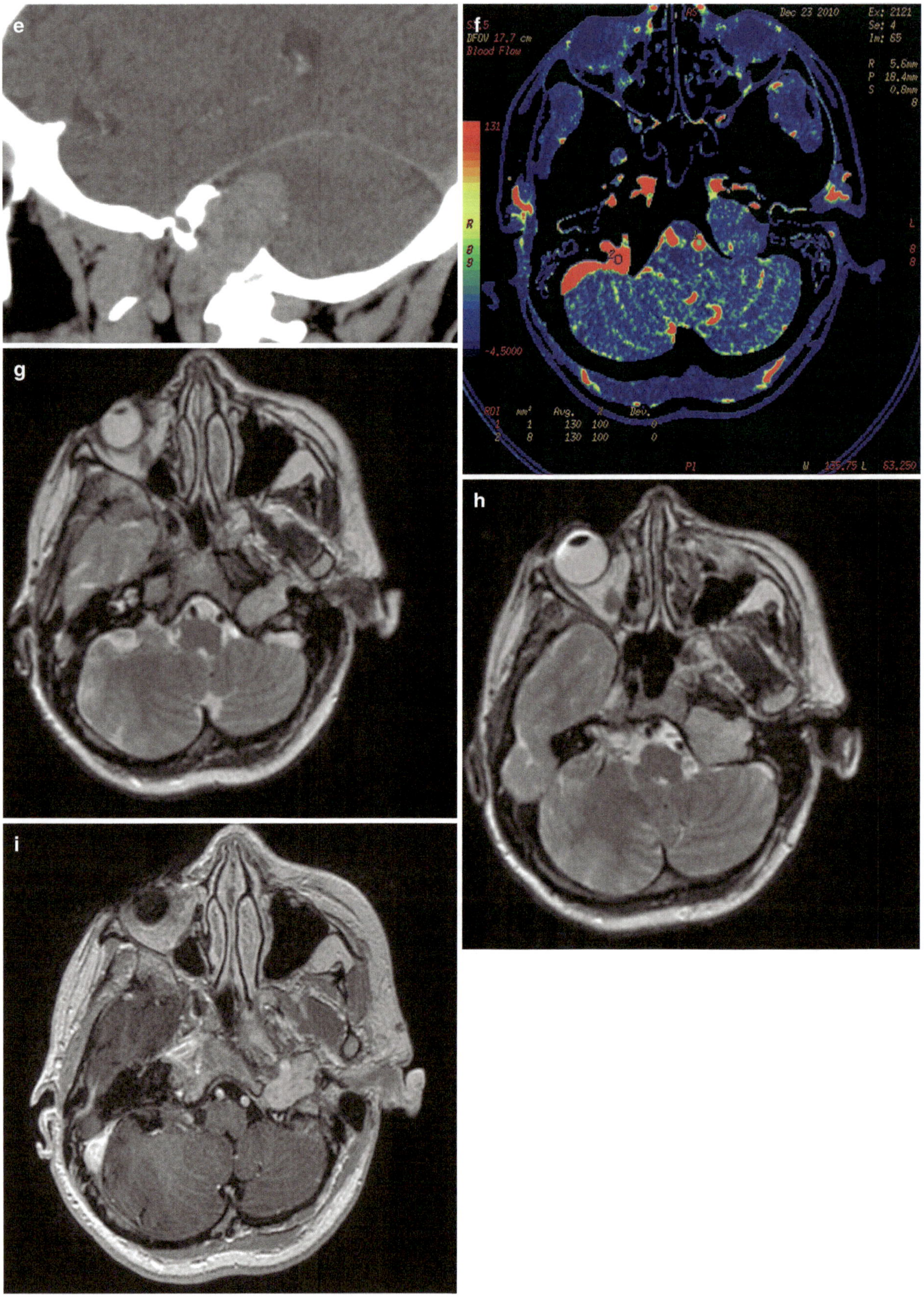

Fig. 23.48 (continued)

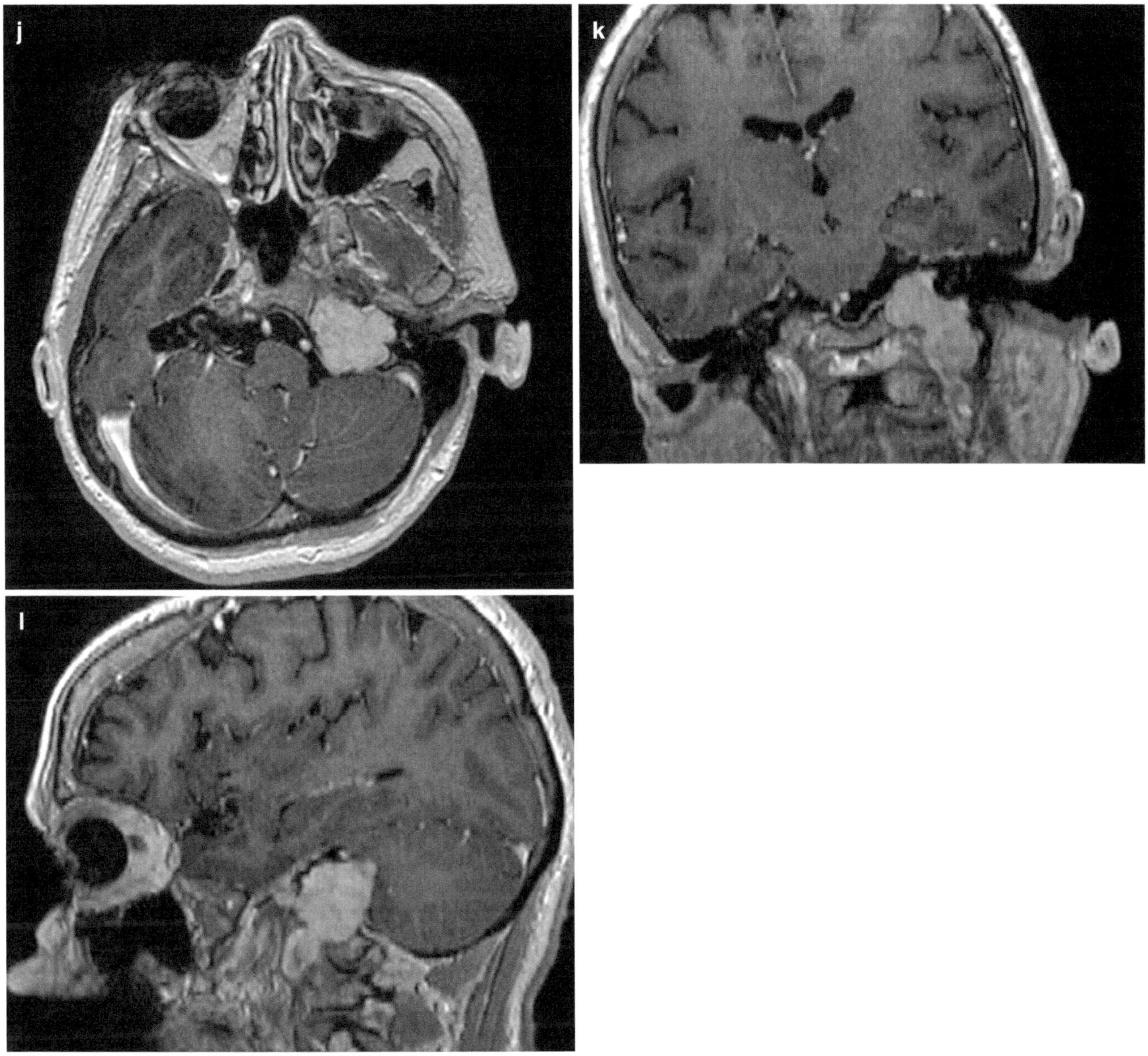

Fig. 23.48 (continued)

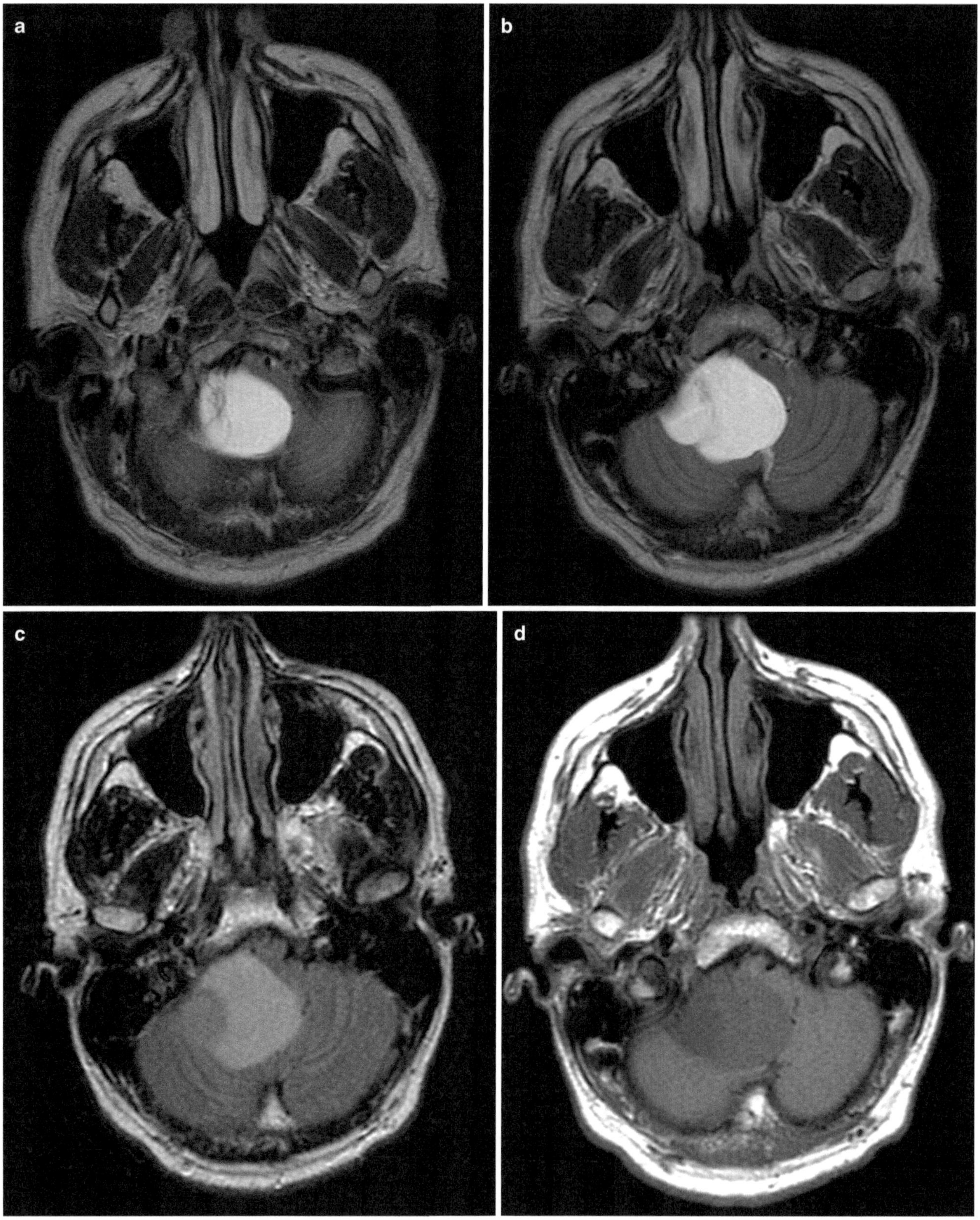

Fig. 23.49 Schwannoma of foramen Magnum (left XIIth cranial nerve). Axial T2- (**a**, **b**), T2-FLAIR- (**c**), and T1(**d**) weighted MR-images demonstrate a heterogeneous and hyperintense on T2 and T2-FLAIR predominantly cystic lesion. Solid mural part of the tumor and capsule are characterized by prominent contrast enhancement improving the visualization of the lesion size and extension (**e**, **f**)

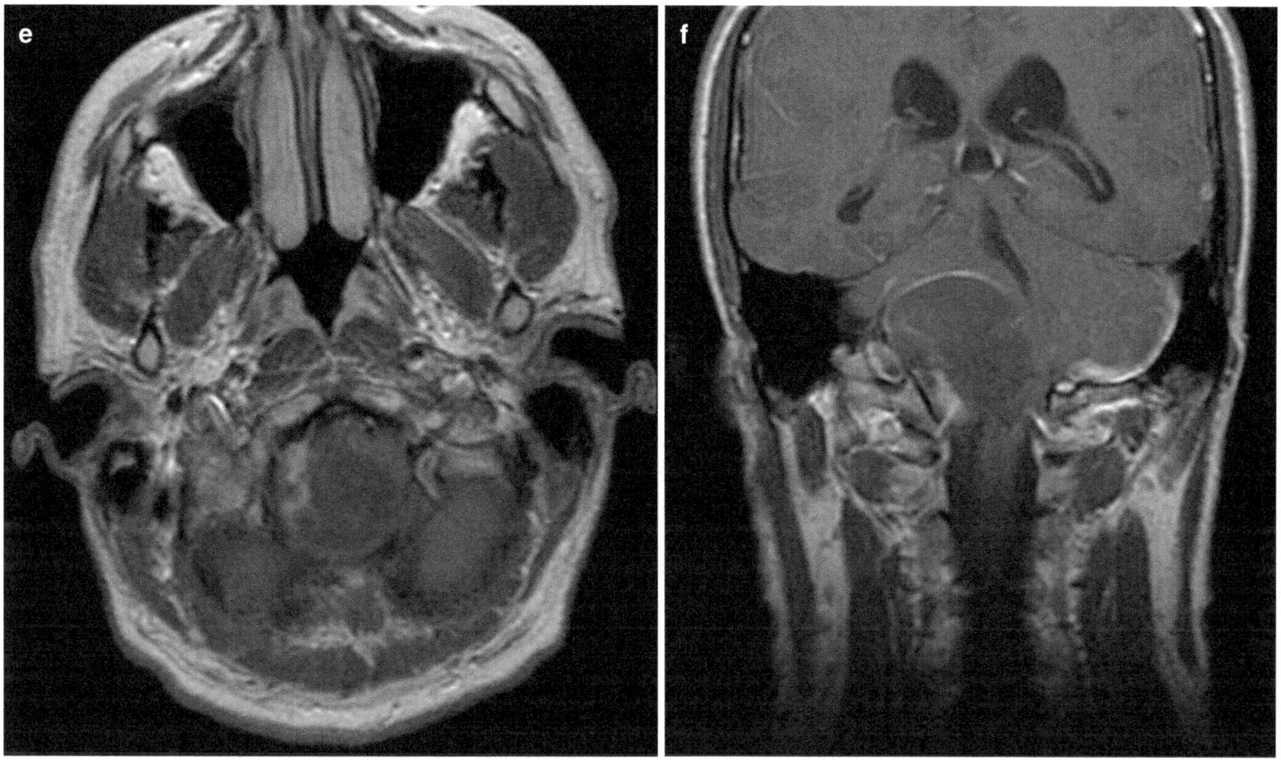

Fig. 23.49 (continued)

appearance on MRI), cholesteatoma (high MR signal on DWI), hemangioblastoma (no relation to the internal auditory meatus, newly formed vessels and often perifocal edema), metastases (usually accompanied by an extensive destruction of the bone structures), enlargement of the jugular vein bulb, etc.

Paragangliomas *(glomus tumors, chemodectomas)* belong to a group of relatively rare neuroendocrine tumors. They comprise 0.6% of all intracranial tumors. This benign slow growing tumor is located mostly at the skull base. It develops from the nerve ganglia (glomus cells and nonchromaffin paraganglia), sympathetic and parasympathetic nervous system. These anatomical structures are responsible for the changes in a ratio of oxygen and carbon dioxide in blood, and are located generally along the carotid artery, the vagus nerve and the jugular foramen around the jugular vein, as well as in cochlear eminence. The most correct is considered the paraganglioma term, as it corresponds to the notion about the histological structure of this tumor and involves common pathogenesis with homologous tumors at other sites, also originating from the paraganglionar tissue, i.e. paragangliomas of the lungs, skin, adrenal gland (pheochromocytoma). Paraganglioma is the most common tumor of the middle ear and is second among the temporal bone tumors after vestibular schwannoma.

In some cases, if the tumor contains chromaffin cells (1% of cases) in its structure, it can have a secretory activity, producing a number of highly active substances such as norepinephrine and dopamine. In rare cases (5%), glomus tumors may become malignant. Women are affected more often than men (3–6:1), and onset of the disease usually falls within the fifth to sixth decades of life.

Depending on a paraganglioma location, they are usually divided into tumors of the bifurcation of the common carotid artery, jugular glomus tumors and tympanic paragangliomas (Weber et al. 2001). These tumors are characterized by an abundant vascular network.

Clinical signs depend on the tumor location and its influence on the surrounding structures. With involvement of the middle ear, a varying degree of hearing loss and pulsating tingling in the ear are observed; if cranial nerves are compressed (especially facial nerve; glossopharyngeal, vagus,

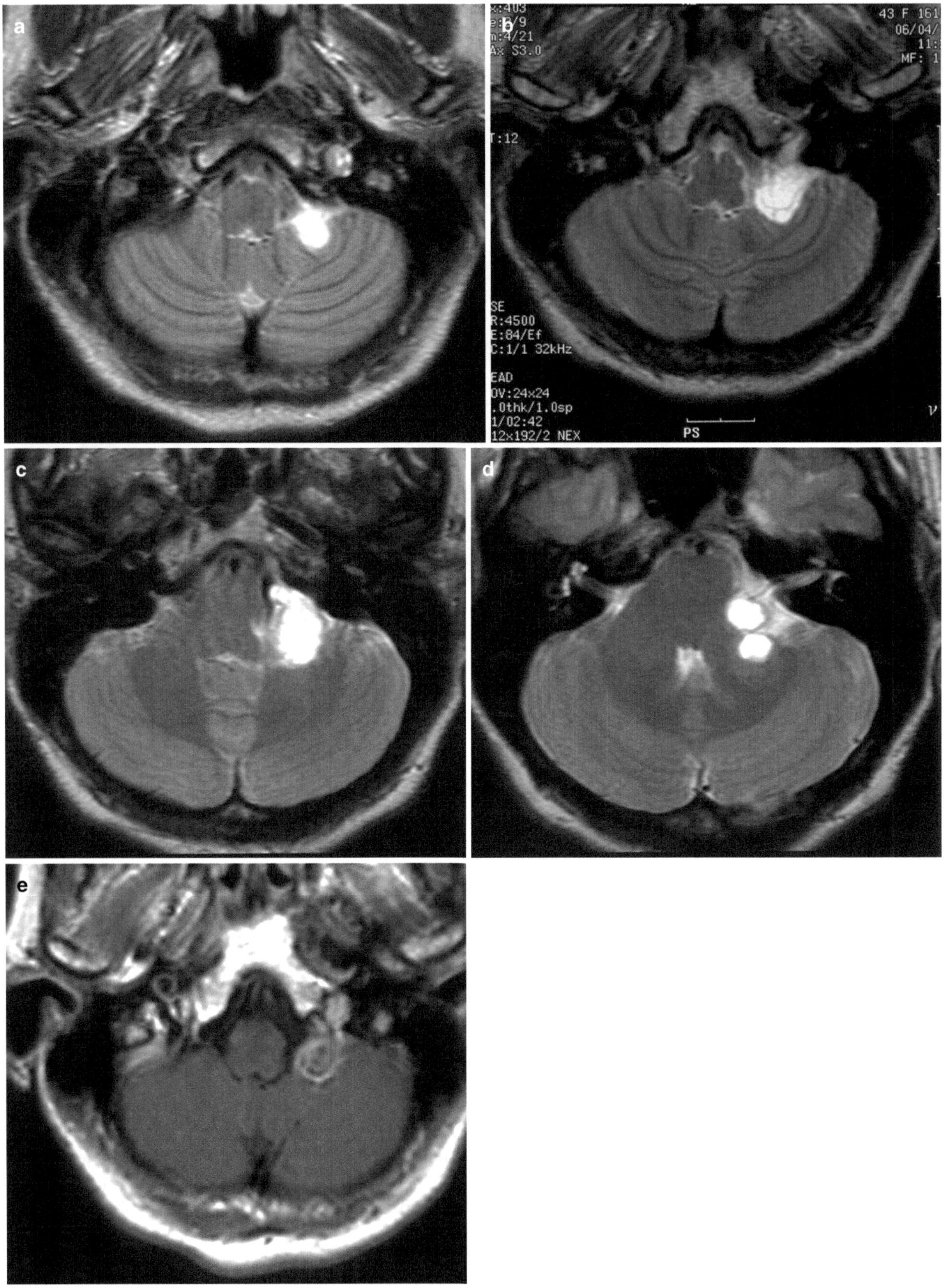

Fig. 23.50 Schwannoma of the left hypoglossal nerve. Series of axial T2- (**a–d**) and postenhanced T1- (**e**) weighted MR-images demonstrate a predominantly cystic lesion with hyperintense MR-signal on T2. Tumor is characterized by prominent contrast enhancement improving the visualization of lesion extension through the hypoglossal nerve bone canal (**e**)

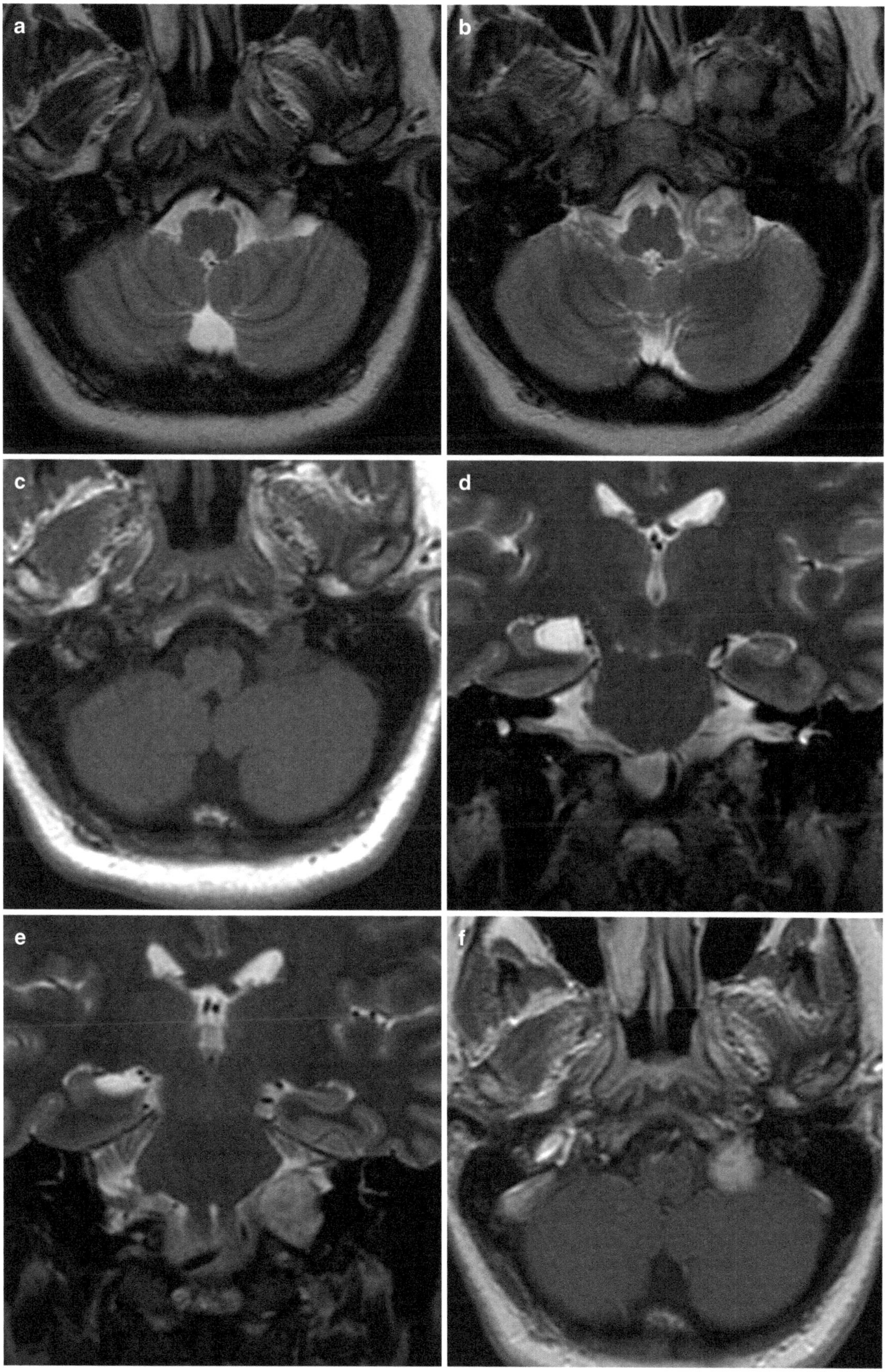

Fig. 23.51 Schwannoma of the left hypoglossal nerve. Series of T2- (**a**, **b**, **d**, **e**), T1- (**c**), and postenhanced T1- (**f**–**i**) weighted MR-images demonstrate a predominantly solid lesion with slightly hyperintense MR-signal on T2. Tumor is characterized by prominent contrast enhancement improving the visualization of lesion extension through the hypoglossal nerve bone canal (**e**)

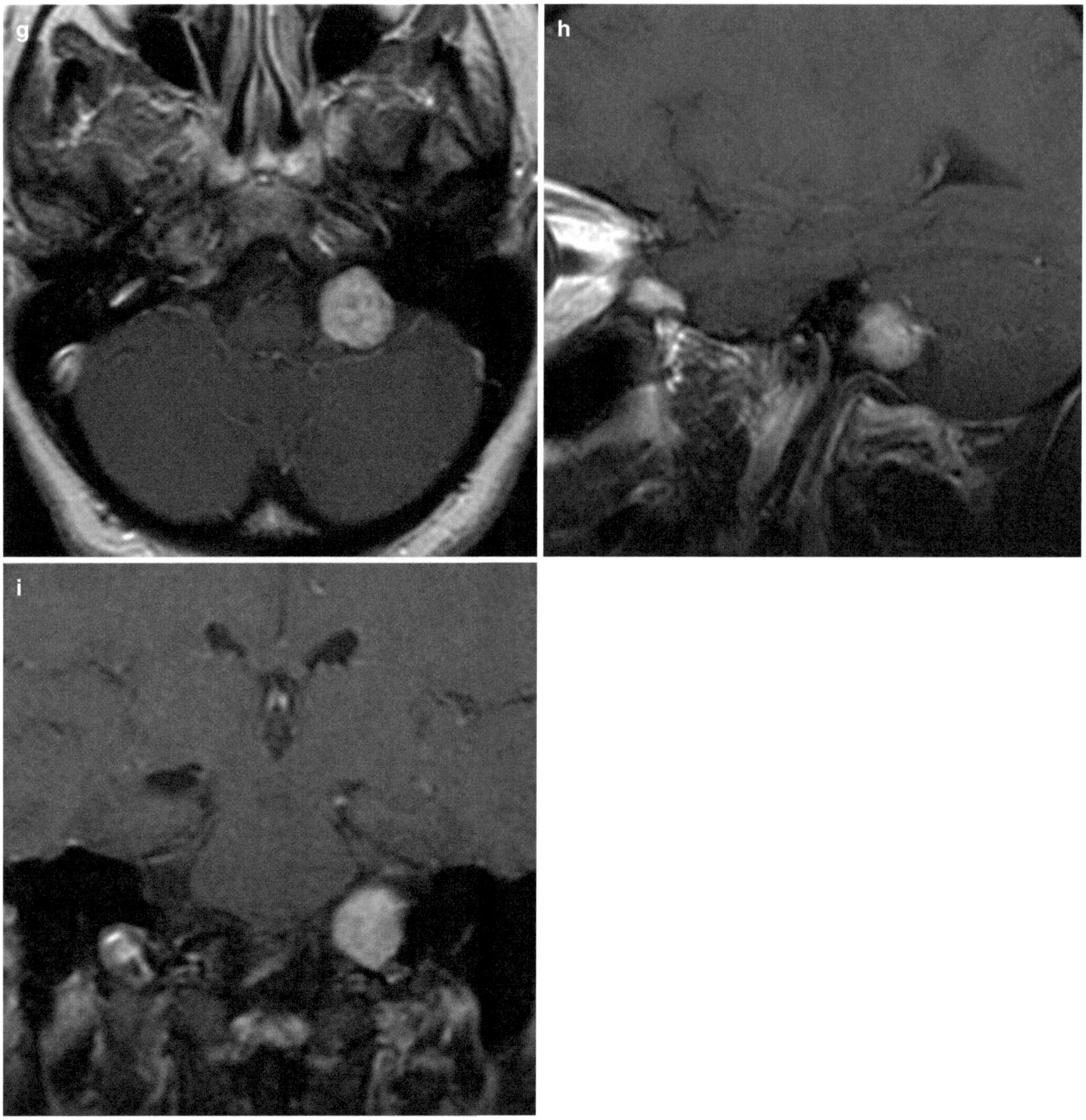

Fig. 23.51 (continued)

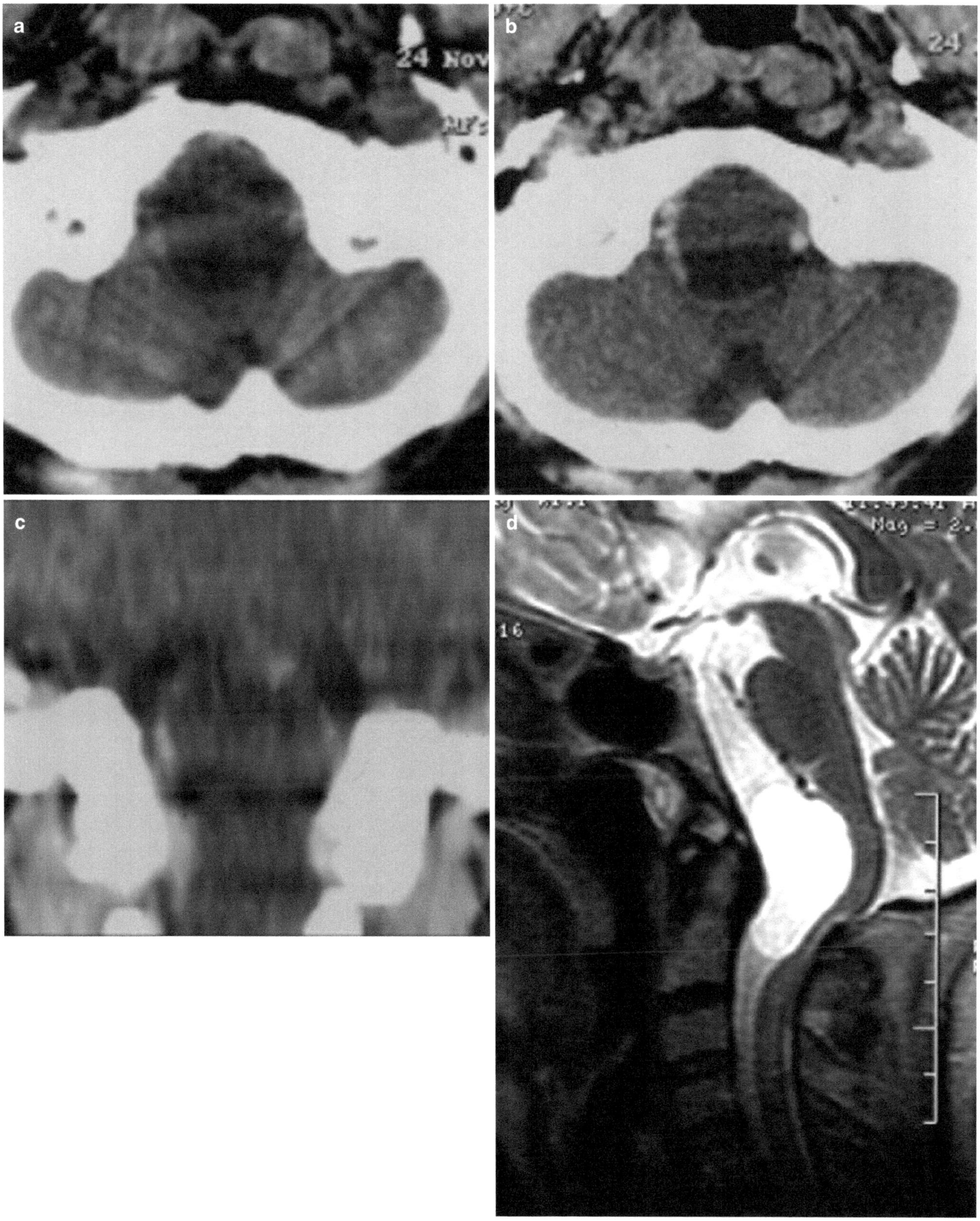

Fig. 23.52 Schwannoma of the right C1 nerve root. Axial and coronal CT scans before (**a**) and after (**b**, **c**) contrast enhancement demonstrate a hypodense predominantly cystic lesion with intermediate enhancement on the periphery. The tumor is located in the area of foramen Magnum, compresses the brain stem and has hyperintense signal on sagittal T2 (**d**)-weighted image, isointense signal on T2-FLAIR (**e**) and shows a hypointensity on T1(**f**)-weighted MR-image

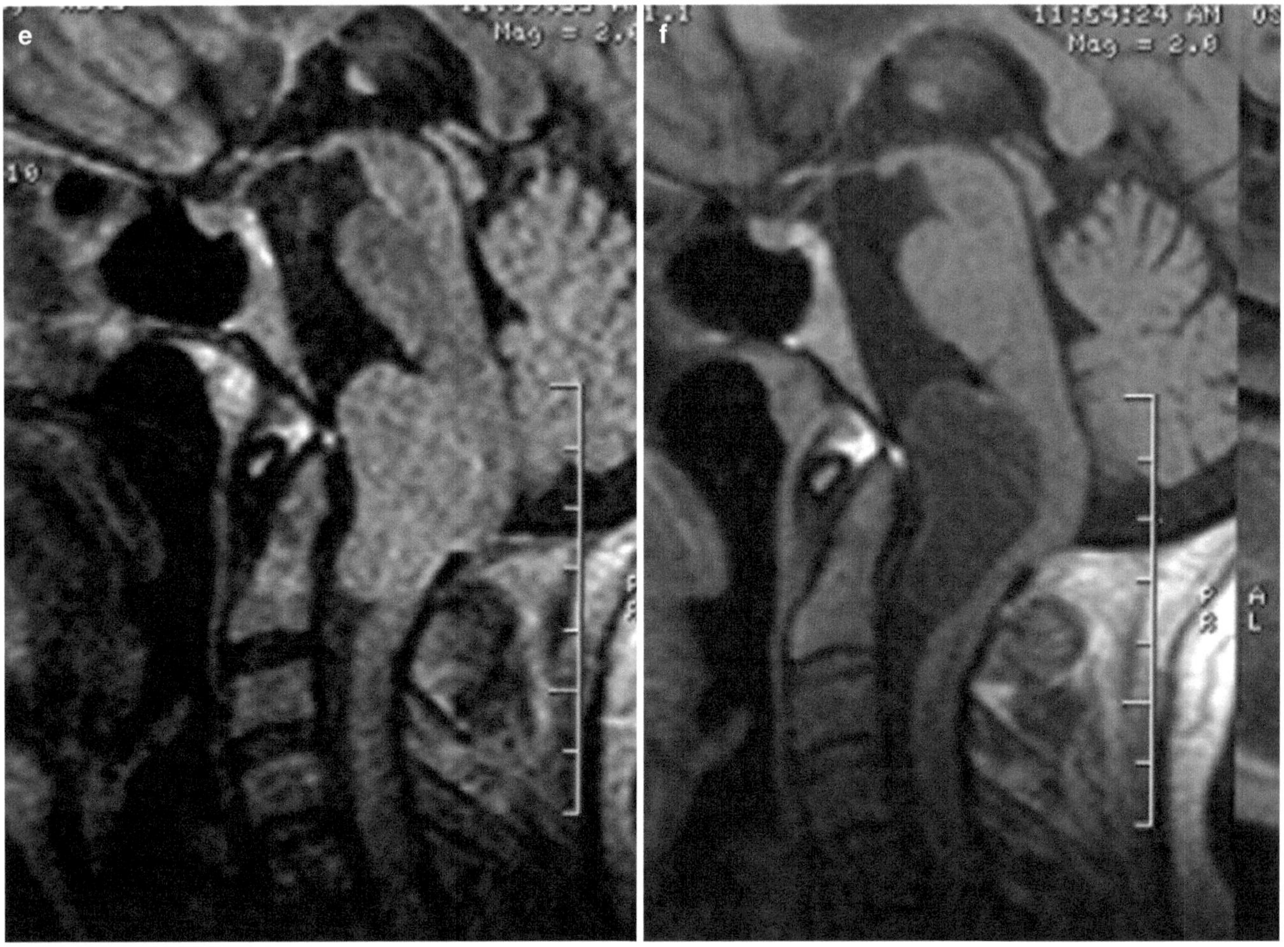

Fig. 23.52 (continued)

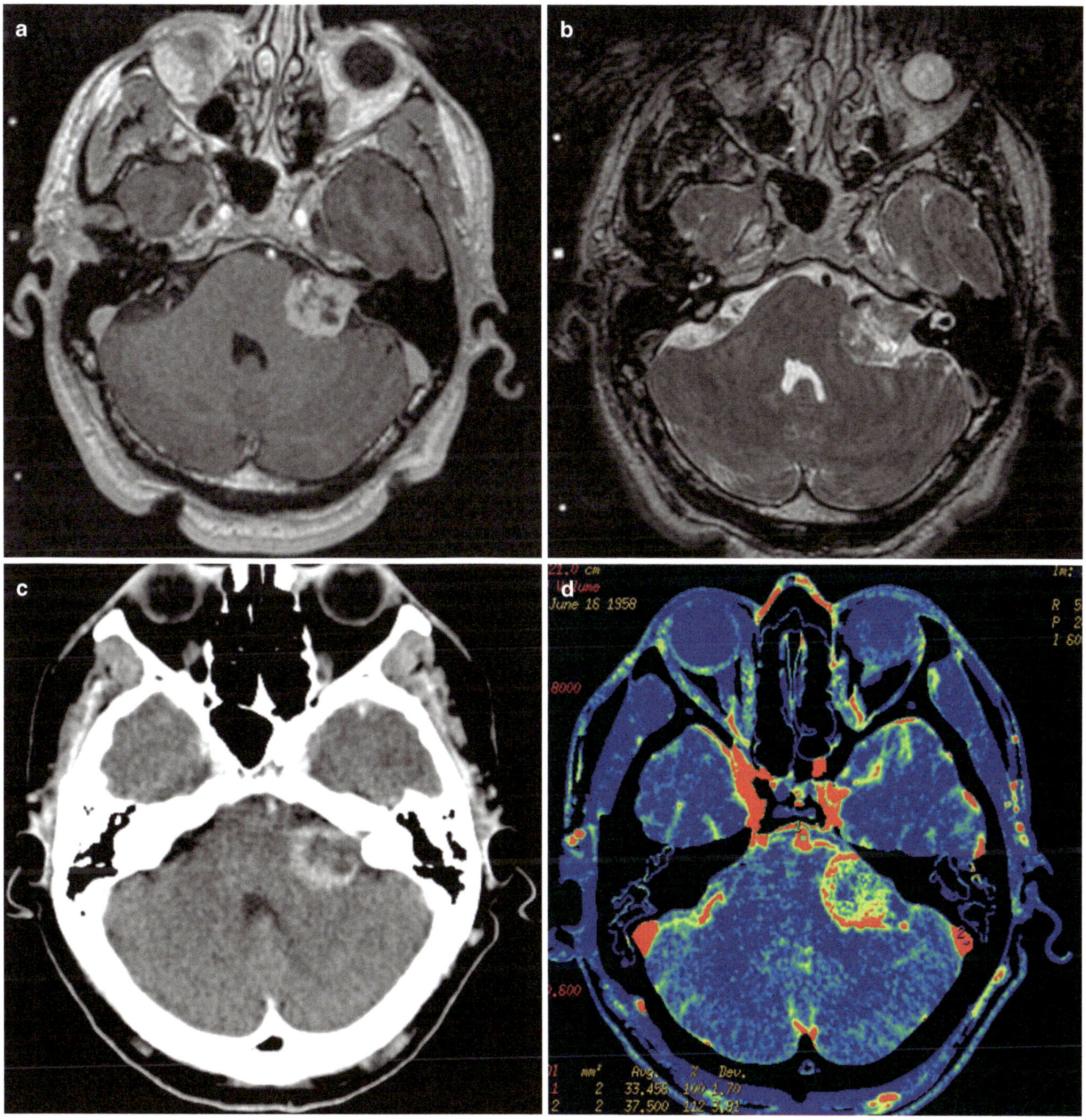

Fig. 23.53 Schwannoma of VIIIth cranial nerve. Axial postenhanced T1-weighted MR-image (**a**), T2- (**b**) weighted MR-image and postenhanced CT scan (**c**) demonstrate a heterogeneously enhancing lesion of left cerebellopontine angle. Tumor has a prominent elevation of CBV values (**d**) with heterogeneous distribution. Follow-up CT-perfusion study performed 1 year after radiosurgery showed the mismatch between size of enhancing tumor and decrease (in two folds) of CBV in lesion (as a result of radiosurgery)

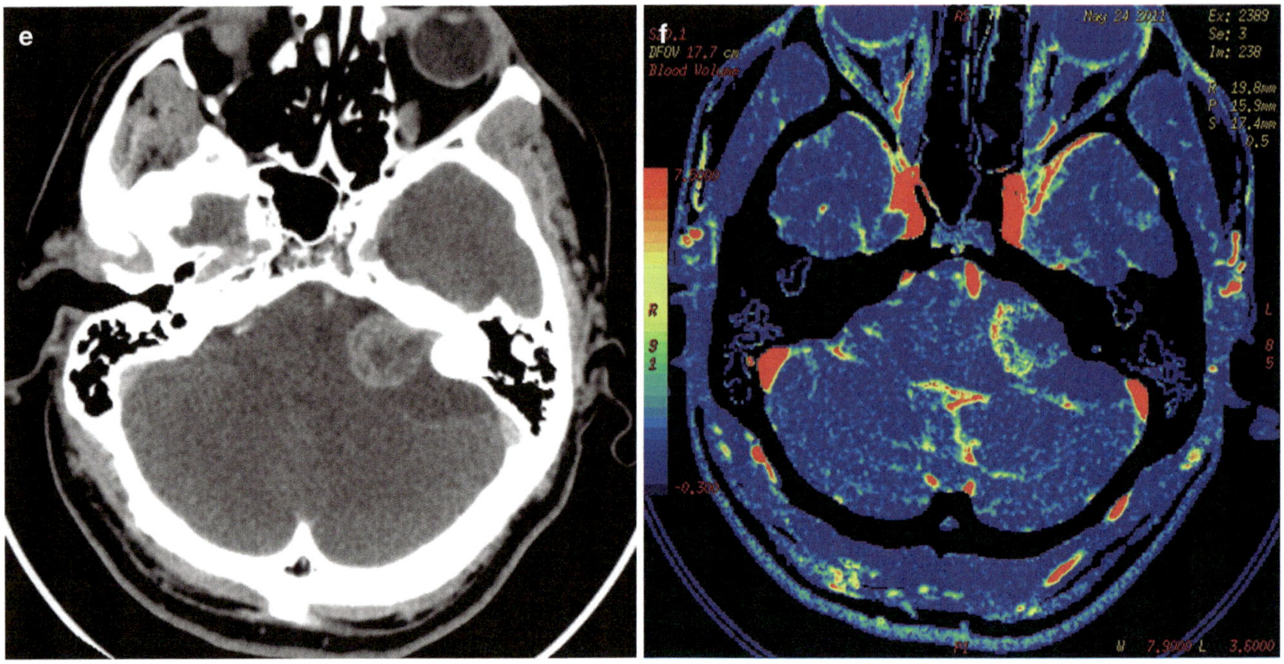

Fig. 23.53 (continued)

accessory nerves in complicated cases; trigeminal and abducent nerves in cases with large tumors), their paresis develops.

Jugular glomus tumors are the most common type of paragangliomas. They arise in the jugular foramen and cause typical destruction of petrous bone structures. They can grow intracranially (extradurally), penetrate into the mastoid, spread extracranially into the soft tissues of the neck (Jackson 2001). Intracranial paragangliomas spread through the jugular foramen, growing over the cranial nerves from the caudal group and venous sinuses. The degree of tumor invasion at the surrounding structures of the skull base, related treatment approach and surgical radicality were the basis of classification of skull base paragangliomas developed by Firch and Mattox (1988), subsequently modified by M. Sanna in 2005. Based on this classification, paragangliomas are divided into four main types (A–D): type A—a tumor within the promontorium, type B—a tumor growing into the hypotympanum, but not destroying the jugular fossa and not spreading into the infralabyrinthine space, type C—a tumor affecting the infralabyrinthine space and the petrous apex, type D—a tumor with intracranial spread (epi- and intradural).

Macroscopically, paraganglioma can be seen during an otoscopic examination as a polypoid reddish-brown mass, penetrating deep into the ear canal, or a pulsatile mass behind the eardrum membrane.

Imaging Direct angiography detects a hypervascular tumor tissue at the projection of the skull base with visualization of multiple hypertrophied arteries in the early arterial phase. Also, a rapid discharge of a contrast agent into the draining veins is noted. The main lesion supply comes from the ascending pharyngeal artery (lower medial tumor segments). Tympanic branches of the internal carotid and meningeal branches of the vertebral artery, anterior tympanic arteries (from the external carotid artery) supply the anterior part of the lesion and the stylomastoid artery (from the external carotid artery system) supplies postero-lateral sections of the tumor (Fig. 23.54).

Paragangliomas as a soft-tissue lesions in the jugular foramen are very well visualized both on CT and MRI. Coronal and oblique reformations of CT row data improve delineating the tumor masses with intranasal and extracranial location and demonstration of the destructive

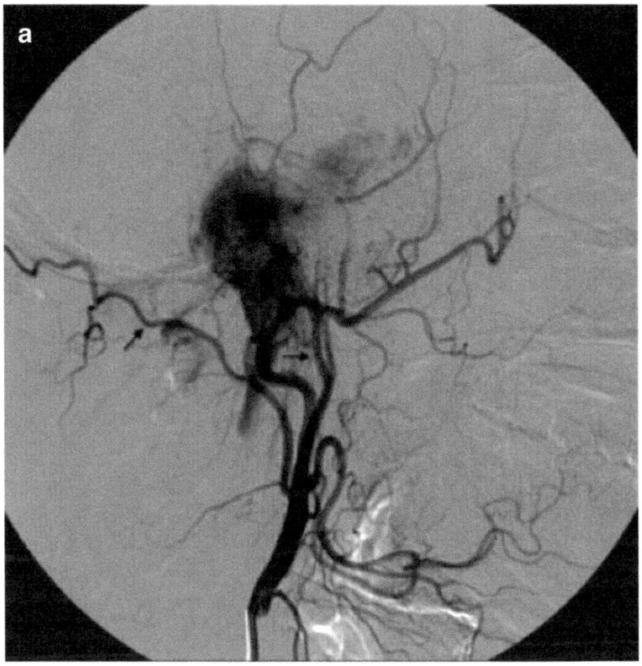

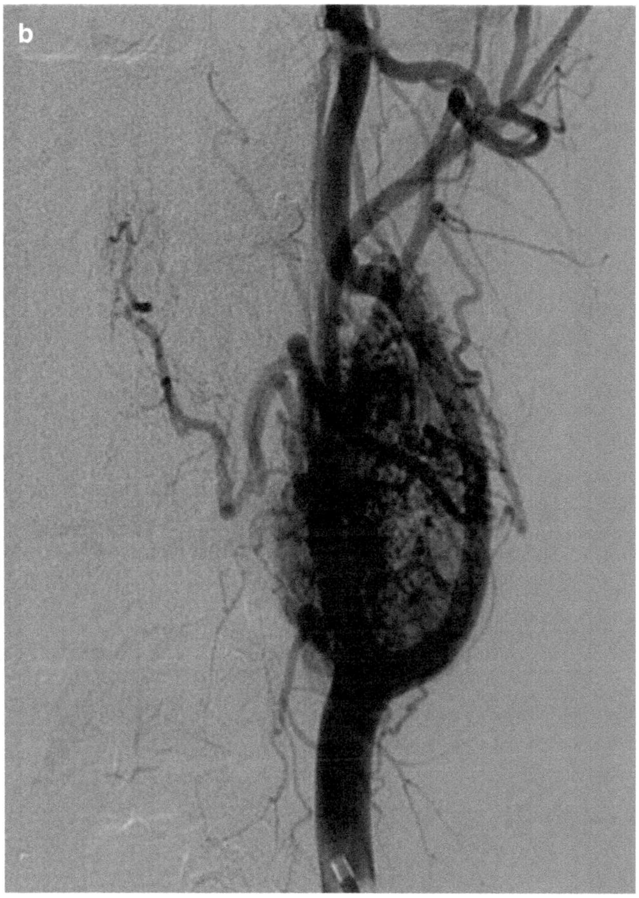

Fig. 23.54 Paraganglioma's vasculature (different patients). Case 1. Paraganglioma of the temporal bone: DSA (lateral view (**a**)) of external carotid artery demonstrates an abundant and multiple blood supply of the lesion (a. auricularis posterior, a. meningeal media and others). Case 2. Paraganglioma of the carotid glomus: DSA (lateral view (**b**)) of common carotid artery demonstrates an abundant and multiple blood supply of the lesion (short branches of external carotid artery) with dislocation of ICA

changes in the bone tissue. Intravenous contrast enhancement is a mandatory attribute of the primary diagnosis. The tumor rapidly and often heterogeneously accumulates contrast media (Figs. 23.55 and 23.56). Following contrast enhancement, the dura separating the tumor and intradural space are well identified. It should be remembered, however, that a CT examination should begin immediately after administration of a contrast agent, so the degree of tumor enhancement will be higher. CT-angiography is a method of choice in complex estimation of paragangliomas of head and neck location.

On MRI, glomus tumors are characterized by a heterogeneous MR-signal and have a mottled appearance that reflects the abundance of newly formed blood vessels, their different caliber, omnidirectional blood flow, and partial thrombosis (Rao et al. 1999; Noujaim et al. 2000; Mafee et al. 2000). The tumors intensely enhance, thus, it is possible to more accurately estimate an extension of the lesion into the cranial cavity, the deformation of the brainstem and the relationship with the large vessels, including venous sinuses. Typical mottled appearance "salt and pepper" pattern persists after contrast enhancement—arterial vessels with rapid blood flow remain hypointense on standard T1-weighted sequences (Figs. 23.57 and 23.58). On SPGR sequence, arterial vessels appear bright, which improves visualization of the overall picture of abnormal tumor's vasculature (Fig. 23.59).

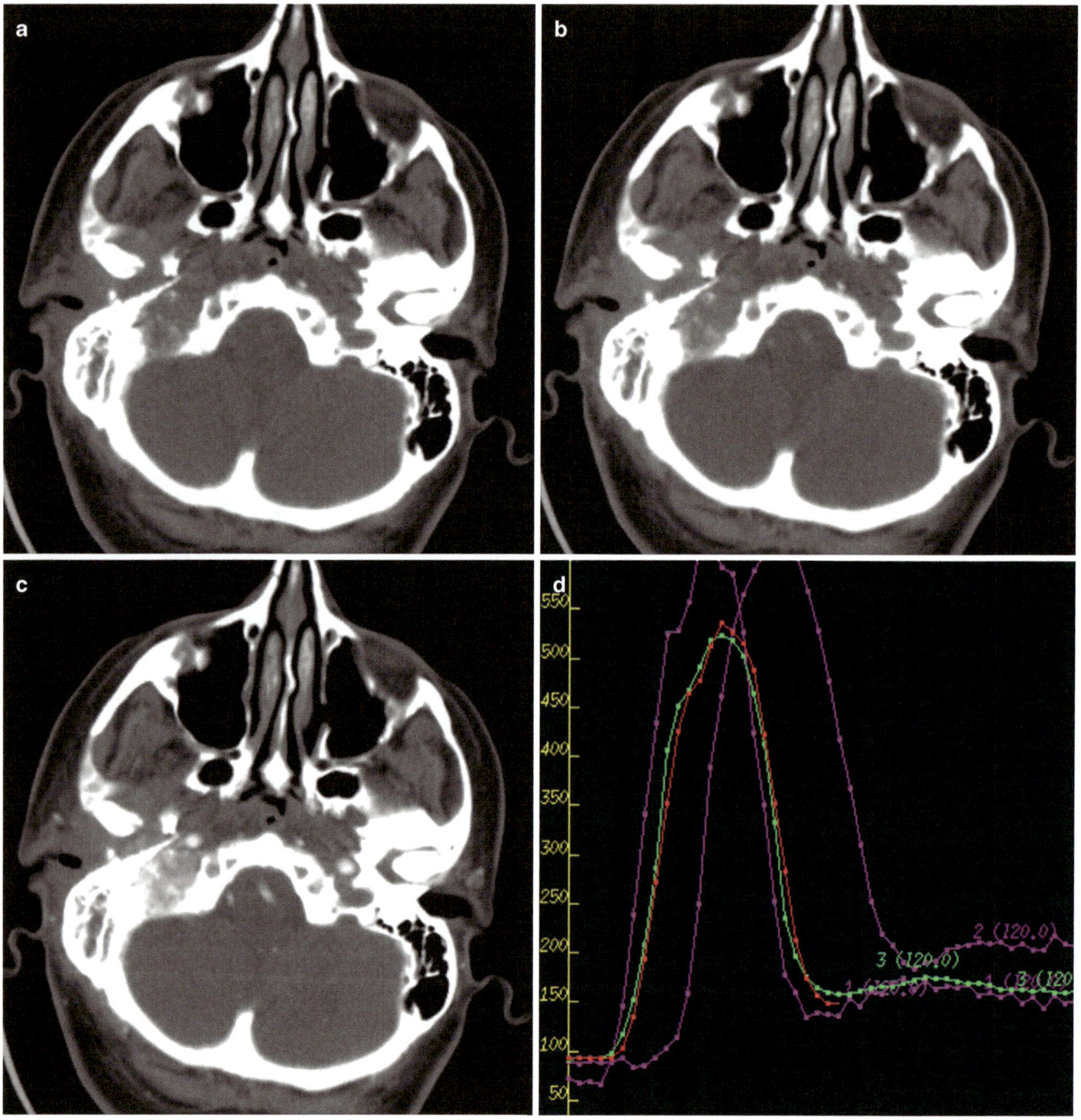

Fig. 23.55 Paraganglioma of the temporal bone. Series of axial CT scans in different contrast enhancement phases during CT-perfusion study demonstrate fast contrast agent accumulation within the tumor (**a**–**c**). (**d**) Dynamic contrast enhancement curves. *Green line* represents the distribution of contrast agent in paraganglioma, 1-artery, 2-vein

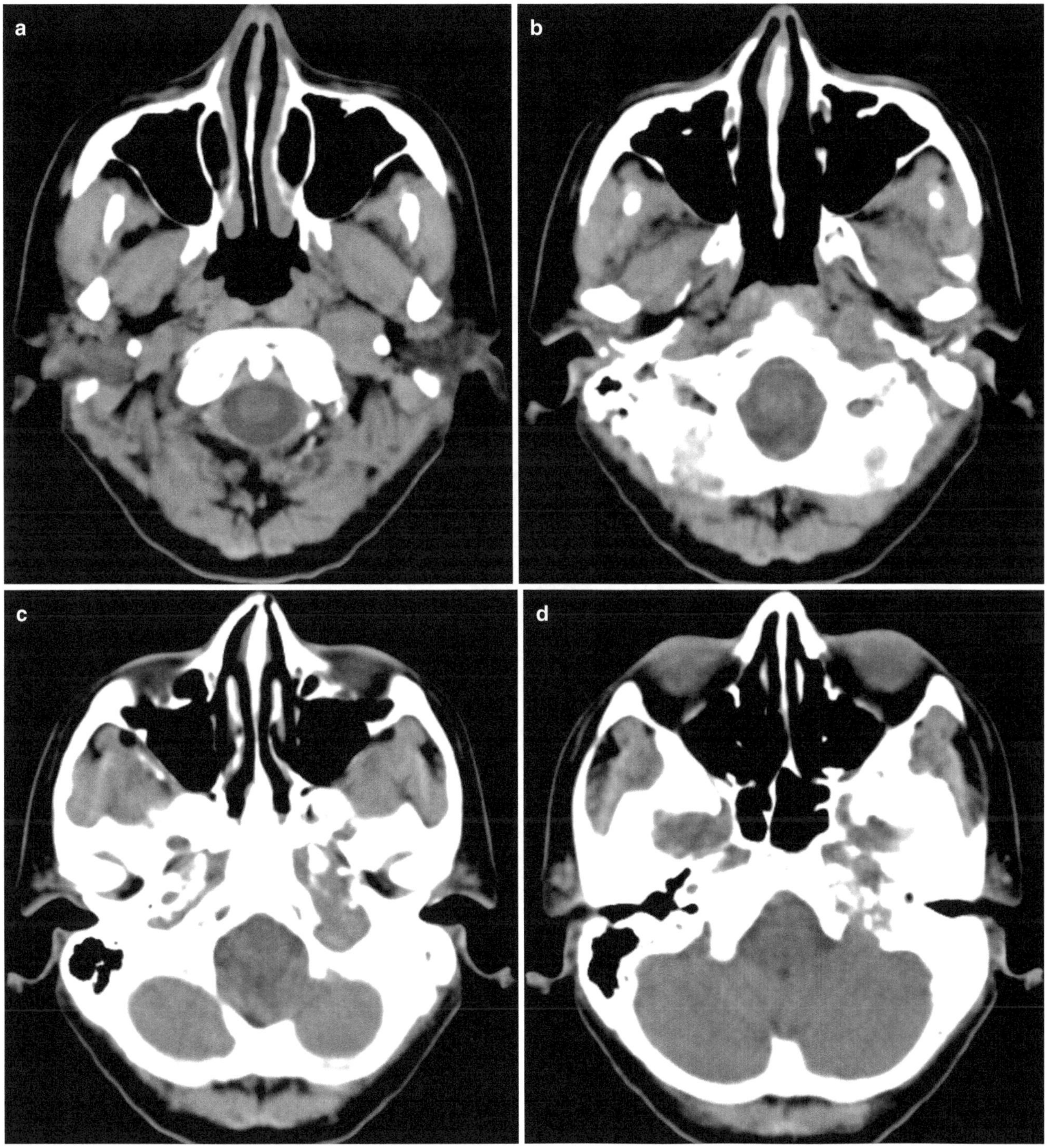

Fig. 23.56 Paraganglioma of the left temporal bone. Axial CT scans before (**a–d**) and after (**e–h**) contrast enhancement demonstrate a strongly enhancing tumor causing the focal bone destruction. Tumor is characterized by prominent elevation the blood flow (CBF map (**i**))

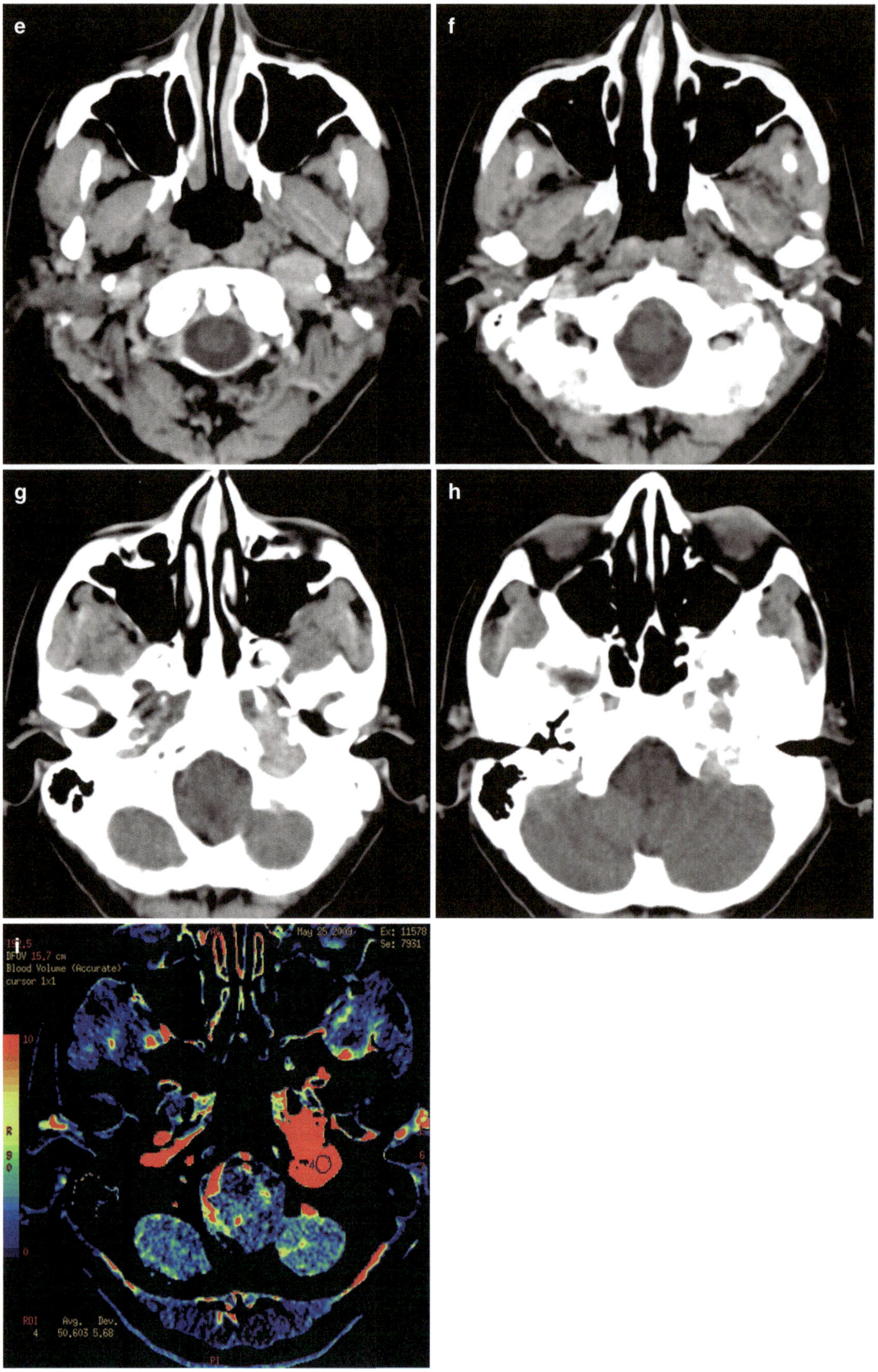

Fig. 23.56 (continued)

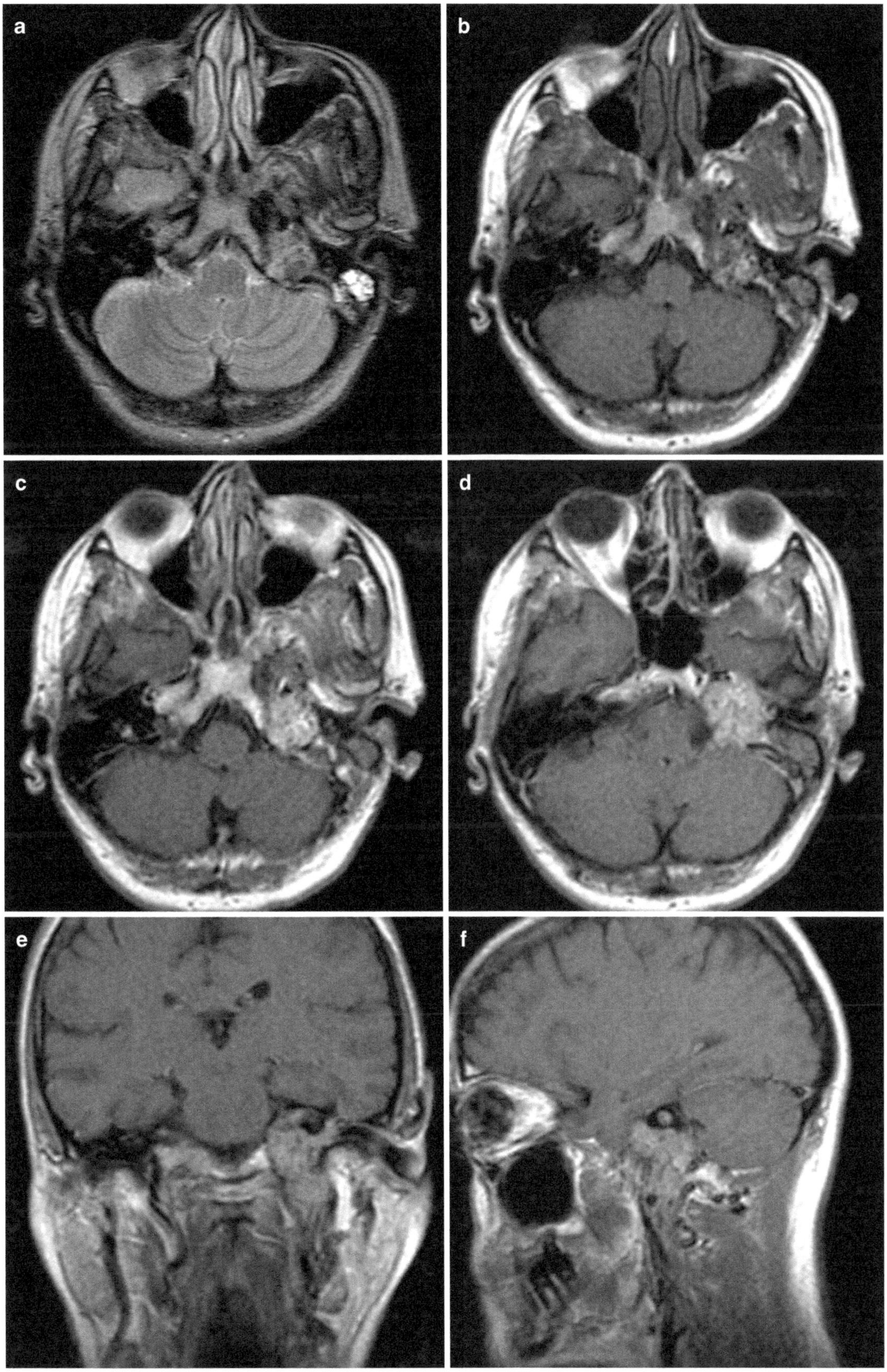

Fig. 23.57 Paraganglioma of the left temporal bone. Axial T2 (**a**)-weighted MR-image, T1 before (**b**)- and T1 after (**c**–**f**) contrast enhancement weighted MR-images demonstrate a strongly enhancing tumor in projection of the left pyramid. Lesion has "speckled" pattern

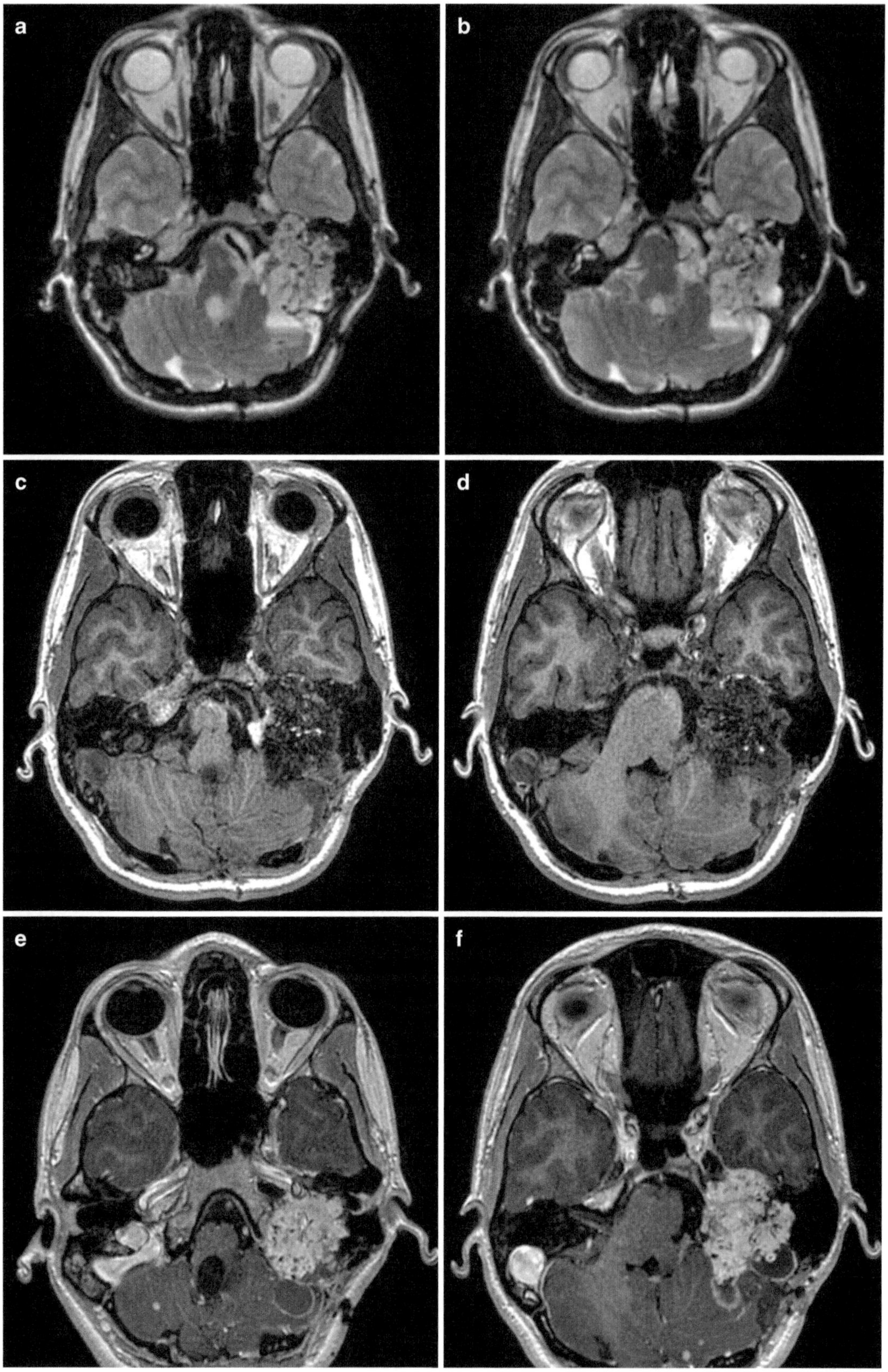

Fig. 23.58 Giant paraganglioma of the left temporal bone. MR imaging using T2-weighted MR-images (**a**, **b**), T1-WI before (**c**, **d**) and T1-WI after (**e**–**i**) contrast enhancement demonstrate a strongly enhancing tumor in projection of left pyramid. Lesion has "speckled" "pepper and salt" pattern

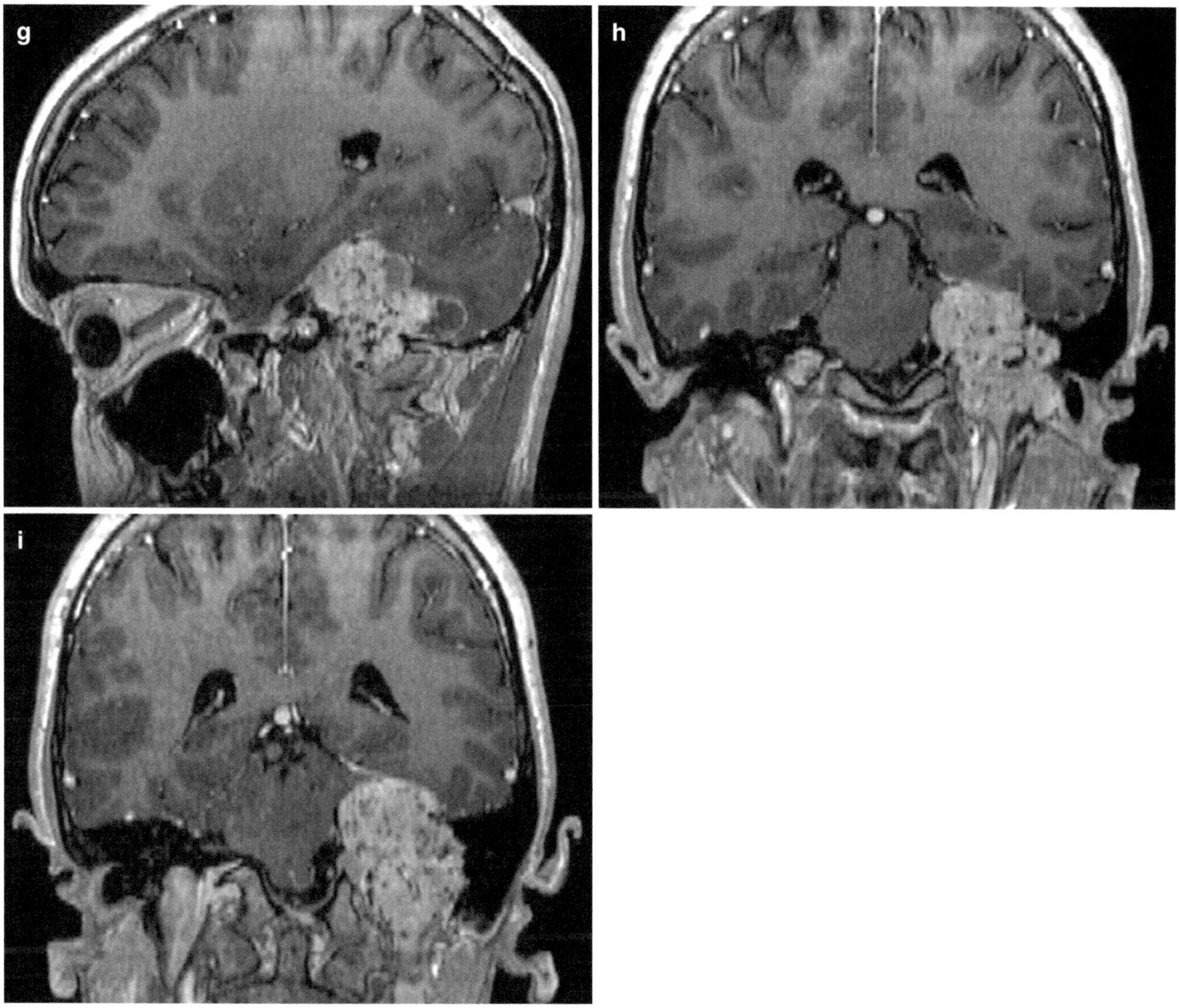

Fig. 23.58 (continued)

2D- and 3D TOF MR angiography, despite their high efficacy in visualizing the arterial and venous components of paraganglioma, currently serves only as a primary diagnostic tool to assess the degree of paraganglioma vasculature, in general (Figs. 23.60 and 23.61). Bolus MR angiography provides greater opportunities in the assessment of the tumor blood flow allowing to visualize not only the arterial, but also the venous component during the diagnostic procedure (Fig. 23.62). However, direct angiography (especially, superselective one), in our opinion, is still a leading method allowing to simultaneously evaluate the nature and extent of tumor blood supply, such as arterial afferents and venous drainage, and to conduct selective embolization of incoming tumor vessels.

Recently, developing CT-perfusion methods allows obtaining the information about the characteristics of the blood supply to paragangliomas, without using invasive and complicated direct angiographic techniques. Even small-sized paragangliomas have characteristic changes in their hemodynamics: these are very high CBV and CBF values, short MTT values (parameters that reliably distinguish them from other tumors at this site, even malignant tumors) (Fig. 23.63).

Differential Diagnosis Meningioma (can have hyperostotic changes in the bone, "dural tail," growth along the dura), schwannoma (a marked enlargement of the jugular foramen, no hypertrophied vessels with direct angiography), metastases and primary cancers of the base (no mottled appearance, moderately increased perfusion rates).

Giant cell tumor (syn. osteoclastoma, osteoblastoclastoma, gigantoma, brown tumor (in case of hemorrhagic inclusions), benign giant cell bone tumor, myeloid tumor) belongs to a group of intraosseous lesions, containing a large number of multinucleated giant cells of osteoclast type. They

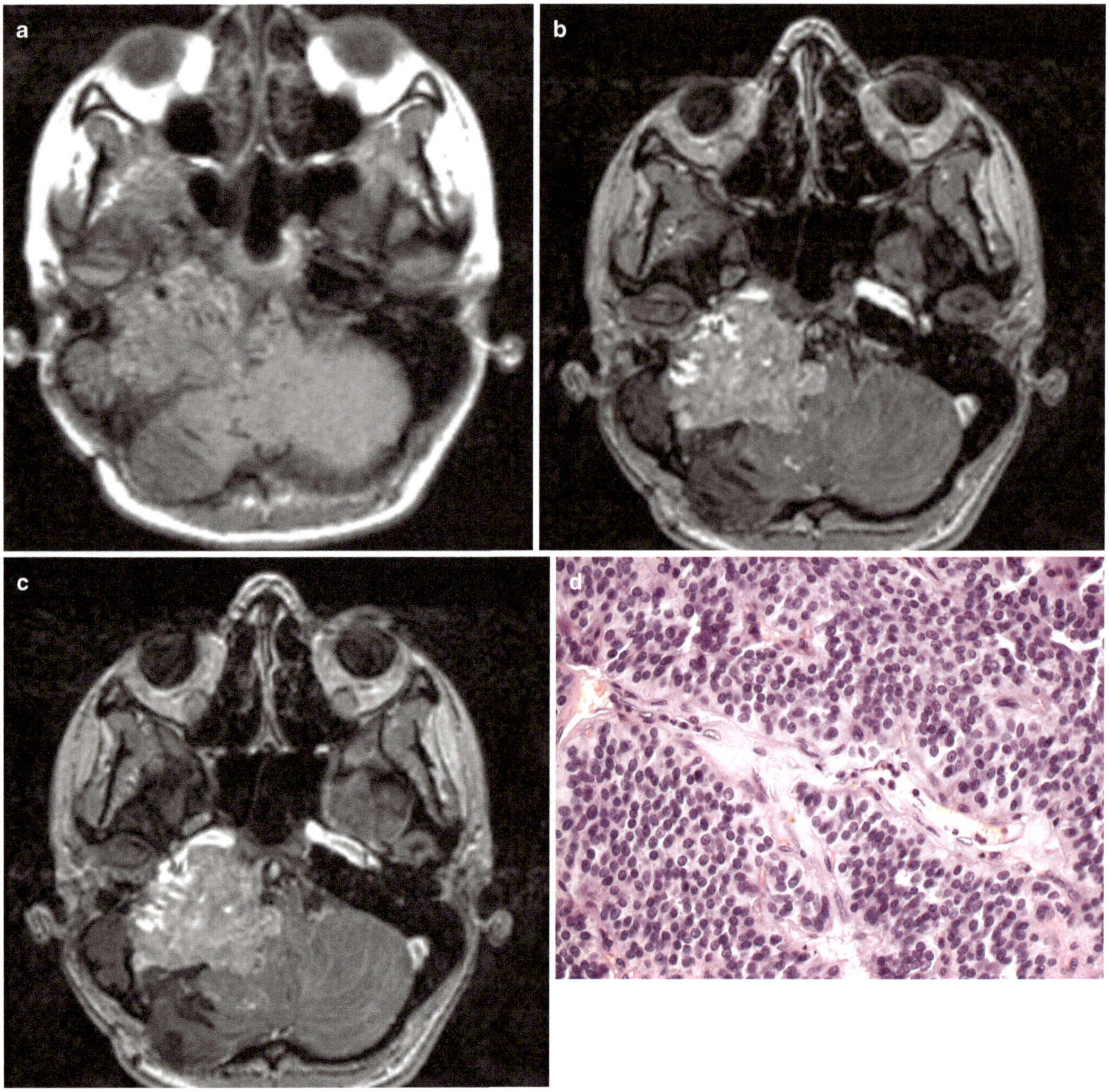

Fig. 23.59 Giant paraganglioma of the right temporal bone. MR imaging before (**a**) and after (**b**, **c**) contrast enhancement demonstrate a strongly enhancing tumor in projection of right pyramid. Lesion has "speckled" "pepper and salt" pattern due to abundant vascular network. (**d**) Histologic specimen

are common located in epiphyses and metaphyses of long bones, and are less common in the skull bones, affecting the sphenoid, temporal and rarely frontal bones. A high frequency of lesions in the maxilla and mandibular bones is noted, accounting for about 65% of all neoplastic processes in the jaws (Tang et al. 2003).

Microscopy of the tumor tissue reveals serous or "bloody" cysts as a result of osteoclastic process, combined with osteoplastic events, such as formation of bone trabeculae.

Giant cell tumors occur mainly in children and adolescents. They can develop as a solitary nodule at the projection of the temporal bone and very rarely multicentric growth occur. If the tumors are located in the mastoid area, a tight knot behind the ear is noted, sometimes combined with facial nerve palsy. The clinical signs are manifested in the form of headaches, local pain, cranial nerve palsies, and visual disturbances, diplopia, ophthalmoplegia, hearing loss in case of lateral tumor growth (Sheikh et al. 1999).

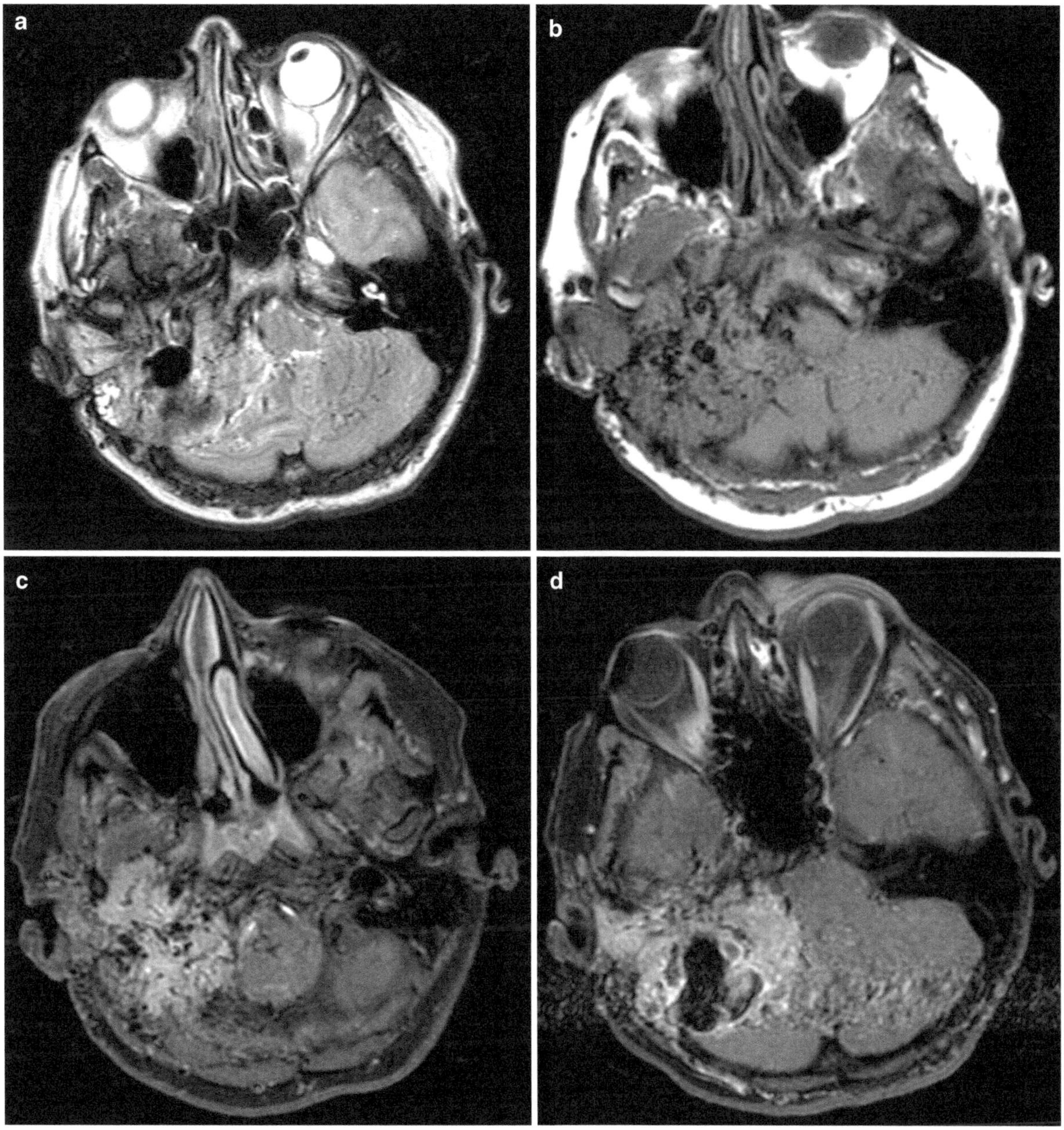

Fig. 23.60 Giant paraganglioma of the right temporal bone with intra- and extracranial extension. MR imaging using T2-weighted MR-image (**a**), T1-WI before (**b**) and T1-WI after (**c**–**f**) contrast enhancement demonstrates a strongly enhancing tumor in projection of right temporal bone with typical "speckled" pattern due to abundant vasculature. Contrast enhanced 3D TOF MR-angiography (**g**–**i**) confirms the abundant vascular network of the paraganglioma

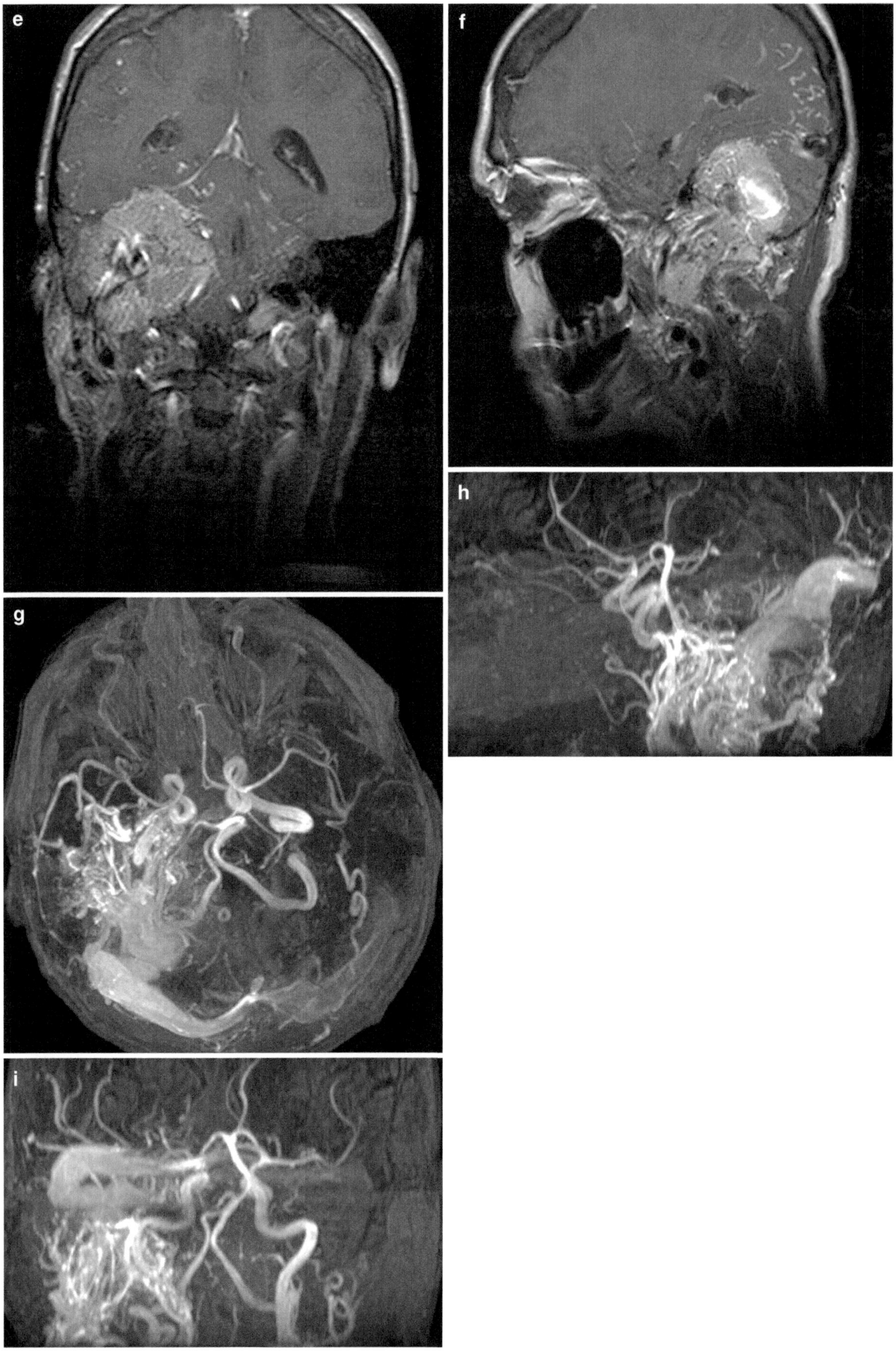

Fig. 23.60 (continued)

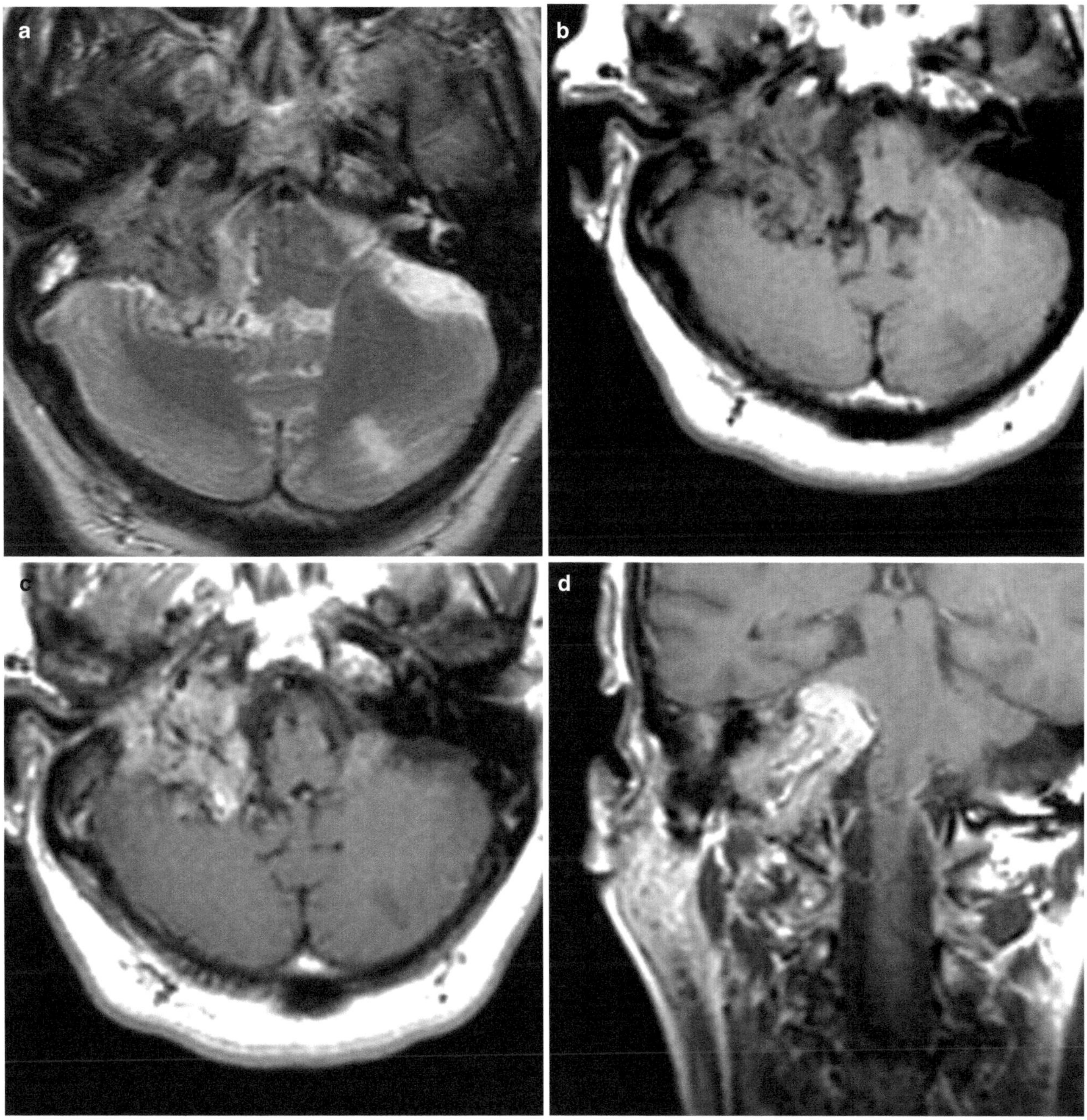

Fig. 23.61 Paraganglioma of the right temporal bone with intracranial extension. MR imaging using T2-weighted MR-image (**a**), T1-WI before (**b**) and T1-WI after (**c**, **d**) contrast enhancement demonstrates a strongly enhancing tumor in the projection of the right temporal bone with typical "speckled" pattern due to abundant vasculature. Contrast enhanced 3D TOF MR-angiography (**e**) confirms the abundant vascular network of the paraganglioma. 2D TOF MR-venography shows the occlusion of the right sigmoid sinus due to tumor spreading (**f**)

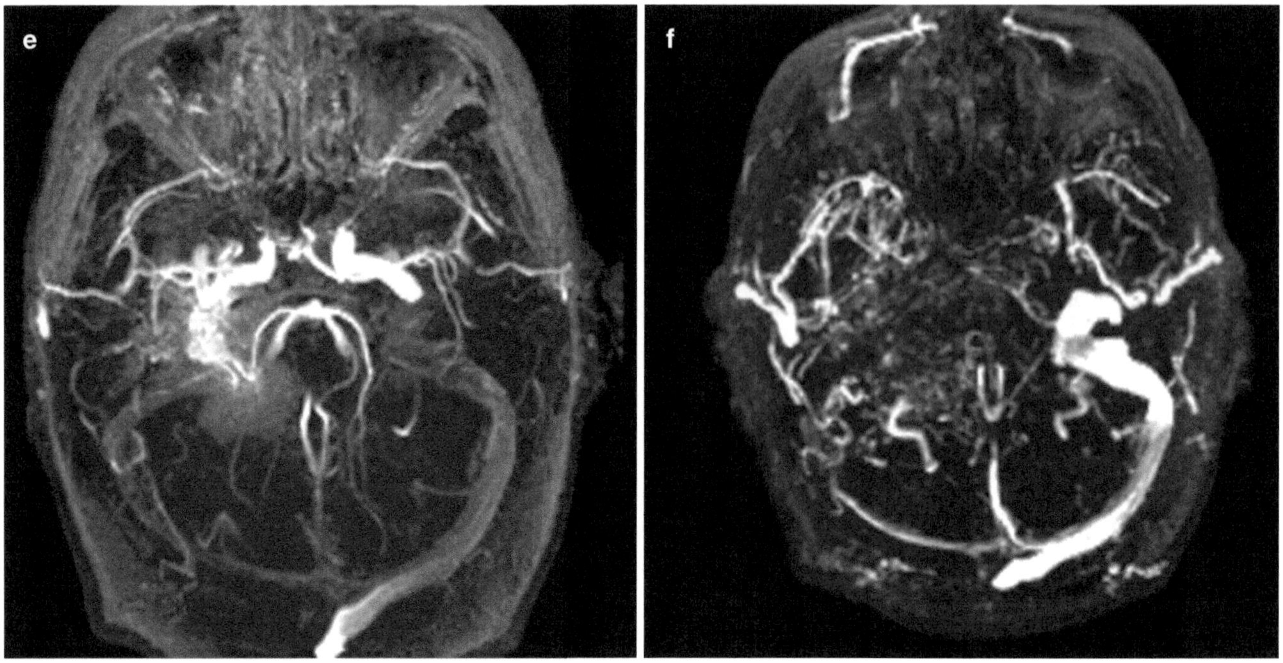

Fig. 23.61 (continued)

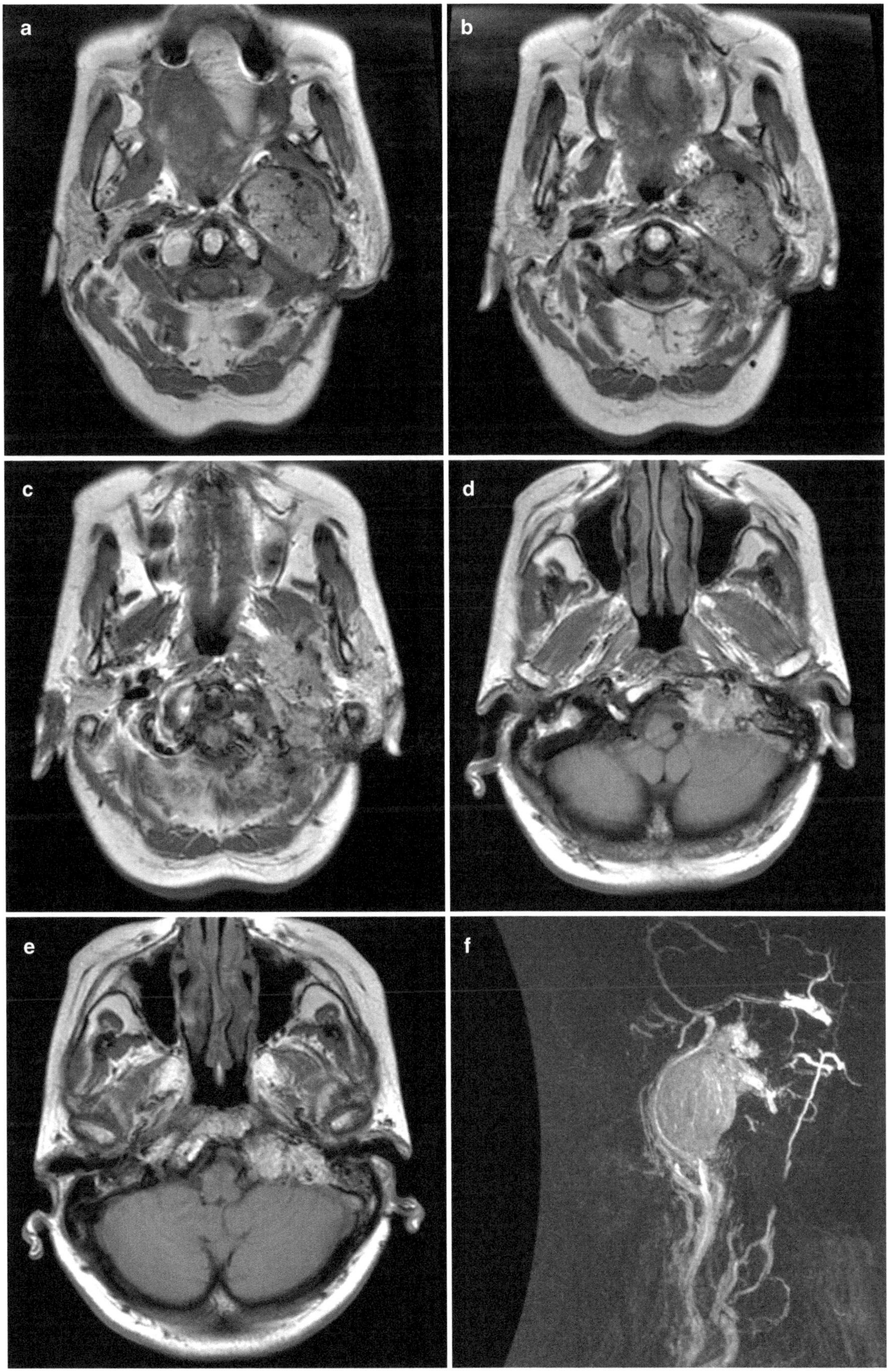

Fig. 23.62 Giant paraganglioma of the left temporal bone with intra- and extracranial extension. On enhanced T1-weighted MR images (**a–e**) a large soft-tissue tumor can be seen. Lesion has typical MR-appearance—"pepper and salt" pattern. Series of TRICKS images demonstrate the abundant tumor vasculature and complex remodel of neck arterial and venous systems (**f–o**)

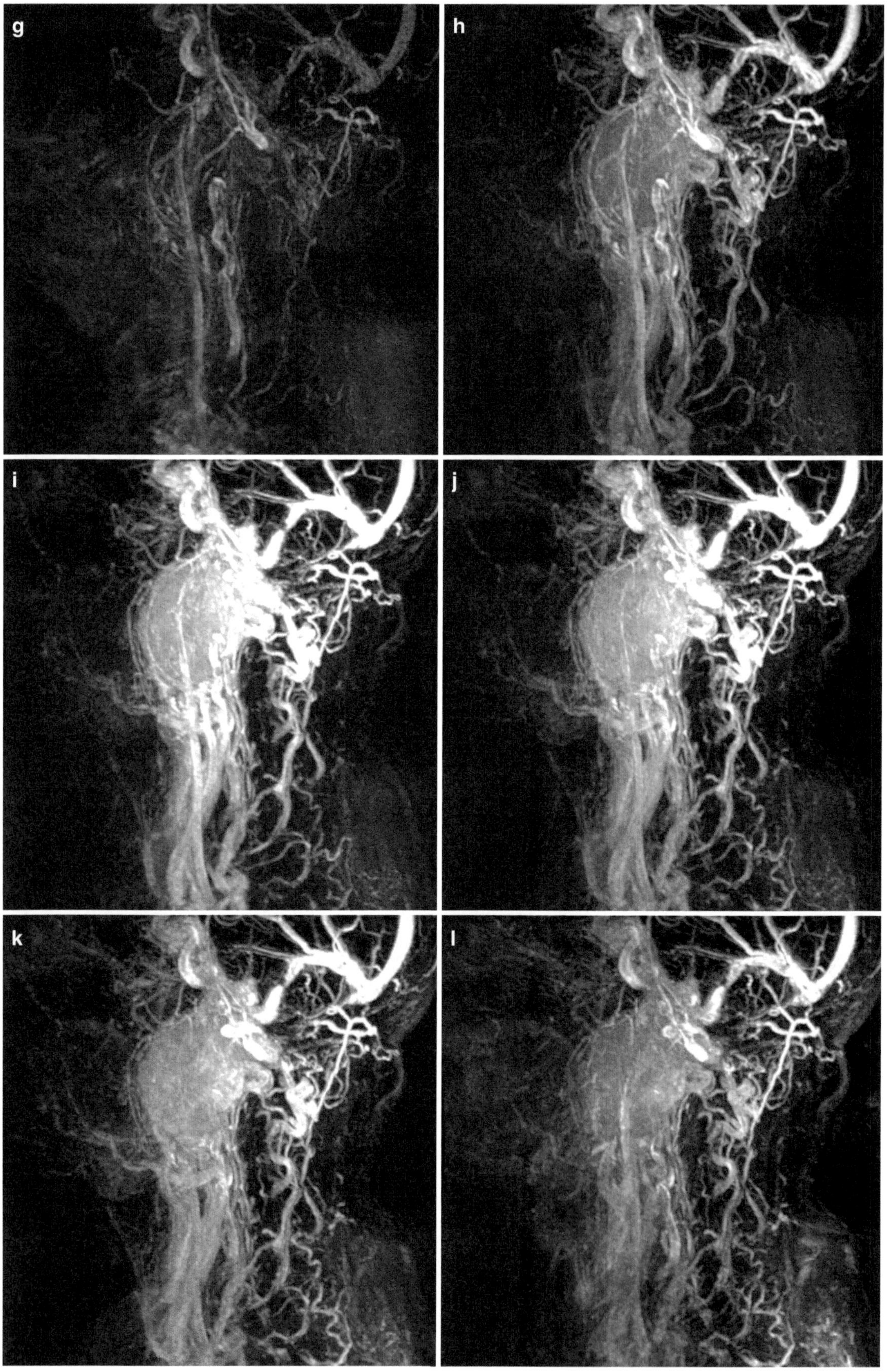

Fig. 23.62 (continued)

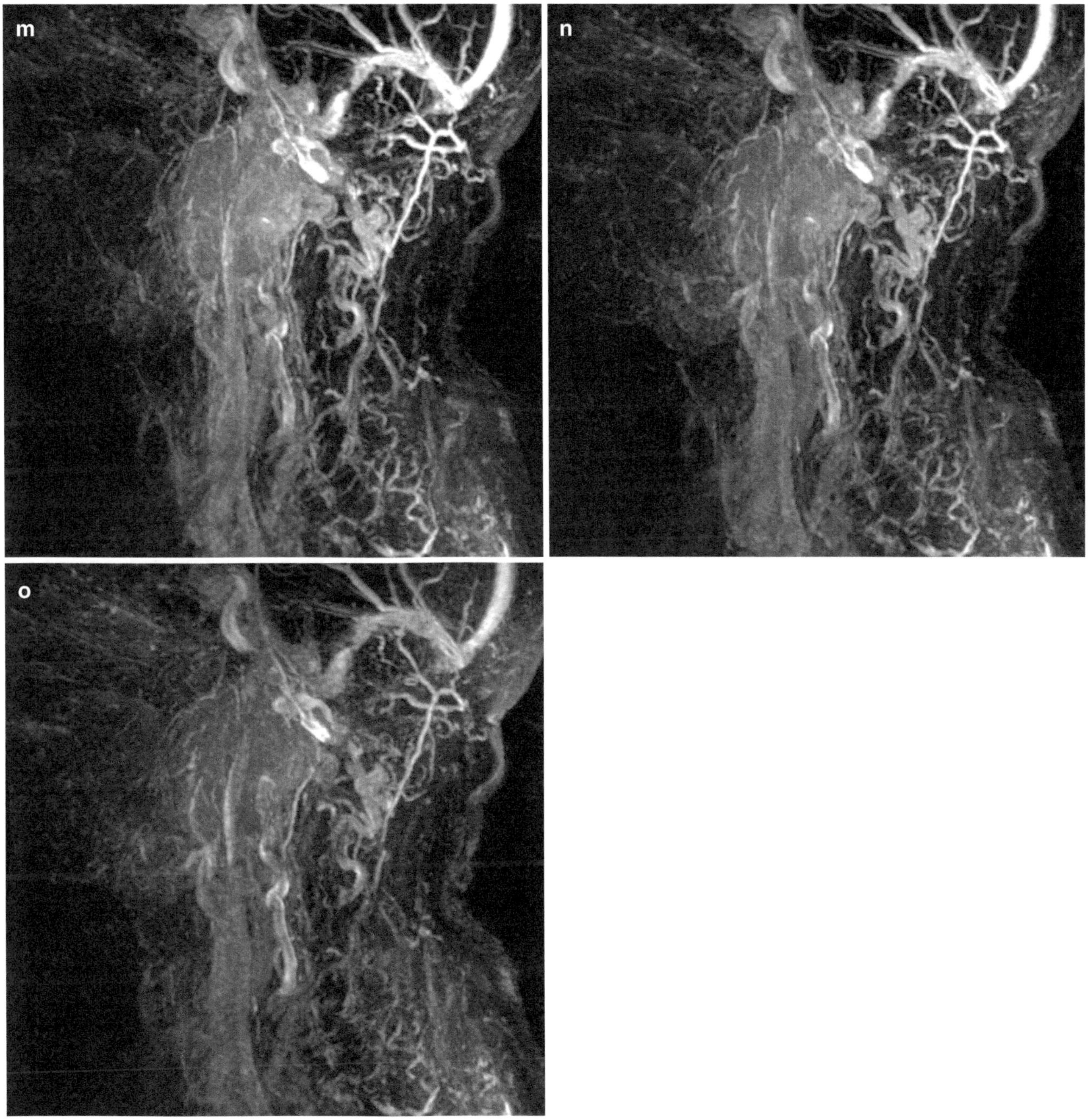

Fig. 23.62 (continued)

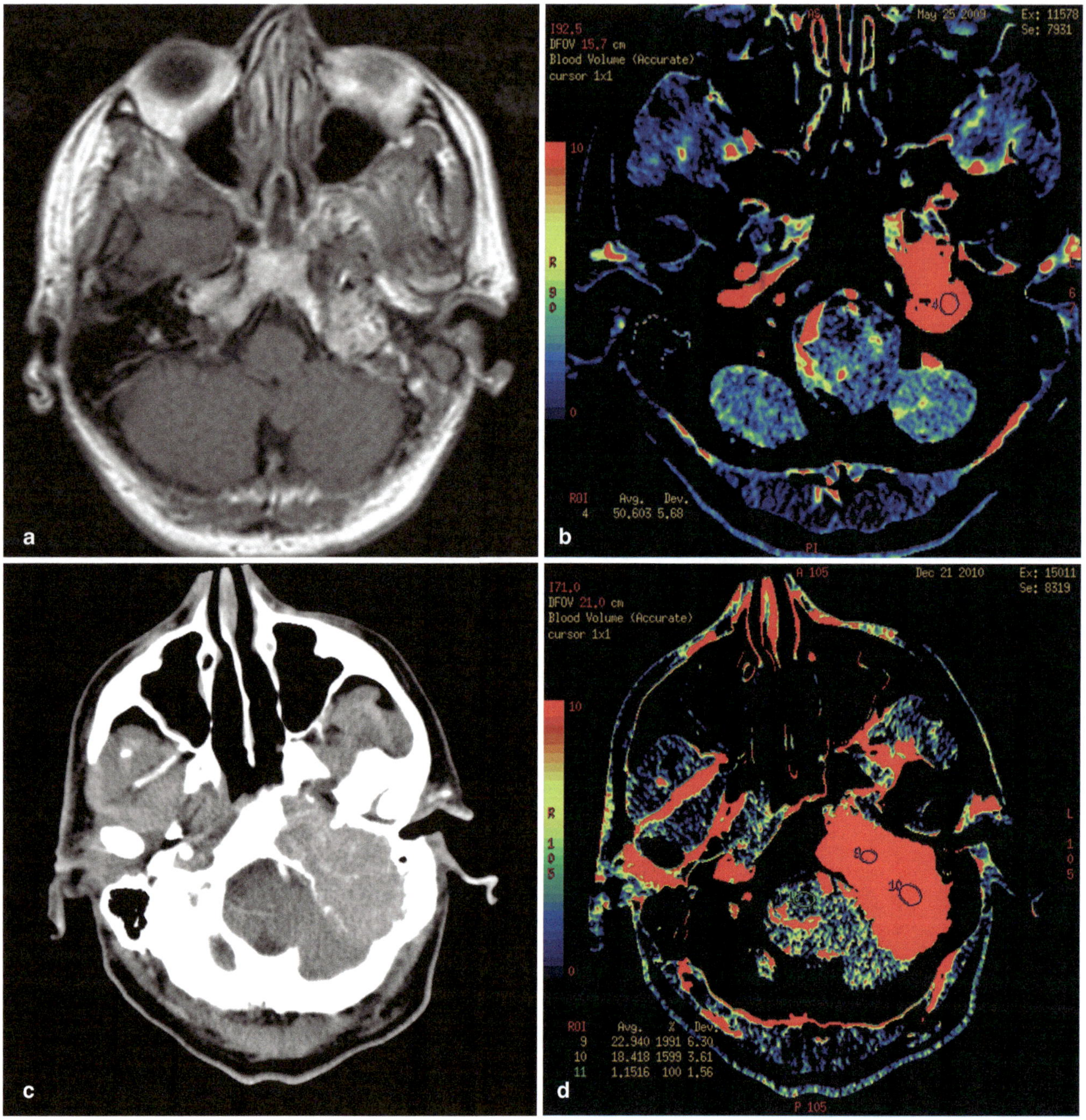

Fig. 23.63 Different patterns of paragangliomas hemodynamics (different patients). Case 1-(**a**, **b**), Case 2-(**c**, **d**), Case 3-(**e**, **f**). In all cases, paragangliomas show an extremely high values of CBV in their structure

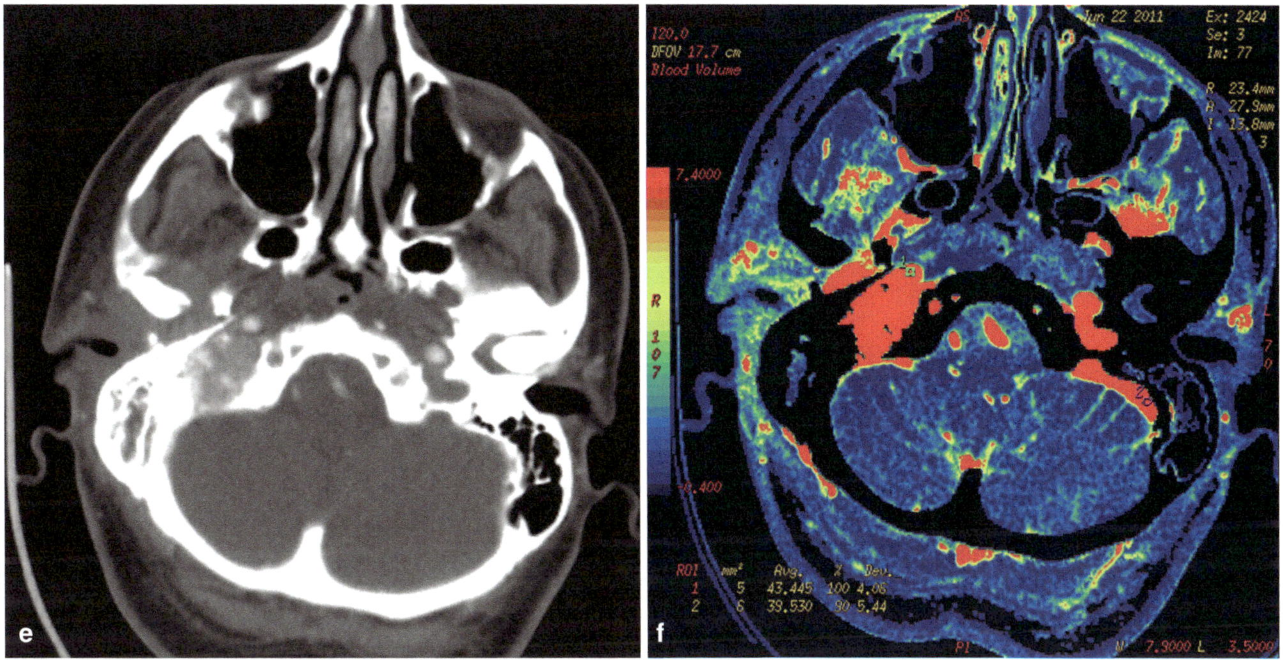

Fig. 23.63 (continued)

Imaging Direct angiography shows moderately vascularized masses with supply frequently from branches of the external carotid artery.

CT scanning demonstrates an intraosseous expansile lesion with thinning of the cortical layer, which may become sclerotic and have local destruction areas. In general, this lesion is moderately hyperdense on non-enhanced scanning. In rare cases, there may be small calcifications in the center. Cellular forms of osteoblastoclastoma contain a large number of smaller and larger cavities delimited from each other by bony partitions. Cystic forms are characterized by oval areas of bone lysis with various sizes. In lytic forms, a bone lesion has no definite shape, which makes it difficult to diagnose the disease. After the process starts to spread into the wall of the auditory meatus and tumor invades the tympanum cavity, the signs of impairment of the sound-conducting system in the form of conductive hearing loss can be diagnosed. Contrast enhancement ranges from homogeneous to heterogeneous, but is always detected by CT (Lee et al. 1998).

On MRI, hemorrhages into the tumor cysts appear by sedimentation of erythrocytes decaying with formation of hemosiderin, which determines its brown color during surgery. If cysts are combined into one cystic cavity, fibrous tissue often grows through them. This is why MR-signal on T1-weighted images can be heterogeneous with hyperintense inclusions, often with a hypointense rim. On T2-weighted images, an isointense or slightly hyperintense MR-signal from the tumor mass is noted. A low MR-signal is rare due to the presence of hemosiderin in the tumor cyst. Also, a peripheral area with low MR-signal is clearly visualized. On post-contrast T1-weighted images, the tumor is characterized by a fairly pronounced, but usually heterogeneous contrast enhancement.

Differential Diagnosis Mucocele (often preceded by allergic sinusitis, is formed in the sinus cavity, typically has a high MR-signal on T1-weighted sequences and heterogeneous signal on T2-weighted images), aneurysmal bone cyst (looks like a "soap bubbles," sedimentations levels can be detected), invasive pituitary macroadenoma (endocrine disturbances, relation to the sella turcica, more homogeneous structure), chordoma, chondrosarcoma, myeloma, plasmacytoma, metastatic lesion, fibrous dysplasia.

***Hemangioblastoma** (HMB)* is a benign rare tumor (1–2.5% of all intracranial tumors). Pediatric population consists of about 20% of all hemangioblastomas. The tumor can be associated with Von Hippel-Lindau disease in up to 10% of cases. It is believed that HMBs originate from primitive mesenchymal vascular cells or hematopoietic stem cells. Microscopically HMBs represent clusters of thin-walled vessels of various calibers. Interstitial cells with lipid-rich, clear cytoplasm are located in intervascular spaces.

Macroscopically HMBs are divided into three types:

1. Solid tumors in the form of a soft, dark-cherry encapsulated nodule with a typical spongy pattern on the histological slice (about 40%);
2. A large smooth-wall cyst with yellowish transparent contents and a small mural nodulus on one of the walls (55%);
3. Mixed tumors, a large tumor nodule with a large cyst (5%).

Most common HMBs site is the cerebellum hemisphere (80–85%) or, less frequently, vermis. They can also affect the spinal cord (3–13%) and medulla oblongata (2–3%), are extremely rare in the supratentorial area. Necrosis and hemorrhage are rarely identified in HMBs.

Imaging A solid HMB nodule is always well-depicted with direct angiography, and its vasculature is visualized up to a late venous phase. In cases with solid forms of HMB arterio-venous shunts can be detected (Figs. 23.64 and 23.65).

Generally, there are two forms of tumors, based on CT and MRI: a nodule with a cyst and nodular form. The first form of the tumor is characterized by a tumor nodule that typically combining with large cyst. A HMB's cyst is usually round or oval, has a lower density on CT (8–14 HU), after administration of contrast medium, the density of the cyst and its walls remain unchanged. The tumor nodule is clearly revealed by CT in the form of a focus with increased, usually inhomogeneous granular density (up to 38–44 HU). It is located on one of the cyst walls, entering into its lumen, intensely enhances (up to 60–85 HU).

In cases with cystic tumors, MRI well visualizes the cystic component, which is characterized by a hypointense MR-signal on T1- and a high MR-signal on T2-weighted images. On this background, a peripheral mural solid nodule of HMB can be seen, typically demonstrating signal characteristics close to those of the brain on T1-weighted images (tumor masses have usually iso- or slightly hyperintense MR-signal on T2 and T2-FLAIR sequences) and rapidly, and pronouncedly accumulates contrast medium (Fig. 23.66).

Fig. 23.64 Hemangioblastoma of the posterior cranial fossa (different patients). Case 1. Hemangioblastoma of the cerebellar vermis is characterized by hypointense MR-signal on DWI (**a**) and an abundant blood supply from the posterior inferior cerebellar artery (PICA) on DSA (**b**, **c**). Case 2. Postenhanced MRI (**d**) reveals a strongly enhancing tumor of the cerebellar vermis with blood supply predominantly from superior cerebellar artery on DSA (**e**, **f**)

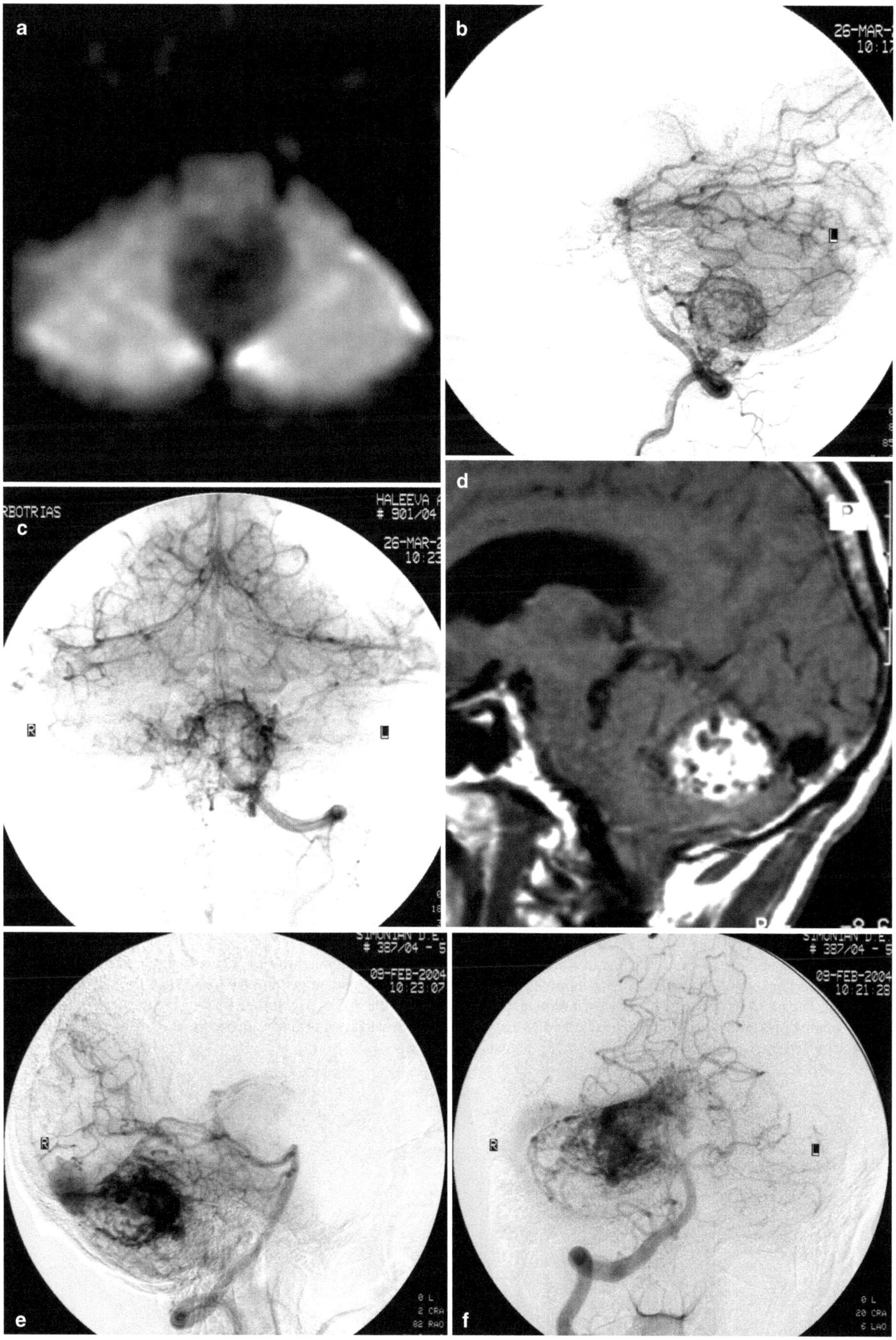
a
b
26-MAR-
L
c
HALEEVA A
901/04
26-MAR-
10:23
R
L
d
P
SIMONIAN D.E.
387/04 - 5
09-FEB-2004
10:23:07
R
0 L
2 CRA
82 RAO
e
SIMONIAN D.E.
387/04 - 5
09-FEB-2004
10:21:28
R
L
0 L
20 CRA
6 LAO
f

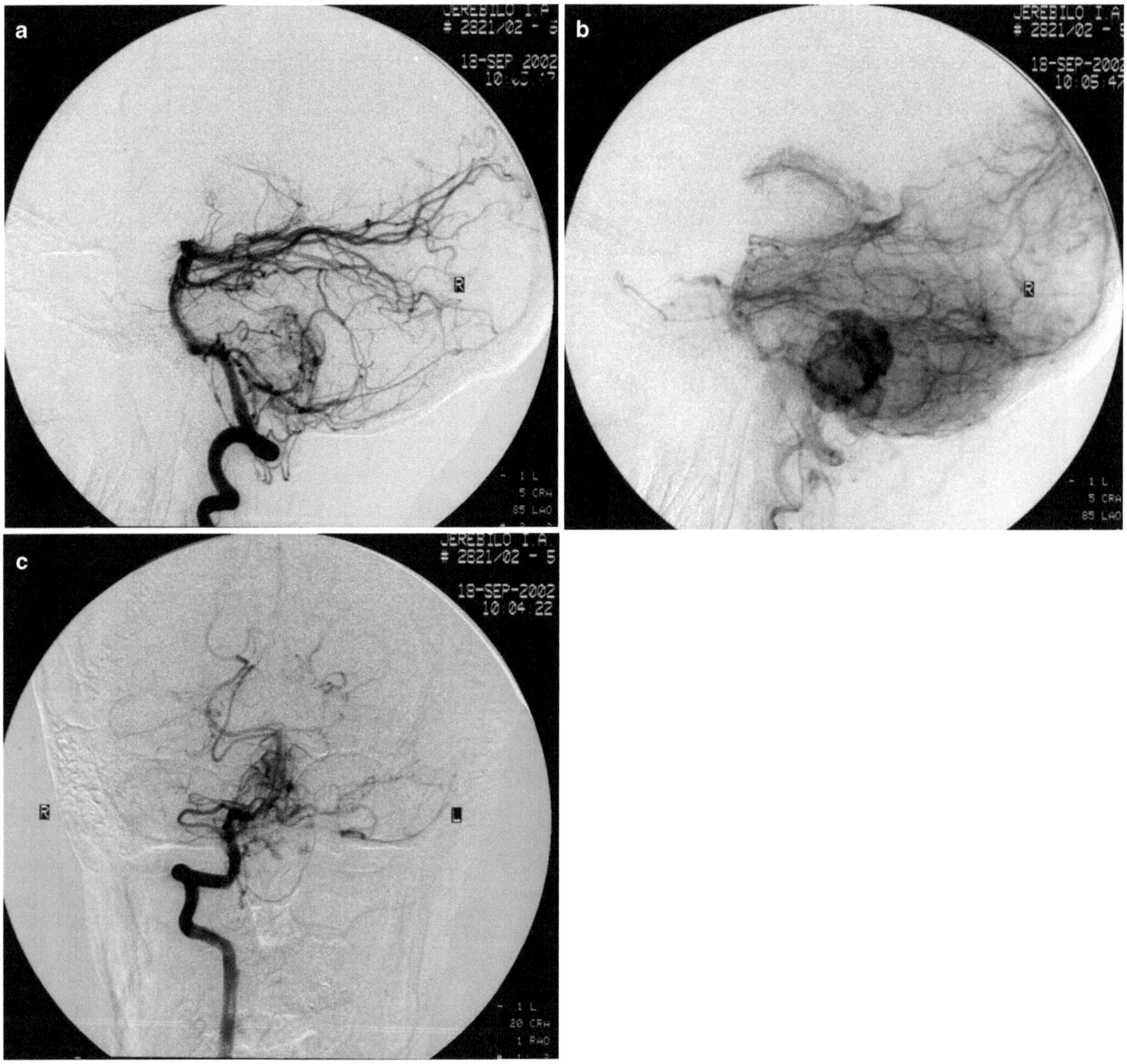

Fig. 23.65 Hemangioblastoma of the cerebellar vermis. DSA (**a–c**) demonstrates an abundant tumoral vasculature with supplying from the PICA. Axial NECT scans show a slightly hyperdense lesion in the middle line with small calcification (**d**). On T2-weighted MR-image (**e**) tumor is characterized by heterogeneous hyperintense MR-signal and shows the hypointensity on T1-weighted image (**f**). There are a lot of dark spots and serpentine dark lines due to abundant arterial supply within the lesion. Tumor has a strong contrast enhancement improving the visualization of the lesion structure (**g–i**)

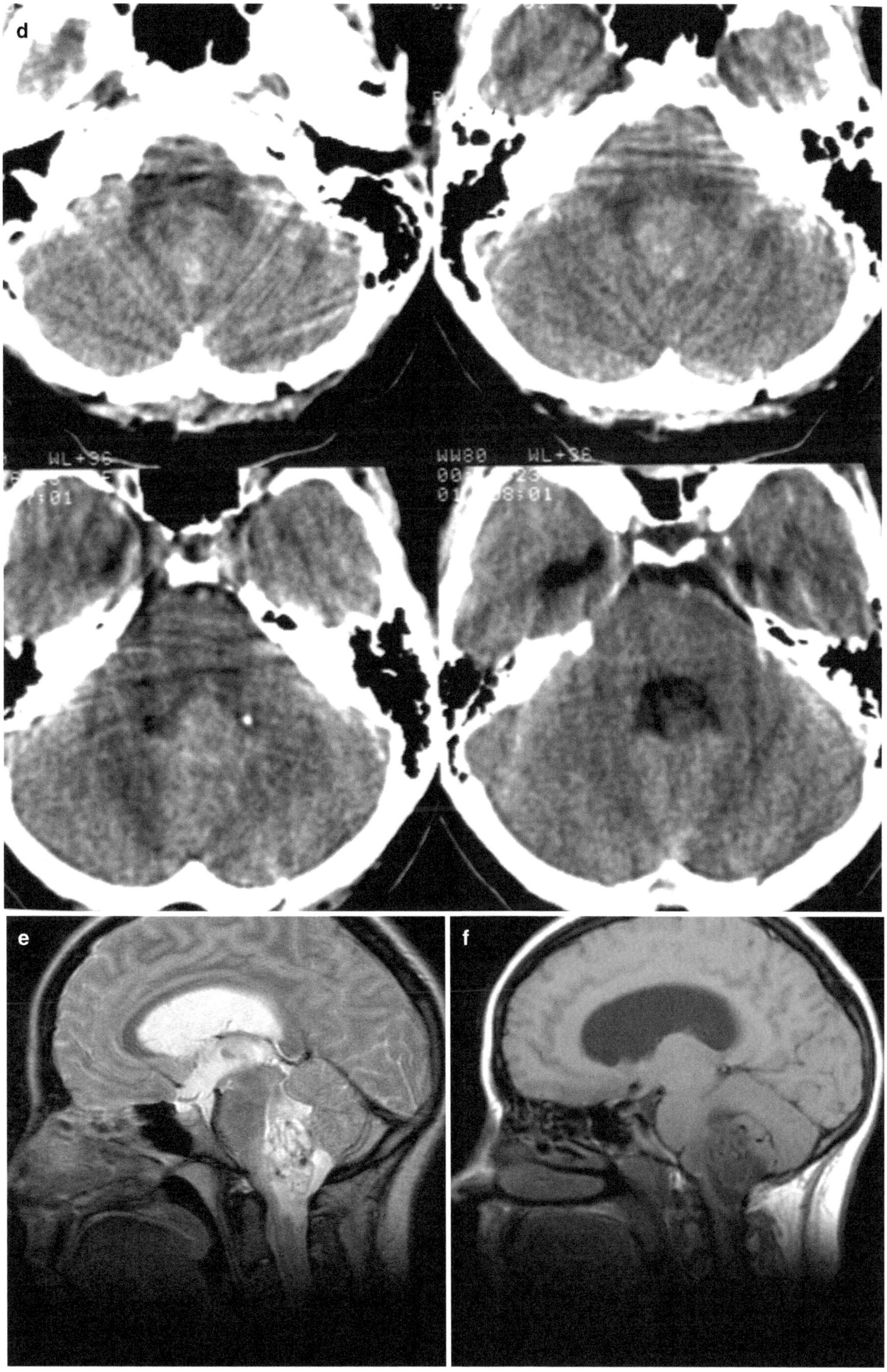

Fig. 23.65 (continued)

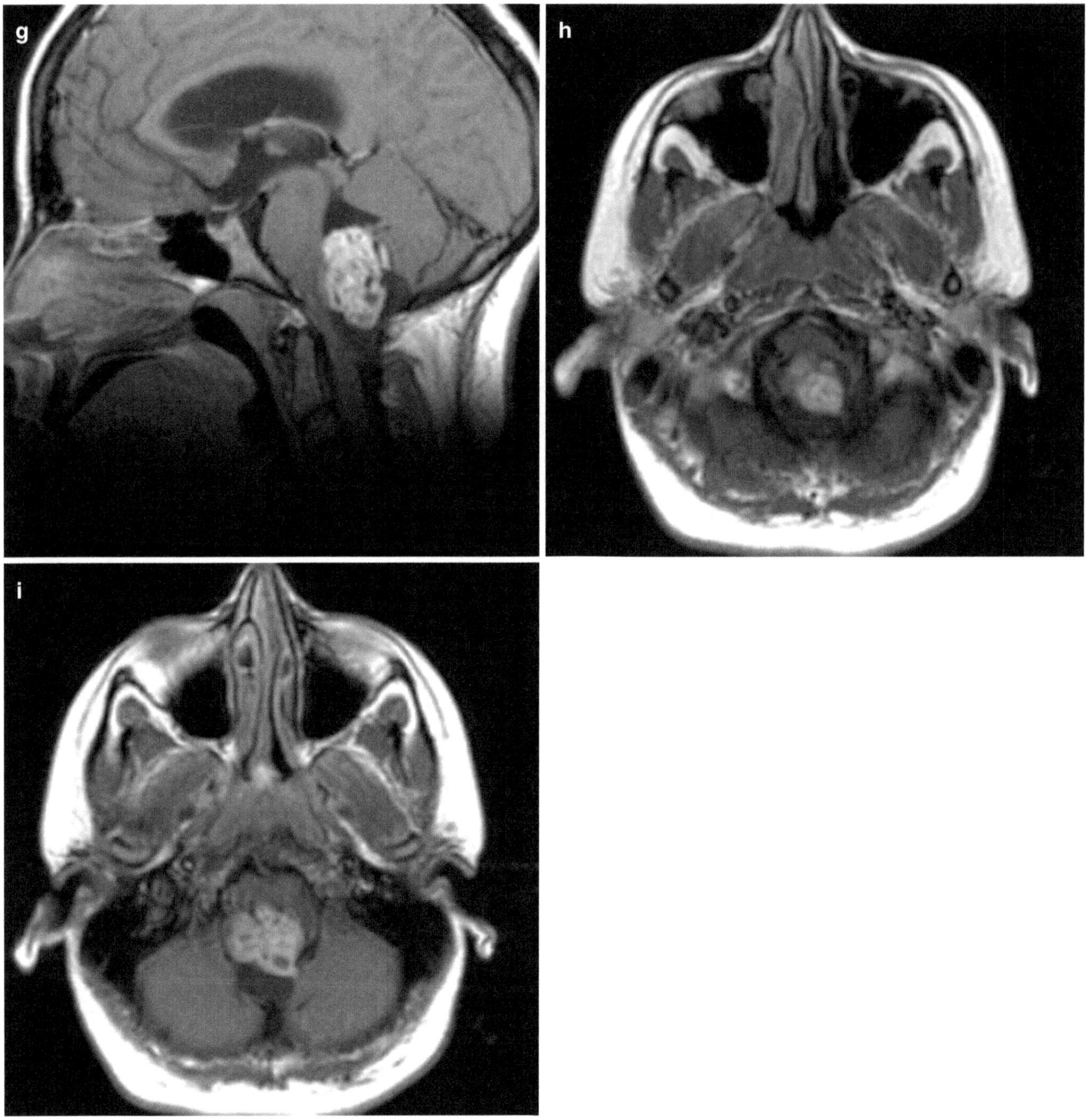

Fig. 23.65 (continued)

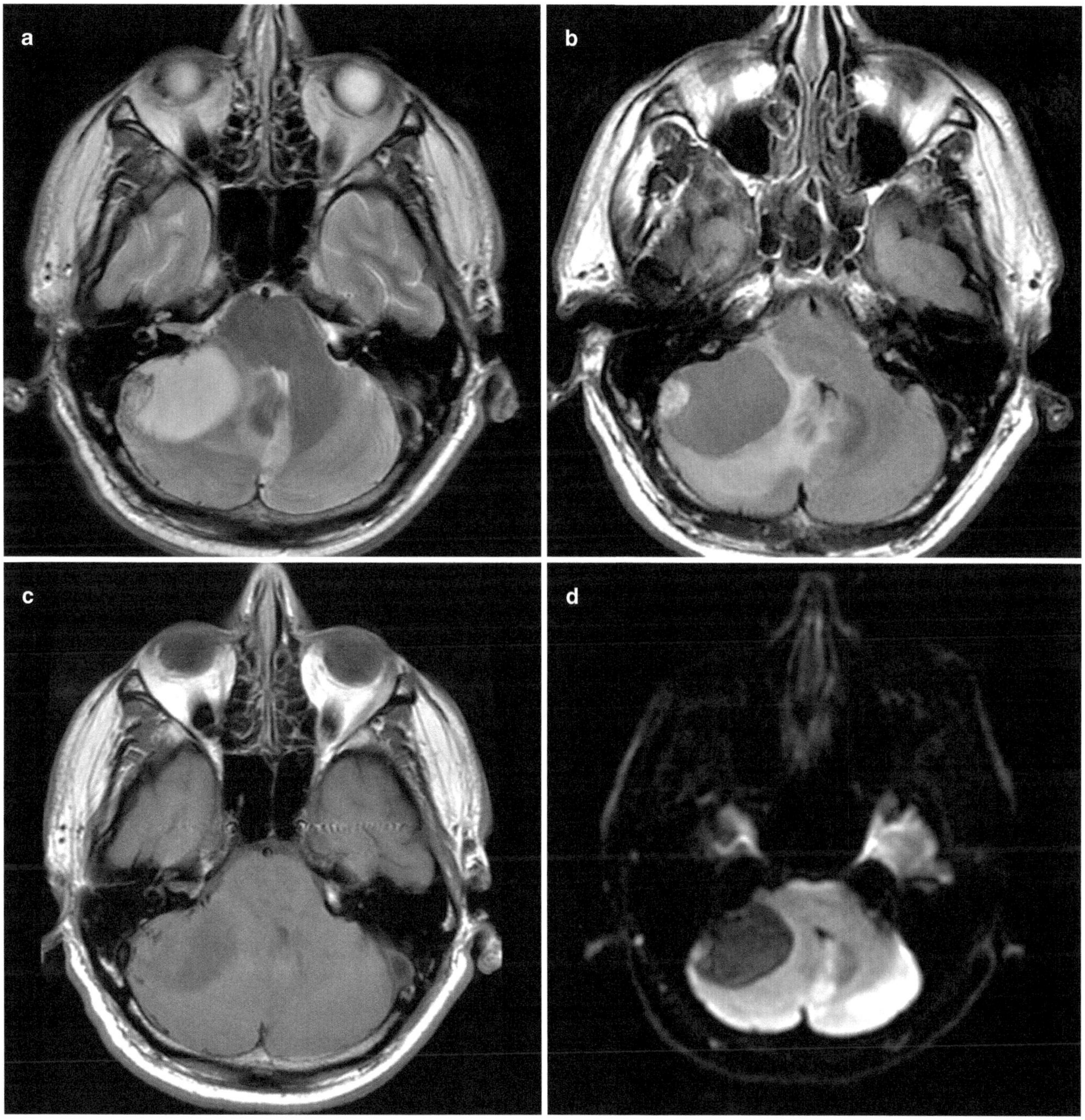

Fig. 23.66 Hemangioblastoma of the right cerebellar hemisphere. Axial T2- (**a**), T2-FLAIR- (**b**), T1- (**c**), DWI- (**d**) and enhanced T1- (**e**) weighted MR-images demonstrate a tumor with strong contrast enhancement improving the visualization of the lesion location on wall of large cystic lesion, surrounded with perifocal edema. (**f**) Histologic specimen

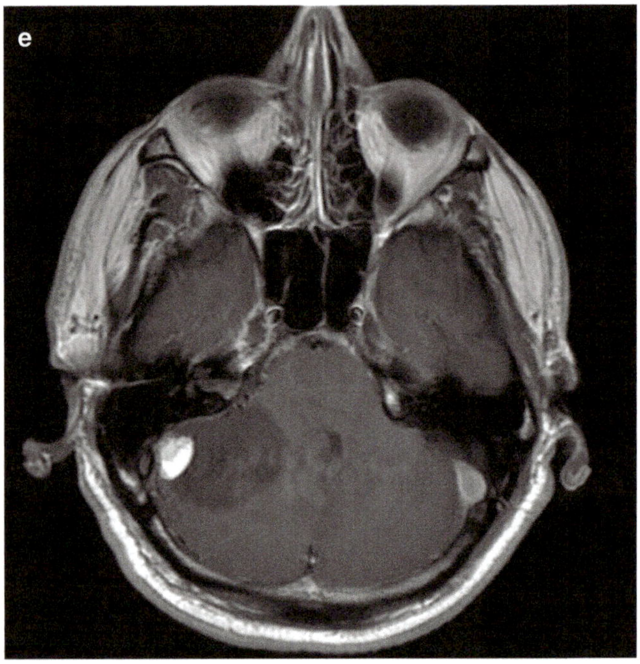

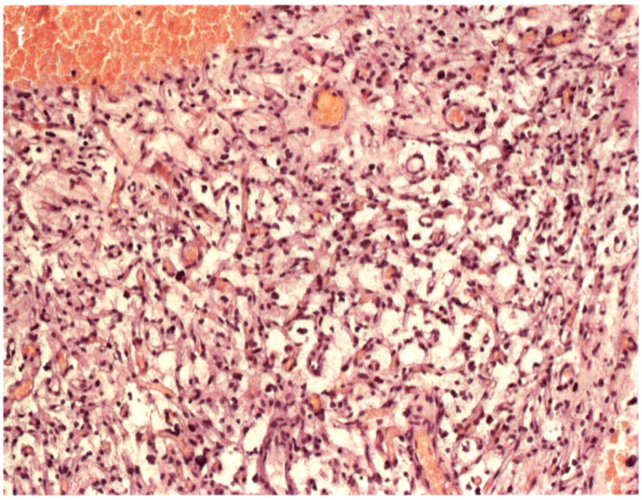

Fig. 23.66 (continued)

Solid HMBs have rounded and convoluted areas of signal loss from the tumor vessels. Presence of a large number of such vessels, better visualized on T2-weighted MR-sequences, in the HMB's structure is highly pathognomonic for this type of lesions. Abundance of blood tumor vessels makes justified the use of non-invasive angiographic techniques during MR-scanning. Most often large tumor afferents can be visualized using 3D TOF sequence (Figs. 23.67 and 23.68). Specificity of diffusion-weighted MRI and MR-spectroscopy findings is low. On DWI, compact solid tumor masses are characterized by reduced MR-signal. Proton MR-spectroscopy most often detects a high lipid-lactate complex with reduction of other metabolites (Figs. 23.69 and 23.70).

CT-perfusion detects a pronounced increase in CBF and CBV in the tumor (Fig. 23.71). Blood flow parameters are practically comparable to those recorded in the lumen of the carotid artery and in the major venous sinuses. Our comparisons have shown that HMBs and paragangliomas have similar hemodynamic blood flow parameters that are the highest among all tumors of the skull base and the posterior cranial

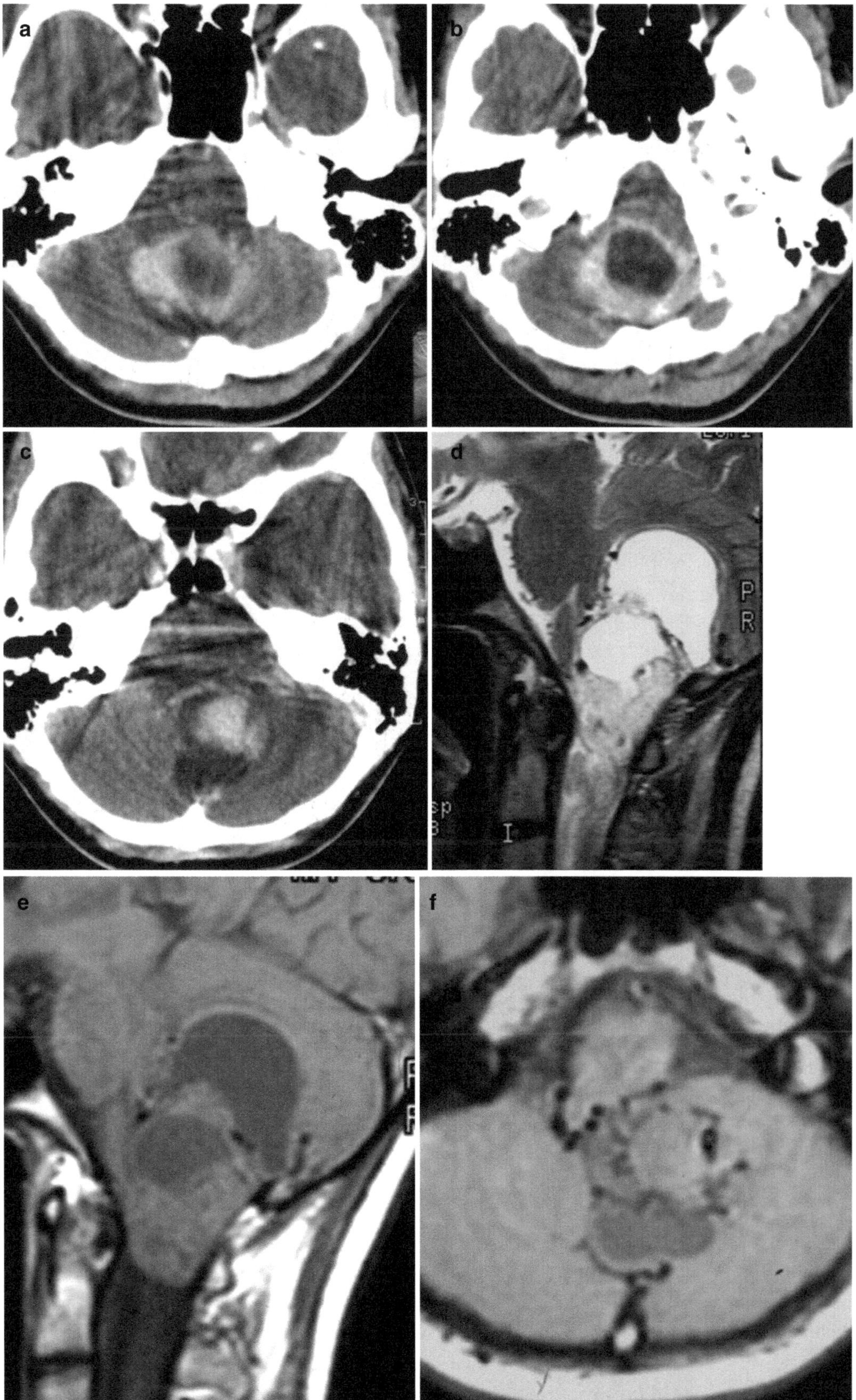

Fig. 23.67 Hemangioblastoma of the foramen magnum. Axial CECT scans show a heterogeneous and strongly enhancing lesion in the projection of cranio-cervical junction with presence of solid as well as cystic components (**a–c**). On sagittal and axial MR scans using T2- (**d**) and T1- (**e**, **f**) weighted images tumor has hyperintense on T2 and isointense on T1 MR-signal. Within the tumor structure plenty of vessels with dark signal can be visualized

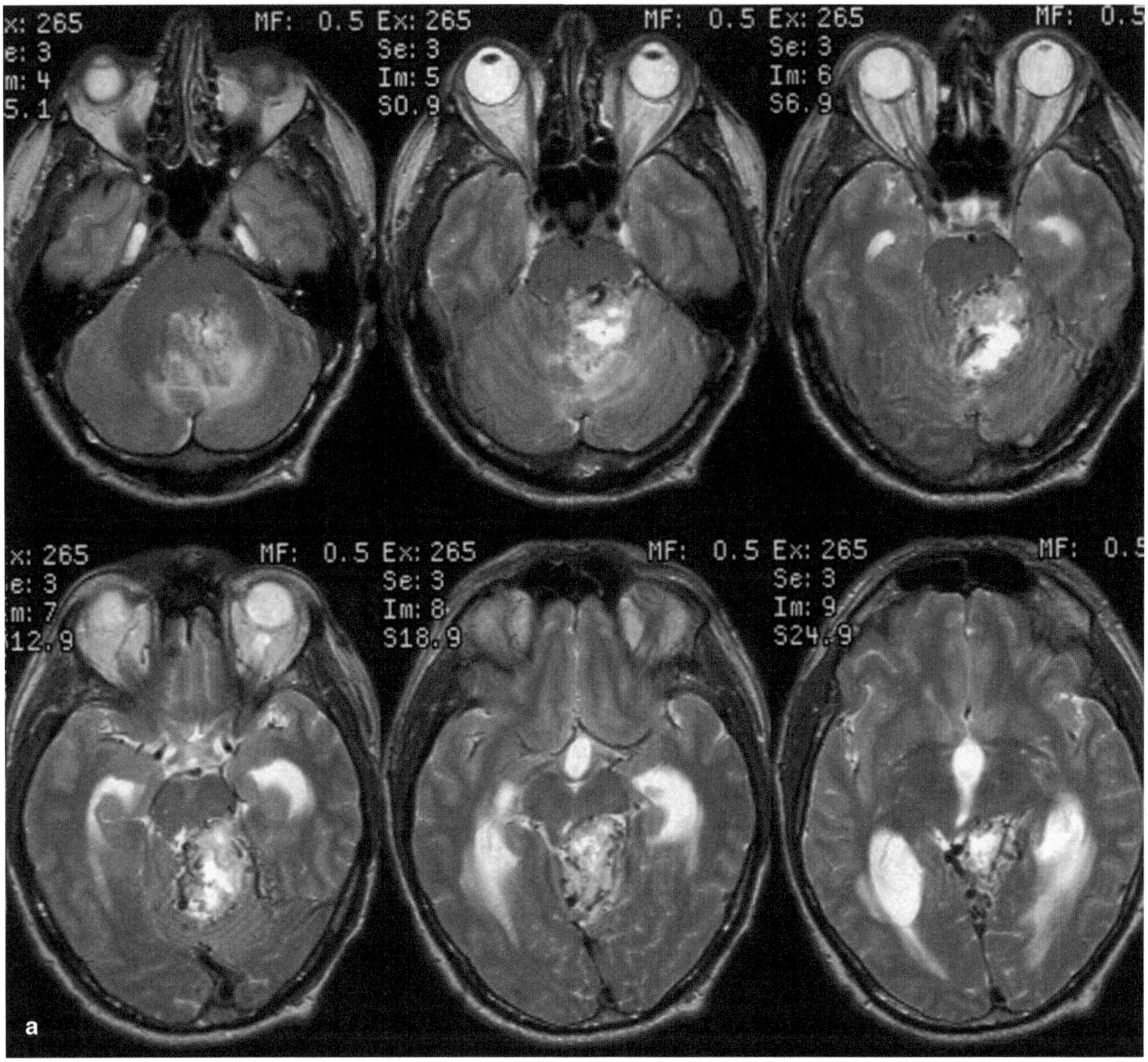

Fig. 23.68 Hemangioblastoma of the vermis and left cerebellar hemisphere. Series of axial T2- (**a**) and T1- (**b**) weighted MR-images demonstrate a tumor with hyperintensity on T2 and isointense signal on T1. Within the tumor structure plenty of vessels with dark signal can be visualized. 3D TOF MR-angiography shows a source of blood supply of the lesion- branches of posterior cerebral artery on the left (**c**)

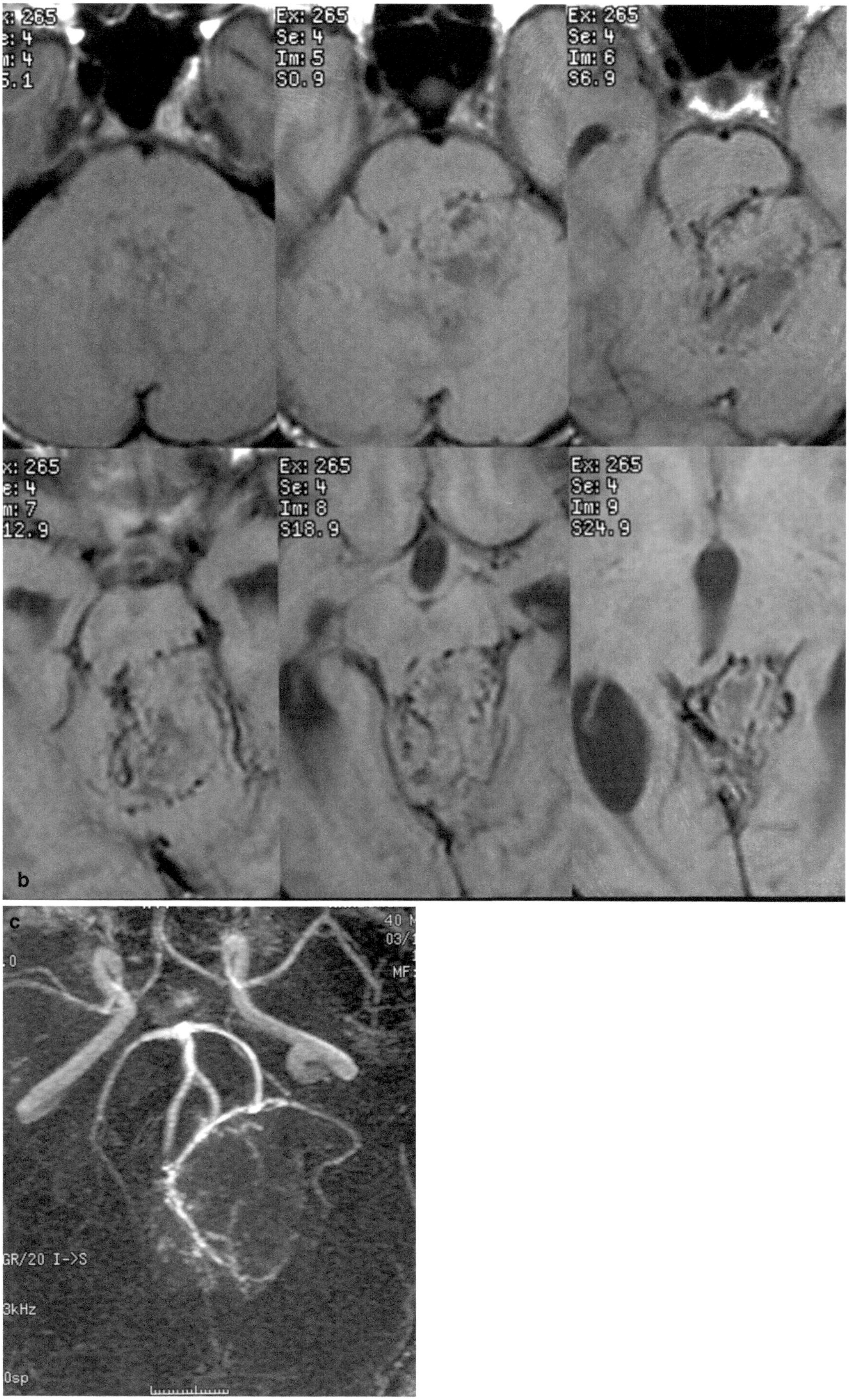

Fig. 23.68 (continued)

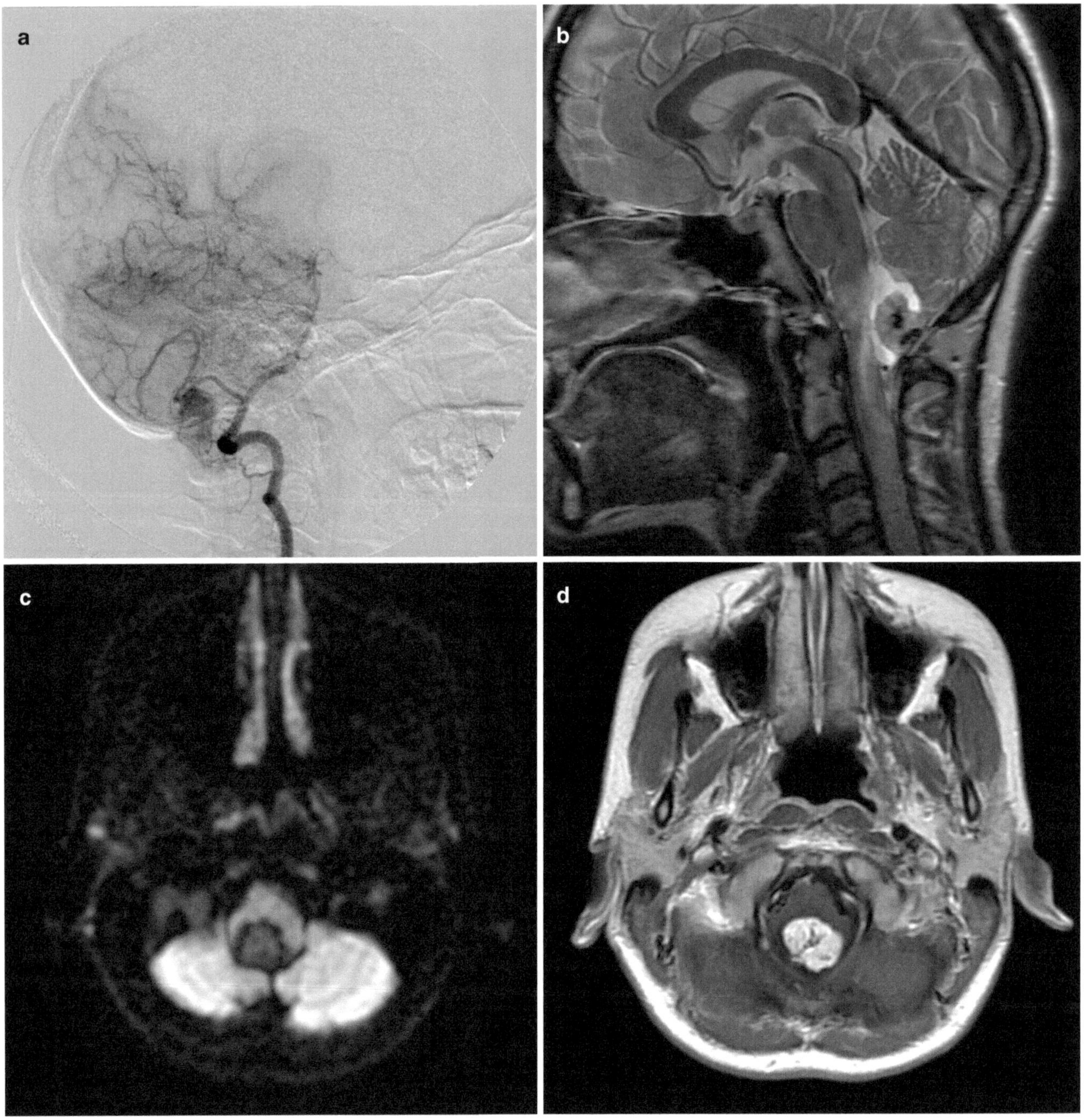

Fig. 23.69 Hemangioblastoma of the foramen magnum. DSA (**a**) demonstrates an abundant tumor vasculature with supplying from the branches of vertebral artery. On T2-weighted MR-image (**b**), DWI (**c**), postenhanced T1-weighted scans (**d**–**g**) tumor is characterized by heterogeneous hyperintense MR-signal on T2, hypointense signal on diffusion-weighted image and strong enhancement. There are a lot of dark spots and serpentine dark lines due to abundant arterial supply within the lesion. 3D TOF MR-angiography shows a source of hemangioblastoma blood supply—both PICA (**h**). Only Lipid-Lactate peak on MR-spectroscopy is visible (**i**)

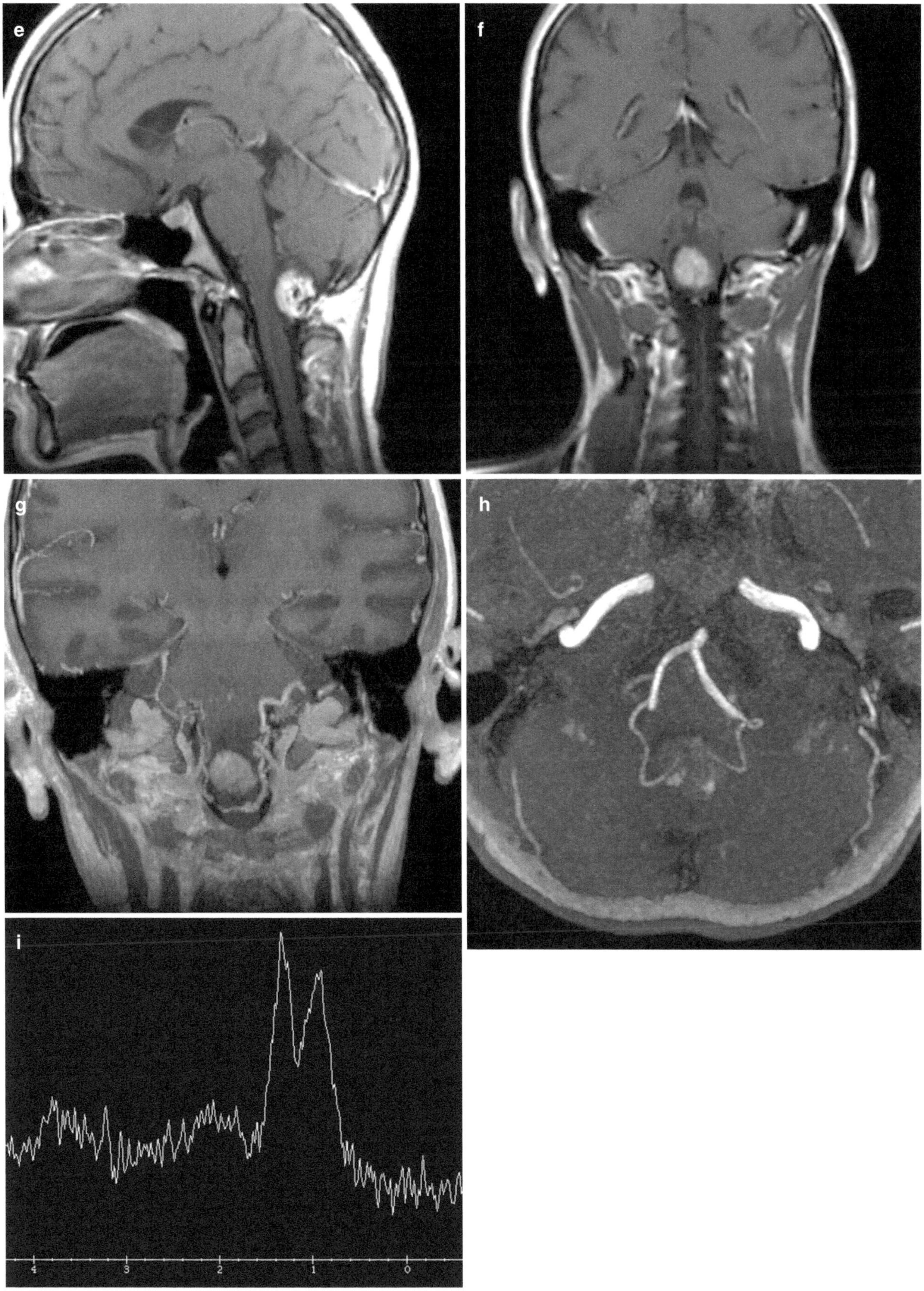

Fig. 23.69 (continued)

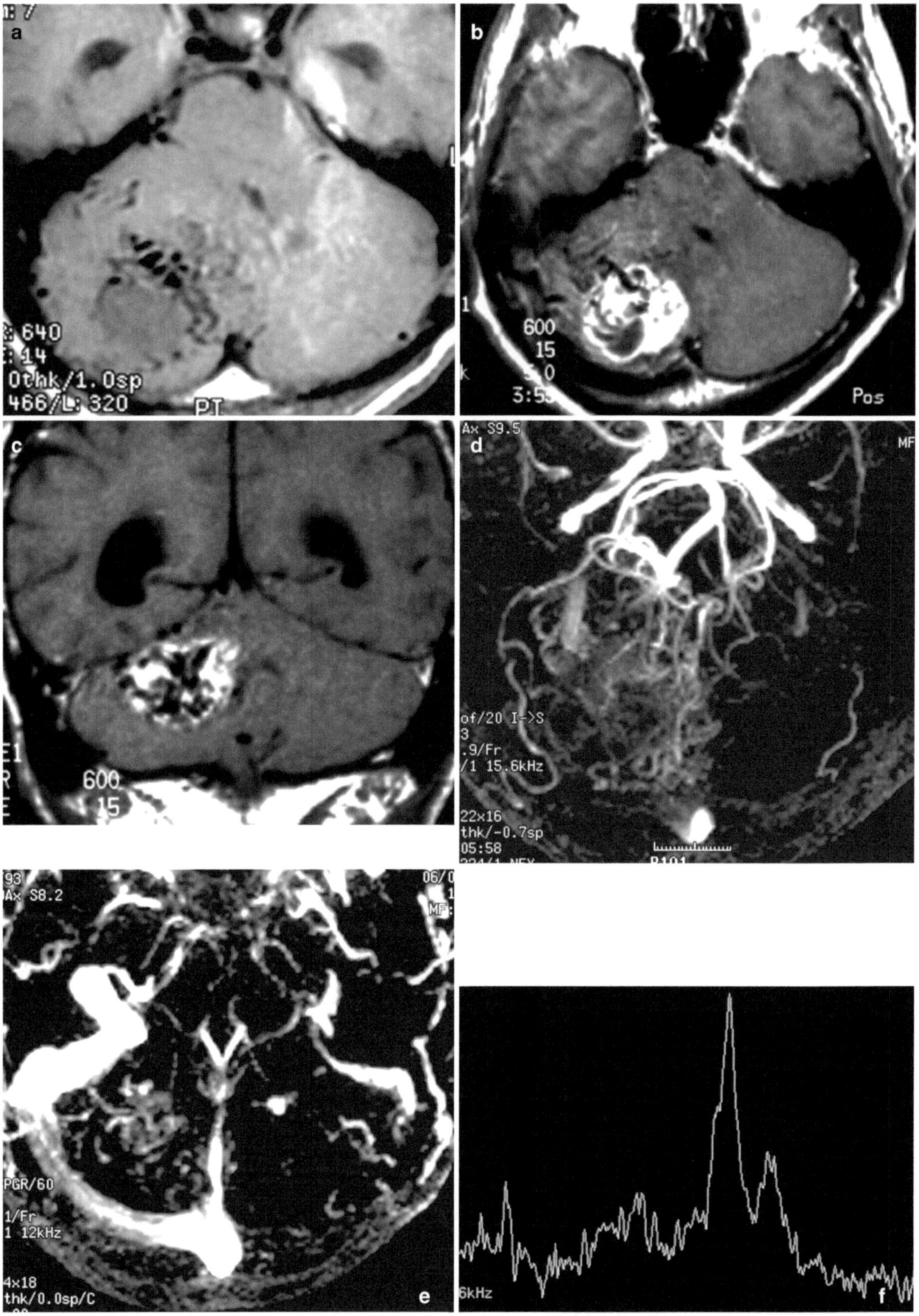

Fig. 23.70 Hemangioblastoma of the right cerebellar hemisphere. On T1-weighted MR-image before (**a**) and postenhanced T1-weighted scans (**b**, **c**) tumor is characterized by heterogeneous and strong enhancement. There are a lot of dark spots and serpentine dark lines due to abundant arterial supply within the lesion. 3D TOF (**d**) and 2D TOF (**e**) MR-angiography shows a source of hemangioblastoma blood supply—right superior cerebellar artery, and venous drainage into sigmoid sinus. Only high Lipid-Lactate peak on MR-spectroscopy is visible (**i**)

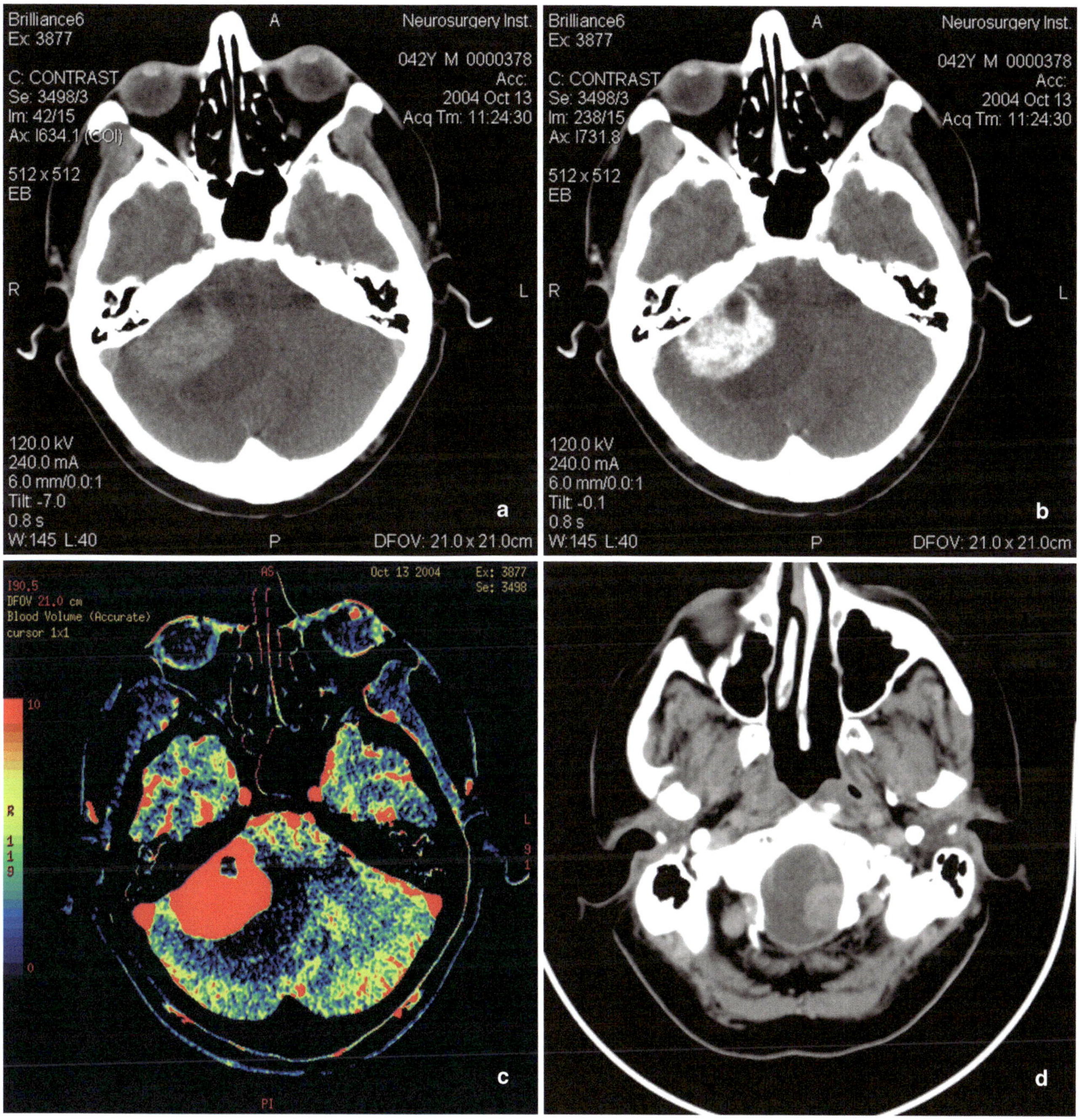

Fig. 23.71 Hemangioblastomas of the posterior fossa (different patients). Case 1. Axial NECT (**a**) and CECT (**b**) scans demonstrate a heterogeneous and strongly enhancing tumor of lateral aspects of right cerebellar hemisphere. On CT-perfusion study (CBV map (**c**)) the lesion is characterized by extremely high CBV values. Case 2. Axial NECT scan (**d**) and sagittal reformat of CECT (**e**) demonstrate a homogeneously and strongly enhancing tumor in the foramen magnum. On CT-perfusion study (CBV map (**f**)) the lesion is characterized by extremely high CBV values

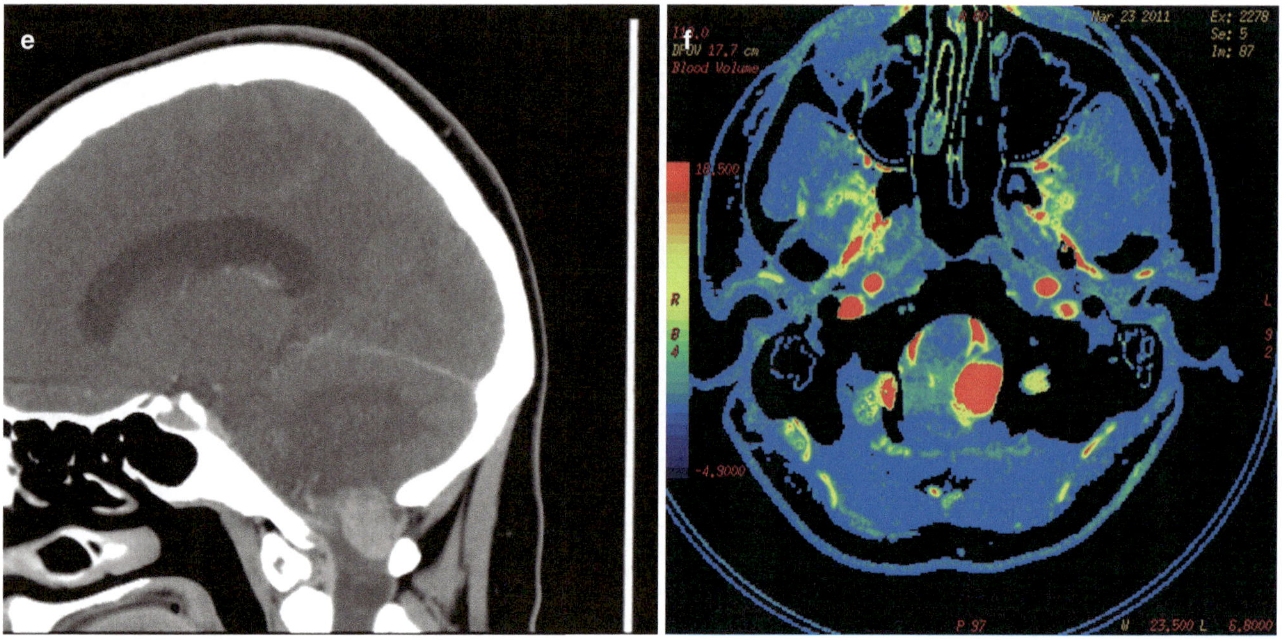

Fig. 23.71 (continued)

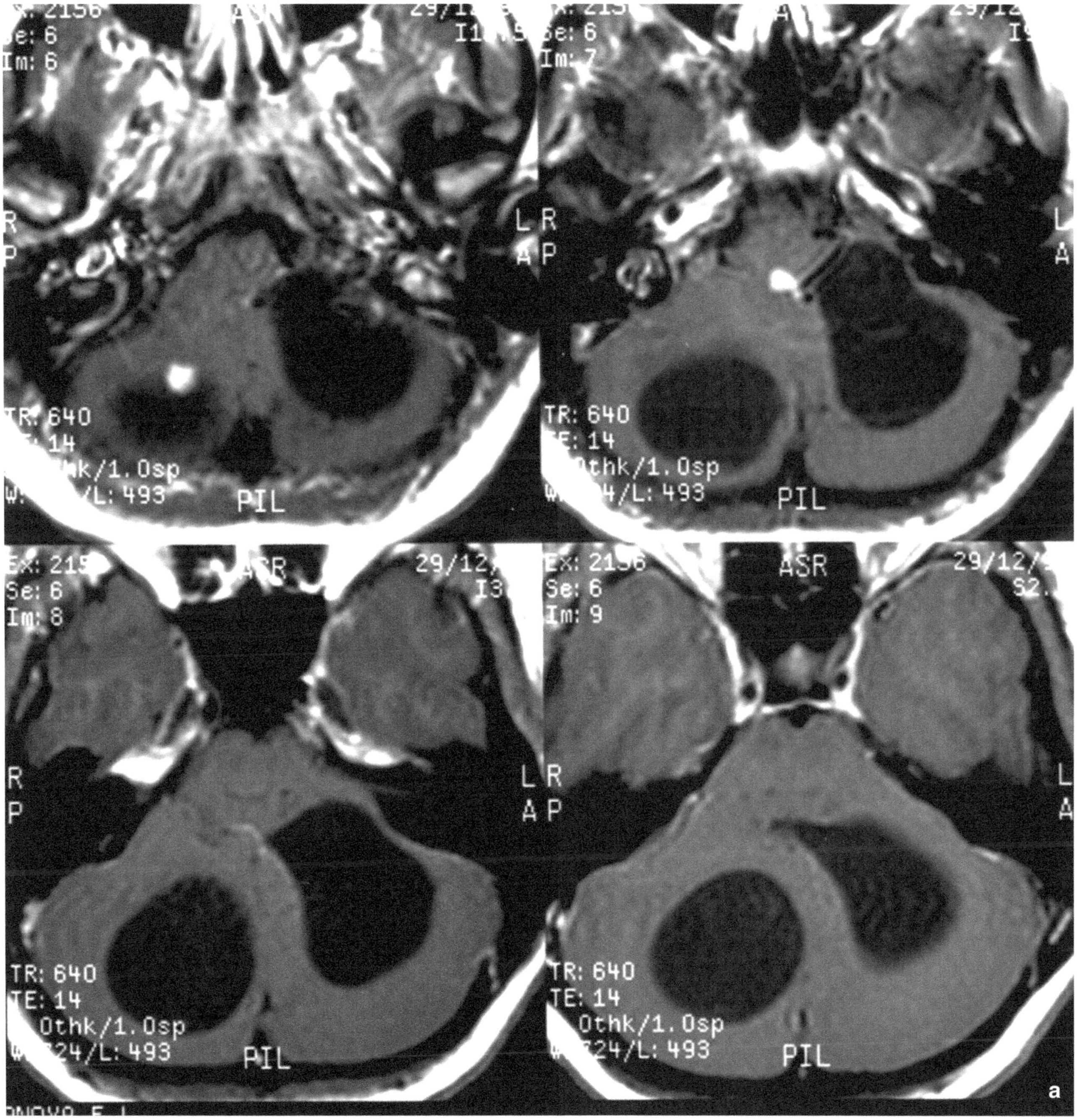

Fig. 23.72 Multiple hemangioblastomas of the posterior fossa (von Hippel-Linday disease). Series of axial (**a**) and coronal (**b**, **c**) postenhanced MR-images demonstrate multiple cystic lesions with mural enhancing nodules in the projection of cerebellar hemispheres and foramen magnum

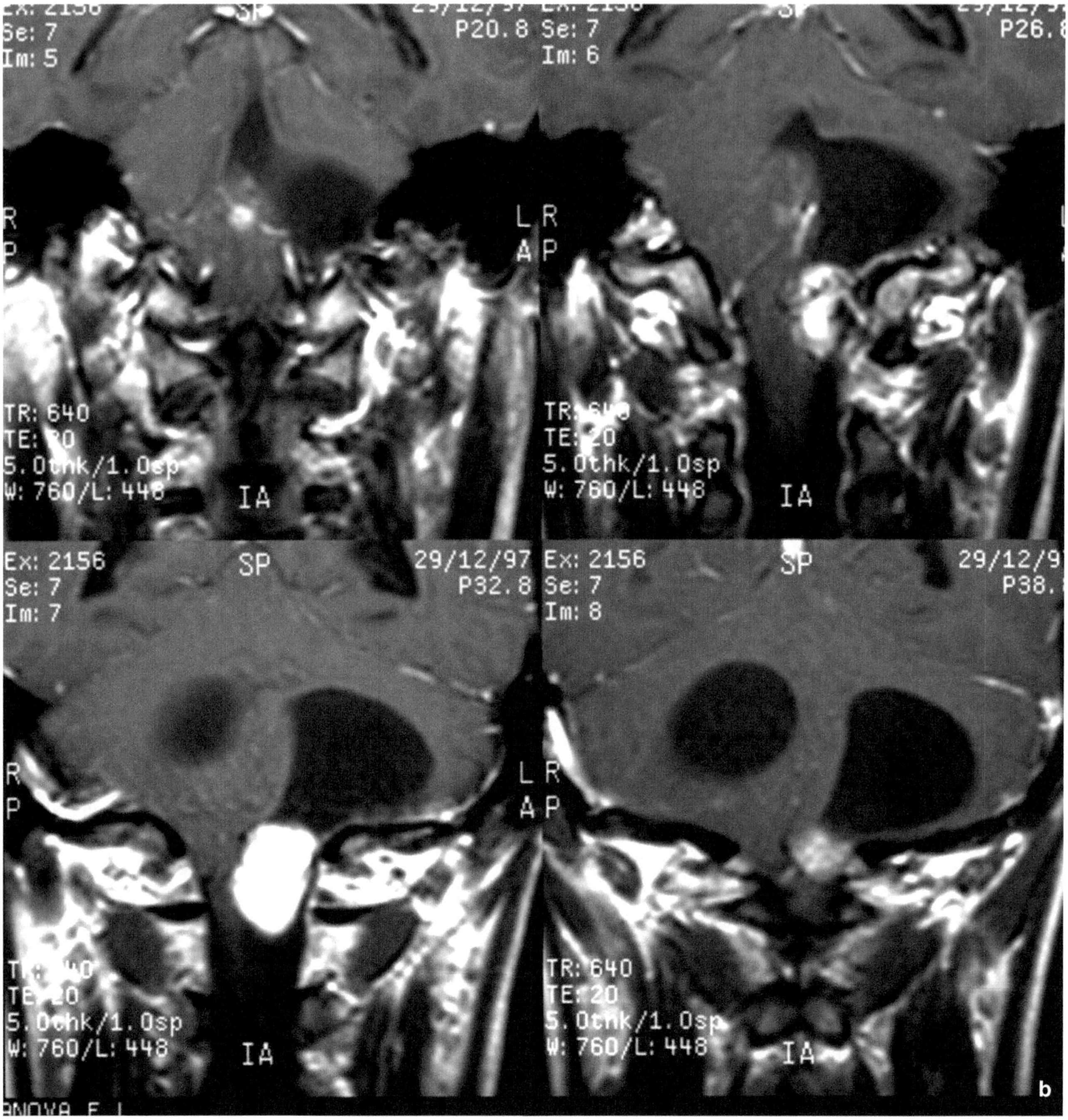

Fig. 23.72 (continued)

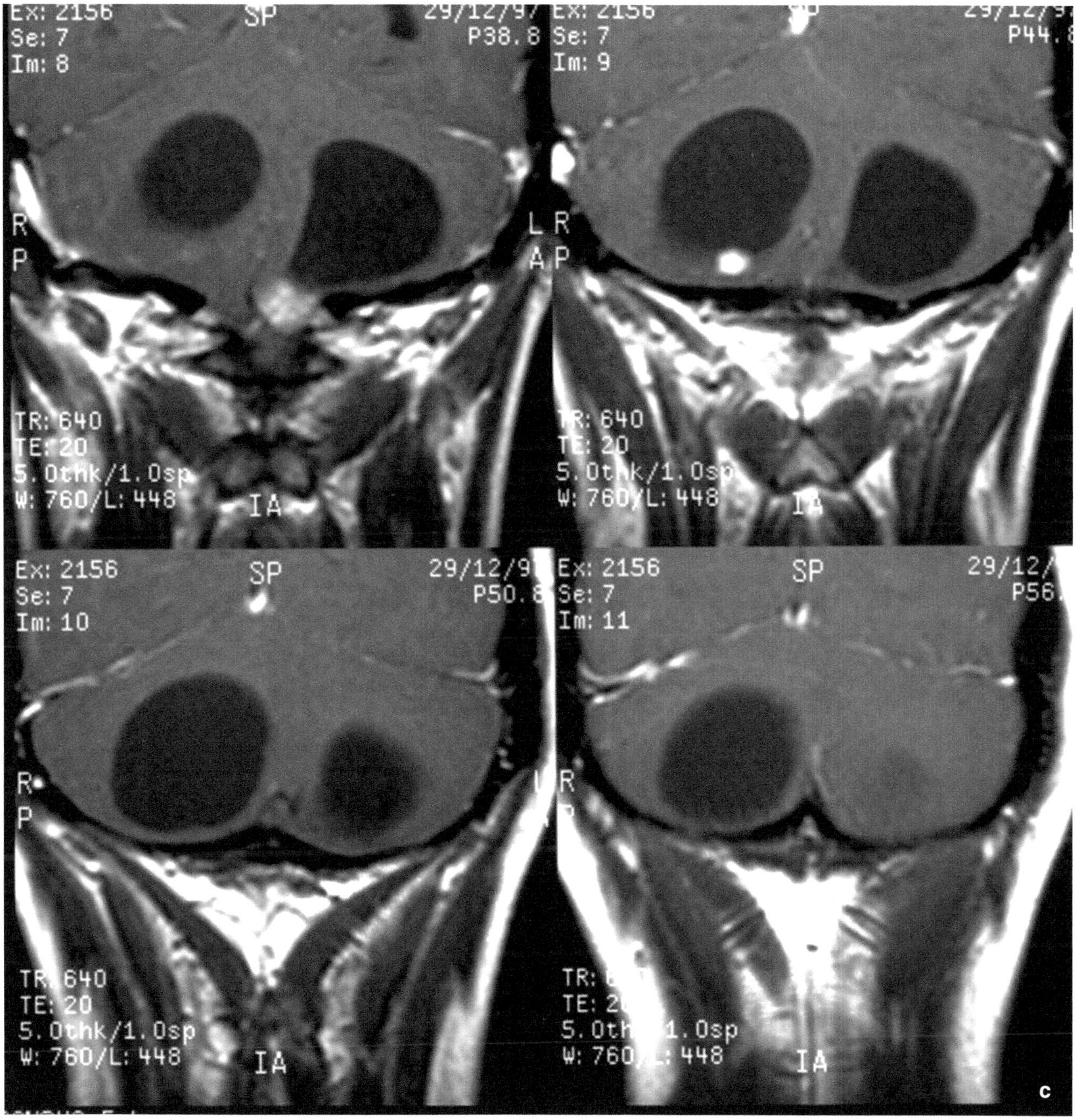

Fig. 23.72 (continued)

fossa. It turned out that other parameters, such as sites of lesions (paraganglioma is located in the petrous pyramid, while HMBs are located in the cerebellar hemisphere) play a more important role in the differential diagnosis between these two histologically different types of tumors. Multiple brain lesions, typical for Von Hippel-Lindau disease, may serve as an additional argument in favor of HMB (Figs. 23.72 and 23.73). It is advisable to make the final decision on surgical approach in cases of PCF HMBs only after a comprehensive analysis of all diagnostic findings, with mandatory direct selective angiography of the vertebral-basilar territory.

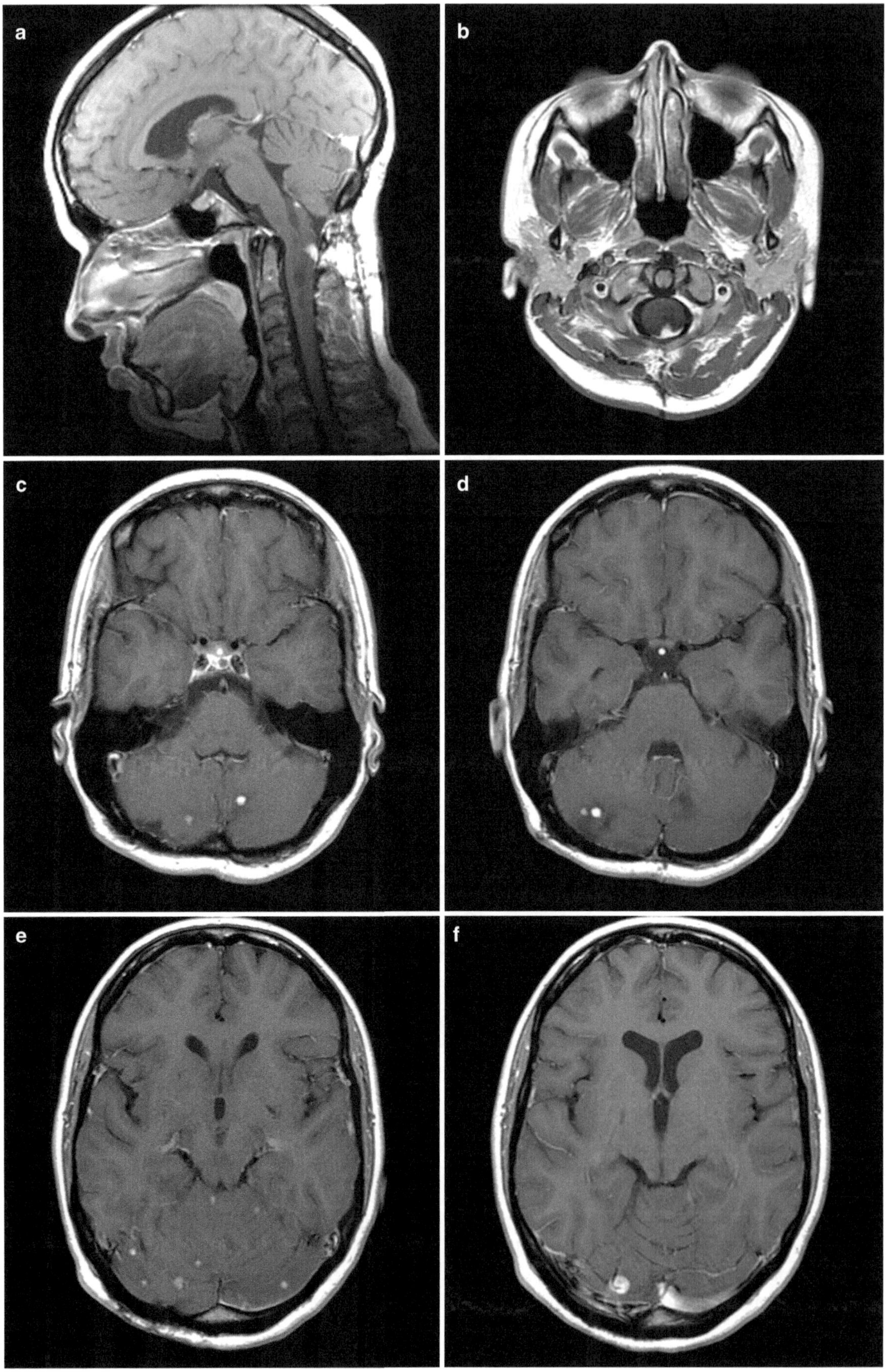

Fig. 23.73 Multiple hemangioblastomas of the posterior fossa (von Hippel-Linday disease). Sagittal (**a**) and axial (**b–f**) postenhanced MR-images demonstrate multiple small solid enhancing lesions in the projection of cerebellar hemispheres and foramen magnum (after partial resection)

Malignant Tumors

24

Content

Chondrosarcoma belongs to a group of primary cartilaginous malignant tumors. Approximately 10–15% of all chondrosarcomas are located in the head and neck, 75%—in the skull base. If chondrosarcomas grow at the projection of the skull base, they are often located in the petro-occipital and petrosphenoidal fissures, less frequently in the sphenoid bone or petrous apex. That is why the important diagnostic feature of these tumors is the lateralization of the lesion. Usually chondrosarcomas locate within the skull base with the involvement of the following regions: MCF—64%, MCF and PCF—14%, ACF—14%, PCF—7%. These tumors account for about 0.15% of all intracranial tumors and 6–10% of skull base tumors. There are five different types of chondrosarcoma structure: true (or conventional), mesenchymal, myxoid, clear cell, and dedifferentiated. The first three types mainly develop in the skull base region (Rosenberg et al. 1999; Neff et al. 2002).

Chondrosarcomas of the skull base are characterized by the slow growth, destruction of tissues in the area of tumor growth, quite rapid development of local recurrence after the treatment. Usually this is a solitary lesion, but cases with multiple localization are also described. Chondrosarcomas with a high degree of malignancy can metastasize to bones and lungs (10% of all chondrosarcoma cases) (Brown et al. 1994).

Clinical signs are associated with the involvement of adjacent cranial nerves and is manifested, at the initial stage, in the form of headaches.

Imaging Direct angiography detects an avascularized or hypovascularized tumor, the internal carotid artery is often displaced laterally and can be included into the tumor.

CT scanning shows chondroid calcifications in the tumor matrix in the form of an arch or a ring, located in the central parts of the petro-occipital fissure. Focal bone destruction without marginal sclerotic changes is visualized in more than 50% of CT studies (Fig. 24.1). Usually, tumor has a slightly hyperdense properties with a variable level of the contrast enhancement.

I. Pronin, V. Kornienko, *CT and MRI of Skull Base Lesions*, https://doi.org/10.1007/978-3-319-65957-2_24

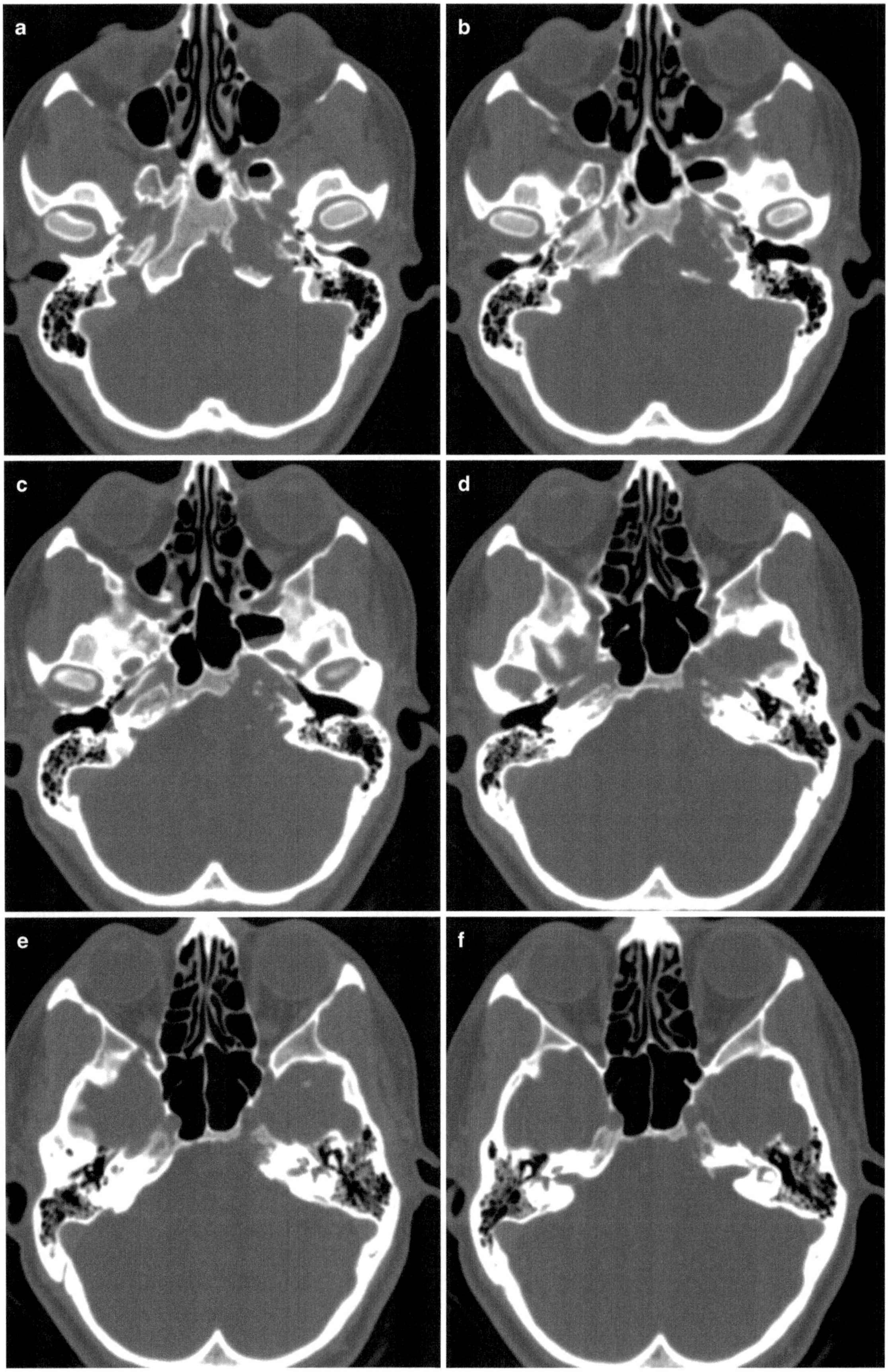

Fig. 24.1 Chondrosarcoma of the skull base. Series of axial NECT scans (**a**–**f**) performed in bone window mode show a focal bone disruption zone in the projection of petrooccipital synchondrosis with involvement of lateral aspects of clivus and petrous apex. There are irregular contours of the bone defect

MR imaging allows to clearly identify the boundaries of the tumor spread within the bones and soft tissues, infiltration of the dura with intracranial growth. On T1-weighted images chondrosarcomas demonstrate a hypointense or isointense MR-signal, while T2 and T2-FLAIR images show a high MR-signal from the tumor soft-tissue component (Fig. 24.2). Hypointense inclusions due to calcifications can be seen inside the lesion. After intravenous contrast enhancement the tumors in majority of the cases demonstrate relatively pronounced and usually heterogeneous enhancement (Fig. 24.3).

Differential Diagnosis Cholesteatoma (low signal on T1 and high on T2, non-enhanced lesion, high MR-signal on DWI), calcified meningioma (hyperostosis, no apparent bone destruction, low MR-signal on T2-WI, enhancing with the presence of a "dural tail" sign), chondromyxoid fibroma (no bone infiltration), chondroma (typically on midline, with bone fragments and calcifications in the tumor tissue), plasmacytoma and metastasis.

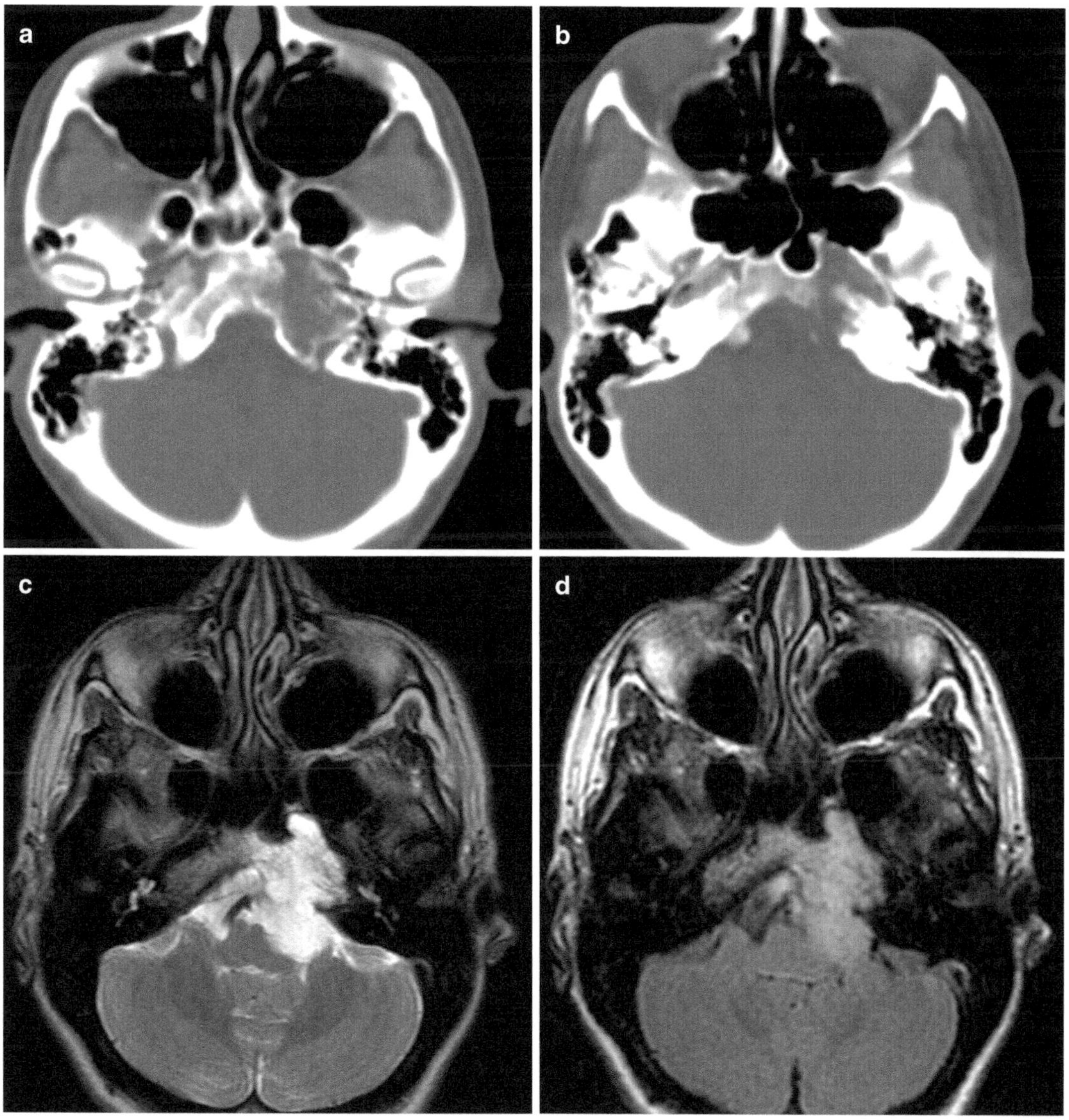

Fig. 24.2 Chondrosarcoma of the skull base. Axial NECT scans (**a**, **b**) performed in bone window mode show a focal bone disruption zone in the projection of petro-occipital synchondrosis with involvement of lateral aspects of clivus and petrous apex. There are irregular contours of the bone defect. On T2- (**c**), T2-FLAIR (**d**) MR images a lesion has hyperintense MR-signal. On T1- (**e**) weighted MRI a tumor is characterized by isointense compared to brain MR-signal. Contrast enhancement study (**f–i**) demonstrates a homogeneously enhancing tumor in the projection of petro-occipital junction with intracranial spreading (**d–f**)

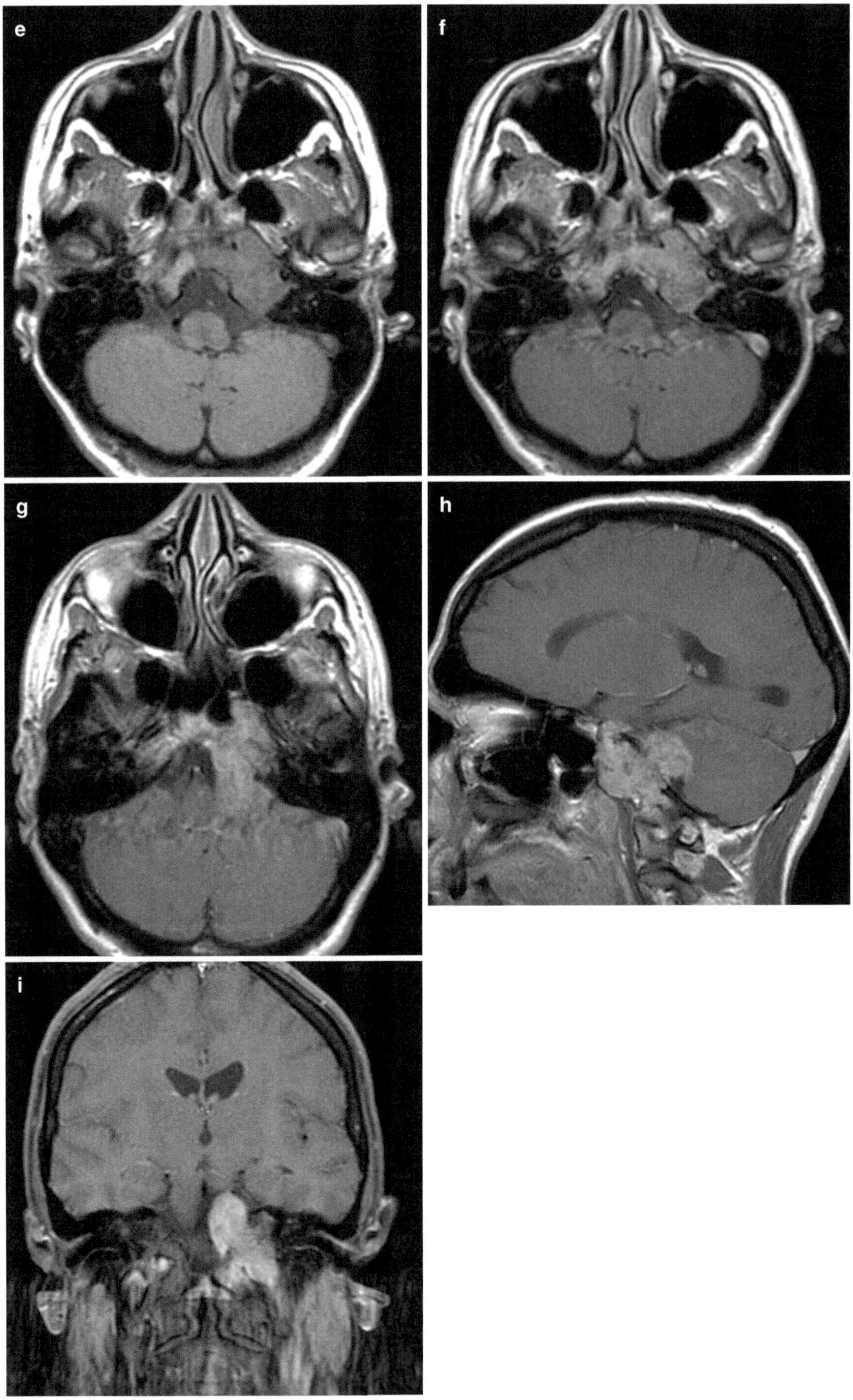

Fig. 24.2 (continued)

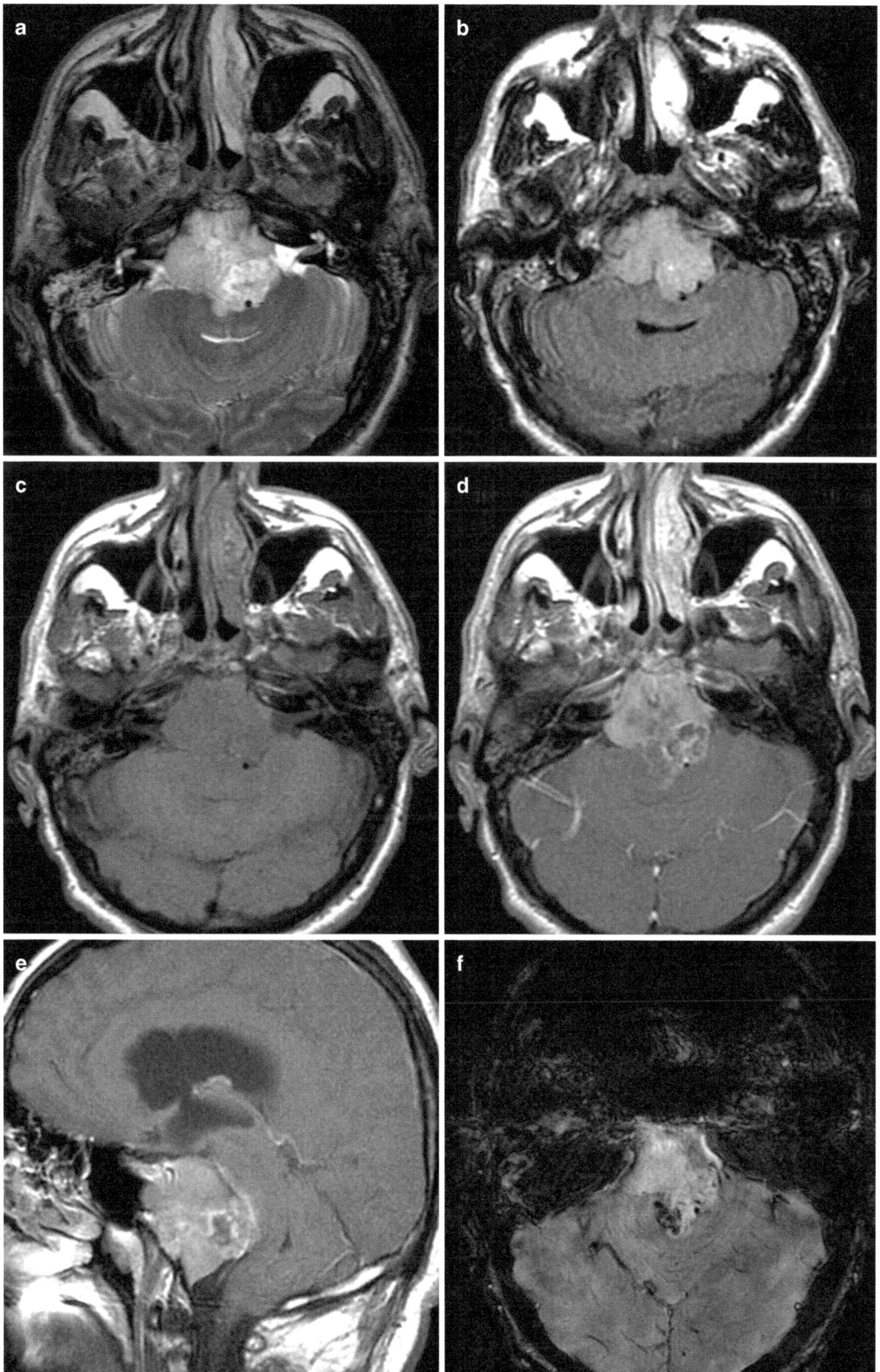

Fig. 24.3 Chondrosarcoma of the clivus. Axial T2 (**a**), T2-FLAIR (**b**), T1 before (**c**) and after (**d**, **e**) of contrast enhancement MR images show a hyperintense (on T2) tumor with clivus involvement and intracranial extension with brain stem compression. Tumor is isointense to brain on T1 MRI. This tumor is significantly enhanced. There are hypointense inclusions within the lesion—microcalcifications in dorsal tumor's aspects on SWAN (**f**)

24.1 Mixed Mesenchymal Tumors

Rhabdomyosarcoma is the most common soft-tissue sarcoma of skeletal muscle derivation, especially in children (up to 75%). But it can appear in any part of the body. Majority of patients with RMS are younger than 12 years (up to 78% of all cases) and it accounts for 4–8% of all malignancies in patients under the age of 15 years (Soule et al. 1968; Sutow et al. 1970). The head and neck is the principal location for childhood rhabdomyosarcoma, especially the orbit; however, this anatomic region is rare in adults RMS (Feldman 1982; Nayar et al. 1993). The ethmoidal sinus is the most common site of origin of head and neck rhabdomyosarcomas in adults (Nayar et al. 1993). The location within petrous bone is extremely rare location of the RMS (Fig. 24.4). Its biological behavior varies widely, and despite the absence of specific clinical or radiological characteristics, rhabdomyosarcoma should be

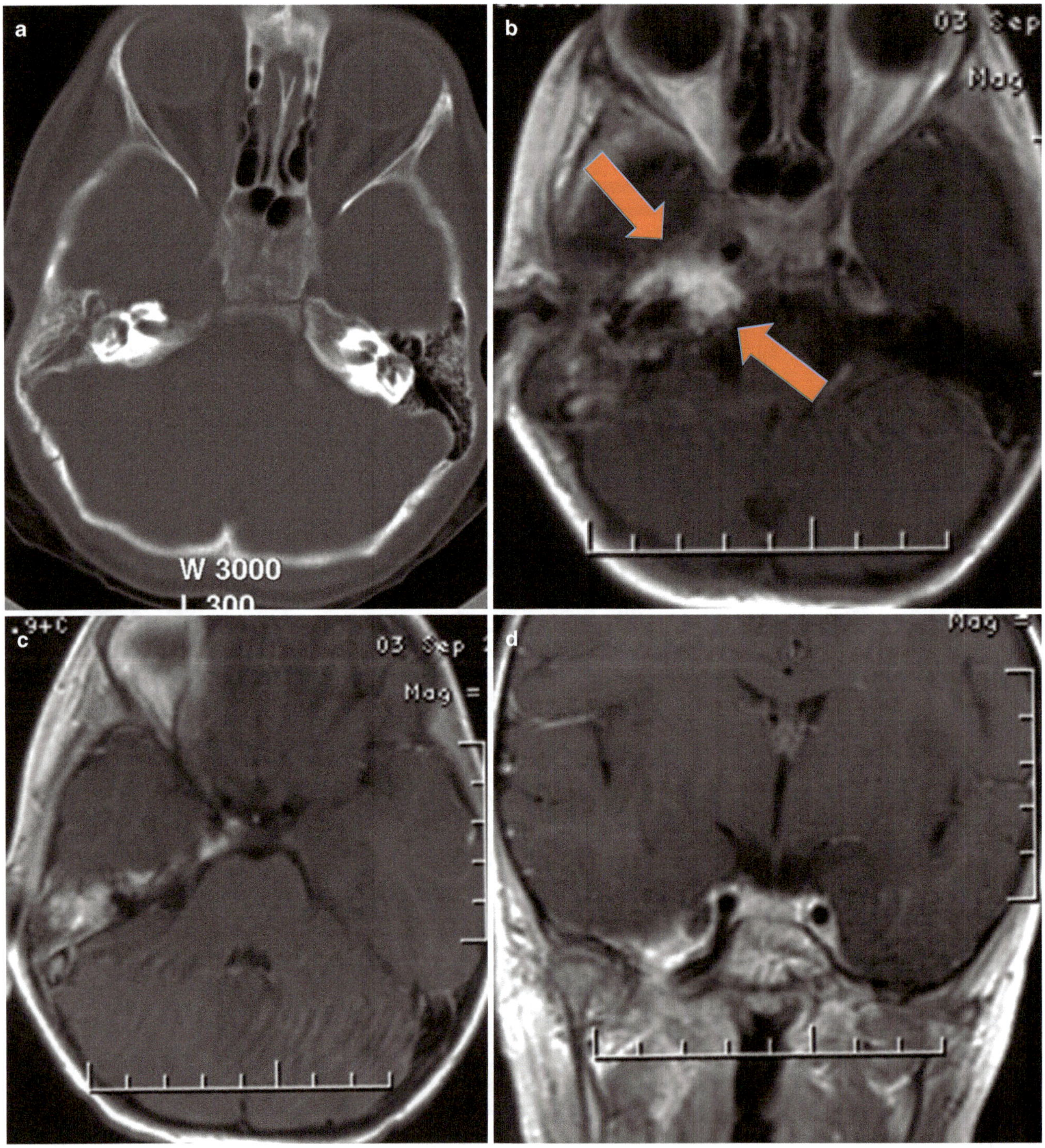

Fig. 24.4 Rhabdomyosarcoma of the petrous bone pyramid apex (child, 5 years old). Axial NECT scan (**a**) shows a focal pyramid apex destruction with effusion of mastoid's cells on the right. Series postenhanced MRI (**b–e**) demonstrate a homogeneously enhancing lesion with involvement of petrous bone and exrtacranial extension (*arrows*). (**f**) Histologic specimen

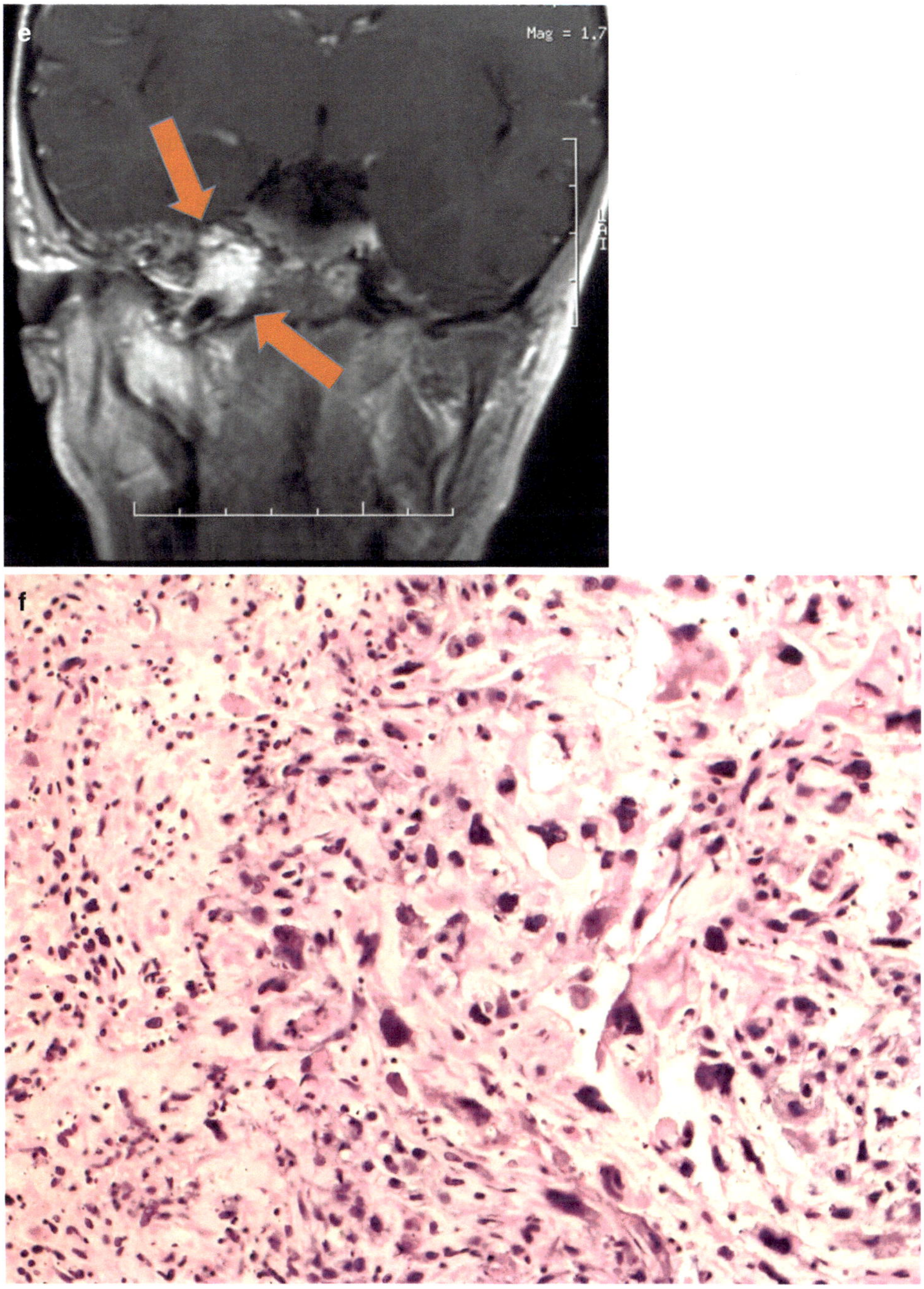

Fig. 24.4 (continued)

taken into account in the differential diagnosis of solid tumors in children.

In case it's located in the head and neck, most common sites of initial growth are the orbit, nasopharynx, area of the mastoid process of the temporal bone, nasal cavity and paranasal sinuses (Dolan 1974; Goepfert et al. 1979; Castillo 1993).

There are several morphological types of the tumors:

- Embryonal rhabdomyosarcoma occurs usually in children and adolescents, in the head and neck, most often in the orbital soft tissues;
- Alveolar rhabdomyosarcoma can occur in any part of the body in young people;
- Botroid alveolar rhabdomyosarcoma is a type of alveolar rhabdomyosarcoma that is distinguished by myxomatosis and a pronounced stromal edema, usually occurs in children with localization in the pelvis, almost never metastasizes;
- Polymorphic cellular rhabdomyosarcoma occurs more often than others and develops mainly in the extremities in elderly people;
- Mixed rhabdomyosarcoma that combines elements of microscopic features of the previously described forms.

Relapses occur in 17–46%, survival rates range from 35–93%.

Leiomyosarcoma is a rare, malignant smooth muscle tumor, most commonly occurs in the uterus and occasionally limbs, very rarely at the projection of the skull base (sinonasal area, etc.). Leiomyosarcoma is often located near the vascular structures. The tumor grows in the form of a nodule with dense or dense-elastic consistency, with indistinct borders, with deep localization in soft tissues. The tumor may involve the skin and/or bones. It is extremely malignant. It recurs, on average, in 35% of cases, metastases occur in 50% of patients, 5-year survival rate is 61% after the combination therapy (Figs. 24.5 and 24.6).

Ewing's sarcoma is a malignant skeletal tumor, by the WHO classification, belongs to a group of mixed bone tumors. The first description of the tumor belongs to James Ewing and dates from 1921. The researcher described it as a tumor mainly affecting long bones. Ewing's sarcoma is one of the most aggressive tumors, which is characterized by the rapid growth with damage to the surrounding tissues and

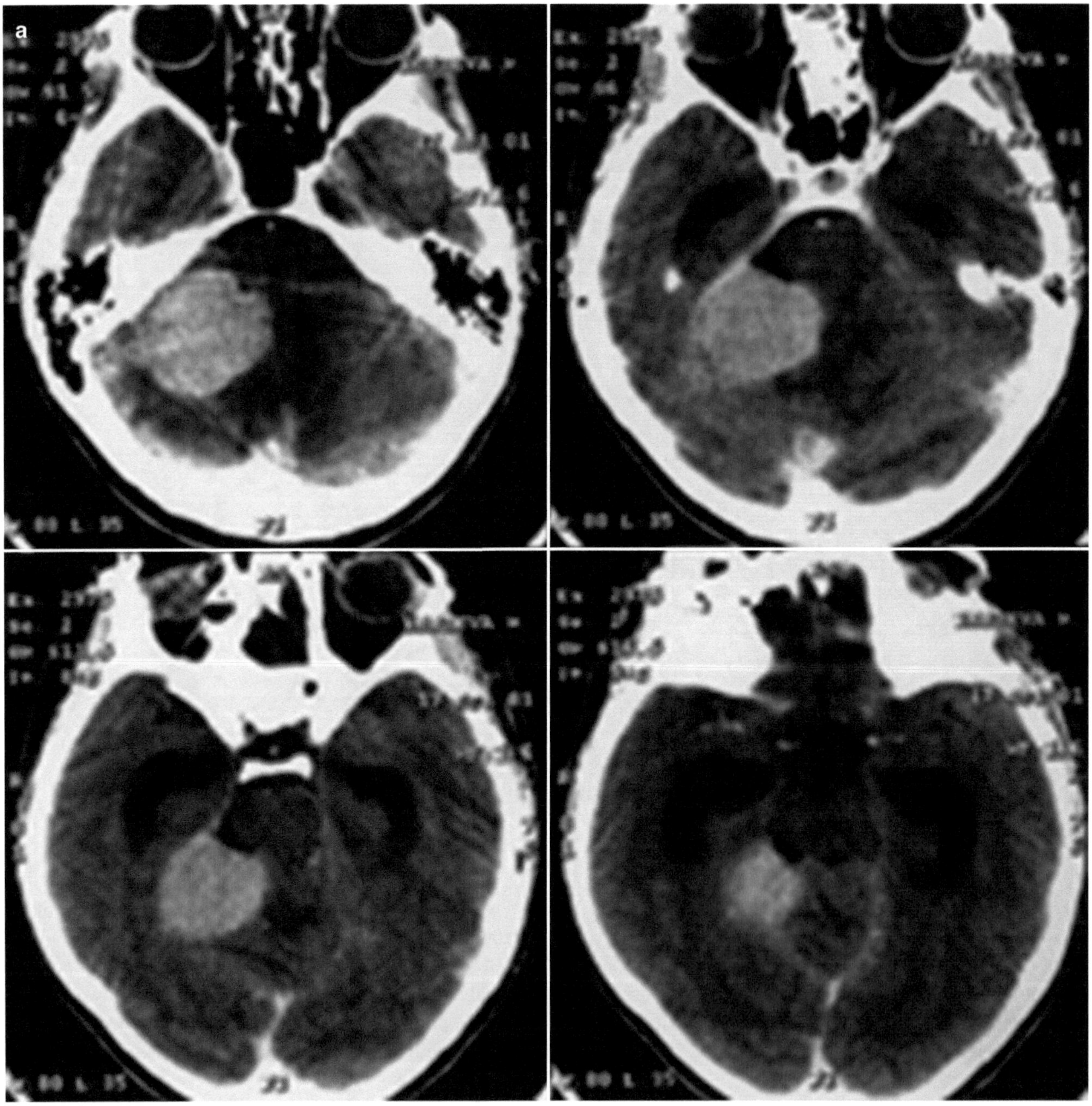

Fig. 24.5 Leiomyosarcoma of the right cerebellar hemisphere. Series of axial postenhanced CT scans demonstrate a homogeneously enhancing lesion in the lateral aspects of cerebellar hemisphere without bone involvement (**a**, **b**). (**c**) Histologic specimen

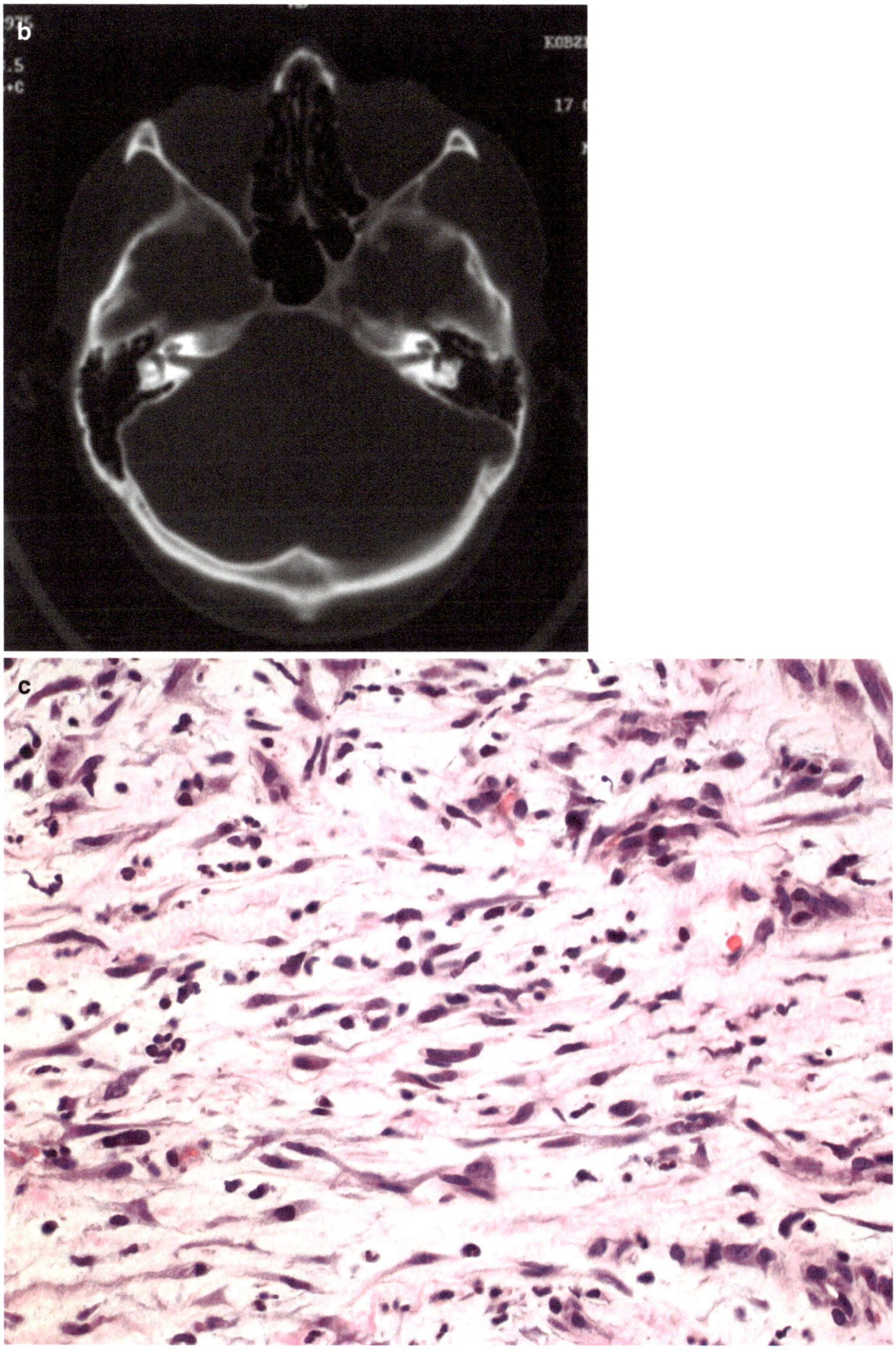

Fig. 24.5 (continued)

early hematogenous metastases. The most frequent sites of metastases at the time of initial diagnosis are lungs and bones (preferred locations are long bones, ribs, pelvis, scapula, spine, and collarbone). Unfortunately, today, despite the higher availability of diagnostic equipment and advances in the treatment of tumors, 14–50% of patients already have metastases at the time of initial diagnosis, which are identified by standard diagnostic examinations, and much more patients have micrometastases. Lymphatic metastatic spread is rare and is always associated with a poor prognosis. Up to 5% of patients have CNS metastases at initial diagnosis (Shuper 1998). It is believed that CNS metastases penetrate

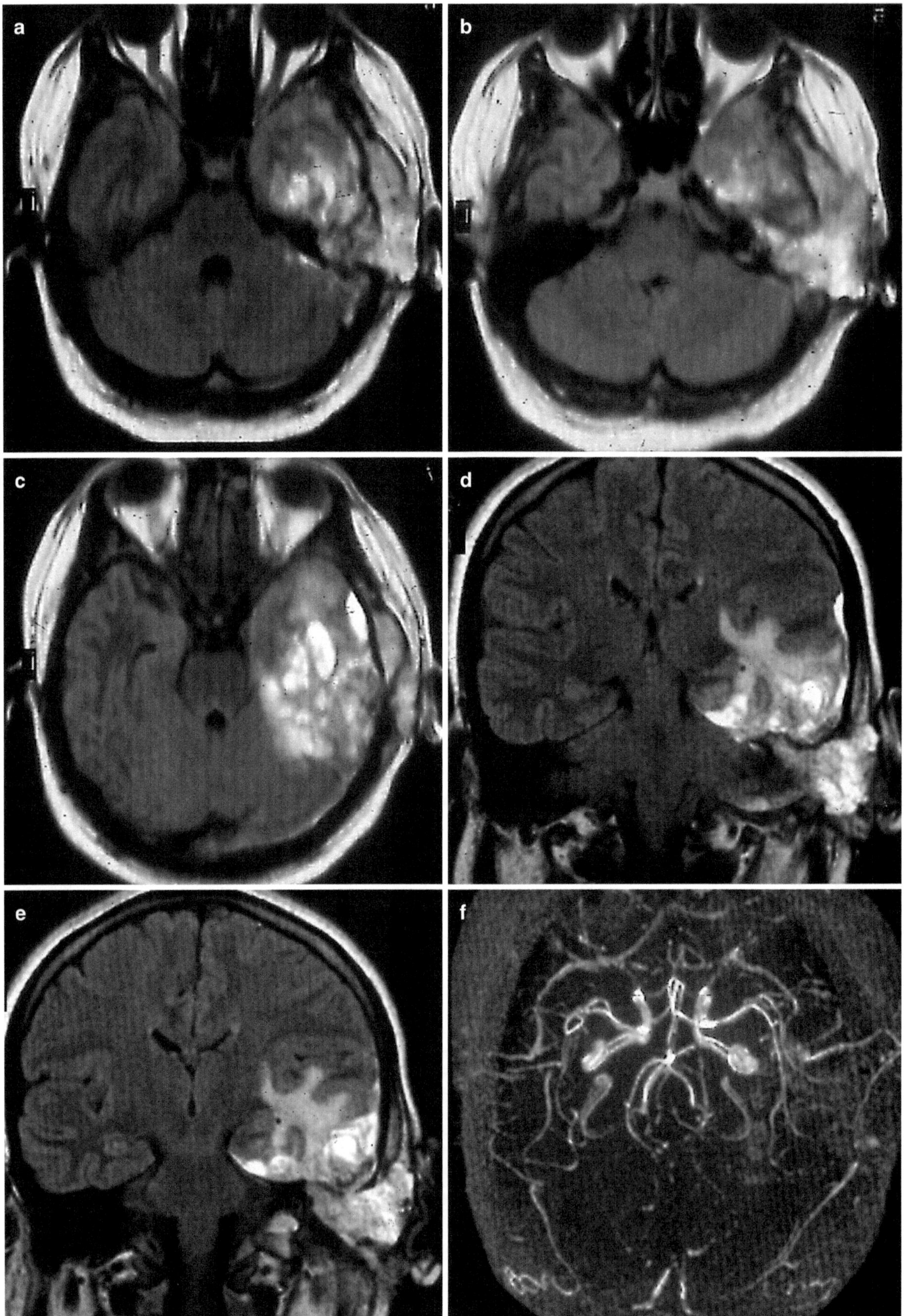

Fig. 24.6 Leiomyosarcoma of the left temporal area. Series of axial (**a**–**c**) and coronal (**d**, **e**) T2-FLAIR MR images demonstrate a heterogeneous hyperintense lesion with intra- and extracerebral extension. There is wide area of temporal bone pyramid destruction. (**f**) 3D TOF MR-angiography shows branches of external carotid artery which are supplied the tumor

directly through the bone tissue and, therefore, are located mainly in the epidural area, hematogenous metastases are considered rare. To date, 10-year survival rate is 50%.

Ewing's sarcoma is the second most common bone malignancy in children and observed in 10–15% of patients. This tumor is rare in children younger than 5 years old and adults over 30 years old. A peak incidence occurs at the age of 10–15 years old. The cause of malignant bone tumors is yet unknown, but it is proved that occurrence of bone sarcoma in 40% is provoked by an injury.

Histologically, Ewing's sarcoma is composed of small round cells with scant cytoplasm, a round nucleus containing delicate chromatin and poorly visualized basophilic nucleoli. These cells acquire blue color following specific staining. Unlike osteosarcoma, it does not produce osteoid.

Although Ewing's sarcoma is a dedifferentiated bone tumor, there is evidence of soft tissues involvement by the tumor. There is even a so-called extraosseous form of Ewing's sarcoma. In specialized literature, the term of "tumour family of Ewing's sarcoma type" appeared.

For the first time, an extraosseous form of Ewing's sarcoma was described by M. Tefft in 1969, who diagnosed five cases of paravertebral soft tissue tumors with histological signs of Ewing's sarcoma. Descriptions of tumors located within the central nervous system are extremely rare in the early radiological literature. The only case of the posterior fossa tumor, which was originally diagnosed as medulloblastoma, is reported by Jay (1999).

In our practice, there was only one case of a 3-year-old child (girl), whose clinical signs manifested by headache, vomiting, followed by subsequent addition of coordination disturbances. There were edema of the optic disc. Brainstem symptoms quickly developed. MRI revealed a large tumor that occupied the right half of the posterior cranial fossa, severely dislocated the cerebellum and brainstem. There were a local destructive bone changes of the pyramid on CT scans (not presented). The lesion itself had a heterogeneous structure with large cysts in its stroma and intensively enhanced with a fairly clear delineation from the brain structures (Fig. 24.7).

Chordoma is a rare tumor (up to 1–2% of all brain tumors), originating from the remnants of the embryonic notochord (cranial and primary notochord). Typical sites of its development are the skull base (clivus) and sacrum. The lesion grows from the cartilage cells on the midline of the sphenopetroclival junction in 35%, has sacrococcygeal location in 50%, and also vertebral involvement is possible in 15% of cases.

The disease occurs in people of all ages, however, is more common in males. Chordomas of the skull base are more common in younger patients, while chordoma of the sacrum are more common in elderly patients. Previously, there was a meaning about its relative benignity, because of its slow growth and relatively rare metastases outside the local area of the primary lesion. However, current clinical and histological studies identify chordoma as a malignant neoplasm with local bone-destructive growth, tendency to relapse and possibility of multiple metastases in the bone, lung, liver, and lymph nodes.

Histologically, there are two types: classic chondroma and chondroid chordoma, the stroma of the latter is similar to the hyaline cartilage with neoplastic cells in lacunae, although there is no cartilage tissue within the tumor itself.

Clinical manifestations of the disease can vary; their severity and type depend predominantly on the tumor location. Typically, clinical manifestations are caused by the involvement of the cranial nerves and brainstem compression. Tumor growth leads to compression or enveloping the arteries. The most common initial symptoms are diplopia and trigeminal neuralgia, ophthalmoplegia, visual disturbances, VII or VIII nerves palsies (Maira et al. 1996).

A typical intracranial chordomas location is a clivus. The growing tumor can invade the cavernous sinus and sella turcica from above, the jugular foramen and the pyramid apex laterally, surrounds the basilar artery and displaces the brain stem. Chordomas can extend into the sphenoid bone and ethmoidal labyrinth in case of anterior growth or the foramen magnum in case of growth downwards (Erdem et al. 2003).

Imaging Direct angiography reveals an avascularized area, large arteries are usually displaced laterally and posteriorly. The typical symptom confirming the intracranial growth is an arched displacement of the basilar artery upwards and posteriorly.

CT examination shows an expansile mass with wide area of bone destruction with bone and calcified fragments in the tumor stroma in 95% of the cases. The tumor has hypo- and isodense CT-characteristics. In same cases the connective-tissue trabeculae within the tumor stroma can give these lesions the lobular structure. A postenhanced CT studies in most cases do not reveal accumulation of contrast media by the tumor or the contrast enhancement may be minimal (Figs. 24.8, 24.9, and 24.10).

On MRI, the tumors have a hypointense MR-signal on T1-weighted images, with various in size areas of hyperintense MR-signal due to hemorrhages. The MR-signal on T2-weighted images is typically hyperintense causes by cystic components (Fig. 24.11). T2*-gradient echo sequences demonstrate the hemorrhagic areas and bone fragments as hypointense foci (Oot et al. 1988; Fischbein et al. 2000). After contrast enhancement, a "honeycomb" pattern is observed (thin contrast enhancement of the cysts contour). On T2-weighted sequences, thin connective-tissue trabeculae with hypointense MR-signal can also be visualized within the tumor. Sphenoid bone involvement in the neoplastic process with the replacement of the bone structure with tumor tissue,

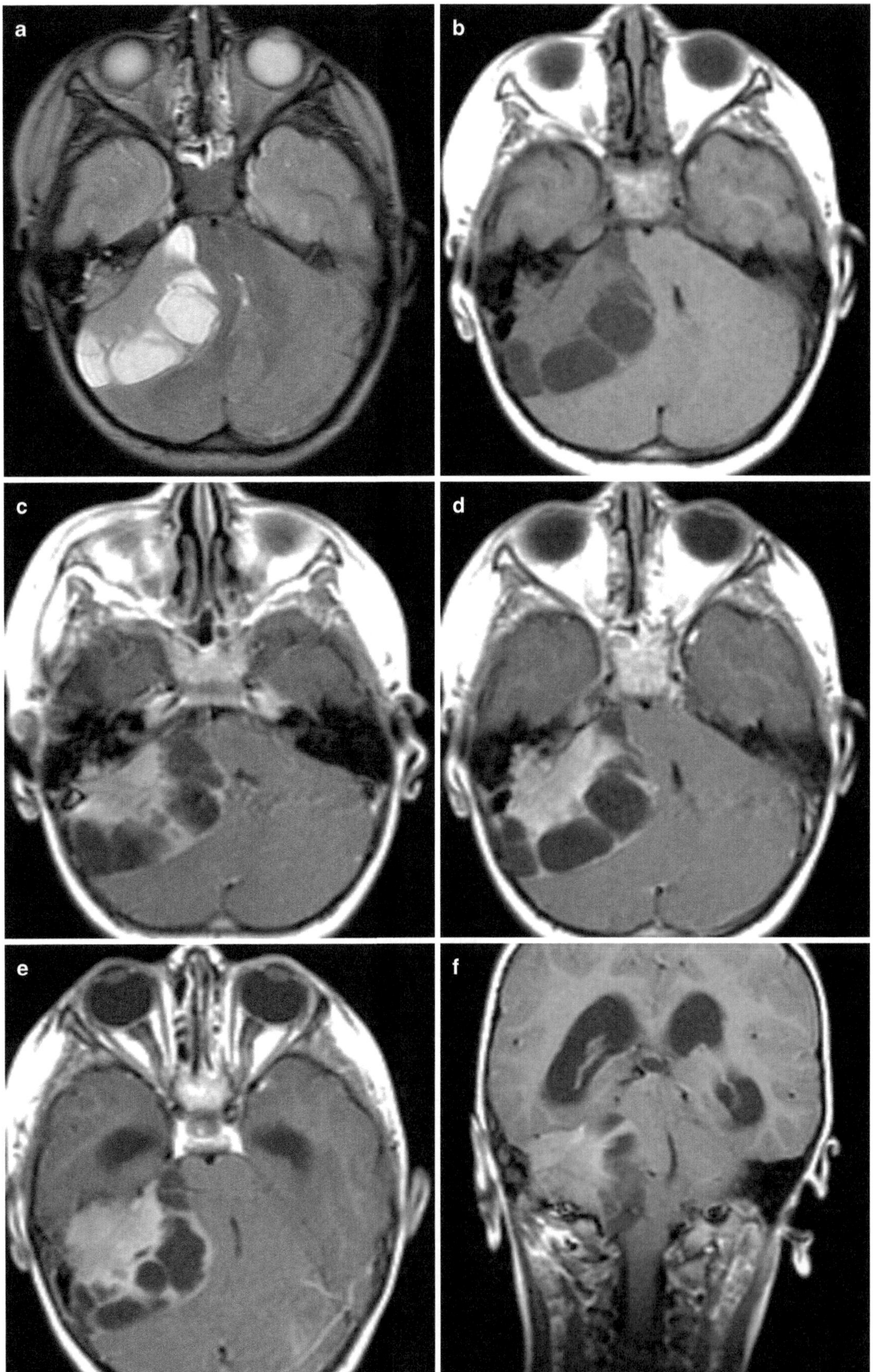

Fig. 24.7 Ewing sarcoma of the right half of posterior cerebral fossa. Axial T2- (**a**), T1-weighted MR images before (**b**) and after (**c**–**f**) contrast enhancement show a heterogeneous isointense (on T2 and T1) from solid part and hyperintense on T2 from cystic parts of the tumor with prominent contrast enhancement. MRI reveals the invasion of petrous pyramid

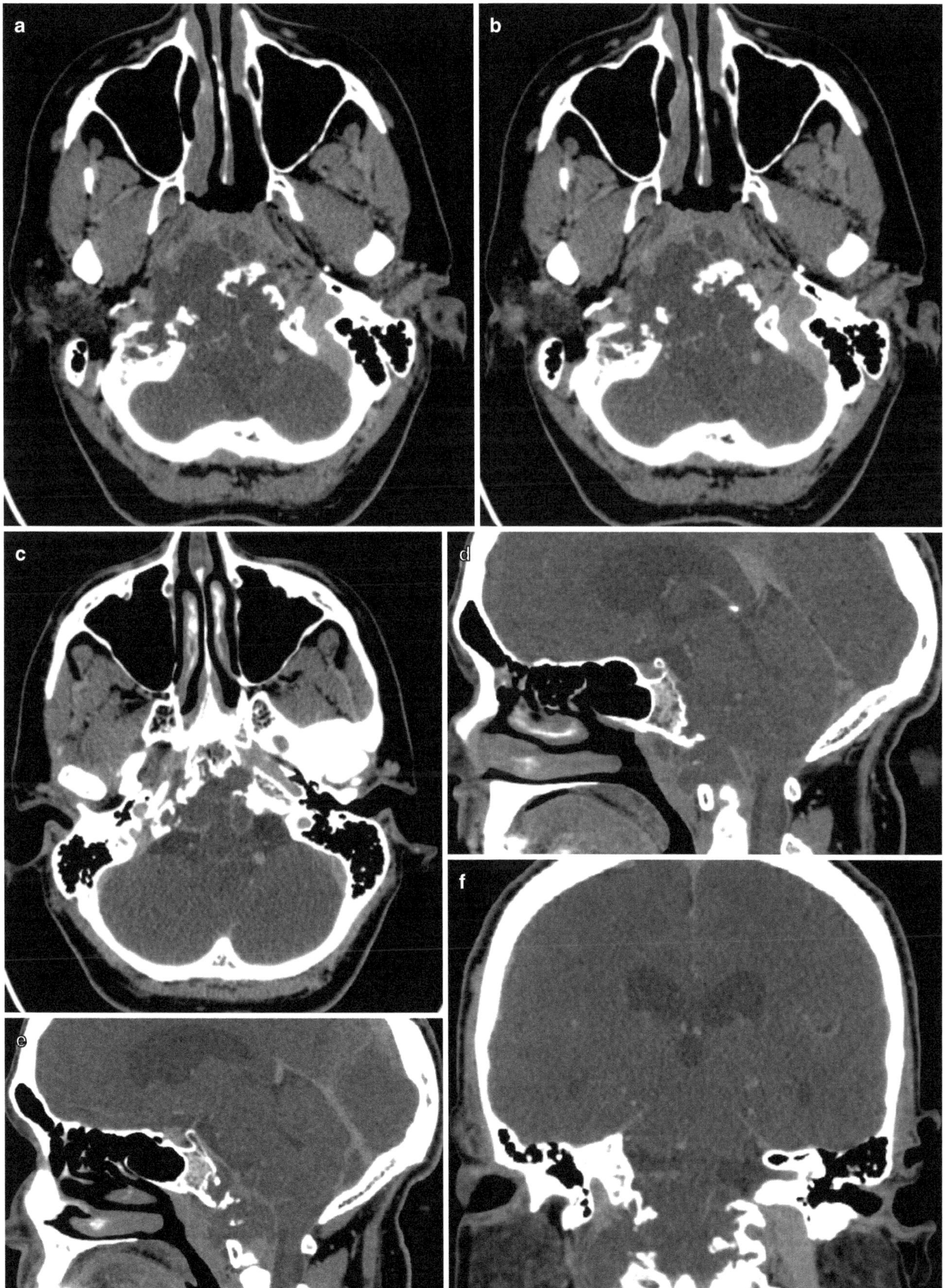

Fig. 24.8 Chordoma of the clivus. Axial CECT scans (**a**–**c**), coronal and sagittal reformats (**d**–**f**) reveal a large expansile tumor, which is located in clivus and lower parts of occipital bone. The tumor heterogeneously accumulates contrast medium and leads to wide destruction of the bones. Sagittal and frontal reformats show an expansion of the tumor in the skull base and its growth into the cranial cavity, spinal canal, and oropharynx

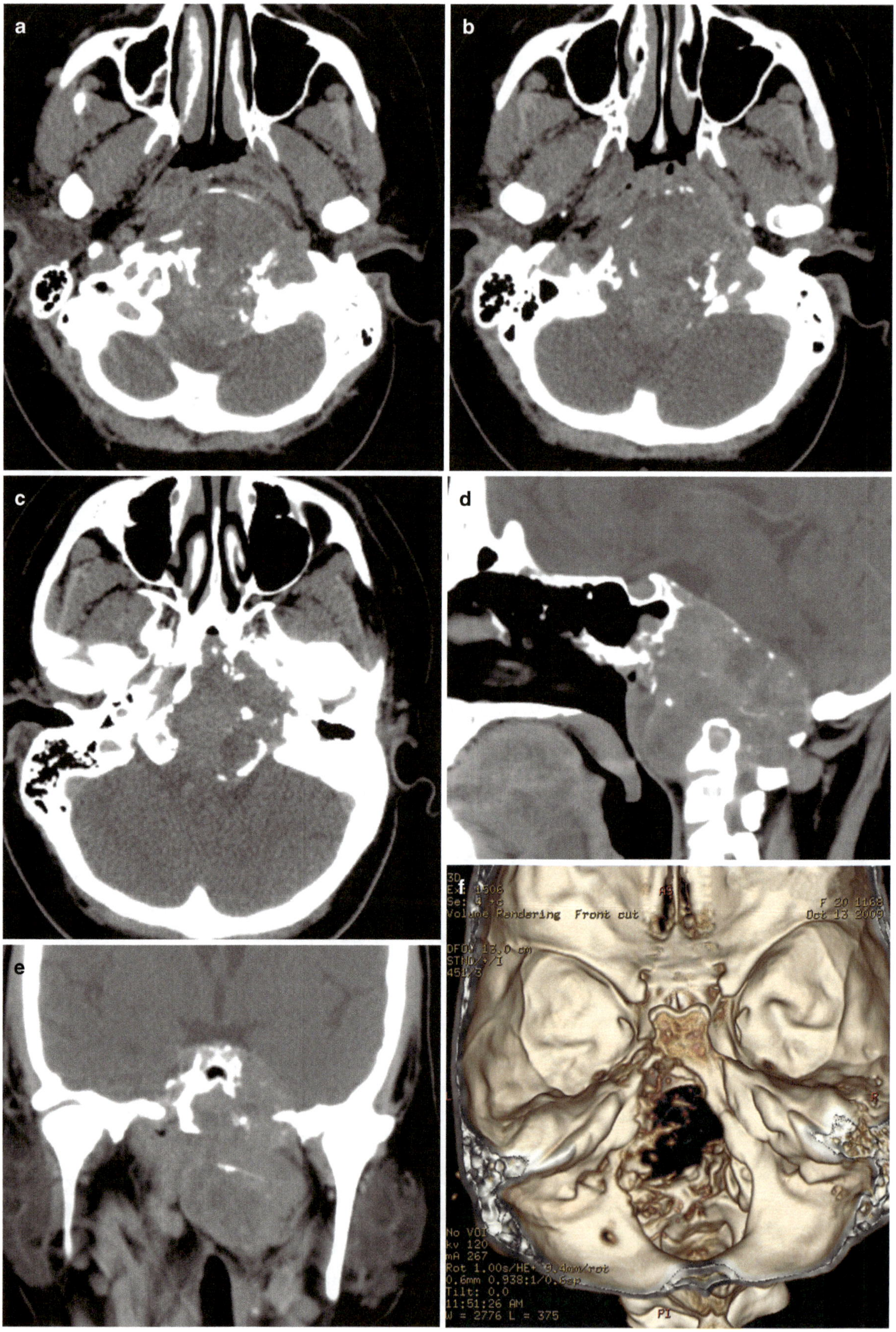

Fig. 24.9 Chordoma of the clivus. Axial CECT scans (**a**–**c**), coronal and sagittal reformats (**d**, **e**) reveal a large expansile tumor, which is located in clivus and sphenoid bone. The tumor heterogeneously accumulates contrast medium and leads to wide destruction of the skull base bones. Sagittal and frontal reformats show an expansion of the tumor in the skull base and its growth into the cranial cavity, spinal canal, and naspharynx. 3D reconstruction demonstrates the extent of skull base destruction (**f**)

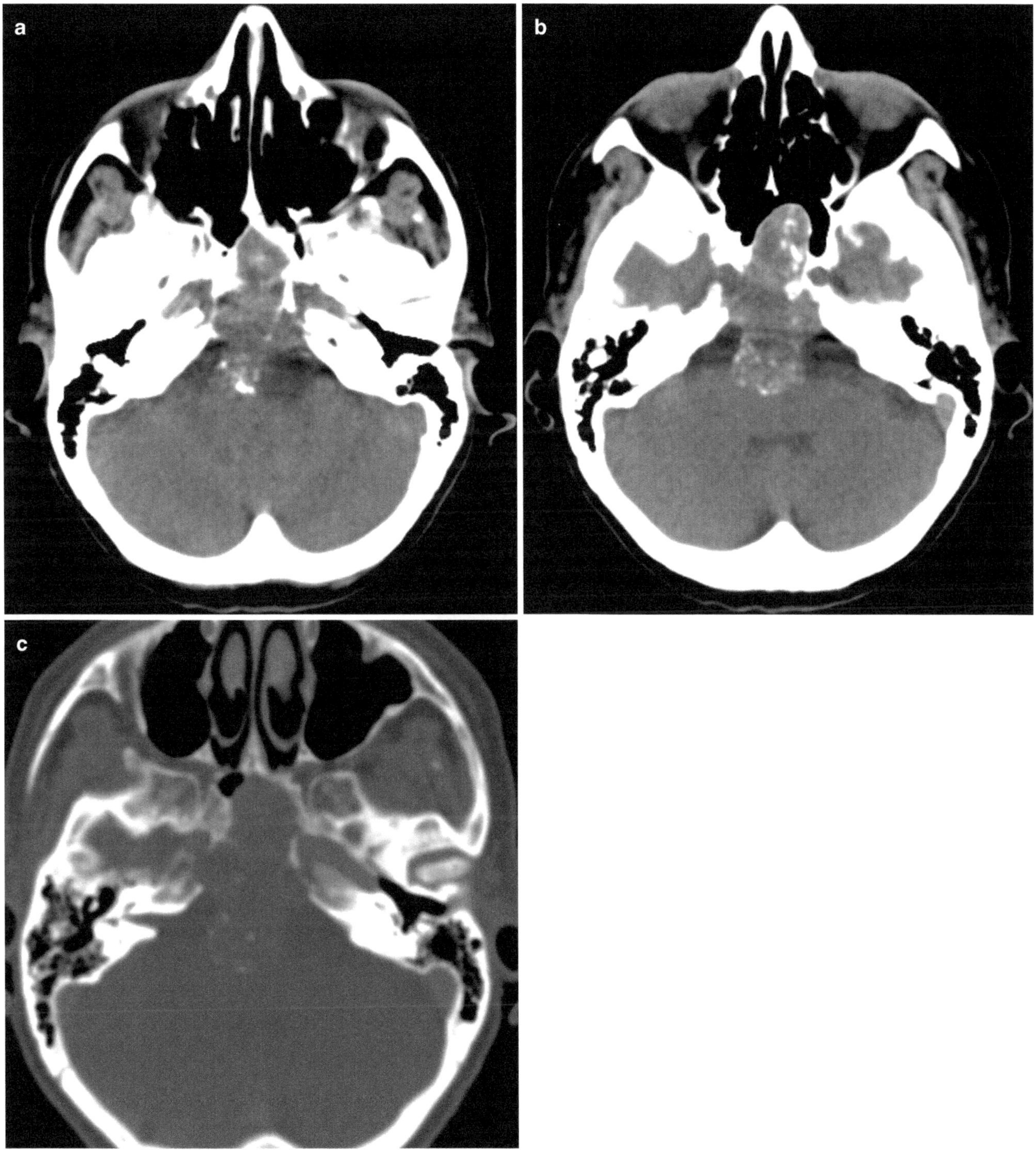

Fig. 24.10 Chordoma of the clivus. Axial NECT (**a**) and CECT scans (**b**, **c**) reveal a large expansile tumor, which leads to wide bone destruction of the clivus and sphenoid bone. The tumor heterogeneously accumulates contrast medium and contains plenty of small calcifications

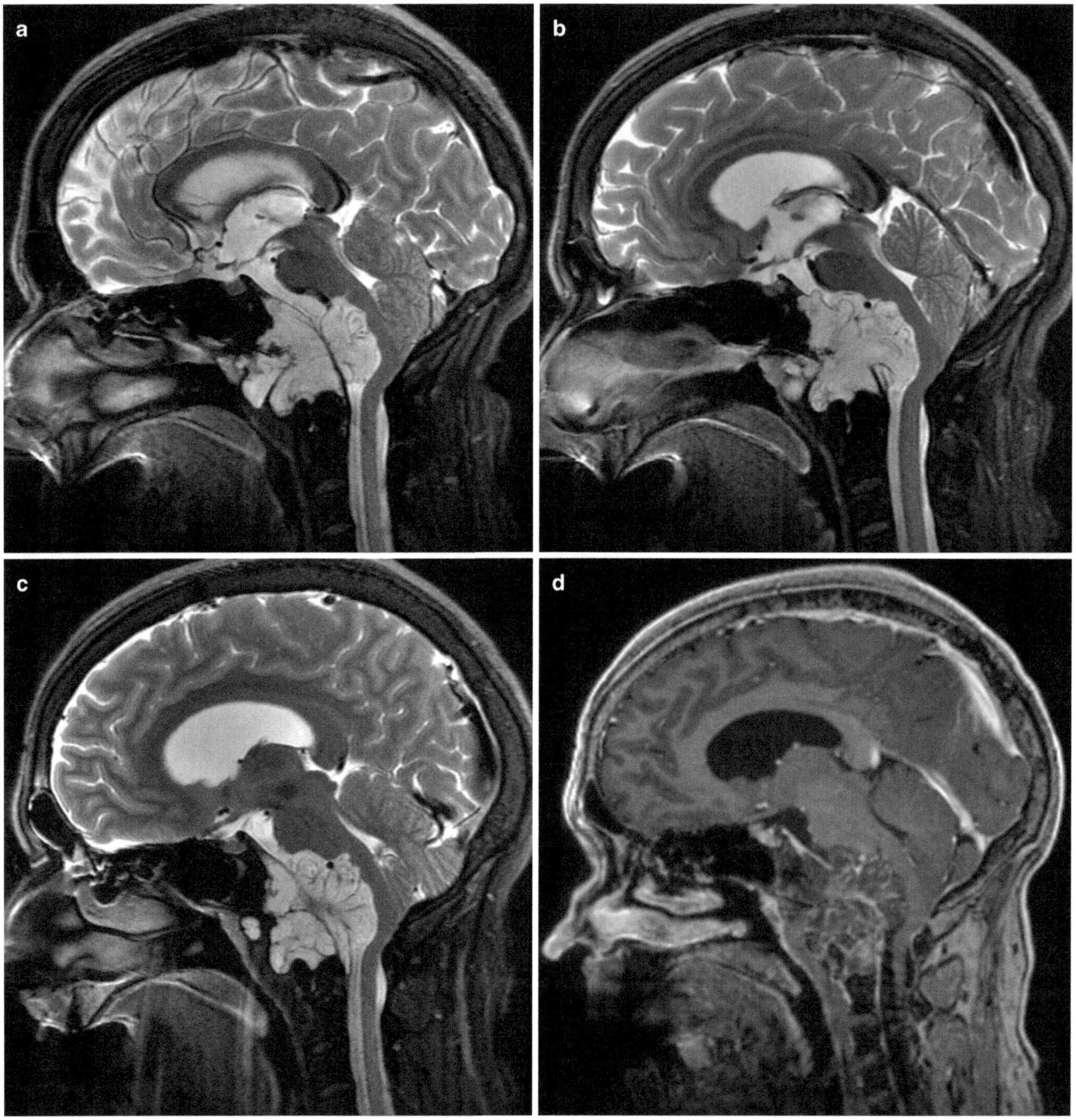

Fig. 24.11 Chordoma of the clivus. Sagittal MR images using T2 (**a**–**c**)- and postenhanced T1-weighted (**d**, **e**) sequences show a heterogeneous hyperintense (on T2) and hypointense on T1 tumor which is located in projection of clivus. Tumor is characterized by heterogeneous contrast enhancement predominantly within intratumoral septa. MRI reveals the tumor extension into nasopharynx and intracranially with brain stem compression. (**f**) Histologic specimen

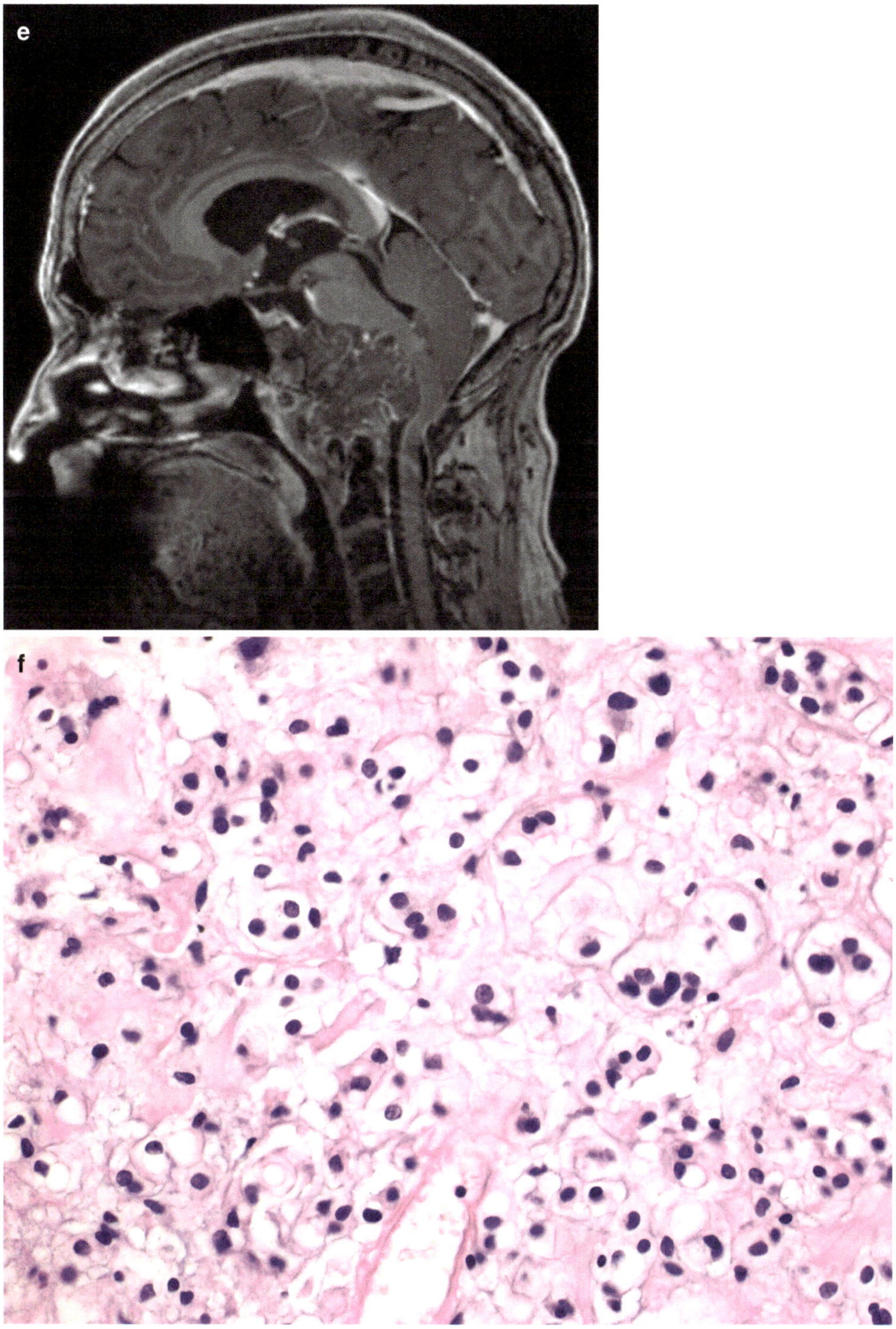

Fig. 24.11 (continued)

which is characterized by lower signal intensity than normal bone, is best detected on sagittal and axial T1-weighted images. T2-STIR sequence is useful in evaluating a chordoma distribution in the bones and soft tissues of the skull base—the tumor has a hyperintense MR-signal, while the surrounding tissue is hypointense (Fig. 24.12). Tumors located laterally from the midline are visualized mainly at the projections of the petrous apex, cavernous sinus and parasellar area. In such cases, the combination of bone destruction and calcification processes in the chordoma stroma can be visible on MRI and CT (Fig. 24.13). CT-perfusion helps to distinguish the tumor from, for example, calcified meningiomas at this location: soft-tissue meningioma component is characterized by high CBV and CBF values, while chordoma is characterized by low values.

Differential Diagnosis Macroadenoma (growth from the sella turcica, more homogeneously enhances), chondrosarcoma, plasmacytoma, metastases, primary cancer of the skull base.

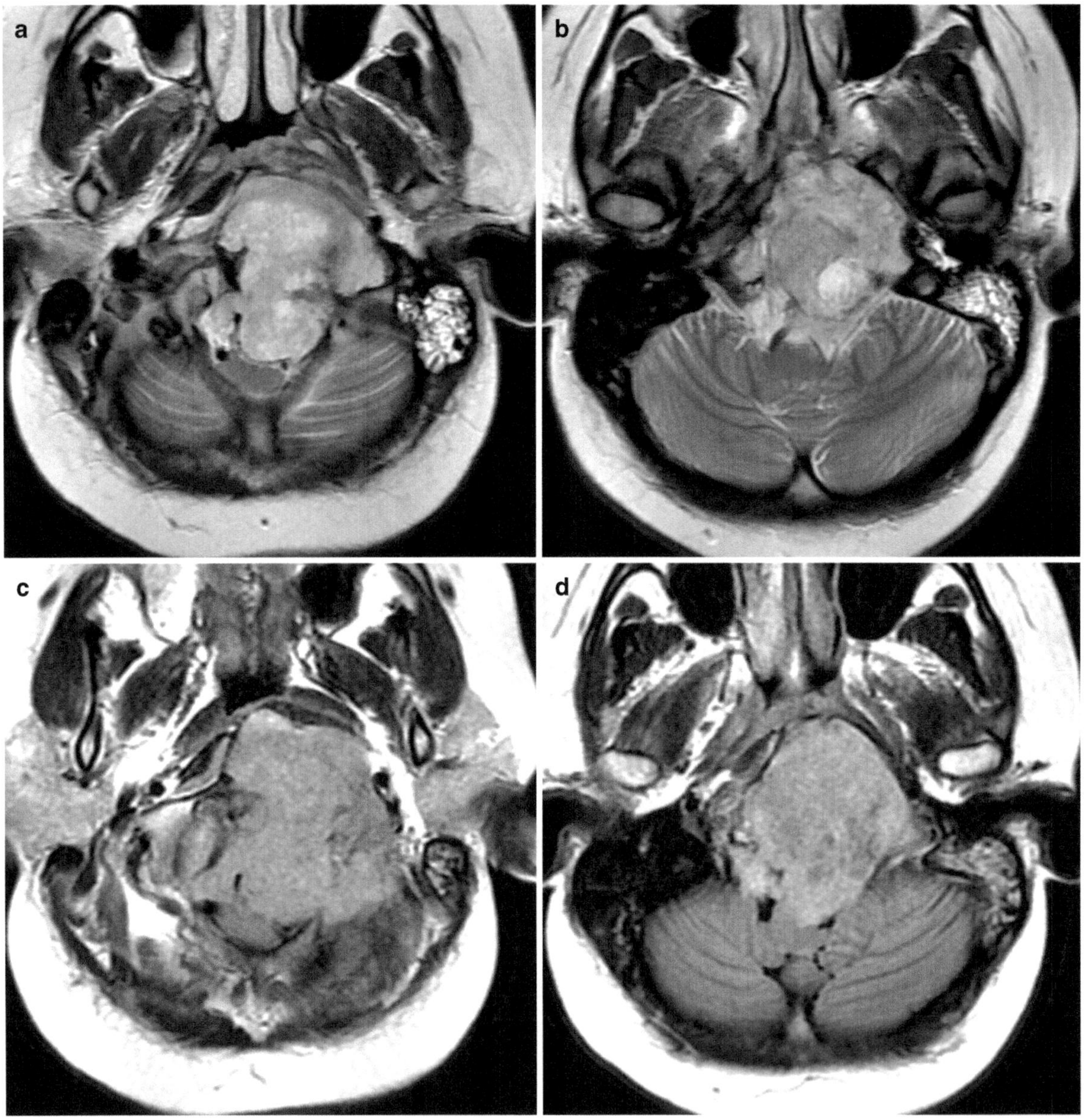

Fig. 24.12 Chordoma of the skull base. Axial T2- (**a**, **b**), T2-FLAIR- (**c**, **d**), T1-weighted MR images before (**e**) and T1 after (**f**–**i**) contrast enhancement show a heterogeneous hyperintense (on T2) and hypointense on T1 tumor which is located in projection of clivus with wide invasion of the bone structures. Tumor is characterized by heterogeneous and prominent contrast enhancement. MRI reveals the tumor extension into nasopharynx, into spinal canal and intracranially with brain stem compression. Fat-Sat technology helps better delineate the tumor's margins (**i**)

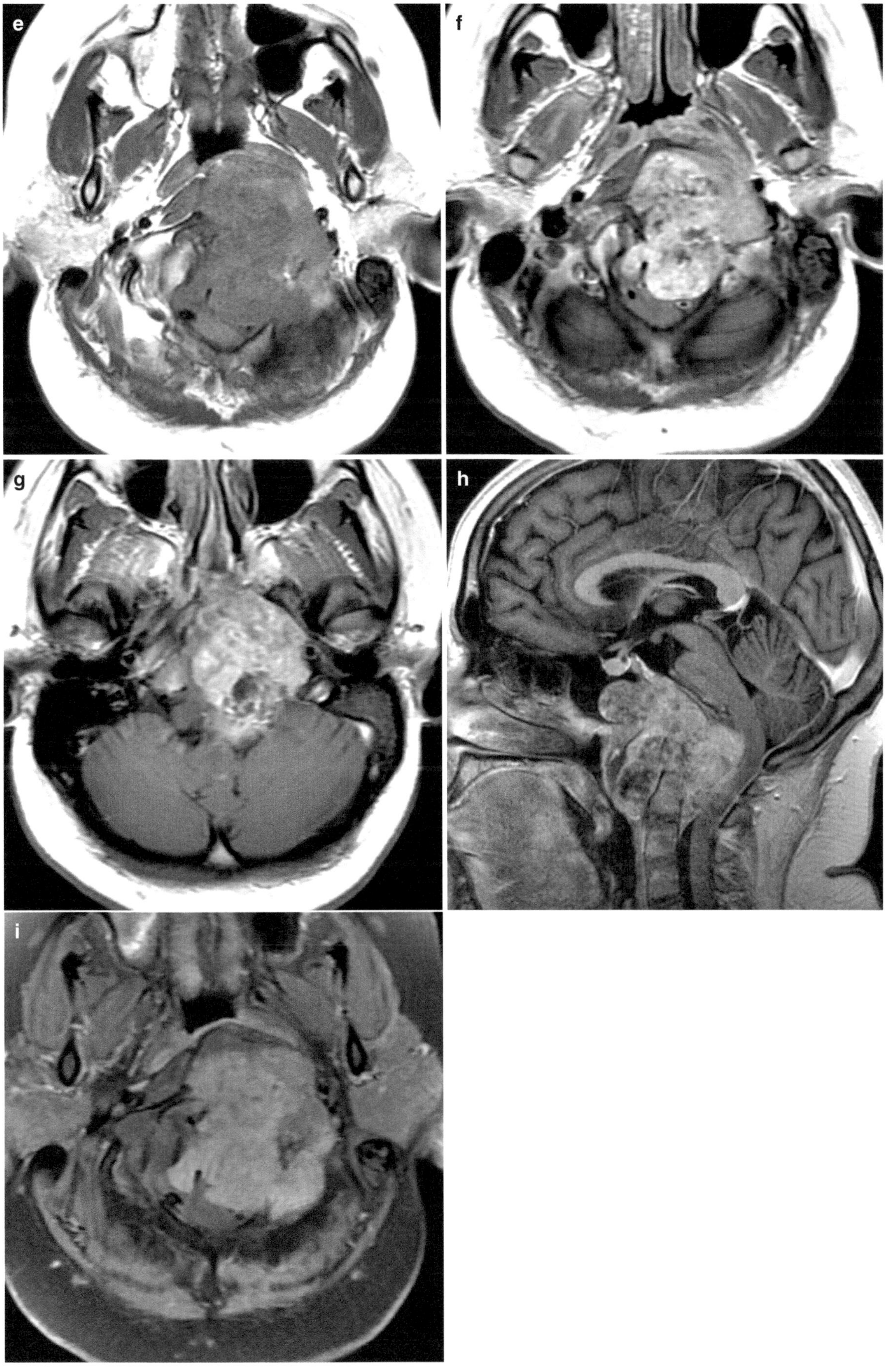

Fig. 24.12 (continued)

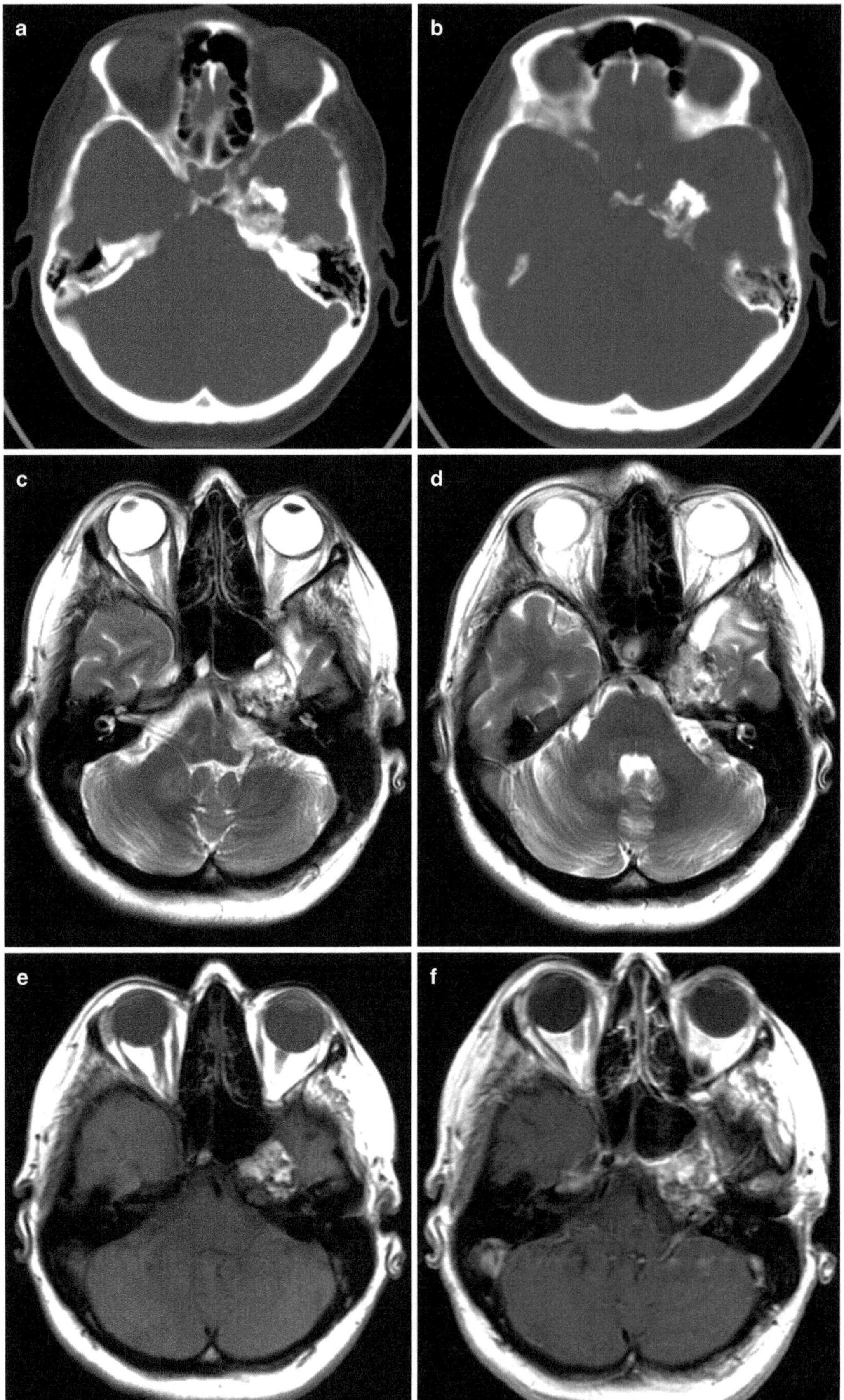

Fig. 24.13 Chordoma of the petrous portion apex on the left. Axial NECT scans (**a**, **b**) detect predominantly calcified tumor in the apex of petrous bone. On T2 MRI (**c**, **d**) the chordoma has heterogeneous hypo-hyperintense MR signal due to presence of cystic component and calcifications. On T1-weighted MR image the tumor is characterized by hyperintense MR-signal (**e**). MRI with contrast enhancement in axial (**f**, **g**), sagittal (**h**), and coronal (**i**) planes improves visualization of the chordoma margins

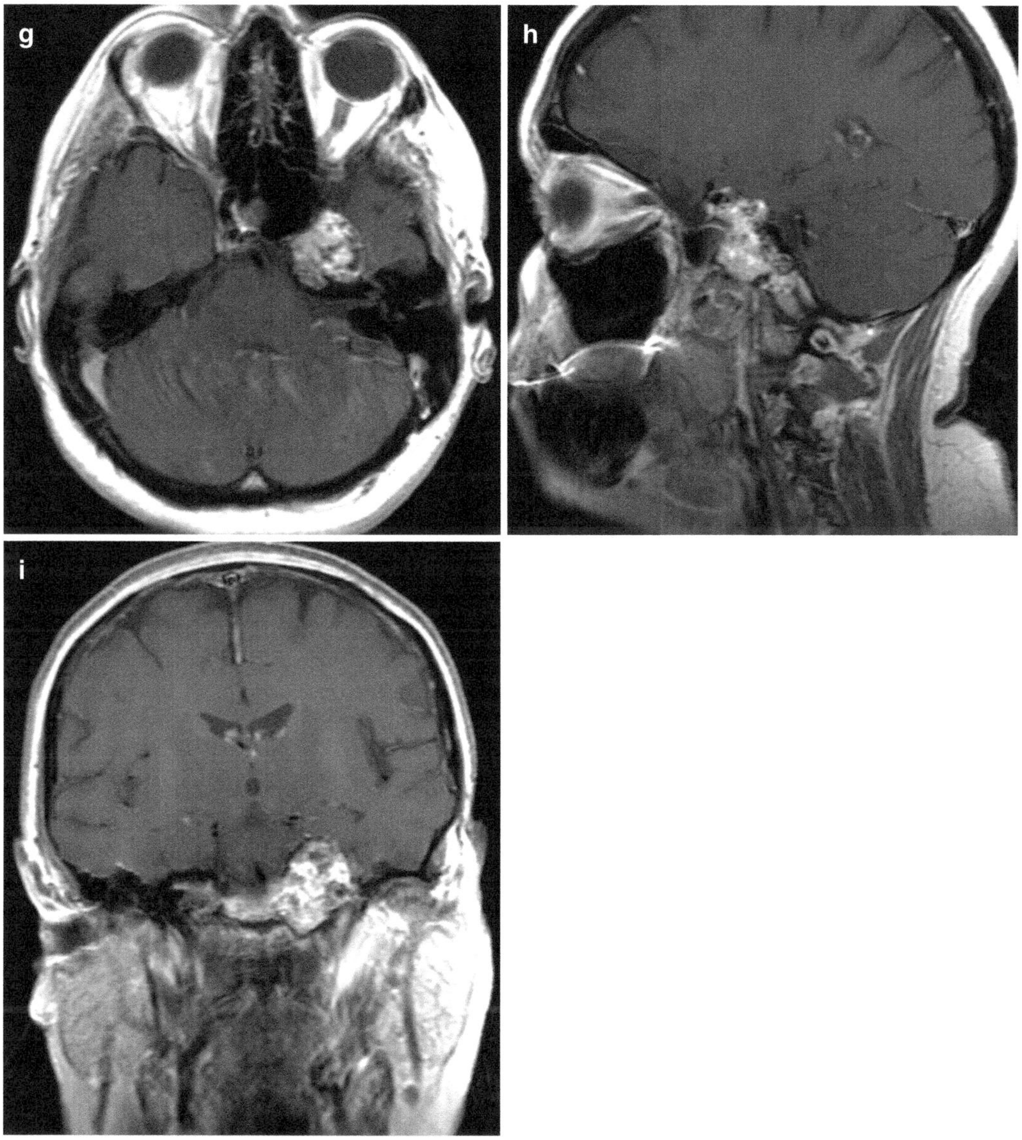

Fig. 24.13 (continued)

Endolymphatic Sac Tumor An aggressive papillary tumor of the endolymphatic sac of the temporal bone (synonyms: low-grade endolymphatic sac adenocarcinoma, tumor of the endolymphatic sac, endolymphatic sac papillary tumor, aggressive papillary tumor of the temporal bone, papillary adenoma) is an epithelial tumor that does not metastasize and has papillary structure with a pronounced local invasive growth. The suspected source of development is epithelium lining up the endolymphatic sac, which is an end section of the vestibular canal of the membranous cochlear labyrinth. The tumor develops on the posterior surface of the petrous portion of the temporal bone, but can occur outside the endolymphatic sac in other parts of the temporal bone: the area of the jugular bulb, middle ear, and mastoid. In case of Von Hippel-Lindau disease, a bilateral lesion is observed. This neoplasm occurs at different ages with the same frequency in both genders.

Microscopically, cystic papillary structures surrounded by fibrovascular stroma are detected. Papillae are lined up by a single layer of low cylindrical or cubical epithelium. Signs of nuclear polymorphism or mitotic activity of epithelial cells are absent.

Imaging CT exam detects a space-occupying lesion located in the posterior surface of the petrous bone with the presence of bone destruction. Soft-tissue tumor nodule usually bulges into the posterior cranial fossa, where it compresses the cerebellum. The tumor nodule heterogeneously accumulates contrast material.

On MR images, the tumor's features depend on the presence of hemorrhages, calcifications, and bone fragments. On T1-weighted sequences, it is characterized by an increased signal from the tumor stroma, sometimes with a peripheral hyperintense rim (Mukherji 1997). On T2-weighted MR-images the lesion has a heterogeneous MR-signal, with hyperintense foci of subacute microhemorrhages, bone fragments being hypointense. The contrast enhancement is heterogeneous, but quite pronounced (Fig. 24.14).

Differential Diagnosis Metastases (especially papillary thyroid cancer), facial nerve schwannoma, laterally located choroid plexus papilloma and meningioma of the cerebellopontine angle.

Plasmacytoma in the form of a solitary *(solitary myeloma)* or multiple tumor in generalized myeloma is a lesion composed of plasma cells, can occur with anemia, an increase in immunoglobulin levels, infections, and kidney disease. The form developing in conjunction with myeloma, which may occur due to its degeneration because of abnormal gammaglobulin synthesis, is called malignant plasmacytoma. The diagnosis requires additional identification of Bence-Jones protein in urinalysis, determination of an increase in the plasma cell amount via bone marrow biopsies (Schwartz et al. 2001; Bret et al. 2002).

At the projection of the skull base, plasmacytoma is commonly located in the sphenoid bone and the petrous apex, rarely in the dura covered the PCF. In cases with multiple tumors abnormal lesions could be simultaneously detected in the ribs, pelvis, spine, long bones, sternum. Craniobasal plasmacytomas are characterized by a worse prognosis compared with plasmacytomas of the cranial vault and commonly progress to multiple myeloma.

Clinical manifestations develop in the form of local pain, headache, neuropathy of VIth nerve, hearing loss (Vijaya-Sekaran et al. 1999).

Imaging Direct angiography reveals a hypervascularized tumor that is mainly supplied from branches of the external carotid artery.

CT scanning shows a solitary intraosseous osteolytic soft-tissue lesion with poorly defined margins and the absence of bone sclerotic edge changes. Calcified fragments within the lesion are typically absent, but bone fragments can be present. Non-enhanced CT scans demonstrate a relatively homogeneous, slightly hyperdense (relative to the brain tissue) lesion in the projection of the underlying bone (Fig. 24.15). Moderated and homogeneous contrast enhancement is typical feature of the plasmacytomas (Randoux et al. 2000).

On MRI, the lesion has a homogeneously iso-hypointense MR-signal (relative to the gray matter) on T1- and T2-weighted images. In the presence of ossified inclusions, hypointense foci can be detected. After administration of contrast agent, homogeneous pronounced contrast enhancement of the tumor is noted, which becomes close to MR signal from the intact bone marrow. Fat-Sat technique allows improving the delineation of an abnormal contrast-enhanced area from the healthy tissue on post-contrast scans. On T2-STIR sequence, this lesion is characterized by an iso-hyperintense signal. On T2-FLAIR images plasmacytoma is iso-hyperintense (Fig. 24.16).

Differential Diagnosis Intraosseous meningioma (accompanied by sclerotic bone changes, intensive enhancement), metastases, myeloma (multifocal lesion), nasopharyngeal carcinoma (growing from the nasopharynx), chordoma (commonly located in the midline, with calcification, hyperintense on T2-weighted images).

Lymphoma of the Skull Base Bone lymphoma is considered an independent nosological form, although it is very similar to Ewing's sarcoma. It is rare than the latter, usually occurs at the age of 20–40 years old and predominantly in males.

Malignant bone lymphoma is a neoplasm from lymphatic and reticulo-endothelial tissues, consisting of immature cells resembling lymphocytes, plasma cells, or histiocytes.

These are the following types of malignant lymphomas with bone involvement:

Fig. 24.14 Tumor of endolymphatic sac. Axial NECT (**a**) and CECT (**b**) scans detect a mix structure tumor invading and eroding the petrous bone in projection of endolymphatic sac. The intracerebral part of the lesion has prominent and heterogeneous enhancement. CT-perfusion study (**c**–**e**) demonstrates prominent elevation of CBF (**c**), CBV (**d**), and PS (**e**) in the tumor. There are calcifications and focal bone destruction of medial margin of the petrous bone in projection of tumor's matrix (**f**). On T2- (**g**), T1- (**h**), T2-FLAIR (**i**) and DWI (**j**) MR images tumor is characterized by heterogeneous MR-signal with focal peripheral hemorrhages (hyperintense signal on T1 and T2-FLAIR). Lesion shows prominent contrast enhancement (**k**). Spinal MRI reveals syringomyelia of the cervical and thoracic spinal cord with small hemangioblastoma on Th1 level (**l**, *arrow*)

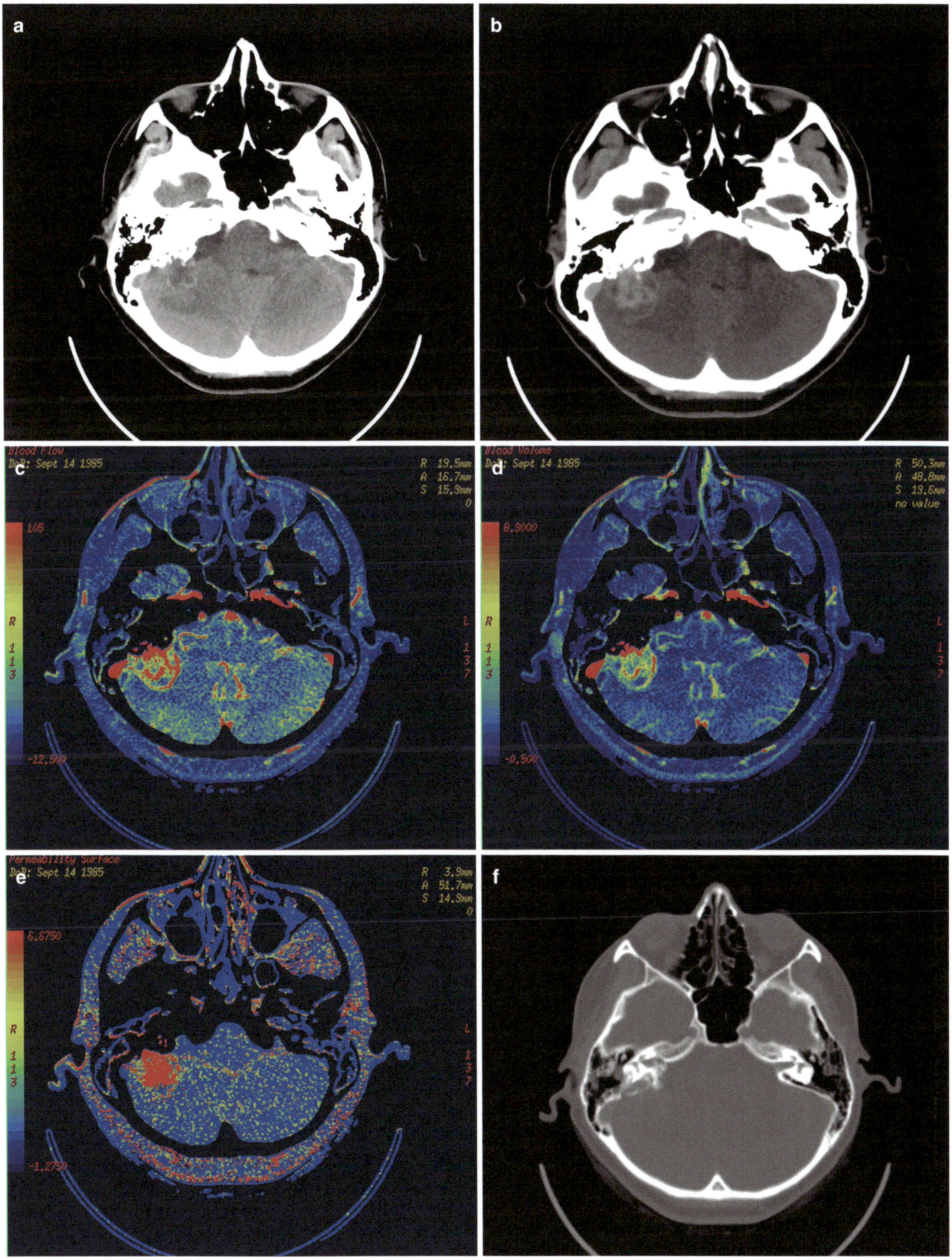
a
b
Blood Flow
c
105
-12.500
Blood Volume
d
8.9000
-0.500
Permeability Surface
e
6.5750
-1.2750
f

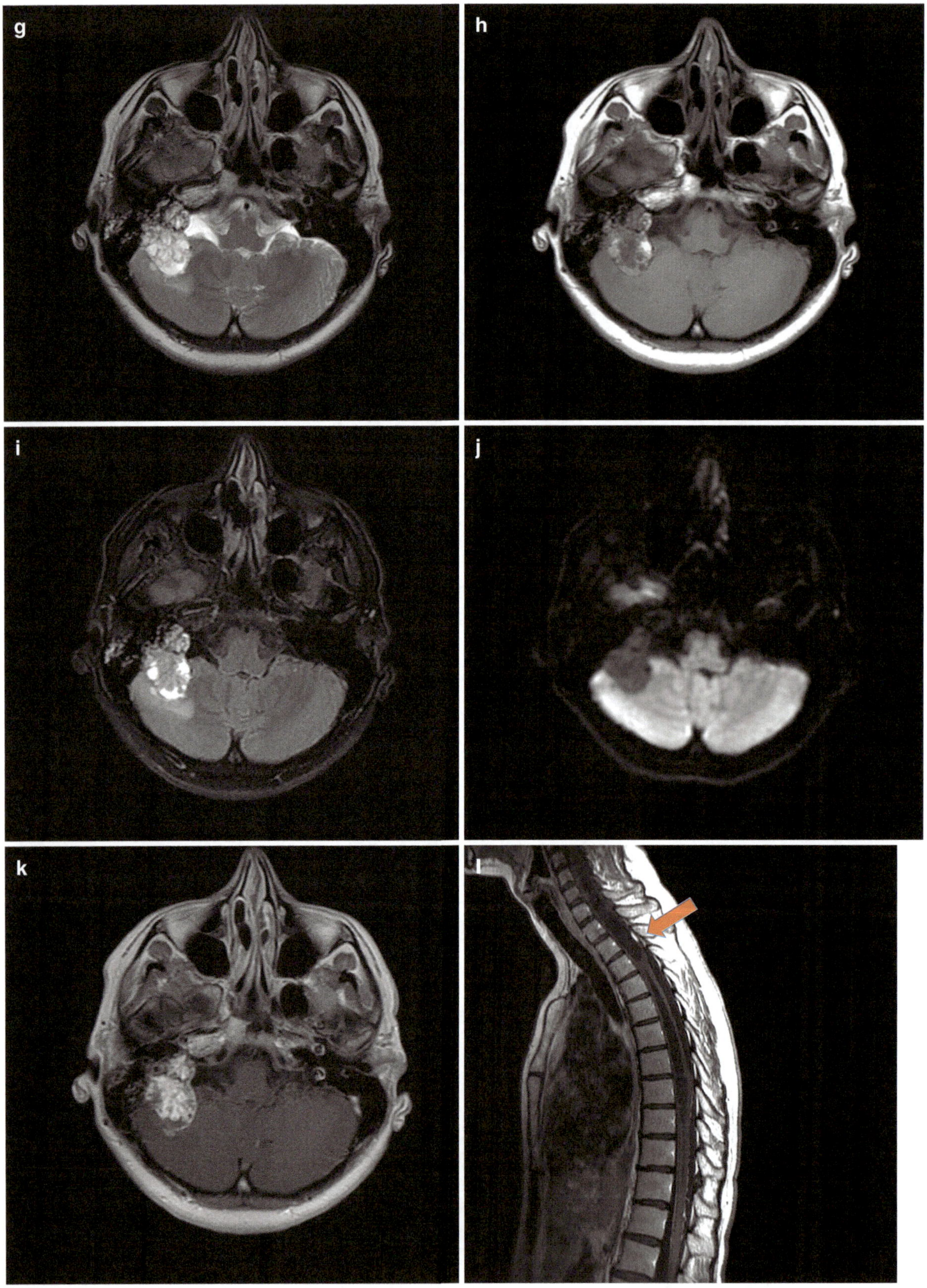

Fig. 24.14 (continued)

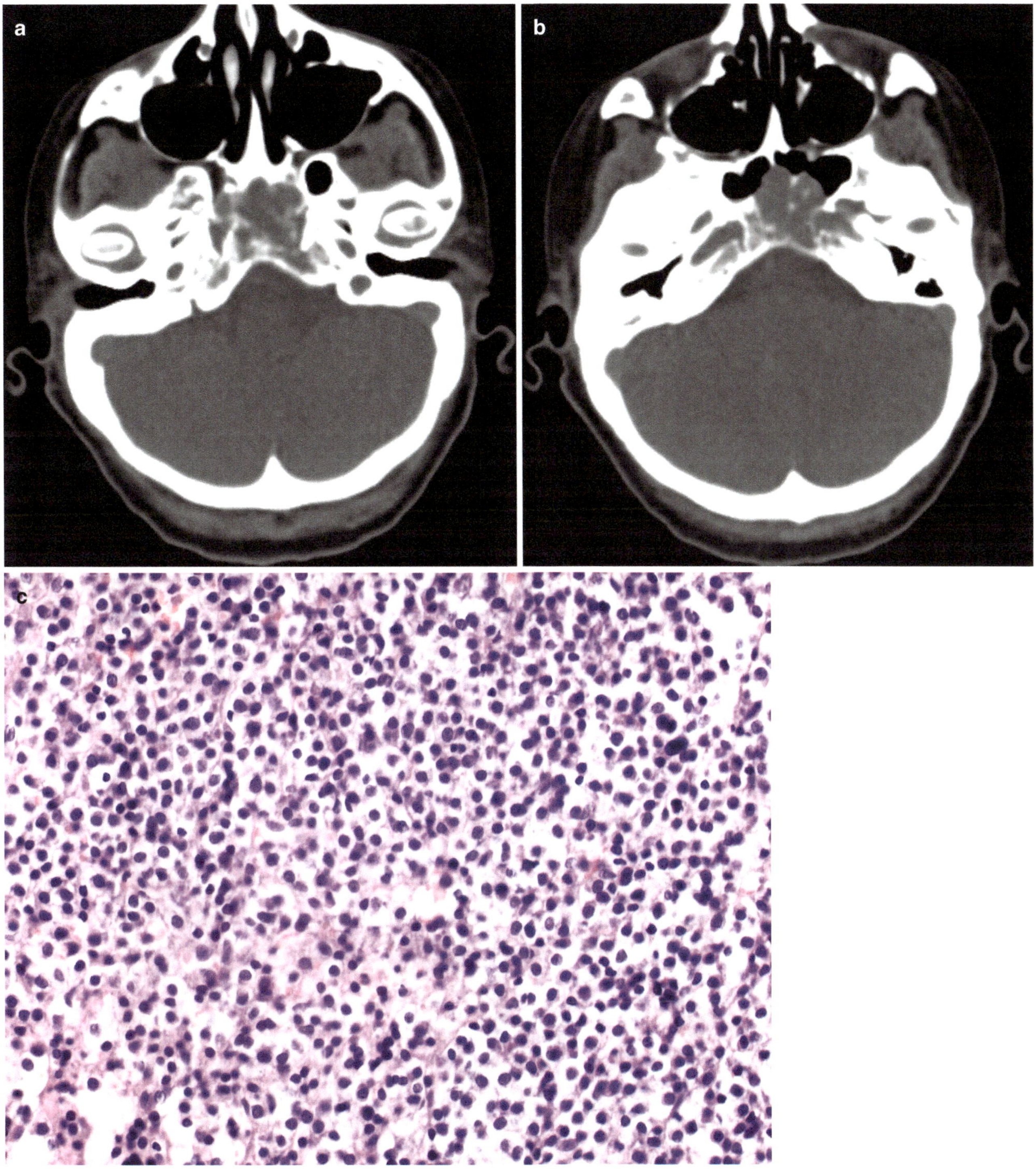

Fig. 24.15 Plasmacytoma of the sphenoid bone. Axial NECT scans (**a**, **b**) demonstrate an expansile isodense lesion in the projection of sphenoid bone, which leads to destruction of surrounding bone structures. Frontal pole of the tumor prolapses into the sphenoid sinus. Histological specimen (**c**)

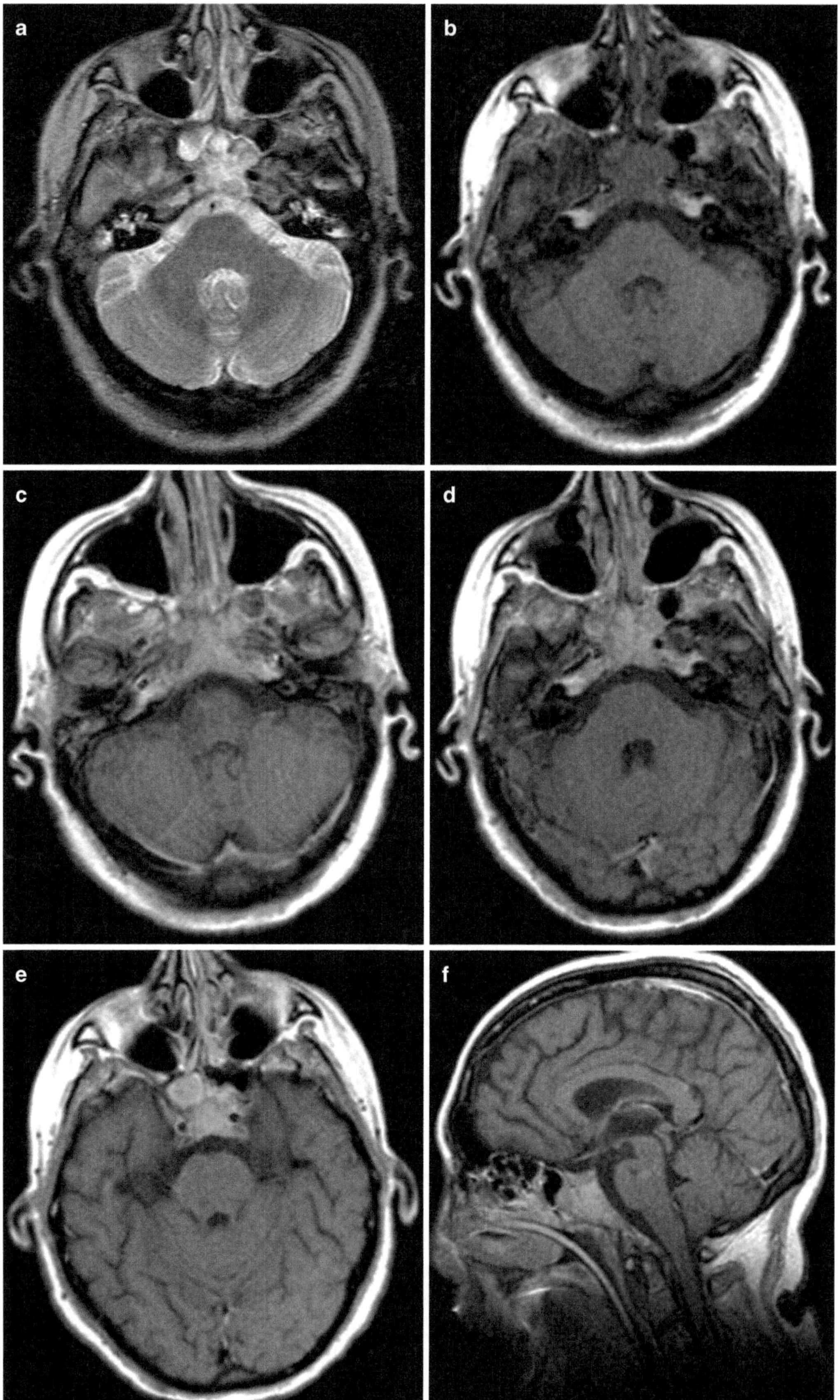

Fig. 24.16 Plasmacytoma of sphenoid bone (CT scans are on Fig. 24.15). Axial T2 (**a**), T1- weighted MR images before (**b**) and after (**c–e**) contrast enhancement show a soft tissue tumor which is hyperintense on T2 and isointense on T1. Contrast enhancement is homogeneous and prominent. Boundaries of the tumor are blurred within bones of the skull base on the standard T1-weighted image (**f**)

1. A primary bone tumor without any evidence of its presence in other tissues;
2. Soft tissue lymphoma;
3. Primary soft tissue lymphomatosis with bone metastases.

The disease usually begins with onset of pain, getting worse at night, often intermittent (Lee et al. 1987; Nathu et al. 1999). Pain can occur in the joints, not in the bones. The process develops for a relatively long time and is more benign than Ewing's sarcoma. Generally, bone lymphomas of the skull base are rare.

Imaging Most authors suggest that bone lymphoma has no pathognomonic radiological features. At the initial phases of the disease, radiologic diagnosis of bone lymphoma is very difficult. Periosteal reaction is rare and does not have any specific features. The cortex is destroyed to greater or lesser extent, but is not melted, as in cases with osteolytic tumors like osteosarcomas. Multiple small-focal destructions are considered as a classic manifestation that creates the picture of porous, mottled bone. Small-focal destructions are a relatively early lymphoma symptom that is not always radiologically visible. With progression of the tumor, small foci coalesce into extensive lytic areas that cause considerable diagnostic difficulties during primary evaluation of patients.

CT scanning detects lytic bone changes as areas of reduced density (Rosenstiel et al. 2001). After administration of contrast agent, lymphoma intensively enhance0s (Fig. 24.17).

Differential Diagnosis Ewing's sarcoma, osteosarcoma (more severe lysis with periosteal reaction), osteoblastoclastoma (only lysis without small focal destruction).

Langerhans cell histiocytosis (synonyms: histiocytosis X, Hand-Schüller-Christian disease, eosinophilic granuloma, Taratynov's disease, Letterer-Siwe disease) is a disease with extremely varied clinical manifestations and course, characterized by the accumulation and/or proliferation of cells with characteristics of epidermal histiocytes, Langerhans cells. This is a very rare disease; its incidence in children is 3–4 cases per one million children per year, being even rarer in adults (Cunningham et al. 1989).

There are single-system (involvement of one organ or organ system) and multi-system (involvement of two or more organs or organ systems) forms of the disease. A single-system disease can occur with a single focus (unifocal) or two or more foci (multifocal), with or without impairment of the function of vital organs.

The etiology and pathogenesis of the disease are still unknown. Immunopathological and oncologic nature of the disease are suggested. The immunopathological nature is evidenced by a high rate of spontaneous remission, low mortality (in children 15%, in adults 3%), and lack of chromosomal abnormalities in cells from the lesions. The oncologic nature is evidenced by clonal proliferation of Langerhans cells in lesions.

Clinical symptoms and outcomes of Langerhans histiocytosis (HLH) range from spontaneously healing isolated lesions to rapidly progressive disseminated forms, leading to multiple organ failure. Isolated or multiple bone lesions are the most frequent, mainly of the cranial vault, legs, ribs, pelvis, vertebrae, lower jaw. Bone disease is manifested by pain and swelling coming from the focus of tissue destruction. If lesions are located in the upper and lower jaws, tooth loss occurs. Involvement of the temporal bone and mastoid process is accompanied by the development of clinical otitis media.

A single lesion form of HLH, also called eosinophilic granuloma, is among the most favorable disease subtype in terms of treatment and prognosis. It is usually diagnosed in children older than 5 years of age. The lesion is located exclusively in the bone structure. These are usually long bones, skull, skull base (mostly temporal bone and mastoid process). The prognosis is good, with possible complete recovery.

Hand-Schüller-Christian disease is a more aggressive form of HLH. It is often revealed in children aged 1–5 years old. The disease involves numerous bone structures, skin, abdomen, and brain. Its clinical signs are characterized by the primary triad of symptoms: diabetes insipidus, exophthalmos, and involvement of skeletal bones. The prognosis is relatively favorable.

An extreme form of HLH is Letterer-Siwe disease, prognosis in most cases being poor with high mortality of children in early childhood. It is usually diagnosed before the age of 3 years old. It is a rapidly progressive multi-system and multi-organ disease affecting the liver, spleen, lymphatic system, lungs, and skeletal bones.

Imaging X-ray examination of bones and lungs is needed to identify and assess the extent of HLH. Typical lesions in the skeleton bones have lytic nature. Mixed, osteolytic, and osteoplastic lesions are rare.

CT and MRI are the most sensitive imaging techniques to visualize lesions of the bone vault and skull base, allowing to identify involvement of skull bone structures at the stages not accessible for visualization by X-ray imaging.

CT scanning detects an area of sharply defined bone-destructive lesion with "beveled" edges in the pyramid and mastoid process. Edges of the destructive area can be sufficiently well-defined ("punched out" lesions) or inhomogeneous, but usually with sclerotic boundary changes. Involvement of middle ear structures is typical. Bone fragments in the structure of a soft-tissue part of the lesion can be observed. After intravenous contrast enhancement, heterogeneous, but quite pronounced contrast enhancement is noted.

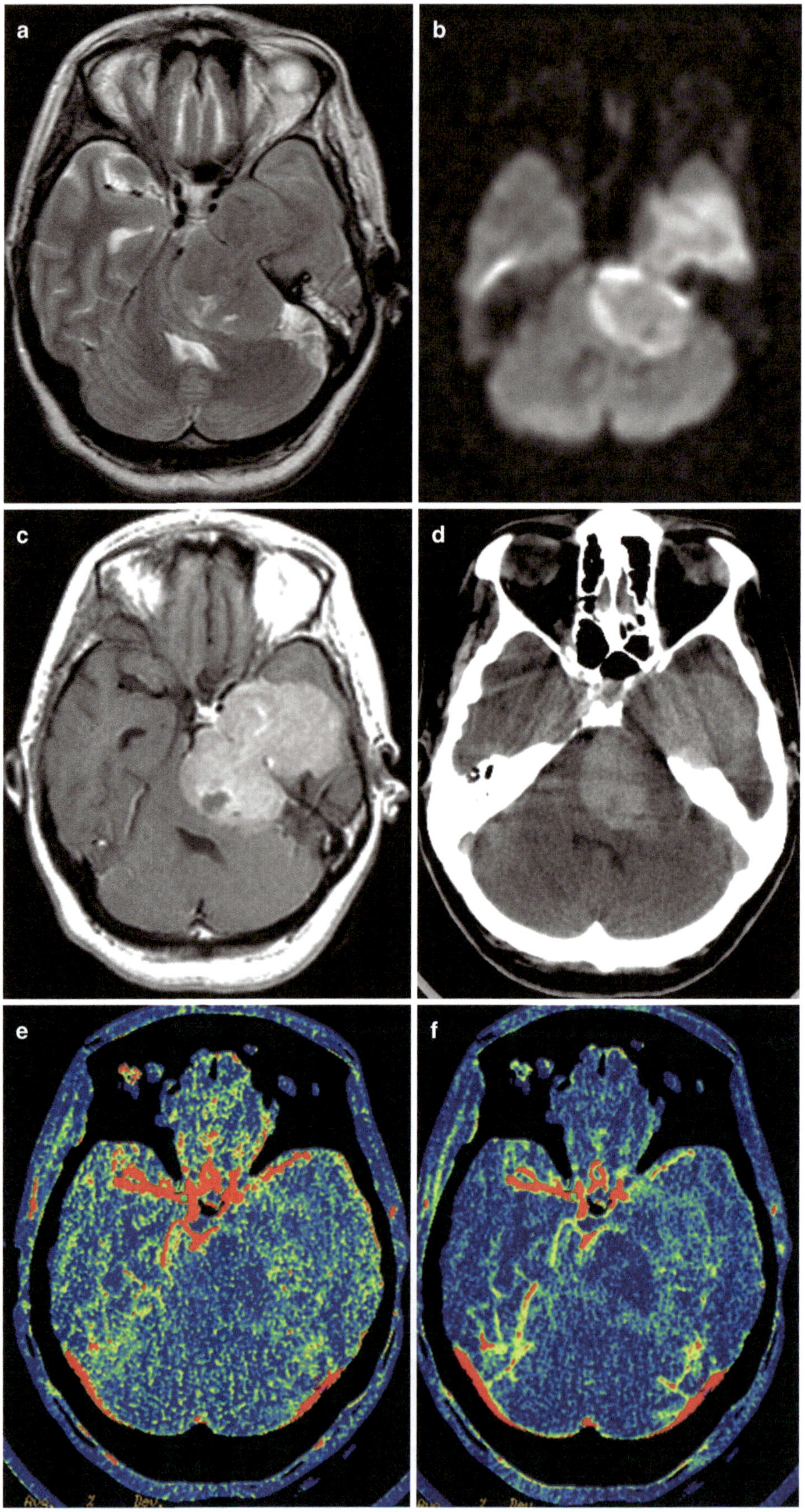

Fig. 24.17 Histiocytic lymphoma of the skull base. Axial T2- (**a**) and diffusion- (**b**) weighted MR images demonstrate a large solid tumor that has supra- and subtentorial spreading. On DWI (**b**) lesion has hyperintense MR-signal and is characterized by strong contrast enhancement as on T1 MRI (**c**) as on CT (**d**). CT-perfusion study (CBF (**e**), CBV (**f**)) demonstrates typical for lymphoma low perfusion parameters

On MRI, eosinophilic granuloma has iso- or hypointense MR-signal on T1-weighted sequences, located in the projection of mastoid process, the middle ear cavity and adjacent parts of the skull base. MR-signal on T2-weighted images is hyperintense or has signal characteristics similar to the gray matter of the brain (Angeli et al. 1996). Foci of low MR-signal (microhemorrhages) may look as black-spot inclusions. Contrast enhancement is pronounced and heterogeneous, improving the assessment of the lesion growth both within the bones of the base, and into the cranial cavity (an epidural extent is typical for eosinophilic granuloma) (Fig. 24.18).

Differential Diagnosis Inflammatory diseases (acute mastoiditis, otitis media), cholesterol granuloma (high MR-signal on T1-weighted sequences and smooth contour), cholesteatoma (high MR-signal on DWI), mesenchymal tumors (rhabdomyosarcoma, leiomyosarcoma, etc.).

Tumor metastases in bones, unfortunately, are quite common in oncology. Most often breast cancer (47–85%), prostate cancer (54–85%), thyroid (28–60%), kidney (33–40%), lung (32–40%), melanoma (12%), ovarian (9%), esophagus (5–7%), rectum (8–13%) cancers metastasize to the skull bones. Skull bones metastases occur in 20% of all bone metastases. Metastasizing to the vertebral bodies and skull bones can occur not via the system blood flow (hematogenously), but through the vertebral venous plexus—a valveless system of venous anastomoses running along the spine from the brain to the pelvis. Tumor cells secrete a variety of factors that start to affect osteoclasts, increasing their activity and accelerating the process of bone destruction (osteolytic metastases). Hence, bone thinning, fractures even at low loads occur. In some tumors (e.g., prostate cancer), osteoblasts are activated, which leads to excessive growth of bone tissue (osteoplastic metastases). The type of metastases, osteolytic or osteoplastic, depends on the ratio of activity of osteoclasts and osteoblasts.

The main clinical manifestation of tumor metastases in the bone is a pain, which occurs in most cases. Pain occurs as a result of tumor infiltration of nerve endings, an increase in intraosseous pressure, fracture, as well as stimulation of nerve endings by the substances secreted by the tumor. Osteolytic metastases are characterized by pathological fractures in the majority of cases (Gautier-Smith 1960).

Imaging The valuable diagnostic method for detecting bone metastases, including the bones of the vault and skull base is scintigraphy, which allows to obtain the overall picture of a skeleton with foci of radiopharmaceutical hyperfixation. If needed, screening may be continued using target radiography. However, current oncologic search for metastases cannot be imagined without the use of advanced neuroimaging techniques. Multi-detector spiral CT scanners provide a high-quality imaging of the bony of skeleton and skull in combination with a short acquisition time, allowing recommend this method as the first line investigation in detection of early stages of metastatic disease (Healy et al. 1981). If the presence of soft tissue component is suspected, the additional intravenous contrast enhancement is needed.

Localization of bone metastases in the skull base area is characterized by destruction of bone tissue, without clear contours and lack of sclerotic boundary changes (Zimmerman and Bilaniuk 1980). On CT scans majority of metastatic nodules moderately or intensely accumulate contrast agent (Figs. 24.19 and 24.20).

On MRI bones metastases are better visualize using the Fat-Sat technique before and after intravenous contrast enhancement. It not only provides visualization of the soft-tissue, extraosseous part of the tumor, but also allows to define intraosseous bone marrow infiltration and the degree of adjacent meninges invasion. When evaluating soft tissues of the skull base, this technology clarifies the degree of infiltration of the muscular structures, tumor extension under the skull base and even regional enlargement of lymph nodes in the neck. At the same time, CT and MRI data do not allow to differentiate the source of metastatic bone lesions of the vault and skull base, firstly because of the diversity of their primary nature, and secondly because of the lack of typical radiological features in most cases. If metastatic lesions are located in the brain (brainstem, cerebellum hemisphere), a detailed complex differential diagnosis has to be conducted based on many factors, including both medical history and imaging data (Figs. 24.21, 24.22, and 24.23).

An important additional diagnostic method in terms of the differential diagnosis between benign and malignant tumors of the skull base, affecting bone structures, is CT-perfusion, which allows to determine increased hemodynamic parameters, typical for some metastatic tumors.

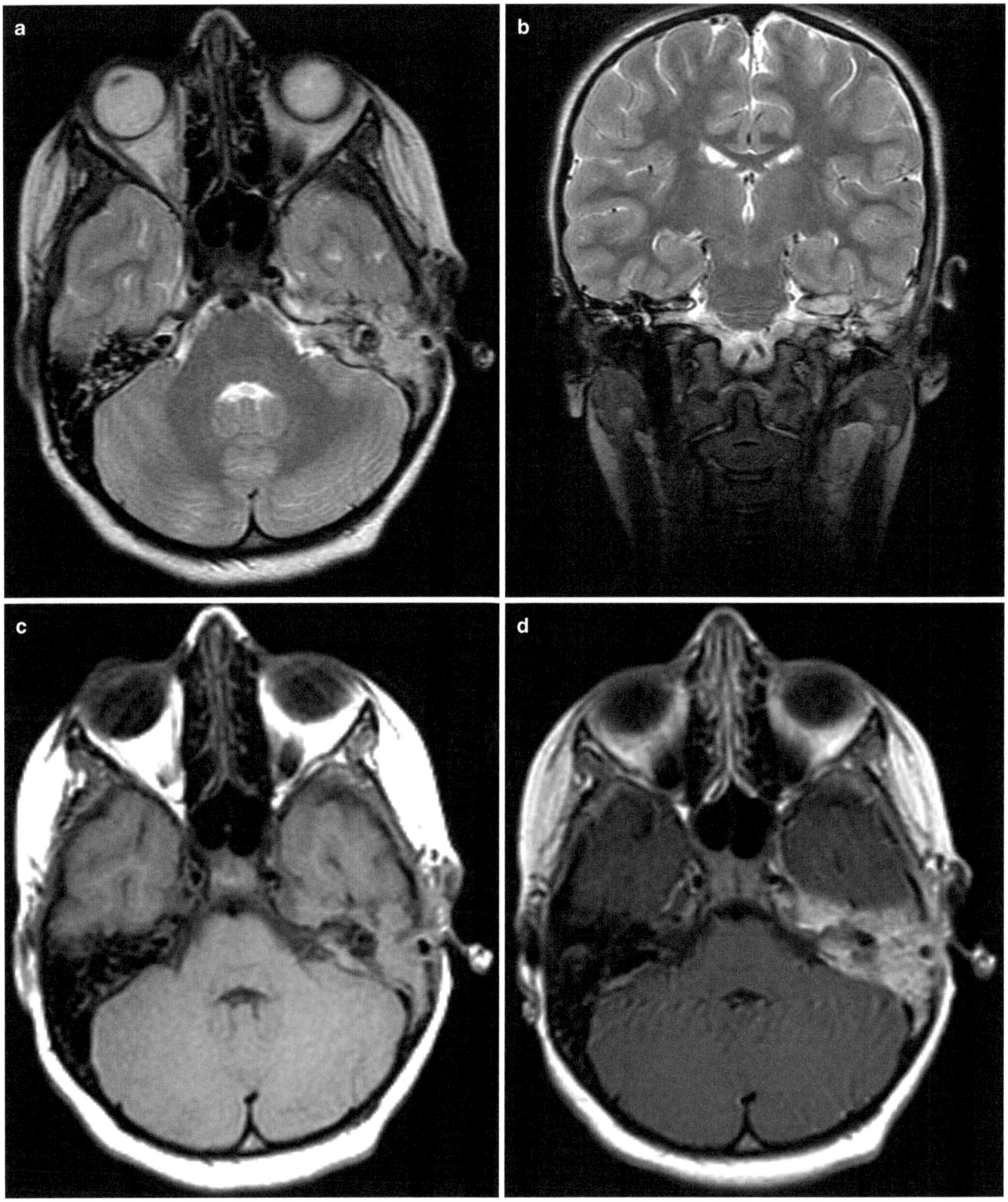

Fig. 24.18 Eosinophilic granuloma of the temporal bone pyramid on the left. On T2 (**a**, **b**)- and T1-weighted MR images before (**c**) and after (**d**, **e**) contrast enhancement the slightly hyperintense area in the projection of the temporal bone pyramid and mastoid cells is visible. The lesion involves the whole pyramid, part of mastoid cells and squamous portion of temporal bone. Lesion is characterized by homogeneous and strong contrast enhancement improving the visualization of the tumor expansion (**d**, **e**). Histological specimen (**f**)

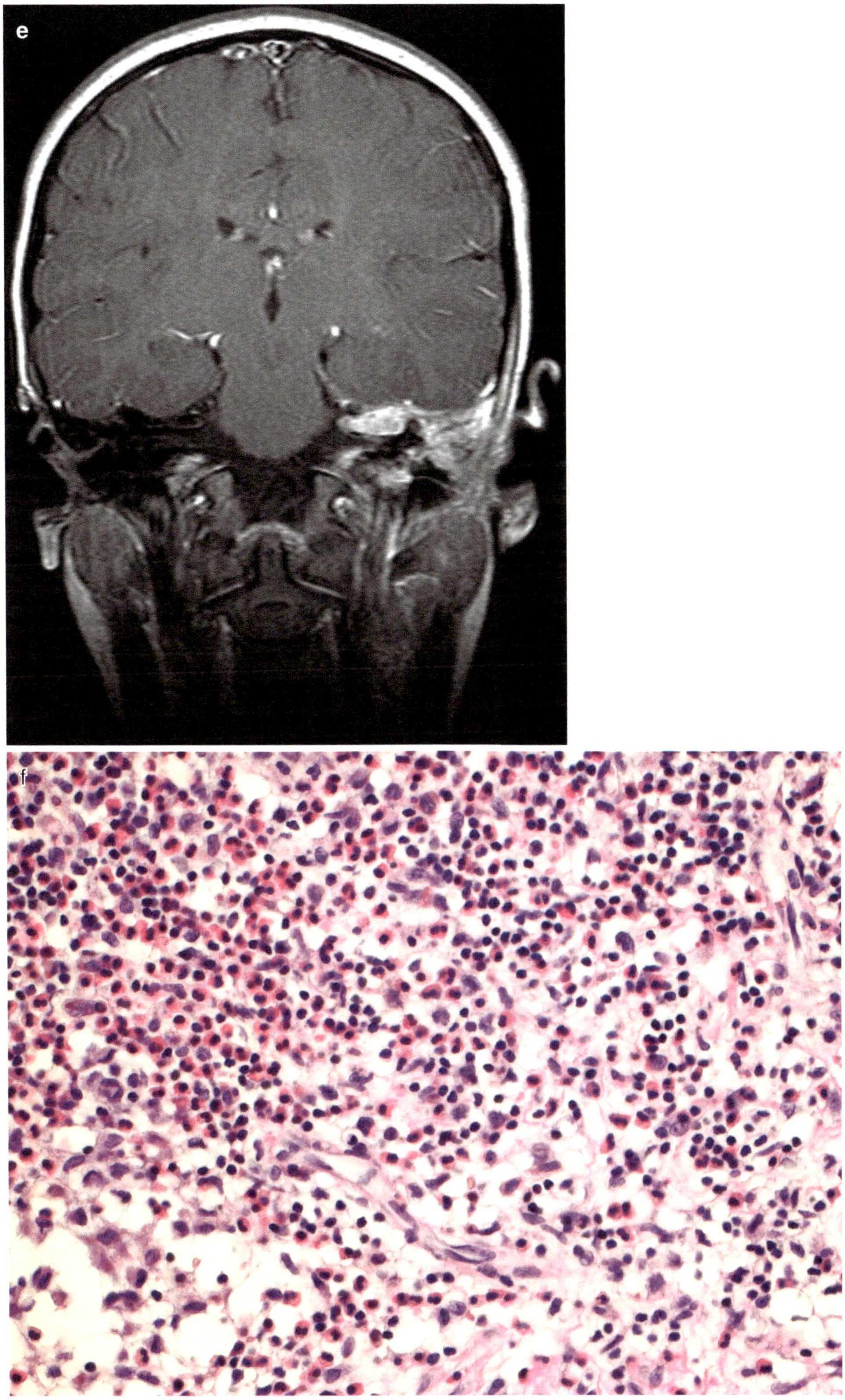

Fig. 24.18 (continued)

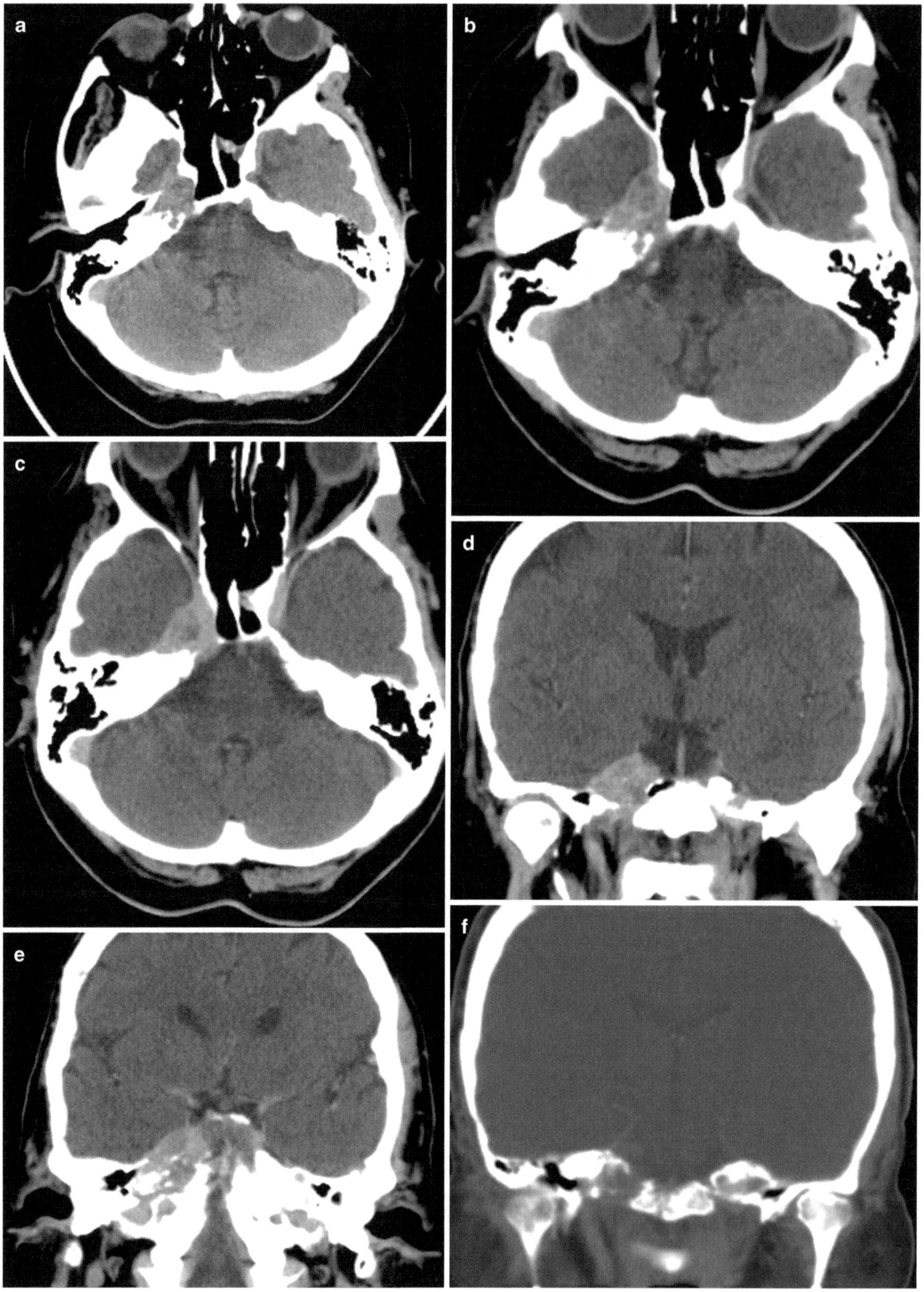

Fig. 24.19 Metastasis of cancer into the skull base on the right. Axial NECT (**a**) and series of CECT scans (**b–f**) demonstrate a soft tissue lesion located in the projection of the right temporal bone apex and in lateral parts of sphenoid bone, which leads to destruction of surrounding bones (**f**). The tumor has a prominent contrast enhancement

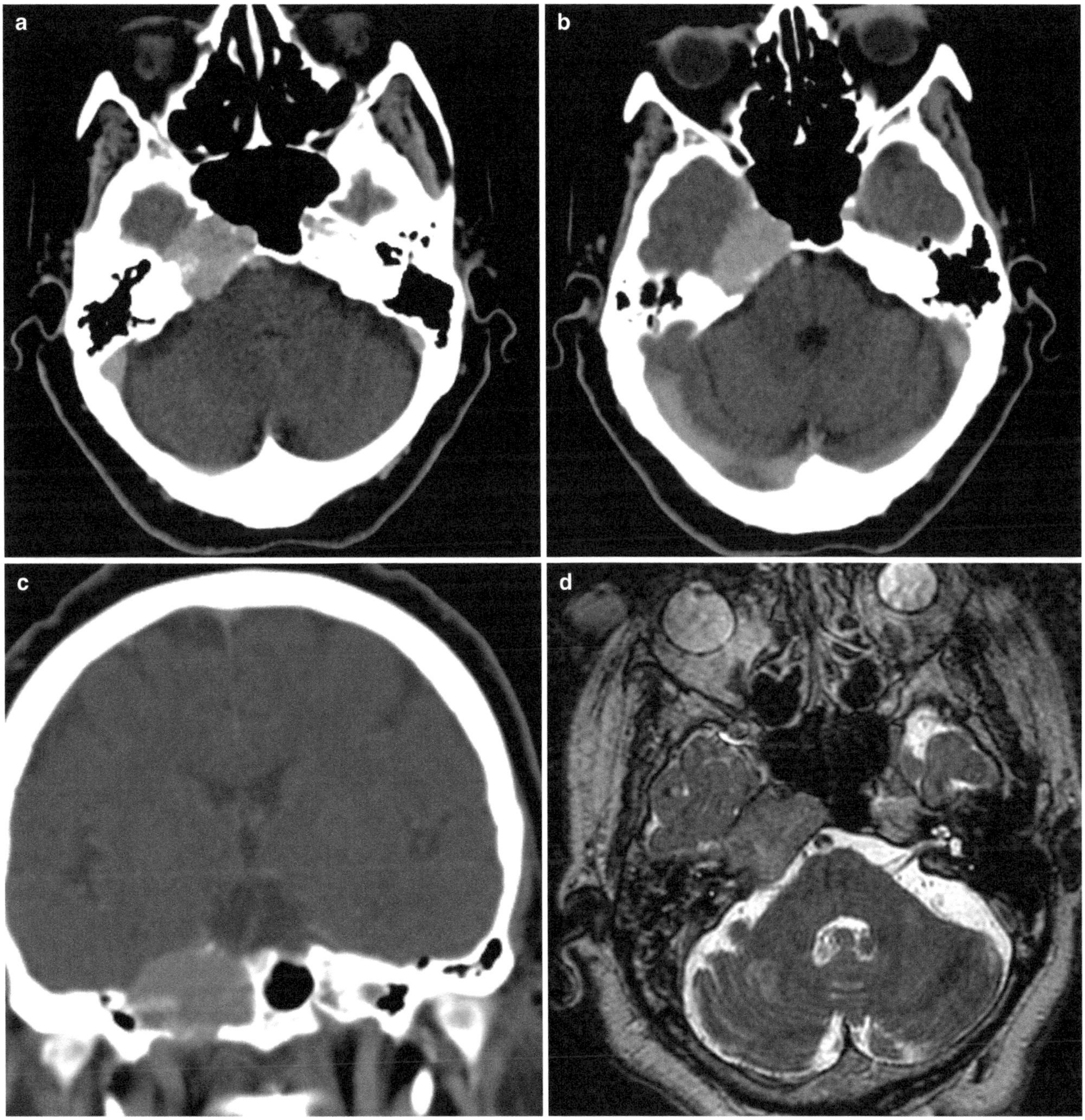

Fig. 24.20 Metastasis of cancer into the skull base on the right. CECT scans (**a–c**) reveal a homogeneously enhancing lesion located in the projection of temporal bone apex and in lateral parts of sphenoid bone, which leads to destruction of surrounding bones. On T2- (**d**) and postenhanced T1- (**e**, **f**) weighted MR images the metastasis has an isointense MR-signal compare to the brain and prominent and homogeneous contrast enhancement

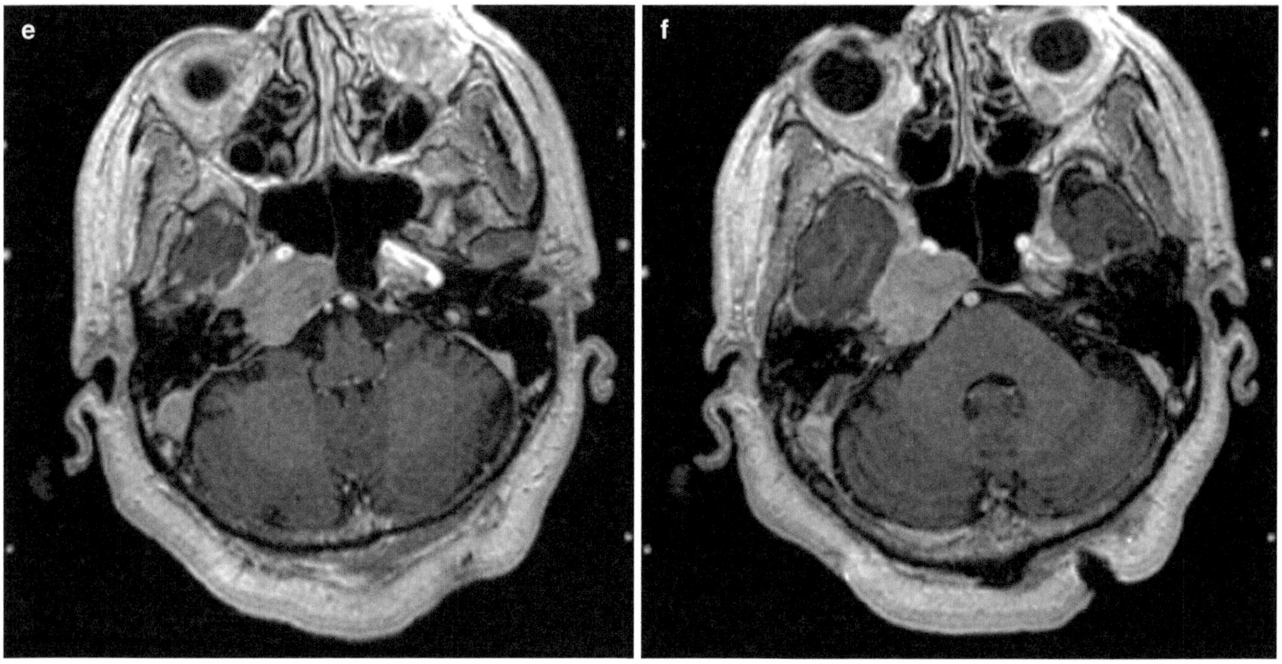

Fig. 24.20 (continued)

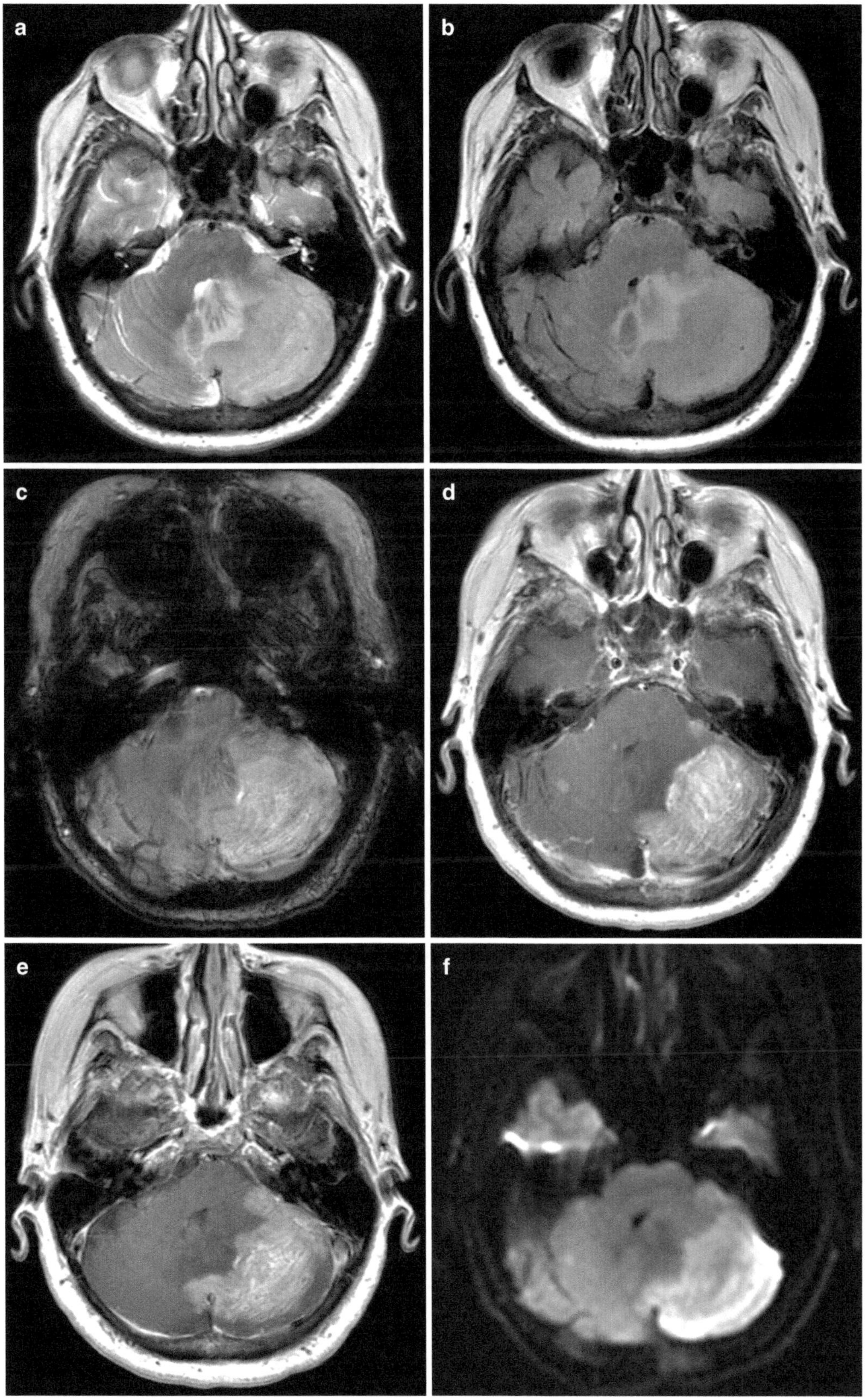

Fig. 24.21 Metastasis of the cancer into the left cerebellar hemisphere. T2- (**a**), T2-FLAIR (**b**), SWAN (**c**)weighted MR images demonstrate an isointense compared to brain MR-signal tumor of the left half of posterior cranial fossa with surrounding edema. A lesion has hyperintense MR-signal on SWAN without evidences for hemorrhages. On post-contrast T1-weighted images (**d**, **e**) tumor is characterized by fairly homogeneous and prominent contrast enhancement. Hyperintense MR-signal on DWI (**f**) simulates the lymphoma or acute ischemia appearance

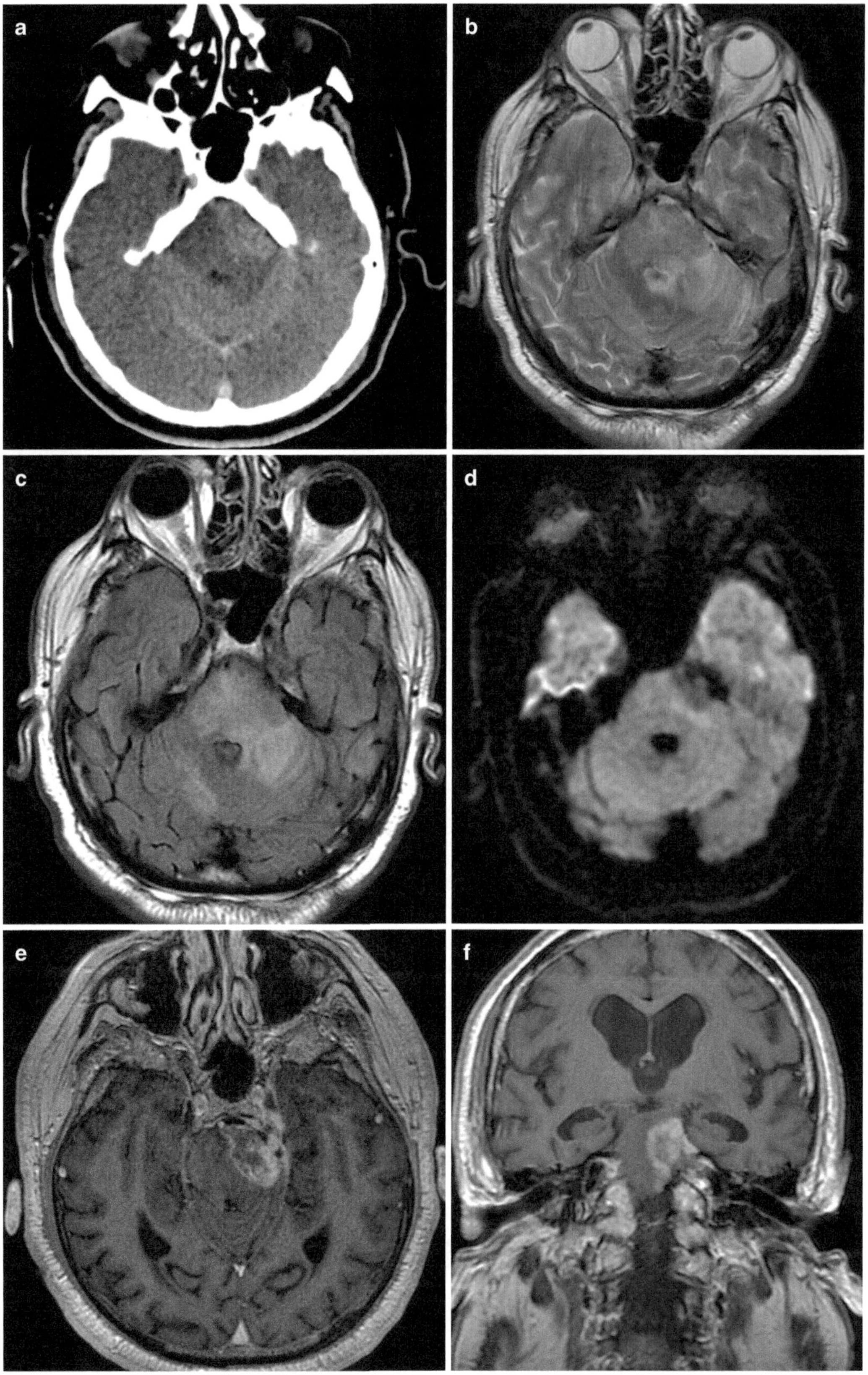

Fig. 24.22 Metastasis of cancer into petroclival area on the left. Axial CECT scan (**a**) shows the solid tumor with intermediate enhancement, border with brainstem is not well-defined. MRI using T2- (**b**) and T2-FLAIR (**c**) sequences demonstrates a poorly delineated tumor of petro-clival region on the left with edema of pons and middle cerebellar peduncle. On DWI (**d**) the tumor has demarcation with brain due to hyperintense perifocal edema. Contrast-enhanced MR imaging allows to improve the delineation of the lesion, estimation of tumor structure and its extension into the left Meckel's cavity (**e**, **f**)

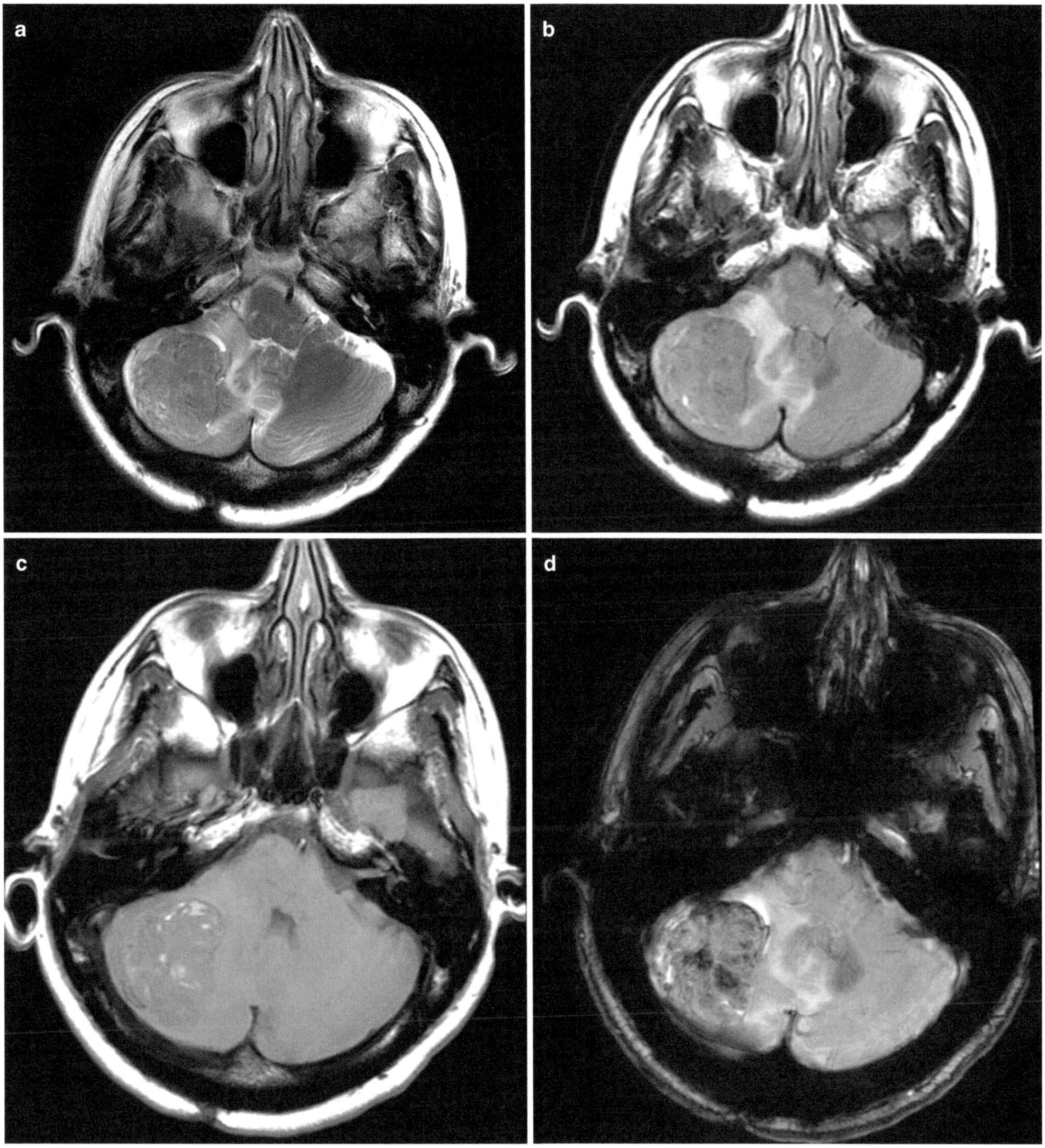

Fig. 24.23 Metastasis of thyroid gland cancer into posterior cranial fossa. Axial T2- (**a**), T2-FLAIR-, (**b**) and T1- (**c**) weighted MR images visualize a solid isointense with brain tumor, which is surrounded with brain edema. The tumor has sharp boundaries due to perifocal edema. In the tumor stroma there are multiple microhemorrhages with high MR-signal on T1 (**c**) and hypointense signal on SWAN (**d**) images. There is a homogeneous and intensive accumulation of contrast medium in the tumor (**e**). H1MR-spectroscopy shows high peaks of myo-inositol and Lipid-Lactate complex with decrease of NAA peak (**f**)

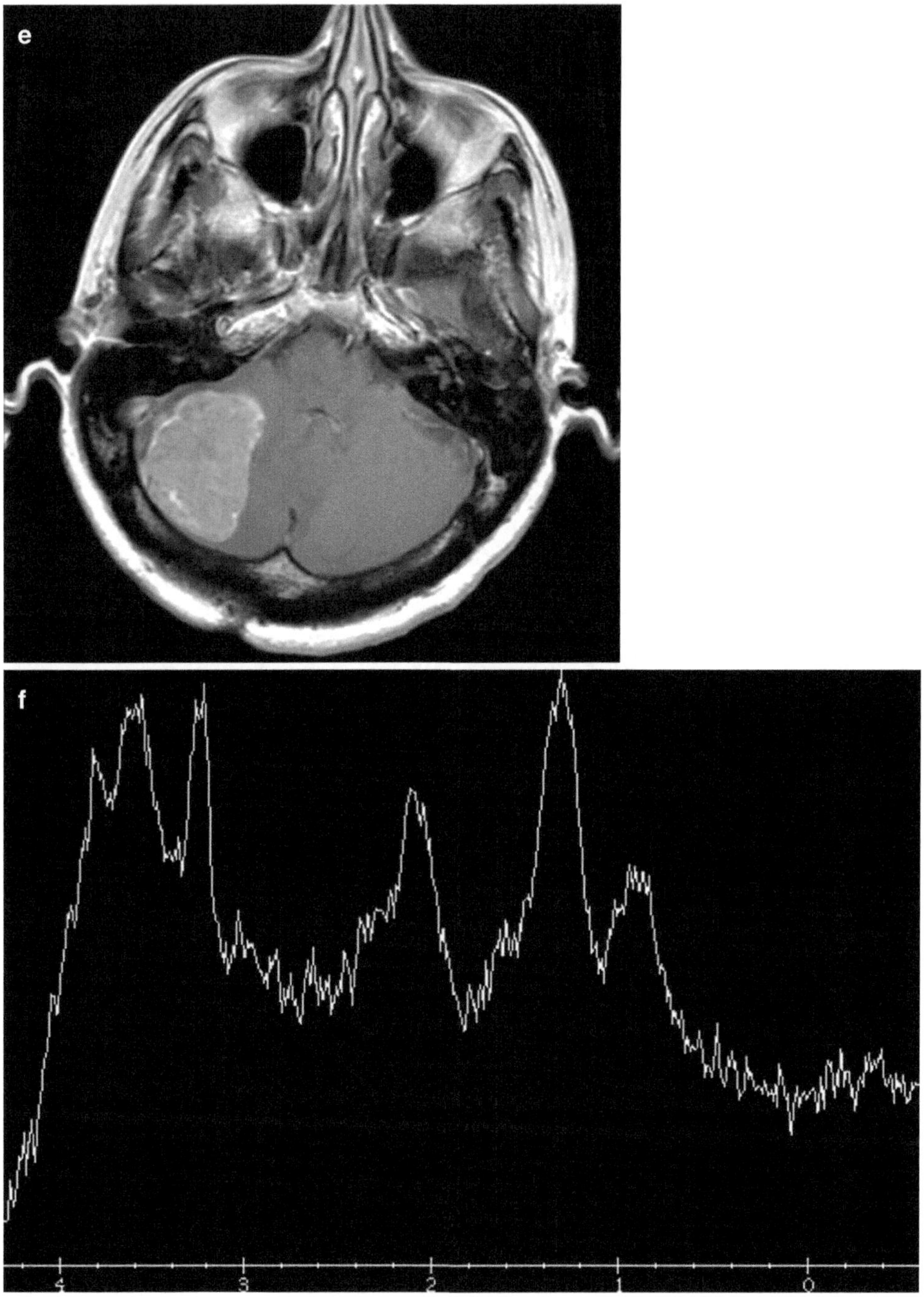

Fig. 24.23 (continued)

Fibro-Osseous Disorders

25

Fibrous dysplasia (FD) (synonyms: fibrous osteodysplasia, fibrous bone dysplasia, Lichtenstein-Braitsev disease) is a benign non-neoplastic tumor-like congenital lesion, manifested as a localized defect in osteoblastic differentiation and maturation with the replacement of normal bone with fibrous stroma and islands of immature bone. The term "fibrous dysplasia" was introduced by Liechtenstein (1938), who first described disorders characterized by progressive replacement of normal bone elements by fibrous tissue. In 70%, there is a local one-sided lesion; spreading to the facial skeleton is observed in 25%. Malignant (sarcomatous) transformation into osteosarcoma occurs in 0.5%.

Reasons for the development of fibrous dysplasia are not clearly understood; the role of heredity is not excluded. It is believed that disease is based on a tumor-like process associated with abnormal development of osteogenic mesenchyme. The disease often begins in childhood, but can occur in the young, middle, and old age. Seventy five percent of patients presenting before the age of 30 years. The disease is prevalent in females (Adada et al. 2003).

Microscopy shows multiple osteoid irregularly shaped trabeculae, lying in the fibrous tissue with a small number of osteoblasts. Osteoid trabeculae represent mostly fibrous, rather than compact bone. Small portions of osteoid may be calcified. Calcium is usually deposited in the center of a trabecula. There are multinuclear cells of osteoclast type bordering some trabeculae. In the peripheral parts, a fibrous dysplasia lesion merges with reactive bone without any sharp borders. Fibrous stroma is collagenized in some places, has myxomatous properties in others, and is rich in cellular elements in some places or almost devoid of them in others. Fibroblasts may have large, oval, or elongated nuclei that look as if shriveled. There are cartilage islets calcified on the periphery between hypertrophied fibrous tissue and osteoid.

Depending on the process growth, there are two forms of fibrous dysplasia: monostotic, affecting only one bone, and polyostotic, affecting several bones, mainly on one side of the body. The polyostotic form of fibrous dysplasia can be combined with skin melanosis and various endocrinopathies (McCune-Albright syndrome). Monoostotic form of fibrous dysplasia can develop at any age, but these are patients under 30 years in 75% of cases. This form comprises up to 70% of all cases of fibrous dysplasia, most often affects the skull base and facial skeleton. By incidence, it is distributed as follows: upper jaw (zygomatic arch), mandible, frontal bone, sphenoid bone and ethmoidal labyrinth, petrous bone. A polyostotic form is often diagnosed in children (mean age of 8 years), so patients with this form of fibrous dysplasia have pronounced diffuse deformation of the skeleton and predisposition to multiple fractures. Skull base and facial skeleton are affected in up to 50% of cases.

According to another approach FD can be divided into four subtypes: monostotic, polyostotic, craniofacial dysplasia (skull and facial bones alone), and cherubism (involving only mandibular and maxilla (considered as a not true FD).

McCune-Albright syndrome is a subtype of the polyostotic form of fibrous dysplasia, and includes the following triad of manifestations: usually unilateral polyostotic form of fibrous dysplasia, endocrine disorders (premature sexual development), and skin hyperpigmentation ("coffee grounds" like spots). It occurs in 2–3% of fibrous dysplasia cases.

Any form of fibrous dysplasia can affect the temporal bone and its elements, such as external auditory canal, middle ear, jugular vein foramina, petrous bone cells with relevant clinical manifestations: tinnitus, conducting or neurosensory hearing loss with satisfactory general health (Sharma et al. 2002; Hullar et al. 2003). The nature of hearing loss is secondary and dependent on the site of the process (in the external auditory canal—conducting hearing loss, in the pyramid—neurosensory hearing loss). In 50% of cases, clinical manifestations are similar to Paget's disease.

Imaging CT shows an abnormally thickened bone area at the projection of the bone marrow with variable density.

I. Pronin, V. Kornienko, *CT and MRI of Skull Base Lesions*, https://doi.org/10.1007/978-3-319-65957-2_25

A sclerotic form (25% of FD) is characterized by a high density on CT described as the ground-glass pattern, with typical swelling of dense bone structures, absence of clear boundaries of the process within the bone, which distinguishes it from osteoma or ossifying fibroma (Fig. 25.1). A Paget-like form of the disease (up to 50% of FD) is manifested by a combination of fields with low and high density of bone tissue, while a cystic form (25%) is manifested only by spread of hypodense areas surrounded by the thin sclerotic bone. Pure cystic dysplasia is difficult to diagnose,

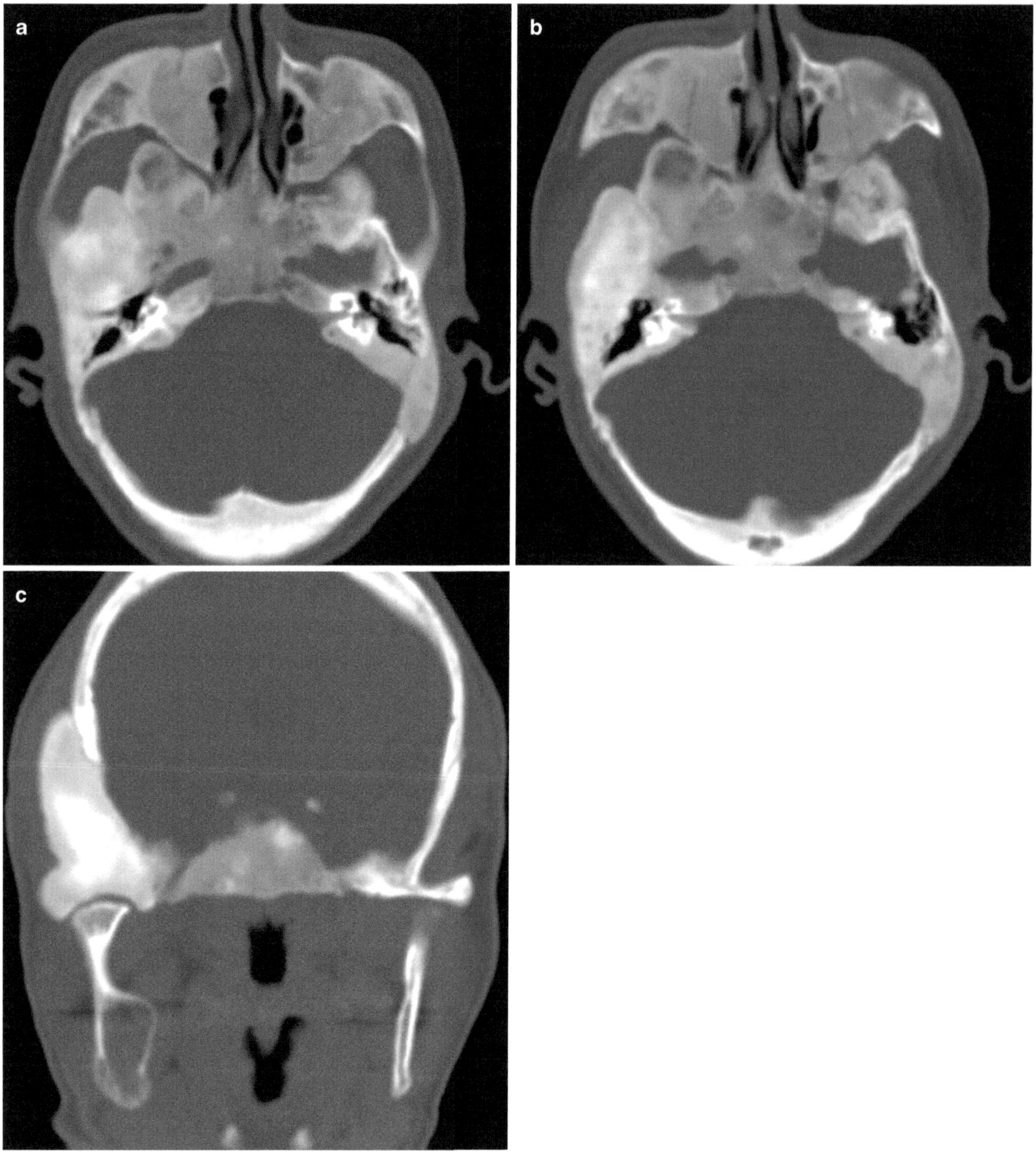

Fig. 25.1 Extensive fibrous dysplasia of the skull base and craniofacial bones. On axial CT scans (**a**, **b**) and with coronal reformation (**c**) the wide involvement of skull base bones is detected. CT imaging demonstrates a pathologic thickening of bone structures, mostly on the right side with "ground glass" pattern. Also there is a disappearance of sphenoid and maxillary sinuses. Dysplasia also affects the temporal bone on the right side and facial bones

because it can mimic manifestations of such aggressive diseases as rhabdomyosarcoma, small cell lung cancer, metastatic disease, which often shows an abrupt border between diseased and healthy bone. When the petrous pyramid is affected in fibrous dysplasia, the eardrum membrane remains intact. The degree of contrast enhancement is always difficult to assess due to the presence of high bone density, with the exception of bone loss area.

MRI shows a hypointense MR-signal on T1-weighted sequence in ossified or fibrous parts of FD. On T2-weighted images, MR-signal is also reduced. Heterogeneity of MR signal is possible; a spotty form precedes a cystic variant. After administration of contrast agent, its accumulation is noted in heterogeneous areas. PET-imaging can show accumulation of C11-methionine, but no accumulation of FDG.

Differential Diagnosis Paget's disease (more diffuse and more symmetrical involvement of bone disease), intraosseous meningioma (presence of enhanced soft tissue component, visualization of a dural "tail" symptom), giant cell tumor, ossifying fibroma (often mimics the cystic form of PD, a low signal on T2-WI due to the presence of hemosiderin, more intensely accumulates contrast agent), metastases, chondrosarcoma (located at the projection of the petro-occipital suture, annular sclerotic edge visualized in 50% of cases).

Paget's disease (also known as osteitis deformans, deforming osteodystrophy) occurs when the bone recovery mechanism is damaged. Bone tissue is composed of organic and inorganic (mineral) parts. The first one includes collagen, albumin, and other proteins. Inorganic part of the bone, which accounts for about 65% of weight, consists of hydroxyapatite (it contains calcium and phosphorus). Bone tissue is constantly regenerating, i.e. restored. Constant bone turnover occurs due to cells destroying the bone (osteoclasts) and cells producing it (osteoblasts). Full bone turnover occurs approximately every 10 years.

Paget's disease can occur in any bone of the skeleton. In one third of patients, only one bone is affected, but the average number of damaged bones is about three. Bones, most often involved in the process, include pelvis, spine, skull, long bones of hands and feet. If the skull bones are affected, the cranial vault, base and temporal bone are involved most often, with relative intactness of the facial skull (Hullar et al. 2003).

Up to 3% of Caucasians over the age of 40 years old have clinical and radiological manifestations of Paget's disease, its incidence increases with age, occurs twice as often in men as in women. Causes of Paget's disease are still unknown. The most common opinion is about the viral nature of the disease (slow viral infection). Measles is considered as one of the most significant viral infection (Donath et al. 2004).

Symptoms of Paget's disease include pain around the damaged bone and osteoarthritis if the disease occurs around the joint. Bones in various parts of the body become greatly thickened and fragile, which leads to the destruction of the bone that supports the body weight. Fractures can occur even with light injuries, the back becomes hunched and deformed, legs get crooked. Overgrowth of bone tissue leads to tension and constant irritation of the periosteum. If a lesion is located in the bones of the skull base, narrowing of the cranial foramina causes compression of the cranial nerves, especially the optic and vestibular-cochlear nerves. Otosclerosis leads to deafness. Lesions in the skull base cause platybasia.

The disease usually develops in three stages: early osteolytic phase, mixed and sclerotic phase.

Imaging X-ray imaging shows broad bands of translucence at the projections of frontal, parietal, and occipital bones of the skull (so-called osteoporosis circumscripta). These bands correspond to areas of active resorption. Serum alkaline phosphatase test, which is produced in the process of bone remodeling, is used for the disease diagnosis.

Bone scintigraphy with 99mTc-labeled diphosphonates reveals areas of increased bone metabolism. Sometimes the isotope is not accumulated in the foci of resorption, detected by X-ray. This usually occurs after exacerbations or in the later stages of disease.

CT determines extensive thickening of the bony structures of the skull base and the vault with low differentiation of the bone marrow and cortical part. Edges of the affected bone are irregular, without clear boundaries (typical only for sclerotic phase).

MRI shows the presence of a heterogeneously modified MR signal with intermediate intensity on T1- and T2-weighted images (Vande Berg et al. 2001). Inhomogeneous contrast enhancement could be observed.

Osteoma is a benign tumor, originating from the bone and consisting of bone tissue. According to WHO classification, it belongs to the group of bone-forming benign tumors, with osteoid osteoma and osteoblastoma. They are the most mature and differentiated neoplasms of the skeleton. There are several types of osteoma: (1) spongy osteoma; (2) osteoma consisting from cortical or spongiosum bone, with cavities resembling the bone marrow, and (3) osteoma from solid compact bone substance (Yegorenkov 2010). It is believed that osteoma with a compact structure typically affects flat bones, and the first two types of osteoma are localized mainly in the long bones. Among the bones of the skull base, it most often affects the occipital and temporal bones, although lesions in the frontal bone and facial skeleton, in general, are more common. Solitary osteomas are usually diagnosed; multiple lesions are typical for Gardner syndrome (a combination of multiple osteomas with intestinal polyposis and soft tissue tumors (fibroma, lipoma, etc.)).

Clinically, in most cases, occipital bone osteomas are asymptomatic. Patients complain of a dense non-movable lump in the occipital region, not altering the adjacent skin.

Rarely local pain associated with compression of the adjacent nerve trunk can be observed in large tumor sizes. Osteomas grow very slowly; the fastest osteoma growth is noted in puberty.

Imaging The diagnosis of osteoma is confirmed radiographically, which allows to determine the form, size of the tumor and its relationship with the surrounding bone structures. Evaluation by multi-plane CT is preferred. Osteoma has high density comparable with the cortical bone layer that limits the tumor. The osteoma structure is, as a rule, homogeneous, without perifocal changes in the soft tissue covering the tumor (Fig. 25.2). MRI is less specific in the diagnosis of osteoma due to low sensitivity to the bone structures with low content of hydrogen protons. However, MRI is useful in assessing the condition of the surrounding adjacent bone structures, especially on T2-STIR sequences. Osteoma is not characterized by the presence of perifocal bone marrow edema in the surrounding bones, low signal characteristics are typical on all scanning sequences (Fig. 25.3). If osteoma is located at the plane of the petrous pyramid, it is very difficult to differentiate it from calcified meningioma.

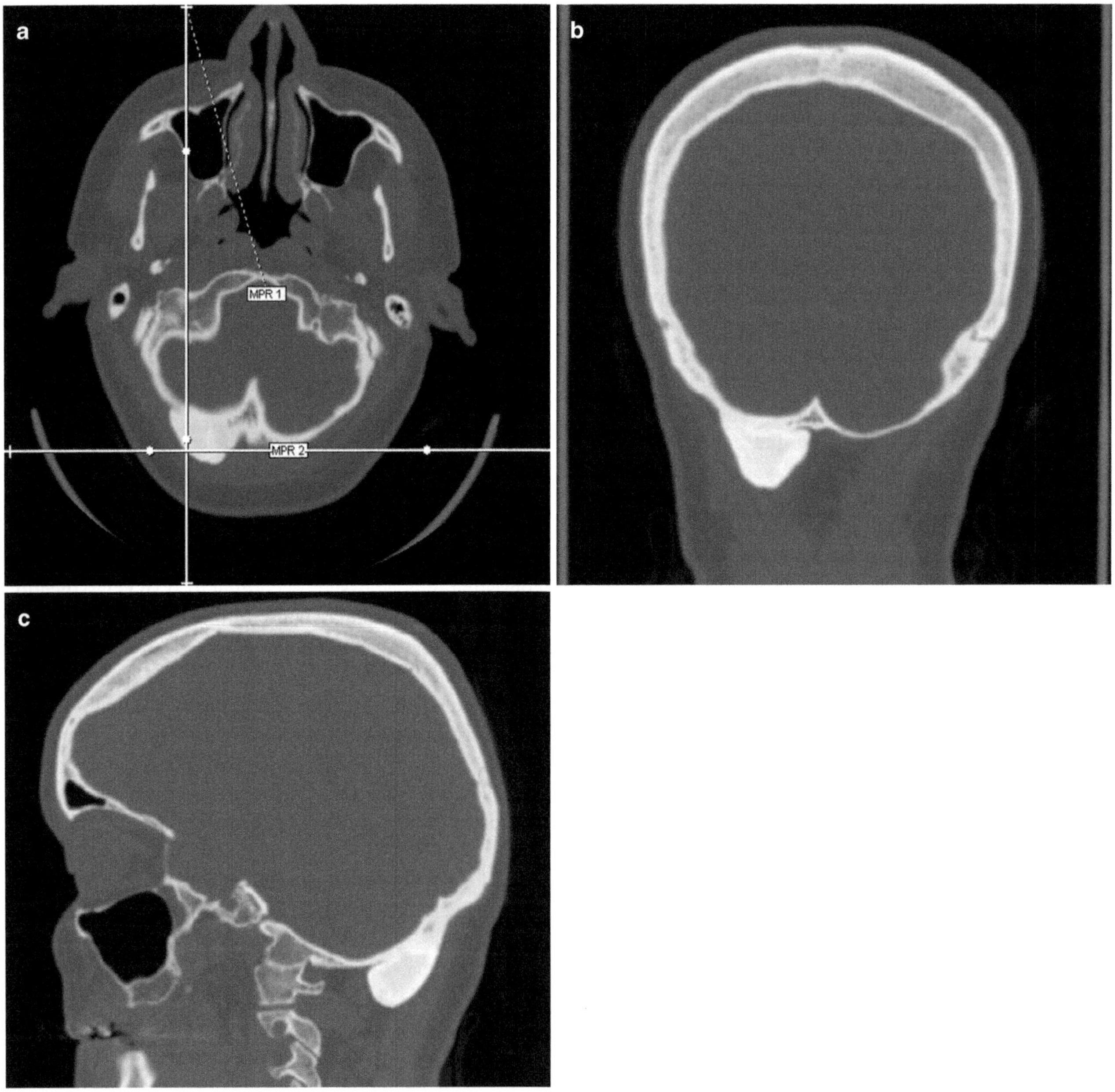

Fig. 25.2 Osteoma of the occipital bone on the right. CT scans in axial (**a**), coronal (**b**), and sagittal (**c**) planes demonstrate a tumor with high density that is equal to cortical bone and grows from the outer cortical layer of the right occipital bone

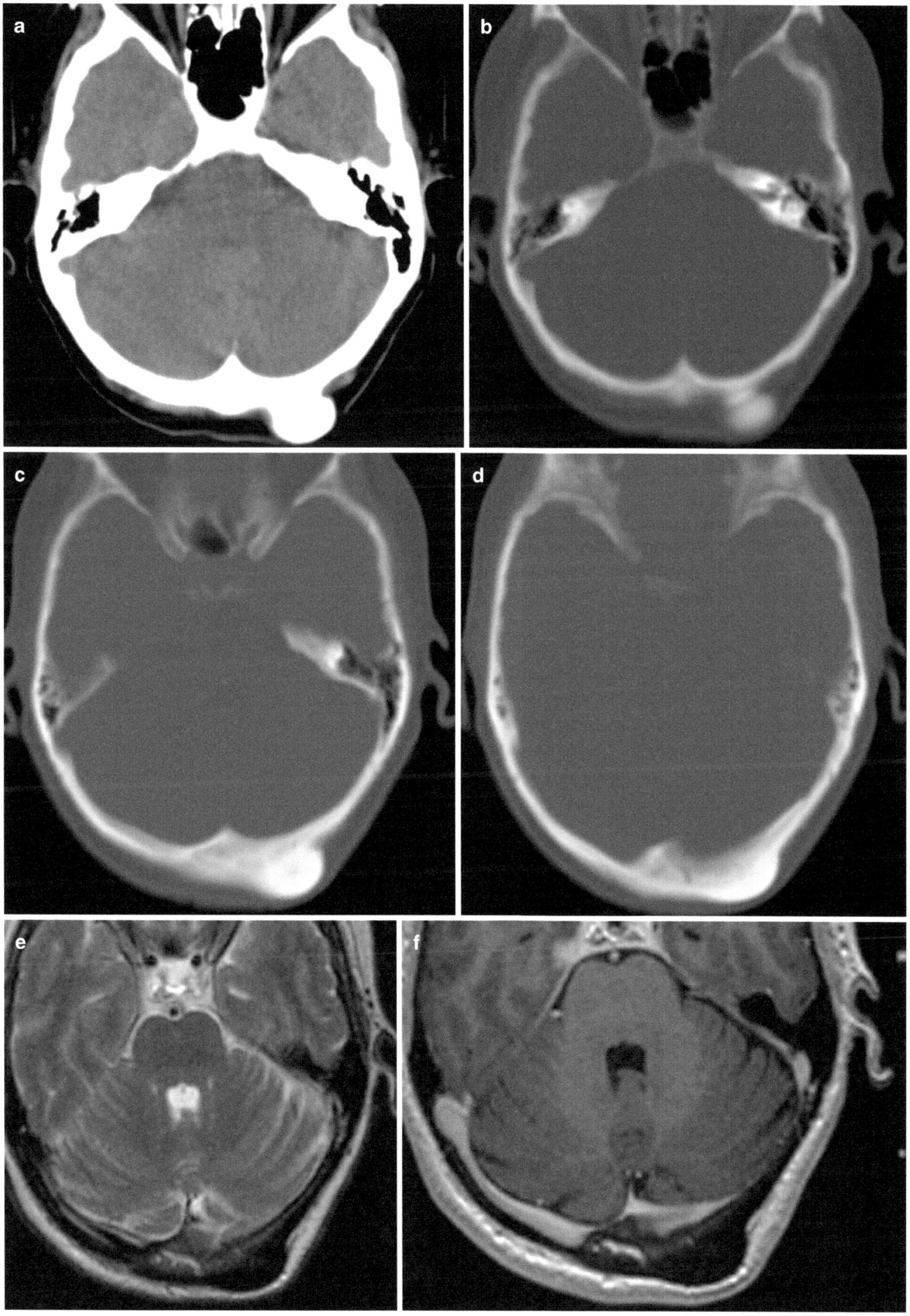

Fig. 25.3 Osteoma of the occipital bone on the left. CT scans (**a–d**) in axial projection reveal an extracranial hyperdense lesion growing from the squamous part of the left occipital bone. Density of the lesion is equal to cortical bone one. MRI (**e**, **f**) demonstrates the lesion with low MR signal on both T2 and T1 sequences

Differential Diagnosis Bone exostosis, periosteal hematoma, meningioma with hyperostosis, fibrolipoma, bone metastases.

Albers-Schonberg disease (synonyms: marble bone disease, osteopetrosis, congenital systemic osteosclerosis) is a rare, inherited disease manifested by diffuse thickened bones of the skeleton with increased bone fragility and deficiency of bone marrow hematopoiesis. The disease was first described by the German surgeon Albers-Schoenberg in 1904. The estimated incidence is 1 in 500 thousand to 5.5 in 100 thousand newborns. In total, about 800 cases were described in literature. There are early infantile and late forms of the disease.

Pathogenesis of the disease is not completely understood. It is believed that the disease disrupts the osteoclast function, which normally resorbs the bone tissue as part of a balanced process between bone formation and lysis in healthy people. In the disease, this balance is disrupted with increased formation of the bone tissue, carbonic anhydrase type II deficiency in osteoclasts, the lack of which causes a defect of osteoclast proton pump. Ultimately, bone resorption is affected with its continuing development, bone tissue gets compressed and becomes redundant.

Clinical Manifestations Despite excess bone tissue, marble bone disease is characterized by increased bone fragility with a tendency to pathological fractures. The most frequently pathological fractures are observed in the femur. Due to intact periosteum, consolidation occurs in a timely manner, however, in some cases, the fusion of bone fragments is slow because endosteum is not involved in the osteogenesis. In connection with sclerosis of the medullary canal and disrupted hematopoietic function, the development of hypochromic anemia, compensatory hepatomegaly, splenomegaly, lymphadenopathy are noted in children.

Excessive bone formation in the vault and mainly the skull base leads to a severe deformation of the skull, a decrease in the intracranial space can be accompanied by signs of intracranial hypertension, there may be a compression of the cranial nerves, especially in their bone canals at the skull base, which leads to paresis and paralysis. Deformation is identified both in the spine and chest. The consequence of early osteosclerosis of the skull base may also be hydrocephalus.

Imaging Diagnosis of marble bone disease is mainly based on radiographic findings demonstrating the systemic nature of bone changes. Skull X-ray and CT, in particular, show thick and dense bones of the vault and skull base (Fig. 25.4). CT clearly visualizes narrowing of bone canals and foramina in the skull base. CT study often diagnoses hydrocephalic enlargement of the ventricular system. Multiple pathological vertebral fractures can be seen on CT as well. On MRI T1- and T2-weighted images, there is no typical characteristics of the bone marrow. The vault bones are thickened and have a heterogeneously altered MR- signal.

Differential Diagnosis Diseases accompanied by osteosclerosis (hypervitaminosis D, hypoparathyroidism, Paget's disease, metastases, Hodgkin's disease, leukemia, chronic renal failure, etc.).

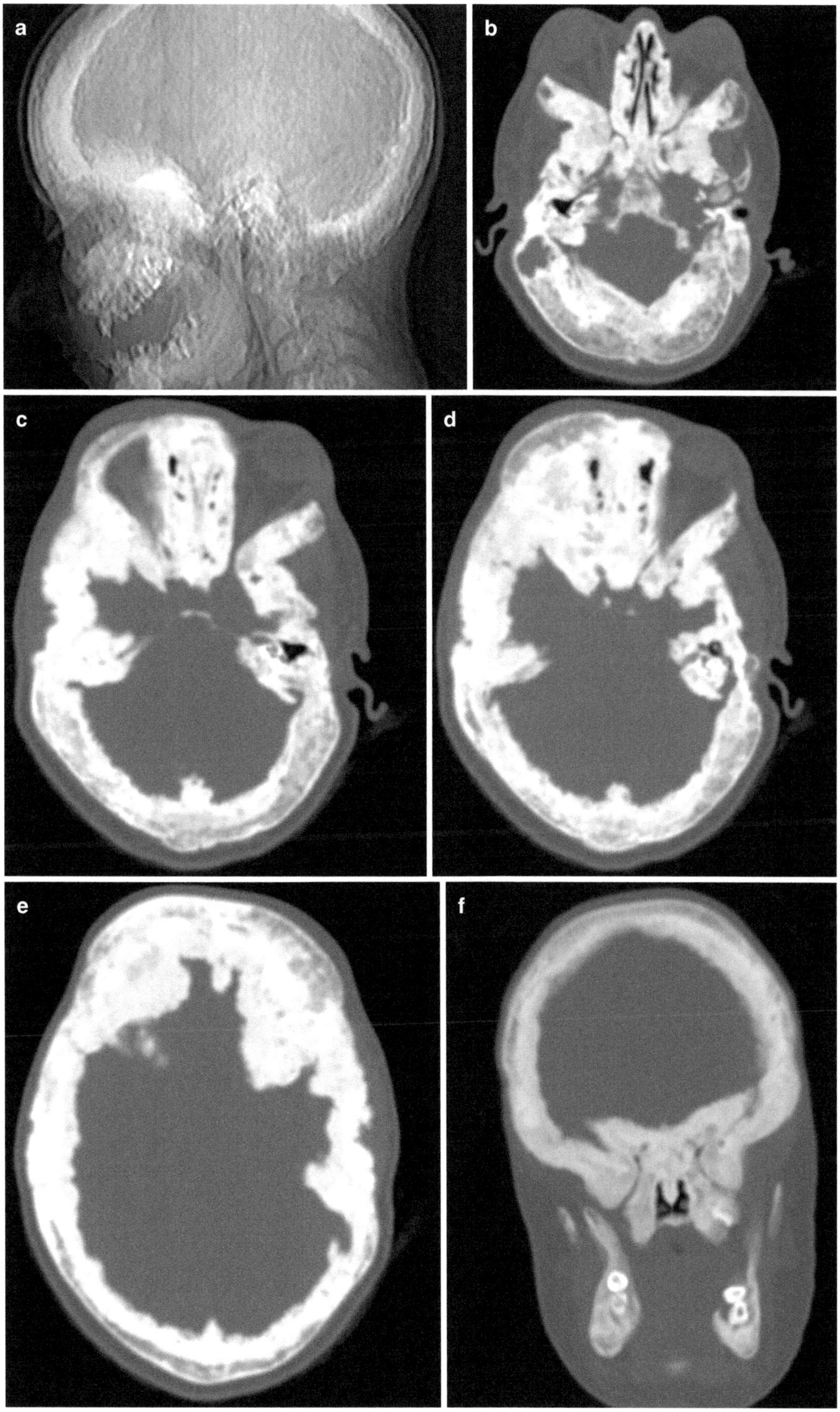

Fig. 25.4 Albers-Schoenberg disease (marble disease). On lateral CT-topogram (**a**) and series of axial NECT scans (**b–e**) with reformations in coronal (**f**, **g**) and sagittal (**h**) planes a diffuse thickening of calvarium and skull base bones are clearly detected. CT can fairly clearly visualize the stenosis of bone channels and foramens in the skull base; (**i**)—3D reformation demonstrates deformation of calvarium and facial bones

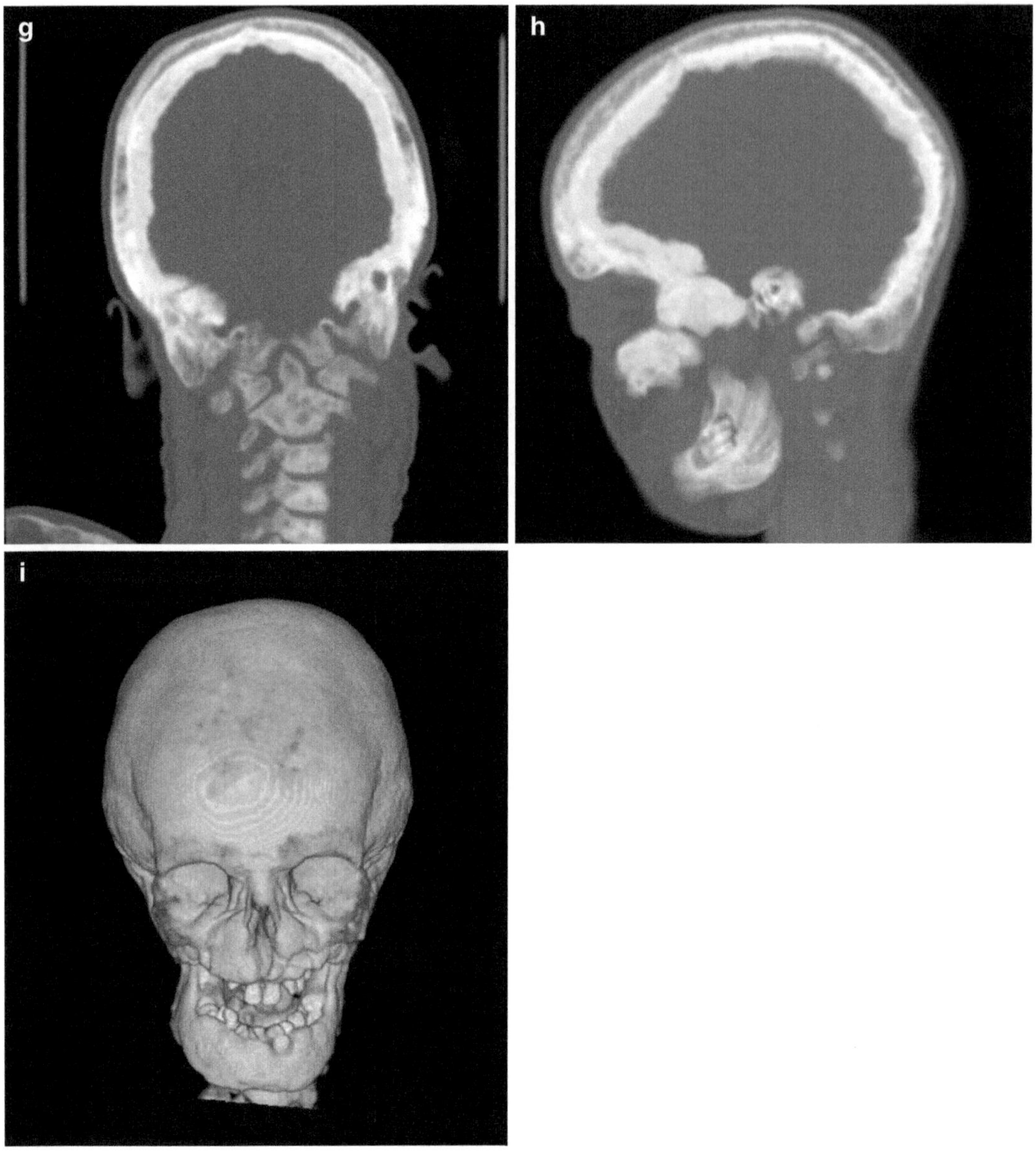

Fig. 25.4 (continued)

26 Inflammatory Disorders

Petrositis is a form of inflammatory lesion in projection of pneumatic cells of the petrous pyramid, especially in cases with its atypically high initial pneumatization.

It occurs relatively rarely. The reason of petrositis both in children and adults in most cases is acute or chronic purulent otitis media and especially epitympanitis. It very rarely occurs due to presence of cholesterol granuloma or congenital cholesteatoma of the middle ear. The inflammatory process is often located in the apex of the pyramid. Spreading of purulent inflammation from the middle ear is facilitated by pneumatization of the mastoid and petrous portion of the temporal bone, when infectious agents (*Streptococcus pneumoniae, Haemophilus influenzae, Staphylococcus aureus*) can penetrate into this area via pneumatic bone cells and vascular canals. As a result of infection spreading to the pyramid, an abscess may occur. Often a more or less wide fistula from the mastoid area or tympanic cavity toward the top of the pyramid is formed. The cases of breakthrough of pus into the sphenoid sinus, the upper and lateral parts of the pharynx are known.

The main clinical *manifestation of the disease* is a long profuse suppuration from the ear. The body temperature is usually subfebrile. The vast majority of patients have intense, often paroxysmal headaches on the affected side, which may radiate to the orbit, the fronto-temporal region, teeth and neck. The occurrence of pain is caused by involvement of the cranial nerves surrounding the apex of the pyramid (trigeminal, vagus, glossopharyngeal nerves) and dura in the inflammatory process. Involvement of other cranial nerves also is noted. If the process involves the abducens nerve, the mobility of the eyeball is limited outwards. The clinical signs of the disease in some cases are similar to manifestations of Gradenigo syndrome: acute purulent otitis media, pain in the face along the course of the trigeminal nerve (V1), abducens nerve paralysis.

If inflammation is located in the anterior upper sections of the pyramid, in addition to abnormalities in the function of the trigeminal and abducens nerves, the oculomotor and trochlear nerves can be affected, which is manifested by limited movements of the eyeball inwards and downwards, or even complete immobility of the eyeball. A major complication of inflammatory changes in the mastoid process (mastoiditis) is retropharyngeal abscesses, which can be observed in the early (more common) and late childhood. Pus, following the sheath of the neck vessels and digastric muscle, may form leakages along the spine.

Imaging Stenvers and Schüller X-ray methods, previously widely used for both temporal bones, and linear tomography allowing to identify the pathological focus in most cases in the petrous pyramid have now almost become a history. CT and MRI have become the main methods in visualization of inflammatory changes at the temporal bone.

CT usually determines filling of hypertrophied cells of the mastoid process and the petrous apex with moderately hyperdense exudate. A marked purulent process leads to destructive changes in bone structures and lysis of bone trabeculae separating the pneumatic cells (Horn 1996; Migirov 2003) (Fig. 26.1).

On MR T2-weighted sequences, a marked increase in MR-signal from both hypertrophic edematous mucosa and inflammatory effusion is noted. On T1-weighted images, the MR-signal is usually isointense relative to the cerebellum (Fig. 26.2). On T2-FLAIR images, MR-signal has hyperintense features. During a long-term course of the disease, congestive changes with an increase in the protein component in the exudate can cause an increase in the MR-signal on T1-weighted images (Fig. 26.3). After administration of contrast agent a moderated contrast enhancement of the affected mucosa is noted (Dobben et al. 2000). In case of abscess formation, the areas of increased MR-signal are identified on DW-sequences (Fig. 26.4). In typical cases of petrositis changes in the MR-signal are not observed on diffusion-weighted images.

I. Pronin, V. Kornienko, *CT and MRI of Skull Base Lesions*, https://doi.org/10.1007/978-3-319-65957-2_26

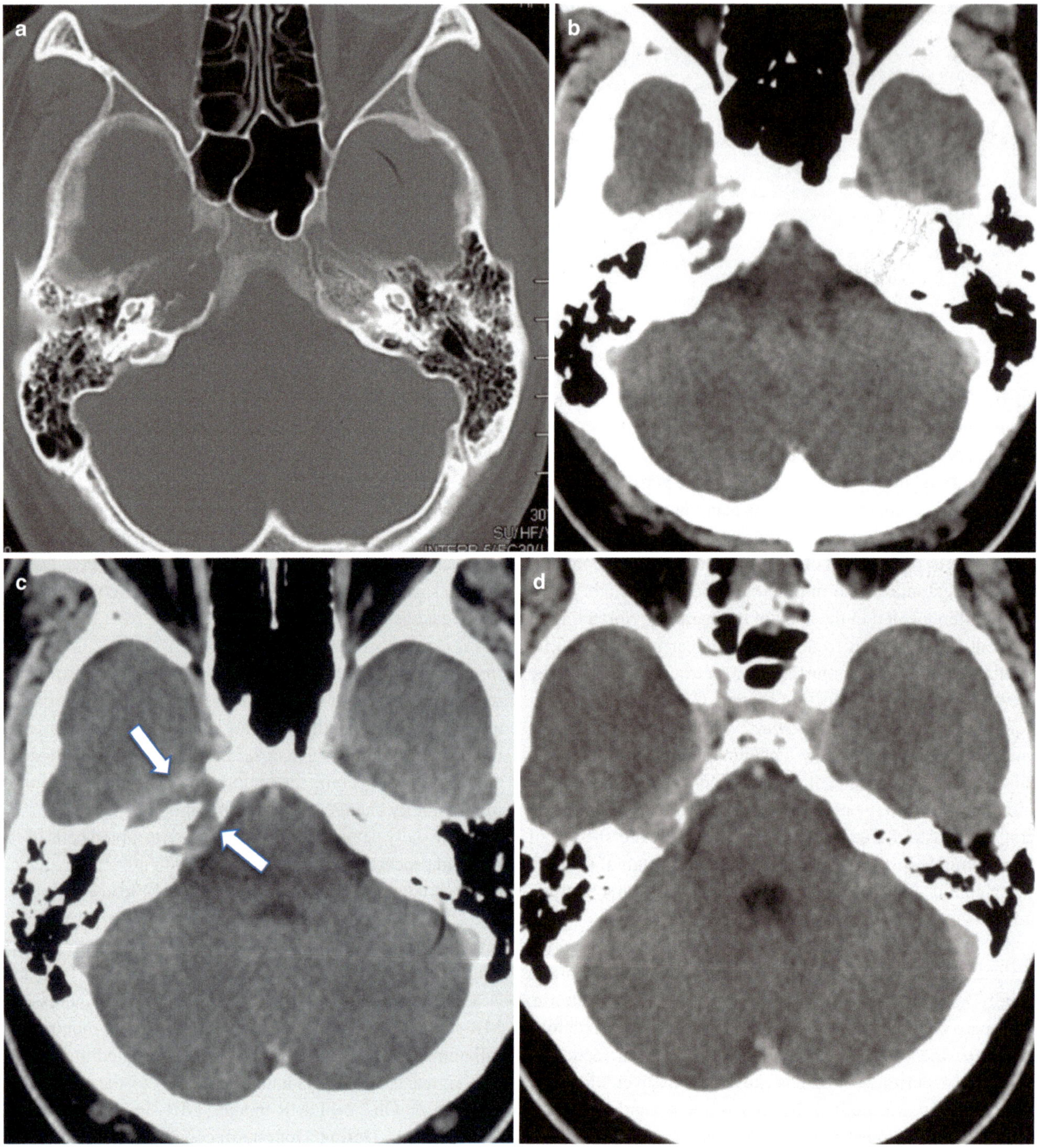

Fig. 26.1 Petrositis of the right temporal bone pyramid. Axial CT scan in "bone window" mode demonstrates lytic changes of bone trabeculae, which split air-bearing cells in the projection of the apex of the temporal bone (**a**). On CT with contrast enhancement (**b**–**d**) the pathologic contrast enhancement of the meninges, which is adjacent to the inflammation (*arrows*) can be seen

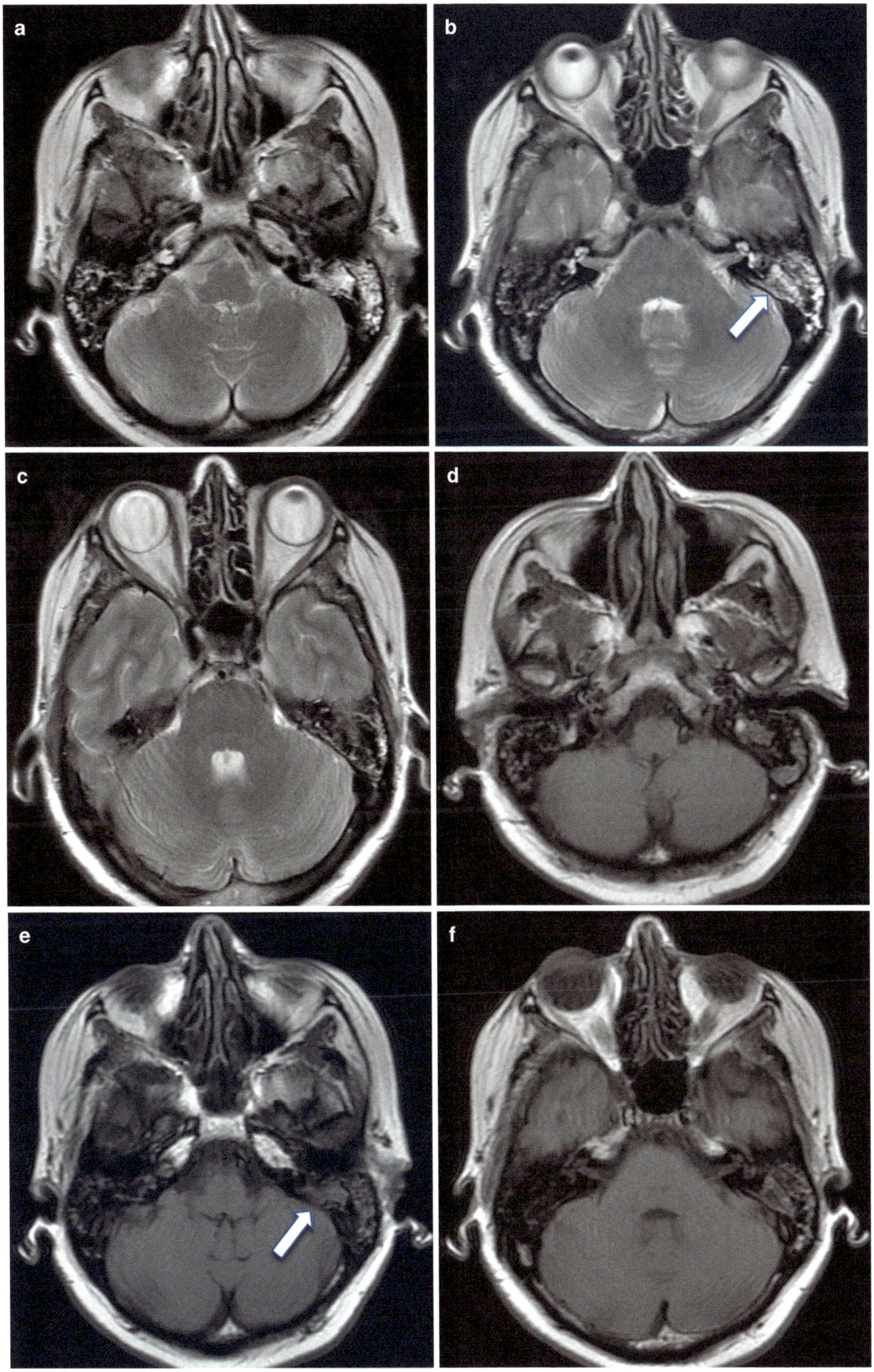

Fig. 26.2 Bilateral mastoiditis. On series of T2- (**a–c**) and T1- (**d–f**) weighted MR images the signal changes in projection of the cells of the mastoid processes on both sides are detected. Inflammatory exudate and thickened mucosa have hyperintense MR-signal on T2 and isointense MR-signal on T1 sequences compared to brain tissue (*arrows*)

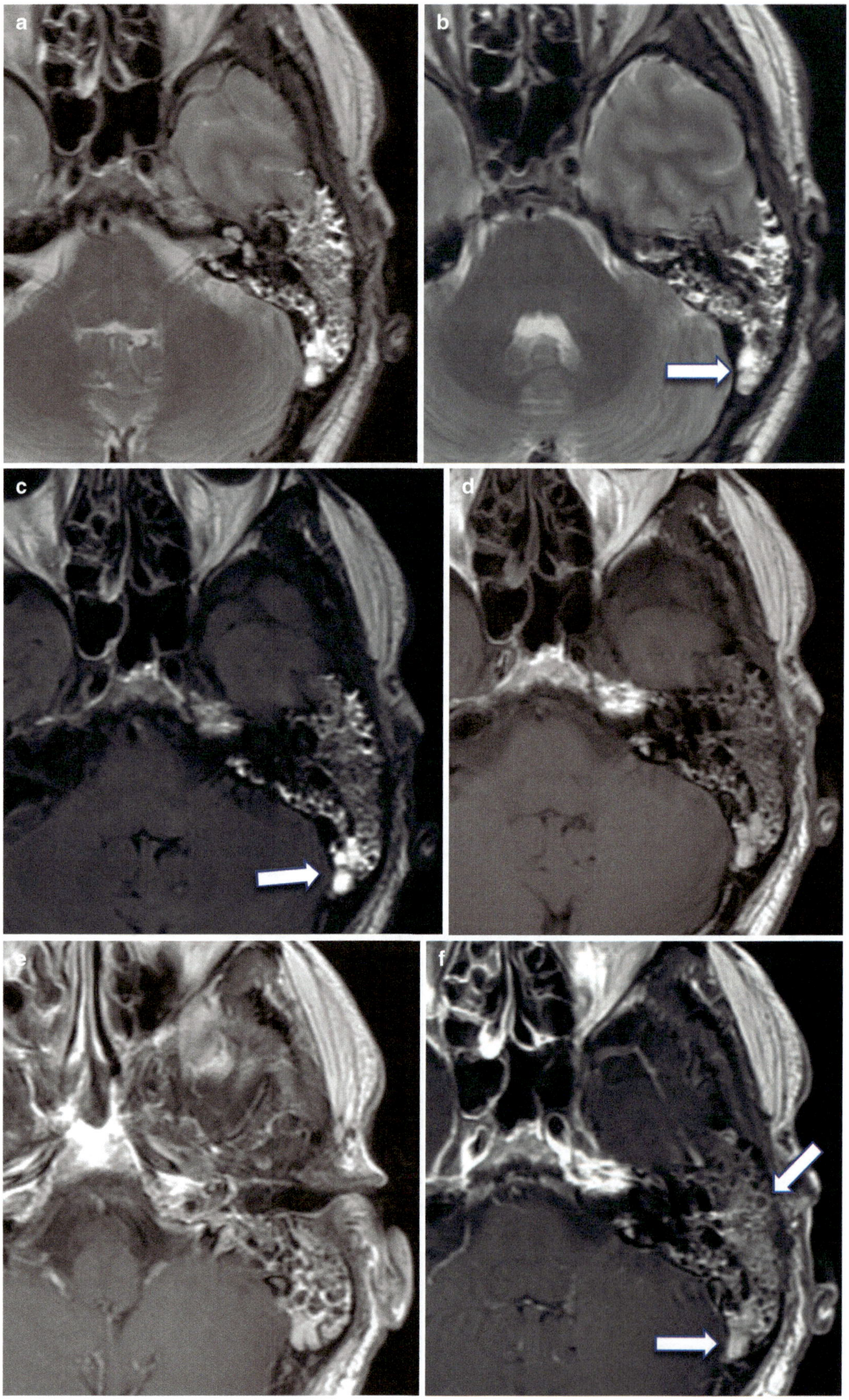

Fig. 26.3 *Left*-sided mastoiditis and otitis media. On T2- (**a**, **b**) and T2-FLAIR- (**c**) weighted MR images an inflammatory thickening of the mucosa with formation of separate areas of exudate accumulation (*arrows*) in the projection of the *left* mastoid cells can be seen. The inflammatory changes have increased MR-signal. Axial T1-weighted images before (**d**) and after (**e**, **f**) contrast enhancement visualize the increased MR-signal from thickened mucosa, which accumulated contrast medium. "Islets" of exudate are saving their hyperintensity due to high protein content (*arrows*)

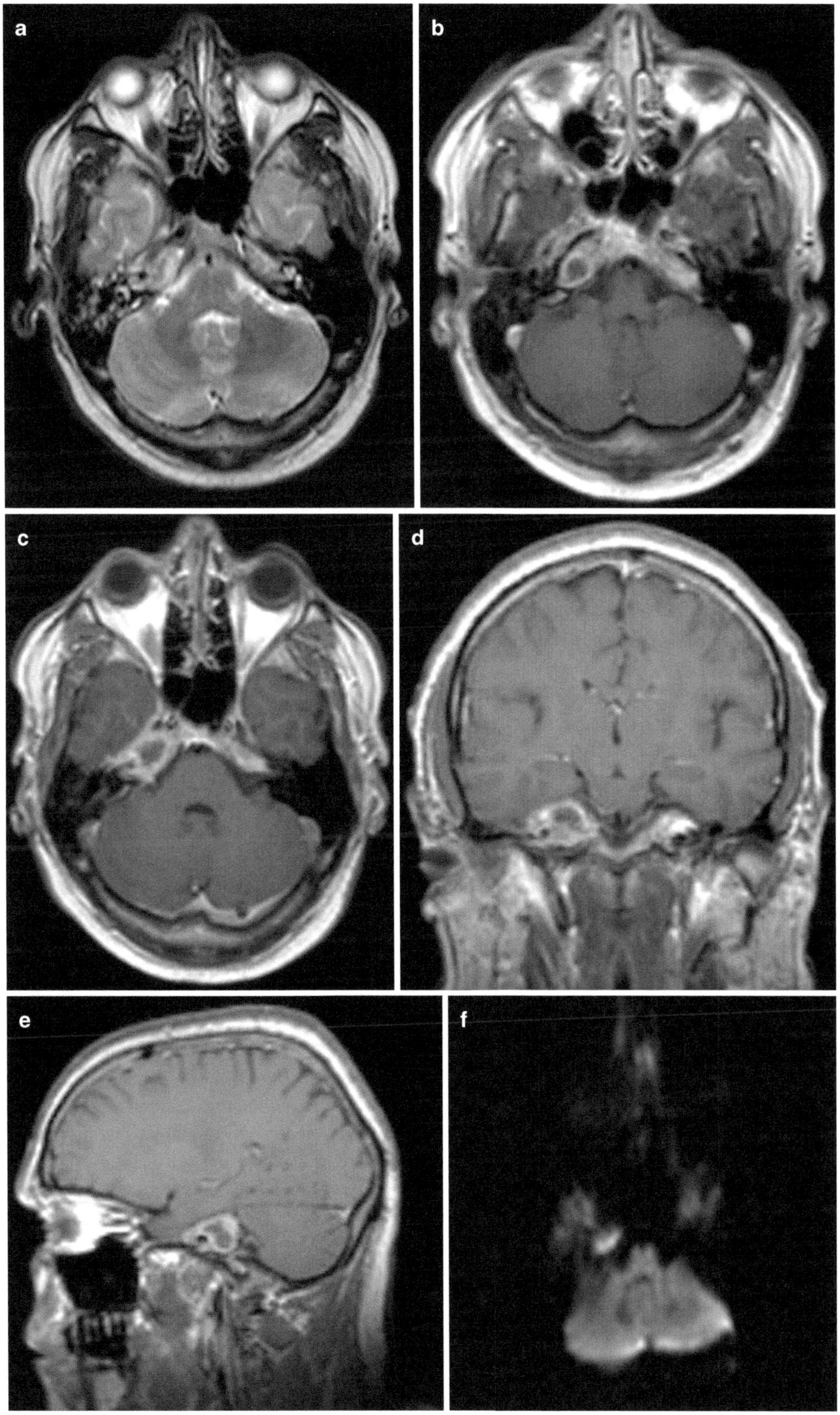

Fig. 26.4 Petrositis with conjunction into abscess of the right temporal bone pyramid. T2- (**a**) weighted axial MR image and series of T1-weighed postenhanced MR scans demonstrate a focal heterogeneously hyperintense area on T2 in projection of the petrous apex of the right temporal bone. MR images with contrast enhancement in axial (**b**, **c**), coronal (**d**), and sagittal (**e**) planes show a region with "ring-like" contrast enhancement in the pyramid apex. There is a moderately increased MR-signal on DWI (**f**), suggesting the initial phase of pus formation

Granulomatous Lesion **Granuloma** is a focus of productive inflammation in the form of a dense nodule resulting from proliferation and transformation of cells capable of phagocytosis.

Morphogenesis of granuloma consists of four stages: (1) accumulation of young monocytic phagocytes in the tissue lesion; (2) maturation of these cells into macrophages and formation of macrophage granuloma; (3) maturation and transformation of monocytic phagocytes and macrophages into epithelioid cells and formation of epithelioid cell granuloma; (4) fusion of epithelioid cells (or macrophages) and formation of giant cells (Pirogov-Langhans) and epithelioid cell granulomas or giant cell granulomas. The granuloma outcome is sclerosis.

Based on morphological features, there are three types of granulomas:

1. Macrophage granuloma;
2. Epithelioid cell granuloma;
3. Giant cell granuloma.

Depending on the level of metabolism, they distinguish granulomas with low and high metabolism. Granulomas with low metabolism develop as a result of an interaction with inert substances (inert foreign bodies). Granulomas with high metabolism appear under the influence of toxic stimuli (mycobacterium tuberculosis, leprosy, etc.) and are presented as epithelioid cell nodules.

There are infectious, non-infectious granulomas and granulomas with unknown origin. Infectious granulomas occur in typhus and typhoid, rheumatism, rabies, viral encephalitis, tularemia, brucellosis, tuberculosis, syphilis, leprosy, scleroma (Paparella et al. 1982). Non-infectious granulomas are found in dust diseases (silicosis, talcosis, asbestosis, byssinosis, etc.), medication effects (granulomatous hepatitis, etc.); they also develop around foreign bodies.

Tuberculous granuloma (or tuberculoma) has the following structure: it contains a necrotic focus in the center and a rim of epithelioid cells and lymphocytes with admixture of macrophages and plasma cells on the periphery. Giant Pirogov-Langhans cells that are very typical for tuberculous granuloma are located between lymphocytes and epithelioid cells.

Syphilitic granuloma (gumma) is presented as an extensive necrotic focus surrounded by cellular infiltrate from lymphocytes, plasma cells, and epithelioid cells; giant Pirogov-Langhans cells are rare.

Leprosy granuloma (leproma) is presented as a nodule, consisting mainly of macrophages, as well as lymphocytes and plasma cells. Macrophages appear as large cells with fat vacuoles, containing *Mycobacterium leprae* packed in the form of balls.

Scleromous granuloma consists of epithelioid and plasma cells, as well as lymphocytes, including many hyaline globes. Occurrence of large macrophages with clear cytoplasm called Mikulicz cells is very typical. Cytoplasm contains the causative agent, Volkovych-Frisch rods. It is also characterized by significant sclerosis and hyalinosis of granulation tissue.

Imaging If granuloma is located in the bone structures at the projection of the mastoid process or more common the temporal bone, X-ray or CT better reveal the bone defect without reactive sclerosis. The defect edges are clear and sharp. If it is located in the brain substance (brain stem, cerebellar hemispheres), CT shows granuloma only after administration of contrast agent. Prior to contrast enhancement, most granulomas (except for calcified ones) are not visualized, having isodense properties. The degree of contrast enhancement varies from slight to moderate, depending on the stage of the inflammatory process. Granulomatous involvement of the brain and leptomeniges at the basal cisterns is better visualized on MRI. Typical for granulomas is the presence of a foci with hypointense MR-signal on T2-weighted sequences, surrounded by a local (sometimes quite pronounced) perifocal edema of adjacent brain tissue (a hyperintense MR-signal). On T1-weighted images, this type of lesions has iso- or slightly increased MR-signal. In case of hemorrhagic inclusions, the signal on T1-weighted sequences is typically increased (Martin et al. 1990). After contrast agent administration, its intense accumulation is noted in a lesion with various shapes (ring, nodule, foci, diffuse) (Fig. 26.5).

Sarcoidosis is a systemic granulomatous disorder affecting many organs (usually the lungs), involving the central nervous system in course of the disease. CNS involvement occurs in 5–10% of cases with systemic disorder, usually in patients aged 20–40 years old and manifests as basal meningitis and granulomatous inflammation in the brain tissue. However, the process can be located in the cerebellopontine angle, around the brain stem, and even in the spinal canal. Most common, patients have lung disease, diabetes insipidus.

Imaging Contrast-enhanced CT and MRI detect irregular thickening of brain leptomeninges and their pronounced

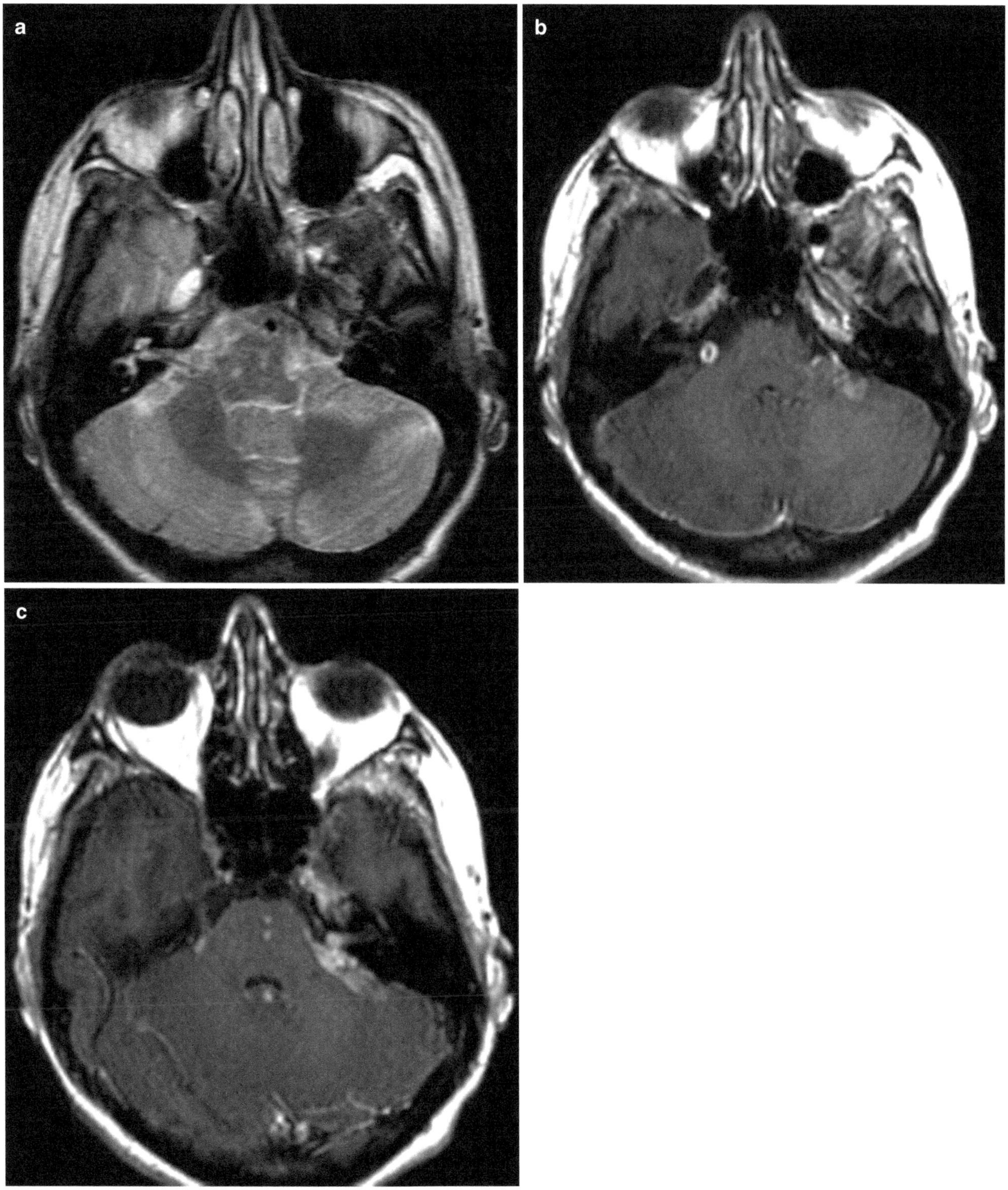

Fig. 26.5 Tuberculosis of CNS. On T2-weighted MR image (**a**) a poorly defined rounded small areas of the hypointense MR-signal can be detected, located in the projection of cerebellopontine angle in both sides. Postenhanced T1-weighted (**b**, **c**) sequences help better recognize the multiple enhancing lesions in cerebellopontine angles with involvement predominantly of the *left* side as well as intrapontine small lesions. Small lesion in the right cerebellopontine angle has ring-like contrast enhancement

enhancement. Sometimes these can be multiple distinct nodules in the meninges. Cranial nerves, pituitary and hypothalamus, third ventricle may be involved in the process. In case of local invasion of the adjacent brain tissue, an increase in MR-signal on T2-weighted images (edema) is observed.

Osteomyelitis of the Skull Base The development of acute inflammation (osteomyelitis) at the skull base is most often caused by spread of infection from the purulent necrotizing otitis externa or due to spreading of thrombophlebitis along the venous plexus in the area of unpneumatized petrous apex.

Imaging CT detects foci of bone fragmentation, erosion, or sclerotic changes depending on the stage of the process. MRI manifestations are limited by a decrease in MR-signal from the skull base that originally had a high MR-signal from the normal fat component of the bone marrow on T1-weighted sequences. On T2-weighted images, MR-signal can be slightly elevated from affected soft-tissue lesions under the skull base. A quite pronounced diffuse contrast enhancement is typical at the projection of the affected skull base bones with involvement of extracranial soft tissues adjacent to the inflammation areas. The best visualization is achieved using Fat-Sat technique with intravenous contrast enhancement. It is believed that technetium 99 m-based SPECT allows to monitor the treatment effectiveness (Rubin et al. 1990; Seabold et al. 1995).

Bell's palsy (facial paralysis) is an acute disease of unknown origin, possibly caused by a virus, presumably herpes family (Varicella-Zoster). Clinical manifestations of this disorder are signs of peripheral facial paralysis expressed as downturned mouth and difficulty speaking, difficulty eating, and difficulty closing the eyelids. Some patients complain of pain behind the ear, in the jaw or the entire affected portion of the face, twitching or contractions of the affected side of the face, salivation and taste changes; an increased sensitivity to sound can occur. Bell's palsy usually begins suddenly, patients notice its appearance on waking. Pain behind the ear usually appears a day or two before the paralysis. Maximum weakness or paralysis may occur within 48 hours after the onset. The incidence is 23:100,000 per year; in other words, one of 60–70 people suffers with Bell's palsy during his life. Bell's palsy can occur at any age, but is most commonly diagnosed between 30 and 60 years old. It requires medical treatment, although it may recover without any treatment. Although impaired mimic muscles movement and downturned mouth can persist for a long time.

Pathogenesis of the disease is unclear. Single pathological study revealed nonspecific (non-inflammatory, as it is commonly believed) changes in the facial nerve. Sometimes it is associated with a middle ear infection. If both sides of the face are affected, the cause may be Lyme disease or sarcoidosis.

Imaging CT study of the petrous bone using standard and bone window modes usually does not detect abnormalities in cases of this disease. An enlargement of the bone canal of the facial nerve is absent. In case of a local enlargement, another cause for development of paralysis should be considered. The role of contrast enhancement in CT is not determined.

Contrast-enhanced MRI is the method of choice in the correct diagnosis. The main diagnostic feature is a local pronounced contrast enhancement at the projection of the ganglion, labyrinthine, and mastoid portions of the facial nerve canal on post-contrast T1-weighted MR images, especially if fat suppression technique with thin slices is used (Fig. 26.6). Contrast enhancement is linear and represented with a micronodule (for example, in neurinomas). On T2-weighted images, obvious changes along the facial nerve canal course are usually not detected, possibly due to the small size of the lesion and insufficiently standard MR equipment.

Differential Diagnosis With asymmetrical contrast enhancement of the tubular portion of the facial nerve (no clinical signs of paralysis, considered as a normal variant), microschwannoma of the facial nerve (most often hearing loss, nodular contrast enhancement), hemangioma of the facial nerve, Ramsay Hunt syndrome (a combination of facial paralysis with herpes at the external auditory meatus).

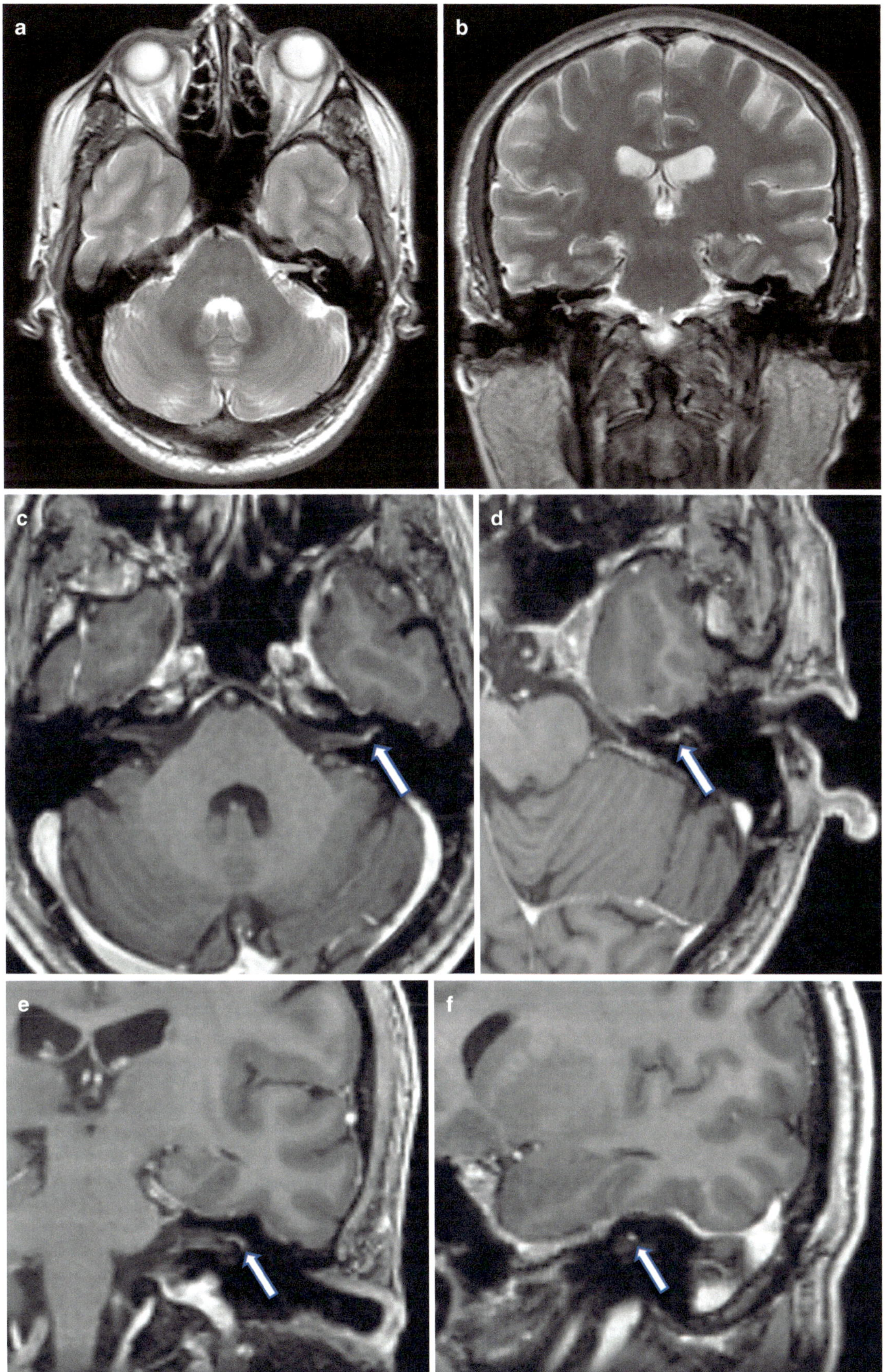

Fig. 26.6 Bell's paralysis on the left. MRI using T2 sequence (**a**, **b**) doesn't reveal any pathology in projection of internal auditory canals and middle ears on both sides. After intravenous contrast enhancement on T1 MR images (**c**–**f**) in labyrinthine and tympanic segments of the facial nerve as well as in the projection of VII-th nerve ganglion an area with prominent contrast enhancement (*arrows*) is detected. This area has linear shape (without the formation of a micro-nodule) along the nerve

Vascular Lesions

27

Dural venous sinus thrombosis *(sinus thrombosis)* belongs to a group of vascular diseases where the clinical syndrome is caused by thrombosis of the venous sinuses of the brain and impairment of the blood outflow from the cranial cavity with the development of rapidly progressive intracranial hypertension. It can have either septic (a complication of purulent otitis media, mastoiditis, sinusitis) or aseptic origin. For example, the cause of the sigmoid sinus thrombosis and subsequent sepsis is usually necrotic inflammation of the middle ear, especially, extending to the mastoid. Osteomyelitis of the petrous part of the temporal bone and other inflammatory diseases of the skull bones in rare cases can cause sinus thrombosis. Trauma, vascular dural fistulas, postoperative complications after posterior fossa surgeries may also be the cause of thrombosis. This disorder can develop during pregnancy and postpartum period, when using oral contraceptives, in coagulopathy and vasculitis, hypercoagulation states in malignant tumors and cyanotic congenital heart disease, cachexia in infants, sickle cell anemia, antiphospholipid syndrome and other lesions. It is believed that the most frequent cause of dural sinus thrombosis are congenital defects of blood clotting (for example, a mutation of the gene encoding coagulation factor V, protein S or C deficiency, antithrombin III deficiency, resistance to activated C protein (the most common cause of spontaneous sinus thrombosis), as well as erythremia or polycythemia, thrombocythemia, paroxysmal nocturnal hemoglobinuria, etc. Approximately 50% sinus thromboses can lead to the formation of venous (hemorrhagic) infarcts in the cerebellum, temporal and occipital lobes of the brain.

Among venous sinuses of the subtentorial area, thrombosis of the sigmoid and transverse sinuses is most frequently observed. Local symptoms are most clearly presented in an infected thrombus. There are marked redness and swelling of the soft tissues over the mastoid, pain in this area and tenderness on palpation, dilation of superficial veins at the posterior edge of the mastoid process. In rare cases a number of patients have changes in the vessels on the neck, which are limited to the jugular vein pain on palpation. At a later stage, the vein is palpated as a solid cord, which is an evidence of its thrombosis. Swollen lymph nodes along the course of the venous vessels occur in case of thrombus spread to the bulb or the jugular vein itself. Over time, the thrombus is replaced with sclerotic tissue. Initially, an increase in body temperature in infectious sinus thrombosis occurs in over half the cases, then, in the first hours and days of the disease, the vast majority of patients develop a picture of sepsis and the temperature curve becomes hectic with a few drops by 1.5–2 °C during 1 day, indicating the development of septicopyemia. Temperatures range from low grade to hectic (37.5–39.5 °C).

Imaging X-ray examination of the temporal bone in cases with inflammatory changes shows the erosion of the mastoid and destruction of pneumatic cells. Direct angiography determines a defect of filling of a corresponding sinus which sometimes spreads to the jugular vein.

CT without contrast enhancement reveals areas of hyperdensity at the projection of the transverse or sigmoid sinus due to acute thrombus. However, density characteristics measured on both sides of the projections of sinuses should be always compared. Intravenous contrast enhancement does not always allow making a correct diagnosis, as contrast agents can mask a blood clot due to high density. A typical symptom of intraluminal thrombus is considered to be a delta symptom («Δ»), a blood clot looking like an area of contrast enhancement defect, especially when the slice is perpendicular to the sinus course. Unfortunately, this symptom occurs in only 25% of all cases. CT-angiography is more informative, especially when scanning at the early venous phase. The study clearly visualizes the blood clot in the sinus lumen, which may spread into the jugular vein (Figs. 27.1 and 27.2). Routine CT may show foci of hemorrhage (venous infarcts) and edema in cerebellar hemispheres, rarely subarachnoid blood location. CT-perfusion studies demonstrate lack of blood flow at the level of sinus thrombosis and hemodynamic changes in the cerebellum and brainstem.

I. Pronin, V. Kornienko, *CT and MRI of Skull Base Lesions*, https://doi.org/10.1007/978-3-319-65957-2_27

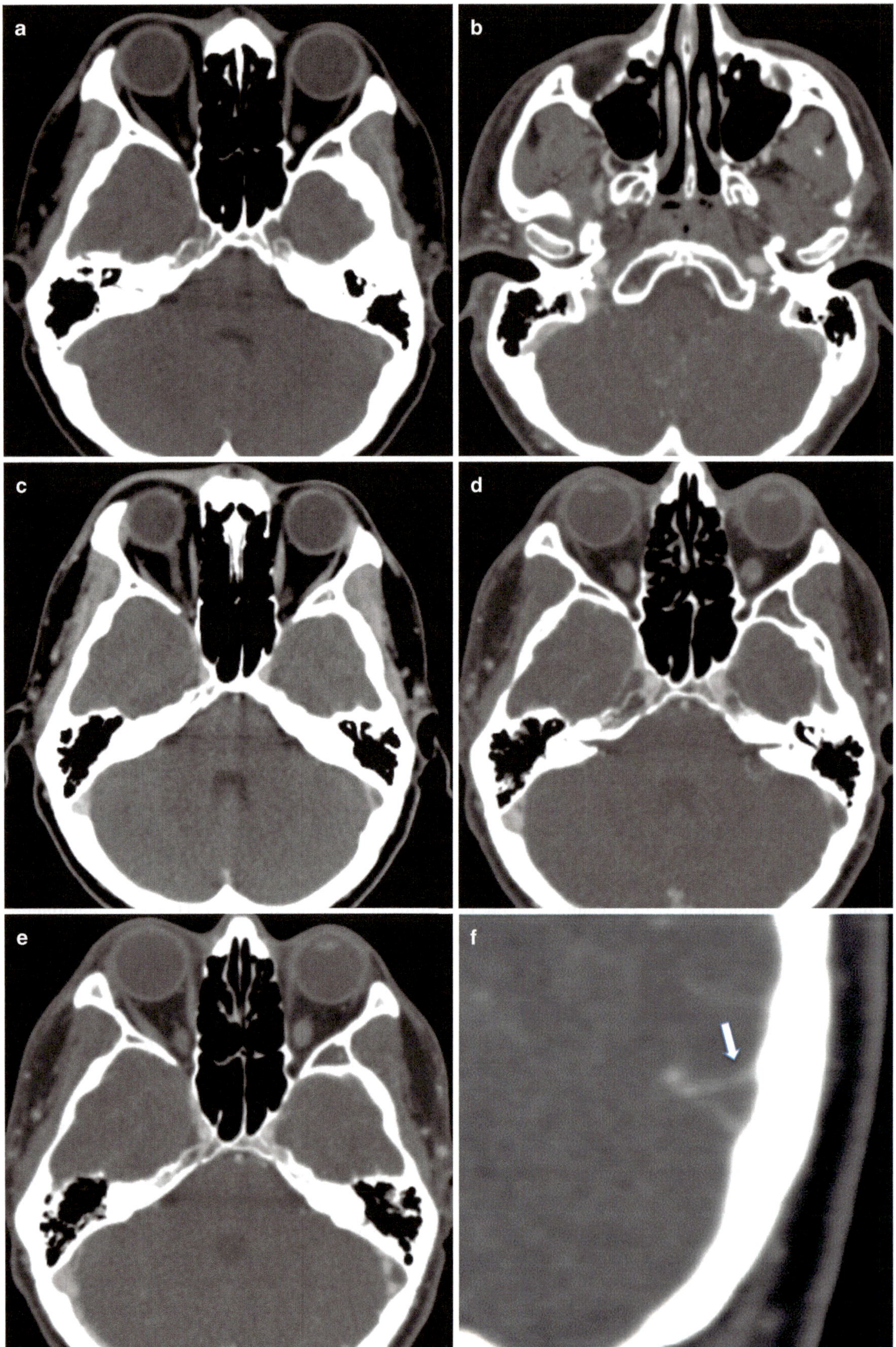

Fig. 27.1 Thrombosis of left transverse and sigmoid sinuses. Axial CT scans before (**a**) and after (**b–e**) intravenous contrast enhancement visualizes a filling defect in lumen of sigmoid sinus, which is located in the center of contrast medium filling. There is no visualization of jugular vein bulb on the *left*. Oblique (perpendicular to the transverse sinus) CT reformation (**f**) demonstrates "Λ" sign (*arrow*) in lumen of this sinus

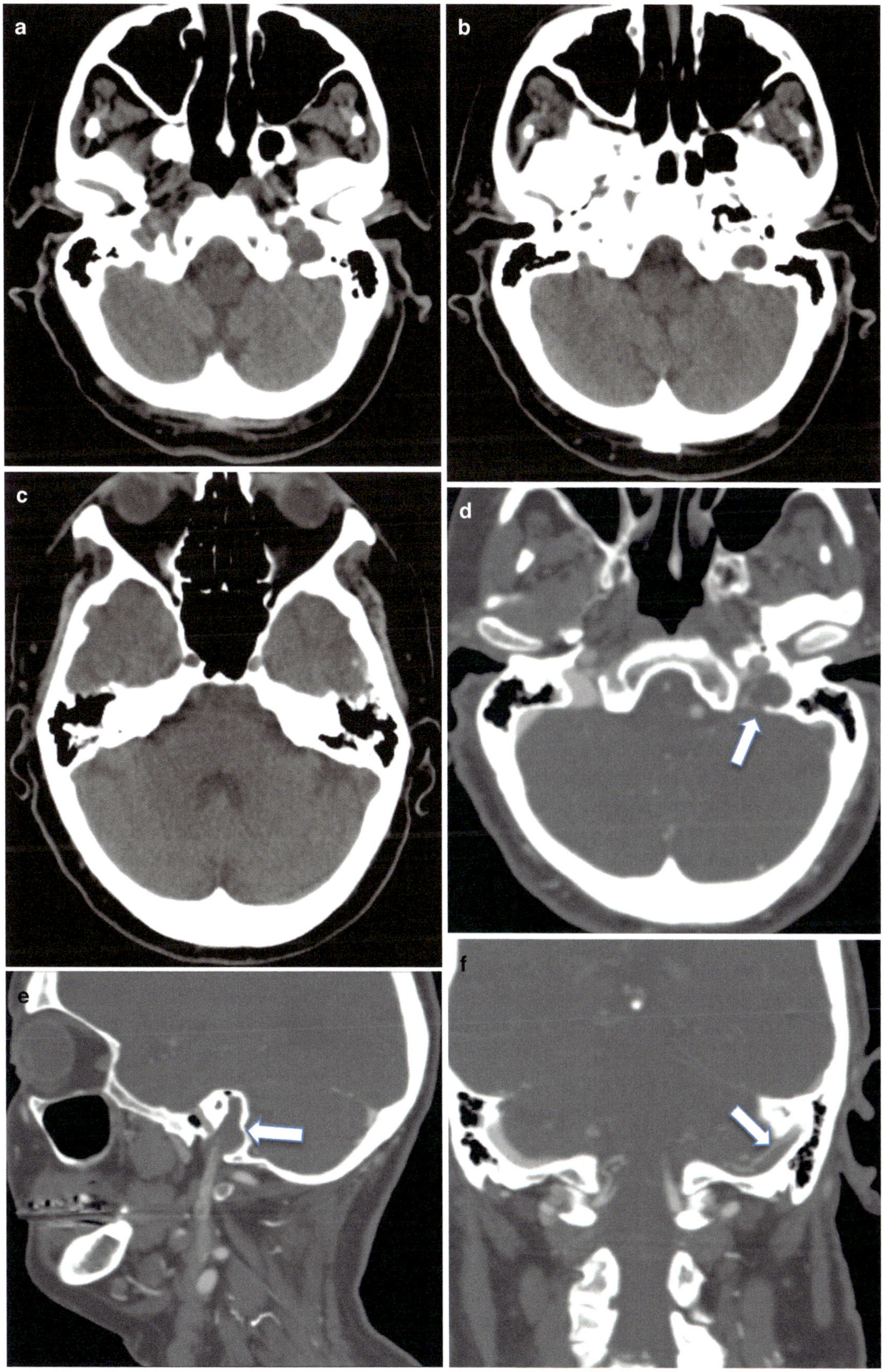

Fig. 27.2 Thrombosis of the left transverse, sigmoid sinuses and jugular vein. On series of CT scans before (**a–c**) and after (**d–f**) intravenous contrast enhancement in lumen of bulb of jugular vein and sigmoid sinus a hypodense area is visualized. After injection of contrast medium the defect of contrast agent filling within the sinuses can be seen. This defect is clearly visible on sagittal and frontal CT reformations in projection of these venous structures (*arrows*)

Visualization of thrombus itself into the sinus lumen with MR imaging depends on the duration of the pathologic process. The thrombus is best seen in the subacute phase as an area of a pronouncedly increased MR-signal on T1-weighted images and a slight hyperintense on T2-weighted images. At this phase T2-FLAIR sequence also demonstrates a hyperintense MR-signal from the thrombus. After administration of a contrast agent, filling defect is observed in the central part of the sinus («Δ» symptom).

Accumulation of contrast material on the periphery of the thrombus may occur due to reactive changes in the dura, or residual, but reduced blood flow (Dormont et al. 1995; Roche et al. 1996) (Figs. 27.3, 27.4, and 27.5).

An increased signal on DWI is noted in cases with a full occlusion. Also, on DWI, a hyperintense signal from cortical regions of the brain indicates ischemic changes due to venous stasis. Cortical and subcortical hemorrhages, edema, subarachnoid hemorrhage are possible, which are better visualized by MRI as hyperintense areas on T1-weighted sequences (methemoglobin phase) as well as T2-FLIAR images.

MR-venography is an important additional method of confirming the absence of blood flow in the lumen of the sinus. It not only determines the lack of blood movement through the sinuses, but also evaluates a comprehensive remodeling of the venous circulation of the brain, which in most cases is an outcome of the disease in the absence of early recanalization (Figs. 27.6 and 27.7).

However, the results of only single venography, excluding standard MRI data should be interpreted with caution. Overestimation in cases of unilateral hypoplasia of the dural sinus is possible. New possibilities of complex assessment of intra- and extracranial arterial and venous blood flow are opened using dynamic contrast-enhanced MR angiographic protocols (bolus MR angiography, TRISKS).

Differential Diagnosis Arachnoid granulation (a local rounded defect entering the sinus, signal intensity may be similar to that of CSF), hypoplasia of the transverse sinus is found in 33% (no signs of pathological changes in the signal on T1, T2, and T2-FLAIR at the projection of the sinus), physiological asymmetry of sinuses, subdural hematoma, subdural empyema (high signal on DWI, low on T1).

Dural arteriovenous fistula *(DAVF)* consists of 10–15% of all intracranial arteriovenous shunts (Lasjaunias et al. 1986). The characteristics of this disease are the presence of arteriovenous shunt in the dura. Most common, these fistulas are formed in the walls of the cavernous, transverse, and sigmoid sinuses. Cases with fistulas formation in other sinuses and dura of the skull base are more rare (Barrow 1985; Terada 1996). Their blood supply is usually multichannel. In addition to the most common sources of blood supply (meningeal arteries), branches of cerebral vessels through the pial dural anastomoses can participate in the blood supply of the dural fistula (Serbinenko et al. 1999). The most common causes are trauma, venous occlusion, and venous hypertension. DAVFs are classified on the basis of a number of parameters: etiology, nature, and location of the arteriovenous shunt, lateralization and prevalence relative to the intracranial space and a variety of other parameters.

The main *clinical manifestation* is pulsating tingling (noise) in postaural and occipital areas, cranial neuropathy, headaches, and progressive dementia. With concomitant sinus thrombosis, clinical symptoms are significantly increased (Lasjaunias et al. 1986; Noguchi et al. 2004).

Imaging A direct angiographic study shows afferent arteries supplying the DAVF, with varying degrees of tortuosity and multiplicity. Afferent vessels come from the dural and transosseous branches of the external carotid artery and tentorial meningeal branches of the internal carotid and vertebral arteries, as well as major branches of the occipital artery (Fig. 27.8).

On CT, the imaging picture can be normal, without pathological changes, especially in case of small-size fistulas. However, with the use of the bone window mode, extended tortuous defects in bones of the cranial vault may occur at the fistula site. Contrast enhancement should be better combined with angiographic mode, which allows to visualize both incoming extracranial arteries and intracranial vascular changes in the meningeal arteries and the area of fistula itself near the dural sinus (Fig. 27.9).

As with CT, MRI patterns strongly depend on the size of DAVF. In the presence of large afferent arteries, T1- and T2-weighted scans can visualize convoluted areas of MR signal loss (flow-void) in subcutaneous fat and intracranial subarachnoid space (best seen on T2-weighted sequences). In cases with sinus thrombosis, the signal is hyperintense at the region of the blood clot on T2-weighted and T2-FLAIR sequences.

CT and MR angiography are an important scanning modes, which allow visualizing the architecture of both arterial and venous parts of the fistula (Figs. 27.10 and 27.11). However, direct angiography remains the main diagnostic and therapeutic method in the treatment of DAVF (Rucker et al. 2003).

Differential Diagnosis Hypoplasia of the transverse sinus, sinus thrombosis, subdural hematoma, enlarged Pacchionian granulations.

Neurovascular conflict occurs as a result of pressure of an artery or, rarer, a vein on the cranial nerves. Several typical symptoms caused by an impact of vessels on nerves located within the posterior cranial fossa are usually distinguished: trigeminal neuralgia and hemifacial spasm.

Trigeminal neuralgia (sharp pain along the branches of the trigeminal nerve on one side) develops as a result of

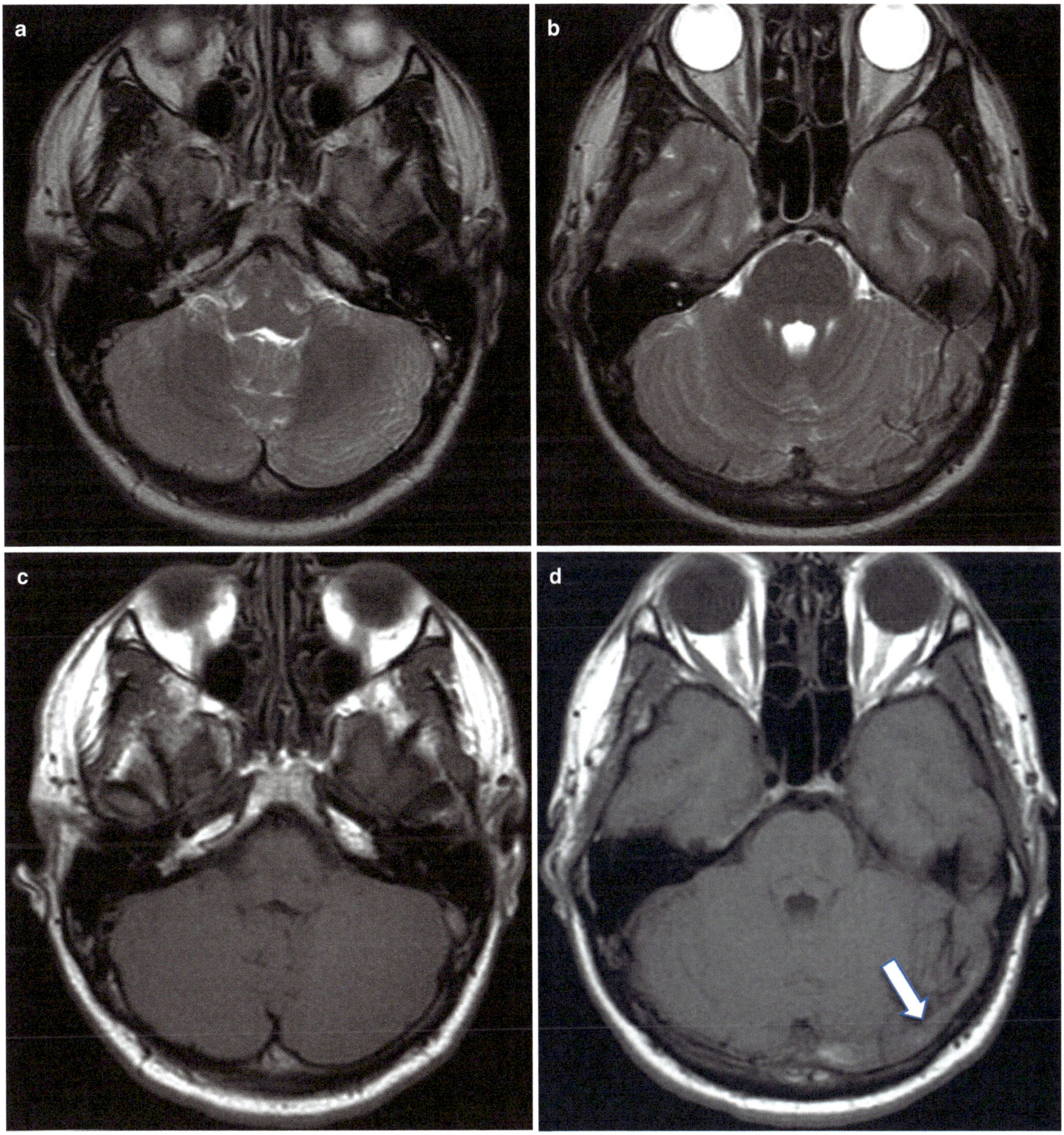

Fig. 27.3 Thrombosis of the superior sagittal sinus with expansion into the *left* transverse and sigmoid sinuses. On T2- (**a**, **b**), T1- (**c**, **d**), and T2-FLAIR- (**e**) weighted MRI an inhomogeneously changed MR-signal in the lumen of the transverse and sigmoid sinuses is visualized (*arrows*). Right transverse sinus is hypoplastic and its lumen isn't clearly visible. Increased MR signal in T1 sequence suggests the appearance of methemoglobin in the thrombus (a subacute phase). MR-angiography with using 2D TOF (**f**, **g**) and 3D PC (**h**) sequences demonstrates the absence of superior sagittal sinus, *left* transverse and sigmoid sinuses visualization. There is a remodel in venous blood circulation of the brain on MR-angiography

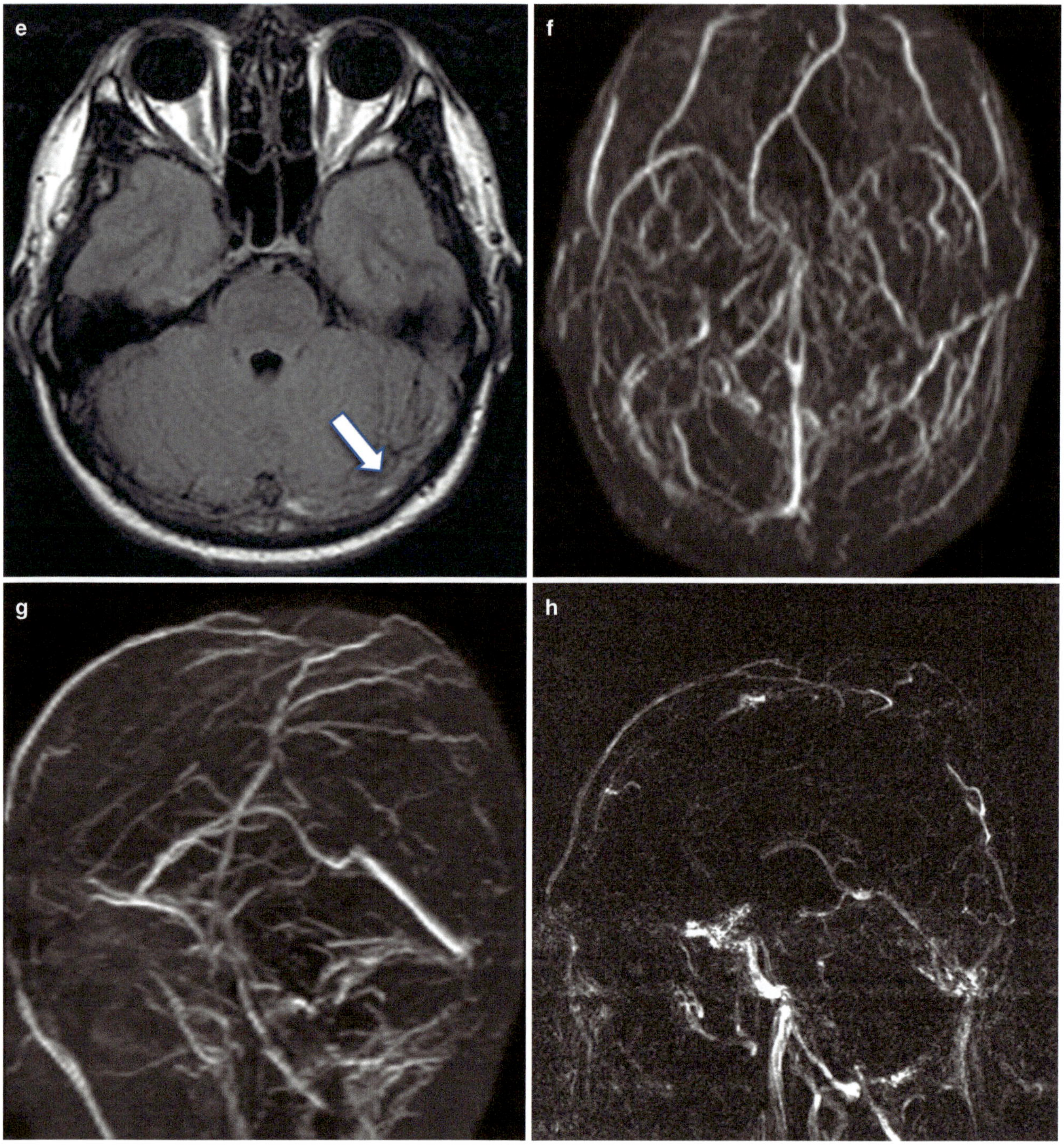

Fig. 27.3 (continued)

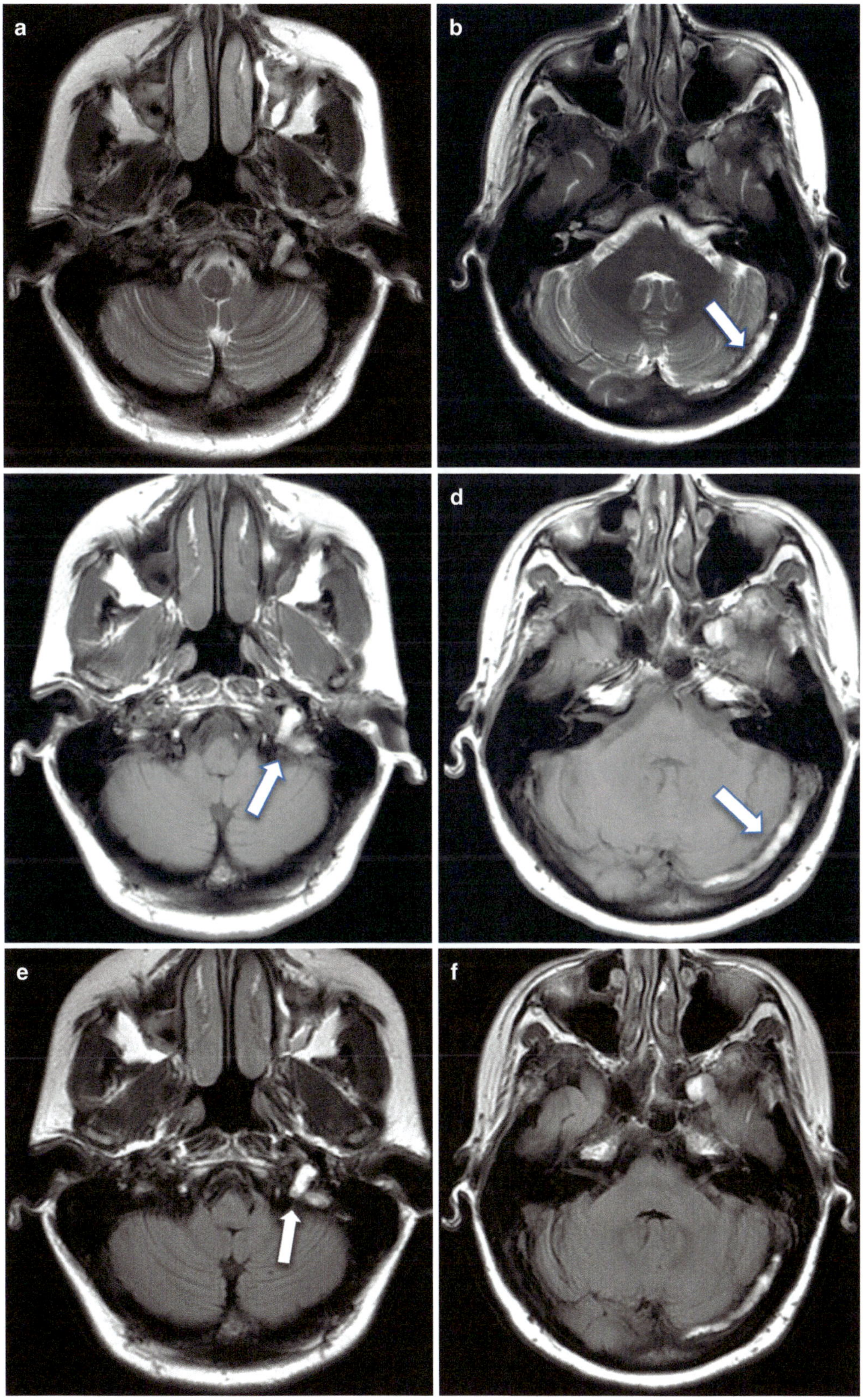

Fig. 27.4 Thrombosis of superior sagittal sinus with expansion into the left transverse and sigmoid sinuses. On T2- (**a**, **b**), T1- (**c**, **d**), and T2-FLAIR- (**e**, **f**) weighted MR images a hyperintensive MR-signal in the lumen of the jugular vein bulb, transverse and sigmoid sinuses on the left due to thrombosis can be visualized (*arrows*). Increased MR-signal in T2 and T1 sequences resembles the extracellular methemoglobin in the thrombus (a late acute phase). In SWAN (**g**) and DWI (**h**) sequences MR-signal from the thrombus is increased. MR-angiography using 2D TOF (**i**, **j**) and 3D PC (**k**, **l**) techniques reveals the absence of the MR-signal from lumens of superior sagittal sinus, left transverse and sigmoid sinuses. The extensive changes in venous blood circulation of the brain can be seen on MR-angiography

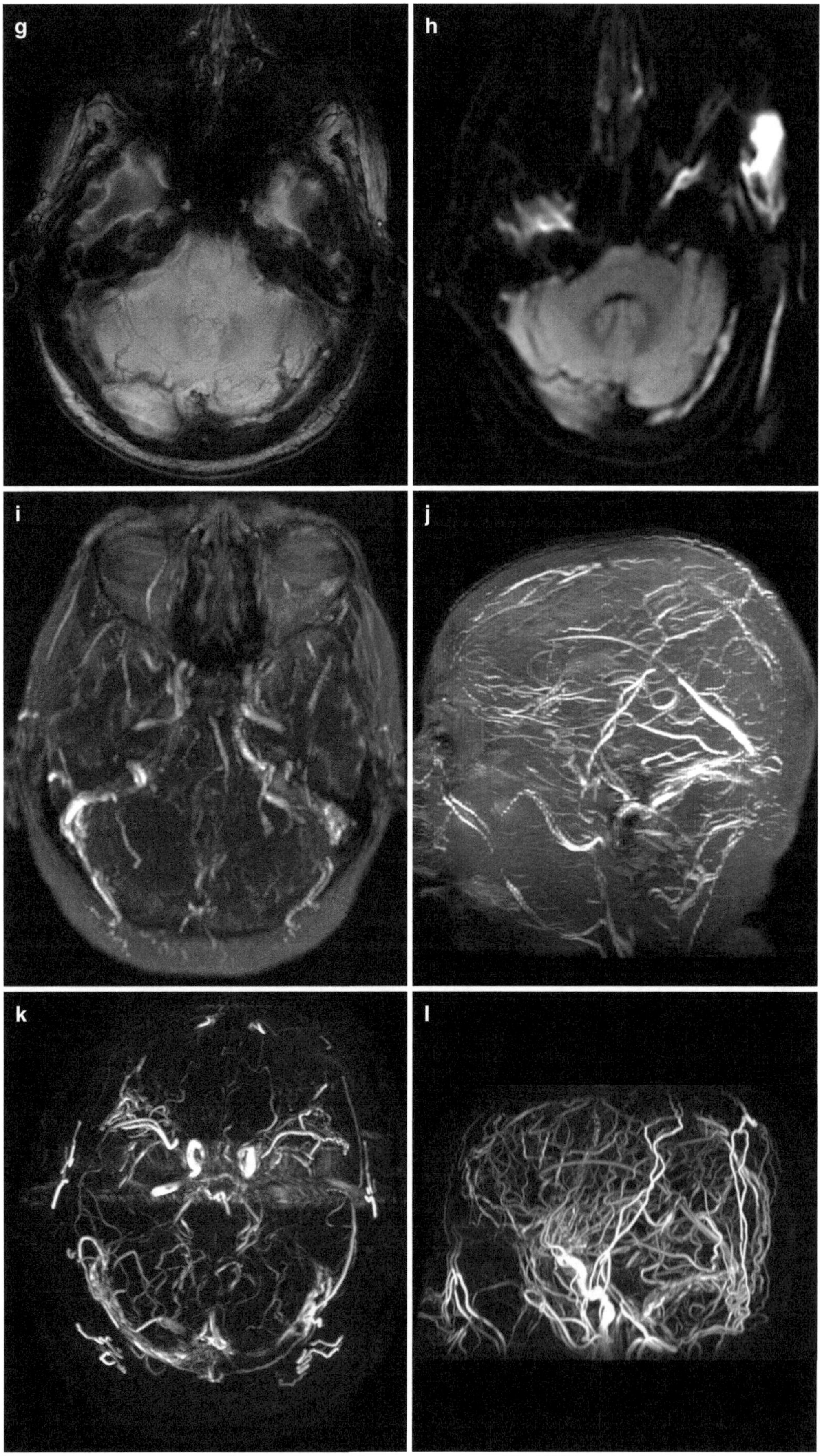

Fig. 27.4 (continued)

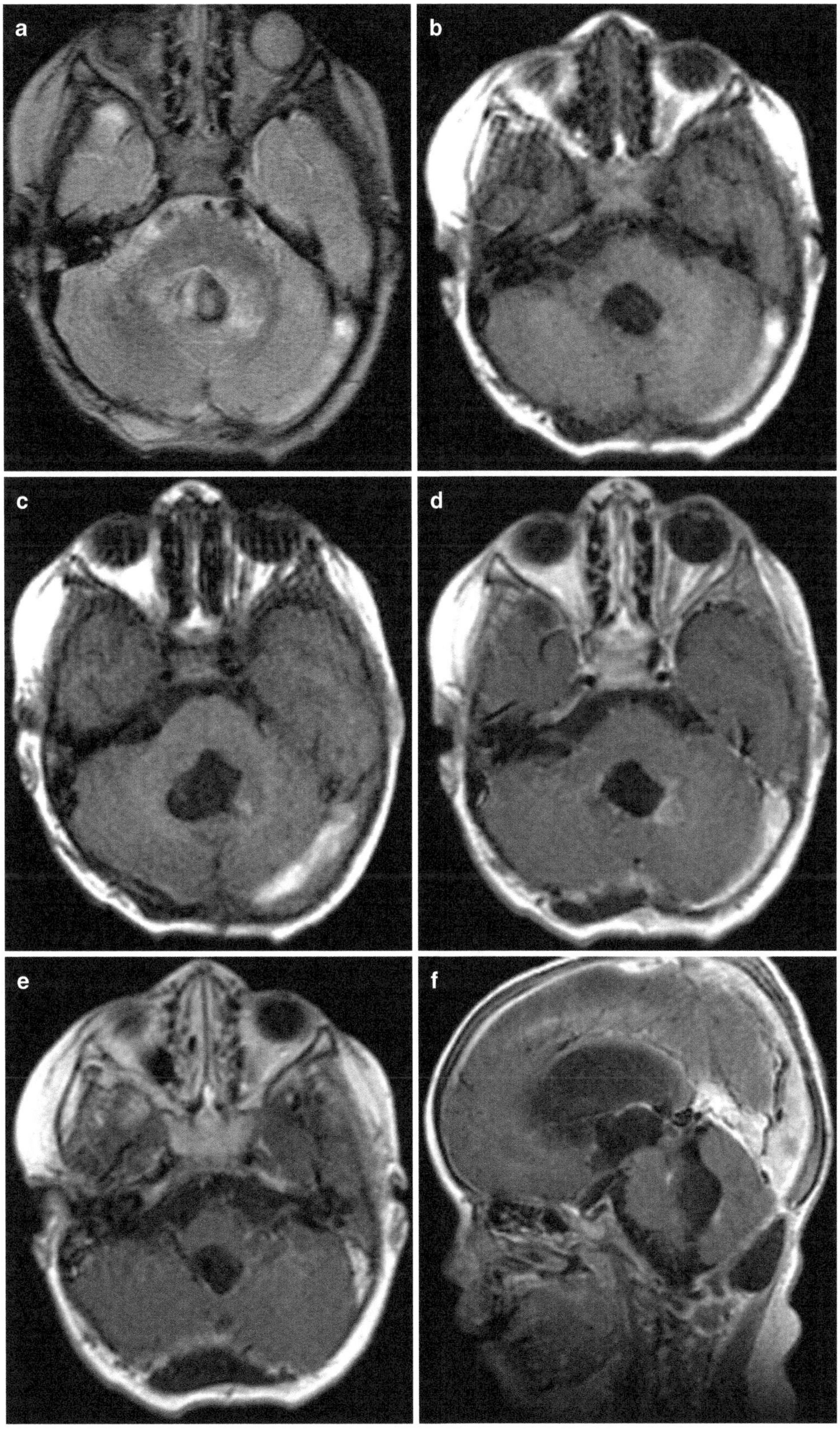

Fig. 27.5 Postoperative thrombosis of superior sagittal sinus with expansion into the left transverse and sigmoid sinuses. Complication after resection of 4th ventricle medulloblastoma. Series of T2- (**a**), T1-weighted MR images before (**b**, **c**) and after (**d**–**f**) intravenous contrast enhancement visualize a hyperintense MR-signal from the intraluminal thrombus of transverse and sigmoid sinuses. On sagittal postenhanced T1-weighted MR image (**f**) a hyperintense MR-signal in lumen of the superior sagittal sinus can be visible

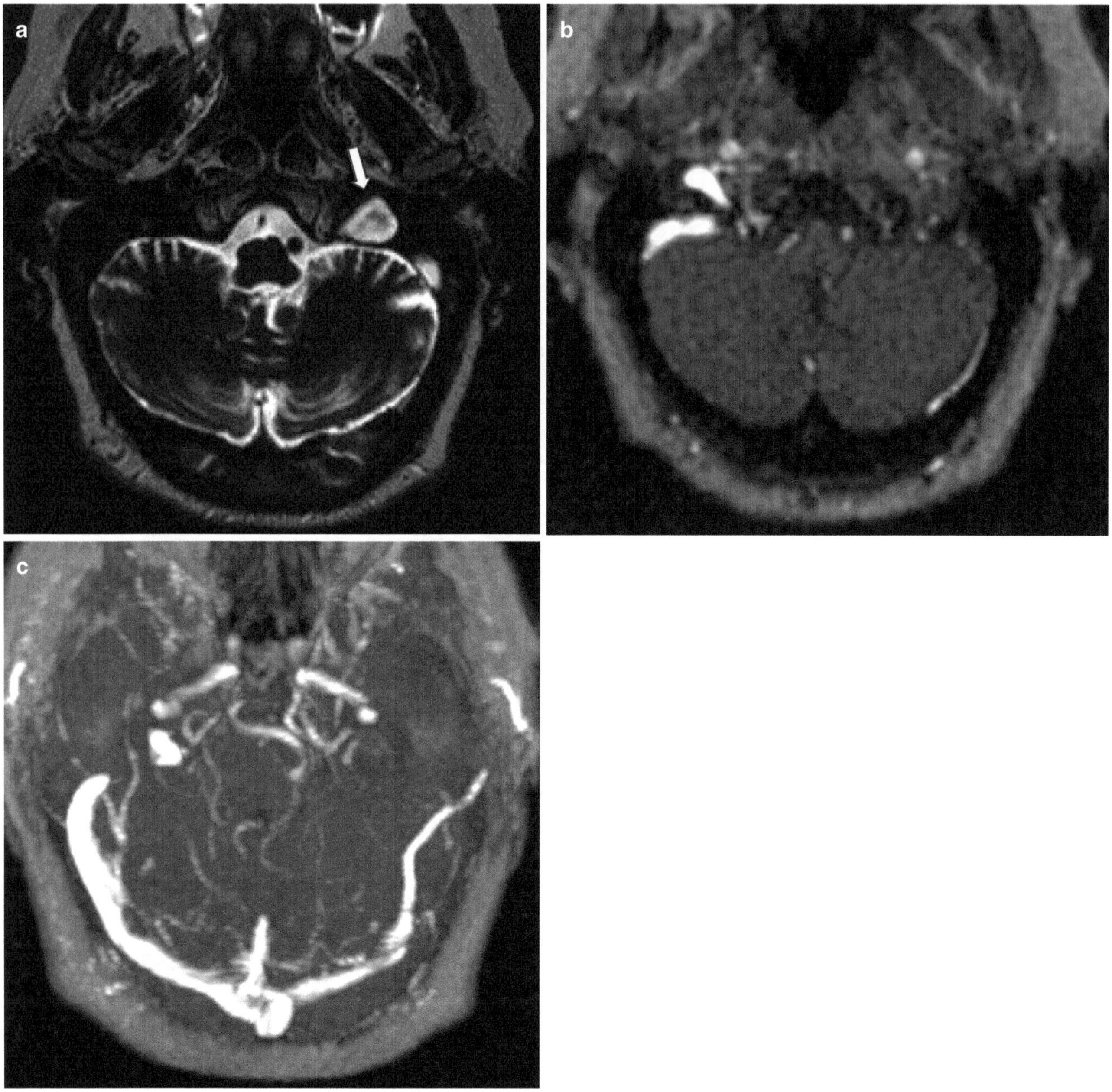

Fig. 27.6 Thrombosis of the jugular vein bulb, sigmoid and transverse sinuses on the left. MRI in T2 mode (**a**) visualizes an increased MR-signal from the thrombus in lumen of the jugular vein bulb (*arrow*). MR-angiography using 2D TOF technique demonstrates the absence on blood flow in the sinuses on the *left*. Additional draining vein at the level of thrombosis (**b**–raw data, **c**–MIP reformation) can be seen

compression on one of the vertebral-basilar system arteries of the trigeminal nerve root (cisternal portion). By frequency, vessels that compress the nerve can be ranged as follows: superior cerebellar artery, anterior inferior cerebellar artery, pontine branches of the basilar artery, posterior inferior cerebellar artery. In addition, the vertebral-basilar dolichoectasia, saccular aneurysms, AVMs and dural arteriovenous fistulas may cause neurovascular conflict. Tumors growing at the projection of the cerebellopontine angle and petroclival area can also cause local neuralgia in many cases. That is why, even with a typical clinical picture of the disease, an extended CT or MRI of the specified area is indicated, usually with the use of intravenous contrast enhancement.

If a vascular loop is located high in the anterior part of the cerebellopontine cistern (usually the superior cerebellar artery), it puts pressure on the proximal preganglionic segment of V-th nerve.

Hemifacial Spasm If a vascular loop is located in the middle of the cerebellopontine cistern (usually the superior

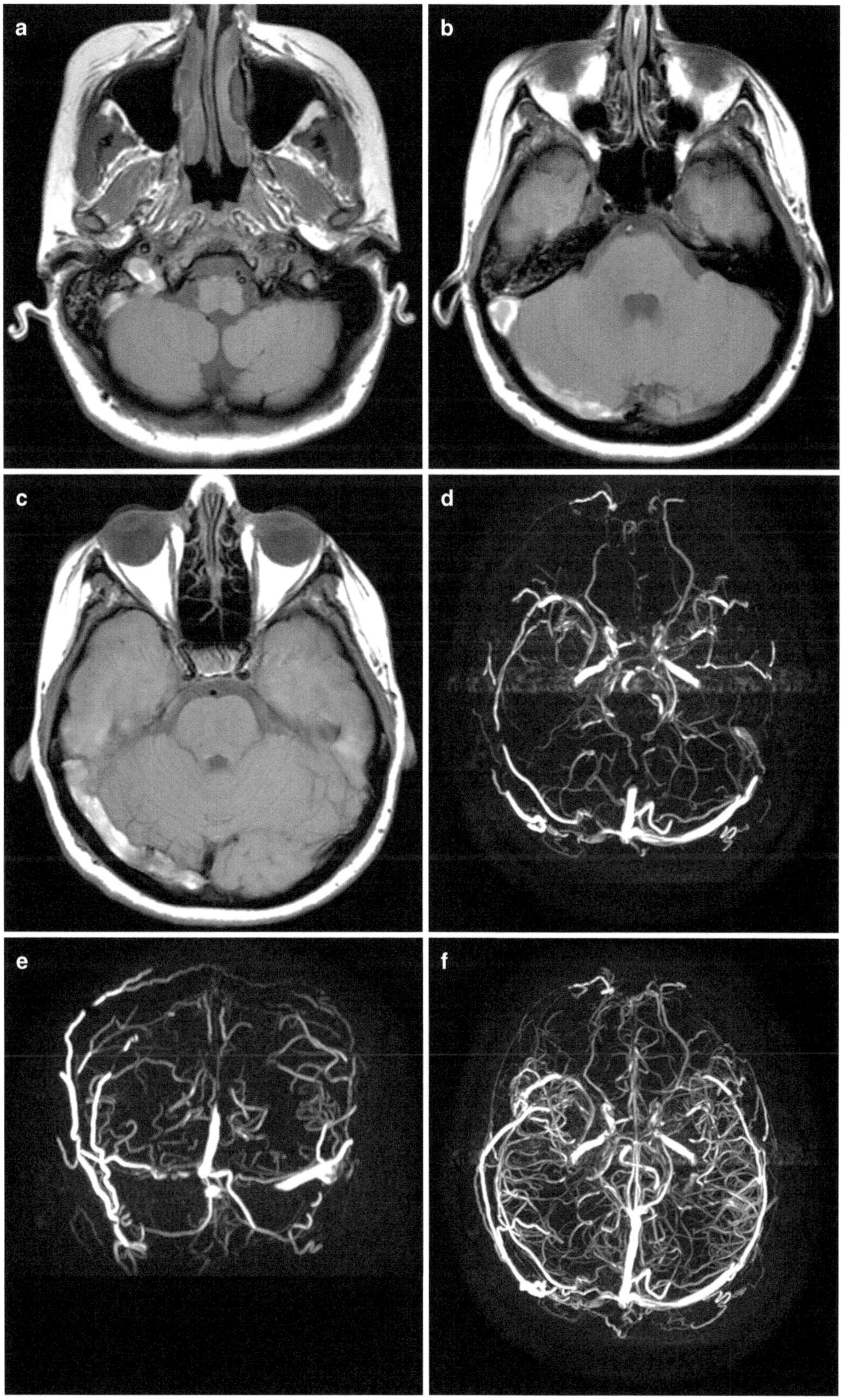

Fig. 27.7 Thrombosis of the jugular vein bulb, sigmoid and transverse sinuses on the right. MRI in T1 sequence (**a–c**) visualizes an increased MR-signal from the thrombus in the lumen of these sinuses. MR-angiography using 3D PC technique (**d–f**) demonstrates the absence of blood flow within the sinuses. Meanwhile an extensive remodel in venous blood circulation both at the level of posterior cranial fossa and whole brain can be detected. Additional draining venous network is appeared at the level of thrombosed sinuses

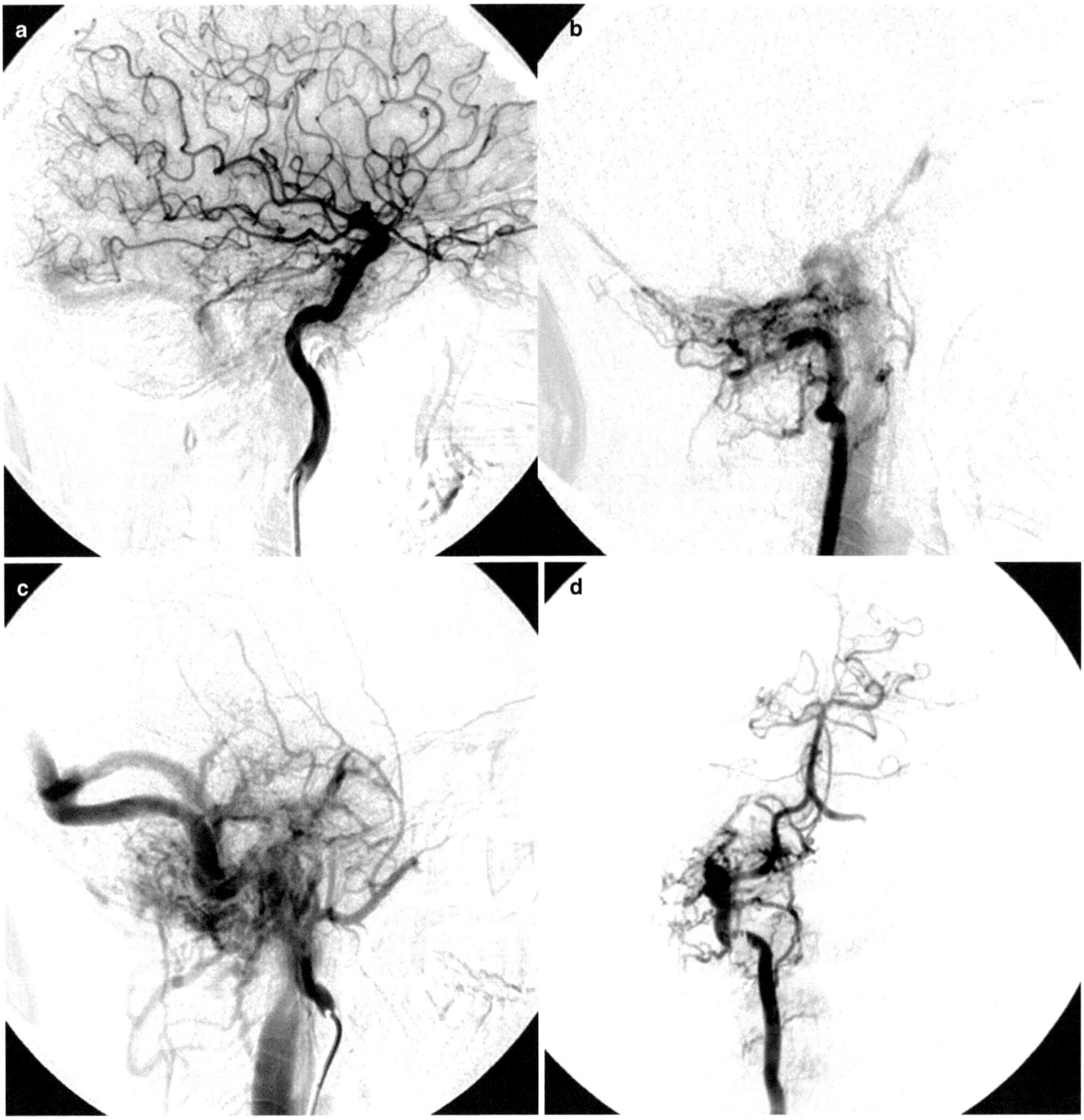

Fig. 27.8 Dural arteriovenous fistula of the right transverse sinus. Direct cerebral selective angiography of the right internal carotid artery (**a**–lateral view) and right vertebral artery (**b**, **c**–lateral views, **d**–coronal view) demonstrates an extensive dural fistula, which is supplied mainly from the vertebral artery system and from meningeal branches of the carotid artery. During venous phase of DSA (**c**) a spreading of pathological fistula network can be estimated

cerebellar artery and anterior inferior cerebellar artery), it puts pressure on the proximal part or base of the root of VII-th cranial nerve. Clinically, it is manifested by the development of hemifacial spasm, which is characterized by sudden unilateral involuntary facial muscles spasm. It occurs as a result of local pressure of anterior inferior, posterior inferior cerebellar or vertebral arteries on VII-th nerve.

Vascular conflict with the vestibular nerve is characterized by staccato-like tingling or typewriter sound in ears and dizziness. The same arteries as in cases with hemifacial spasm are responsible for this. Neuralgia of the caudal group of nerves is much rare. Vascular compression of IX-th pair is characterized by unilateral paroxysmal pain arising during swallowing and irradiating from the oropharynx to the ear. In case of Eagle syndrome, the cause of

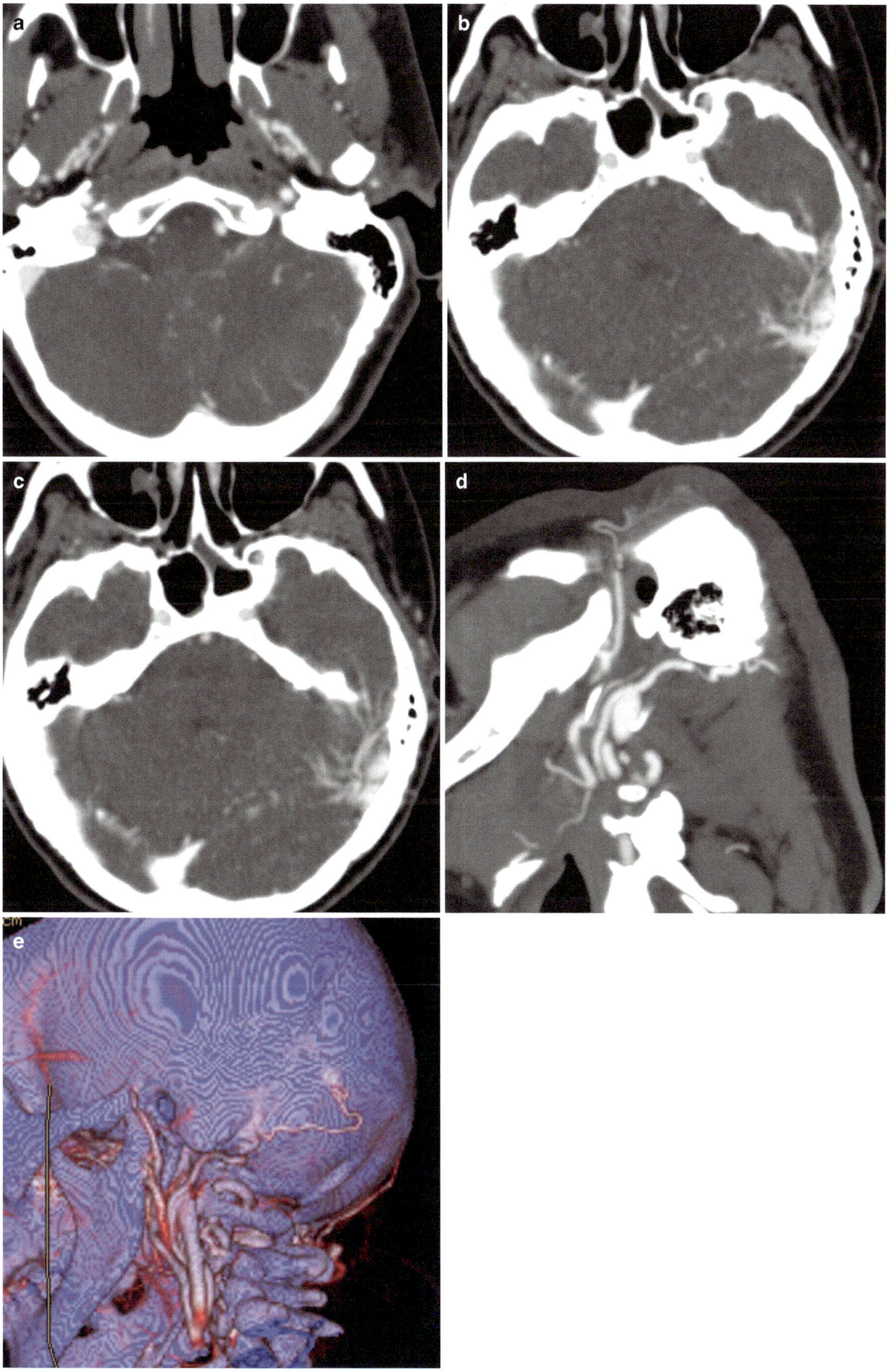

Fig. 27.9 Dural arteriovenous fistula of the left transverse sinus. CT-angiography series (**a**–**c**) demonstrates a large pathological arterial network in projection of the left transverse sinus. Fistula is supplied from the occipital branch of the external carotid artery (**d**–2D reformation, **e**–3D view)

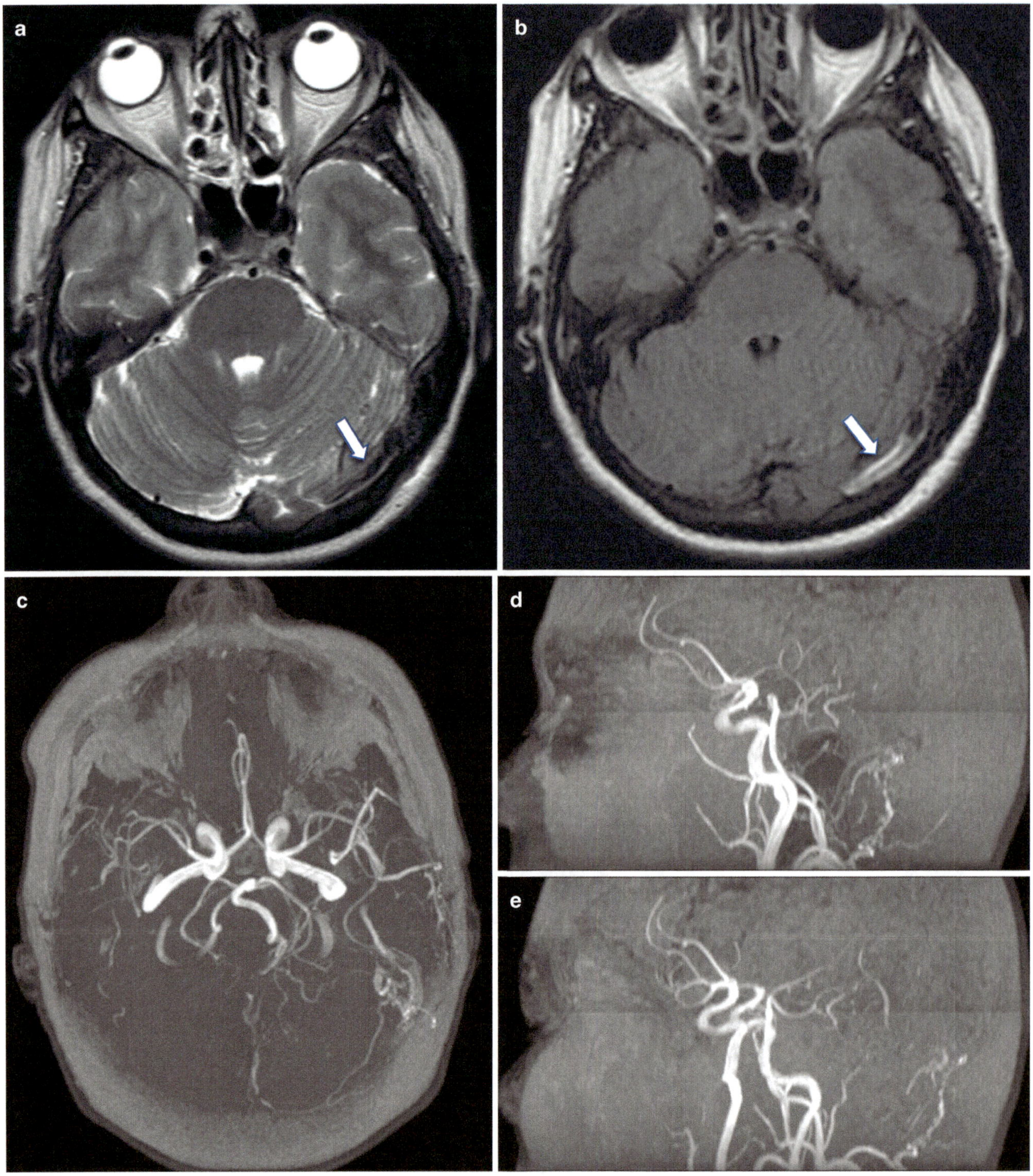

Fig. 27.10 Dural arteriovenous fistula of the left transverse sinus. On axial MR images in T2 (**a**) and T2-FLAIR (**b**) sequences a hyperintense MR-signal due to acute thrombosis in the lumen of the left transverse sinus is visualized (*arrows*). MR-angiography using 3D TOF technique with reformation in different planes (**c**–**i**) demonstrates pathological vessel network of the fistula. Blood supply is coming from the occipital and the middle meningeal arteries (branches of the external carotid artery)

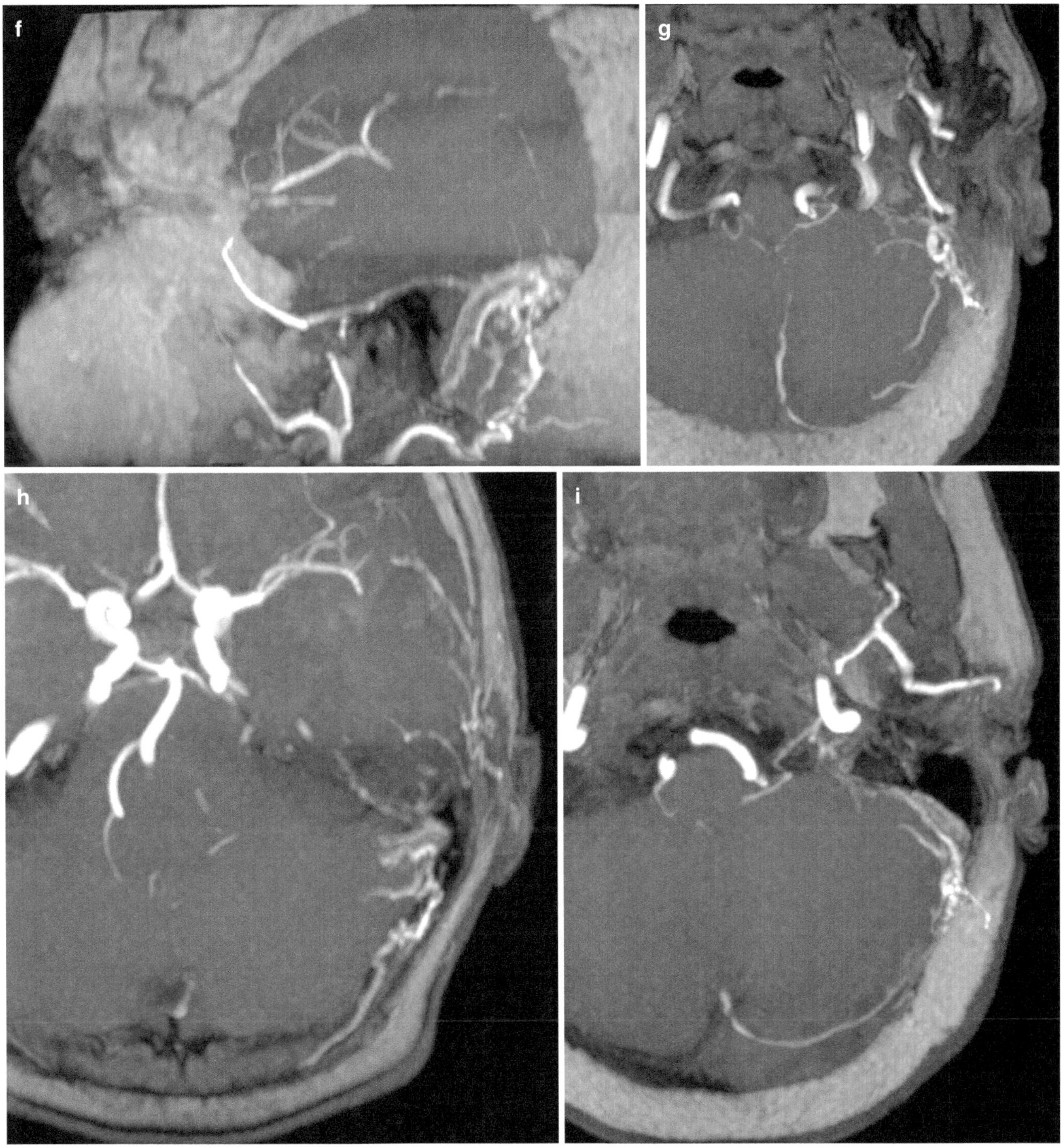

Fig. 27.10 (continued)

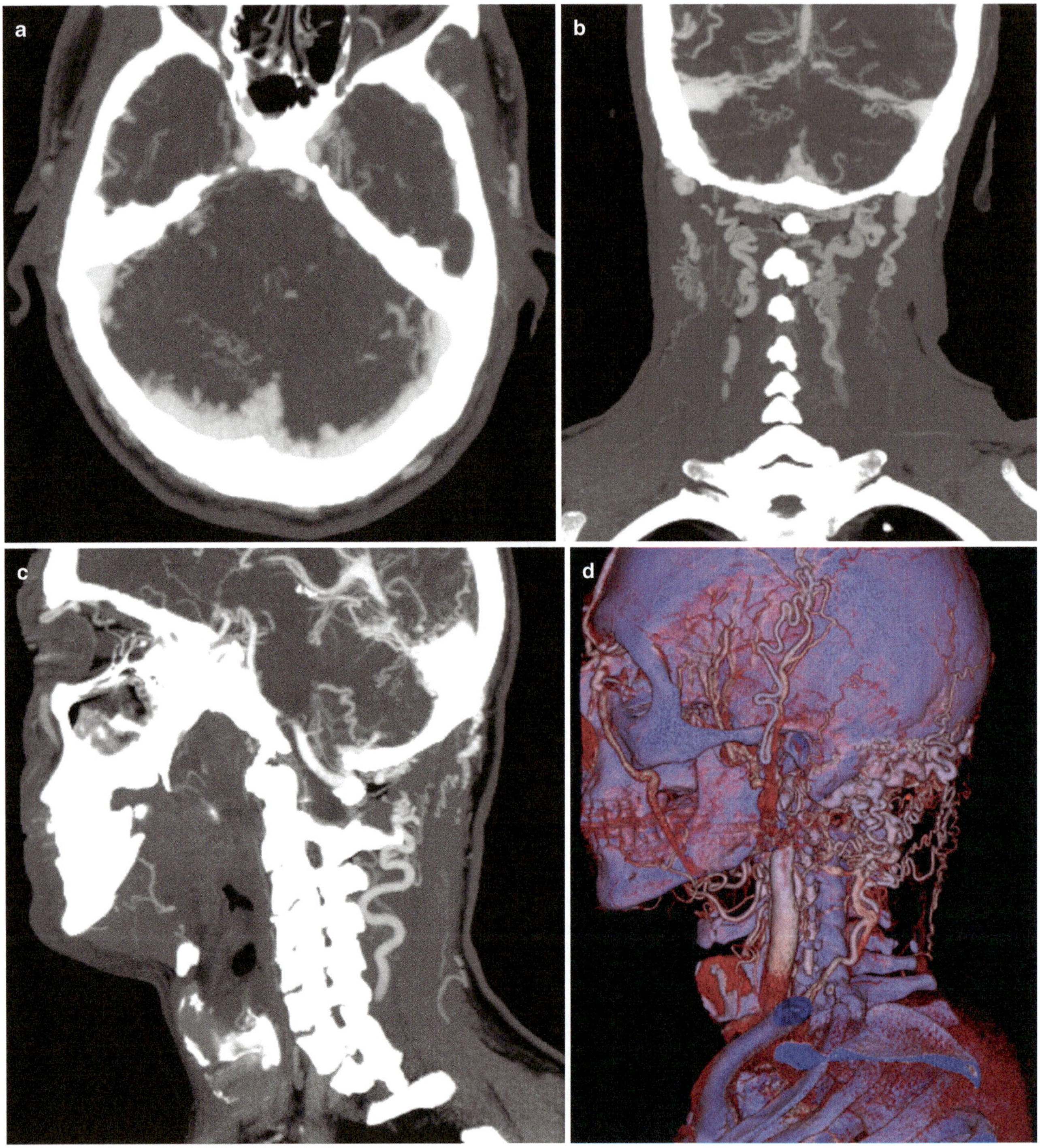

Fig. 27.11 Extensive dural arteriovenous fistula of transverse sinuses on both sides. CT-angiograms in axial projection (**a**), coronal (**b**) and sagittal (**c**) reformations, 3D reconstructions (**d**, **e**) demonstrate a large dural arteriovenous fistula in the occipital area. The fistula extends into posterior cranial fossa. On MRI using T2- (**f**, **g**), SWAN- (**h**) weighted sequences and 3D TOF MR-angiography (**i**) a dural fistula, which is supplied from branches of the right vertebral, *left* middle meningeal artery and both occipital arteries is clearly depicted

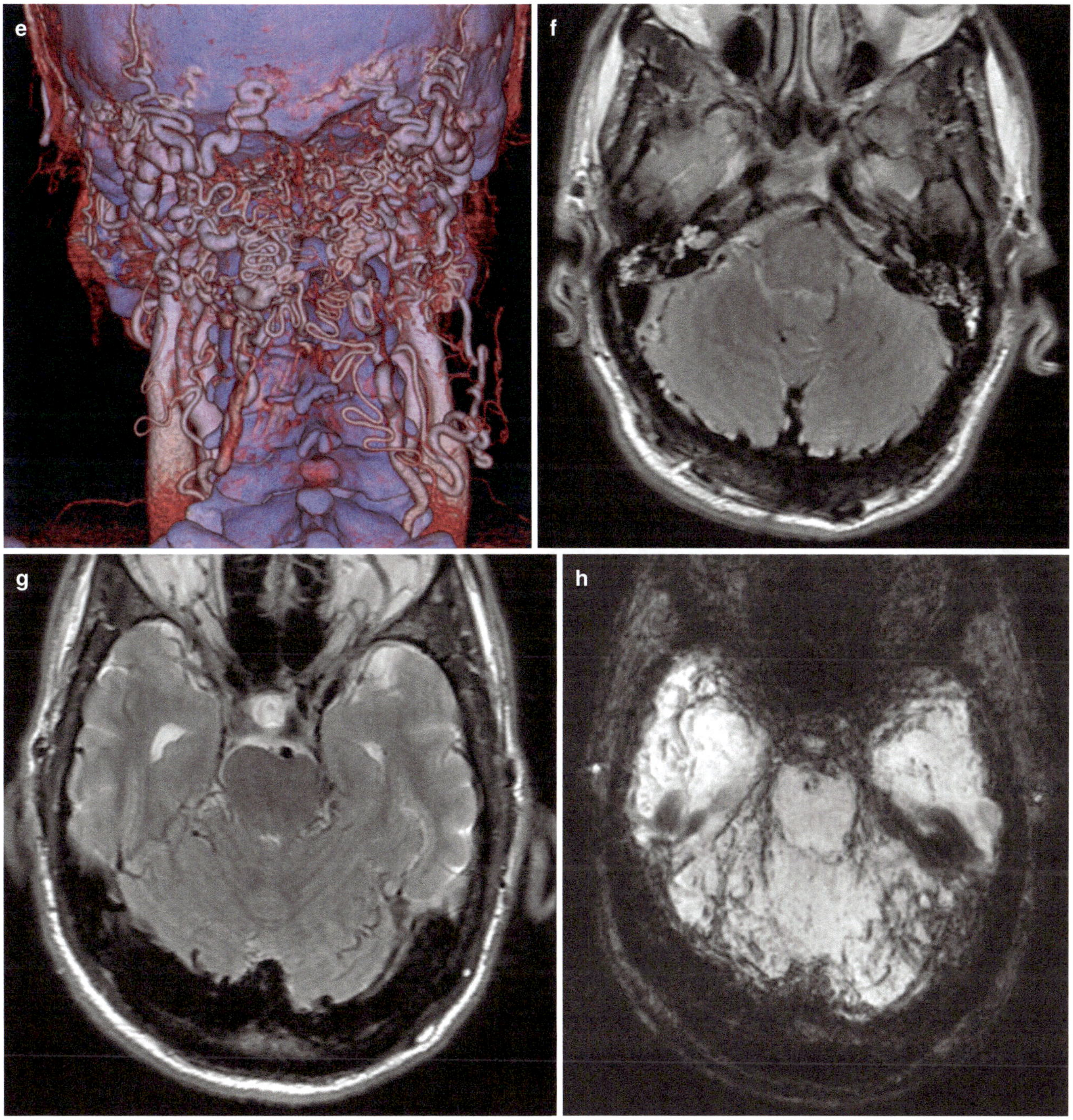

Fig. 27.11 (continued)

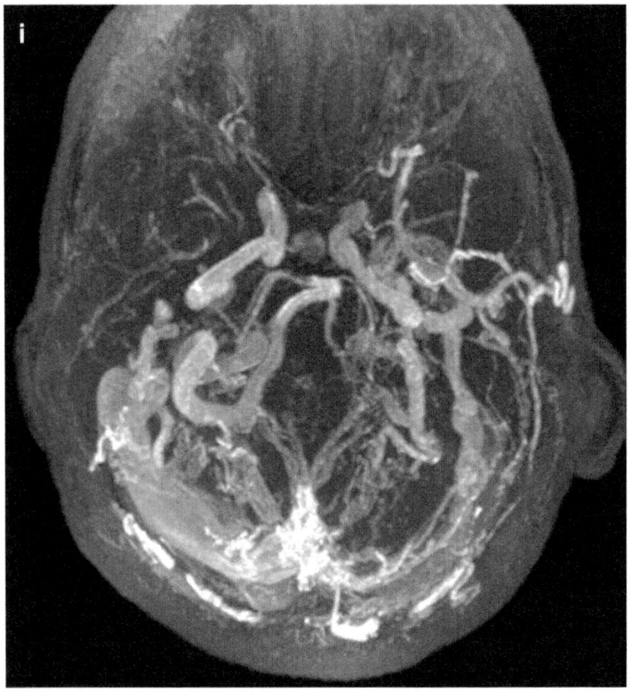

Fig. 27.11 (continued)

glossopharyngeal neuralgia is elongated styloid process of the temporal bone.

Imaging CT scan is usually negative. Attention should be paid to the position of the vertebral and basilar arteries, which are usually visible without the contrast enhancement. The best method for diagnosing neurovascular conflict is MR imaging using high resolution technique. Thin slices (no more than 1–3 mm for T2- and T1-weighted sequences) and myelographic sequences (strongly T2-weighted sequence, FIESTA, and other similar protocols) are better to use, since they better identify the relationship of the arteries and nerves in the basilar cisterns of the brain. The use of multiplanar MR-reformation (along the course of an artery or a nerve) provides the possibility to detect not only the proximity of the nerve and artery, but even deviation and compression of the corresponding nerve trunk. The preferred scanning sequences include 3D SPGR (slice thickness of 1 mm, isotropic voxel), FIESTA (GE), which uses suppression of pulsation artifacts from CSF with slice thickness 0.6–0.8 mm, and 3D TOF angiography before and after administration of contrast medium (Figs. 27.12 and 27.13). 3D additional post-processing of data obtained from MRI allows displaying the picture close to data from a direct microsurgical (or endoscopic) intervention (Fig. 27.14).

Arterial Aneurysms (AA) Almost all major arteries located within the posterior cranial fossa or in its close proximity can be an initial site of formation of an arterial aneurysm and both clinically and radiologically simulate a tumor of the clivus, petrous apex, and cerebellopontine angle. In general, AAs are not very common, accounting for about 1% of the posterior cranial fossa space-occupying lesions. Most often, AAs are formed at the projection of the basilar artery bifurcation and the distal segment of the vertebral artery, followed by the posterior inferior and anterior inferior cerebellar artery as well. AAs from the internal carotid artery siphon can bulge out into the subtentorial area. Sometimes pseudotumor clinical course is observed in fusiform aneurysms of the basilar artery (Hwang et al. 2003).

Most AAs are round or oval lesions with sizes from a few millimeters to several centimeters (giant). Larger AAs can clinically occur as space-occupying lesions with mass effect, especially on the brain stem. Fusiform aneurysms of the basilar artery characterized by elongated shapes sometimes similar to a muff, sometimes occupying the entire run of the artery.

Imaging The method of choice in the diagnosis of arterial aneurysms is still considered direct selective angiography, which demonstrates main topical features of the all anatomical aneurysm peculiarities in relation to the "mother" vessel. At the same time, the method does not visualize concomitant changes in the surrounding brain tissue (extent of the thrombosed part, extent of SAH, ischemic and other changes in the brain). Modern neuroradiological diagnosis of AAs cannot be performed without the use of CT and MRI (Coley et al. 1998; Depauw et al. 2003).

Routine CT of fully functioning AAs shows moderately increased density within the aneurysm sac (adequate visualization is available in sizes greater than 1 cm). In large and giant aneurysms, calcifications in their walls are often found, which are easily identified with non-enhanced CT (Fig. 27.15). Moreover, CT helps assess intracerebral or even intrathecal hemorrhages, concomitant to most AAs, determines the degree of internal hydrocephalus and dem-

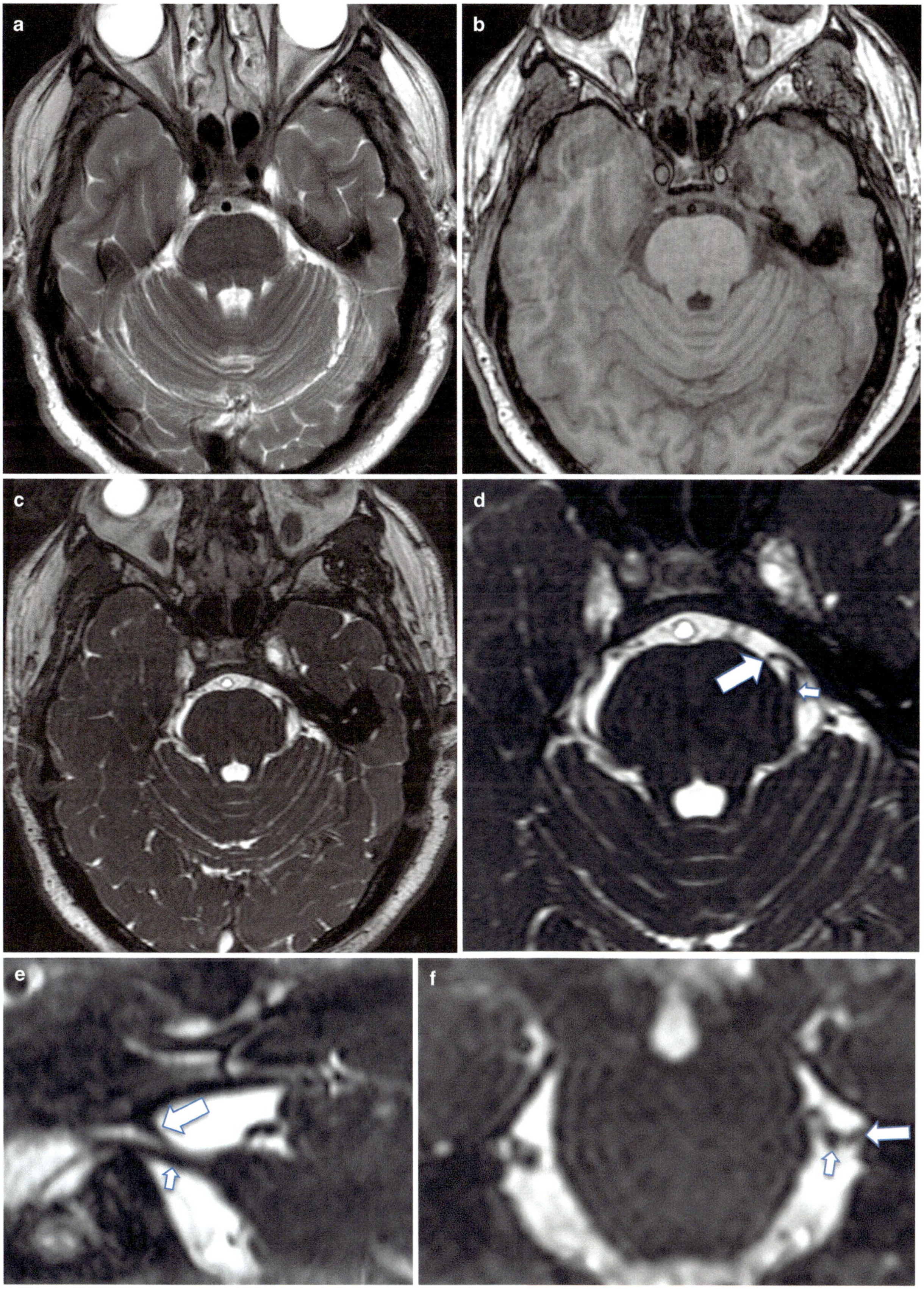

Fig. 27.12 Trigeminal neuralgia on the left side due to neurovascular conflict. Series MRI using T2- (**a**), SPGR- (**b**), FIESTA (**c**–**f**) techniques with reformations detect a close vicinity of superior cerebellar artery (*large arrow*) to the root of the V nerve with its dislocation (*small arrow*)

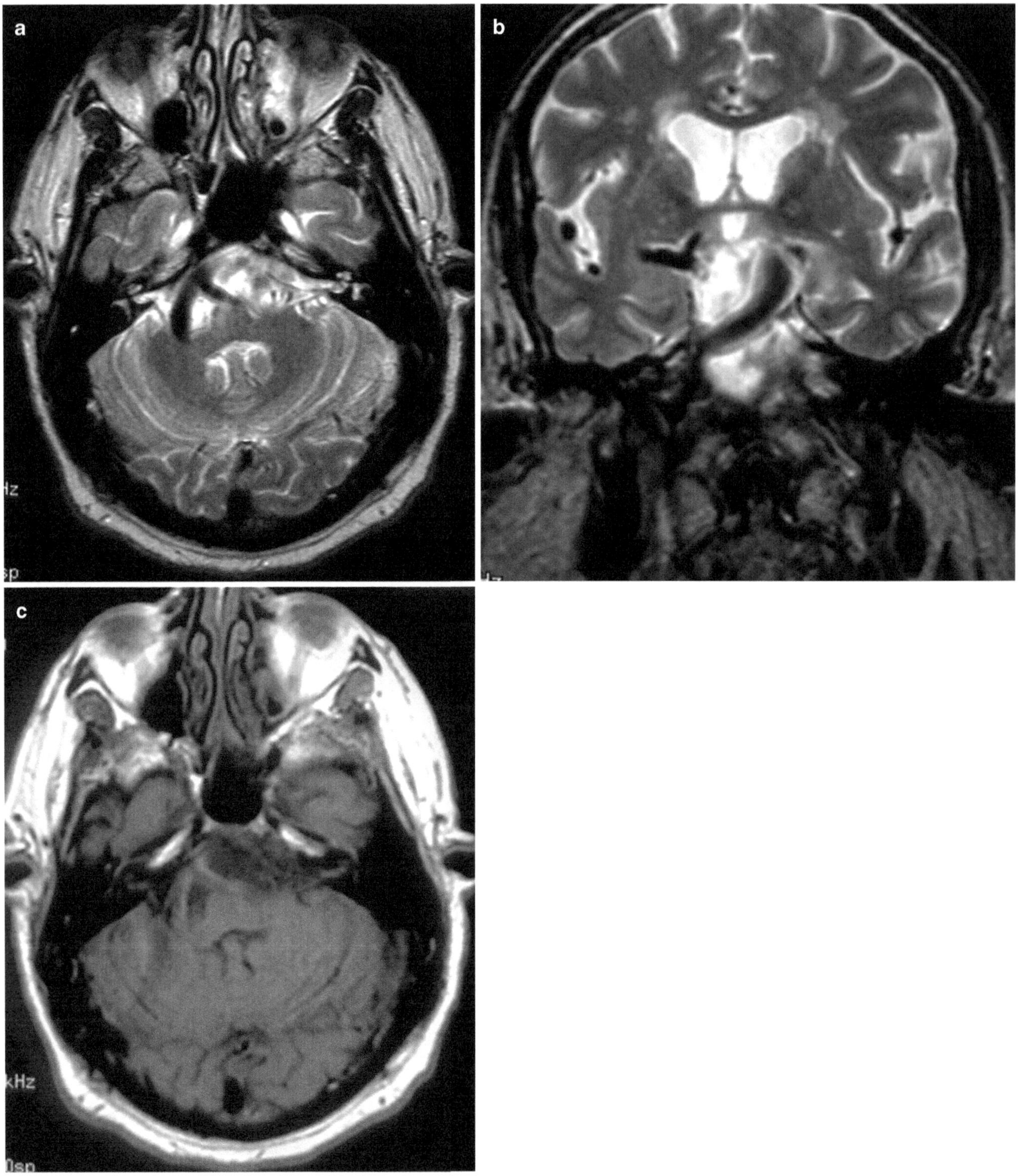

Fig. 27.13 Trigeminal neuralgia on the right side due to neurovascular conflict. Clinical symptoms are caused by the compression and dislocation of the brain stem due to enlarged and fusiform basilar artery. The artery has a wide lumen and compresses brain stem. T2- (**a**, **b**) and T1- (**c**) weighted MRI

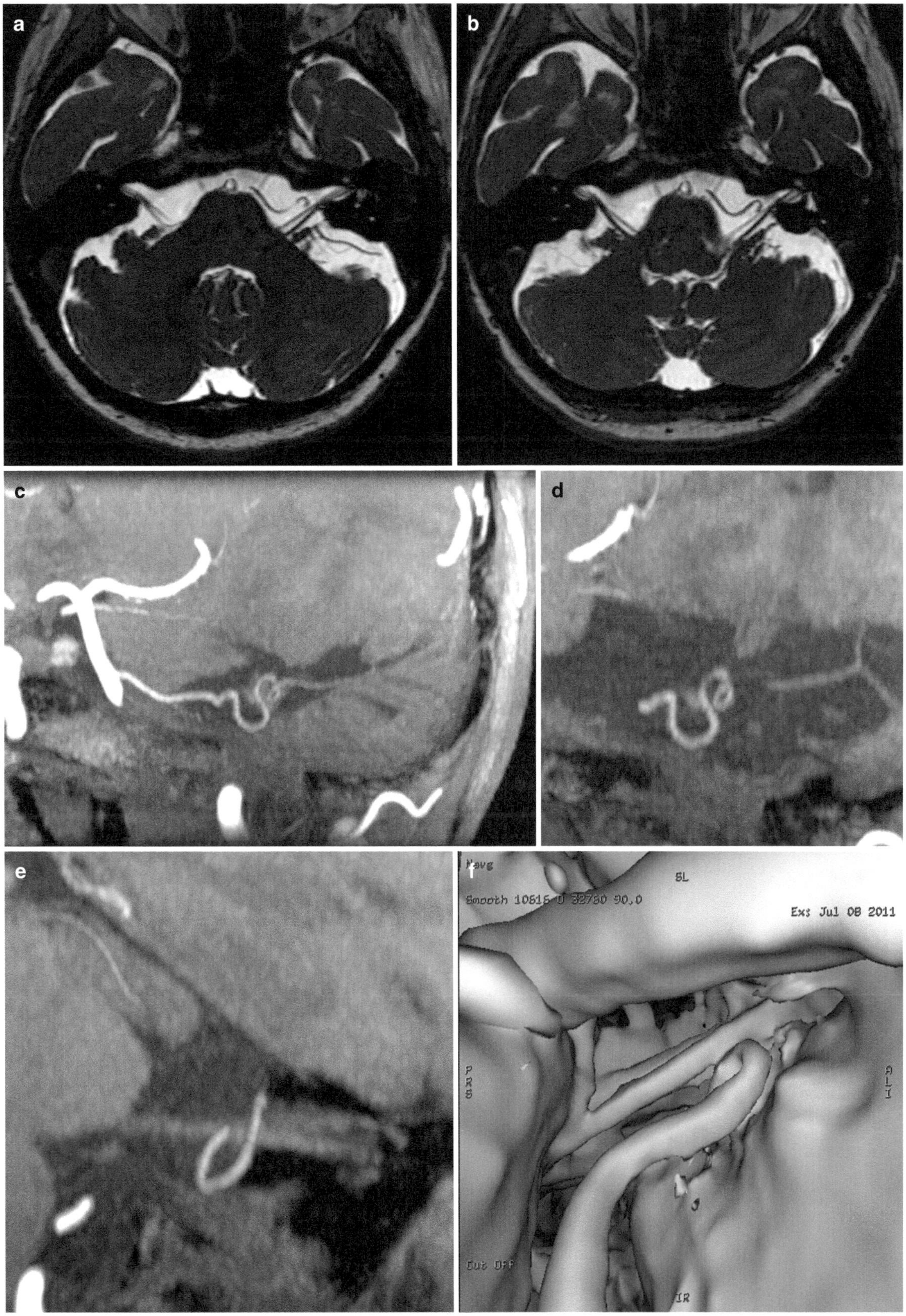

Fig. 27.14 Facial nerve neuralgia on the left side due to neurovascular conflict. MRI using FIESTA sequence (**a**, **b**), 3D TOF MR-angiography with following 2D reformations (**c**–**e**) and 3D reconstructions (**f**–**i**—from FIESTA, Navigator, GE) visualizes an atypical shape and pathway of the anterior inferior cerebellar artery. The artery forms loop at the level of cerebellopontine angle. The artery adjacent to the root of the facial nerve (*arrows*)

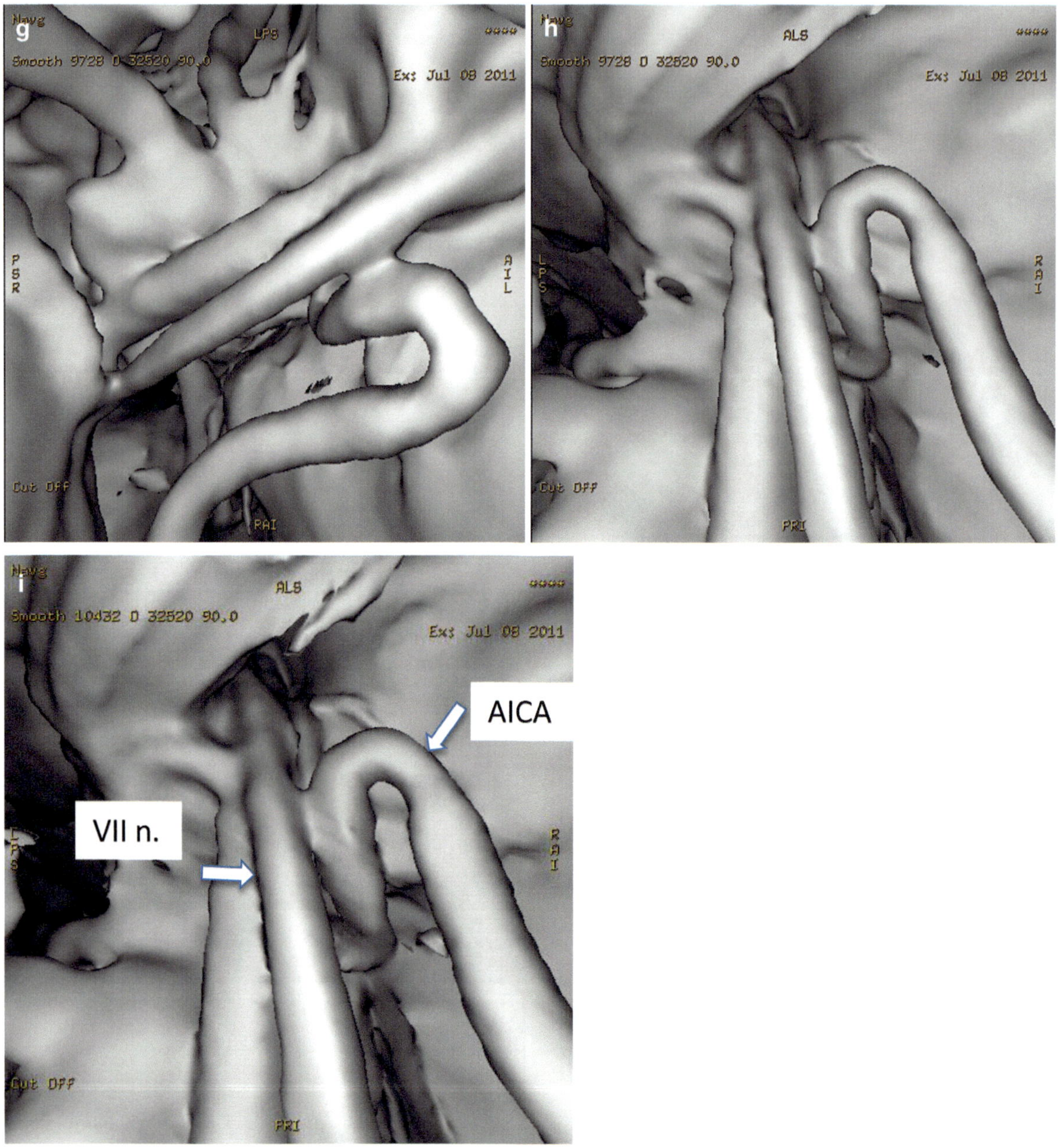

Fig. 27.14 (continued)

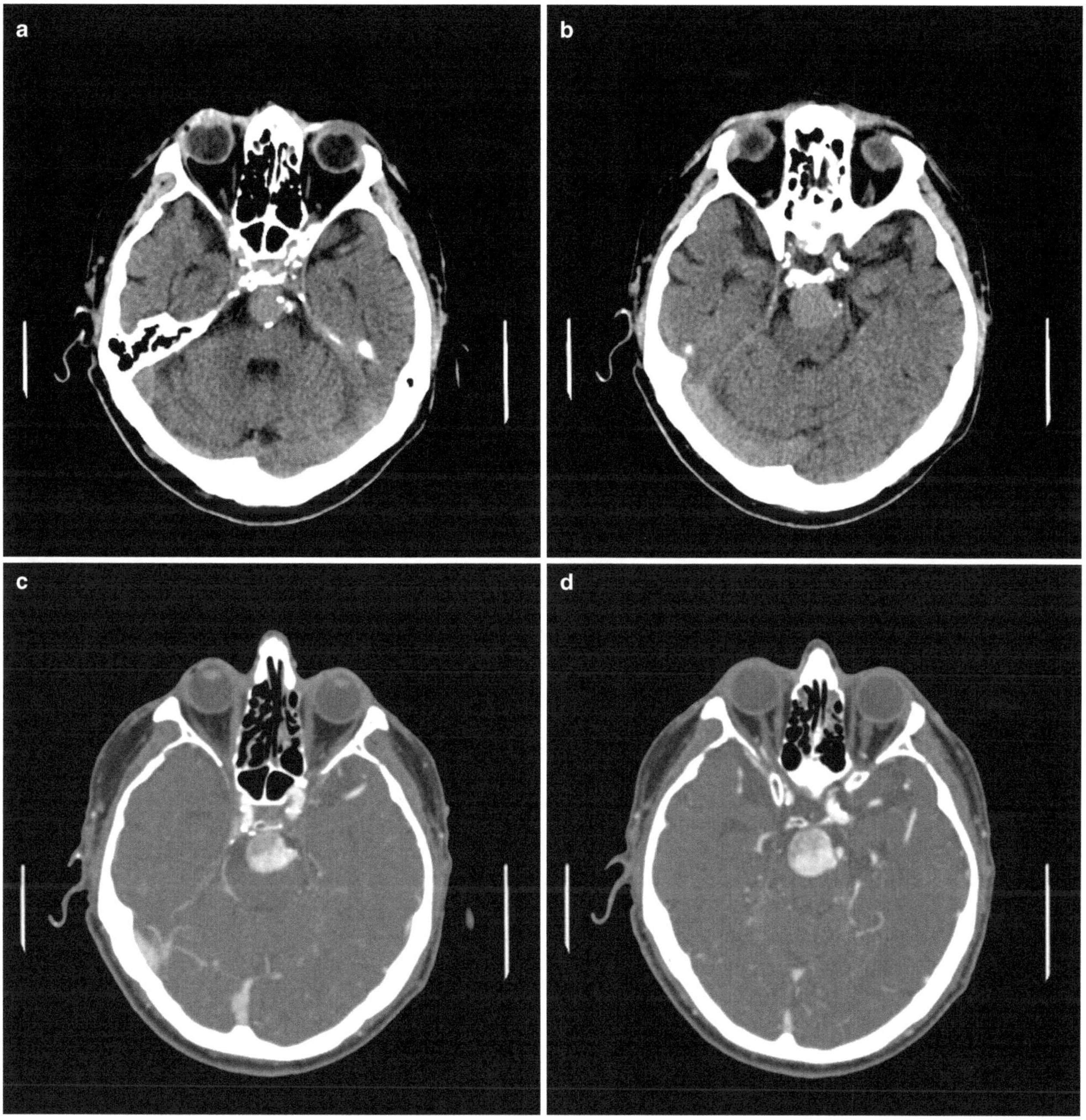

Fig. 27.15 Saccular arterial aneurysm of the basilar artery. Axial CT scans with contrast enhancement (**a**, **b**) demonstrate a hyperdense enhancing lesion, which has round shape and retrosellar location. There are small calcifications in the capsule. CT angiography (**c**, **d**) shows a partially functioning arterial aneurism with thrombosed ventral part of the basilar artery top. 3D reconstructions demonstrate a large saccular aneurysm of the top of basilar artery (**e**, **f**)

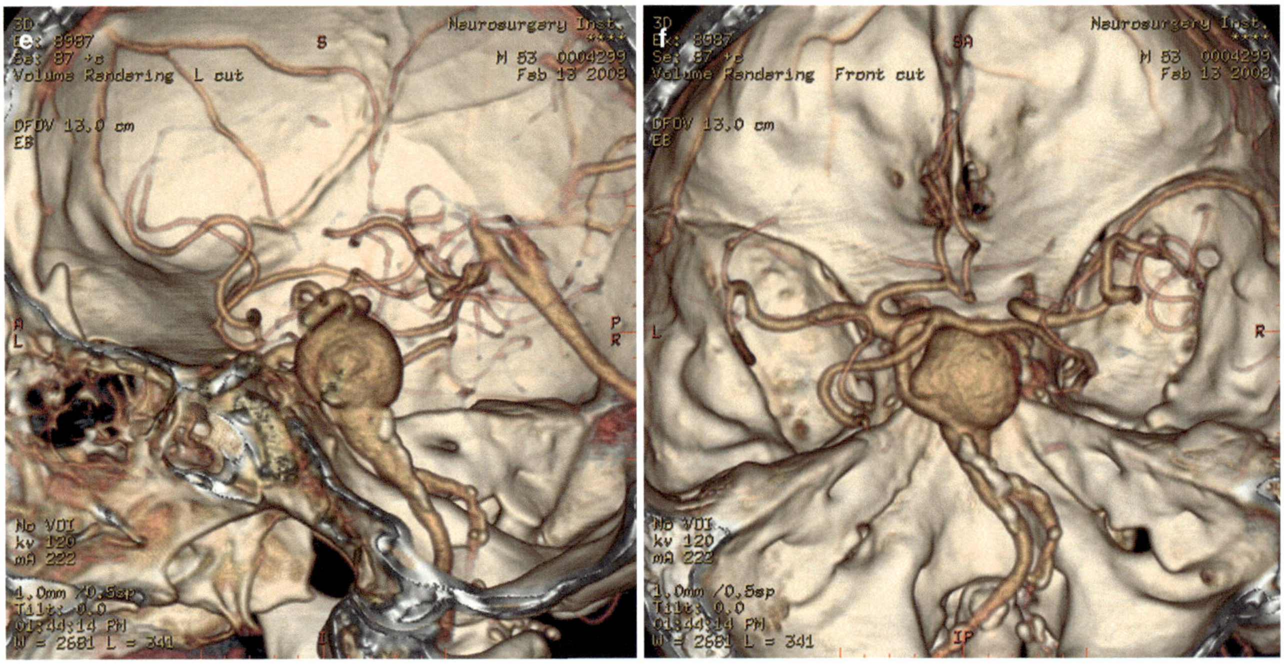

Fig. 27.15 (continued)

onstrates ischemic foci in the brain tissue both in close proximity and at a distance from an AA. Long-term, large AAs located at the base of the brain can cause expansive changes in the skull base bones (clivus, apex of the pyramid of the temporal bone). CT with bone window mode clearly visualizes these features, without revealing the destructive and infiltrative changes typical for tumor growth (Fig. 27.16).

Best differentiation of functioning and thrombosed parts of AAs is achieved using CT angiography. Subsequent 2D reformation and 3D reconstruction (the use of virtual endoscopy mode is possible) allows answering basic questions of preoperative diagnosis (Figs. 27.17 and 27.18).

MRI appearance of AAs depends mainly on the ratio between the thrombosed and functioning parts of an aneurysm. Fully functioning AAs are characterized by loss of MR-signal (flow-void) on all scanning sequences (T1, T2, T2-FLAIR, DWI). Only a giant aneurysm can manifest as heterogeneous round space-occupying lesions. A pathognomonic MR-sign of AA is the presence of pulsation artifacts in the direction of the phase-encoding gradient. The MR-signal from the thrombosed portion may range from hypo- to hyperintensity according to the degree of clot retraction. Layering of MR-signal from the thrombus is another very typical AA characteristic. Simultaneous total thrombosis of an arterial aneurysm sac is an exception rather than a rule; however, this event occurred in our clinical practice (Figs. 27.19, 27.20, 27.21, and 27.22).

Intravenous administration of contrast agent significantly increases AAs density on CT and their MR-signal on T1-weighted images (marked heterogeneity of MR-signal due to rapid blood flow in the AA's sac).

The diagnosis of AA can be confirmed by MR angiography using 3D TOF or 3D PC sequences. Rarely, in case of full thrombosis of the aneurysm, they cannot be enhanced with direct and CT-angiography, and be invisible on MR angiography protocol (if the MR-signal on T1-weighted sequence is isointense in relation to the brain).

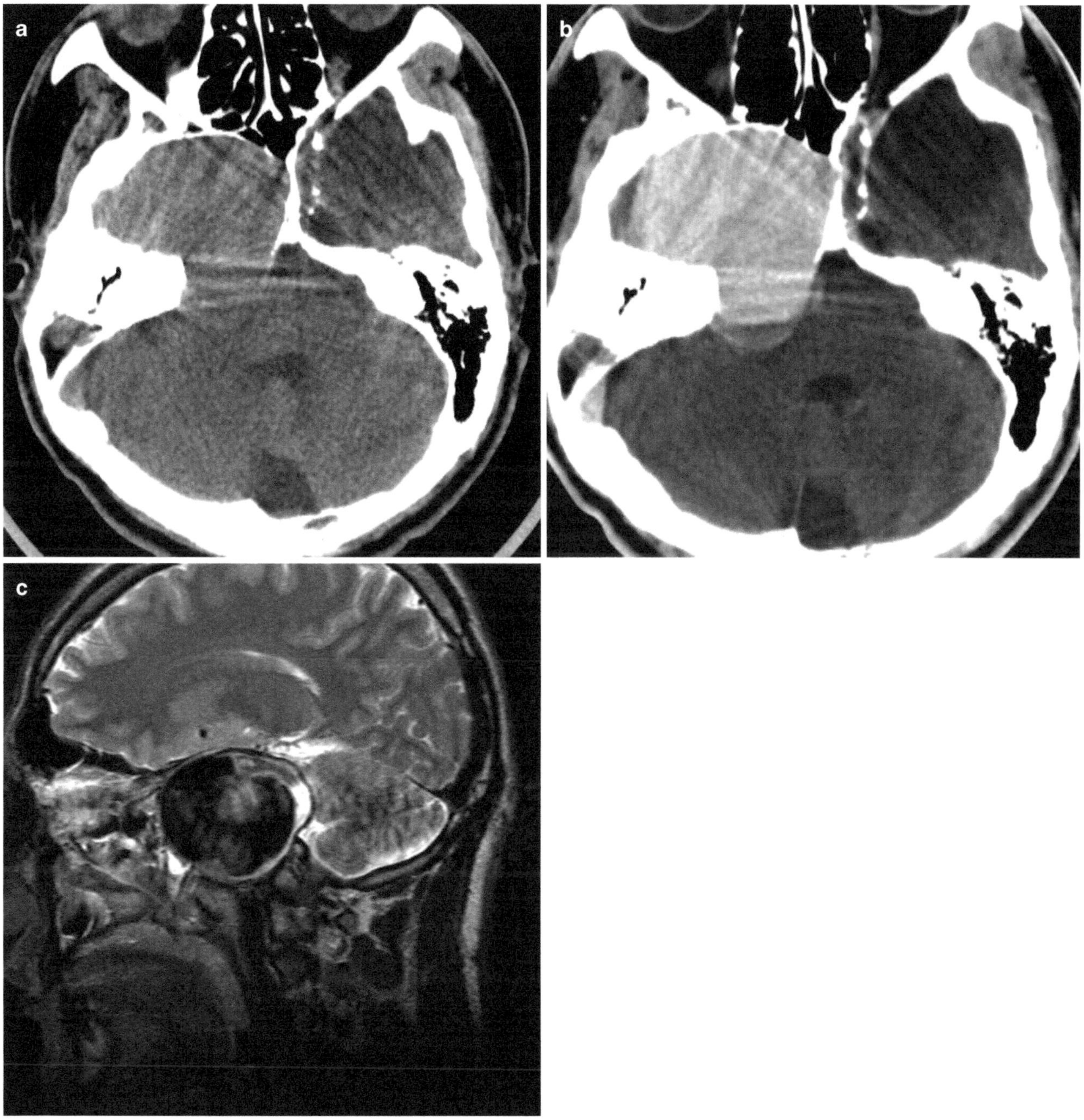

Fig. 27.16 Giant arterial aneurysm of the internal carotid artery. Axial CT scans before (**a**) and after (**b**) contrast enhancement demonstrate a huge in size and strongly enhanced lesion in the projection of the right middle cranial fossa, which leads to prominent and expansive bone deformations. On MRI in T2 sequence the lesion has a hypointense MR-signal typical for aneurism (**c**)

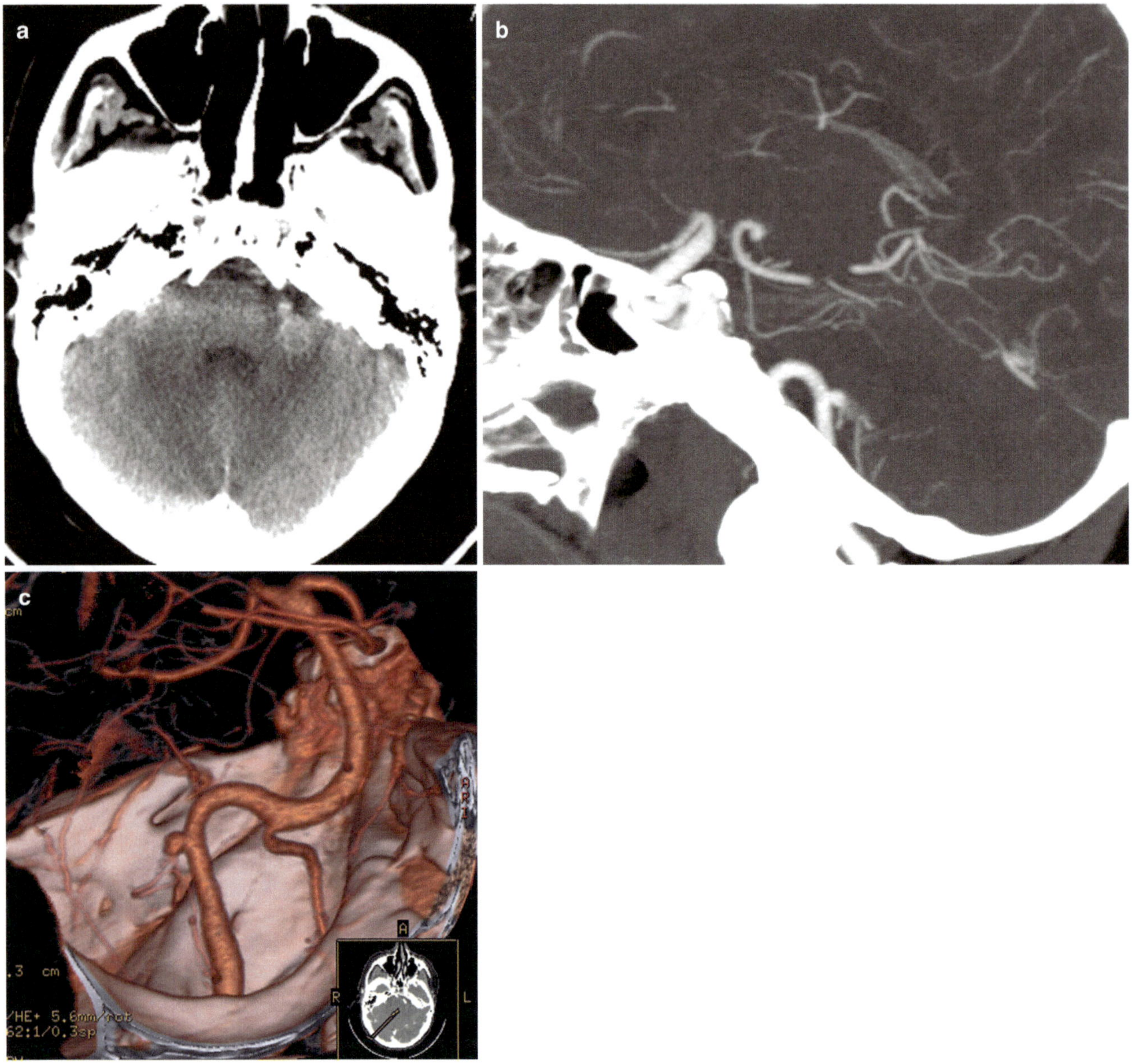

Fig. 27.17 Partially thrombosed aneurysm of the *left* vertebral artery. Axial NECT scan (**a**) shows hyperdense lesions that are located in the projection of cerebellopontine angle. This lesion consists of two nodules with round shape. CT angiography with 3D reconstruction (**b**, **c**) demonstrates a partially thrombosed arterial aneurism growing from the origin of left PICA

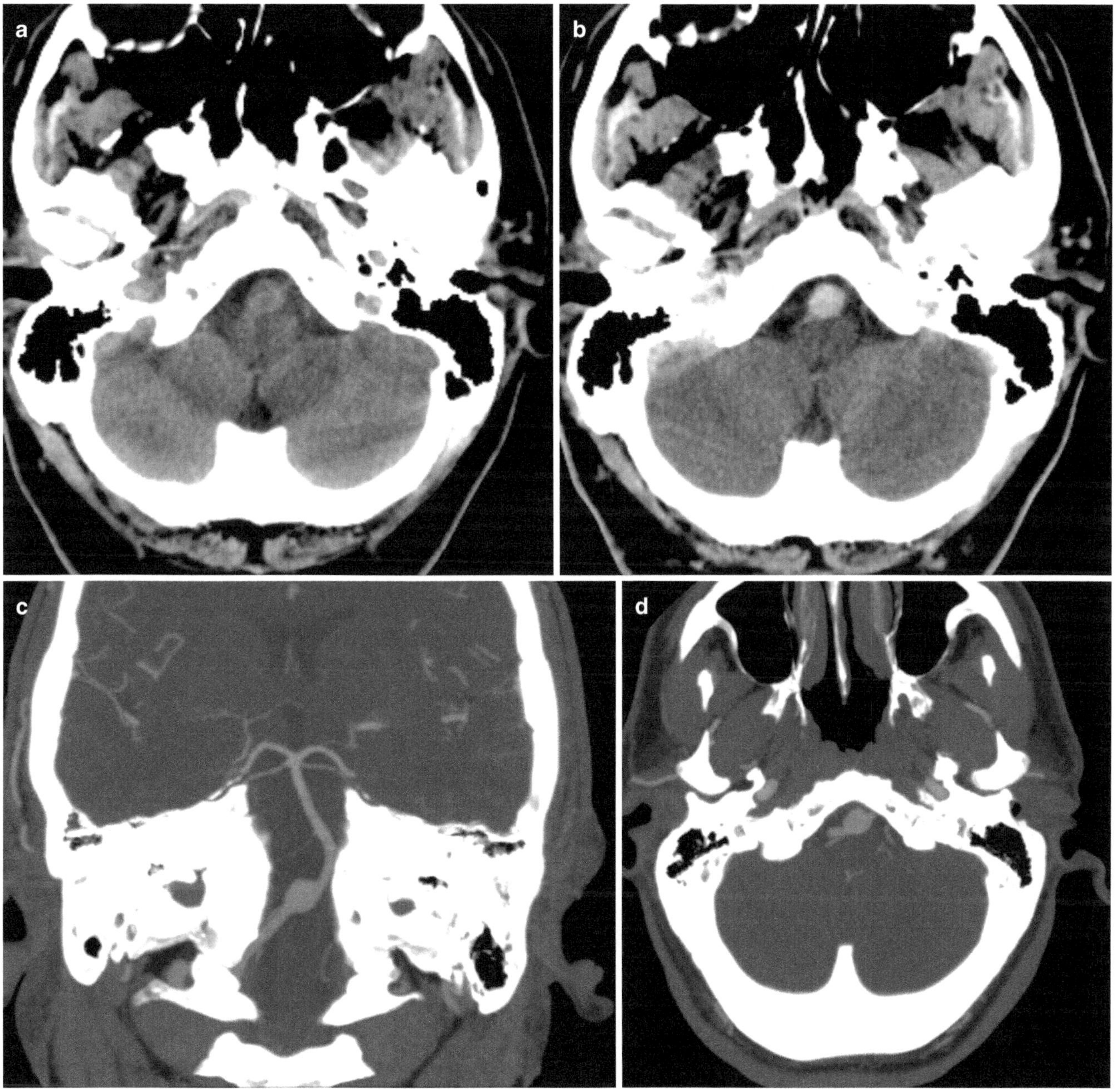

Fig. 27.18 Fusiform aneurysm of the right vertebral artery. On axial CT scans before (**a**) and after (**b**) intravenous injection a small oval enhancing lesion located anteriorly to the medulla oblongata can be seen. CT angiography with reformation in coronal (**c**), axial (**d**), and sagittal (**e**) projections demonstrates a typical imaging pattern for fusiform aneurism, which is located above the level of PICA origin. 3D reconstruction (**f**, **g**) and virtual endoscopy angiography (**h**, **i**) demonstrate both external and internal view of the aneurysm's walls

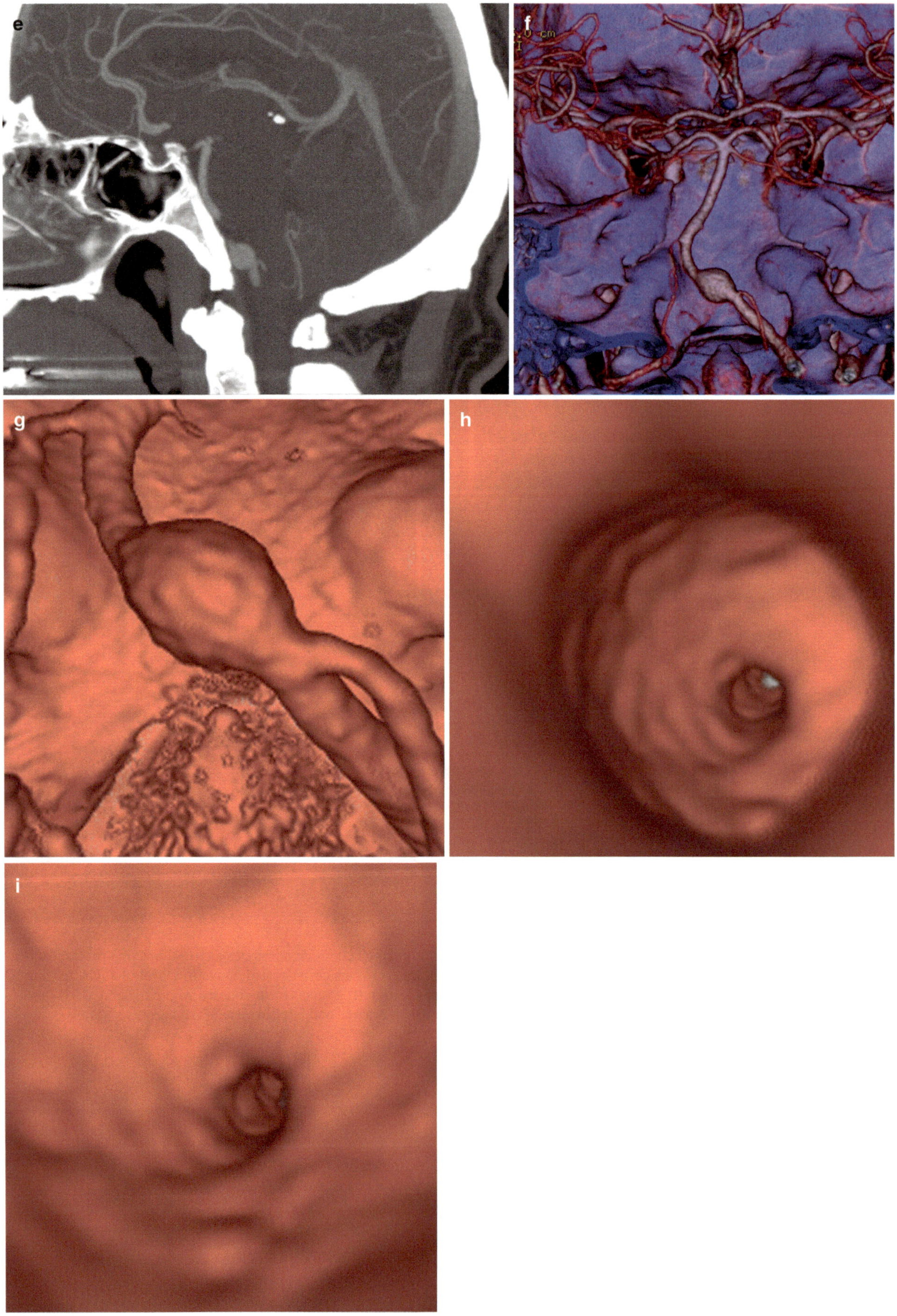

Fig. 27.18 (continued)

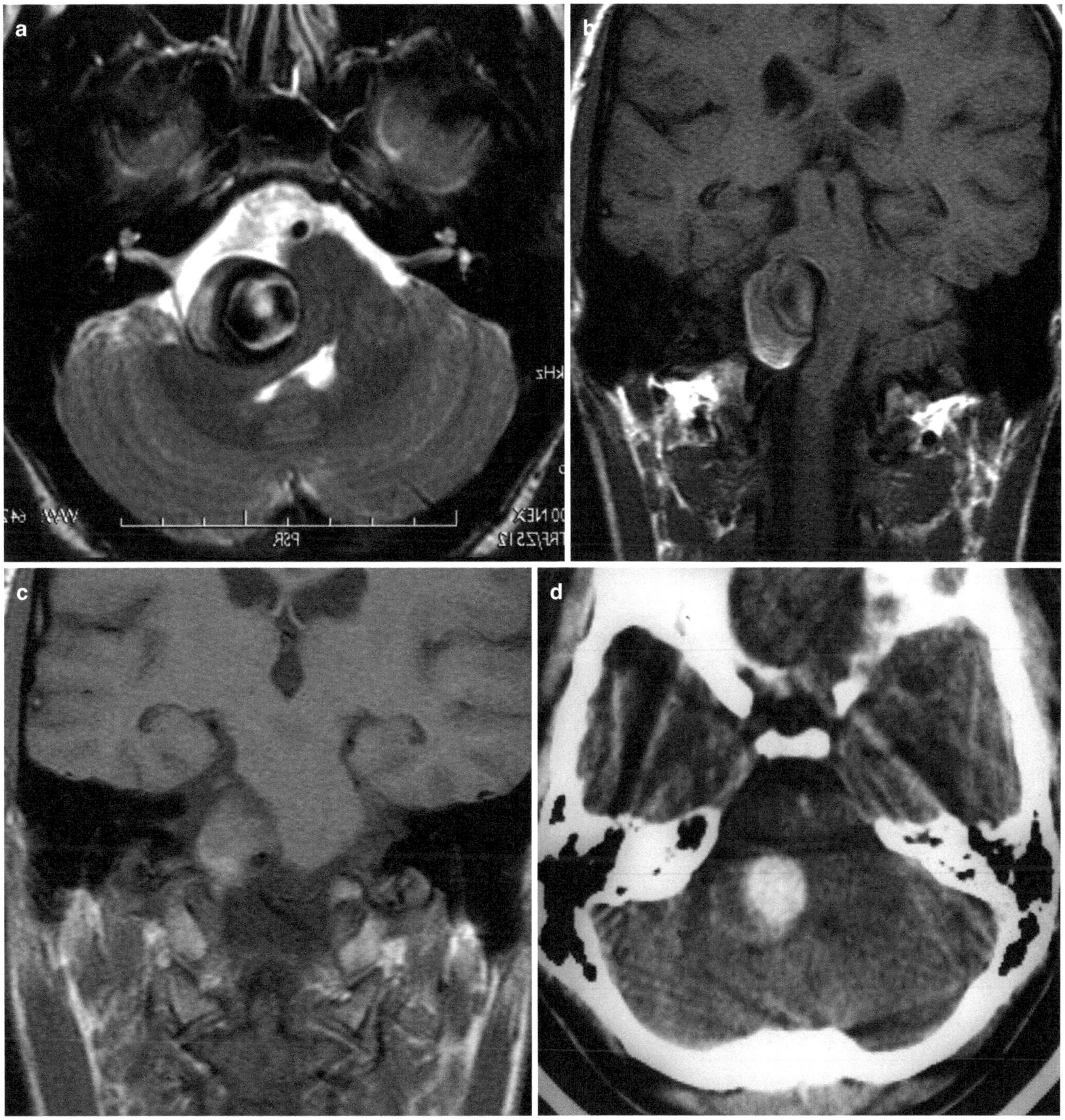

Fig. 27.19 Partially thrombosed aneurysm of the right vertebral artery. MR imaging using T2- (**a**) and T1- (**b**, **c**) weighted sequences reveals a hypointense round shaped vascular lesion with signs of intraluminal thrombosis and brain stem compression. The thrombus has layered structure and hyperintense MR-signal on T1-weighted images. Axial postenhanced CT scan shows an intensive contrast agent accumulation in the medial functioning part of the aneurysm (**d**). On 3D TOF MR-angiography (**e**, **f**) the aneurysm has increased MR-signal

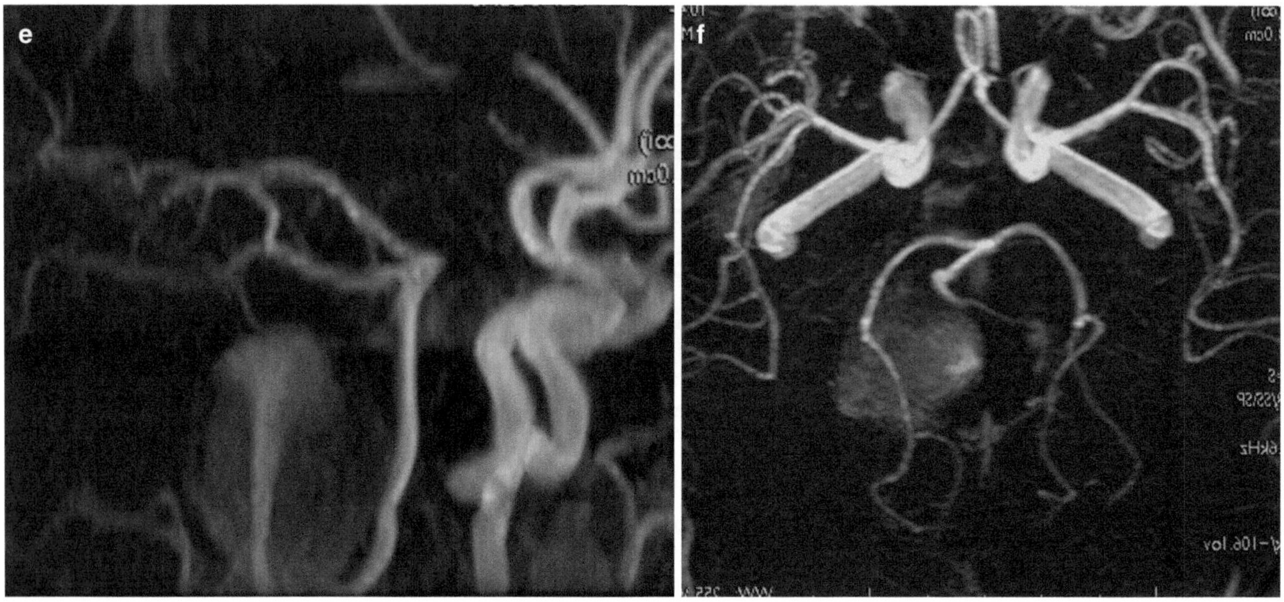

Fig. 27.19 (continued)

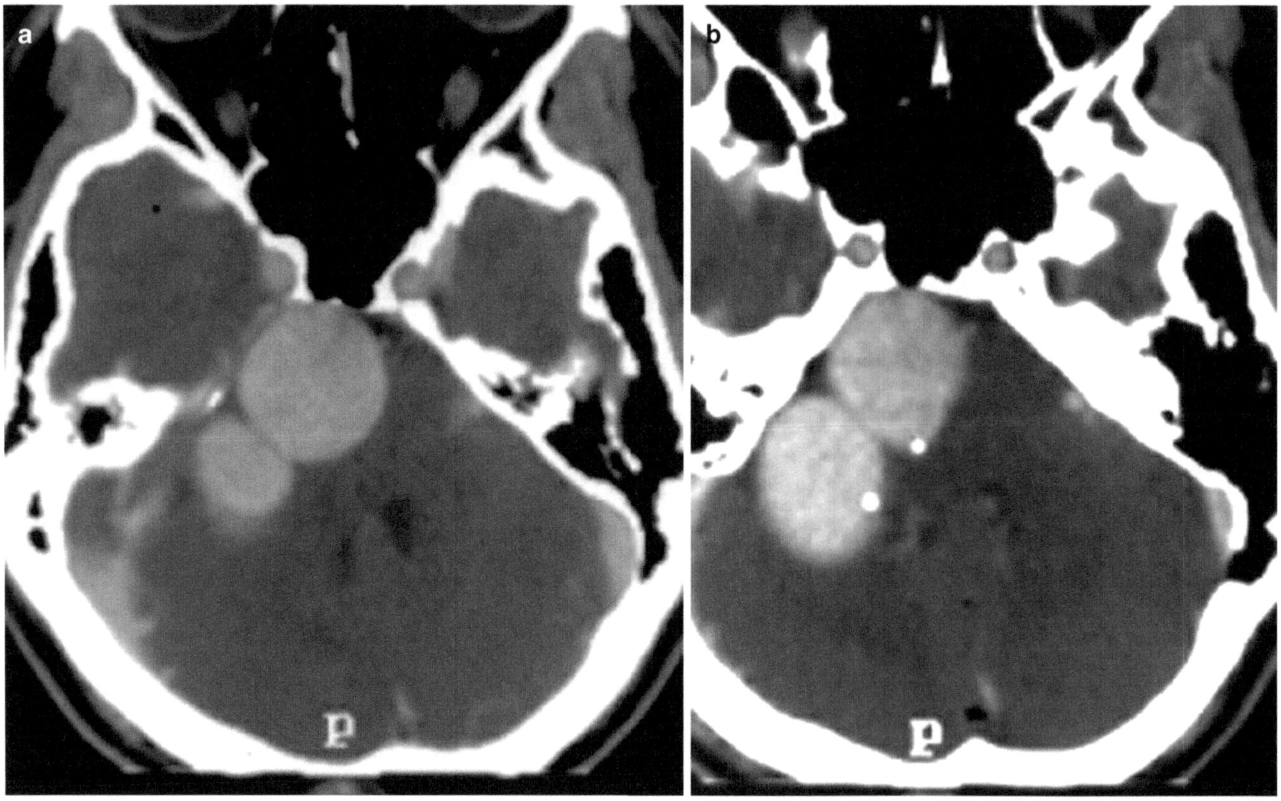

Fig. 27.20 Multiple arterial aneurysms of the vertebrobasilar system. On axial CT-angiograms (**a**, **b**), sagittal reformations (**c**, **d**) and 3D images (**e**, **f**) large saccular aneurysms of the right vertebral artery are detected. There is another (third) saccular aneurysm in the projection of the right posterior cerebral artery on MR-angiography

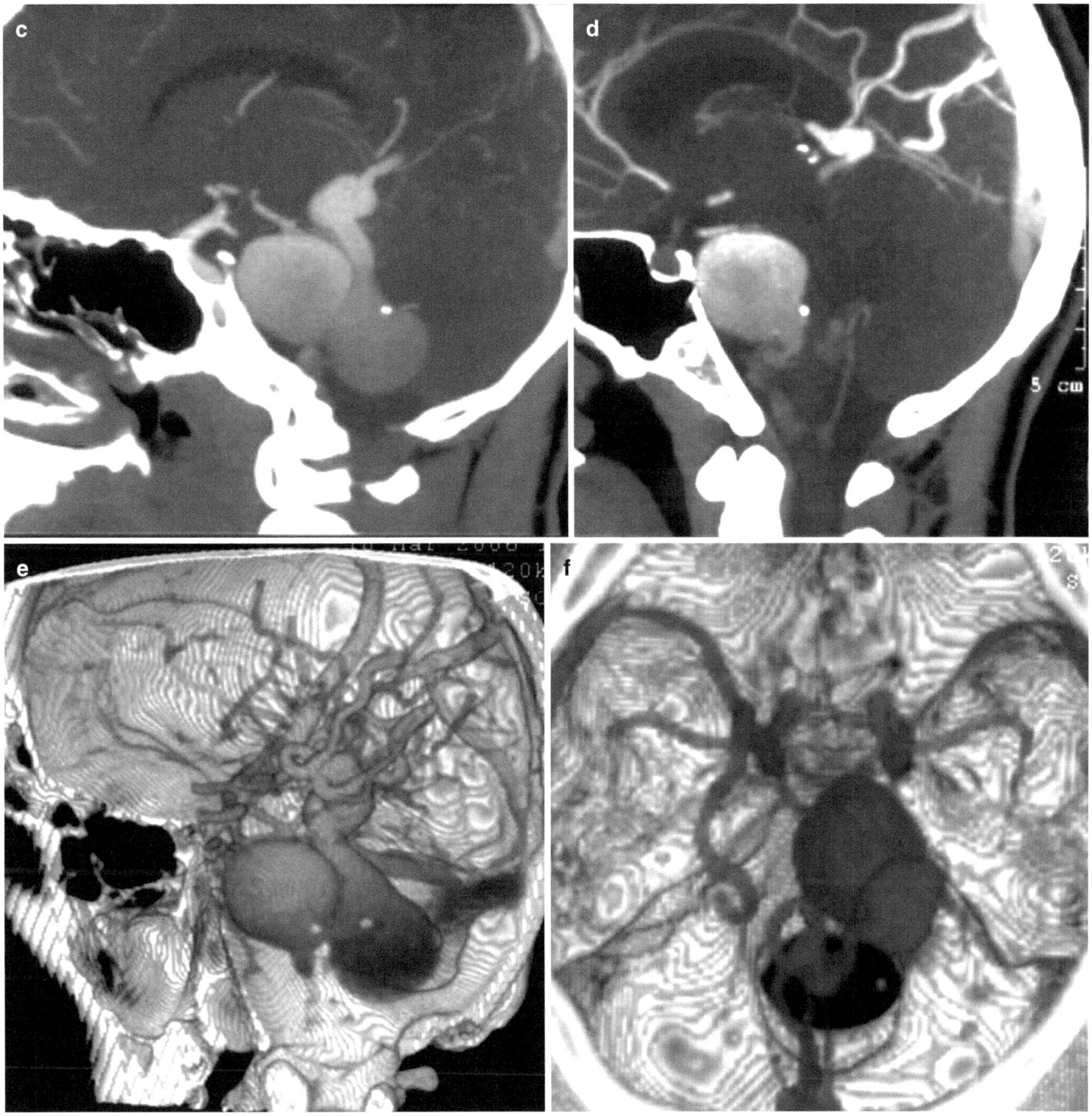

Fig. 27.20 (continued)

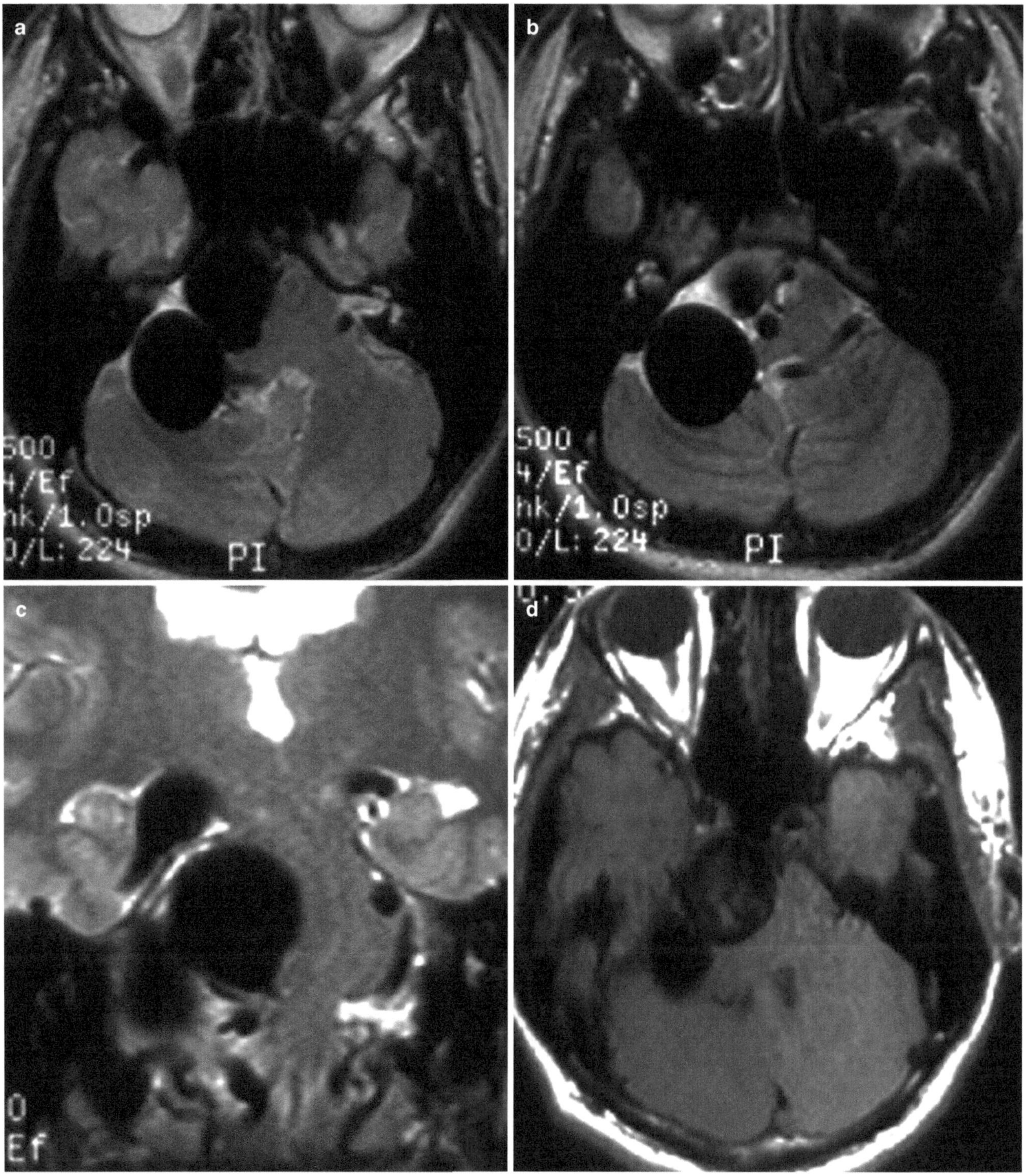

Fig. 27.21 Multiple arterial aneurysms of the vertebrobasilar system (CT images are presented in Fig. 27.19). T2- (**a**–**c**) and T1- (**d**, **e**) weighted MR images demonstrate a large rounded shape hypointense (on T2) vascular lesions. These lesions have a typical for the fast blood flow—"flow-void" signal. Turbulent blood flow in the aneurysm in T1 sequence leads to inhomogeneities within the aneurysms with a hypo-hyperintense MR-signal. 3D TOF MRI (**f**) in axial plane shows functioning aneurysms of the right vertebral and right posterior cerebral arteries

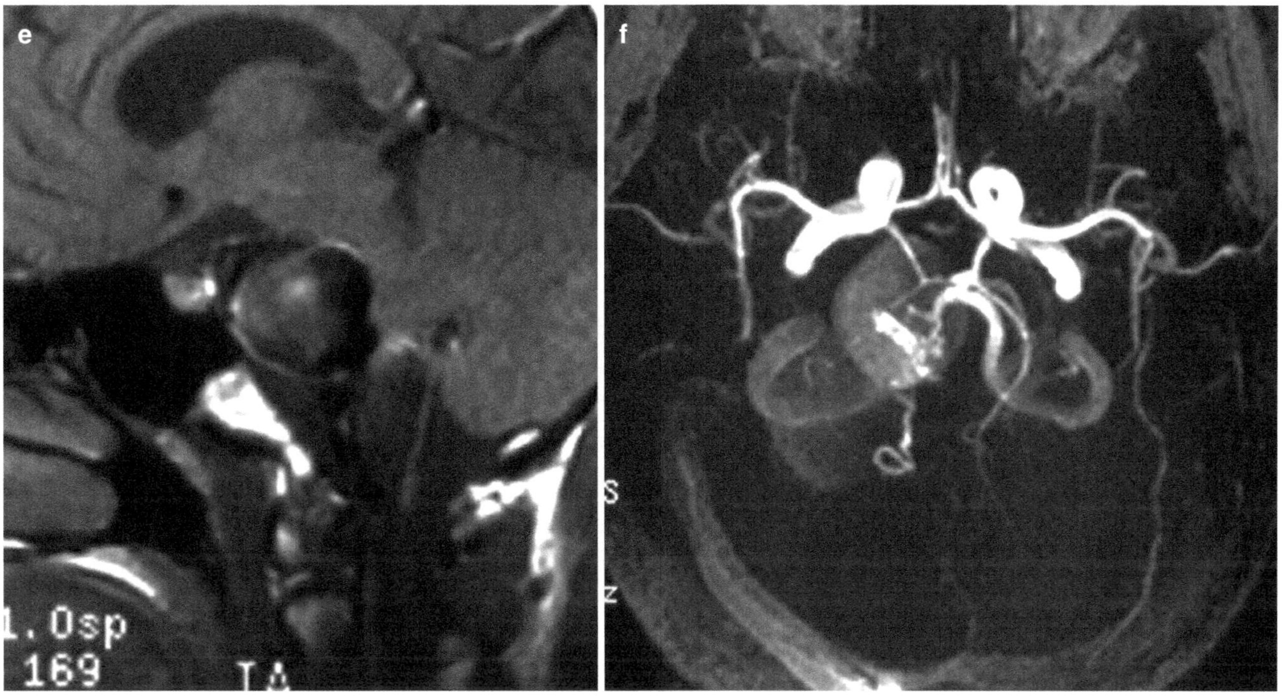

Fig. 27.21 (continued)

Venous malformations *(venous angioma)* represent venous developmental defect, which is characterized by formation of abnormally enlarged and branched microvenous vasculature in the brain tissue of cerebellar hemispheres. This venous net is typically drained into a single hypertrophied vein, which normally runs in the radial direction towards the surface of the cerebellar hemisphere and subsequently may be located in the cisterns of the brain base. Most often, this vein falls into one of the sinuses (transverse, sigmoid) of the dura. Sometimes venous angioma has such an unusual shape and large size, that some researchers call such malformations with specific names, such as "head of Medusa," etc.

A typical anatomical feature of venous angiomas is a lack of arterial blood inflow (or shunting), which distinguishes them from arteriovenous malformations.

Imaging Direct angiography is able to visualize an angioma only at a very late phase (10–12 s) of angiography. It usually appears as a small venous vasculature, collecting into one larger vein, which flows into the venous sinus.

Non-enhanced CT does not visualize venous angioma. Post-contrast CT series often detect linear portions of contrast enhancement at the projection of a cerebellar hemisphere, which are difficult to analyze without the use of multi-plane processing. Only CT-angiography is an adequate method for displaying anatomy of venous angioma within the posterior fossa. The study clearly visualizes all structural features of abnormal venous vasculature, including visualization of microphleboliths (calcifications) in the walls of varicose veins (Fig. 27.23).

MRI with standard T2, T2-FLAIR, and T1-weighted sequences is able to demonstrate venous angioma better than

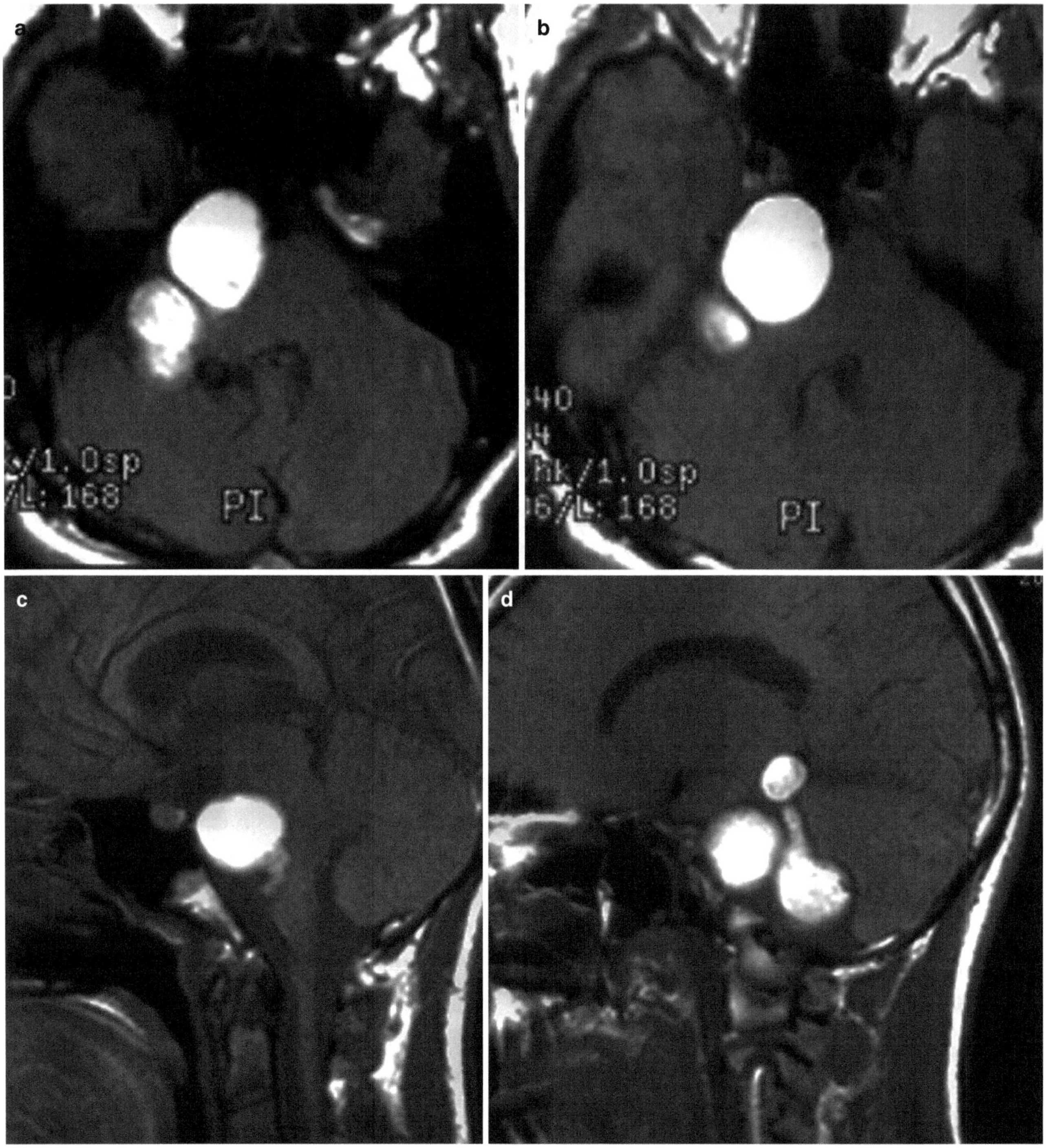

Fig. 27.22 Multiple arterial aneurysms of the vertebrobasilar system (CT and MRI images are presented in Figs. 27.19 and 27.20). Dynamic MRI series were obtained 6 months later after balloon occlusion of aneurysms. This study demonstrates a high homogeneous MR-signal from intraluminal thrombus on T1-weighted images (**a**–**d**). On 3D TOF MR-angiography these lesions are characterized by hyperintense signal due to effect of methemoglobin appearance in the thrombus (**e**, **f**). Functioning parts of aneurysms were not found

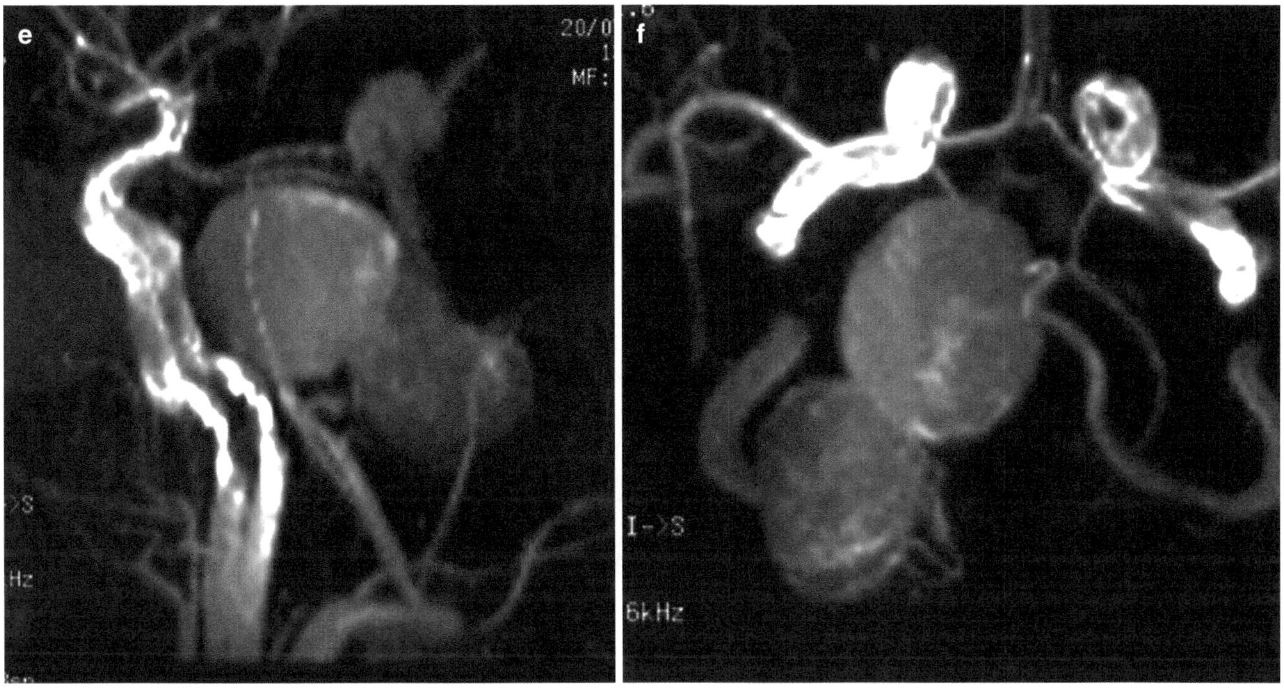

Fig. 27.22 (continued)

CT, determining linear areas of low MR-signal from blood flow along the draining vein. Primary venous vasculature itself on MRI is usually not detected. Visualization of venous angioma vasculature is improved in association with edema of surrounding brain tissue on T2 and T2-FLAIR sequences. The method of choice in the diagnosis of venous malformations is MRI with intravenous contrast enhancement, especially if 3D protocols are used in T1-weighted sequences (FSPGR, BRAVO, etc.). Subsequent reformation allows for clear visualization of abnormal venous vasculature and draining vein (Fig. 27.24).

Differential Diagnosis AVM, multiple sclerosis foci, hemangioblastoma, metastases.

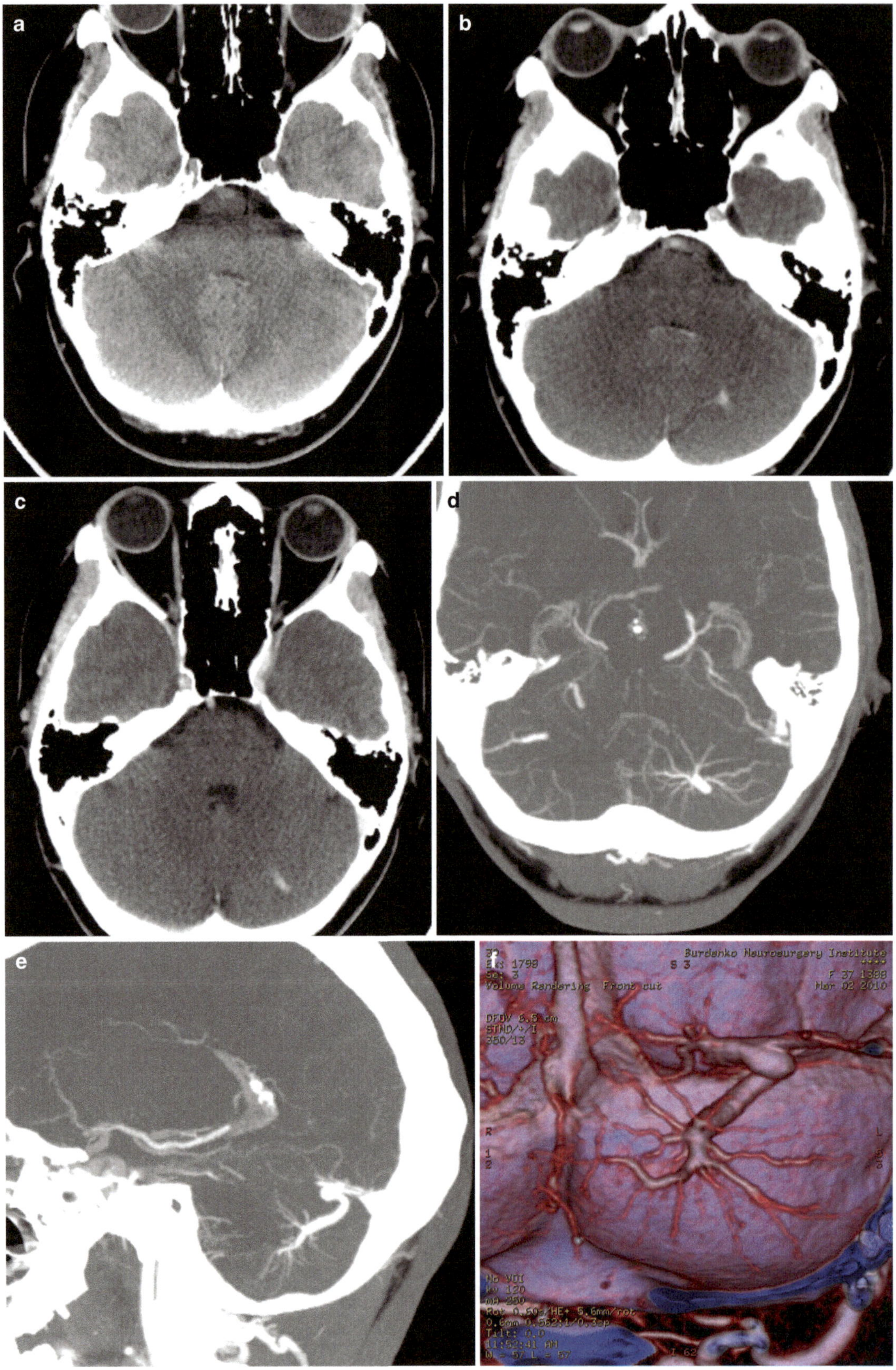

Fig. 27.23 Venous angioma of the left cerebellar hemisphere. Axial CT scans before (**a**) and after contrast enhancement (**b**, **c**) demonstrate a small linear in shape area with prominent contrast enhancement in the projection of the *left* cerebellar hemisphere. On CT angiography with 2D reformations (**d**, **e**) and 3D reconstruction (**f**) venous angioma has fairly clear appearance (like a "tree-roots") with drainage of blood into transverse sinus

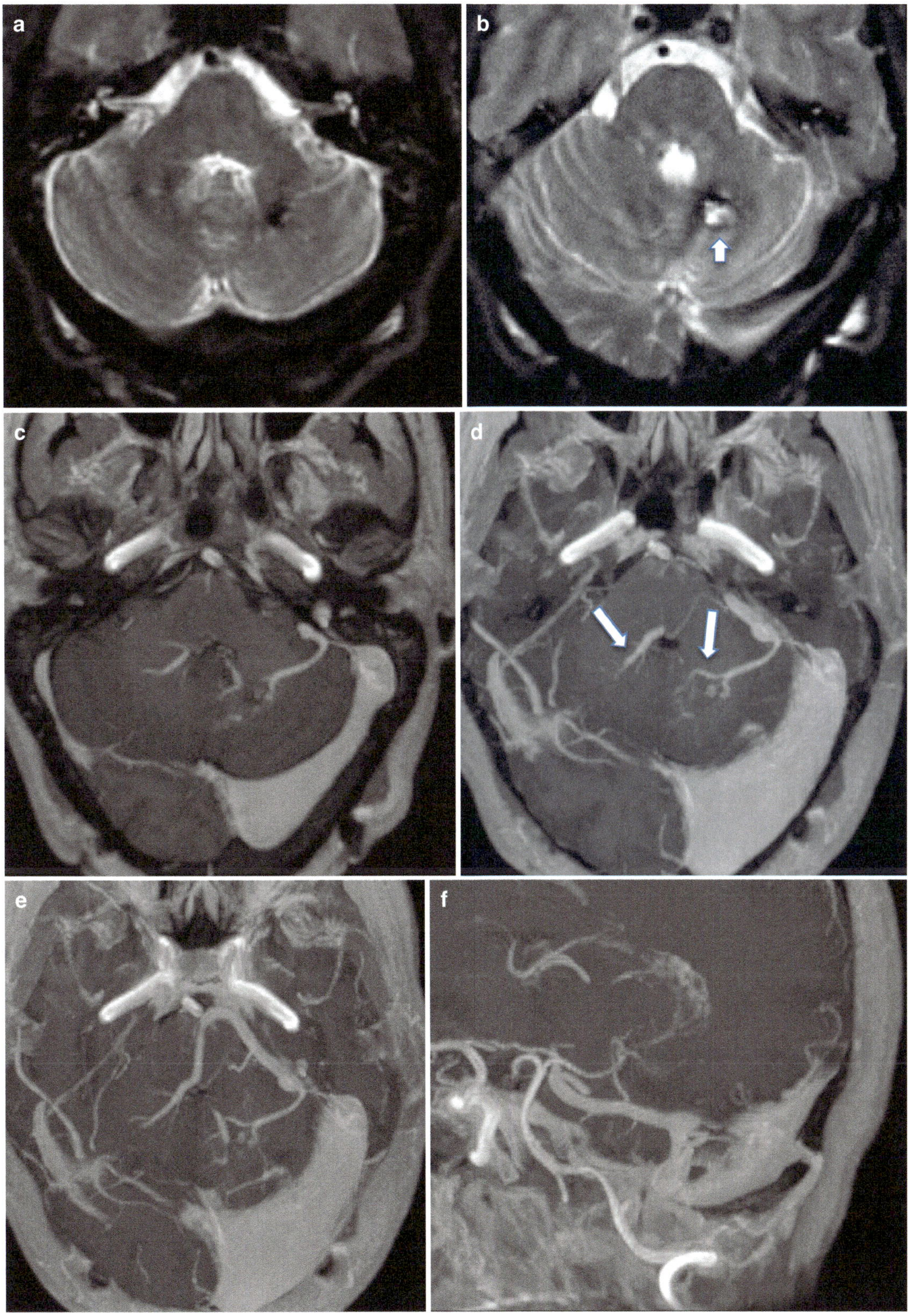

Fig. 27.24 Venous angioma of the left cerebellar hemisphere. MRI using T2 (**a**, **b**) and postenhanced T1-SPGR-weighted MR-sequences (2D–reformations with different thickness, **c**–**f**) demonstrates two venous angiomas in the depth of the left cerebellar hemisphere (*arrows*) associated with a small cavernous angioma (*small arrow*)

Presentation of Rare Cases of Posterior Cranial Fossa and Skull Base Lesions

28

Contents

I. Pronin, V. Kornienko, *CT and MRI of Skull Base Lesions*, https://doi.org/10.1007/978-3-319-65957-2_28

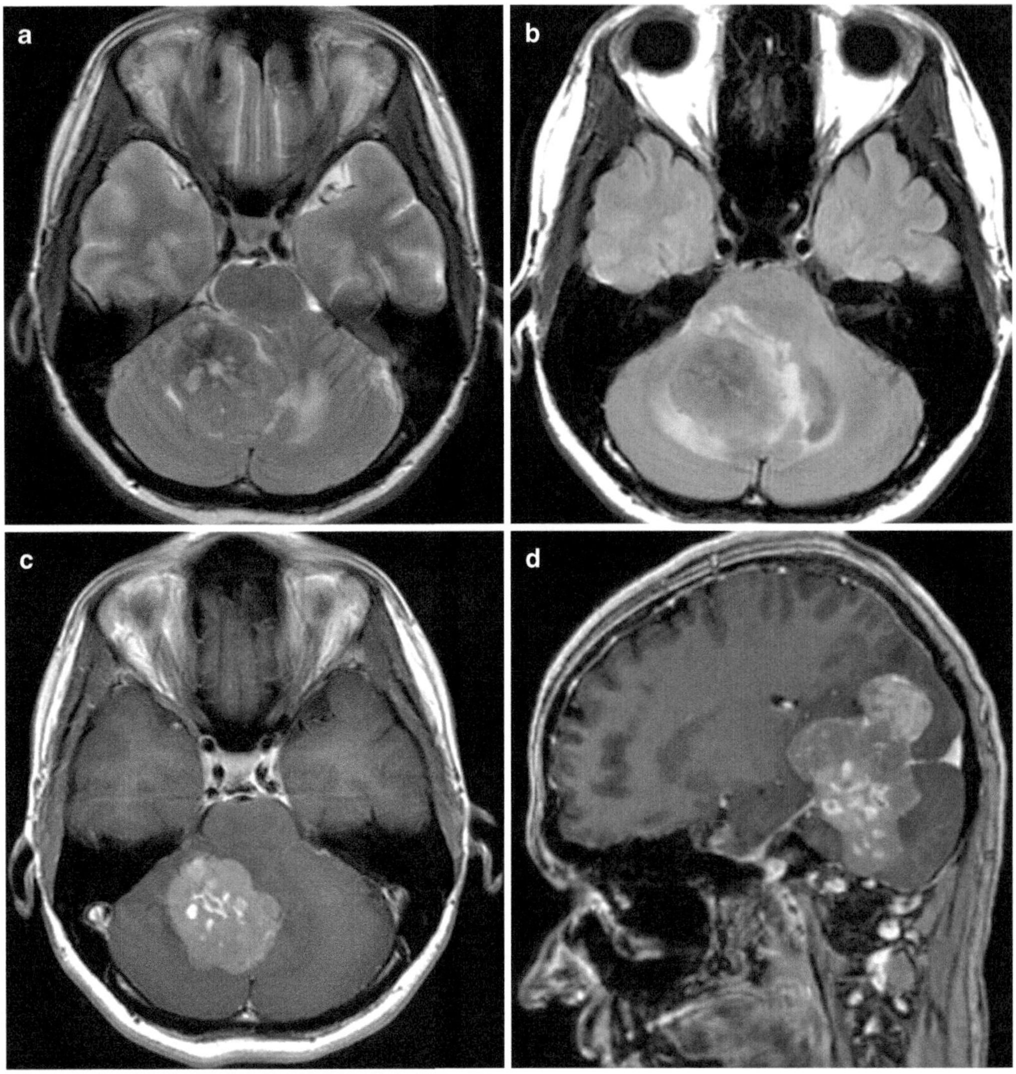

Fig. 28.1 Hemangiopericytoma of the cerebellar tentorium with sub- and supratentorial growth. Axial T2- (**a**), T2-FLAIR- (**b**), and T1-weighted MR images with contrast enhancement (**c**, **d**) demonstrate a large solid predominantly hypointense (on T2) tumor surrounded with perifocal edema of the brain. Tumor has a strong and heterogeneous contrast enhancement. There are "islands" with increased contrast enhancement in comparison with common tumor tissue. 3D PC MR-angiography visualizes the blood supply of the tumor from the tentorial branches of the internal carotid artery (**e**). MR-perfusion (ASL) demonstrates very high values of blood flow in the tumor (**f**)

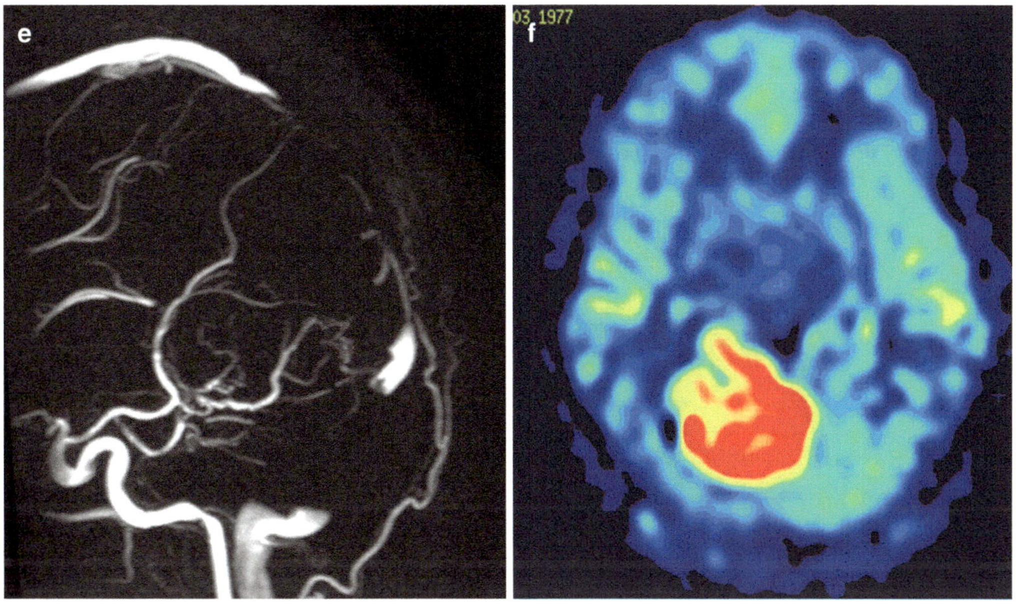

Fig. 28.1 (continued)

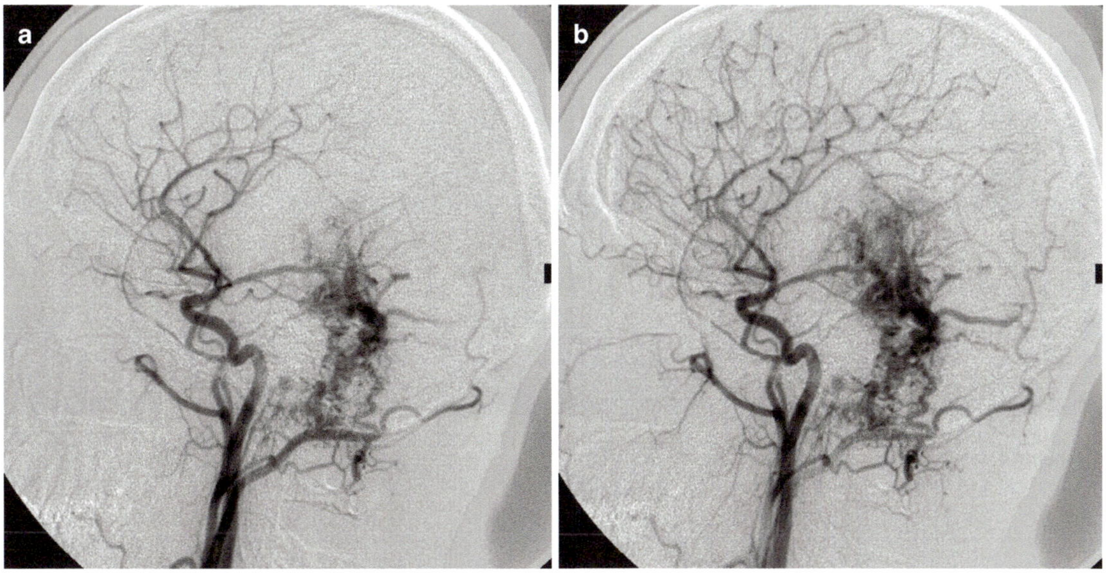

Fig. 28.2 Hemangiopericytoma of the cerebellar tentorium with sub- and supratentorial growth. Direct cerebral angiography (**a**–**c**) of the right common carotid artery reveals an abundant vascularity of the tumor, which is supplied from the external carotid artery (superficial temporal artery, occipital artery, and others). There are plenty of arteriovenous shunts in the arterial phase within the lesion. On axial CT scans with contrast enhancement (**d**–**f**) the tumor has strong enhancement. There are foci of temporal bone pyramid and occipital bone destruction. Coronal (**g**) and sagittal (**h**) CT-reformations visualize clearly supratentorial growth of the tumor. CBF CT-perfusion map (**i**) demonstrates extremely high values of blood flow in the tumor

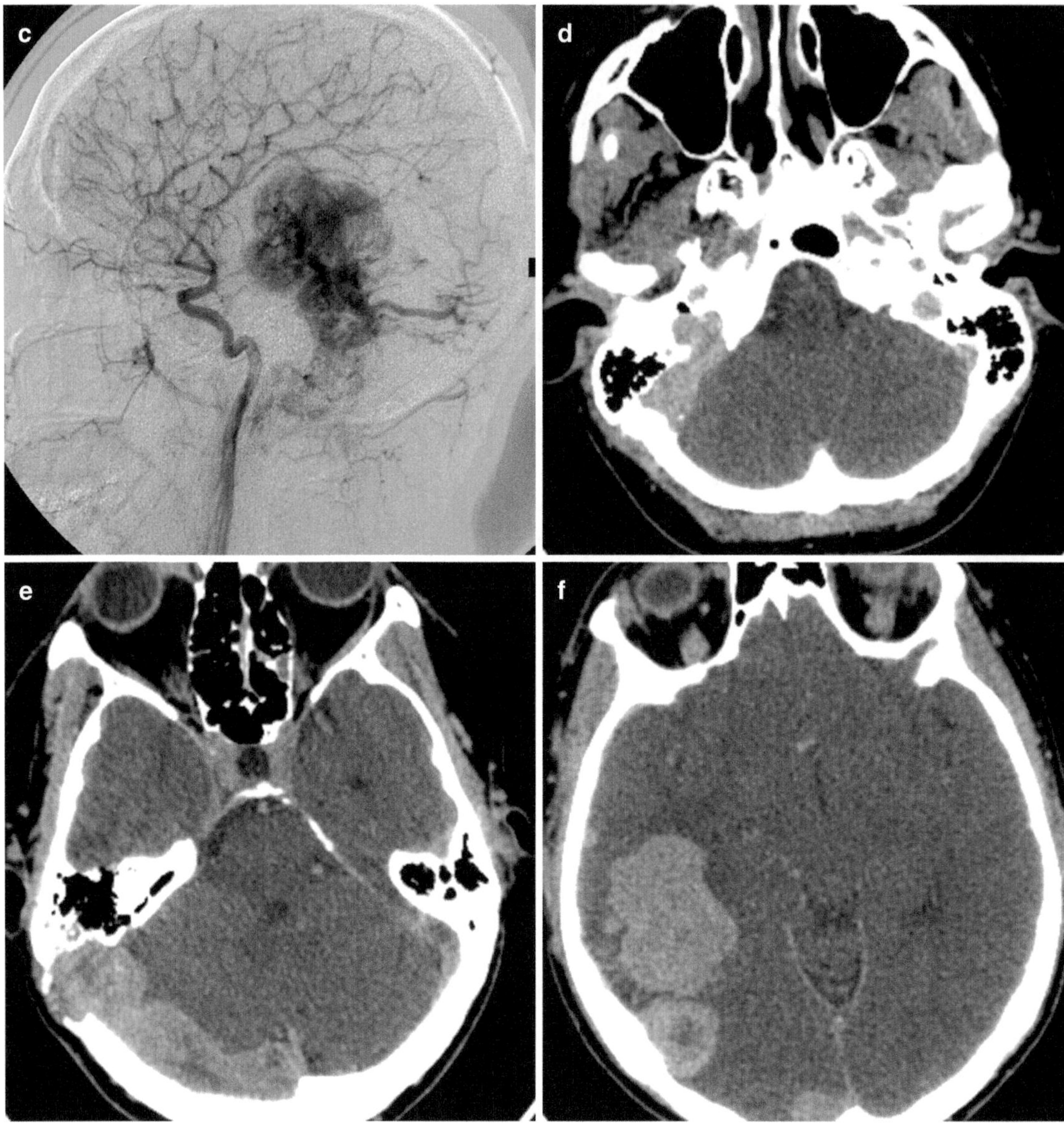

Fig. 28.2 (continued)

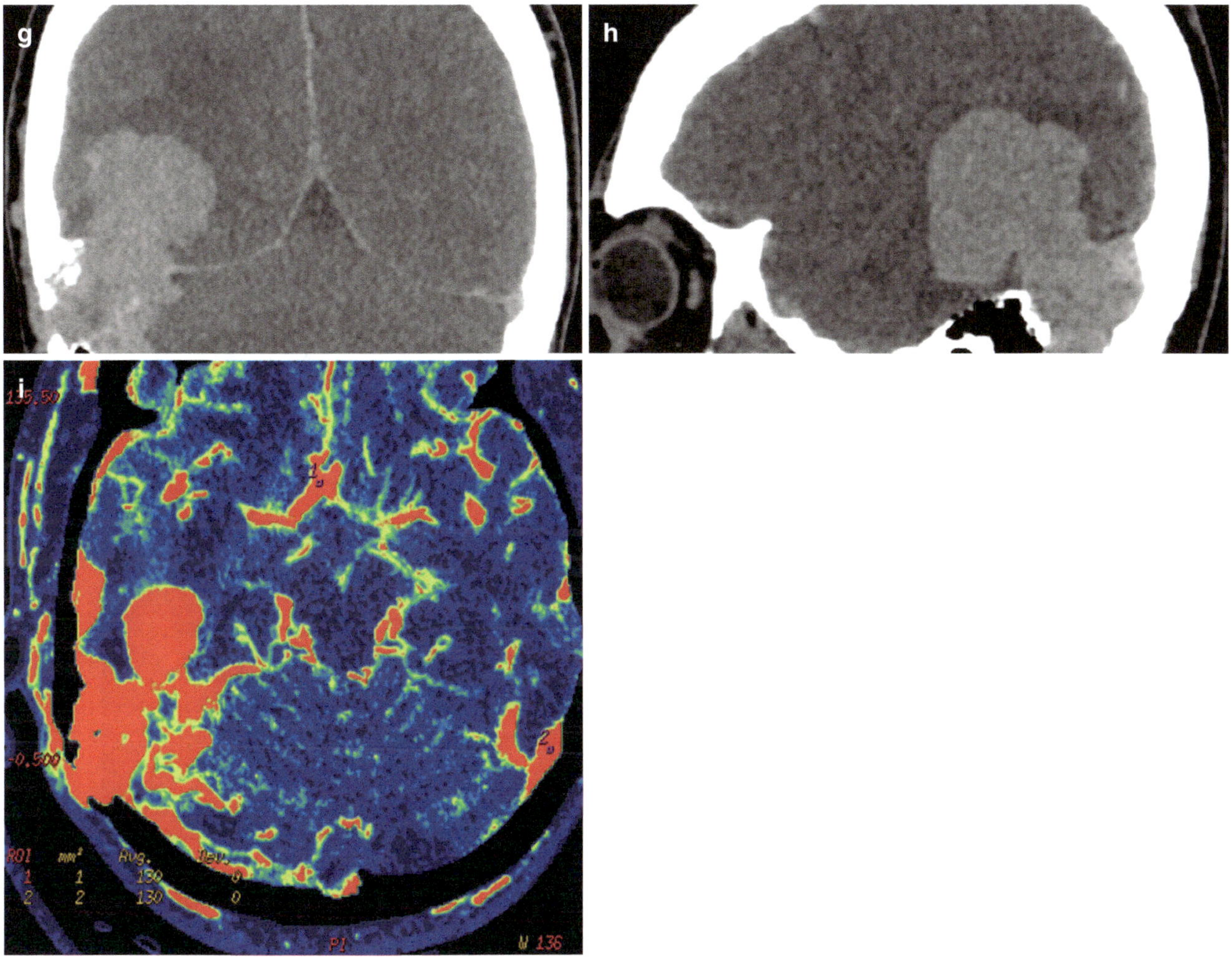

Fig. 28.2 (continued)

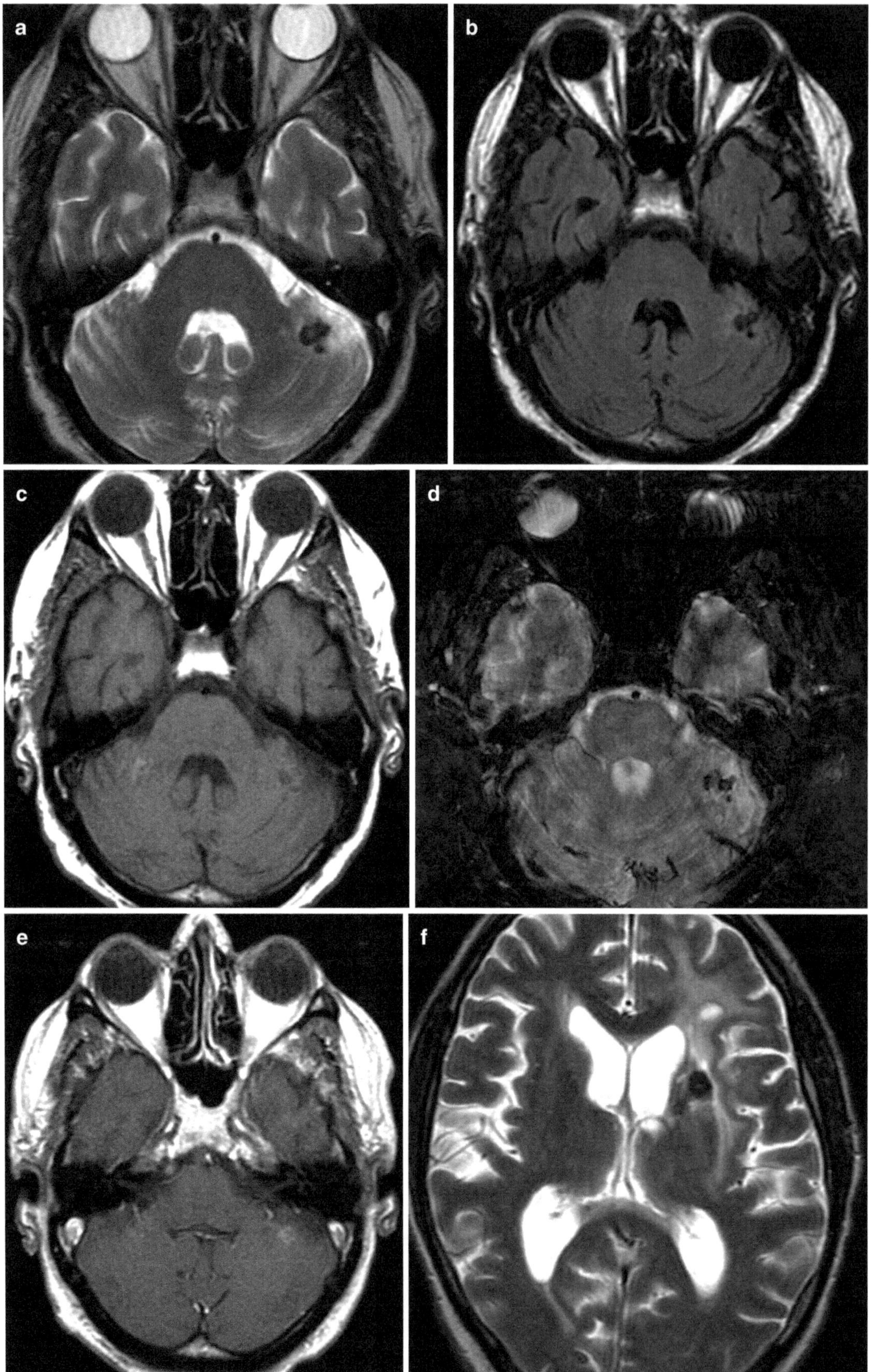

Fig. 28.3 Fungal granulomas. Axial T2- (**a**), T2-FLAIR- (**b**), T1- (**c**), and SWAN- (**d**) weighted MR images demonstrate a small area of hypointense MR-signal in lateral parts of the left cerebellar hemisphere with perifocal edema. Granuloma has intermediate contrast enhancement (**e**). Axial T2 MR image on the level of lateral ventricles (**f**) reveals second hypointensive area in left basal ganglia

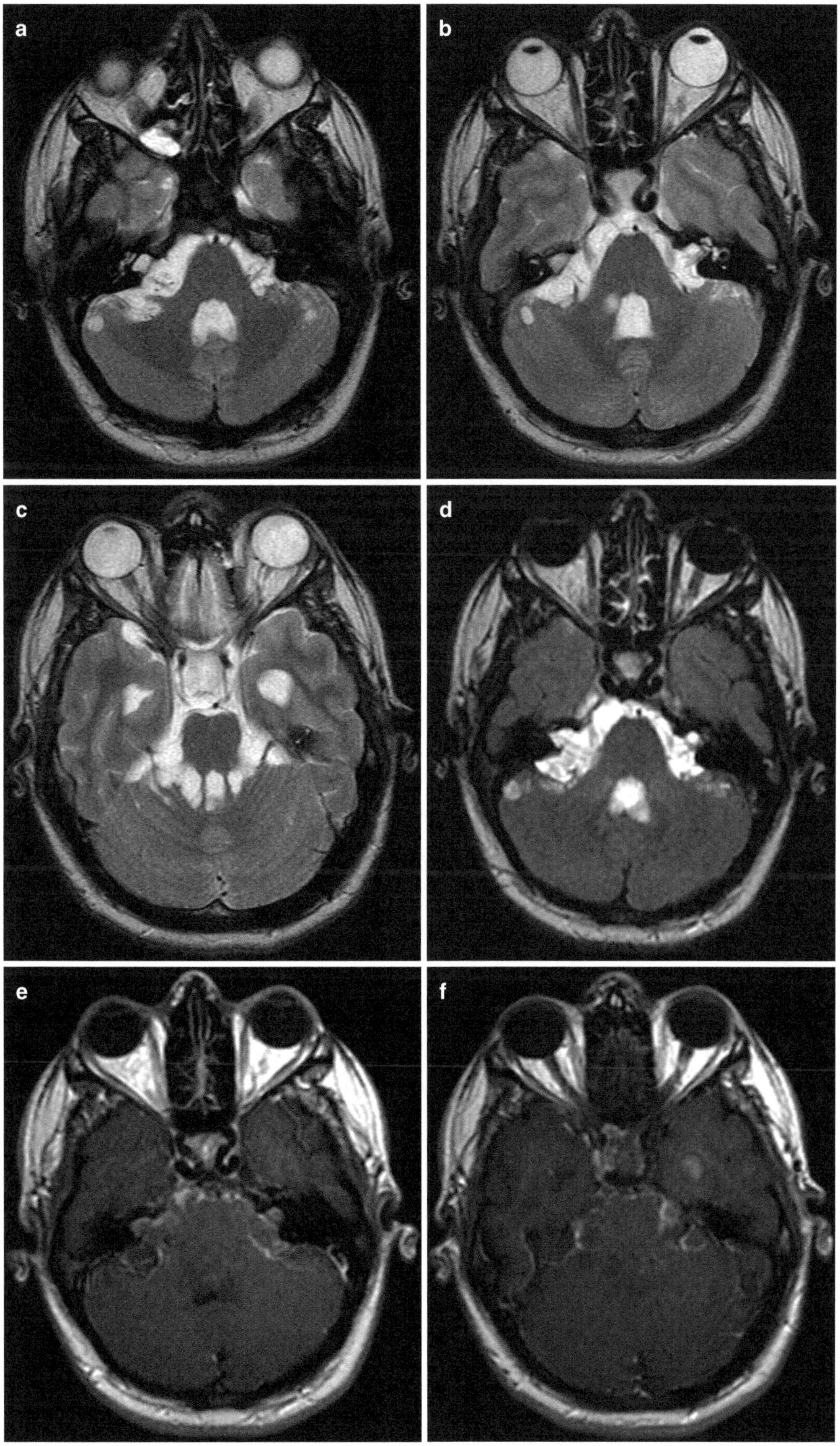

Fig. 28.4 Fibrosarcoma of the skull base. Series of axial, coronal, sagittal T2- (**a–c**), T2-FLAIR- (**d**), and postenhanced T1- (**e–i**) weighted MR images demonstrate a widespreading along basal cisterns lesion with hyperintense MR-signal on T2 and T2-FLAIR sequences. There are also visible multiple foci with hyperintense signal in cerebellar hemispheres and cerebellar peduncles. MRI with contrast enhancement (**e–i**) shows a pathological heterogeneous contrast enhancement of extensive lesion

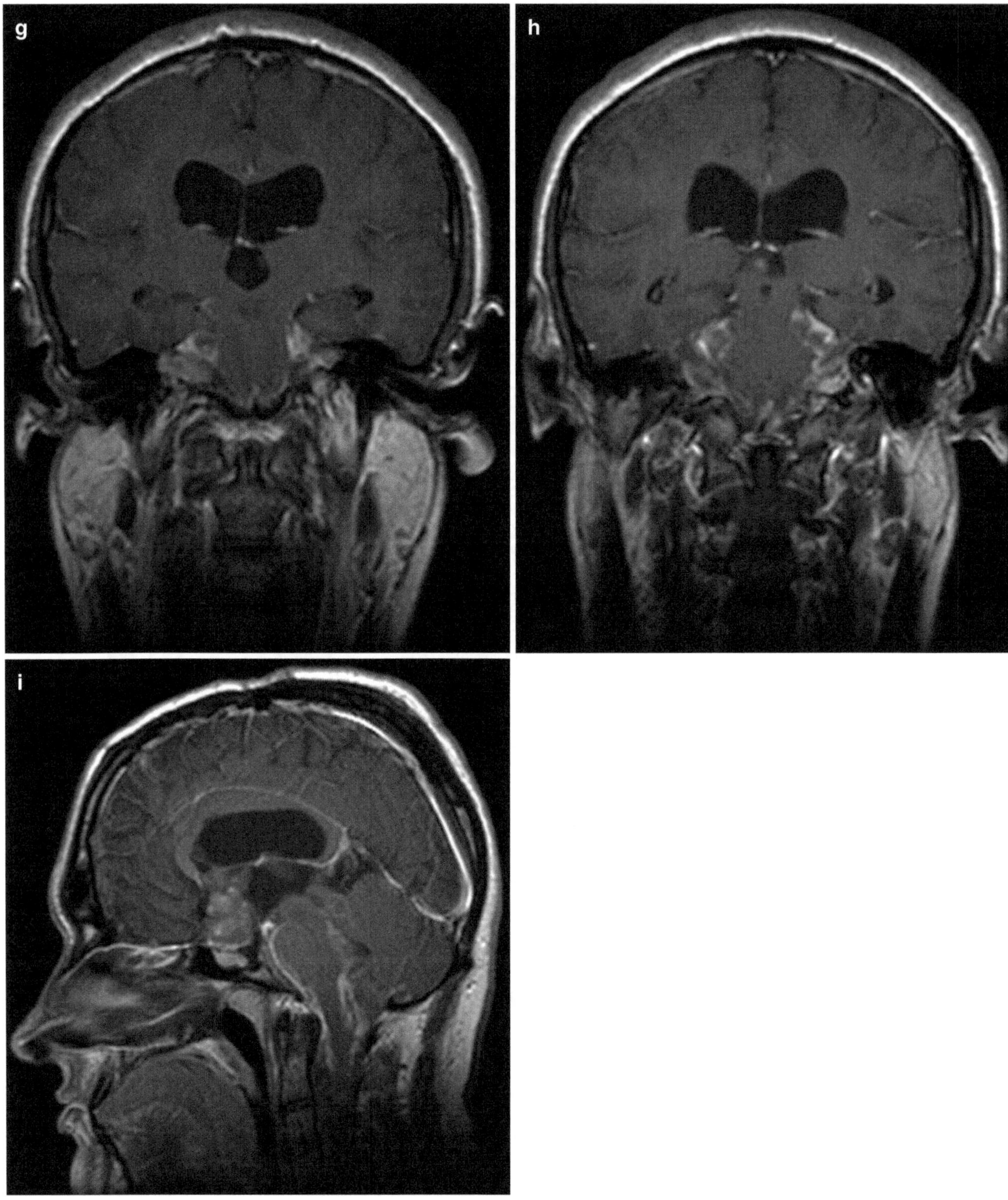

Fig. 28.4 (continued)

Bibliography

Abe T et al (2002) Evaluation of pituitary adenomas by multidetectional multislice dynamic CT. Acta Radiol 43:556–559

Abramson D et al (2003) Adult ophthalmic oncology. In: Kufe DW, Pollock RE, Weichselbaum RR et al (eds) Holland-Frei Cancer Medicine, 6th edn. BC Decker, Hamilton, ON

Adada B et al (2003) Fibrous dysplasia of the clivus. Neurosurgery 52(2):318–322

Ahmadi J et al (1985) Cavernous sinus invasion by pituitary adenomas. AJNR 6:893–899

Alawi F (2002) Benign fibro-osseous disease of the maxillofacial bones. A review and differential diagnosis. Am J Clin Pathol 118(Suppl):50–70

Alkonyi B et al (2015) Differential imaging characteristics and dissemination potential of pylomyxoid astrocytomas versus pilocytic astrocytomas. Neuroradiology 57(6):625–638

Angeli S et al (1996) Magnetic resonance imaging in the evaluation of Langerhan's cell histiocytosis. Otolaryngol Head Neck Surg 114:120–124

Arat Y, Mawad M, Boniuk M (2004) Orbital venous malformations: current multidisciplinary treatment approach. Arch Ophthalmol 122:1151–1158

Aron-Rosa D, Doyon D, Salamon G et al (1978) Tolosa-Hunt syndrome. Ann Ophthalmol 10:1161–1168

Asa S (2008) Practical pituitary pathology: what does the pathologist need to know? Arch Pathol Lab Med 132:1231–1240

Asaumi J, Matsuzaki H, Hisatomi M et al (2002) Application of dynamic MRI to differentiating odontogenic myxomas from ameloblastomas. Eur J Radiol 43(1):37–41

Astafyeva L et al (2009) Decision making in the treatment of the giant prolactin-secreting pituitary adenomas. Vopr Neurochirurgii NN Burdenko 2:23–28. (in Russian)

Astafyeva L et al (2011) Giant prolactin-secreting pituitary adenomas. In: Dedov I (ed) Clinical endocrinology. UP Print, Moscow, pp 127–136. (in Russian)

Atlas S (ed) (2009) MR imaging of the brain and spine. Wolters Kluwer/Lippincott, Philadelphia, p 1086

Atlas S, Grossman R et al (1987) MR imaging of metastatic melanoma. Radiology 3:577–582

Baert A, Sartor K (2006) Imaging of orbital and visual pathway pathology. Springer, Berlin, p 429

Balcer L, Liu G, Heller G et al (2001) Visual loss in children with neurofibromatosis type 1 and optic pathway gliomas: relation to tumor location by magnetic resonance imaging. Am J Ophthalmol 131:442–445

Balmer A, Zografos L, Munier F (2006) Diagnosis and current management of retinoblastoma Oncogene 25:5341–5349. doi:10.1038/sj.onc.1209622

Barath K et al (2011) Neuroradiology of Cholesteatomas. AJNR 32(2):221–229

Barnes L (1985) Diseases of the nose, paranasal sinuses and nasopharynx. In: Barnes L (ed) Surgical pathology of the head and neck, vol 2. Marcel Dekker, New York, pp 1045–1209

Barnes L, Kanbour A (1988) Malignant fibrous histiocytoma of the head and neck. A report of 12 cases. Arch Otolaryngol Head Neck Surg 114(10):1149–1156

Barnes L, Verbin R, Appel B et al (2000) Tumor and tumor-like lesions of the soft tissue. In: Barnes L (ed) Surgical pathology of the head and neck, vol 2, 2nd edn. Marcel Dekker, New York, p 1084

Barsi P, Kenéz J, Várallyay G, Gergely L et al (1992) Unusual origin of free subarachnoid fat drops: a ruptured spinal dermoid tumour. Neuroradiology 34:343–344

Barrow et al (1985) Classification and treatment of spontaneous carotid cavernous sinus fistulas. J Neurosurg 62:248–256

Battineni ML et al (2007) Idiopathic hypereosinophilic syndrome with skull base involvement. AJNR 28(5):971–973

Beardsley T, Brown S, Sydnor C et al (1984) Eleven cases of sarcoidosis of the optic nerve. Am J Ophthalmol 97(1):62–77

Beltran J, Simon D, Levy M, Herman L et al (1986) Aneurysmal bone cysts: MR imaging at 1.5T. Radiology 158:689–690

Bencherif B, Zouaoui A, Chedid G et al (1993) Intracranial extension of an idiopathic orbital inflammatory pseudotumor. AJNR 14:181–184

Benninger M, Ferguson B, Hadley J, Hamilos D et al (2003) Adult chronic rhinosinusitis: definitions, diagnosis, epidemiology and pathophysiology. Otolaryngol Head Neck Surg 129(Suppl):1–32

Berlit P, Fedel C et al (1996) Bacterial brain abscess: experiences with 67 patients. Fortschr Neurol Psychiatr 64(8):297–306

Bernal-Sprekelsen M, Vazquez A, Pueyo J et al (1998) Endoscopic resection of juvenile nasopharyngeal fibromas. HNO 46(2):172–174. (German)

Bertelmann E, Hartmann C, Minko N (2011) Intraorbital cavernous hemangiomas: symptoms, diagnostics and surgical approaches. Klin Monbl Augenheilkd 228(1):49–53. (in German)

Bilgen C et al (2003) Jugular bulb diverticula: clinical and radiologic aspects. Otolaryngol Head Neck Surg 128(3):382–386

Boellis A et al (2014) Pituitary apoplexy: an update on clinical and imaging features. Insights Imaging 5(6):753–762

Boonvisut S, Ladpil S, Sujatanond M et al (1998) Morphologic study of 120 skull base defects in frontoethmoidal encephalomeningoceles. Plast Reconstr Surg 101(7):1784–1795

Bradly P, Jones N et al (2003) Diagnosis and management of esthesioneuroblastoma. Curr Opin Otolaryngol Head Neck Surg 11(2):112–118

Bret P et al (2002) Solitary plasmacytoma of the sphenoid. Neurochirurgie 48(5):431–435

Britt R, Enzmann D et al (1984) Experimental anaerobic brain abscess. Computerized tomographic and neuropathological correlations. J Neurosurg 60(6):1148–1159

I. Pronin, V. Kornienko, *CT and MRI of Skull Base Lesions*, https://doi.org/10.1007/978-3-319-65957-2

Brook I (2003) Acute and chronic frontal sinusitis. Curr Opin Pulm Med 9(3):171–174

Brovkina AF (2002) Ophtalmooncology: Guideline for medical doctors. Medicine Moscow, p 420 (in Russian)

Brovkina AF (2004) Endicrine ophtalmopathy. Medicine: GEOTAR-Media Moscow, p 174 (in Russian)

Brovkina AF (2008) Diseases of the orbit. Medicine: Medical News Agency Moscow, p 256 (in Russian)

Brown R, Sage MR et al (1990) CT and MR findings in patients with chordomas of the petrous apex. Am J Neuroradiol 11:121

Brown E et al (1994) Chondrosarcoma of the skull base. Neuroimag Clin N Am 4(3):529–541

Buetow M, Burton P, Smirniotopoulos J (1991) Typical, atypical and misleading features in meningioma. Radiographics 11:1087–1100

Cabanis E, Bourgeois H, Iba-Zizen M (1996) Imagerie en ophtalmologie. Masson, Paris, pp 408–666

Caldemeyer K et al (1997) The jugular foramen: a review of anatomy, masses, and imaging characteristics. Radiographics 17(5):1123–1139

Camody R, Mafee M, Goodwin J et al (1994) Orbital and optic pathway sarcoidosis: MR findings. AJNR 15:775–783

Cantore W (2000) Neural orbital tumors. Curr Opin Ophthalmol 11:367–371

Carmel P (1985) The empty sella syndrome. In: Wilkins R, Reganchary S (eds) Neurosurgery. McGraw-Hill, New York, pp 884–888

Carmel P, Antunes J, Chang C (1982) Craniopharyngiomas in children. Neurosurgery 11:382–389

Carrol G, Haik B, Fleming J et al (1999) Peripheral nerve tumors of the orbit. Radiol Clin N Am 37(1):195–202

Castillo M (1993) Rhabdomyosarcoma of the middle ear: imaging features in two children. AJNR 14:730–733

Castillo M (2002) Neuroradiology. Lippincott Williams &Wilkins, Philadelphia, p 493

Castillo B, Kaufman L (2003) Pediatric tumors of the eye and orbit. Pediatr Clin N Am 50:149–172

Charabi S et al (1995) Acoustic neuroma (vestibular schwannoma). Growth and surgical and nonsurgical consequences of the wait–and–see policy. Otolaryngol Head Neck Surg 113:5–14

Chen C, Ying S, Yao M et al (2008) Sphenoid sinus osteoma at the sella turcica associated with empty sella. AJNR 29:550–551

Chena X et al (2011) Clival invasion on multi-detector CT in 390 pituitary macroadenomas: correlation with sex, subtype and rates of operative complication and recurrence. AJNR 32:785–789

Cherekaev V, Korshunov A, Pronin I et al (2001) Extensive craniofacial chondrosarcoma. J Voprosi Neurosurg 4:28–31. (in Russian)

Cherekaev V, Makhmudov U et al (1998) Variants in the growth of meningiomas of the base of the skull spreading into the orbit and paranasal sinuses. Zh Vopr Neirokhir Im NNBurdenko 2:45–50

Chung S, Chang B, Dhong H (2002) Surgical, radiological, and histological findings of the antrochoanal polyp. Am J Rhinol 16(2):71–76

Chung S et al (1998) Facial nerve schwannomas: CT and MR findings. Yonsei Med J 39(2):148–153

Ciricillo S et al (1991) Intracranial arachnoid cysts in children: a comparison of the effects of fenestration and shunting. J Neurosurg 74:230–235

Citardi M, Janjua T, Abrahams J et al (1996) Orbitoethmoid aneurysmal bone cyst. Otolaryngol Head Neck Surg 114:466–470

Cohen T, Powers S, Williams D (1992) MR appearance of intracanalicular eight nerve lipoma. AJNR 13:1188–1190

Coley S et al (1998) Giant aneurysm of the petrous internal carotid artery: diagnosis and treatment. J Laryngol Otol 112(2):196–198

Collins VP et al (2015) Pilocytic astrocytoma: pathology, molecular mechanisms and markers. Acta Neuropathol 129(6):775–788

Constantinidis J, Steinhart H, Koch M et al (2004) Olfactory neuroblastoma: the University of Erlangen–Nuremberg experience 1975–2000. Otolaryngol Head Neck Surg 130(5):567–574

Coupland S, Hummel M et al (2002) Ocular adnexal lymphomas: five case presentations and a review of the literature. Surv Ophthalmol 47:470–490

Crabtree J (1983) Acute otitis media and mastoiditis. In: English GM (ed) Otolaryngology. Harper & Row, Hagerstown

Cummings T, Provenzale J, Hunter S et al (2000) Gliomas of the optic nerve: histological, immunohistochemical (MIB-1 and p53), and MRI analysis. Acta Neuropathol 99:563–570

Cunnane M, Sepahdari A, Gardier M, Mafee M (2011) Pathology of the eye and orbit. In: Som P, Cutrin H (eds) Head and neck imaging, vol 1, 5th edn. Mosby, Maryland Heights, MI, pp 591–756

Cunningham M et al (1989) Otologic manifestations of Langerhans' cell histiocytosis. Arch Otolaryngol Head Neck Surg 115:807–813

Curati W et al (1986) Acoustic neuromas: Gd-DTPA enhancement in MR imaging. Radiology 158:447–451

Curin H, Cunnane M (2009) The skull base. In: Magnetic resonance imaging of the brain and spine. Wolters Kluwer/Lippincott Williams & Wilkins, Philadelphia, pp 1088–1119

D'Ambrosio N et al (2008) Craniofacial and intracranial manifestations of langerhans cell histiocytosis: report of findings in 100 patients. AJR 191(2):589–597

Daemerel P, Wilms G, Lammeus M (1991) Intracranial meningiomas: correlation between MRI and histology in fifty patients. J Comput Assist Tomogr 15:45–51

Dalley R et al (1986) Case report: computed tomography of anterior inferior cerebellar artery aneurysm mimicking an acoustic neuroma. J Comput Assist Tomogr 10:881–884

Daningue J, Wilson C (1977) Pituitary abscesses: report of 7 cases and review of the literature. J Neurosurg 46:601–608

Darrouzet V et al (2002) Congenital middle ear cholesteatomas in children. Our experience in 34 cases. Arch Otolaryngol Head Neck Surg 126(1):34–40

Daughaday W (1985) The anterior pituitary. In: Wilson J, Foster D (eds) Willian's textbook of endocrinology, 7th edn. Saunders, Philadelphia, pp 568–612

de Graaf P, Barchov F et al (2005) Retinoblastoma: MR Imaging parameters in detection of tumor extent. Radiology 235:197–207

De Potter P, Shields J, Shields C (1995) MRI of the eye and orbit. Lippencott, Philadelphia

Dedov I (ed) (1997) MRI in diagnostics of hypothalamic-pituitary system and adrenal gland disease. Medicine, Moscow. (in Russian)

Deen H, Sheithauer B, Ebersold M (1982) Clinical and pathological study of meningiomas of the first two decade of life. J Neurosurg 56:317–322

Delfini R et al (1993) Mucoceles of the paranasal sinuses with intracranial and intraorbital extension: report of 28 cases. Neurosurgery 32:901–906

Demirci H (2002) Orbital tumors in the older adults population. Ophthalmology 109(2):243

Depauw P et al (2003) Endovascular treatment of a giant petrous internal carotid artery aneurysm. Case report and review of the literature. Minim Invasive Neurosurg 46(4):250–253

Djindjian R et al (1973) Internal carotid-cavernous sinus, arteriovenous fistulae: current radio-anatomic aspects and therapeutic perspectives. Neurochirurgie 19(1):75–80

Dolan K (1974) Malignant lesions of the ear. Radiol Clin N Am 12:585–600

Donath J et al (2004) Effect of bisphosphonate treatment in patients with Paget's disease of the skull. Rheumatology (Oxford) 43(1):89–94

Donnet A, Metellus P, Levrier O et al (2008) Endovascular treatment of idiopathic intracranial hypertension: clinical and radiologic outcome of 10 consecutive patients. Neurology 70(8):641–647

Dormont D et al (1995) Gadolinium-enhanced MR of chronic dural sinus thrombosis. AJNR 16:1347–1352

Ducrey N, Spahn B (2002) Emergencies in nontraumatic orbital diseases. J Fr Ophtalmol 25:927–930

Dulguerov P, Allal A, Calcaterra T (2001) Esthesioneuroblastoma: a meta-analysis and review. Lancet Oncol 2(11):683–690
Dutton J (1994) Gliomas of the anterior visual pathway. Surv Ophthalmol 38:427–452
Dobben G et al (2000) Otogenic intracranial inflammations: role of magnetic resonance imaging. Top Magn Reson Imaging 11(2):76–86
Eagle R (1999) Eye pathology. In: An atlas and basic text. WB Saunders, Philadelphia, pp 247–283
Earwaker J (1993) Paranasal sinus osteomas: a review of 46 cases. Skelet Radiol 22:417–423
Eckardt A, Lemound J, Gellrich N (2013) Orbital lymphoma: diagnostic approach and treatment outcome. World J Surg Oncol 11:73
Egan R, Lessell S (2002) A contribution to the natural history of optic nerve sheath meningiomas. Arch Ophthalmol 120:1505–1508
Egorenkov VV (2010) Boundary and benign bone tumours. J Pract Oncol 11(1):37–44. (in Russian)
Elster A et al (1989) Meningiomas: MR and histopathological features. Radiology 170:857–862
Engelbrecht V, Preis S, Hassler W, Lenard H et al (1999) CT and MRI of congenital sinonasal ossifying fibroma. Neuroradiology 41(7):526–529
Enzinger F (1965) Intramuscular myxoma:a review and follow-up study of 34 cases. Am J Clin Pathol 43:104–113
Enzinger F, Weiss S (1988) Rhabdomyosarcoma. In: Soft tissue tumors, 2nd edn. Mosby, St Louis, MO, pp 448–488
Erdem E et al (2003) Comprehensive review of intracranial chordoma. Radiographics 23(4):995–1009
Essuman V, Ntim-Amponsah C, Akafo S (2010) Presentation of retinoblastoma at a pediatric eye clinic in Ghana. Ghana Med J 44(1):5–10
Esteves C et al (2015) Pituitary incidentalomas: analysis of a neuroradiological cohort. Pituitary 18(6):777–781
Eustis H et al (1998) MR imaging and CT of orbital infections and complications in acute rhinosinusitis. Radiol Clin N Am 36:1165–1183
Feldman BA (1982) Rhabdomyosarcoma of the head and neck. Laryngoscope 92:424–440
Fellbaum C, Hansmann M, Lennert K (1989) Malignant lymphomas of the nasal and paranasal sinuses. Virchows Arch A Pathol Anat Histopathol 414:399–405
Fischbein N et al (2000) Recurrence of clival chordoma along the surgical pathway. AJNR 21(3):578–583
Fisch, Mattox (1988) Microsurgery of the skull base. Stutgart Georg Thieme, Verlag
Freeman JL et al (2004) MR imaging and spectroscopic study of epileptogenic hypothalamic hamartomas: analysis of 72 cases. AJNR 25:450–462
Frezza A, Cesari M, Baumhoer D et al (2015) Mesenchymal chondrosarcoma: Prognostic factors and outcome in 113 patients. A European Musculoskeletal Oncology Society study. Eur J Cancer 51:374–381
Friedrich R et al (2010) Dysplasia of the orbit and adjacent bone associated with plexiform neurofibroma and ocular disease in 42 NF-1 patients. Anticancer Res 30(5):1751–1764
Frierson H, Mills S, Fechner R et al (1986) Sinonasal undifferentiated carcinoma : an aggressive neoplasm derived from Schneiderian epithelium and distinct from olfactory neuroblastoma. Am J Pathol 10:771–779
Fujisawa I et al (1987) Transection of the pituitary stalk: development of an ectopic posterior lobe assessed with MRI. Radiology 165:487–489
Fusco N, Guerini-Rocco E, Schultheis A et al (2015) The birth of an adenoid cystic carcinoma. Int J Surg Pathol 23(1):26–27
Gabibov G (1993) Meningiomas of the anterior skull base expanding into orbit, paranasal sinuses, nasopharynx, and oropharynx. J Craniofac Surg 4(3):124–127
Gadwal S, Fanburg-Smith J, Gannon F et al (2000) Primary chondrosarcoma of the head and neck in pediatric patients: a clinicopathologic study of 14 cases with a review of the literature. Cancer 88:2181–2188
Garcia Santos J et al (1993) Arachnoid cysts of the middle fossa: a consideration of their origin based on imaging. Neuroradiology 39:395–358
Gautier-Smith P (1960) Bilateral pulsating exophthalmos due to metastases from carcinoma of prostate. Br Med J 1:330
Goepfert H et al (1979) Rhabdomyosarcoma of the temporal bone: is surgical resection necessary? Arch Otolaryngol 105(6):301–313
Gordon L (2003) Diagnostic dilemmas in orbital inflammatory disease. Ocul Immunol Inflamm 11:3–15
Graham D, Lantos P (1997) Greenfield's neuropathology, vol 2, 6th edn. Arnold, London, pp 583–795
Gray B et al (1995) Spontaneous meningocele, a rare middle ear mass. AJNR 16:203–207
Greenberg J et al (1988) Cholesterol granuloma of the petrous apex: MR and CT evaluation. AJNR 9(6):1205–1214
Griffeth M, Dailey R, Ofner S (1997) Bilateral spontaneous subperiosteal hematoma of the orbit: a case report. Arch Ophthalmol 115(5):679–680
Griffin C et al (1987) MR and CT correlation of cholesterol cysts of the petrous bone. AJNR. 8:825–829
Grossman R, Davis KR (1981) Cranial computed tomographic appearance of chondrosarcoma of the base of the skull. Radiology 141:403–408
Grossman R, Yousem D (1994) Neuroradiology. Chapter 13. In: Sinonasal disease. Mosby, St. Louis, pp 359–376
Gualdi G et al (1991) Unusual MR and CT appearance of an epidermoid tumor. AJNR 12:711–772
Gupta R (1989) Sellar abscess associated with tuberculous osteomyelitis of skull: MR findings. AJNR 10:448–454
Gupta S, Gupta RK et al (1993) Signal intensity patterns in intraspinal dermoids and epidermoids on MR imaging. Clin Radiol 48:405–413
Gupta A et al (2011) Carcinoid tumor metastases to the extraocular muscles: MR imaging and CT findings and review of the literature. AJNR 32:1208–1211
Hamilos D, Lund VJ et al (2004) Etiology of chronic rhinosinusitis: the role of fungus. Ann Otol Rhinol Laryngol Suppl 193:27–30
Harcourt J, Gallimore A (1993) Leiomyoma of the paranasal sinuses. J Laryngol Otol 107:740–741
Har-El G (2001) Endoscopic management of 108 sinus mucoceles. Laryngoscope 111(12):2131–2134
Harnsberger H, GlastonburyChristine M, MichelMichelle A et al (2004) Diagnostic imaging. Head and neck. Section 2. In: Nose and sinus. Amyrsys, Manitoba, pp II-2-2–II-2-98
Harnsberger R, Wiggins R et al (2004) Head and neck, vol 1. Amirsys, Salt Lake City, pp 3–75
Harris G (1999) Orbital vascular malformations: a consensus statement on terminology and its clinical implications—orbital society. Am J Ophthalmol 127:453–455
Hasso A et al (1988) Normal anatomy and pathology of the temporal bone and mastoid. In: Newton TH, Hasso AN, Dilon WP (eds) Computed tomography of the head and neck. Raven Press, New York
Haynes R et al (1988) Asymmetric temporal bone pneumatization: an MR imaging pitfall. AJNR 9:699
Healy J, Bishop J, Rosenkrantz H (1981) Cranial computed tomography in the detection of dural, orbital, and skull involvement in metastatic neuroblastoma. J Comput Tomogr 5:319–323
Heffelfinger M, David C, Dahlin MD et al (1973) Chordomas and cartilaginous tumors at the skull base. Cancer 32:410–420
Henderson J (1994) Orbital tumors, 3rd edn. Raven Press, New York, p 440

Hermans R, De Vuysere S, Marchal G et al (1999) Squamous cell carcinoma of sinonasal cavities. Semin Ultrasound CT MRI 20:150–161
Hillstrom R, Zarbo R, Jacobs J (1990) Nerve sheath tumors of the paranasal sinuses: electron microscopy and histopathologic diagnosis. Otolaryngol Head Neck Surg 102:257–263
Hoffman H et al (1992) Aggressive surgical management of craniopharyngiomas in children. J Neurosurg 76:47–52
Horn K et al (1996) Supportive petrous apicitis: osteitis or osteomyelitis: an imaging case report. Am J Otolaryngol 17:54–57
Horowitz B et al (1990) MR in intracranial epidermoid tumors: correlation of in vitro imaging with in vitro 13C spectroscopy. AJNR 11:299–302
Howell M, Branstetter BF IV, Snyderman C (2011) Patterns of regional spread for esthesioneuroblastoma. AJNR 32:929–933
Hoyt W et al (1970) Septo-optic dysplasia and pituitary dwarfism. Lancet 1:893–894
Huang C, Chien C, Su C et al (2000) Leiomyoma of the inferior turbinates. J Otolaryngol 29:55–56
Hughes C, Wilson WR, Olding M et al (1999) Giant ameloblastoma: report of an extreme case and description of its treatment. Eur Nose Throat J 78(8):570–574
Huh W, Beverly R (2006) Orbital metastasis in patients with rhabdomyosarcoma: case series and review of the literature. J Pediatr Hematol Oncol 28(10):684–687
Huk W, Cademann G, Friedmann G (1990) MRI of central nervous system diseases. Springer-Verlag, Berlin
Hullar T et al (2003) Paget's disease and fibrous dysplasia. Otolaryngol Clin North Am 36(4):707–732
Hwang C et al (2003) Bilateral petrous internal carotid artery pseudoaneurysms presenting with sensorineural hearing loss. AJNR 24(6):1139–1141
Iannetti G, Cascone P, Valentini V, Agrillo A (1997) Paranasal sinus mucocele: diagnosis and treatment. J Craniofacial Surg 8(5):391–398
Ing E, Garrity J, Cross S et al (1997) Sarcoid masquerading as optic nerve sheath meningioma. Mayo Clin Proc 72:38–43
Jackler R et al (2003) A new theory to explain the genesis of petrous apex cholesterol granuloma. Otol Neurotol 24(1):96–106
Jackson C (2001) Glomus tympanicum and glomus jugulare tumors. Otolaryngol Clin North Am 34(5):941–970
Jacobs D, Galetta S (2002) Diagnosis and management of orbital pseudotumor. Curr Opin Ophthalmol 13:347–351
Jakovlev SB (1997) Arteriosinus anastomosis between the middle meningeal artery and cavernous sinus. Surgical treatment using ballooncatheter. Vopr Neurochirurgii NN Burdenko 2:31–33. (in Russian)
Jay V et al (1999) An unusual cerebellar primitive neuroectodermal tumor with t(11;22) translocation: pathological and molecular analysis. Pediatr Pathol Lab Med 16:119–128
Jee WH, Choi KH, Choe BY, Park JM, Shinn KS (1996) Fibrous dysplasia: MR imaging characteristics with radiopathologic correlation. AJNR 167(7):1523–1527
Jethanamest D, Morris L, Sikora A (2007) Esthesioneuroblastoma: a population-based analysis of survival and prognostic factors. Arch Otolaryngol Head Neck Surg 133:1571–1576
Jiltsova MG, Kaplina AV (2010) Malignant neoplasms. Vestnik Ophthalmol 6:9–17. (in Russian)
Johnson D, Chandra R et al (1985) Trilateral retinoblastoma: ocular and pineal retinoblastoma. J Neurosurg 63:367–370
Kadashev B (2007) Pituitary adenomas: clinical features, diagnostics, treatment. Triada, Tver. (in Russian)
Kaffe I, Naor H, Calderon S et al (1999) Radiological and clinical features of aneurysmal bone cyst of the jaws. Dentomaxillofac Radiol 28:167–172
Kahana A, Lucarelli M, Grayev A et al (2007) Noninvasive dynamic magnetic resonance angiography with time-resolved imaging of contrast kinetics (TRICKS) in the evaluation of orbital vascular lesions. Arch Ophtalmol 125(12):1635–1642
Kallmes D, Provenzale J, Cloft H et al (1997) Typical and atypical MR imaging features of intracranial epidermoid tumors. AJNR 169:883–887
Kaplan R, Coon S, Drayer B (1992) MR characteristics of meningioma subtypes at 1.5 Tesla. J Comput Assist Tomogr 16:366–371
Kapur R et al (2009) MR imaging of orbital inflammatory syndrome, orbital cellulitis, and orbital lymphoid lesions: the role of diffusion-weighted imaging. AJNR 30:64–70
Kato T, Sawamura Y, Tada M et al (1998) Occult neurohypophyseal germinomas in patients presenting with central diabetes insipidus. Neurosurg Focus 5:1–6
Katsuta T, Rhoton A (1997) The jugular foramen: microsurgical anatomy and operative approaches. Neurosurgery 41(1):149–202
Kelly W et al (1988) Posterior pituitary ectopia: an MR feature of pituitary dwarfism. AJNR 9:453–460
Kendler DL, Lippa J, Rootman J (1993) The initial clinical characteristics of Graves'orbitopathy vary with age and sex. Arch Ophtalmol 111(2):197–201
Khoury N, Naffaa L, Shabb N et al (2002) Juvenile ossifying fibroma: CT and MR findings. Eur Radiol 12(Suppl 3):109–113
Kim D, Choi J, Yang K et al (2002) Optic sheath schwannomas: report of two cases. Childs Nerv Syst 18:684–689
Kim J et al (2004) Surgical treatment symptomatic Rathke cleft cysts: clinical features and results with special attention to recurrence. J Neurosurg 100:33–40
Klein M et al (1989) Heterotopic brain in the middle ear: CT findings. J Comput Assist Tomogr 13(6):1058–1060
Kline LB, Hoyt WE (2001) The Tolosa-hunt syndrome. J Neurol Neurosurg Psychiatry 71(5):577–582
Klintenberg C, Olofsson J, Hellquist H et al (1984) Adenocarcinoma of the ethmoid sinuses:a review of 38 cases with special reference to wood dust exposure. Cancer 31:482–488
Kondo M, Hashimoto S, Inuyama Y (1986) Extramedullary plasmacytoma of the sinonasal cavities: CT evaluation. J Comput Assist Tomogr 10:841–844
Konovalov A, Kornienko V (1985) Computerized tomography in neurosurgical clinics. Medicine, Moscow. (in Russian)
Konovalov A, Kornienko V, Ozerova V (1983) Modern possibilities of radiological diagnostics of craniopharyngiomas. Vestn Roentgol Radiol 3:5–12. (in Russian)
Konovalov A, Kornienko V, Pronin I (1997) Magnetic resonance tomography in neurosurgery. Vidar, Moscow. (in Russian)
Kopylov M (1968) Radiological diagnostic basics of brain disease. Medicine, Moscow. (in Russian)
Kornienko V, Ozerova V (1993) Childhood neuroradiolsogy. Medicine, Moscow. (in Russian)
Kornienko V, Pronin I (2009) Diagnostic neuroradiology. Springer-Verlag, Berlin, p 1288
Korshunov AG, Shishkina LV (2009) Histobiological characteristic of the posterior cranial fossa meningiomas and its impact on the remote treatment results. Vopr Neurochirurgii NN Burdenko 4:3–7. (in Russian)
Kozlov A (2001) Biology of meningiomas: state-of-art. Vopr Neurochirurgii NN Burdenko 1:32–37. (in Russian)
Kucharczyk W, Montanera W (1991) The sella and parasellar region. In: Atlas SW (ed) MRI of the brain and spine. Raven Press, New York
Kujas M, Faillot T, Van Effenterre R et al (1999) Bone gaint cell tumour in neuropathologic practice. A fifty years overview. Arch Anat Cytol Pathol 47:7–12
Kuruvilla A, Wenig B, Humphery D et al (1990) Leiomyosarcoma of the sinonasal tract: a clinicopathologic study of nine cases. Arch Otolaryngol Head Neck Surg 116:1278–1286
Kuta J, Worley C, Kaugars G et al (1995) Central cementoossifying fibroma of the maxillary sinus: a review of six cases. AJNR 16:1282–1286

Kwan E, Wolpert S, Hedges TR et al (1987) Tolosa-Hunt syndrome revisited: not necessarily a diagnosis of exclusion. AJNR 8:1067–1072

Lanzieri C, Shah M, Krauss D, Lavertu P (1991) Use gadolinium-enhanced MR imagines for differentiating mucoceles from neoplasms in the paranasal sinuses. Radiology 178:425–428

Lasjaunias P, Burrows P, Planet C (1986) Developmental venous anomalies (DVA). The so-called venous angioma. Neurosurg Rev 9:233–244

Latack J, Hutchinson R, Heyn R (1987) Imaging of rhabdomyosarcomas of the head and neck. AJNR Am J Neuroradiol 8:353–359

Leavitt R, Fauci A, Bloch D et al (1990) The American College of Rheumatology criteria for the classification of Wegener's granulomatosis. Arthritis Rheum 33:1101–1107

Leddy L, Holmes R (2014) Chondrosarcoma of bone. Cancer Treat Res 162:117–130

Lee J et al (1998) Giant cell tumor of the skull. Radiographies 18(5):1295–1302

Lee J et al (1979) Computed tomography of arachnoid cysts. Radiology 130:675–680

Lee J et al (1987) Lymphomas of the head and neck: CT findings at initial presentation. AJNR 8:665–671

Lee HJ et al (2015) Pretreatment diagnosis of suprasellar papillary craniopharyngioma and germ cell tumors of adult patients. AJNR 36(3):508–517

Levine PA, Frierson HF Jr, Stewart FM et al (1987) Sinonasal undifferentiated carcinoma: a distinctive and highly aggressive neoplasm. Laryngoscope 97:905–908

Levine S et al (1988) Lymphocytic hypophysitis: clinical, radiological, and magnetic resonance imaging characterization. Neurosurgery 22:937–941

Li C, Yousem DM, Hayden R et al (1993) Olfactory neuroblastoma. MR evaluation. AJNR 14(5):1167–1171

Lieb W et al (2010) Tumors and tumor-like lesions of the orbit. HNO 58(7):661–671

Liechtenstein (1938) Polyostotic fibrous dysplasia. Arch Surg 36(1): 874–898

Lippert B, Godbersen G, Luttges J et al (1996) Leiomyosarcoma of the nasal cavity. Case report and literature review. ORL J Otolaryngol Relat Spec 58:115–120

Liu R et al (2001) Facial nerve schwannoma: surgical excision versus conservative management. Ann Otol Rhinol Laryngol 110(11):1025–1029

Liu Z et al (2015) Imaging characteristics of primary intracranial teratoma. Acta Radiol 55(7):874–881

Lloyd G, Howard D, Phelps P et al (2000) Imaging for juvenile angiofibroma. J Laryngol Otol 114(9):727–730

Lloyd G, Lund V, Savy L, Howard D et al (2000) Optimum imaging mucoceles. J Laryngol Otol 114(3):233–236

Lloyd G, Phelps P (1986) Juvenile angiofibroma: imaging by magnetic resonance, CT and conventional techniques. Clin Otolaryngol Allied Sci 11:247–259

Lloyd G, Wright J, Morgan G (1971) Venous malformations in the orbit. Br J Ophthalmol 55:505–508

Loevner L, Sonners A (2002) Imaging of neoplasms of the paranasal sinuses. Magn Reson Imaging Clin N Am 10(3):467–493

Lopez F, Triantafyllou A, Snyderman C et al (2017) Nasal juvenile angiofibroma: current perspectives with emphasis on management. Head Neck 39(5):1033–1045. https://doi.org/10.1002/hed.24696

Mafee M (1998) Uveal melanoma, choroidal hemagioma, and simulating lesions. Role of MR imaging. Radiol Clin N Am 36(6):1083–1099

Mafee M, Dorodi S (1999) Sarcoidosis of the eye, orbit and central nervous system: role of MR imaging. Radiol Clin N Am 37: 73–87

Mafee M, Goodwin J, Dorodi S (1999) Optic nerve sheath meningioma: role of MR imaging. Radiol Clin North Am 37(1):37–58

Mafee M, Jampol L, Lager B et al (1987) CT of optic nerve colobomas, morning glory anomaly, and colobomatous cyst. Radiol Clin N Am 25(4):693–699

Mafee M et al (2000) Glomus faciale, glomus jugulare, glomus tympanicum, glomus vagale, carotid body tumors, and simulating lesions. Role of MR imaging. Radiol Clin North Am 38(5): 1059–1076

Maghnie M et al (1992) MR of the hypothalamic-pituitary axis in Langerhans cell histiocytosis. AJNR 13(5):1365–1371

Mahapatra A, Suri A et al (2002) Anterior encephalocele: a study of 92 cases. Pediatr Neurosurg 36(3):113–118

Maira G et al (1996) Surgical treatment of clival chordomas: the transsphenoidal approach revisited. J Neurosurg 85(5):784–792

Mann W, Jecker P, Amedee RG et al (2004) Juvenile angiofibromas: changing surgical concept over the last 20 years. Laryngoscope 114(2):291–293

Marchiò C, Weigelt B, Reis-Filho J (2010) Adenoid cystic carcinomas of the breast and salivary glands (or 'The strange case of Dr Jekyll and Mr Hyde' of exocrine gland carcinomas). J Clin Pathol 63(3):220–228

Markus H, Kendall BE (1993) MRI of a dermoid cyst containing hair. Neuradiology 35:256–257

Marova E (1996) Nelson syndrome. In: Starkova N (ed) Guidelines for the clinical endocrinology. American Association of Clinical Endocrinologists, St. Petersburg, pp 78–83. (in Russian)

Martin N et al (1989) Cholesterol granuloma of the middle ear cavities: MR imaging. Radiology 172:521–525

Martin N et al (1990) Chronic inflammatory disease of the middle ear cavities. Gd-DTPA-enhanced MR imaging. Radiology 176:399–405

Matsko D, Korshunov A (1998) Atlas of tumours of the central nervous system (the histological structure). RNSI AL Poloenov, St. Peterburg, p 200 (in Russian)

MacDonald A et al (2004) Primary jugular foramen meningioma. Imaging appearance and differentiating features. AJR 182(2):373–377

Mehhlisch D, Dahlin D, Masson J (1972) Ameloblastoma: a clinicopathologic report. J Oral Surg 30:9–22

Melero G et al (2000) Facial paralysis. An unusual presentation of congenital cholesteatoma. Otolaryngol Head Neck Surg 122(4):615–616

Menor F et al (1991) Imaging consideration of central nervous system manifestations in pediatric patients with neurofibromatosis type I. Pediatr Radiol 21:389–394

Meyer M, Hahn C (2011) Intraosseous cavernous hemangioma of the bony orbit. Ugeskr Laeger 173(5):360–361

Meyers S, Hirsch W Jr, Curtin H et al (1992) Chondrosarcomas of the skull base: MR imaging features. Radiology 184:103–108

Migirov L (2003) Computed tomographic versus surgical findings in complicated acute otomastoiditis. Ann Otol Rhinol Laryngol 112(8):675–677

Miller DC (1994) Pathology of craniopharyngiomas: clinical import of pathological findings. Pediatr Neurosurg 21:11–17

Miro J, Videgain G, Petrenas E et al (1998) Chordoma of the ethmoidal sinus. A case report. Acta Otorrinolaringol Esp 49:66–69

Mittal S et al (2013) Hypothalamic hamartomas. Part 1. Clinical, neuroimaging and neurophysiological characteristics. Neurosurg Focus 34(6):E6

Moore K et al (2001) Petrous Apex Cephaloceles. AJNR. 22(10): 1867–1871

Motoyama S, Maruyama K, Sato Y (2011) A case of recurrent malignant melanoma of esophagus responsive to combined chemotherapy, radiotherapy and cellular immunotherapy. Gan To Kadaku Ryoho 38(4):639–642

Mukherji et al (1997) Papillary endolymphatic sac tumors: CT, MR imaging, and angiographic findings in 20 patients. Radiology 202:801–808

Muller HL (2013) Childhood craniopharyngioma. Pituitary 16(1):56–67

Muller-Forell W (2006) Imaging of orbital abd visual pathway pathology. Springer-Verlag, Berlin, p 448

Murphree A (2005) Intraocular retinoblastoma: the case for a new group classification. Ophtalmol Clin North Am 18(1):41–53

Naidich T et al (1983) Midline craniofacial dysraphism: midline cleft upper lip, basal encephalocele, callosal agenesis, and optic nerve dysplasia. Concepts Pediatr Neurosurg 4:186–207

Nathu R et al (1999) Non–Hodgkin's lymphoma of the head and neck: a 30-year experience at the University of Florida. Head Neck 21(3):247–254

Nayar R, Prudhomme F, Parise O Jr et al (1993) Rhabdomyosarcoma of the head and neck in adults: a study of 26 patients. Laryngoscope 103:1362–1366

Neff B et al (2002) Chondrosarcoma of the skull base. Larhyngoscop 112(1):134–139

Ng Y, Kingston J, Perry N (1990) The role of computerized tomographic scanning in the management of rhabdomyosarcoma in non-orbital head and neck sites. Pediatr Hematol Oncol 7:149–157

Noguchi K et al (2004) Intracranial dural arteriovenous fistulas: evaluation with combined 3D time-of-flight MR angiography and MR digital subtraction angiography. AJR 182(1):183–190

Noujaim S et al (2000) Paraganglioma of the temporal bone. Role of magnetic resonance imaging versus computed tomography. Top Magn Reson Imaging 11(2):108–122

Oberman H, Sullenger G (1967) Neurogenous tumors of the head and neck. Cancer 20:1992–2001

Oot R et al (1988) The role of MR and CT in evaluating clival chordomas and chondrosarcomas. AJR 151(3):567–575

Orrison W, Hart B (2000) Intraaxsial brain tumors. In: Neuroimaging. W.B. Saunders Company, Philadelphia, pp 583–611

Osborn A (2004a) Brain diagnostic imaging. Amirsys, Salt Lake City, p 936

Osborn A (2004b) Diagnostic Imaging: Brain 1ed Amirsys, Salt Lake City, p 992

Osborn A, Salzman K, Jhaveri M (eds) (2016) Diagnostic imaging: brain, 3rd edn. Elsevier, Philadelphia, p 1197

Ottaviani G, Jaffe N (2009) The epidemiology of osteosarcoma. Cancer Treat Res 152:3–13

Ozdek A et al (2002) Antrochoanal polyps in children. Int J Pediatr Otorhinolaryngol 65(3):213–218

Paparella M et al (1982) Clinical significance of granulation tissue of chronic otitis media. In: Sade J (ed) Cholesteatoma and mastoid surgery. Kugler, Amsterdam, pp 387–395

Pawha P (2009) Neoplastic disease of the spine and spinal cord. Chapter 26. In: Magnetic resonance imaging of the brain and spine. Wolters Kluwer/Lippincott Williams & Wilkins, Philadelphia, p 1521

Petruson K, Rodriguez-Catarino M, Petruson B, Finizia C (2002) Juvenile nasopharyngeal angiofibroma: long-term results in preoperative embolized and non-embolized patients. Acta Otolaryngol 122(1):96–100

Peyster R, Augsburger J (1985) Choroidal melanoma: comparison of CT funduscopy and US. Radiology 156:675–680

Phillips C et al (2002) The facial nerve: anatomy and common, pathology. Semin Ultrasound CT MR 23(3):202–217

Pinker K et al (2005) The value of high-field MRI (3T) in the assessment of sellar lesions. Eur J Radiol 54:327–361

Presutti L et al (1991) Jugular bulb diverticula. ORL J Otorhinolaryngol Relat Spec 53(1):57–60

Quencer R (1980) Lymphocytic adenohypophysitis: autoimmune disorder of the pituitary gland. AJNR 1:343–349

Randoux B et al (2000) Solitary plasmacytoma of the calvarium. Neuroradiology 27(4):278–281

Rang T et al (2002) Evaluation of pituitary microadenomas with dynamic MRI. Eur J Radiol 41:131–135

Rao V, Sharma D, Madan A et al (2001) Imaging of frontal sinus disease: concepts, interpretation, and technology. Otolaryngol Clin N Am 34(1):23–39

Rao A et al (1999) Paragangliomas of the head and neck. Radiologic-pathologic correlation. Radiographics 19:1605–1632

Rassekh C, Nuss D, Kapadia S et al (1996) Chondrosarcoma of the nasal septum: skull base imaging and clinicopathologic correlation. Otolatyngol Head Neck Surg 115:29–37

Regenbogen V, Zinreich S, Kim K, Kuhajda F, Applebaum B et al (1988) Hyperostotic esthesioneuroblastoma: CT and MR findings. J Comput Assist Tomogr 12:52–56

Ren X et al (2012) Clinical, radiological, and pathological features of 24 atypical intracranial epidermoid cysts. J Neurosurg 116(3):611–621

Rice C, Brawn H (1990) Primary orbital melanoma associated with orbital melanocytosis. Arch Ophthalmol 108(8):1130–1134

Roberti F et al (2001) Posterior fossa meningiomas: surgical experience in 161 cases. Surg Neurol 56(1):8–20

Robertson J, Hugh B (2000) Cranial base surgery. Churchill Livingston, London, p 688

Roche J et al (1996) Arachnoid granulations in the transverse and sigmoid sinuses: CT, MR and MR angiographic appearance of a normal anatomic variation. AJNR 17:677–683

Rock J (1986) Arachnoid cysts of the posterior fossa. Neurosurgery 18:176–179

Roeder M, Bazan C, Jinkins J et al (1995) Ruptured spinal dermoid cyst with chemical arachnoiditis and disseminated intracranial lipid droplets. Neuroradiology 37:146–147

Rohr A, Riedel C, Fruehauf M et al (2011) MR imaging findings in patients with secondary intracranial hypertension. AJNR 32(6):1021–1209

Rojvachiranonda N, David D, Moore M, Cole J (2003) Frontoethmoidal encephalomeningocele: new morphological findings and a new classification. J Craniofac Surg 14(6):847–858

Rootman S (ed) (1988) Diseases of the orbit, 1st edn. Lippincott, New York, p 565

Rosenberg A et al (1999) Chondrosarcoma of the base of the skull. A clinicopathologic study of 200 cases with emphasis on its distinction from chordoma. Am J Surg Pathol 23:1370–1378

Rosenstiel O et al (2001) MALT lymphoma presenting as a cystic salivary gland mass. Head Neck 23(3):254–258

Ross DA, Norman D, Wilson CB (1992) Radiologic characteristics and results of surgical management of Rathke's cysts in 43 patients. Neurosurgery 30:173–179

Rozhinskaya L (2011) Nelson syndrome. In: Dedov I (ed) Clinical neuroendocrinology. UP Print, Moscow, pp 79–94. (in Russian)

Rubin J et al (1990) Malignant external otitis: utility of CT in diagnosis and follow-up. Radiology 174:391–394

Rucker J et al (2003) Diffuse dural enhancement in cavernous sinus dural arteriovenous fistula. Neuroradiology 45(2):88–89

Russell D, Rubinstein L (1989) Pathology of tumors of the nervous system, 5th edn. Williams and Wilkins, Baltimore

Saito K, Unni K, Wollan P et al (1995) Chondrosarcoma of the jaw and facial bones. Cancer 76:1550–1558

Sakamoto Y et al (1991) Normal and abnormal pituitary glands: gadopentetate dimeglumine-enhanced MR imaging. Radiology 178:441–445

Schaerer J, Whitney R (1953) Prostatic metastases simulating intracranial meningioma. Neurosurgery 10:546–549

Schmerber S et al (2002) Endolymphatic duct obstruction related to a jugular bulb diverticulum: high resolution CT and MR imaging findings. Clin Radiol 57(5):424–428

Scholl R, Kellett H, Neumann D, Lurie A (1999) Cysts and cystic lesions of the mandible: clinical and radiologic-histopathologic review. Radiographics 19:1107–1124

Schuknecht H et al (1986) Anatomy of the temporal bone with surgical implications. Lea and Febiger, Philadelphia

Schwartz T et al (2001) Association between intracranial plasmacytoma and multiple myeloma. Clinicopathological outcome study. Neurosurgery 49(5):1039–1044

Scott T (1993) Neurosarcoidosis: progress and clinical aspects. Neurology 43(1):8–12

Seabold J et al (1995) Cranial osteomyelitis: diagnosis and follow-up with In-111 white blood cell and Tc-99m methylene diphosphonate bone SPECT, CT, and MR imaging. Radiology 196:779–788

Seidenwurm DJ (2008) Neuroendocrine imaging. AJNR 29(3):613–615

Selosse P, Mahler C, Klaes R (1980) Pituitary abscess: case report. J Neurosurg 53:851–852

Sepahdari A et al (2014) Diffusion-weighted imaging of orbital masses: multi-institutional data support a 2-ADC threshold model to categorize lesions as benign, malignant, or indeterminate. AJNR 35:170–175

Serbinenko FA (1968) Carotid-cavernous fistulae. Neurosurgery 2:651–660

Serbinenko FA (1974) Clinics, diagnosis and surgical treatment of arterio-sinusal fistulas. In: Neurosurgical pathology of cerebral vessels, Medicine, Moscow, pp 334-339

Serbinenko F et al (1999) Anastomoses between meningeal arteries and cavernous sinus. Clinics, diagnostics, treatment. Vopr Neurochirurgii NN Burdenko 4:2–7. (in Russian)

Sergides I et al (2007) Pituitary apoplexy can mimic subarachnoid haemorrhage clinically and radiologically. Emerg Med J 24(4):308

Shady J, Bland LI, Kazee A, Pilcher W (1994) Osteoma of the frontoethmoidal sinus with secondary brain abscess and intracranial mucocele. Neurosurgery 34(5):920–923

Shapiro R, Janzen A (1959) Osteoblastic metastases to floor of skull simulating meningioma en plaque. Am J Roentgenol 81:964–966

Sharma R et al (2002) Symptomatic cranial fibrous dysplasias. Clinico-radiological analysis in a series of eight operative cases with follow-up results. J Clin Neurosci 9(4):381–390

Sheehan A, Stanford J (1961) The pathogenesis of post-partum a pituitary necrosis of the anterior lobe of the pituitary gland. Acta Endocrinol 37:479–510

Sheikh M et al (1999) Giant cell tumor of the temporal bone: case report and review of the literature. Australas Radiol 43(1):113–115

Shields J, Shields C et al (2004) Survey of 1264 patients with orbital tumors and simulating lesions: the 2002 Montgomery lecture, part 1. Ophthalmology 111:997–1008

Shugar J, Som P, Krespi Y (1980) Primary chordoma of the maxillary sinus. Laryngoscope 90:1825–1830

Shuper A et al (1998) Metastatic brain involvement in Ewing family of tumors in children. Neurology 51:1336–1338

Sidorkin D (2009) Surgical treatment of the skull base chordomas. Vopr Neurochirurgii NN Burdenko 2:15–23. (in Russian)

Sigal R, Monnet O, Baere T et al (1992) Adenoid cystic carcinoma of the head and neck: evaluation with MR imaging and clinical-pathologic correlation in 27 patients. Radiology 184:95–10

Sklar E, Pizarro J (2003) Sinonasal intestinal-type adenocarcinoma involvement of the paranasal sinuses. AJNR 24(6):1152–1155

Smith A et al (1991) Diagnosis of ruptured intracranial dermoid cyst: value of MR over CT. AJNR 12:75–180

Som P, Bradwein-Gensler M, Kassel E, Gender E (2011) Tumors and tumor-like conditions of the sinonasal cavities. In: Som P, Cutrin H (eds) Head and neck imaging, vol 1, 5th edn. Mosby-Elsevier, St. Louis, pp 253–410

Som P, Dillon W, Fullerton G et al (1989) Chronically obstructed sinonasal secretions: observations on T1 and T2 shortening. Radiology 172:515–520

Som P, Lidov M, Catalano P, Biller H (1994) Sinonasal esthesioneuroblastoma with intracranial extension: marginal tumor cysts as a diagnostic MR finding. AJNR 15:1259–1262

Som P, Schatz C, Flaum E et al (1991) Aneurysmal bone cyst of the paranasal sinuses associated with fibrous dysplasia: CT and MR findings. J Comput Assist Tomogr 15:513–515

Som P, Shapiro M, Biller H et al (1988) Sinonasal tumors and inflammatory tissues: differentiation with MR imaging. Radiology 167:803–808

Sorensen T, Fredericson J et al (1999) Optic neuritis as onset manifestation of multiple sclerosis. Neurology 53:473–478

Soule E, Mahour G, Mills S, Lynn H (1968) Soft tissue sarcomas of infants and children: a clinicopathologic study of 135 cases. Mayo Clin Proc 43:313–326

Spreer J (2009) Pyogenic cerebritis and brain abscess. In: Hahnel S (ed) Inflammatory diseases of the brain. Springer-Verlag, Berlin, pp 55–70

Stankewich JA (1989) Sphenoid sinus mucocele. Arch Otolaryngol Head Neck Surg 115:735–740

Stout AP (1948) Mesenchymoma, the mixed tumot mesenchymal derivation. Ann Surg 127:278–290

Strasser M, Gleich L, Hakim S et al (1998) Pathologic quiz case 2. Nasal leiomyosarcoma, low grade. Arch Otolaryngol Head Neck Surg 124:715–717

Sutow W, Sullivan M, Ried H et al (1970) Prognosis in childhood rhabdomyosarcoma. Cancer 25:1384–1390

Sze G et al (1988) Chordomas: MR imaging. Radiology 166:187–191

Taban M, Perry J (2007) Classification of orbital tumors. In: Singh A et al (eds) Clinical ophthalmic oncology. Lippincott Williams &Wilkins, Philadelphia, pp 517–519

Tailor T, Gupta D et al (2013) Orbital neoplasms in adults: clinical, radiologic, and pathologic review. Radiographics 33(6):1739–1758

Tampieri D, Melanson D, Ethie R (1989) MR imaging of epidermoid cysts. AJNR 10:351–356

Tanaka A, Mihara F et al (2004) Differentiation of cavernous hemangioma from schwannoma of the orbit: a dynamic MRI study. AJR 183(6):1799–1804

Tang J et al (2003) MRI appearance of giant cell tumor of the lateral skull base. A case report. Clin Imaging 27(1):27–30

Tarasova LN, Drozdova EA (2005) Inflammatory disorders of the orbit. In: Diseases, neoplasms and trauma of the orbit. Medicine. Russian Edition. M., pp 145–149

Tatler G, Kendall B (1991) The radiological diagnosis of epidermoid tumors. Neuroradiology 33(Suppl):324–325

Terada et al (1996) Clinical use of mechanical detachable coils for dural arteriovenous fistulas. AJNR 17(7):134–138

Teramoto A, Hirakawa K, Sanno N et al (1994) Incidental pituitary lesions in 1,000 unselected autopsy specimens. Radiology 193:161–164

Thiagalingam S, Flaherty M, Billson F et al (2004) Neurofibromatosis type 1 and optic pathway gliomas: follow-up of 54 patients. Ophthalmology 111:568–577

Tien RD et al (1990) Thickened pituitary stalk on MR images in patients with diabetes insipidus and Langerhans cell histiocytosis. AJNR 11:703–308

Tokumaru A, O'uchi T, Eguchi T et al (1990) Prominent meningeal enhancement adjacent to meningioma on Gd-DTPA-enhanced MR images: histopathologic correlation. Radiology 175:431–433

Toro J, Travis L, Wu H et al (2006) Incidence patterns of soft tissue sarcomas, regardless of primary site, in the surveillance, epidemiology and end results program, 1978–2001: an analysis of 26,758 cases. Int J Cancer 119(12):2922–2930

Tow S, Chandela S, Miller N et al (2003) Long-term prognosis in children with gliomas of the anterior visual pathway. Pediatr Neurol 28:262–270

Trombly R, Sandberg D et al (2006) High-flow orbital arteriovenous malformation in a child: current management and options. J Craniofac Surg 17:779–782
Tsuruda J, Chew W, Moseley M et al (1990) Diffusion-weighted MR imaging of the brain: value of differentiating between extraaxial cysts and epidermoid tumors. AJNR 155:1059–1068
Tufan K et al (2005) Intracranial meningiomas of childhood and adolescence. Pediatr Neurosurg 41:1–7
Turbin R, Pokorny K (2004) Diagnosis and treatment of orbital optic nerve sheath meningioma. Cancer Control 11(5):334–341
Uehara F, Ohba N (2002) Diagnostic imaging in patients with orbital cellulitis and inflammatory pseudotumor. Int Ophthalmol Clin 42:133–142
Ulivieri S, Oliveri G, Motolese I (2001) Supero-lateral orbitotomy for resection of spheno-orbital meningioma: a case report. Radiol Clin N Am 42(3):118–119
Valvassori G, Sabnis S, Mafee R et al (1999) Imaging of orbital lymphoproliferative disorders. Radiol Clin N Am 37(1):135–150
Van Effenterre R et al (2002) Craniopharyngioma in adults and children: a study of 122 surgical cases. J Neurosurg 97:3–11
Vande Berg B et al (2001) Magnetic resonance appearance of uncomplicated Paget's disease of bone. Semin Musculoskelet Radiol 5(1):69–77
Veselinović D, Krasić D, Stefanović I (2010) Orbital dermoid and epidermoid cysts: case study. J Plast Reconstr Aesthet Surg 10:755–759
Vidal R, Devaney K, Ferlito A et al (1999) Sinonasal malignant lymphomas: a distinct clinicopathological category. Ann Otol Rhinol Laryngol 108:411–419
Vijaya-Sekaran S et al (1999) Solitary plasmacytoma of the skull base presenting with unilateral sensorineural hearing loss. Laryngol Otol 113(2):164–166
Voelker J, Campbell R, Muller J (1991) Clinical radiographic and pathological features of Rathke's cleft cysts. J Neurosurg 74:535–544
Walia R et al (2010) An uncommon cause of recurrent pyogenic meningitis: pituitary abscess. BMJ Case Rep. https://doi.org/10.1136/bcr0620091945
Wasmeier C, Pfadenhauer K, Rosler A (2002) Idiopathic inflammatory pseudotumor of the orbit and Tolosa-Hunt syndrome—are they the same disease? J Neurol 249:1237–1241
Weber A, Romo L (1999) Pseudotumor of the orbit. Radiol Clin N Am 37:151–158
Weber P et al (2001) Jugulotympanic paragangliomas. Otolaryngol Clin North Am 34(6):1231–1240
Weissman J, Snyderman C, Youesm S, Cutrin H (1993) Ameloblastoma of the maxilla: CT and MR appearance. AJNR 14(1):223–226
Wenig B, Mafee M, Ghosh L (1988) Fibro-osseous, osseous and cartilagenous lesions of the orbit and paraorbital region. Radiol Clin N Am Imag Ophtalmol I:1241–1259
Wester K (1992) Gender distribution and sidedness of middle fossa arachnoid cysts: a review of cases diagnosed with computed imaging. Neurosurgery 31:940–944
Wiener SN, Pearlstein AE, Eiber A (1987) MRI of intracranial arachnoid cysts. J Comput Assist Tomogr 11:236–241
Wilms G et al (1991) CT and MRI of ruptured intracranial dermoids. Neuroradiology 33:149–151
Wolfsberger S et al (2004) Application of three-Tesla magnetic resonance imaging for diagnosis and surgery of sellar lesions. J Neurosurg 100:278–286
Woo M et al (2000) MR imaging findings of Rathke's cleft cysts: significance of intracystic nodules. AJNR 21:485–488
Xu W, Zhang M, Wei R (2010) Clinical analysis of ocular adnexal MALT lymphoma. Zhonghua Yan Ke Za Zhi 46(4):299–303
Yadav S, Singh I, Chanda R et al (2002) Nasopharyngeal angiofibroma. J Otolaryngol 31(6):346–350
Yamaguchi S, Nagasawa H, Suzuki T et al (2004) Sarcomas of the oral and maxillofacial region: a review of 32 cases in 25 years. Clin Oral Investig 8(2):52–55
Yan J, Wu Z (2004) Cavernous hemangioma of the orbit: analysis of 214 cases. Orbit 23(1):33–40
Yan J, Wu Z, Li Y (2000) A clinical analysis of idiopathic orbital inflammatory pseudotumor. Yan Ke Xue Bao 16:208–213
Yan J, Wu Z, Li Y (2004) The differentiation of idiopathic inflammatory pseudotumor from lymphoid tumors of orbit: analysis of 319 cases. Orbit 23:245–254
Yegorenkov (2010) Boundary and bening bone tumors. Practical Oncology 1:37–44. (in Russian)
Yousem D, Lexa F, Bilaniuk L (1990) Rhabdomyosarcoma in the head and neck: MR imaging evaluation. Radiology 177:683–686
Yousem D et al (1989) MR imaging of Tolosa-Hunt syndrome. AJNR 10:1181–1184
Yuen S, Rubin P (2003) Idiopathic orbital inflammation: distribution, clinical features, and treatment outcome. Arch Ophthalmol 121(4):491–499
Yuh W, Flickinger F, Barloon T (1985) MR imaging of unusual chordomas. J Comput Assist Tomogr 12:30–35
Yuh W et al (1988) MR imaging of primary tumor of trigeminal nerve and Meckel's cave. AJNR 9:665–670
Zimmer W, Berquist T, Sim F et al (1984) Magnetic resonance imaging of aneurysmal bone cyst. Mayo Clin Proc 59:633–636
Zimmerman R, Bilaniuk L (1980) CT of primary and secondary craniocerebral neuroblastoma. AJR 135:1239–1242
Zinreich S (2004) Imaging for staging of rhinosinusitis. Ann Otol Rhinol Laryngol Suppl 193:19–23
Zygourakis CC et al (2015) Pituicytoma and spindle cell oncocytomas: modern case series from the University of California, San Francisco. Pituitary 18(1):150–158

Index

I. Pronin, V. Kornienko, *CT and MRI of Skull Base Lesions*, https://doi.org/10.1007/978-3-319-65957-2

N

GPSR Compliance

The European Union's (EU) General Product Safety Regulation (GPSR) is a set of rules that requires consumer products to be safe and our obligations to ensure this.

If you have any concerns about our products, you can contact us on ProductSafety@springernature.com

In case Publisher is established outside the EU, the EU authorized representative is:

Springer Nature Customer Service Center GmbH
Europaplatz 3
69115 Heidelberg, Germany

Batch number: 10731648

Printed by Printforce, the Netherlands